MW00757366

Students Synthesize Information

At the end of each body system, a capstone Build Your Knowledge System Integrator helps students understand how body systems work together.

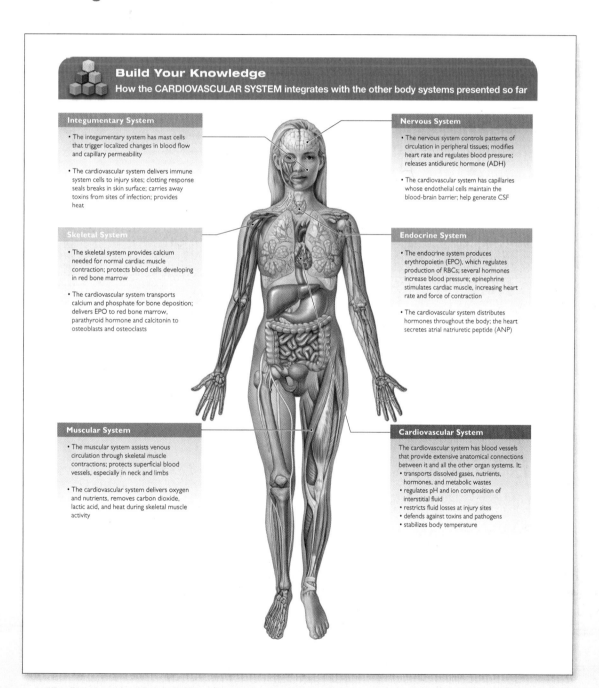

Build Your Knowledge
How the CARDIOVASCULAR SYSTEM integrates with the other body systems presented so far

Integumentary System
- The integumentary system has mast cells that trigger localized changes in blood flow and capillary permeability
- The cardiovascular system delivers immune system cells to injury sites; clotting response seals breaks in skin surface; carries away toxins from sites of infection; provides heat

Skeletal System
- The skeletal system provides calcium needed for normal cardiac muscle contraction; protects blood cells developing in red bone marrow
- The cardiovascular system transports calcium and phosphate for bone deposition; delivers EPO to red bone marrow, parathyroid hormone and calcitonin to osteoblasts and osteoclasts

Muscular System
- The muscular system assists venous circulation through skeletal muscle contractions; protects superficial blood vessels, especially in neck and limbs
- The cardiovascular system delivers oxygen and nutrients, removes carbon dioxide, lactic acid, and heat during skeletal muscle activity

Nervous System
- The nervous system controls patterns of circulation in peripheral tissues; modifies heart rate and regulates blood pressure; releases antidiuretic hormone (ADH)
- The cardiovascular system has capillaries whose endothelial cells maintain the blood-brain barrier; help generate CSF

Endocrine System
- The endocrine system produces erythropoietin (EPO), which regulates production of RBCs; several hormones increase blood pressure; epinephrine stimulates cardiac muscle, increasing heart rate and force of contraction
- The cardiovascular system distributes hormones throughout the body; the heart secretes atrial natriuretic peptide (ANP)

Cardiovascular System
The cardiovascular system has blood vessels that provide extensive anatomical connections between it and all the other organ systems. It:
- transports dissolved gases, nutrients, hormones, and metabolic wastes
- regulates pH and ion composition of interstitial fluid
- restricts fluid losses at injury sites
- defends against toxins and pathogens
- stabilizes body temperature

MORE! SPOTLIGHT FIGURES Teach

Spotlight Figures provide highly visual one- and two-page presentations of tough topics in the book. Brief text and related figures and photos communicate information in a visually effective and student-friendly format.

In the Third Edition, there is now at least one Spotlight Figure in every chapter.

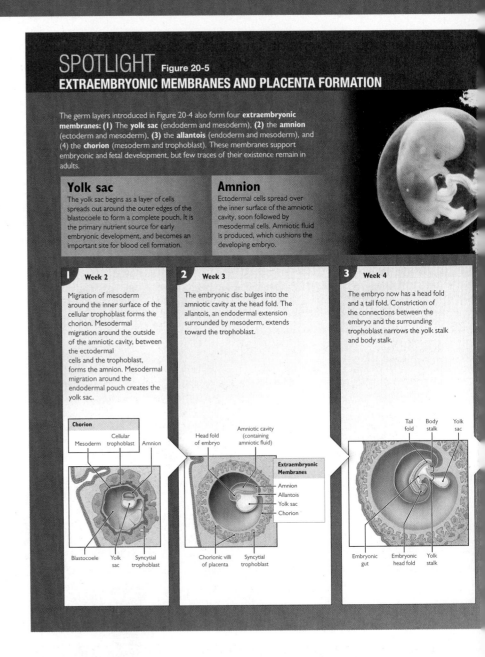

SPOTLIGHT Figure 20-5
EXTRAEMBRYONIC MEMBRANES AND PLACENTA FORMATION

The germ layers introduced in Figure 20-4 also form four **extraembryonic membranes**: (1) The **yolk sac** (endoderm and mesoderm), (2) the **amnion** (ectoderm and mesoderm), (3) the **allantois** (endoderm and mesoderm), and (4) the **chorion** (mesoderm and trophoblast). These membranes support embryonic and fetal development, but few traces of their existence remain in adults.

Yolk sac
The yolk sac begins as a layer of cells spreads out around the outer edges of the blastocoele to form a complete pouch. It is the primary nutrient source for early embryonic development, and becomes an important site for blood cell formation.

Amnion
Ectodermal cells spread over the inner surface of the amniotic cavity, soon followed by mesodermal cells. Amniotic fluid is produced, which cushions the developing embryo.

1 Week 2
Migration of mesoderm around the inner surface of the cellular trophoblast forms the chorion. Mesodermal migration around the outside of the amniotic cavity, between the ectodermal cells and the trophoblast, forms the amnion. Mesodermal migration around the endodermal pouch creates the yolk sac.

2 Week 3
The embryonic disc bulges into the amniotic cavity at the head fold. The allantois, an endodermal extension surrounded by mesoderm, extends toward the trophoblast.

3 Week 4
The embryo now has a head fold and a tail fold. Constriction of the connections between the embryo and the surrounding trophoblast narrows the yolk stalk and body stalk.

NEW SPOTLIGHT FIGURES IN THE THIRD EDITION

Tough Topics

Allantois

The allantois begins as an outpocket of the endoderm near the base of the yolk sac. The free endodermal tip then grows toward the wall of the blastocyst, surrounded by a mass of mesodermal cells. The base of the allantois eventually gives rise to the urinary bladder.

Chorion

The mesoderm associated with the allantois spreads around the entire blastocyst, separating the cellular trophoblast from the blastocoele. The appearance of blood vessels in the chorion is the first step in the creation of a functional placenta. By the third week of development, the mesoderm extends along the core of each trophoblastic villus, forming chorionic villi in contact with maternal tissues and blood vessels. These villi continue to enlarge and branch, forming the placenta, the exchange platform between mother and fetus for nutrients, oxygen, and wastes.

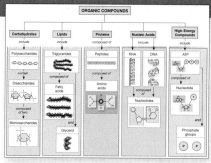

An Overview of the Structures of Organic Compounds in the Body, p. 51

4	Week 5

The developing embryo and extraembryonic membranes bulge into the uterine cavity. The trophoblast pushing out into the uterine cavity remains covered by endometrium but no longer participates in nutrient absorption and embryo support. The embryo moves away from the placenta, and the body stalk and yolk stalk fuse to form an umbilical stalk.

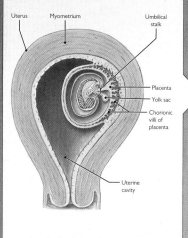

5	Week 10

The amnion has expanded greatly, filling the uterine cavity. The fetus is connected to the placenta by an elongated umbilical cord that contains a portion of the allantois, blood vessels, and the remnants of the yolk stalk.

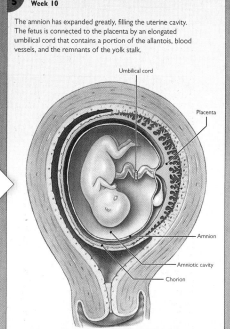

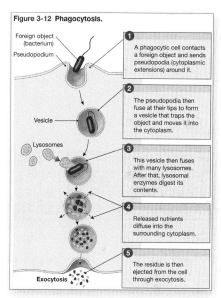

Stepwise illustration of Phagocytosis, p. 74

NEW SPOTLIGHT FIGURES IN THE THIRD EDITION

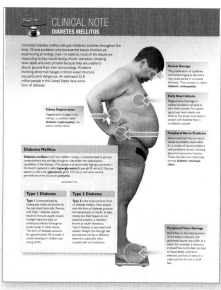

Full-page Clinical Note on Diabetes Mellitus, p. 416

Instructor Supplements

To access supplementary materials online from Pearson's Instructor Resource Center (IRC), instructors will need to use their IRC login credentials. If they don't have IRC login credentials they will need to request an instructor access code. Go to www.pearsonhighered.com/irc to register for an instructor access code. Within 48 hours of registering, you will receive a confirming e-mail including an instructor access code. Once you have received your code, locate your book in the online catalog and click on the Instructor Resources button on the left side of the catalog product page. Select a supplement, and a login page will appear.

Once you have logged in, you can access instructor material for all Pearson textbooks. If you have any difficulties accessing the site or downloading a supplement, please contact Customer Service at http://support.pearson.com/getsupport. This book has the following instructor's resources.

- Instructor's Manual
- PowerPoint lecture slides
- TestGen
- Image Library

Student Supplements

Workbook—The Student Workbook contains exercises that test students' knowledge of the key concepts presented in the core textbook.

- Student Resource Website: To access the material on student resources that accompany this book, visit www.pearsonhighered.com/bradyresources.

Click on view all resources and select Emergency Medical Services from the choice of disciplines. Find this book and you will find the complimentary study materials.

ANATOMY & PHYSIOLOGY for EMERGENCY CARE

THIRD EDITION

Bryan E. Bledsoe, D.O., F.A.C.E.P., F.A.E.M.S.
Frederic H. Martini, Ph.D.
Edwin F. Bartholomew, M.S.

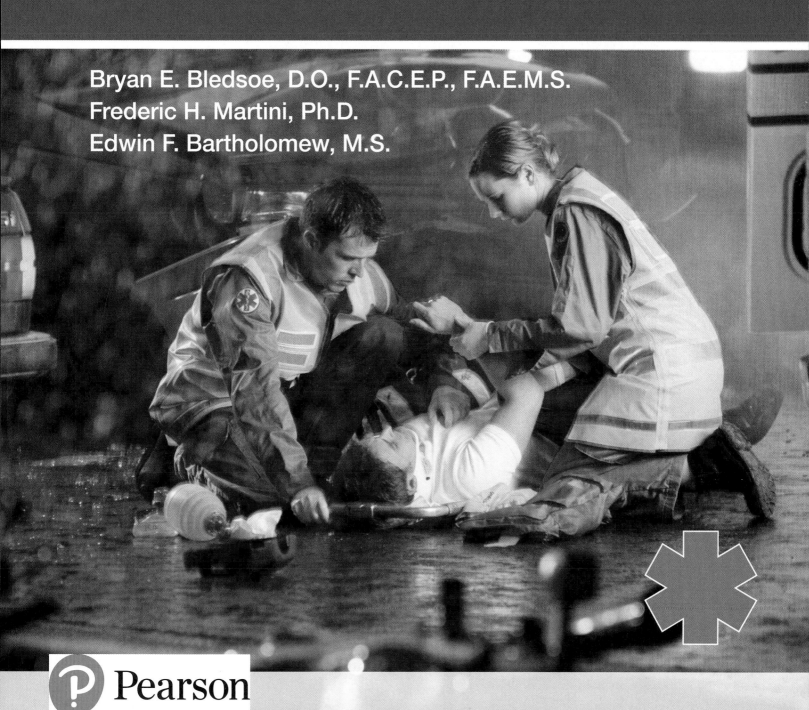

Pearson

SVP, Product Management: Adam Jaworski
Director Product Management - Health Sciences: Katrin Beacom
Content Manager - Health Professions & Nursing: Kevin Wilson
Associate Sponsoring Editor: Zoya Zaman
Product Marketing Manager: Brian Hoehl
Vice President, Digital Studio and Content Production: Paul DeLuca
Director, Digital Studio and Content Production: Brian Hyland
Managing Producer: Jennifer Sargunar

Content Producer (Team Lead): Faraz Sharique Ali
Content Producer: Neha Sharma
DGM, Global R&P: Tanvi Bhatia
Project Manager, Global R&P: Anjali Singh
Operations Specialist: Maura Zaldivar-Garcia
Cover Design: SPi Global
Cover Photo: Taxi/Getty Images
Full-Service Project Management and Composition: Ashwina Ragounath, Integra Software Services Pvt. Ltd.
Printer/Binder: LSC Communications
Cover Printer: LSC Communications
Text Font: Garamond LT Std

Copyright © 2020, 2008, 2002 by Pearson Education, Inc. 221 River Street, Hoboken, NJ 07030. All rights reserved. Manufactured in the United States of America. This publication is protected by Copyright, and permission should be obtained from the publisher prior to any prohibited reproduction, storage in a retrieval system, or transmission in any form or by any means, electronic, mechanical, photocopying, recording, or otherwise. For information regarding permissions, request forms, and the appropriate contacts within the Pearson Education Global Rights and Permissions department, please visit www.pearsoned.com/permissions/.

Acknowledgments of third-party content appear on the appropriate page within the text.

Unless otherwise indicated herein, any third-party trademarks, logos, or icons that may appear in this work are the property of their respective owners, and any references to third-party trademarks, logos, icons, or other trade dress are for demonstrative or descriptive purposes only. Such references are not intended to imply any sponsorship, endorsement, authorization, or promotion of Pearson's products by the owners of such marks, or any relationship between the owner and Pearson Education, Inc., authors, licensees, or distributors.

Library of Congress Cataloging-in-Publication Data

Names: Bryan E. Bledsoe, author. | Frederic H. Martini, author. | Edwin F. Bartholomew, author.
Title: Anatomy & physiology for emergency care/Bryan E. Bledsoe, D.O., F.A.C.E.P., F.A.E.M.S., Frederic H. Martini, Ph.D., Edwin F. Bartholomew, M.S.
Other titles: Anatomy and physiology for emergency care
Description: Third edition. | Hoboken, New Jersey: Pearson, 2020. | Includes bibliographical references and index.
Identifiers: LCCN 2019013335| ISBN 9780135211458 | ISBN 013521145X
Subjects: LCSH: Human physiology–Textbooks. | Human anatomy–Textbooks. | Emergency medical services–Textbooks.
Classification: LCC QP36 .M42 2019 | DDC 612–dc23
    LC record available at https://lccn.loc.gov/2019013335
Pearson Education Australia Pty. Ltd.

1 2019

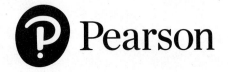

ISBN 10:   0-13-521145-X
ISBN 13: 978-0-13-521145-8

Text and Illustration Team

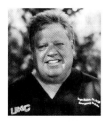

BRYAN BLEDSOE, DO, FACEP, FAEMS, is Professor of emergency medicine and surgery (trauma) at the University of Nevada, Las Vegas School of Medicine and an attending emergency physician at University Medical Center of Southern Nevada in Las Vegas, Nevada. He also serves as the System EMS Medical Director for Texas Health Resources. A former EMT, paramedic and firefighter, Bledsoe is the author of numerous textbooks, as well as journal and magazine articles. In 2008 he was named a "Hero of Emergency Medicine" by the American College of Emergency Physicians and one of twenty "Heroes of Health and Fitness" by *Men's Health* magazine. In 2014, he received the John P. Pryor, MD Award for exemplary service to EMS. He lives in Nevada and Texas.

FREDERIC (RIC) MARTINI, PH.D. (Author), earned his Ph.D. from Cornell University. In addition to his technical and journal publications, he has been the lead author of 10 undergraduate texts on anatomy and physiology or anatomy. He is currently affiliated with the University of Hawaii at Manoa and has a long-standing bond with the Shoals Marine Laboratory, a joint venture between Cornell University and the University of New Hampshire. He has been active in the Human Anatomy and Physiology Society (HAPS) for 26 years and is a President Emeritus of HAPS. He is also a member of the American Physiological Society, the American Association of Anatomists, the Society for Integrative and Comparative Biology, the Australia/New Zealand Association of Clinical Anatomists, and the International Society of Vertebrate Morphologists.

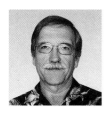

EDWIN F. BARTHOLOMEW, M.S. (Author), earned his undergraduate degree from Bowling Green State University in Ohio and his M.S. from the University of Hawaii. His interests range widely, from human anatomy and physiology to the marine environment, "backyard" aquaculture, and oil and watercolor painting. He has taught human anatomy and physiology at both the secondary and undergraduate levels. In addition, he has taught a range of other science courses (from botany to zoology) at Maui Community College (now the University of Hawaii Maui College). For many years, he taught at historic Lahainaluna High School, the oldest high school west of the Rockies, where he assisted in establishing an LHS Health Occupations Students of America (HOSA) chapter. He has written journal articles, a weekly newspaper column, and many magazine articles. Working with Dr. Martini, he coauthored *Structure & Function of the Human Body* and *The Human Body in Health and Disease* (Pearson). Along with Dr. Martini and Dr. Judi Nath, he coauthored *Fundamentals of Anatomy & Physiology*, 11th edition. He also coauthored *Visual Anatomy & Physiology*, 3rd edition, with Dr. Martini, Dr. William Ober, Dr. Judi Nath, and Dr. Kevin Petti. He is a member of the Human Anatomy and Physiology Society, National Science Teachers Association, and the American Association for the Advancement of Science.

WILLIAM C. OBER, M.D. (Art Coordinator and Illustrator), earned his undergraduate degree from Washington and Lee University and his M.D. from the University of Virginia. While in medical school, he also studied in the Department of Art as Applied to Medicine at Johns Hopkins University. After graduation, he completed a residency in Family Practice and later was on the faculty at the University of Virginia in the Department of Family Medicine. He was Chief of Medicine at Martha Jefferson Hospital and was an Instructor in the Division of Sports Medicine at UVA. He also was part of the Core Faculty at Shoals Marine Laboratory for 22 years, where he taught Biological Illustration every summer. He is currently a visiting professor of Biology at Washington and Lee University. The textbooks illustrated by his company Medical & Scientific Illustration have won numerous design and illustration awards.

CLAIRE E. OBER, R.N. (Illustrator), practiced pediatric and obstetric nursing before turning to medical illustration as a full-time career. She earned her degree at Mary Baldwin College with distinction in studio art. Following a five-year apprenticeship, she has worked as Dr. Ober's partner in Medical & Scientific Illustration since 1986. She was on the Core Faculty at Shoals Marine Laboratory and co-taught the Biological Illustration course.

KATHLEEN WELCH, M.D. (Clinical Consultant), earned her M.D. from the University of Washington in Seattle and did her residency at the University of North Carolina in Chapel Hill. For two years, she served as Director of Maternal and Child Health at the LBJ Tropical Medical Center in American Samoa and subsequently was a member of the Department of Family Practice at the Kaiser Permanente Clinic in Lahaina, Hawaii. She was in private practice from 1987 until her retirement in 2012. She has been the Clinical Consultant for nine textbooks and the coauthor of one textbook and several clinical supplements. She is a Fellow of the American Academy of Family Practice and a member of the Hawaii Medical Association, the Maui County Medical Association, the American Medical Association, and the Human Anatomy and Physiology Society.

 RALPH T. HUTCHINGS (Biomedical Photographer), was associated with the Royal College of Surgeons for 20 years. An engineer by training, he has focused for years on photographing the structure of the human body. The result has been a series of color atlases, including the *Color Atlas of Human Anatomy*, *The Color Atlas of Surface Anatomy*, and *The Human Skeleton* (all published by Mosby-Yearbook Publishing). For his anatomical portrayal of the human body, the International Photographers Association chose Mr. Hutchings as the best photographer of humans in the twentieth century. He lives in North London, where he tries to balance the demands of his photographic assignments with his hobbies of early motorcars and airplanes.

Brief Contents

Contents

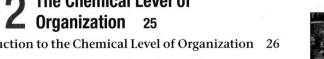

4 The Tissue Level of Organization   96

5 The Integumentary System   128

6 The Skeletal System 156

7 The Muscular System 212

8 The Nervous System 269

9 The General and Special Senses 343

10 The Endocrine System 386

13 The Cardiovascular System: Blood Vessels and Circulation   489

14 The Lymphatic System and Immunity   536

15 The Respiratory System 575

An Introduction to the Respiratory System 576

18 The Urinary System 693

19 The Reproductive System 734

20 Development and Inheritance 770

Preface

Before one can learn the various aspects of prehospital emergency care, one must first learn and understand normal human anatomy and physiology. This text, *Anatomy and Physiology for Emergency Care*, Third Edition, provides the necessary anatomy and physiology instruction to embark upon prehospital emergency care studies.

This text is based upon the popular college text *Essentials of Anatomy and Physiology* by Fredric H. Martini and Edwin F. Bartholomew, Seventh Edition. We have taken this work and added clinical correlations and applications specific to emergency care. Now, as an emergency medical services student, you can begin to learn selected disease processes and injury patterns while you learn normal human anatomy and physiology.

This text has three primary goals:

1. **Build a foundation of essential knowledge in human anatomy and physiology.** Constructing this knowledge requires answers to questions such as: What structure is that? How does it work? What happens when it does not work?

2. **Provide a framework for interpreting and applying information that can be used in problem-solving.** This framework is based on the fact that certain themes and patterns appear again and again in the study of anatomy and physiology. These themes and patterns provide the hooks on which to organize and hang the information you will find in the text. Problems that require interpreting and applying information include such general questions as: How does a change in one body system affect the others? How does aging affect body systems?

3. **Provide an introduction to common injuries and illnesses in a manner that will reinforce basic anatomy and physiology principles.** You will tend to remember material better if presented in a context that directly relates to your interest and field of study. In this text we have taken selected anatomy and physiology principles and carefully integrated clinical concepts, usually of an emergency nature, that will help you to retain the material and see how abnormal anatomy and physiology (pathophysiology) are directly related to normal anatomy and physiology.

In addition, the need for well-trained professionals in the allied health field is greater than ever. To succeed in an allied health career, you must master the same skills that you need to succeed in this course. You must do more than develop a large technical vocabulary and retain a large volume of detailed information. You must learn how to learn—how to organize new information, connect it to what you already know, and then apply it as needed.

Can a text simplify this process? No textbook can give you more time. A text can, however, help you make better use of your time. By presenting the material in a clear, logical way that stresses concept organization, this textbook provides you with a strong foundation of essential knowledge and a framework for integrating and applying that knowledge. For example, certain themes and patterns appear again and again in the study of anatomy and physiology. The conceptual material will be much easier to deal with if you learn to recognize those patterns and organize the information accordingly. With this realization in mind, we have taken extra care to highlight the important patterns, create a sensible framework, and organize new information around that framework.

The User's Guide that follows this page describes the many learning aids that are built into this text. If you use them, they will help you improve your study skills and will make you more efficient at learning and integrating new information. These features were developed through feedback from students and instructors on campuses across the United States, Canada, Australia, New Zealand, and Europe. Many students, in person or by phone or e-mail, have told us that this system really works for them when other presentation styles have not. Take the time to examine this User's Guide carefully, and ask your instructor if you have questions about any of the book's learning aids. If you invest the time now, you can learn to use the book properly from the outset. Doing so will ensure that you will get the most from the time you invest in this course. In addition, becoming a more efficient learner will set you forth on a lifetime of learning that will make you a more valuable future professional, constantly improving and growing long after you've taken your last exam.

New to This Edition

Anatomy and Physiology for Emergency Care, Third Edition, has been extensively revised and updated. Most important, the clinical correlation material has been placed throughout the text next to the related topic being discussed.

Numerous new clinical discussions have been added as well as new art and photographs. The practice of prehospital care is always changing and the text has been updated to reflect these changes.

Chapter-by-Chapter Changes in the Third Edition

This annotated Table of Contents provides select examples of revision highlights in each chapter of the Third Edition.

Chapter 1 An Introduction to Anatomy and Physiology

- New Spotlight Figure 1-1 Levels of Organization
- Figure 1-2 The Organ Systems of the Human Body revised
- Updated discussion on Homeostasis and Disease
- New Figure 1-3 The Control of Room Temperature
- New Figure 1-4 Negative Feedback in Thermoregulation
- New Figure 1-8 Directional References (incorporates former Table 1-1 Directional Terms)
- New Figure 1-9 Sectional Planes (incorporates former Table 1-2 Terms That Indicate Sectional Planes)
- Figure 1-11 Relationships among the Subdivisions of the Body Cavities of the Trunk revised
- New Clinical Note: Imaging Techniques (added PET scan of the brain; replaces Spotlight Figure 1-9 Imaging Techniques)

Chapter 2 The Chemical Level of Organization

- Figure 2-4 Ionic Bonding revised (new part c)
- Spotlight Figure 2-7 Chemical Notation revised ("reactants" and "product" labels added)
- Updated discussion on Understanding pH
- Figure 2-11 The Structures of Glucose revised (new part c replaced former part c)
- Figure 2-17 Amino Acids and the Formation of Peptide Bonds revised
- New Figure 2-18 Protein Structure
- Figure 2-20 The Structure of Nucleic Acids revised

Chapter 3 Cell Structure and Function

- Figure 3-1 The Diversity of Cells in the Human Body revised
- Spotlight Figure 3-2 Anatomy of a Model Cell revised (distinguishes primary and motile cilia)
- Figure 3-4 Diffusion revised (Step art [1–4] added)
- Enhanced discussion of fluid movement
- Figure 3-7 Osmotic Flow across a Plasma Membrane

- New Figure 3-13 Phagocytosis
- Figure 3-15 The Endoplasmic Reticulum revised
- New Figure 3-16 The Golgi Apparatus
- Updated information on prehospital IV fluids
- Spotlight Figure 3-17 Protein Synthesis, Processing, and Packaging revised
- Figure 3-18 Mitochondria revised (added ribosome label)
- New Figure 3-22 Translation
- Figure 3-25 Interphase, Mitosis, and Cytokinesis revised

Chapter 4 The Tissue Level of Organization

- New Figure 4-1 An Orientation to the Tissues of the Body
- Figure 4-2 Cell Junctions revised
- Figure 4-4 Simple Epithelia revised
- Figure 4-5 Stratified Epithelia revised
- Figure 4-6 Modes of Glandular Secretion revised
- New Figure 4-7 Major Types of Connective Tissue
- Enhanced discussion of obesity and impact on EMS
- Figure 4-8 Cells and Fibers of Connective Tissue Proper revised (added Fibrocyte)
- Figure 4-9 Loose Connective Tissues revised
- Figure 4-10 Dense Connective Tissues revised
- Figure 4-11 Types of Cartilage revised
- Figure 4-13 Tissue Membranes revised (text in part b)
- Figure 4-14 Muscle Tissue revised
- Figure 4-15 Neural Tissue revised

Chapter 5 The Integumentary System

- New Terminology: added keratinocytes
- Figure 5-1 The General Structure of the Integumentary System revised (now includes papillary plexus)
- New Spotlight Figure 5-4 The Epidermis
- Figure 5-8 Hair Follicles and Hairs revised
- Figure 5-11 The Structure of a Nail revised (added cross-sectional view)
- New Figure 5-25 A Keloid
- Updated discussion of skin conditions
- New Clinical Note: Dermatitis
- Clinical Note: Hair Loss revised (new discussion of hair loss due to chemotherapy and radiation)
- New Clinical Note: Traumatic Conditions of the Skin
- Updated discussion of soft-tissue injuries

- New Build Your Knowledge: How the INTEGUMENTARY SYSTEM integrates with the other body systems presented so far

Chapter 6 The Skeletal System

- Figure 6-2 The Structure of a Long Bone revised (added periosteum art)
- Figure 6-8 The Microscopic Structure of a Typical Bone revised (added Types of Bone Cells art)
- Figure 6-11 Appositional Bone Growth revised
- Updated information on intraosseous infusion
- New Figure 6-22 An Introduction to Bone Markings
- Figure 6-25 The Adult Skull, Part I revised (added color-coded labels)
- Figure 6-26 The Adult Skull, Part II revised
- Figure 6-27 Sectional Anatomy of the Skull revised
- Updated discussion of skeletal injuries
- Figure 6-30 The Skull of an Infant revised
- Figure 6-31 The Vertebral Column revised (added text to labels)
- Figure 6-34 The Sacrum and Coccyx revised (added a lateral view)
- Figure 6-35 The Thoracic Cage revised
- Figure 6-40 The Bones of the Wrist and Hand revised
- Figure 6-41 The Hip Bones and the Pelvis revised (added a lateral view)
- Figure 6-45 The Bones of the Ankle and Foot revised (added arches and a lateral view)
- Figure 6-46 The Structure of a Synovial Joint revised
- Spotlight Figure 6-50 Synovial Joints revised (added descriptions of types of synovial joints)
- Figure 6-55 The Knee Joint revised (boxed ligament labels)
- New Clinical Note: Types of Fractures and Steps in Repair
- New Clinical Note: Osteoporosis
- New Build Your Knowledge: How the SKELETAL SYSTEM integrates with the other body systems presented so far

Chapter 7 The Muscular System

- Figure 7-2 The Organization of a Skeletal Muscle Fiber revised (added titin label)
- Spotlight Figure 7-4 Events at the Neuromuscular Junction revised
- Enhanced discussion of neuromuscular blockade

- New Figure 7-6 Steps Involved in Skeletal Muscle Contraction and Relaxation
- Figure 7-10 Muscle Metabolism revised
- New Figure 7-12 An Overview of the Major Skeletal Muscles
- Figure 7-14 Muscles of the Anterior Neck revised (added omohyoid muscle and boxed labels)
- Table 7-3 Muscles of the Head and Neck revised
- Figure 7-15 Muscles of the Spine revised
- Figure 7-16 Oblique and Rectus Muscles and the Diaphragm revised (parts b and c captions)
- Figure 7-19 Muscles That Move the Arm revised (added identification of rotator cuff muscles)
- New Figure 7-20 Muscles That Move the Forearm and Wrist
- Figure 7-22 Muscles That Move the Leg revised (added identification of hamstring muscles)
- Figure 7-23 Muscles That Move the Foot and Toes revised (added new anterior view and fibularis tertius muscle)
- Table 7-12 Muscles That Move the Foot and Toes revised (added fibularis tertius, brevis, and longus muscles)
- Clinical Note: Interference at the NMJ and Muscular Paralysis revised
- Clinical Note: Rigor Mortis revised
- Clinical Note: Tetanus revised
- Updated discussion of rhabdomyolysis
- Clinical Note: Intramuscular Injections revised
- New Build Your Knowledge: How the MUSCULAR SYSTEM integrates with the other body systems presented so far
- Updated discussion of emergency laboratory testing in heart attack

Chapter 8 The Nervous System

- Figure 8-1 A Functional Overview of the Nervous System revised (new art is added and definitions are added for the CNS, PNS, Receptors, and Effectors)
- Figure 8-2 The Anatomy of a Representative Neuron revised (new three-dimensional neuron art)
- Figure 8-4 Neuroglia in the CNS revised (added descriptions of neuroglia to correlate the art with text)
- New Figure 8-7 The Resting Membrane Potential
- Spotlight Figure 8-8 The Generation of an Action Potential revised

- New Spotlight Figure 8-9 Propagation of an Action Potential
- Figure 8-11 The Events at a Cholinergic Synapse revised
- Updated discussion of organophosphate poisoning
- Figure 8-13 The Meninges of the Brain and Spinal Cord revised (art moved for label sharing and correlation between similar structures)
- New Figure 8-14 Gross Anatomy of the Spinal Cord
- Figure 8-16 The Brain revised (labels boxed to better correlate art and text)
- Updated and enhanced epidural and subdural hemorrhages
- Figure 8-18 The Formation and Circulation of Cerebrospinal Fluid revised (added new art for part a and steps to improve correlation between art and text)
- Figure 8-19 Motor and Sensory Regions of the Cerebral Hemispheres revised (labels boxed to better correlate art and text)
- Figure 8-22 The Basal Nuclei revised (labels boxed to better correlate art and text)
- Figure 8-24 The Diencephalon and Brain Stem revised (labels boxed to better correlate art and text)
- Figure 8-25 The Cranial Nerves revised (incorporated table of cranial nerves to better correlate art and text)
- New Figure 8-26 Peripheral Nerves and Nerve Plexuses
- Figure 8-27 Dermatomes revised (added color-coded art and key to better correlate art and text)
- Figure 8-30 The Flexor Reflex, a Type of Withdrawal Reflex revised (step art added to better correlate art and text)
- Figure 8-31 The Posterior Column Pathway revised (step art added to better correlate art and text)
- Figure 8-32 The Corticospinal Pathway revised (step art added to better correlate art and text)
- Figure 8-34 The Sympathetic Division revised (shading added to spinal cord to better correlate art and text)
- Figure 8-35 The Parasympathetic Division revised (shading added to brain stem and spinal cord to better correlate art and text)
- Updated discussion of stroke
- Clinical Note: Epidural and Subdural Hemorrhages revised (added photograph)
- Clinical Note: Aphasia and Dyslexia revised
- Clinical Note: Alzheimer's Disease revised
- New Build Your Knowledge: How the NERVOUS SYSTEM integrates with the other body systems presented so far

Chapter 9 The General and Special Senses

- Figure 9-1 Receptors and Receptive Fields revised
- Figure 9-2 Referred Pain revised
- Updated discussion of pain management from a prehospital perspective
- Figure 9-3 Tactile Receptors in the Skin revised (boxed text added to better correlate art and text)
- Figure 9-4 Baroreceptors and the Regulation of Autonomic Functions revised
- Figure 9-5 Locations and Functions of Chemoreceptors revised
- Figure 9-6 The Olfactory Organs revised (changed olfactory cilia label to olfactory dendrites)
- Figure 9-7 Gustatory Receptors revised (changed supporting cell label to transitional cell)
- Figure 9-10 The Sectional Anatomy of the Eye revised
- Updated discussion of eye injuries and conditions
- Figure 9-13 The Circulation of Aqueous Humor revised (enhanced color of arrow showing circulation route)
- Figure 9-14 Focal Point, Focal Distance, and Visual Accommodation revised
- Spotlight Figure 9-16 Refractive Problems revised (title corrected from Accommodation Problems)
- Figure 9-19 Bleaching and Regeneration of Visual Pigments revised (added step art and text to improve topic comprehension)
- Figure 9-22 The Middle Ear revised
- New Figure 9-23 The Internal Ear
- New Figure 9-24 The Semicircular Ducts
- New Figure 9-25 The Utricle and Saccule
- Figure 9-27 Sound and Hearing revised (added diagram to better correlate step art and text)
- Clinical Note: Cataracts revised (added photograph)

Chapter 10 The Endocrine System

- Figure 10-1 Organs and Tissues of the Endocrine System revised (new art)
- Figure 10-2 The Role of Target Cell Receptors in Hormone Action revised (added step art and text)
- Figure 10-3 Processes of Hormone Action revised (added step art and text to improve topic comprehension)
- Figure 10-5 The Location and Anatomy of the Pituitary Gland revised (new photomicrograph)

- Figure 10-6 The Hypophyseal Portal System and the Blood Supply to the Pituitary Gland revised (added boxed text to improve topic comprehension)
- Figure 10-9 The Thyroid Gland revised (added new diagram to clarify histological details in photomicrograph)
- New Figure 10-10 The Homeostatic Regulation of Calcium Ion Concentrations
- New Figure 10-12 The Adrenal Gland and Adrenal Hormones (added new photomicrograph and incorporated former Table 10-3 The Adrenal Hormones)
- Enhanced discussion of adrenal disorders
- New Figure 10-14 The Regulation of Blood Glucose Concentrations
- New Clinical Note: Diabetes Mellitus
- Updated discussion of diabetes mellitus
- New Clinical Note: Endocrine Disorders
- Updated discussion of the stress response
- New Build Your Knowledge: How the ENDOCRINE SYSTEM integrates with the other body systems presented so far

Chapter 11 The Cardiovascular System: Blood

- Spotlight Figure 11-1 The Composition of Whole Blood revised
- Figure 11-4 The Origins and Differentiation of RBCs, Platelets, and WBCs revised (replaced specific names of developing WBCs with "Developmental stages")
- New Figure 11-5 The Role of EPO in the Stimulation of Erythropoiesis
- Figure 11-7 Blood Type Testing revised (part of text, no longer within a Clinical Note)
- Updated discussion of the emergency blood transfusion
- New Figure 11-9 The Vascular, Platelet, and Coagulation Phases of Hemostasis
- New Figure 11-10 The Structure of a Blood Clot
- Updated information on fibrinolytic therapy
- Clinical Note: Hemolytic Disease of the Newborn revised (added new art)
- Clinical Note: Abnormal Hemostasis revised (added new thrombus art)

Chapter 12 The Cardiovascular System: The Heart

- New Figure 12-1 An Overview of the Cardiovascular System
- Figure 12-3 The Position and Surface Anatomy of the Heart revised (added new part b of cadaver dissection)

- Figure 12-4 The Heart Wall and Cardiac Muscle Tissue revised (improved correlation between parts a and c)
- New Spotlight Figure 12-5 The Heart: Internal Anatomy and Blood Flow
- Updated discussion of coronary artery disease
- Figure 12-8 Action Potentials and Muscle Cell Contraction in Skeletal and Cardiac Muscle revised
- Updated discussion factors causing decreased cardiac output
- Figure 12-9 The Conducting System of the Heart revised (new three-dimensional art in part b)
- Figure 12-10 An Electrocardiogram revised (new three-dimensional art in part b)
- Figure 12-11 The Cardiac Cycle revised (art enlarged)
- New Figure 12-12 Heart Sounds
- Figure 12-13 Autonomic Innervation of the Heart revised
- Clinical Note: Heart Valve Disorders revised (added photograph of bioprosthetic valve)

Chapter 13 The Cardiovascular System: Blood Vessels and Circulation

- Figure 13-1 A Comparison of a Typical Artery and a Typical Vein revised (clarified thickness of artery wall)
- New Figure 13-2 The Structure of the Various Types of Blood Vessels
- Figure 13-5 Pressures within the Systemic Circuit revised (clarified pulse pressure within the diagram)
- Figure 13-6 Forces Acting across Capillary Walls revised (added tissue cells to highlight capillary surroundings)
- New Figure 13-7 Short-Term and Long-Term Cardiovascular Responses
- New Figure 13-8 The Baroreceptor Reflexes of the Carotid and Aortic Sinuses
- New Figure 13-9 The Chemoreceptor Reflexes
- New Figure 13-10 The Hormonal Regulation of Blood Pressure and Blood Volume
- New Spotlight Figure 13-13 Major Vessels of the Systemic Circuit
- New Figure 13-14 Arteries of the Chest and Upper Limb (incorporates former art and flowchart)
- Figure 13-16 Major Arteries of the Trunk revised (added boxed labels to better correlate art and text)
- Figure 13-19 A Flowchart of the Tributaries of the Superior and Inferior Venae Cavae revised

- Figure 13-20 The Hepatic Portal System revised (added boxed labels to better correlate art and text)
- Clinical Note: Arteriosclerosis revised (added photomicrograph of a normal coronary artery for comparison)
- Updated discussion of vascular trauma
- New Build Your Knowledge: How the CARDIOVASCULAR SYSTEM integrates with the other body systems presented so far

Chapter 14 The Lymphatic System and Immunity

- Figure 14-1 The Components of the Lymphatic System revised (added art depicting lymph and lymphocyte and red bone marrow)
- New Spotlight Figure 14-4 Origin and Distribution of Lymphocytes
- Figure 14-5 The Tonsils revised (added photomicrograph of pharyngeal tonsil)
- Figure 14-9 The Body's Innate Defenses revised
- Figure 14-11 Forms of Immunity revised
- Figure 14-13 Antigen Recognition and Activation of Cytotoxic T Cells revised (added costimulation to step 2 to correlate with text description)
- Figure 14-14 The B Cell Response to Antigen Exposure revised (added costimulation to step 2 art)
- Table 14-2 Cells That Participate in Tissue Defenses revised
- Figure 14-17 A Summary of the Immune Response and Its Relationship to Innate (Nonspecific) Defenses revised
- Clinical Note: "Swollen Glands" revised (added photograph)
- Updated discussion of allergies and allergic reactions
- New Build Your Knowledge: How the LYMPHATIC SYSTEM integrates with the other body systems presented so far

Chapter 15 The Respiratory System

- New Figure 15-1 The Structures of the Respiratory System
- Figure 15-2 The Respiratory Mucosa revised (mucous gland added to part a to better correlate art and text)
- Figure 15-4 The Anatomy of the Larynx and Vocal Cords revised (corrected shared labeling between art in part d and photograph in part e)
- Figure 15-6 The Bronchi and Lobules of the Lung revised (improved clarity of pulmonary lobule anatomy in part b)
- Figure 15-7 Alveolar Organization revised (replaced part a art and part b SEM of lung tissue with photomicrograph)

- New Figure 15-8 The Gross Anatomy of the Lungs
- New Spotlight Figure 15-10 Pulmonary Ventilation
- Updated discussion of respiratory system interventions
- Figure 15-12 An Overview of Respiratory Processes and Partial Pressures in Respiration revised
- Figure 15-14 A Summary of Gas Transport and Exchange revised (added partial pressures of oxygen and carbon dioxide to improve interpretation of the diagram)
- New Spotlight Figure 15-16 The Control of Respiration
- Clinical Note: Tracheal Blockage revised (added photograph of Heimlich maneuver)
- Clinical Note: Emphysema and Lung Cancer revised (added photographs of healthy lung and smoker's lung)
- Updated information on carbon monoxide poisoning
- New Build Your Knowledge: How the RESPIRATORY SYSTEM integrates with the other body systems presented so far

Chapter 16 The Digestive System

- Figure 16-1 The Components of the Digestive System revised (Teeth and Tongue moved to Accessory Organs of the Digestive System box)
- Figure 16-5 The Salivary Glands revised
- Figure 16-7 The Swallowing Process revised
- New Spotlight Figure 16-9 Regulation of Gastric Activity
- Figure 16-10 The Segments of the Small Intestine revised (new gross anatomy of the jejunum photograph)
- New Figure 16-12 The Activities of Major Digestive Tract Hormones
- Updated discussion of Upper GI bleeding
- Figure 16-13 The Pancreas revised (added a new part b diagram to improve interpretation of part c photomicrograph)
- Updated discussion of pancreatitis
- Figure 16-15 Liver Histology revised
- Figure 16-17 The Large Intestine revised (added new part b cadaver photo of cecum and appendix)
- Clinical Note: Liver Disease revised (added cirrhosis of the liver art)
- New Build Your Knowledge: How the DIGESTIVE SYSTEM integrates with the other body systems presented so far

Chapter 17 Metabolism and Energetics

- Figure 17-3 Glycolysis revised (clarified text in Step 5)
- New Spotlight Figure 17-5 The Electron Transport System and ATP Formation

- Figure 17-6 A Summary of the Energy Yield of Aerobic Metabolism revised (clarified ATP gain per glucose molecule based on recently accepted lower conversion ratios of ATP per NADH and $FADH_2$)
- Updated discussion of the diabetes complications
- Updated discussion of ketoacidosis
- Figure 17-9 Lipoproteins and Lipid Transport revised
- Figure 17-10 A Summary of Catabolic and Anabolic Pathways for Lipids, Carbohydrates, and Proteins revised

Chapter 18 The Urinary System

- Figure 18-3 The Structure of the Kidney revised (changed renal lobe to kidney lobe in part a, added papillary duct label to part c)
- Figure 18-5 A Representative Nephron and the Collecting System revised (added boxed text into the art)
- Figure 18-6 The Renal Corpuscle revised (boxed labels added to better correlate art and text)
- Figure 18-8 The Effects of ADH on the DCT and Collecting Duct revised (added compulsory water reabsorption and variable water reabsorption)
- Spotlight Figure 18-9 A Summary of Kidney Function revised (added art showing urea transporter)
- Updated discussion of kidney stones
- New Figure 18-10 The Renin-Angiotensin-Aldosterone System and Regulation of GFR
- Figure 18-11 Organs for the Conduction and Storage of Urine revised (clarified center of trigone in part c)
- Table 18-4 Water Balance revised (added percentages)
- Updated discussion of renal trauma
- New Build Your Knowledge: How the URINARY SYSTEM integrates with the other body systems presented so far

Chapter 19 The Reproductive System

- Figure 19-1 The Male Reproductive System revised (boxed labels added to better correlate art and text)
- Figure 19-2 The Scrotum, Testes, and Seminiferous Tubules revised (boxed label added to better correlate art and text)
- Figure 19-5 The Ductus Deferens revised (added ampulla of ductus deferens label)
- Figure 19-6 The Penis revised (new terminology: changed glans to glans penis)
- Figure 19-8 The Female Reproductive System revised (boxed labels added to better correlate art and text)

- Figure 19-9 Oogenesis revised
- Figure 19-10 Follicle Development and the Ovarian Cycle revised (added new photomicrograph of secondary follicle and corrected image magnifications)
- Figure 19-11 The Uterus revised
- Figure 19-12 The Female External Genitalia revised (caption now clarifies that left labium minus has been removed to show erectile tissue)
- Spotlight Figure 19-14 Regulation of Female Reproduction revised (clarifies that tertiary follicles are involved in step 2 Follicular Phase of the Ovarian Cycle)
- Table 19-1 Hormones of the Reproductive System revised (new terminology: changed progestins to progesterone.)
- Clinical Note: Birth Control Strategies revised (new photograph of contraceptive devices)
- New Build Your Knowledge: How the REPRODUCTIVE SYSTEM integrates with the other body systems presented so far

Chapter 20 Development and Inheritance

- Figure 20-1 Fertilization revised (step 5 title)
- New Spotlight Figure 20-5 Extraembryonic Membranes and Placenta Formation
- Figure 20-7 Development during the First Trimester revised
- Figure 20-8 The Second and Third Trimesters revised (added new ultrasound photograph in part b)
- Table 20-2 An Overview of Prenatal and Early Postnatal Development revised (includes revised sizes and weights at different gestational ages)

Appendix 1 Roles and Responsibilities of Emergency Medical Services Personnel
- Updated overview of the House of Medicine

Appendix 2 A Periodic Chart of the Elements

Appendix 3 Weights and Measures
- Updated nomenclature changes to help avoid medication errors

Appendix 4 Normal Physiologic Values

We hope that you find *Anatomy and Physiology for Emergency Care*, Third Edition, a valuable tool for your prehospital care and allied health education. Your ability to work as a member of the health care team is dependent upon you having an excellent understanding of human anatomy and physiology.

Acknowledgments
Reviewers for the Third Edition

Andrew Appleby, RN
Western Wyoming Community College
Rock Springs, WY

Kevin Collopy, BA, FP-C, CCEMT-P, NRP, CMTE
Cape Fear Community College
Wilmington, NC

Frank Killebrew
Paramedic, EMS Program Instructor
Ogeechee Technical College
Statesboro, GA

Corey Martin, NRP, CCEMT-P, Texas EMS-C
MedTrust Medical, Sweeny EMS
Bastrop, TX

Aaron Nafziger, AAS, BS, NRP
Jefferson State Community College
Birmingham, AL

Rintha Simpson, BS, NRP, NCEE
Baton Rouge Community College
Baton Rouge, LA

An Introduction to Anatomy and Physiology

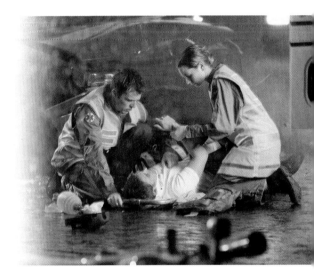

Learning Objectives

These objectives tell you what you should be able to do after completing the chapter. They correspond by number to this chapter's sections.

1-1 Describe the basic functions of living organisms.

1-2 Explain the relationship between anatomy and physiology, and describe various specialties of each discipline.

1-3 Identify the major levels of organization in organisms, from the simplest to the most complex.

1-4 Identify the 11 organ systems of the human body and contrast their major functions.

1-5 Explain the concept of homeostasis.

1-6 Describe how negative feedback and positive feedback are involved in homeostatic regulation.

1-7 Use anatomical terms to describe body regions, body sections, and relative positions.

1-8 Identify the major body cavities of the trunk and the subdivisions of each.

1

An Introduction to Studying the Human Body

In this text, we will introduce you to the essential, inner workings of your body—giving information about its structure (anatomy) and function (physiology). As a human, you are most likely very curious, and few subjects arouse so much curiosity as our own bodies. You will discover how your body works under normal and abnormal conditions, and how it maintains an internal state of balance. As we proceed, you will see how your body deals with injury, disease, or anything that threatens that crucial balance in a changing environment.

 Build Your Knowledge

Throughout each chapter, you will find Build Your Knowledge boxes that will coach you through anatomy and physiology concepts. This feature will help you connect new material with what you already know. At the end of each chapter that closes a body system, you will see a "capstone" Build Your Knowledge page that will illustrate the integration of the body system with the other body systems presented up to that point in the book. Be sure to read every Build Your Knowledge box or page so that you can build your knowledge—and confidence!

1-1 All living things display responsiveness, growth, reproduction, movement, and metabolism

Learning Objective Describe the basic functions of living organisms.

We live in a world containing an amazing diversity of living organisms that vary widely in appearance and lifestyle. One aim of **biology**—the study of life—is to discover the common patterns that underlie this diversity. Such discoveries show that all living things share these common functions:

- *Responsiveness.* Organisms respond to changes in their immediate environment. This property is also called *irritability*. You move your hand away from a hot stove, your dog barks at approaching strangers, fish are alarmed by loud noises, and tiny amoebas glide toward potential prey. Organisms also make longer-term changes as they adjust to their environments. For example, an animal may grow a heavier coat of fur as winter approaches, or it may migrate to a warmer climate. The capacity to make such adjustments is termed *adaptability*.

- *Growth.* Organisms increase in size through the growth or addition of **cells**, the simplest units of life. Single-celled creatures grow by getting larger. More complex organisms grow primarily by increasing the number of cells. Familiar organisms, such as dogs, cats, and humans, are made up of trillions of cells. As such multicellular organisms develop, individual cells become specialized to perform particular functions. This specialization is called *differentiation*.

- *Reproduction.* Organisms reproduce, creating new generations of similar, but not identical, organisms.

- *Movement.* Organisms can move. Their movement may be internal (transporting food, blood, or other materials within the body) or external (moving through the environment).

- *Metabolism.* Organisms rely on complex chemical reactions to provide the energy required for responsiveness, growth, reproduction, and movement. They also build complex chemicals, such as proteins. *Metabolism* refers to all the chemical operations in the body.

For normal metabolic operations, organisms must absorb materials from the environment. To generate energy efficiently, most cells require various nutrients they obtain in food, as well as oxygen, a gas. *Respiration* refers to the absorption, transport, and use of oxygen by cells. Metabolic operations often generate unneeded or potentially harmful waste products that must be eliminated through the process of *excretion*.

For very small organisms, absorption, respiration, and excretion involve the movement of materials across exposed surfaces. But creatures larger than a few millimeters across seldom absorb nutrients directly from their environment. For example, humans cannot absorb steaks, apples, or ice cream without processing them first. That processing, called *digestion*, takes place in specialized structures in which complex foods are broken down into simpler components that can be transported and absorbed easily.

Respiration and excretion are also more complicated for large organisms. Humans have specialized structures for gas exchange (lungs) and excretion (kidneys). Digestion, respiration, and excretion occur in different parts of the body, but the cells of the body cannot travel to one place for nutrients, another for oxygen, and a third to get rid of waste products. Instead, individual cells remain where they are but communicate with other areas of the body through an internal transport system—the circulation. For example, the blood absorbs the waste products released by each of your cells and carries those wastes to the kidneys for excretion.

Biology includes many subspecialties. In this text, we consider two biological subjects: anatomy (ah-NAT-o-mē) and physiology (fiz-ēOL-o-jē). Over the course of this book, you will become familiar with the basic anatomy and physiology of the human body.

> ### CHECKPOINT
>
> 1. How do vital functions such as responsiveness, growth, reproduction, and movement depend on metabolism?
>
> See the blue Answers tab at the back of the book.

1-2 Anatomy is structure, and physiology is function

Learning Objective Explain the relationship between anatomy and physiology, and describe various specialties of each discipline.

The word *anatomy* has Greek origins, as do many other anatomical terms and phrases. **Anatomy**, which means "a cutting open," is the study of internal and external structure and the physical relationships between body parts. **Physiology**, also derived from Greek, is the study of how living organisms carry out their vital functions. The two subjects are interrelated. Anatomical information provides clues about probable functions. Physiological processes can be explained only in terms of their underlying anatomy.

The link between structure and function is always present but not always understood. For example, the anatomy of the heart was clearly described in the 15th century, but almost 200 years passed before anyone realized that it pumped blood. This text will familiarize you with basic anatomy and give you an appreciation of the physiological processes that make human life possible. The information will help you

to understand many diseases to make informed decisions about your own health.

Anatomy

We can divide anatomy into gross (macroscopic) anatomy and microscopic anatomy. We do so on the basis of the degree of structural detail under consideration. Other anatomical specialties focus on specific processes, such as respiration, or on medical applications, such as developing artificial limbs.

Gross Anatomy

Gross anatomy, or *macroscopic anatomy*, considers features visible with the unaided eye. We can approach gross anatomy in many ways. **Surface anatomy** is the study of general form and superficial markings. **Regional anatomy** considers all the superficial and internal features in a specific region of the body, such as the head, neck, or trunk. **Systemic anatomy** considers the structure of major *organ systems*, which are groups of organs that work together in a coordinated manner. For example, the heart, blood, and blood vessels form the *cardiovascular system*, which circulates oxygen and nutrients throughout the body.

Microscopic Anatomy

Microscopic anatomy concerns structures that we cannot see without magnification. The boundaries of microscopic anatomy are set by the limits of the equipment used. A light microscope reveals basic details about cell structure, but an electron microscope can visualize individual molecules only a few nanometers (nm, 1 millionth of a millimeter) across. In this text, we will consider details at all levels, from macroscopic to microscopic.

We can subdivide microscopic anatomy into specialties that consider features within a characteristic range of sizes. **Cytology** (sī-TOL-o-jē) analyzes the internal structure of individual *cells*. The trillions of living cells in our bodies are made up of chemical substances in various combinations. Our lives depend on the chemical processes taking place in those cells. For this reason, we consider basic chemistry (Chapter 2: The Chemical Level of Organization) before looking at cell structure (Chapter 3: Cell Structure and Function).

Histology (his-TOL-o-jē) takes a broader perspective. It examines **tissues**, groups of specialized cells and cell products that work together to carry out specific functions (Chapter 4). Tissues combine to form **organs**, such as the heart, kidney, liver, and brain. We can examine many organs without a microscope, so at the organ level we cross the boundary into gross anatomy.

Physiology

Physiology is the study of functions in living organisms. **Human physiology** is the study of the functions of the human body. These functions are complex and much more difficult to examine than most anatomical structures. As a result, the science of physiology includes even more specialties than does the science of anatomy.

The cornerstone of human physiology is **cell physiology**, the study of the functions of living cells. Cell physiology includes events at the chemical or molecular levels—chemical processes both within cells and between cells. **Special physiology** is the study of the physiology of specific organs. Examples include renal physiology (kidney function) and cardiac physiology (heart function). **Systemic physiology** considers all aspects of the function of specific organ systems. Respiratory physiology and reproductive physiology are examples. **Pathological physiology**, or **pathology** (pah-THOL-o-jē), is the study of the effects of diseases on organ or system functions. (The Greek word *pathos* means "disease.") Modern medicine depends on an understanding of both normal and pathological physiology, to know not only what has gone wrong but also how to correct it.

Special topics in physiology address specific functions of the human body as a whole. These specialties focus on functional relationships among multiple organ systems. Exercise physiology, for example, studies the physiological adjustments to exercise.

CHECKPOINT

2. Describe how anatomy and physiology are closely related.

3. Would a histologist more likely be considered a specialist in microscopic anatomy or in gross anatomy? Why?

See the blue Answers tab at the back of the book.

1-3 Levels of organization progress from atoms and molecules to a complete organism

Learning Objective Identify the major levels of organization in organisms, from the simplest to the most complex.

To understand the human body, we must examine how it is organized at several different levels, from the submicroscopic to the macroscopic. **Spotlight Figure 1-1** presents the relationships among the various levels of organization, using the cardiovascular system as an example.

- **Chemical level.** *Atoms*, the smallest stable units of matter, combine to form *molecules* with complex shapes. Even at this simplest level, a molecule's specialized shape determines its function. This is the chemical level of organization.

- **Cellular level.** Different molecules can interact to form larger structures. Each type of structure has a specific function in a cell. For example, different types of protein filaments interact to produce the contractions of muscle cells in the heart. *Cells*, the smallest living units in the body, make up the cellular level of organization.

- **Tissue level.** A *tissue* is composed of similar cells working together to perform a specific function. Heart muscle cells form *cardiac muscle tissue*, an example of the tissue level of organization.

- **Organ level.** An *organ* consists of two or more different tissues working together to perform specific functions. An example of the organ level of organization is the *heart*, a hollow, three-dimensional organ with walls composed of layers of cardiac muscle and other tissues.

- **Organ system level.** Organs interact in *organ systems*. Each time it contracts, the heart pushes blood into a network of blood vessels. Together, the heart, blood, and blood vessels form the *cardiovascular system*, an example of the organ system level of organization.

- **Organism level.** All the organ systems of the body work together to maintain life and health. The highest level of organization is the *organism*—in this case, a human.

The organization at each level determines both the structural characteristics and the functions of higher levels. As **Spotlight Figure 1-1** shows, the arrangement of atoms and molecules at the chemical level creates the protein filaments that, at the cellular level, give cardiac muscle cells the ability to contract. At the tissue level, these cells are linked, forming cardiac muscle tissue. The structure of the tissue ensures that the contractions are coordinated, producing a heartbeat. When that beat occurs, the internal anatomy of the heart, an organ, enables it to function as a pump. The heart is filled with blood and connected to the blood vessels, and the pumping action circulates blood through the vessels of the cardiovascular system. Through interactions with the respiratory, digestive, urinary, and other systems, the cardiovascular system performs a variety of functions essential to the survival of the organism.

Something that affects a system will ultimately affect each of the system's components. For example, the heart cannot pump blood effectively after massive blood loss. If the heart

Our understanding of how the human body works is based on investigations of its different levels of organization. Interacting atoms form molecules that combine to form the protein filaments of a heart muscle cell. Such cells interlock, creating heart muscle tissue, which makes up most of the walls of the heart, a three-dimensional organ. The heart is only one component of the cardiovascular system, which also includes the blood and blood vessels. The various organ systems must work together to maintain life at the organism level.

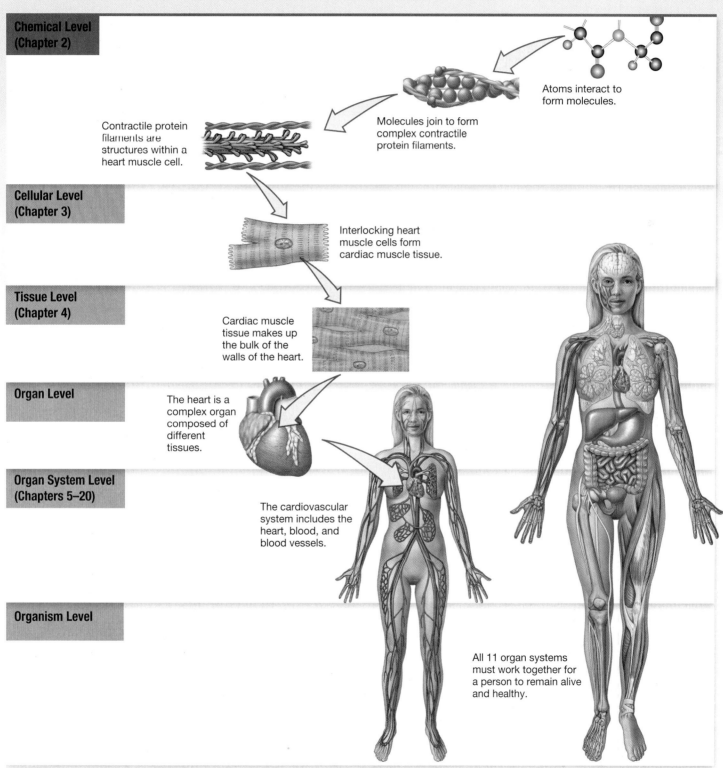

Chemical Level (Chapter 2)

Atoms interact to form molecules.

Molecules join to form complex contractile protein filaments.

Contractile protein filaments are structures within a heart muscle cell.

Cellular Level (Chapter 3)

Interlocking heart muscle cells form cardiac muscle tissue.

Tissue Level (Chapter 4)

Cardiac muscle tissue makes up the bulk of the walls of the heart.

Organ Level

The heart is a complex organ composed of different tissues.

Organ System Level (Chapters 5–20)

The cardiovascular system includes the heart, blood, and blood vessels.

Organism Level

All 11 organ systems must work together for a person to remain alive and healthy.

cannot pump and blood cannot flow, oxygen and nutrients cannot be distributed. Very soon, the cardiac muscle tissue begins to break down as its individual muscle cells die from oxygen and nutrient starvation. These changes will also take place beyond the cardiovascular system: cells, tissues, and organs throughout the body will be damaged.

CHECKPOINT

> 4. Identify the major levels of organization of the human body from the simplest to the most complex.
>
> See the blue Answers tab at the back of the book.

1-4 The human body consists of 11 organ systems

Learning Objective Identify the 11 organ systems of the human body and contrast their major functions.

Figure 1-2 introduces the 11 organ systems in the human body and their major functions and components. The body's organ systems are (1) the integumentary system, (2) the skeletal system, (3) the muscular system, (4) the nervous system, (5) the endocrine system, (6) the cardiovascular system, (7) the lymphatic system, (8) the respiratory system, (9) the digestive system, (10) the urinary system, and (11) the reproductive system.

CHECKPOINT

> 5. Identify the organ systems of the body and list their major functions.
>
> 6. Which organ system includes the pituitary gland and directs long-term changes in the activities of the body's other systems?
>
> See the blue Answers tab at the back of the book.

1-5 Homeostasis is the state of internal balance

Learning Objective Explain the concept of homeostasis.

Organ systems are interdependent, interconnected, and take up a relatively small space. The cells, tissues, organs, and organ systems of the body function together in a shared environment. Just as the people in a large city breathe the same air and drink water from the local water company, the cells in the human body absorb oxygen and nutrients from the body fluids that surround them. All living cells are in contact with blood or some other body fluid. Any change in the composition of these fluids will affect the cells in some way. For example, changes in the temperature or salt content of the blood could cause anything from a minor adjustment (heart muscle tissue contracts more often, and the heart rate goes up) to a total disaster (the heart stops beating altogether).

Various physiological responses act to prevent potentially dangerous changes in the environment inside the body. **Homeostasis** (hō-mē-ō-STĀ-sis; *homeo*, unchanging + *stasis*, standing) refers to a stable internal environment. To survive, every living organism must maintain homeostasis. The term **homeostatic regulation** refers to the adjustments in physiological systems that preserve homeostasis.

Homeostatic regulation usually involves

1. a **receptor** that is sensitive to a particular environmental change or *stimulus*;

2. a **control center**, or *integration center*, which receives and processes information from the receptor; and

3. an **effector**, a cell or organ that responds to the commands of the control center and whose activity opposes or enhances the stimulus.

You are probably already familiar with several examples of homeostatic regulation, although not in those terms. As an example, think about the operation of the thermostat in a house or apartment (**Figure 1-3**).

CLINICAL NOTE

Homeostasis and Disease

The human body is amazingly effective in maintaining homeostasis. Nevertheless, an infection, an injury, or a genetic abnormality can sometimes have effects so severe that homeostatic responses cannot fully compensate for these. One or more characteristics of the internal environment may then be pushed beyond normal limits. When this occurs, organ systems begin to malfunction, producing a state we know as illness or disease.

An understanding of normal homeostatic responses usually aids in thinking about what might be responsible for the signs and symptoms that are characteristic of many diseases. Symptoms are subjective—things that a person experiences and describes but that are not otherwise detectable or measurable. Pain, nausea, and anxiety are examples of symptoms. A sign, by contrast, is an objectively observable or measurable physical indicator of a disease or injury. Examples include a rash, a swelling, fever, or sounds of abnormal breathing. Technology can reveal many additional signs that would not be evident to a physician's unaided senses: an unusual shape on an X-ray or MRI scan or an elevated concentration of a particular chemical in a blood test. We describe many aspects of human health, disease, and treatment in this textbook.

Figure 1-2 The Organ Systems of the Human Body.

The Integumentary System

Protects against environmental hazards; helps control body temperature; provides sensory information

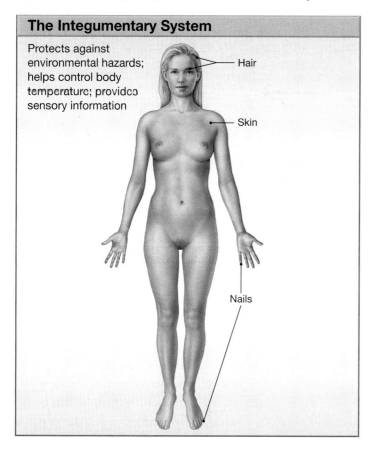

Hair

Skin

Nails

The Skeletal System

Provides support; protects tissues; stores minerals; forms blood cells

AXIAL SKELETON

APPENDICULAR SKELETON

Skull

Supporting bones (scapula and clavicle)

Sternum

Ribs

Upper limb bones

Vertebrae

Sacrum

Pelvis (supporting bones plus sacrum)

Lower limb bones

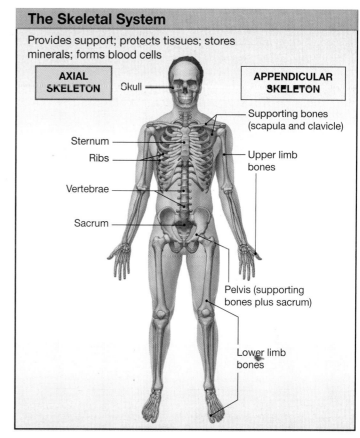

The Muscular System

Provides movement; provides protection and support for other tissues; produces heat

Axial muscles

Appendicular muscles

Tendons

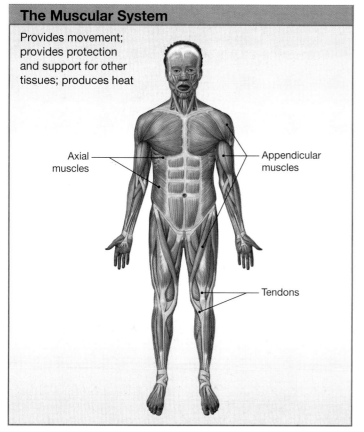

The Nervous System

Directs immediate responses to stimuli, usually by coordinating the activities of other organ systems; provides and interprets sensory information about internal and external conditions

CENTRAL NERVOUS SYSTEM

Brain

Spinal cord

PERIPHERAL NERVOUS SYSTEM

Peripheral nerves

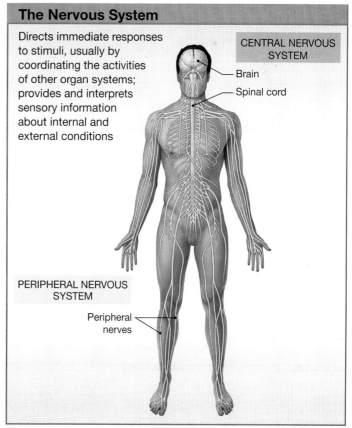

(continued)

Figure 1-2 The Organ Systems of the Human Body. (continued)

The Endocrine System

Directs long-term changes in activities of other organ systems

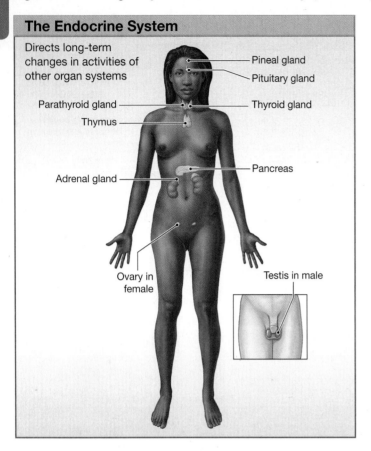

- Pineal gland
- Pituitary gland
- Parathyroid gland
- Thymus
- Thyroid gland
- Adrenal gland
- Pancreas
- Ovary in female
- Testis in male

The Cardiovascular System

Transports cells and dissolved materials, including nutrients, wastes, oxygen, and carbon dioxide

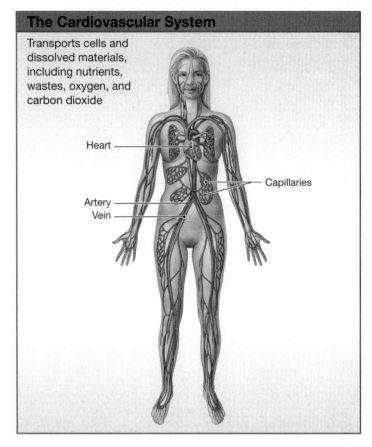

- Heart
- Capillaries
- Artery
- Vein

The Lymphatic System

Defends against infection and disease; returns tissue fluids to the bloodstream

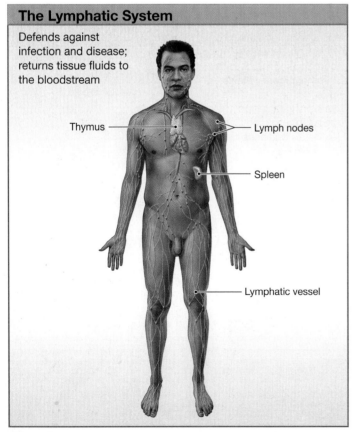

- Thymus
- Lymph nodes
- Spleen
- Lymphatic vessel

The Respiratory System

Delivers air to sites in the lungs where gas exchange occurs between the air and bloodstream; produces sound for communication

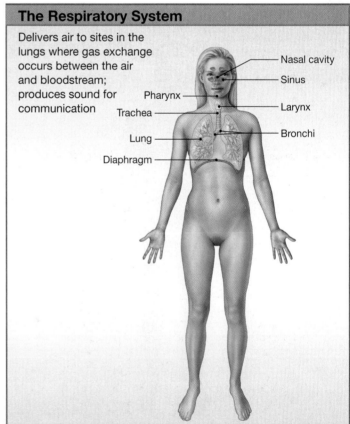

- Nasal cavity
- Sinus
- Pharynx
- Larynx
- Trachea
- Bronchi
- Lung
- Diaphragm

The Digestive System

Processes food and absorbs nutrients

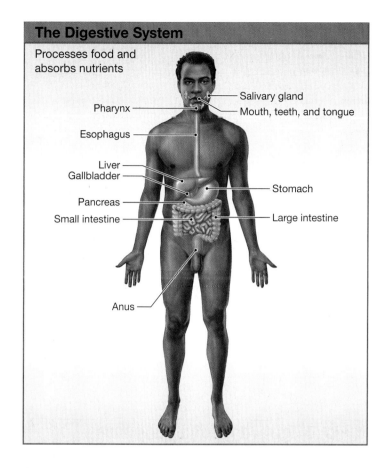

Pharynx —
Salivary gland
Mouth, teeth, and tongue

Esophagus —

Liver —
Gallbladder —

Stomach

Pancreas —
Small intestine —

Large intestine

Anus —

The Urinary System

Eliminates waste products from the blood; controls water balance by regulating the volume of urine produced

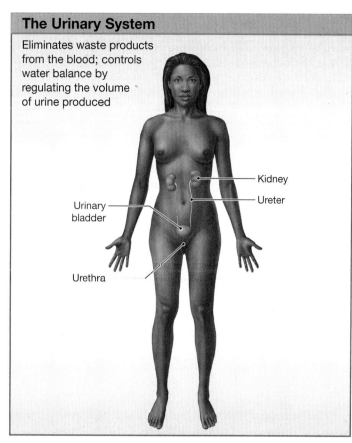

Kidney

Ureter

Urinary bladder —

Urethra —

The Male Reproductive System

Produces male sex cells (sperm) and hormones

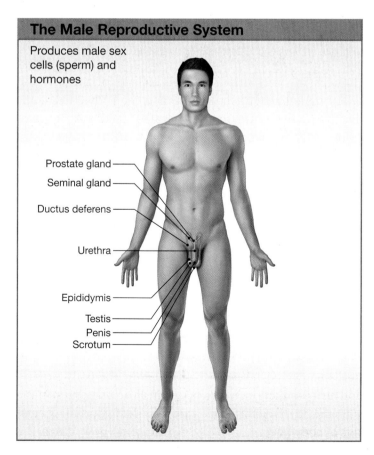

Prostate gland —
Seminal gland —
Ductus deferens —

Urethra —

Epididymis —
Testis —
Penis —
Scrotum —

The Female Reproductive System

Produces female sex cells (oocytes, or immature eggs) and hormones; supports embryonic and fetal development from fertilization to birth

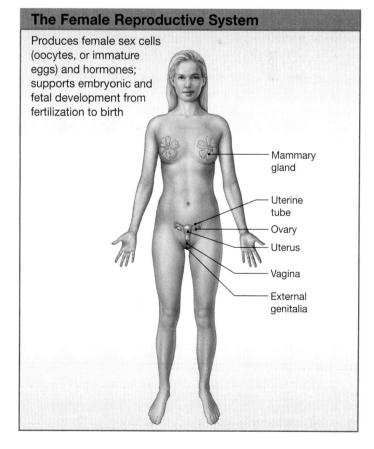

Mammary gland

Uterine tube
Ovary
Uterus

Vagina

External genitalia

1

Figure 1-3 The Control of Room Temperature. In response to input from a receptor (a thermometer), a thermostat (the control center) triggers a response from an effector (in this case, an air conditioner) that restores normal temperature. When room temperature rises above the set point, the thermostat turns on the air conditioner, and the temperature returns to normal.

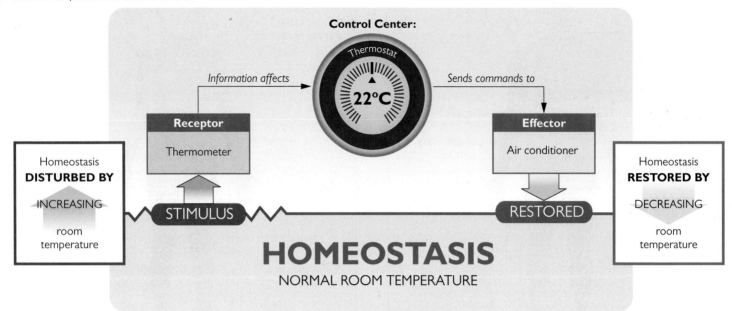

The thermostat is a control center that monitors room temperature. The thermostat shows the set point, the "ideal" room temperature—in this example, 22°C (about 72°F). The function of the thermostat is to keep room temperature within acceptable limits, usually within a degree or so of the set point. The thermostat receives information from a receptor, a thermometer exposed to air in the room, and it controls one of two effectors: a heater or an air conditioner. In the summer, for example, a rise in temperature above the set point causes the thermostat to turn on the air conditioner, which then cools the room (**Figure 1-3**). When the temperature at the thermometer returns to the set point, the thermostat turns off the air conditioner.

We can summarize the essential feature of temperature control by a thermostat very simply: A variation outside the desired range triggers an automatic response that corrects the situation. This method of homeostatic regulation is called *negative feedback*, because an effector activated by the control center opposes, or *negates*, the original stimulus.

CHECKPOINT

7. Define homeostasis.

8. Why is homeostatic regulation important to an organism?

9. What happens to the body when homeostasis breaks down?

See the blue Answers tab at the back of the book.

1-6 Negative feedback opposes variations from normal, whereas positive feedback exaggerates them

Learning Objective Describe how negative feedback and positive feedback are involved in homeostatic regulation.

Homeostatic regulation controls aspects of the internal environment that affect every cell in the body. Most commonly, such regulation uses negative feedback. Positive feedback is less frequent because it tends to produce extreme responses.

Negative Feedback

The essential feature of **negative feedback** is this: Regardless of whether the stimulus (such as temperature) rises or falls at the receptor, *a variation outside normal limits triggers an automatic response that corrects the situation.*

Most homeostatic responses in the body involve negative feedback. For example, consider the control of body temperature, a process called *thermoregulation* (**Figure 1-4**). Thermoregulation involves altering the relationship between heat loss, which takes place primarily at the body surface, and heat production, which occurs in all active tissues. In the human body, skeletal muscles are the most important generators of body heat.

Figure 1-4 Negative Feedback in Thermoregulation. In negative feedback, a stimulus produces a response that opposes the original stimulus. Body temperature is regulated by a control center in the brain that functions as a thermostat with a set point of 37°C.

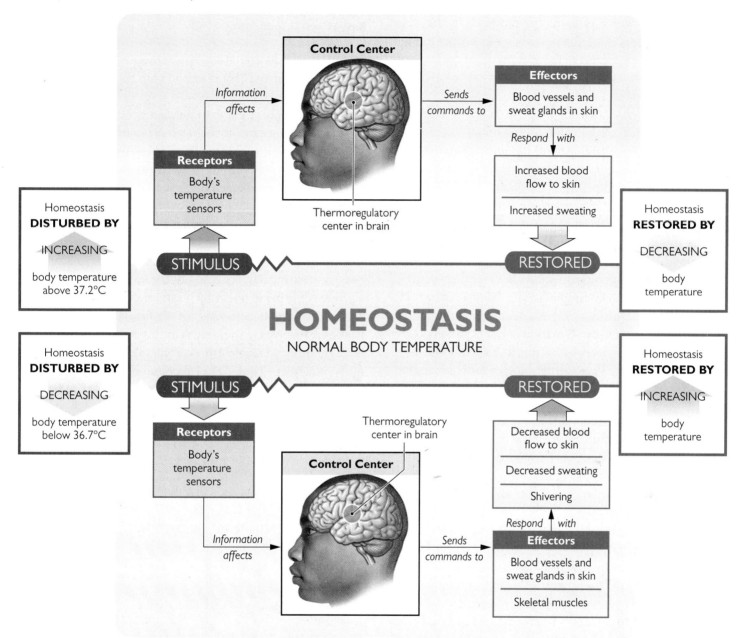

The thermoregulatory control center is located in the brain. This control center receives information from temperature receptors located in the skin and in cells in the control center. At the normal set point, body temperature is approximately 37°C (98.6°F).

If body temperature rises above 37.2°C (99°F), activity in the control center targets two effectors: (1) smooth muscles in the walls of blood vessels supplying the skin and (2) sweat glands. The muscle tissue relaxes and the blood vessels widen, or dilate, increasing blood flow at the body surface.

The sweat glands accelerate, or speed up, their secretion. The skin then acts like a radiator, losing heat to the environment, and the evaporation of sweat speeds the process. When body temperature returns to normal, the control center becomes inactive. Superficial blood flow and sweat gland activity then decrease to normal resting levels.

If temperature at the control center falls below 36.7°C (98°F), the control center targets the same two effectors and skeletal muscles. This time, blood flow to the skin declines, and sweat gland activity decreases. This combination reduces the rate of heat loss to the environment. However, body temperature gradually rises because skeletal muscles continue to produce heat. (Additional heat may be generated by *shivering*, which is caused by random contractions of skeletal muscles.) Once the body has warmed to the set point, the thermoregulatory center turns itself "off." Both blood flow and sweat gland activity in the skin then increase to normal resting levels.

Homeostatic responses using negative feedback maintain a normal range, not a fixed value. In the previous example, body temperature oscillates around the ideal set-point temperature. Thus, for any single individual, any measured value (such as body temperature) can vary from moment to moment or day to day. The variability among individuals is even greater, for each person has a slightly different homeostatic set point. It is, therefore, impractical to define "normal" homeostatic conditions very precisely.

By convention, physiological values are reported either as average values obtained by sampling a large number of individuals or as a range that includes 95 percent or more of the sample population. For example, for 95 percent of healthy adults, body temperature ranges between 36.7°C and 37.2°C (98°F and 99°F, respectively). The other 5 percent of healthy adults have resting body temperatures outside the "normal" range (below 36.7°C or above 37.2°C). Still, these temperatures are perfectly normal for them, and the variations have no clinical significance.

Positive Feedback

In **positive feedback**, *an initial stimulus produces a response that reinforces that stimulus.* For example, suppose a thermostat were wired so that when the temperature rose, the thermostat would turn on the heater rather than the air conditioner. In that case, the initial stimulus (rising room temperature) would cause a response (heater turns on) that strengthens the stimulus. Room temperature would continue to rise until someone switched off the thermostat, unplugged the heater, or intervened in some other way before the house caught fire and burned down. This kind of escalating cycle is called a *positive feedback loop.*

In the body, positive feedback loops are involved in the regulation of a potentially dangerous or stressful process that must be completed quickly. For example, the immediate danger from a severe cut is blood loss, which can lower blood pressure and reduce the pumping efficiency of the heart. The positive feedback loop involved in the body's clotting response to blood loss is diagrammed in **Figure 1-5**. (We will examine blood clotting more closely in Chapter 11.) Labor and delivery (discussed in Chapter 20) is another example of positive feedback in action.

Figure 1-5 Positive Feedback. In positive feedback, a stimulus produces a response that reinforces the original stimulus. Positive feedback is important in accelerating processes that must proceed to completion rapidly. In this example, positive feedback accelerates blood clotting until bleeding stops.

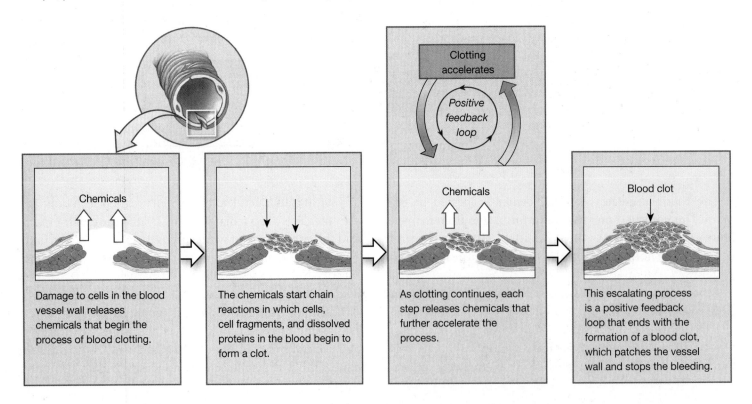

Damage to cells in the blood vessel wall releases chemicals that begin the process of blood clotting.

The chemicals start chain reactions in which cells, cell fragments, and dissolved proteins in the blood begin to form a clot.

As clotting continues, each step releases chemicals that further accelerate the process.

This escalating process is a positive feedback loop that ends with the formation of a blood clot, which patches the vessel wall and stops the bleeding.

CHECKPOINT

10. Explain the function of negative feedback systems.

11. Why is positive feedback helpful in blood clotting but unsuitable for the regulation of body temperature, as with a fever?

See the blue Answers tab at the back of the book.

1-7 Anatomical terms describe body regions, anatomical positions and directions, and body sections

Learning Objective Use anatomical terms to describe body regions, body sections, and relative positions.

Early anatomists faced serious communication problems. For example, stating that a bump is "on the back" does not give very precise information about its location. So anatomists created maps of the human body. Prominent anatomical structures serve as landmarks, distances are measured (in centimeters or inches), and specialized directional terms are used. In effect, anatomy uses a language of its own, called *medical terminology*, that you must learn almost at the start of your study.

Anatomical terms are easier to understand if you are familiar with Latin and Greek word roots and their combinations. As new terms are introduced in the text, we will provide notes on their pronunciation and the relevant word roots. Look inside the back cover for additional information on foreign word roots, prefixes, suffixes, and combining forms.

Latin and Greek terms are not the only foreign words imported into the anatomical vocabulary over the centuries, and the vocabulary continues to expand. Many anatomical structures and clinical conditions were first named after either the discoverer or, in the case of diseases, the most famous victim. Most such commemorative names, or *eponyms*, have been replaced by more precise terms, but many are still in use.

Surface Anatomy

With the exception of the skin, none of the organ systems can be seen from the body surface. For this reason, you must create your own mental maps, basing your information on the terms given in **Figures 1-6** and **1-7**. Learning these terms now will make material in subsequent chapters easier to understand.

Anatomical Landmarks

Standard anatomical illustrations show the human form in the **anatomical position**. When the body is in this position, the hands are at the sides with the palms facing forward,

and the feet are together (**Figure 1-6**). A person lying down in the anatomical position is said to be **supine** (soo-PĪN) when face up and **prone** when face down.

Important anatomical landmarks are also presented in **Figure 1-6**. The anatomical terms are in boldface, the common names in plain type, and the anatomical adjectives in parentheses. Understanding these terms and their origins will help you remember both the location of a particular structure and its name. For example, the term *brachium* refers to the arm. Later chapters will discuss the *brachialis muscle* and the *brachial artery*, which are in the arm, as their names suggest.

Anatomical Regions

Major regions of the body, such as the *brachial region*, are referred to by their anatomical adjectives, as shown in **Figure 1-6**. To describe a general area of interest or injury, anatomists and clinicians often need to use broader terms in addition to specific landmarks. Two methods are used to map the surface of the abdomen and pelvis.

Clinicians refer to four **abdominopelvic quadrants** formed by a pair of imaginary perpendicular lines that intersect at the *umbilicus* (navel). This simple method, shown in **Figure 1-7a**, is useful for describing the location of aches, pains, and injuries, which can help a doctor determine the possible cause. For example, tenderness in the right lower quadrant is a symptom of appendicitis. Tenderness in the right upper quadrant may indicate gallbladder or liver problems.

Anatomists like to use more precise regional terms to describe the location and orientation of internal organs. They recognize nine **abdominopelvic regions** (Figure 1-7b). **Figure 1-7c** shows the relationships among quadrants, regions, and internal organs.

Anatomical Directions

Figure 1-8 presents the principal directional terms and some examples of their use. There are many different terms, and some can be used interchangeably. For example, *anterior* refers to the front of the body, when viewed in the anatomical position. In humans, this term is equivalent to *ventral*, which refers to the belly. Likewise, the terms *posterior* and *dorsal* refer to the back of the human body. Remember that *left* and *right* always refer to the left and right sides of the *subject*, not of the observer.

Sectional Anatomy

Sometimes the only way to understand the relationships among the parts of a three-dimensional object is to slice through it and look at the internal organization. An understanding of

1

Figure 1-6 Anatomical Landmarks. Anatomical terms are in boldface type, common names are in plain type, and anatomical adjectives (referring to body regions) are in parentheses.

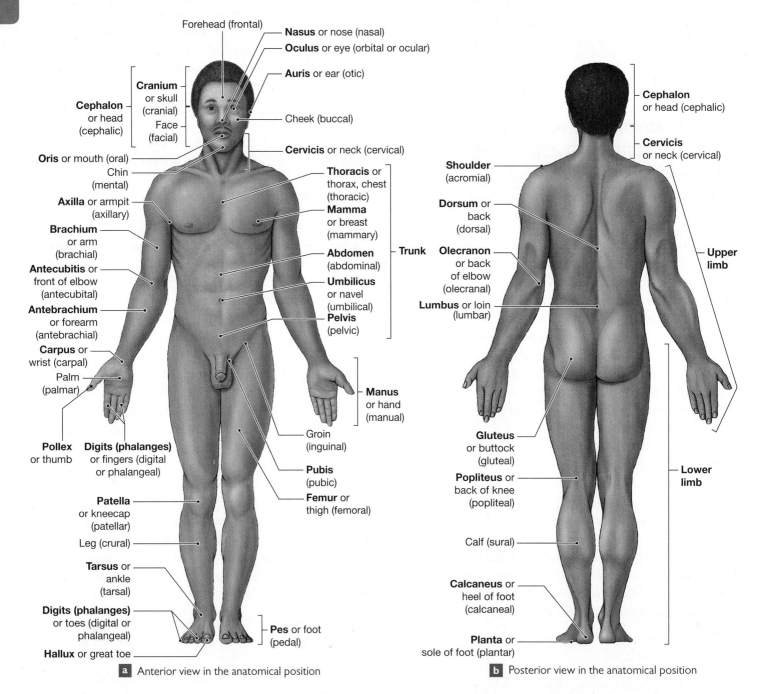

Forehead (frontal)
Nasus or nose (nasal)
Oculus or eye (orbital or ocular)
Auris or ear (otic)

Cranium or skull (cranial)
Face (facial)

Cephalon or head (cephalic)

Cheek (buccal)

Cervicis or neck (cervical)

Oris or mouth (oral)
Chin (mental)

Axilla or armpit (axillary)

Brachium or arm (brachial)

Antecubitis or front of elbow (antecubital)

Antebrachium or forearm (antebrachial)

Carpus or wrist (carpal)

Palm (palmar)

Pollex or thumb

Digits (phalanges) or fingers (digital or phalangeal)

Patella or kneecap (patellar)

Leg (crural)

Tarsus or ankle (tarsal)

Digits (phalanges) or toes (digital or phalangeal)

Hallux or great toe

Thoracis or thorax, chest (thoracic)
Mamma or breast (mammary)

Abdomen (abdominal)

Umbilicus or navel (umbilical)

Pelvis (pelvic)

Trunk

Manus or hand (manual)

Groin (inguinal)

Pubis (pubic)

Femur or thigh (femoral)

a Anterior view in the anatomical position

Cephalon or head (cephalic)

Cervicis or neck (cervical)

Shoulder (acromial)

Dorsum or back (dorsal)

Olecranon or back of elbow (olecranal)

Lumbus or loin (lumbar)

Upper limb

Gluteus or buttock (gluteal)

Popliteus or back of knee (popliteal)

Calf (sural)

Calcaneus or heel of foot (calcaneal)

Planta or sole of foot (plantar)

Lower limb

b Posterior view in the anatomical position

sectional views is particularly important because imaging techniques now enable us to see inside the living body without resorting to surgery. Any slice (or section) through a three-dimensional object can be described with reference to three primary **sectional planes**, indicated in **Figure 1-9.**

1. ***Frontal plane.*** The **frontal plane**, or *coronal plane*, runs along the long axis of the body. The frontal plane extends laterally (side to side), dividing the body into **anterior** and **posterior** portions.

2. ***Sagittal plane.*** The **sagittal plane** also runs along the long axis of the body, but it extends anteriorly and posteriorly (front to back). A sagittal plane divides the body into *left* and *right* portions. A cut that passes along the body's midline and divides the body into left and right halves is a **midsagittal section**. (Note that a midsagittal section does not cut through the legs.)

3. ***Transverse plane.*** The **transverse plane** lies at right angles to the long (head-to-foot) axis of the body,

Figure 1-7 Abdominopelvic Quadrants and Regions.

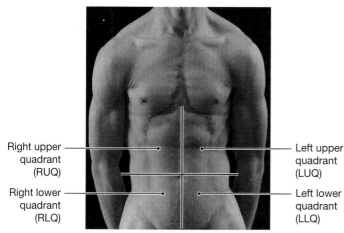

a **Abdominopelvic quadrants**. The four abdominopelvic quadrants are formed by two perpendicular lines that intersect at the navel (umbilicus). The terms for these quadrants, or their abbreviations, are most often used in clinical discussions.

Right upper quadrant (RUQ)
Left upper quadrant (LUQ)
Right lower quadrant (RLQ)
Left lower quadrant (LLQ)

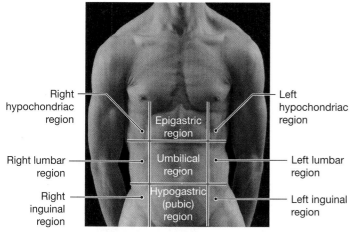

Right hypochondriac region
Left hypochondriac region
Epigastric region
Right lumbar region
Umbilical region
Left lumbar region
Right inguinal region
Hypogastric (pubic) region
Left inguinal region

b **Abdominopelvic regions**. The nine abdominopelvic regions provide more precise regional descriptions.

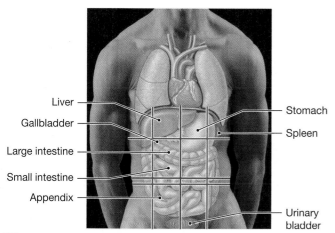

Liver
Gallbladder
Large intestine
Small intestine
Appendix
Stomach
Spleen
Urinary bladder

c **Anatomical relationships**. The relationship between the abdominopelvic quadrants and regions and the locations of the internal organs are shown here.

dividing the body into **superior** and **inferior** portions. A cut in this plane is called a **transverse section**, or *cross section*. (Unless otherwise noted, in this book all anatomical diagrams that present cross-sectional views of the body are oriented as though the subject were supine, with the observer standing at the subject's feet and looking toward the head.)

CHECKPOINT

12. What is the purpose of anatomical terms?

13. Describe an anterior view and a posterior view in the anatomical position.

14. What type of section would separate the two eyes?

See the blue Answers tab at the back of the book.

1-8 Body cavities of the trunk protect internal organs and allow them to change shape

Learning Objective Identify the major body cavities of the trunk and the subdivisions of each.

The body's trunk is subdivided into three major regions established by the body wall: thoracic, abdominal, and pelvic (**Figure 1-6**). Most of the vital organs of the body are located within these regions. The true **body cavities** are closed, fluid-filled spaces lined by a thin tissue layer called a *serous membrane*. The vital organs of the trunk are *suspended* within these body cavities. They do not simply lie there.

Early anatomists began using the term "cavity" when referring to internal regions. For example, they considered everything deep to the chest wall of the thoracic region to be within the thoracic cavity. They also considered all of the structures deep to the abdominal and pelvic walls to be within the abdominopelvic cavity. Internally, these two anatomical regions are separated by the **diaphragm** (DĪ-uh-fram), a flat muscular sheet.

The boundaries of the regional "cavities" and the true body cavities of the trunk are not identical, however. For example, the thoracic cavity contains two pleural cavities (each surrounding a lung), a pericardial cavity (surrounding the heart), and a large tissue mass, the mediastinum. Also, the peritoneal cavity extends only partway into the pelvic cavity. The boundaries between the subdivisions of the thoracic cavity and abdominopelvic cavity are shown in **Figure 1-11** (p. 18).

1

Figure 1-8 Directional References.

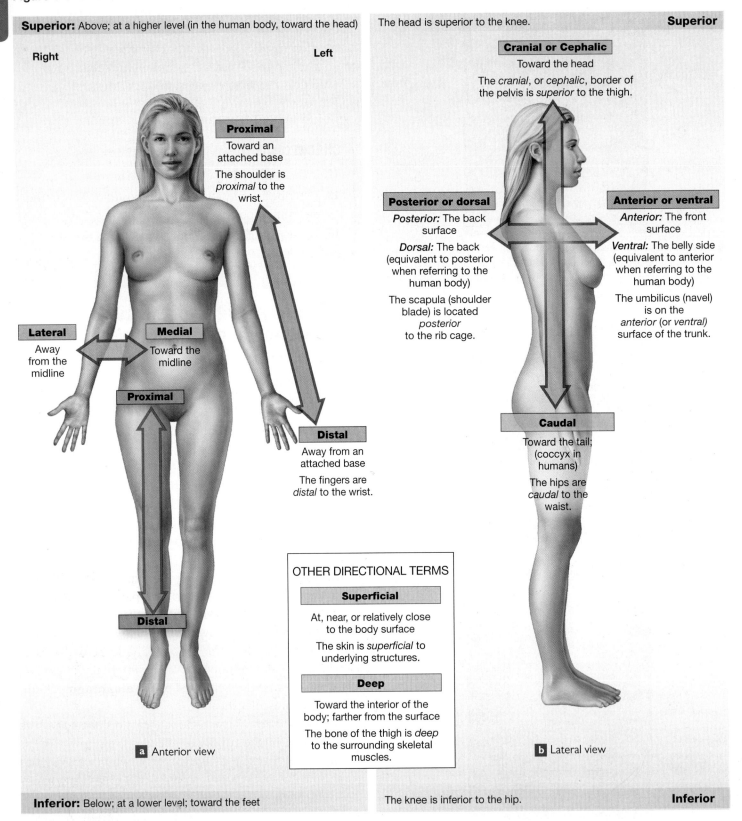

Superior: Above; at a higher level (in the human body, toward the head)

The head is superior to the knee.   **Superior**

Right   Left

Cranial or Cephalic
Toward the head

The *cranial*, or *cephalic*, border of the pelvis is *superior* to the thigh.

Proximal
Toward an attached base

The shoulder is *proximal* to the wrist.

Posterior or dorsal

Posterior: The back surface

Dorsal: The back (equivalent to posterior when referring to the human body)

The scapula (shoulder blade) is located *posterior* to the rib cage.

Anterior or ventral

Anterior: The front surface

Ventral: The belly side (equivalent to anterior when referring to the human body)

The umbilicus (navel) is on the *anterior* (or *ventral*) surface of the trunk.

Lateral
Away from the midline

Medial
Toward the midline

Proximal

Distal
Away from an attached base

The fingers are *distal* to the wrist.

Caudal
Toward the tail; (coccyx in humans)

The hips are *caudal* to the waist.

Distal

OTHER DIRECTIONAL TERMS

Superficial

At, near, or relatively close to the body surface

The skin is *superficial* to underlying structures.

Deep

Toward the interior of the body; farther from the surface

The bone of the thigh is *deep* to the surrounding skeletal muscles.

a Anterior view

b Lateral view

Inferior: Below; at a lower level; toward the feet   The knee is inferior to the hip.   **Inferior**

Figure 1-9 Sectional Planes.

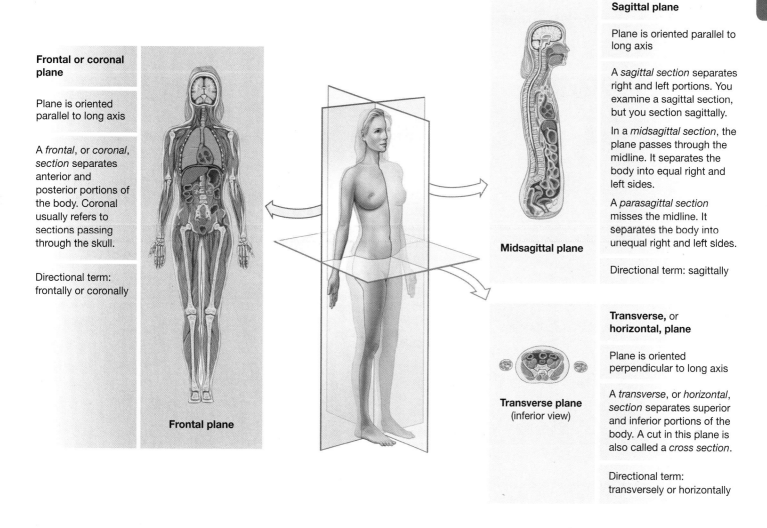

Frontal or coronal plane

Plane is oriented parallel to long axis

A *frontal*, or *coronal*, *section* separates anterior and posterior portions of the body. Coronal usually refers to sections passing through the skull.

Directional term: frontally or coronally

Frontal plane

Sagittal plane

Plane is oriented parallel to long axis

A *sagittal section* separates right and left portions. You examine a sagittal section, but you section sagittally.

In a *midsagittal section*, the plane passes through the midline. It separates the body into equal right and left sides.

A *parasagittal section* misses the midline. It separates the body into unequal right and left sides.

Directional term: sagittally

Midsagittal plane

Transverse, or **horizontal, plane**

Plane is oriented perpendicular to long axis

A *transverse*, or *horizontal*, *section* separates superior and inferior portions of the body. A cut in this plane is also called a *cross section*.

Directional term: transversely or horizontally

Transverse plane (inferior view)

CLINICAL NOTE

Surface Anatomy

It is essential that emergency personnel have a good grasp of human surface anatomy. First, such knowledge will help determine what underlying structures might be injured. Second, using standard surface anatomical terms will allow the paramedic to describe an injury accurately to the receiving facility (**Figure 1-10**). Finally, post-call documentation requires a detailed report of the call and the care delivered. It is not uncommon for prehospital personnel to be questioned about a particular call months or years after it occurred. Only through use of proper anatomical terms and documentation can you accurately recall the circumstances of the encounter and the patient's injuries.

Figure 1-10 Gunshot Wounds to the Torso.

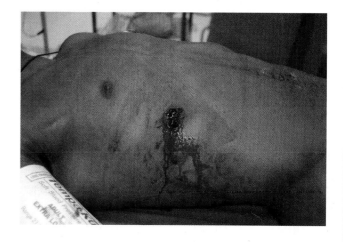

Figure 1-11 Relationships among the Subdivisions of the Body Cavities of the Trunk.

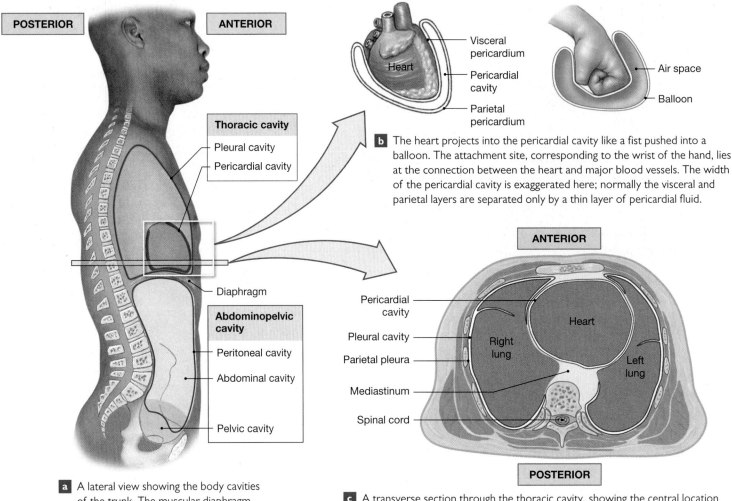

b The heart projects into the pericardial cavity like a fist pushed into a balloon. The attachment site, corresponding to the wrist of the hand, lies at the connection between the heart and major blood vessels. The width of the pericardial cavity is exaggerated here; normally the visceral and parietal layers are separated only by a thin layer of pericardial fluid.

a A lateral view showing the body cavities of the trunk. The muscular diaphragm subdivides them into a superior thoracic cavity and an inferior abdominopelvic cavity. Three of the four adult true body cavities are shown and outlined in red; only one of the two pleural cavities can be shown in a sagittal section.

c A transverse section through the thoracic cavity, showing the central location of the pericardial cavity. The mediastinum and pericardial cavity lie between the two pleural cavities. Note that this transverse or cross-sectional view is oriented as though the observer were standing at a supine subject's feet and looking toward the subject's head. This inferior view of a transverse section is the standard presentation for clinical images. Unless otherwise noted, transverse or cross-sectional views in this text use this same orientation (see *Clinical Note: Imaging Techniques*).

The body cavities of the trunk have two essential functions: (1) They protect delicate organs from accidental shocks and cushion them from the jolting that occurs when we walk, jump, or run; and (2) they permit significant changes in the size and shape of internal organs they surround. For example, the lungs, heart, stomach, intestines, urinary bladder, and many other organs can expand and contract without distorting surrounding tissues or disrupting the activities of nearby organs.

The internal organs that are enclosed by these cavities are called **viscera** (VIS-e-ruh). A delicate serous membrane lines the walls of these internal cavities and covers the surfaces of the enclosed viscera. Serous membranes produce a watery fluid that moistens the opposing surfaces and reduces friction. The portion of a serous membrane that covers a visceral organ is called the *visceral* layer. The opposing portion that lines the inner surface of the body wall or chamber is called the *parietal* layer. Because these opposing portions are usually in direct contact, the body cavities are called *potential spaces.*

The Thoracic Cavity

The thoracic cavity contains three internal chambers: a single *pericardial cavity* and a pair of *pleural cavities*—one for each lung (**Figure 1-11a,c**). Each of these three cavities is lined by shiny, slippery serous membranes. The heart projects into a space known as the **pericardial cavity**. The relationship between the heart and the pericardial cavity resembles that of a fist pushing into a balloon (**Figure 1-11b**). The wrist corresponds to the *base* (attached portion) of the heart. The balloon corresponds to the serous membrane lining the pericardial cavity. The serous membrane is called the **pericardium** (*peri-*, around + *cardium*, heart). The layer covering the heart is the **visceral pericardium**, and the opposing surface is the **parietal pericardium**.

The pericardium lies within the **mediastinum** (mēdē-a-STĪ-num) (**Figure 1-11c**). The connective tissue of the mediastinum surrounds and stabilizes the pericardial cavity and heart, the large arteries and veins attached to the heart, and the thymus, trachea, and esophagus.

Each **pleural cavity** surrounds a lung. The serous membrane lining a pleural cavity is called a **pleura** (PLOOR-ah). The *visceral pleura* covers the outer surfaces of a lung. The *parietal pleura* covers the opposing surface of the mediastinum and the inner body wall.

The Abdominopelvic Cavity

The abdominopelvic cavity extends from the diaphragm to the pelvis. It is subdivided into a superior **abdominal cavity** and an inferior **pelvic cavity** (**Figure 1-11a**). The abdominopelvic cavity contains the **peritoneal (per-i-tō-NĒ-al) cavity**, a chamber lined by a serous membrane known as the **peritoneum** (per-i-tō-NĒ-um). The *parietal peritoneum* lines the inner surface of the body wall. A narrow space containing a small amount of fluid separates the parietal peritoneum from the *visceral peritoneum*, which covers the enclosed organs.

The abdominal cavity extends from the inferior (toward the feet) surface of the diaphragm to the level of the superior (toward the head) margins of the pelvis. This cavity contains the liver, stomach, spleen, small intestine, and most of the large intestine. The organs are partially or completely enclosed by the peritoneal cavity. A few organs, such as the kidneys and pancreas, lie between the peritoneal lining and the muscular wall of the abdominal cavity. Those organs are said to be *retroperitoneal* (*retro*, behind).

Build Your Knowledge

Recall that two methods are used to refer to the locations of aches, pains, injuries, and internal organs of the abdomen and pelvis. Clinicians refer to four abdominopelvic quadrants. Anatomists refer to nine abdominopelvic regions. ↺ **p. 13**

The Clinical Note: Imaging Techniques highlights some noninvasive clinical tests commonly used for viewing the interior of the body.

The pelvic cavity is inferior to the abdominal cavity. The pelvic cavity contains the distal portion of the large intestine, the urinary bladder, and various reproductive organs. It also contains the inferior portion of the peritoneal cavity.

The true body cavities of the trunk in the adult share a common embryonic origin. The term "dorsal body cavity" is sometimes used to refer to the internal chamber of the skull (cranial cavity) and the total space enclosed by the vertebrae (vertebral cavity). These chambers, which are defined by bony structures, are structurally and developmentally distinct from true body cavities.

Many chambers, or spaces, within the body are not true body cavities. A partial list would include the cranial cavity, vertebral cavity, oral cavity, digestive cavity, orbits (eye sockets), tympanic cavity of each middle ear, nasal cavities, and paranasal sinuses (air-filled chambers within some cranial bones that are connected to the nasal cavities). We discuss these structures in later chapters.

CHECKPOINT

15. Describe two essential functions of body cavities.

16. Describe the various body cavities of the trunk.

17. If a surgeon makes an incision just inferior to the diaphragm, which body cavity will be opened?

See the blue Answers tab at the back of the book.

RELATED CLINICAL TERMS

auscultation (aws-kul-TĀ-shun): Listening to a patient's body sounds using a stethoscope.

pathologist (pa-THOL-o-jist): A physician who specializes in the study of disease processes.

radiologist: A physician who specializes in performing and analyzing radiological procedures.

radiology (rā-dē-OL-o-jē): The study of radioactive energy and radioactive substances and their use in the diagnosis and treatment of disease.

Over the past several decades, rapid progress has been made in discovering more accurate and more detailed ways to image the human body, in both healthy and disease conditions.

X-rays

X-rays are the oldest and still the most common method of imaging. X-rays are a form of high-energy radiation that can penetrate living tissues. An x-ray beam travels through the body before striking a photographic plate. Not all of the projected x-rays arrive at the film. The body absorbs or deflects some of those x-rays. The ability to stop the passage of x-rays is referred to as **radiopacity**. When taking an x-ray, these areas that are impenetrable by x-rays appear light or white on the exposed film and are said to be **radiopaque**. In the body, air has the lowest radiopacity. Fat, liver, blood, muscle, and bone are increasingly radiopaque. As a result, radiopaque tissues look white, and less radiopaque tissues are in shades of gray to black.

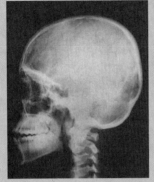

An x-ray of the skull, taken from the left side

To use x-rays to visualize soft tissues, a very radiopaque substance must be introduced. To study the upper digestive tract, a radiopaque barium solution is ingested to the patient. The resulting x-ray shows the contours of the stomach and intestines.

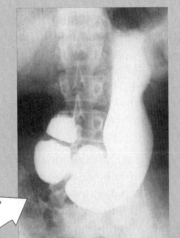

A **barium-contrast x-ray** of the upper digestive tract

Standard Scanning Techniques

More recently, a variety of **scanning techniques** dependent on computers have been developed to show the less radiopaque, soft tissues of the body in much greater detail.

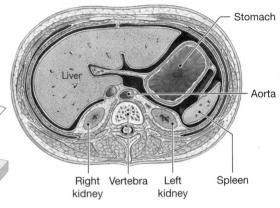

Diagrammatic views showing the relative position and orientation of the CT scan below and the MRI to the right.

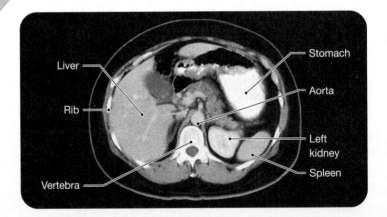

Computed tomographic scan of the abdomen

Computed tomographic (**CT**) **scans** use computers to reconstruct sectional views. A single x-ray source rotates around the body, and the x-ray beam strikes a sensor monitored by the computer. The x-ray source completes one revolution around the body every few seconds. It then moves a short distance and repeats the process. The result is usually displayed as a sectional view in black and white, but it can be colorized for visual effect. CT scans show three-dimensional relationships and soft tissue structures more clearly than do standard x-rays.

- Note that when anatomical diagrams or scans present cross-sectional views, the sections are presented from an inferior perspective, as though the observer were standing at the feet of a person in the supine position and looking toward the head of the subject.

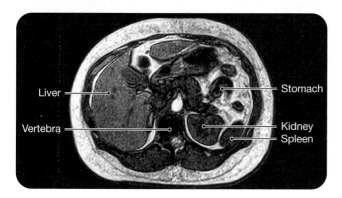

Magnetic resonance imaging scan of the abdomen

A magnetic resonance imaging (**MRI**) of the same region (in this case, the abdomen) can show soft tissue structure in even greater detail than a CT scan. MRI surrounds part or all of the body with a magnetic field 3000 times as strong as that of Earth. This field causes particles within atoms throughout the body to line up in a uniform direction. Energy from pulses of radio waves is absorbed and released by the different atoms. The released energy is used to create a detailed image of the soft tissue structure.

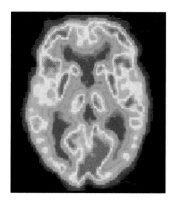

Positron emission tomographic scan of the brain

Positron emission tomography (**PET**) is an imaging technique that assesses metabolic and physiological activity of a structure. A PET scan is an important tool in evaluating healthy and diseased brain function.

Ultrasound of the uterus

In **ultrasound** procedures, a small transmitter contacting the skin broadcasts a brief, narrow burst of high-frequency sound and then detects the echoes. The sound waves are reflected by internal structures, and a picture, or **echogram**, is assembled from the pattern of echoes. These images lack the clarity of other procedures, but no adverse effects have been reported, and fetal development can be monitored without a significant risk of birth defects. Special methods of transmission and processing permit analysis of the beating heart without the complications that can accompany dye injections.

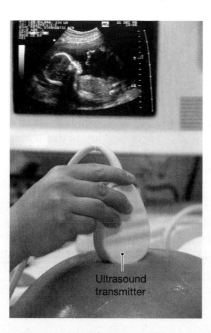

Ultrasound transmitter

Special Scanning Methods

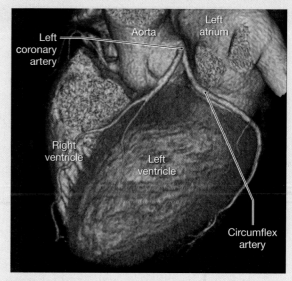

Spiral scan of the heart

A **spiral CT scan** is a form of three-dimensional imaging technology that is becoming increasingly important in clinical settings. During a spiral CT scan, the patient is on a platform that advances at a steady pace through the scanner while the imaging source, usually x-rays, rotates continuously around the patient. Because the x-ray detector gathers data quickly and continuously, a higher quality image is generated, and the patient is exposed to less radiation as compared to a standard CT scanner, which collects data more slowly from only one slice of the body at a time.

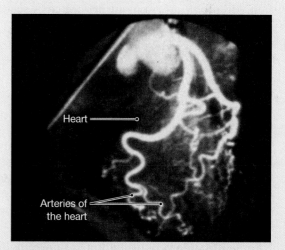

Digital subtraction angiography of coronary arteries

Digital subtraction angiography is used to monitor blood flow through specific organs, such as the brain, heart, lungs, and kidneys. X-rays are taken before and after radiopaque dye is administered, and a computer "subtracts" details common to both images. The result is a high-contrast image showing the distribution of the dye.

1 Chapter Review

Summary Outline

1-1 All living things display responsiveness, growth, reproduction, movement, and metabolism *p. 2*

1. **Biology** is the study of life; one of its goals is to discover the patterns that underlie the diversity of living organisms.

2. All living things, from single **cells** to large multicellular organisms, perform the same basic functions: They respond to changes in their environment; they grow and reproduce to create future generations; they are capable of producing movement; and they carry out the complex chemical reactions of metabolism. They absorb materials from the environment. Organisms absorb and consume oxygen during respiration, and they discharge waste products during excretion. Digestion occurs in specialized body structures that break down complex foods. The circulation forms an internal transportation system between areas of the body.

1-2 Anatomy is structure, and physiology is function *p. 3*

3. **Anatomy** is the study of internal and external structure and the physical relationships among body parts. **Physiology** is the study of how living organisms function. All specific functions are performed by specific structures.

4. **Gross (macroscopic) anatomy** considers features visible without a microscope. It includes *surface anatomy* (general form and superficial markings), *regional anatomy* (superficial and internal features in a specific area of the body), and *systemic anatomy* (structure of major organ systems).

5. The boundaries of **microscopic anatomy** are established by the equipment used. **Cytology** analyzes the internal structure of individual *cells*. **Histology** examines **tissues** (groups of similar cells that have specific functional roles). Tissues combine to form organs, anatomical units with specific functions.

6. **Human physiology** is the study of the functions of the human body. It is based on **cell physiology**, the study of the functions of living cells. *Special physiology* studies the physiology of specific organs. *System physiology* considers all aspects of the function of specific organ systems. *Pathological physiology* **(pathology)** studies the effects of diseases on organ or system functions.

1-3 Levels of organization progress from atoms and molecules to a complete organism *p. 4*

7. Anatomical structures and physiological mechanisms are arranged in a series of interacting levels of organization (*Figure 1-1*).

1-4 The human body consists of 11 organ systems *p. 6*

8. The major organs of the human body are arranged into 11 organ systems. The organ systems of the human body are the *integumentary, skeletal, muscular, nervous, endocrine, cardiovascular, lymphatic, respiratory, digestive, urinary*, and *reproductive systems (Figure 1-2)*.

1-5 Homeostasis is the state of internal balance *p. 6*

9. **Homeostasis** is the existence of a stable internal environment within the body. Physiological systems preserve homeostasis through **homeostatic regulation**.

10. Homeostatic regulation usually involves a **receptor** sensitive to a particular stimulus; a **control center**, which receives and processes the information from the receptor, and then sends out commands; and an **effector** whose activity either opposes or enhances the stimulus (*Figures 1-3* and *1-4*).

1-6 Negative feedback opposes variations from normal, whereas positive feedback exaggerates them *p. 10*

11. **Negative feedback** is a corrective response involving an action that directly opposes a variation from normal limits (*Figures 1-3* and *1-4*).

12. In **positive feedback** the initial stimulus produces a response that reinforces the stimulus (*Figure 1-5*).

13. Symptoms of **disease** appear when failure of homeostatic regulation causes organ systems to malfunction.

1-7 Anatomical terms describe body regions, anatomical positions and directions, and body sections *p. 13*

14. Standard anatomical illustrations show the body in the **anatomical position**. If the figure is shown lying down, it can be either **supine** (face up) or **prone** (face down) (*Figure 1-6*).

15. Abdominopelvic quadrants and **abdominopelvic regions** represent two different approaches to describing anatomical regions of the body *(Figure 1-7).*

16. The use of special directional terms provides clarity when describing anatomical structures *(Figure 1-8).*

17. The three **sectional planes** (**frontal** or **coronal plane,** **sagittal plane,** and **transverse plane**) describe relationships between the parts of the three-dimensional human body *(Figure 1-9).*

1-8 Body cavities of the trunk protect internal organs and allow them to change shape *p. 15*

18. Body cavities protect delicate organs and permit significant changes in the size and shape of visceral organs. The body cavities of the trunk surround organs of the respiratory, cardiovascular, digestive, urinary, and reproductive systems *(Figure 1-11).*

19. The **diaphragm** divides the (superior) **thoracic** and (inferior) **abdominopelvic cavities.** The thoracic cavity includes two **pleural cavities** (each surrounding a lung) with a central mass of tissue known as the mediastinum. Within the mediastinum is the **pericardial cavity,** which surrounds the heart. The abdominopelvic cavity consists of the **abdominal cavity** and the **pelvic cavity.** It contains the *peritoneal cavity,* a chamber lined by *peritoneum,* a *serous membrane (Figure 1-11).*

20. Important **radiological procedures** (which can provide detailed information about internal systems) include **X-rays, CT** and **spiral CT scans, MRI, PET scans,** and **ultrasound.** Each of these noninvasive techniques has advantages and disadvantages *(Clinical Note: Imaging Techniques).*

Review Questions

See the blue Answers tab at the back of the book.

Level 1 Reviewing Facts and Terms

Match each item in column A with the most closely related item in column B. Place letters for answers in the spaces provided.

COLUMN A

_____ **1.** Cytology
_____ **2.** Physiology
_____ **3.** Histology
_____ **4.** Metabolism
_____ **5.** Homeostasis
_____ **6.** cardiac muscle
_____ **7.** Heart
_____ **8.** Integumentary
_____ **9.** Temperature regulation
_____ **10.** Blood clot formation
_____ **11.** Supine
_____ **12.** Prone
_____ **13.** Serous membranes
_____ **14.** Mediastinum
_____ **15.** Pericardium

COLUMN B

a. Study of tissues
b. Stable internal environment
c. Face up
d. Study of vital body functions
e. Positive feedback
f. Organ system that has the skin
g. Study of cells
h. Negative feedback
i. Between pleural cavities
j. All chemical activity in body
k. Line true body cavities
l. Tissue
m. Serous membrane
n. Organ
o. Face down

16. Label the three sectional planes in the figure below.

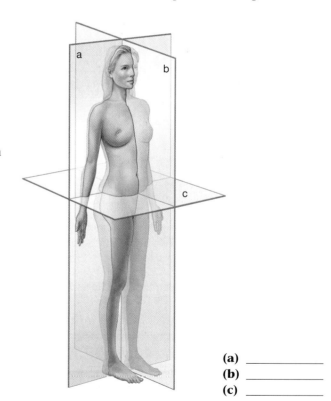

(a) _____
(b) _____
(c) _____

17. Label the directional terms in the figure below.

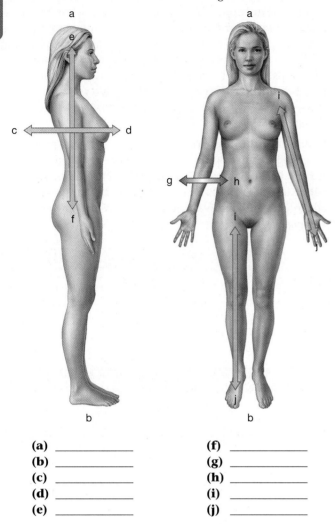

(a) _____	**(f)** _____
(b) _____	**(g)** _____
(c) _____	**(h)** _____
(d) _____	**(i)** _____
(e) _____	**(j)** _____

18. The process by which an organism increases the size and/or number of its cells is called
  (a) reproduction.
  (b) adaptation.
  (c) growth.
  (d) metabolism.

19. When a variation outside normal limits triggers a response that restores the normal condition, the regulatory process involves
  (a) negative feedback.
  (b) positive feedback.
  (c) compensation.
  (d) adaptation.

20. The terms that apply to the front of the body in the anatomical position are
  (a) posterior, dorsal.
  (b) back, front.
  (c) medial, lateral.
  (d) anterior, ventral.

21. The diaphragm, a flat muscular sheet, separates the superior _____ cavity and inferior _____ cavity.
  (a) pleural, pericardial
  (b) abdominal, pelvic
  (c) thoracic, abdominopelvic
  (d) cranial, thoracic

Level 2 Reviewing Concepts

22. What basic functions are common to all living things?

23. Beginning with atoms, list in correct sequence the levels of organization of your body, from the simplest level to the most complex.

24. Define homeostatic regulation in a way that states its physiological importance.

25. How does negative feedback differ from positive feedback?

26. Describe the position of the body when it is in the anatomical position.

27. As a surgeon, you perform an invasive procedure that involves cutting through the peritoneum. Are you more likely to be operating on the heart or on the stomach?

28. In which regional body cavity, or cavities, of the trunk would each of the following organs or systems be found?
  (a) Cardiovascular, digestive, and urinary systems
  (b) Heart, lungs
  (c) Stomach, intestines

Level 3 Critical Thinking and Clinical Applications

29. A hormone called *calcitonin*, produced by the thyroid gland, is released in response to increased levels of calcium ions in the blood. If this hormone acts through negative feedback, what effect will its release have on blood calcium levels?

30. An anatomist wishes to make detailed comparisons of medial surfaces of the left and right sides of the brain. This work requires sections that show the entire medial surface. Which kind of sections should be ordered from the lab for this investigation?

The Chemical Level of Organization

2

Learning Objectives

These objectives tell you what you should be able to do after completing the chapter. They correspond by number to this chapter's sections.

2-1 Describe an atom and how atomic structure affects interactions between atoms.

2-2 Compare the ways in which atoms combine to form molecules and compounds.

2-3 Distinguish among the three major types of chemical reactions that are important for studying physiology.

2-4 Describe the crucial role of enzymes in metabolism.

2-5 Distinguish between organic and inorganic compounds.

2-6 Explain how the chemical properties of water make life possible.

2-7 Describe the pH scale and the role of buffers in body fluids.

2-8 Describe the functional roles of acids, bases, and salts.

2-9 Discuss the structures and functions of carbohydrates.

2-10 Discuss the structures and functions of lipids.

2-11 Discuss the structures and functions of proteins.

2-12 Discuss the structures and functions of nucleic acids.

2-13 Discuss the structures and functions of high-energy compounds.

2-14 Explain the relationship between chemicals and cells.

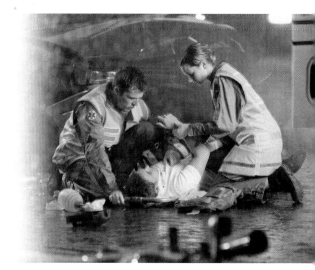

2

An Introduction to the Chemical Level of Organization

We begin our study of the human body with individual atoms and molecules. As you have seen, they are the body's most basic level of organization. All living and nonliving things—people, elephants, oranges, oceans, rocks, and air—get their characteristics from the types of atoms involved and the ways those atoms combine and interact. **Chemistry** is the science that investigates *matter* and its interactions. A familiarity with basic chemistry will help you understand how atoms can affect the anatomy and physiology of the cells, tissues, organs, and organ systems that make up the human body.

Build Your Knowledge

The Build Your Knowledge feature reminds you of what you already know and prepares you to learn new material. Be sure to read every Build Your Knowledge box or page so that you can build your knowledge—and confidence!

Recall that atoms are the smallest stable units of matter (as you saw in **Chapter 1: An Introduction to Anatomy and Physiology**). Atoms combine to form larger structures, such as molecules or groups of molecules, with complex shapes.

Similar to how anatomy and physiology are interrelated, a molecule's specialized shape ("anatomy") determines its function ("physiology"). In turn, its functional role in body processes is affected by its molecular structure. ⊃**pp. 4, 5**

2-1 Atoms are the basic particles of matter

Learning Objective Describe an atom and how atomic structure affects interactions between atoms.

Matter is anything that takes up space and has mass. *Mass* is the amount of matter that an object contains. Mass is a physical property that determines the weight of an object in Earth's gravitational field. On our planet, the weight of an object is essentially the same as its mass. However, the two are not always the same: In orbit you would be weightless, but your mass would remain unchanged. Matter occurs in one of three familiar states: solid (such as a rock), liquid (such as water), or gas (such as the atmosphere).

All matter is composed of substances called **elements**. Elements cannot be changed or broken down into simpler substances, whether by chemical processes, heating, or other ordinary physical means. The smallest stable unit of matter is an **atom**. Atoms are so small that atomic measurements are typically reported in billionths of a meter or *nanometers* (NAN-ō-mē-terz) (nm). The very largest atoms are almost half of one-billionth of a meter (0.5 nm) in diameter. One million atoms placed side by side would span a period on this page, but the line would be far too thin for you to see with anything but the most powerful of microscopes.

Atomic Structure

Atoms contain three major types of subatomic particles: protons, neutrons, and electrons. Protons and neutrons are similar in size and mass, but **protons** (p^+) have a positive electrical charge, and **neutrons** (n or n^0) are neutral—that is, uncharged. **Electrons** (e^-) are much lighter than protons—only 1/1836 as massive—and have a negative electrical charge. **Figure 2-1** is a diagram of a simple atom: the element *helium*. This atom contains two protons, two neutrons, and two electrons.

All atoms contain protons and electrons, normally in equal numbers. The number of protons in an atom is known as its **atomic number**. Each element includes all the atoms that have the same number of protons and thus the same

Figure 2-1 A Diagram of Atomic Structure. The atom shown here—helium—contains two of each type of subatomic particle: two protons, two neutrons, and two electrons.

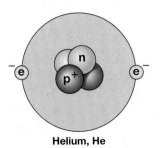

Helium, He

atomic number. For example, all atoms of the element helium contain two protons.

Table 2-1 lists the 13 most abundant elements in the human body. Each element is universally known by its own abbreviation, or chemical symbol. Most of the symbols are easily connected with the English names of the elements. A few; such as Na for sodium, are abbreviations of their original Latin names—in this case, *natrium.*

Hydrogen is the simplest element. It has an atomic number of 1 because its atom contains one proton (**Figure 2-2**). The proton is located in the center of the atom and forms the **nucleus**. Hydrogen atoms seldom contain neutrons, but whenever neutrons are present in any type of atom, they are also located in the nucleus. In a hydrogen atom, a single electron orbits the space around the nucleus at high speed, forming an **electron cloud** (**Figure 2-2a**). Why does the negatively charged electron stay in the electron cloud? One reason is because it is attracted to the positively charged proton. The cloud is usually represented as a spherical **electron shell** (**Figure 2-2b**).

Figure 2-2 Hydrogen Atom Models. A typical hydrogen atom consists of a nucleus containing one proton and no neutrons, and a single electron orbiting around the nucleus.

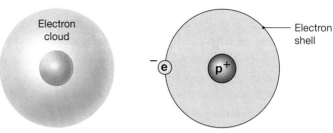

a **Space-filling model.** This space-filling model of a hydrogen atom depicts the three dimensional electron cloud formed by the single orbiting electron.

b **Electron-shell model.** In a two-dimensional electron-shell model, it is easier to visualize the atom's components.

Isotopes

The atoms of an element can differ in the number of neutrons in the nucleus. Such atoms of an element are called **isotopes**. The presence or absence of neutrons generally has no effect on the chemical properties of an atom of a particular element. As a result, isotopes can be distinguished from one another only by their **mass number**—the total number of protons and neutrons in the nucleus.

The nuclei of some isotopes may also be unstable. Unstable isotopes are radioactive: They spontaneously emit subatomic particles or radiation in measurable amounts. Weak *radioisotopes* are sometimes used in diagnostic procedures.

Atomic Weight

Atomic mass numbers are useful because they tell us the number of protons and neutrons in the nuclei of different atoms. However, they do not tell us the *actual* mass of an atom, because they do not account for the masses of electrons and the slight difference between the masses of a proton and neutron. They also don't tell us the mass of a "typical" atom, since any element consists of a mixture of isotopes. Yet we can determine the *average mass* of an element's atoms, a value known as **atomic weight**. Atomic weight takes into account the mass of the subatomic particles and the relative proportions of any isotopes.

For example, even though the mass number of hydrogen is 1, the atomic weight of hydrogen is 1.0079. In this case, the mass number and atomic weight differ primarily because a few hydrogen atoms have a mass number of 2 (one proton plus one neutron), and an even smaller number have a mass number of 3 (one proton plus two neutrons).

Table 2-1	Principal Elements in the Human Body
Element (% of Body Weight)	**Significance**
Oxygen, O (65)	A component of water and other compounds; oxygen gas is essential for respiration
Carbon, C (18.6)	Found in all organic molecules
Hydrogen, H (9.7)	A component of water and most other compounds in the body
Nitrogen, N (3.2)	Found in proteins, nucleic acids, and other organic compounds
Calcium, Ca (1.8)	Found in bones and teeth; important for membrane function, nerve impulses, muscle contraction, and blood clotting
Phosphorus, P (1.0)	Found in bones and teeth, nucleic acids, and high-energy compounds
Potassium, K (0.4)	Important for membrane function, nerve impulses, and muscle contraction
Sodium, Na (0.2)	Important for membrane function, nerve impulses, and muscle contraction
Chlorine, Cl (0.2)	Important for membrane function and water absorption
Magnesium, Mg (0.06)	Required for activation of several enzymes
Sulfur, S (0.04)	Found in many proteins
Iron, Fe (0.007)	Essential for oxygen transport and energy capture
Iodine, I (0.0002)	A component of hormones of the thyroid gland

Electron Shells

Atoms are electrically neutral. Every positively charged proton is balanced by a negatively charged electron. For this reason, each increase in the atomic number has a comparable increase in the number of electrons. These electrons occupy an orderly series of electron shells around the nucleus, and only the electrons in the outer shell can interact with other atoms. *The number of electrons in an atom's outer electron shell determines the chemical properties of that element.*

Atoms with an unfilled outer electron shell are unstable—that is, they will react with other atoms, usually in ways that give them full outer electron shells. An atom with a filled outer shell is stable and will not interact with other atoms. The first electron shell (the one closest to the nucleus) is filled when it contains two electrons. A hydrogen atom has one electron in this electron shell (**Figure 2-2b**), and thus hydrogen atoms can react with many other atoms. A helium atom has two electrons in this electron shell (**Figure 2-1**). Because its outer electron shell is full, a helium atom is stable. Elements that do not readily take part in chemical processes are said to be *inert*. The gaseous element, helium, is called an *inert gas* because its atoms will neither react with one another nor combine with atoms of other elements.

The second electron shell can contain up to eight electrons. Carbon, with an atomic number of 6, has six electrons. In a carbon atom, the first shell is filled (two electrons), and the second shell contains four electrons (**Figure 2-3a**). In

Figure 2-3 The Electron Shells of Two Atoms. The first electron shell of any atom can hold only two electrons. The second shell can hold up to eight electrons.

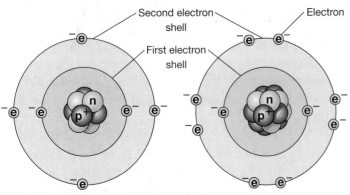

a Carbon (C). In a carbon atom, which has six protons and six electrons, the first shell is full, but the second shell contains only four electrons

b Neon (Ne). In a neon atom, which has 10 protons and 10 electrons, both the first and second electron shells are filled. Notice that the nuclei of carbon and neon contain neutrons as well as protons.

a neon atom (atomic number 10), the second shell is filled (**Figure 2-3b**). Neon is another inert gas.

CHECKPOINT

1. Define atom.

2. How is it possible for two samples of hydrogen to contain the same number of atoms but have different weights?

See the blue Answers tab at the back of the book.

2-2 Chemical bonds are forces formed by interactions among atoms

Learning Objective Compare the ways in which atoms combine to form molecules and compounds.

An atom with a full outer electron shell is very stable and not reactive. The atoms that are most important to biological systems are *un*stable. For this reason, these atoms can interact to form larger structures (see **Table 2-1**). Atoms with unfilled outer electron shells can become stable by sharing, gaining, or losing electrons through chemical reactions with other atoms. They often form **chemical bonds**, which are forces that hold the participating atoms together once the reaction has ended.

Chemical bonding produces *molecules* and *compounds*. **Molecules** are chemical structures that contain more than one atom bonded together by shared electrons. A **compound** is any chemical substance made up of atoms of two or more different elements in a fixed proportion, regardless of the type of bond joining them. A compound is a new chemical substance. Its properties can be quite different from those of its component elements. For example, a mixture of hydrogen and oxygen gases is highly flammable, but chemically combining hydrogen and oxygen atoms produces a compound—water—that can put out a fire's flames.

Ionic Bonds

Atoms are electrically neutral because the number of protons (each with a +1 charge) equals the number of electrons (each with a −1 charge). If an atom loses an electron, it then has a charge of +1 because there is one proton without a corresponding electron. Losing a second electron would leave the atom with a charge of +2. Similarly, adding one or two extra electrons to the atom gives it a charge of −1 or −2, respectively. Atoms or molecules that have an electric charge are called **ions**. Ions with a positive charge (+) are **cations** (KAT-ī-onz). Ions with a negative charge (−) are **anions** (AN-ī-onz). **Table 2-2** lists several common ions in body fluids.

Table 2-2	The Most Common Ions in Body Fluids	
Cations	**Anions**	
Na$^+$ (sodium)	Cl$^-$ (chloride)	
K$^+$ (potassium)	HCO$_3^-$ (bicarbonate)	
Ca^{2+} (calcium)	HPO$_4^{2-}$ (biphosphate)	
Mg^{2+} (magnesium)	SO$_4^{2-}$ (sulfate)	

Ionic (ī-ON-ik) **bonds** are chemical bonds created by the electrical attraction between anions and cations. Ionic bonds are formed in a process called *ionic bonding*, as shown in **Figure 2-4a**. In the example shown, a sodium atom donates an electron to a chlorine atom. This loss of an electron creates a *sodium ion* with a +1 charge and a *chloride ion* with a −1 charge. The two ions do not move apart after the electron transfer because the positively charged sodium ion is attracted to the negatively charged chloride ion. In this case, the combination of oppositely charged ions forms the *ionic compound* **sodium chloride**, the chemical name for the crystals we know as table salt (**Figure 2-4b,c**).

Covalent Bonds

Another way atoms can fill their outer electron shells is by sharing electrons with other atoms. The result is a molecule held together by **covalent** (kō-VĀ-lent) **bonds** (**Figure 2-5**).

As an example, consider hydrogen. Individual hydrogen atoms, as diagrammed in **Figure 2-2**, are not found in nature. Instead, we find hydrogen molecules (**Figure 2-5**). In chemical shorthand, molecular hydrogen is indicated by H$_2$. The H is the chemical symbol for hydrogen, and the subscript 2 indicates the number of atoms. Molecular hydrogen is a gas present in the atmosphere in very small quantities. The two hydrogen atoms share their electrons, with each electron whirling around both nuclei. The sharing of one pair of electrons (one electron from each atom) creates a **single covalent bond**.

Oxygen, with an atomic number of 8, has two electrons in its first electron shell and six in the second. Oxygen atoms (**Figure 2-5**) become stable by sharing two pairs of electrons (two electrons from each atom), forming a **double covalent bond**. Molecular oxygen (O$_2$) is an atmospheric gas that is very important to living organisms. Our cells would die without a constant supply of oxygen.

Figure 2-4 Ionic Bonding.

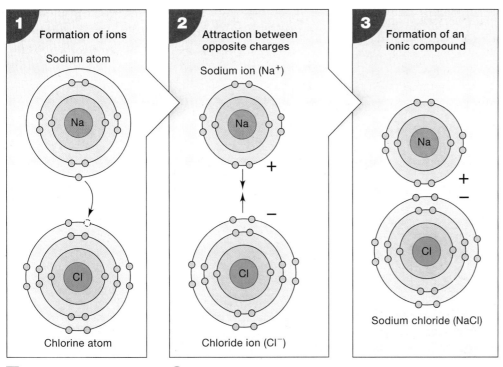

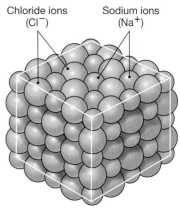

b **Sodium chloride crystal.** Large numbers of sodium and chloride ions form a crystal of sodium chloride (table salt).

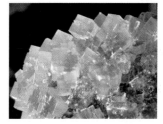

a **Formation of an ionic bond.** ❶ A sodium (Na) atom loses an electron, which is accepted by a chlorine (Cl) atom. ❷ Because the sodium ion (Na$^+$) and chloride ion (Cl$^-$) have opposite charges, they are attracted to one another. ❸ The association of sodium and chloride ions forms the ionic compound sodium chloride.

c **Photo of sodium chloride crystals.** (magnified 0.5X)

Figure 2-5 Covalent Bonds in Three Common Molecules. In a molecule of hydrogen, two hydrogen atoms share their electrons such that each has a filled outer electron shell. This sharing of a pair of electrons creates a single covalent bond (—). A molecule of oxygen consists of two oxygen atoms that share two pairs of electrons. The result is a double covalent bond (=). In a molecule of carbon dioxide, a central carbon atom forms double covalent bonds with a pair of oxygen atoms.

Molecule	Electron Shell Model and Structural Formula		Space-filling Model
Hydrogen (H_2)		H−H	
Oxygen (O_2)		O=O	
Carbon dioxide (CO_2)		O=C=O	

In our bodies, the chemical processes that consume oxygen also produce carbon dioxide (CO_2) as a waste product. In a carbon dioxide molecule, two oxygen atoms form double covalent bonds with the carbon atom, as shown in **Figure 2-5**.

Covalent bonds are very strong because the shared electrons tie the atoms together. When the electrons are shared equally, the bound atoms remain electrically neutral. Such covalent bonds are called **nonpolar covalent bonds**. Nonpolar covalent bonds between carbon atoms create the stable framework of the large molecules that make up most of the structural components of the human body.

Elements differ in how strongly they hold or attract shared electrons. An unequal sharing between atoms of different elements creates a **polar covalent bond**. Such bonding often forms a *polar molecule* because one end, or pole, has a slight negative charge and the other a slight positive charge. For example, in a molecule of water, an oxygen atom forms covalent bonds with two hydrogen atoms. However, the oxygen atom has a much stronger attraction for the shared electrons than do the hydrogen atoms, so those electrons spend most of their time with the oxygen atom. Because of the two extra electrons, the oxygen atom develops a slight negative charge (**Figure 2-6a**). At the same time, the hydrogen atoms each develop a slight positive charge because their electrons are away part of the time.

Hydrogen Bonds

In addition to ionic and covalent bonds, weaker attractive forces act between adjacent molecules and between atoms within a large molecule. The most important of these weak attractive forces is the hydrogen bond. A **hydrogen bond** is the attraction between a slight positive charge on the hydrogen atom of one polar covalent bond and a slight negative charge on an

Figure 2-6 Hydrogen Bonds between Water Molecules.

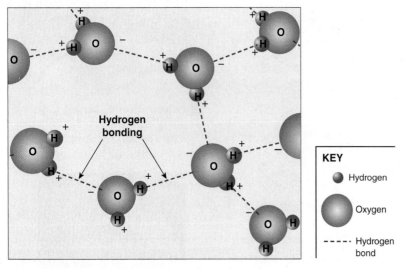

KEY
- Hydrogen
- Oxygen
- - - - Hydrogen bond

a The unequal sharing of electrons in a water molecule causes each of its two hydrogen atoms to have a slight positive charge and its oxygen atom to have a slight negative charge. Attraction between a hydrogen atom of one water molecule and the oxygen atom of another is a hydrogen bond (indicated by dashed lines).

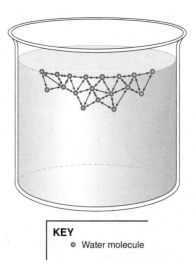

KEY
- Water molecule

b Hydrogen bonding between water molecules at a free surface creates surface tension and slows evaporation.

oxygen or nitrogen atom of another polar covalent bond. The polar covalent bond containing the oxygen or nitrogen atom can be in a different molecule from the hydrogen atom, or in the same molecule. For example, water molecules are attracted to each other through hydrogen bonding (**Figure 2-6a**).

Hydrogen bonds are too weak to create molecules, but they can alter the shapes of molecules or pull molecules closer together. For example, the attraction between water molecules at a free surface slows evaporation and creates what is known as **surface tension** (**Figure 2-6b**). Surface tension acts as a barrier that keeps small objects from entering the water. It is the reason that insects can walk across the surface of a pond or puddle. Similarly, a layer of watery tears keeps small dust particles from touching the surface of our eyes.

CHECKPOINT

3. Define chemical bond, and identify several types of chemical bonds.

4. Oxygen and neon are both gases at room temperature. Why does oxygen combine readily with other elements, but neon does not?

5. Which kind of bond holds atoms in a water molecule together? What attracts water molecules to each other?

See the blue Answers tab at the back of the book.

2-3 Decomposition, synthesis, and exchange reactions are important chemical reactions in physiology

Learning Objective Distinguish among the three major types of chemical reactions that are important for studying physiology.

Cells stay alive by controlling chemical reactions. In a **chemical reaction**, existing bonds between atoms are broken or new chemical bonds form between atoms. These changes occur as atoms in the reacting substances, or **reactants**, are rearranged to form different substances, or **products** (**Spotlight Figure 2-7**).

In effect, each cell is a chemical factory. For example, growth, maintenance and repair, secretion, and muscle contraction all involve complex chemical reactions. Cells use chemical reactions to provide the energy required to maintain homeostasis and to perform essential functions. **Metabolism** (me-TAB-ō-lizm; *metabole*, change) refers to all the chemical reactions in the body.

Basic Energy Concepts

Knowing some basic relationships between matter and energy is essential for discussing chemical reactions. **Work** is the movement of an object or a change in the physical structure of matter. In your body, work includes movements like walking or running and also the building of complex molecules and the conversion of liquid water to water vapor (evaporation). **Energy** is the capacity to perform work. There are two major types of energy: *kinetic energy* and *potential energy*.

Kinetic energy is the energy of motion—energy that can be transferred to another object and do work. When you fall off a ladder, it is kinetic energy that does the damage. **Potential energy** is stored energy. It may result from an object's position (you standing on a ladder) or from its physical or chemical structure (a stretched spring or a charged battery). Kinetic energy must be used in climbing the ladder, in stretching the spring, or in charging the battery. The potential energy is converted back into kinetic energy when you fall, the spring recoils, or the battery discharges. The kinetic energy can then be used to perform work.

Energy cannot be destroyed; it can only be converted from one form to another. A conversion between potential energy and kinetic energy is never 100 percent efficient. Each time an energy conversion takes place, some of the energy is released as heat. *Heat* is an increase in random molecular motion, and the temperature of an object is directly related to the average kinetic energy of its molecules. Heat can never be completely converted to work or to any other form of energy. Cells cannot capture it or use it to perform work.

Cells do work as they build complex molecules and move materials into, out of, or within the cell. As they perform such work and convert energy from one form to another, heat is produced. For example, when skeletal muscle cells contract, they perform work. Potential energy (the positions of protein filaments and the covalent bonds between molecules inside the cells) is converted into kinetic energy, and heat is released. The amount of heat is related to the amount of work done. As a result, when you exercise, your body temperature rises.

Types of Reactions

Three types of chemical reactions are important to the study of physiology: *decomposition reactions, synthesis reactions*, and *exchange reactions*.

Decomposition Reactions

A **decomposition reaction** breaks a molecule into smaller fragments. Such reactions take place during digestion, when food molecules are broken into smaller pieces. You could diagram a typical decomposition reaction as:

$$AB \longrightarrow A + B$$

Decomposition reactions involving water are important in the breakdown of complex molecules in the body. In **hydrolysis**

Before we can consider the specific compounds that occur in the human body, we must be able to describe chemical compounds and reactions effectively. The use of sentences to describe chemical structures and events often leads to confusion. A simple form of "chemical shorthand" makes communication much more efficient. The chemical shorthand we will use is known as **chemical notation**. Chemical notation enables us to describe complex events briefly and precisely; its rules are summarized as follows.

VISUAL REPRESENTATION

Atoms

The symbol of an element indicates one atom of that element. A number preceding the symbol of an element indicates more than one atom of that element.

one atom of hydrogen

one atom of oxygen

two atoms of hydrogen

two atoms of oxygen

=

H
one atom of hydrogen

O
one atom of oxygen

2H
two atoms of hydrogen

2O
two atoms of oxygen

Molecules

A subscript following the symbol of an element indicates a molecule with that number of atoms of that element.

hydrogen molecule
composed of two hydrogen atoms

oxygen molecule
composed of two oxygen atoms

water molecule
composed of two hydrogen atoms and one oxygen atom

=

H_2
hydrogen molecule

O_2
oxygen molecule

H_2O
water molecule

Reactions

In a description of a chemical reaction, the participants at the start of the reaction are called reactants, and the reaction generates one or more products. Chemical reactions are represented with chemical equations. An arrow indicates the direction of the reaction, from reactants (usually on the left) to products (usually on the right). In the following reaction, two atoms of hydrogen combine with one atom of oxygen to produce a single molecule of water.

 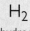

reactants → product

Chemical reactions neither create nor destroy atoms; they merely rearrange atoms into new combinations. Therefore, the numbers of atoms of each element must always be the same on both sides of the chemical equation for a chemical reaction. When this is the case, the equation is balanced.

=

$$2H + O \longrightarrow H_2O$$
Balanced equation

$$2H + 2O \longrightarrow H_2O$$
Unbalanced equation

Ions

A superscript plus or minus sign following the symbol of an element indicates an ion. A single plus sign indicates a cation with a charge of +1. (The original atom has lost one electron.) A single minus sign indicates an anion with a charge of −1. (The original atom has gained one electron.) If more than one electron has been lost or gained, the charge on the ion is indicated by a number preceding the plus or minus sign.

sodium ion
the sodium atom has lost one electron

chloride ion
the chlorine atom has gained one electron

calcium ion
the calcium atom has lost two electrons

=

Na^+
sodium ion

Cl^-
chloride ion

Ca^{2+}
calcium ion

A sodium atom becomes a sodium ion

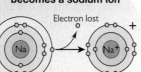

Electron lost

Sodium atom (Na)

Sodium ion (Na^+)

CLINICAL NOTE

Kinetic Energy and Injury

Kinetic energy is the energy contained by a body in motion. The kinetic energy of an object is directly proportional to the square of its speed. That is, for a twofold increase in speed, the kinetic energy will increase by a factor of four. For a threefold increase in speed, the kinetic energy will increase by a factor of nine. For a fourfold increase in speed, the kinetic energy will increase by a factor of 16. The kinetic energy is dependent upon the square of the speed of the object in motion.

A moving automobile has a tremendous amount of kinetic injury. The energy can be released slowly as occurs when the driver applies the brakes and stops in 100 meters. Or, the energy can be released rapidly when the vehicle strikes a bridge and stops in less than one meter. Thus, not only speed can cause injury, but stopping can also cause injury. In a motor vehicle collision, some of the kinetic energy is transferred to the occupants. Likewise, something that stops the car, such as a bridge or a pedestrian, absorbs massive amounts of kinetic energy.

There is a limit on the amount of kinetic energy a human body can absorb. Small amounts of kinetic energy, as occur with walking, are readily absorbed and do not cause injury. As the energy increases, as occurs in a fall from a bicycle, the body may sustain damage from the energy. However, it may not be fatal. Absorbing large quantities of kinetic energy, as occurs in a high-speed motor vehicle collision, can cause severe injuries. At a certain energy level, the forces that result are fatal.

(hī-DROL-i-sis; *hydro-*, water + *lysis*, a loosening), one of the bonds in a complex molecule is broken, and the parts of a water molecule (H and OH) are added to the resulting fragments:

$$A—B + H_2O \longrightarrow A—H + HO—B$$

Catabolism (kah-TAB-ō-lizm; *katabole*, a throwing down) refers to the decomposition reactions of complex molecules within cells. A covalent bond is a form of potential energy. When the bond is broken, it releases kinetic energy that can perform work. Cells can harness some of that energy to power essential functions such as growth, movement, and reproduction.

Synthesis Reactions

Synthesis (SIN-the-sis) is the opposite of decomposition. A synthesis reaction assembles larger molecules from smaller parts. These relatively simple reactions could be diagrammed as:

$$A + B \longrightarrow AB$$

A and B could be individual atoms that combine to form a molecule, or they could be individual molecules combining to form even larger products. Synthesis always involves the formation of new chemical bonds, whether the reactants are atoms or molecules.

Dehydration synthesis, or *condensation reaction*, is the formation of a complex molecule by the removal of water:

$$A—H + HO—B \longrightarrow A—B + H_2O$$

Dehydration synthesis is the opposite of hydrolysis. We will encounter examples of both reactions in later sections.

Anabolism (a-NAB-ō-lizm; *anabole*, a building up) is the synthesis of new compounds in the body. Because it takes energy to create a chemical bond, anabolism is usually an "uphill" process. Living cells are constantly balancing their chemical activities, with catabolism providing the energy needed to support anabolism as well as other vital functions.

Exchange Reactions

In an **exchange reaction**, parts of the reacting molecules are shuffled as follows:

$$AB + CD \longrightarrow AD + CB$$

The reactants and products contain the same components (A, B, C, and D), but the components are present in different combinations. In an exchange reaction, the reactant molecules AB and CD break apart (a decomposition), and then the resulting components interact to form AD and CB (a synthesis).

Reversible Reactions

Many important biological reactions are freely reversible. Such reactions can be diagrammed as:

$$A + B \rightleftharpoons AB$$

This equation indicates that two reactions are occurring at the same time. One is a synthesis (A + B $\longrightarrow$ AB), and the other is a decomposition (AB $\longrightarrow$ A + B). At **equilibrium** (ē-kwi-LIB-rē-um), the rates of the two reactions are balanced. As fast as a molecule of AB forms, another degrades into A + B. As a result, the numbers of A, B, and AB molecules present at any given moment do not change. Altering the concentrations of one or more of these molecules will temporarily upset the equilibrium, shifting the reaction either toward product synthesis or decomposition. For example, adding additional molecules of A and B will accelerate the synthesis reaction (A + B $\longrightarrow$ AB). As the concentration of AB rises, however, so does the rate of the decomposition reaction (AB $\longrightarrow$ A + B), until a new equilibrium is established.

CHECKPOINT

6. Using the rules for chemical notation, write the molecular formula for glucose, a compound composed of 6 carbon atoms, 12 hydrogen atoms, and 6 oxygen atoms.

7. Identify and describe three types of chemical reactions important to human physiology.

8. In living cells, glucose, a six-carbon molecule, is converted into two three-carbon molecules. What type of chemical reaction is this?

9. If the product of a reversible reaction is continuously removed, what will be the effect on the equilibrium of the reaction?

See the blue Answers tab at the back of the book.

2-4 Enzymes catalyze specific biochemical reactions by lowering a reaction's activation energy

Learning Objective Describe the crucial role of enzymes in metabolism.

Most chemical reactions do not occur spontaneously, or they occur so slowly that they would be of little value to cells. Before a reaction can begin, enough energy must be provided to activate the reactants. The amount of energy required to start a reaction is called the **activation energy**.

Many reactions can be activated by changes in temperature or pH, but such changes are deadly to cells. For example, to break down a complex sugar in the laboratory, you must boil it in an acid solution. Cells would not survive such extreme measures. Instead, cells use special molecules called **enzymes** to speed up the reactions that support life. Enzymes belong to a class of substances called **catalysts** (KAT-uh-lists; *katalysis*, dissolution), which accelerate (speed up) chemical reactions without themselves being permanently changed. Cells make an enzyme molecule to promote each specific reaction. Most enzyme reactions are reversible reactions.

Enzymes promote chemical reactions by lowering the activation energy needed (**Figure 2-8**). Lowering the activation energy affects only the rate of a reaction, not the direction of the reaction or the products that are formed. An enzyme cannot bring about a reaction that would otherwise be impossible.

It takes activation energy to start a chemical reaction, but once it has begun, the reaction as a whole may absorb or release energy, generally in the form of heat. If the amount of energy released is greater than the activation energy needed to start the reaction, there will be a net release of energy. Reactions that release energy are said to be **exergonic** (*exo-*, outside). If more energy is needed to begin the reaction than is released as it proceeds, the reaction as a whole will absorb energy. Such reactions are called **endergonic** (*endo-*, inside). Exergonic reactions are relatively common in the body. They generate the heat that maintains our body temperature.

Figure 2-8 The Effect of Enzymes on Activation Energy.
Enzymes lower the activation energy required for a reaction to proceed readily (in order, from 1 to 4) under conditions in the body.

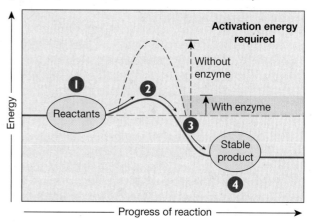

CHECKPOINT

10. What is an enzyme?

11. Why are enzymes needed in our cells?

See the blue Answers tab at the back of the book.

2-5 Inorganic compounds usually lack carbon, and organic compounds always contain carbon

Learning Objective Distinguish between organic and inorganic compounds.

In the rest of this chapter we focus on nutrients and metabolites. **Nutrients** are the substances from food that are necessary for normal physiological functions. They include carbohydrates, proteins, fats, vitamins, minerals, and water. **Metabolites** (me-TAB-ō-līts) are substances that are involved in, or a by-product of, metabolism.

Like all chemical substances, nutrients and metabolites can be broadly categorized as inorganic or organic. **Inorganic compounds** are substances that generally do not contain carbon and hydrogen. (If present, they do not form $C-H$ bonds.) They include small molecules and ionic compounds. **Organic compounds** are substances that contain carbon covalently bonded with one or more other elements. Their molecules can be much larger and more complex than inorganic compounds.

The most important inorganic substances in the human body are water, carbon dioxide, oxygen, and ionic compounds, such as acids, bases, and salts. Water is the primary component of our body fluids and an essential compound for many chemical reactions. Most of the inorganic molecules and compounds in the human body exist in association with water. Carbon dioxide and oxygen are important gases dissolved in body fluids.

Build Your Knowledge

Recall that carbon is the second most common element in our body and is found in all organic molecules. Recall too that carbon atoms contain four electrons in their outer electron shell. With this number of electrons, carbon atoms may form up to four single covalent bonds. Because these bonds may also include other C atoms, a very large number of different carbon frameworks can exist. These frameworks, in turn, provide many bonding sites for hydrogen, as well as oxygen, two other elements found in abundance in the human body and other living things. ⤴ **pp. 27, 29**

Cells produce carbon dioxide (CO_2) through normal metabolic activity. It is transported in the blood and released as a gas into the air in the lungs. Oxygen (O_2), an atmospheric gas, is absorbed at the lungs, transported in the blood, and consumed by cells throughout the body. The chemical structures of these key substances were introduced earlier in the chapter. ⤴ p. 30

CHECKPOINT

12. Distinguish between inorganic compounds and organic compounds.

See the blue Answers tab at the back of the book.

2-6 Physiological systems depend on water

Learning Objective Explain how the chemical properties of water make life possible.

Water (H_2O) is the most important substance in the body, making up to two-thirds of total body weight. A change in the body's water content can have fatal consequences because virtually all physiological systems will be affected.

Three general properties of water are particularly important to the human body:

- **Water is an essential reactant in the chemical reactions of living systems.** Chemical reactions in our bodies take place in water, and water molecules also participate in some reactions. During the dehydration synthesis of large molecules, water molecules are released. During hydrolysis, complex molecules are broken down by the addition of water molecules. ⤴ p. 33

- **Water has a very high heat capacity.** *Heat capacity* is the ability of a substance to absorb and retain heat. It takes a lot of heat energy to change the temperature of a quantity of water. Why? The reason is that water molecules in the liquid state are linked to one another by hydrogen bonding. This bonding interferes with the random motion, or kinetic energy, of the water molecules. (Recall that an object's temperature depends directly on the kinetic energy of its molecules. ⤴ p. 31) So, an increase in water temperature depends on breaking up hydrogen bonds between water molecules. Water retains heat and will change temperature only slowly. As a result, body temperature is stabilized, and the water in our cells remains a liquid over a wide range of environmental temperatures. Hydrogen bonding also explains why a large amount of heat energy is required to change liquid water to a gas, or ice to liquid. When water finally changes from a liquid to a gas, all the hydrogen bonds are broken and the escaping water molecules carry away a great deal of heat. This feature accounts for the cooling effect of perspiration on the skin.

- **Water is an excellent solvent.** A remarkable number of inorganic and organic substances are water *soluble*, meaning they will dissolve in water. As the substances dissolve, their released ions or smaller molecules become uniformly dispersed throughout the water, creating a *solution*. The chemical reactions within living cells take place in solution. The watery component of blood, called plasma, carries dissolved nutrients and waste products throughout the body.

Most chemical reactions in the body take place in **solutions**, which consist of a uniform mixture of a fluid **solvent** and dissolved **solutes**. The solvent in organisms is usually water, forming an *aqueous solution*. The solutes may be inorganic or organic. Inorganic compounds held together by ionic bonds undergo **dissociation** (di-sō-sē-Ā-shun), or **ionization** (ī-on-i-ZĀ-shun) in water. In this process, ionic bonds are broken as individual ions interact with the positive or negative ends of polar water molecules (**Figure 2-9a**). As shown in **Figure 2-9b**, the result is a mixture of cations and anions, each surrounded by so many water molecules that they are unable to re-form their original bonds. Some organic molecules contain polar covalent bonds, which also attract water molecules. An example is glucose, an important soluble sugar in the body (**Figure 2-9c**).

An aqueous solution containing anions and cations can also conduct an electrical current. Substances that release ions when dissolved in water are called *electrolytes*. Electrical forces across cell membranes affect the functioning of all cells. As we will see, small electrical currents carried by ions are essential to muscle contraction and nerve function. (Chapters 7 and 8 discuss these processes in more detail.)

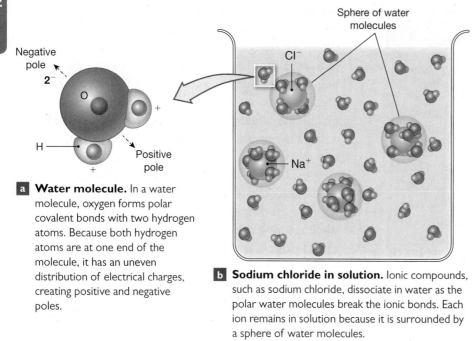

Sphere of water molecules

Glucose molecule

Negative pole

2⁻

O

H

Positive pole

a **Water molecule.** In a water molecule, oxygen forms polar covalent bonds with two hydrogen atoms. Because both hydrogen atoms are at one end of the molecule, it has an uneven distribution of electrical charges, creating positive and negative poles.

b **Sodium chloride in solution.** Ionic compounds, such as sodium chloride, dissociate in water as the polar water molecules break the ionic bonds. Each ion remains in solution because it is surrounded by a sphere of water molecules.

c **Glucose in solution.** Water molecules are also attracted to an organic molecule containing polar covalent bonds. If the molecule binds water strongly, as does glucose, it will be carried into solution—in other words, it will dissolve. Note that the molecule does not dissociate, as occurs for ionic compounds.

Figure 2-9 The Role of Water Molecules in Aqueous Solutions.

CHECKPOINT

13. List the chemical properties of water that make life possible.

14. Why does water resist changes in temperature?

See the blue Answers tab at the back of the book.

2-7 Body fluid pH is vital for homeostasis

Learning Objective Describe the pH scale and the role of buffers in body fluids.

A hydrogen atom involved in a chemical bond or participating in a chemical reaction can easily lose its electron, to become a hydrogen ion (H^+). The concentration of hydrogen ions in blood or other body fluids is important because hydrogen ions are extremely reactive. In excessive numbers, they will break chemical bonds, change the shapes of complex molecules, and disrupt cell and tissue functions. For this reason, the concentration of hydrogen ions must be precisely regulated.

Hydrogen ions are normally present even in pure water because some water molecules dissociate spontaneously, releasing a hydrogen ion and a hydroxide (hī-DROK-sīd) ion (OH^-). The concentration of hydrogen ions is usually reported as the **pH** of the solution. The pH value is a number between 0 and 14. Pure water has a pH of 7. A solution with a pH of 7 is called *neutral* because it contains equal numbers of hydrogen ions and hydroxide ions. A difference of one pH unit equals a tenfold change in H^+ concentration. A solution with a pH below

7 is *acidic* (a-SI-dik) because there are more hydrogen ions than hydroxide ions. A pH above 7 is called *basic*, or *alkaline* (AL-kuh-lin), because hydroxide ions outnumber hydrogen ions.

The pH values of some common liquids are given in **Figure 2-10**. The pH of blood and most body fluids normally ranges from 7.35 to 7.45. Variations in pH outside this range can damage cells and disrupt normal cellular functions. For example, a blood pH below 7 can produce coma. A blood pH higher than 7.8 usually causes uncontrollable, sustained muscular contractions.

CHECKPOINT

15. Define pH, and explain how the pH scale relates to acidity and alkalinity.

16. Why is an extreme change in pH of body fluids undesirable?

See the blue Answers tab at the back of the book.

2-8 Acids, bases, and salts have important physiological roles

Learning Objective Describe the functional roles of acids, bases, and salts.

An **acid** (*acere*; sour) is any substance that breaks apart (dissociates) in solution to *release* hydrogen ions. (Because a hydrogen ion consists solely of a proton, hydrogen ions are often referred to simply as protons, and acids as "proton donors.") Acids and bases are often identified in terms of *strength*. Strength is a measure

Figure 2-10 pH and Hydrogen Ion Concentration. An increase or decrease of one pH unit corresponds to a tenfold change in H$^+$ concentration.

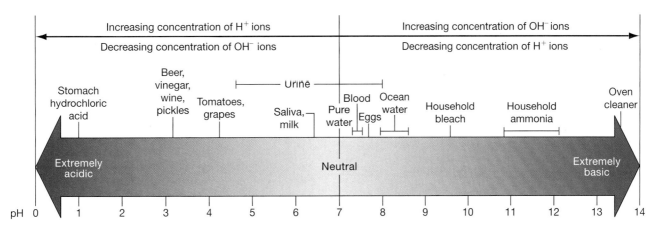

of the degree of dissociation of either an acid or a base when it is in solution. A *strong acid* dissociates completely in solution. Hydrochloric acid (HCl) is an excellent example:

$$HCl \longrightarrow H^+ + Cl^-$$

The stomach produces this powerful acid to help break down food.

A **base** is a substance that removes hydrogen ions from a solution. Many common bases are compounds that dissociate in solution to release a hydroxide ion (OH$^-$). Hydroxide ions have a strong affinity, or attraction, for hydrogen ions and quickly react with them to form water molecules. A *strong base* dissociates completely in solution. For example, sodium hydroxide (NaOH) dissociates in solution as follows:

$$NaOH \longrightarrow Na^+ + OH^-$$

Strong bases have a variety of industrial and household uses. Drain openers and lye are two familiar examples.

Weak acids and *weak bases* do not dissociate completely in solution. The human body contains both weak acids and bases. Weak bases are important in counteracting acids produced during cellular metabolism. For example, active muscle tissues generate *lactic acid*, which can cause potentially dangerous pH changes in body fluids.

Salts

A **salt** is an ionic compound consisting of any cation except a hydrogen ion and any anion except a hydroxide ion. Salts are held together by ionic bonds. In water they dissociate, releasing cations and anions. For example, table salt (NaCl) in solution dissociates into Na$^+$ and Cl$^-$ ions. These two ions are also the most abundant ones in body fluids.

The dissociation of table salt does not affect the concentrations of hydrogen ions or hydroxide ions, so NaCl, like many

salts, is a "neutral" solute. Through their interactions with water molecules, however, other salts may indirectly affect the concentrations of hydrogen ions and hydroxide ions. The dissociation of such salts makes a solution slightly acidic or slightly basic.

Electrolytes (e-LEK-trō-līts) are substances whose ions can conduct an electrical current in solution. They include acids, bases, and salts. All of the examples we discussed above—hydrochloric acid (HCl), sodium hydroxide (NaOH), and sodium chloride (NaCl)—are electrolytes. Examples of ions released by the dissociation of important electrolytes in blood and other body fluids include sodium ions (Na$^+$), potassium ions (K$^+$), calcium ions (Ca^{2+}), chloride ions (Cl$^-$), and bicarbonate ions (HCO$_3^-$). Alterations in the concentrations of these ions in body fluids will disturb almost every vital function. For example, decreasing potassium concentrations will lead to general muscular paralysis. Rising potassium concentrations will cause weak and irregular heartbeats.

Buffers and pH

Buffers are compounds that stabilize pH by either removing or replacing hydrogen ions. Antacids such as Alka-Seltzer, Rolaids, and Tums are buffers that tie up excess hydrogen ions in the stomach. A variety of buffers, including sodium bicarbonate (also known as baking soda), are responsible for stabilizing the pH of most body fluids between 7.35 and 7.45. (We will consider the role of buffers and pH control in Chapter 18.)

CHECKPOINT

17. Define the following terms: acid, base, and salt.

18. How does an antacid help decrease stomach discomfort?

See the blue Answers tab at the back of the book.

CLINICAL NOTE

Understanding pH

Acid-base balance is a dynamic relationship that reflects the relative concentration of hydrogen ions (H^+) in the body. Hydrogen ions are acidic, and their concentration must be maintained within fairly strict limits. Any deviation in the hydrogen ion concentration adversely affects all of the biochemical events in the body. Because of this, determination of the body's hydrogen ion concentration is important in emergency care.

Water molecules have a slight tendency to undergo reversible ionization to yield a *hydrogen ion* (H^+) and a *hydroxide ion* (OH^-) to form the following equilibrium:

$$H_2O \rightleftharpoons H^+ + OH^-$$

The ionization of water is very weak. In fact, only 1 out of every 10 million molecules of water is ionized at any given moment. Although water has only a very slight tendency to ionize, the products of ionization (H^+ and OH^-) have profound biological effects. The number of hydrogen ions and hydroxide ions in an aqueous (water) solution at 25°C (77°F) always equals the fixed number 1.0×10^{-14} M. When the concentrations of both hydrogen ions and hydroxide ions are exactly equal, as in pure water, the solution is said to be *neutral*. When neutral, the number of hydrogen ions equals 1.0×10^{-7} M and the number of hydroxide ions equals 1.0×10^{-7} M. Because of this, we know that when the number of hydrogen ions present is very high, then the concentration of hydroxide ions must be very low. Likewise, when the concentration of hydroxide ions is high, then the concentration of hydrogen ions must be low. Again, regardless of the balance between hydrogen ions and hydroxide ions, the total number of ions must be 1.0×10^{-14}M.

The need for a much simpler system of describing hydrogen ion concentrations quickly became evident. In 1909, the Swedish chemist H.P.L Sørenson proposed that the hydrogen ion concentration be expressed in terms of the logarithm (log) of the reciprocal of the number. This system allows simple numbers to represent extremely large numbers of hydrogen ions. The system was called the pH system, which is an abbreviation for *potential of hydrogen*. Because of the large numbers involved, the use of logarithms simplifies discussion of hydrogen ion concentrations. It is important to remember that the pH system represents the reciprocal of the hydrogen ion concentration. Thus, the greater the number of hydrogen ions, the lower the pH. Conversely, the fewer the number of hydrogen ions, the higher the pH. The pH scale can be defined as:

$$pH = \log 1/[H^+]$$

Because the logarithm of 1 is 0, the equation can be simplified as:

$$pH = -\log[H^+]$$

In precisely neutral solution at 25°C (77°F), where the hydrogen ion concentration equals 1.0×10^{-7} M, the pH would be calculated as:

$$pH = \log 1/1.0 \times 10^{-7} = \log[1.0 \times 10^{-7}] = \log 1.0 + \log 10^{-7}$$

$$pH = 0 + 7$$

$$pH = 7$$

Remember, the value of 7.0 for the pH of a precisely neutral solution is not an arbitrary number but is derived from the absolute value of the hydrogen ion concentration at 25°C. The pH scale varies from 0 to 14. A pH of 14 indicates that only hydroxide ions are present, while a pH of 0 indicates that only hydrogen ions are present.

Any pH greater than 7.0 is considered *alkaline* while any pH less than 7.0 is considered *acidic*. It is also important to note that the pH scale is logarithmic, not arithmetic. For example, if two solutions differ in pH by 1 pH unit, then one solution has 10 times the hydrogen ion concentration of the other. Thus, small changes in pH reflect massive changes in the number of hydrogen ions present.

Occasionally, the *pOH* is used to denote the alkalinity of a solution. The pOH is similar to pH, except that it represents the number of hydroxide ions present, not hydrogen ions (**Table 2-3**). It is helpful to remember that pH and pOH are related to each other in a very simple way:

$$pH + pOH = 14$$

The pH of the body is closely regulated between 7.35 and 7.45. Thus, alkalosis is a pH greater than 7.45, while acidosis is a pH of less than 7.35. Small changes in pH are corrected by the body's compensatory mechanisms, but significant changes are poorly tolerated. In fact, a change in pH of 0.5 units can be fatal.

Table 2-3	The pH Scale		
ACIDIC CONCENTRATIONS		**ALKALINE CONCENTRATIONS**	
[H⁺], Moles	**pH**	**[OH⁻], Moles**	**pOH**
1.0	0	10^{-14}	14
0.1	1	10^{-13}	13
0.01	2	10^{-12}	12
0.001	3	10^{-11}	11
10^{-4}	4	10^{-10}	10
10^{-5}	5	10^{-9}	9
10^{-6}	6	10^{-8}	8
10^{-7}	7	10^{-7}	7
10^{-8}	8	10^{-6}	6
10^{-9}	9	10^{-5}	5
10^{-10}	10	10^{-4}	4
10^{-11}	11	0.001	3
10^{-12}	12	0.01	2
10^{-13}	13	0.1	1
10^{-14}	14	1.0	0

In medical practice, the pH values of blood and urine are measured most frequently. Blood pH is obtained through an arterial blood gas (ABG) sample. For this, a small amount of arterial blood is removed from the radial, brachial, or femoral artery. This is quickly introduced into a blood gas machine where the pH is carefully measured. In the blood gas machine, a special glass electrode selectively measures hydrogen ion concentration. The signal from this electrode is amplified and compared with the signal generated by a control solution having a known pH. Based on this comparison, the pH can be determined. Because of this, it is important for ABG machines to be carefully maintained and calibrated with the control solutions checked on a daily basis. In addition to pH, an ABG analysis measures the partial pressure of oxygen and carbon dioxide in the blood. Also, some machines will measure the bicarbonate concentration and the amount of hemoglobin present. A more detailed discussion of acid-base balance and the body's compensatory buffering mechanisms is presented in Chapter 18.

What Is a Logarithm?

A *logarithm* in mathematics is the *exponent*, or power, to which a stated number, called the *base*, must be raised to yield a specific number. For example, in the expression $10^2 = 100$, the logarithm of 100 to the base 10 is 2. This is properly written as $\log_{10} 100 = 2$. Logarithms were initially created to help simplify arithmetical operations that involve very large numbers. *Common logarithms* use the number 10 as the base number. However, logarithms can be used with base numbers other than 10. This can be illustrated by considering a sequence of powers to the number 2: 2^1, 2^2, 2^3, 2^4, 2^5, and 2^6, which correspond to the sequence of numbers 2, 4, 8, 16, 32, and 64. The exponents 1, 2, 3, 4, 5, and 6 are the logarithms of these numbers to the base 2.

In medicine, logarithms are used to describe chemical concentrations. Unless specified otherwise, always assume that a logarithm is in base 10 ($\log_{10}$). If another logarithm is used, it will be specified in the notation (e.g., $\log_5$). The most frequent use of logarithms in medicine is in the pH system that describes the hydrogen ion concentration of a solution. In pure water, the hydrogen ion concentration is equal to 0.0000001, or 10^{-7} moles per liter. Because the pH scale describes the reciprocal of the hydrogen ion concentration, the numbers are positive even though the concentration of hydrogen ions is less than 1. This simplifies discussion and calculations. Thus, a pH of 3.0 reflects a hydrogen ion concentration of 0.001, or 10^{-3} moles per liter. Likewise, a pH of 10 reflects a hydrogen ion concentration of 0.0000000001, or 10^{-10} moles per liter. A change in pH of 1 unit reflects a tenfold change in hydrogen ion concentration. Likewise, a change of 2 pH units indicates a hundredfold change in hydrogen ion concentration. Thus, the use of logarithms simplifies descriptions and calculations of these extremely large or small numbers.

2-9 Carbohydrates contain carbon, hydrogen, and oxygen in a 1:2:1 ratio

Learning Objective Discuss the structures and functions of carbohydrates.

Carbohydrates are one of the four major classes of organic compounds. Organic compounds always contain the elements carbon and hydrogen. ⟲ p. 34 Many organic molecules are made up of long chains of carbon atoms linked by covalent bonds. These carbon atoms often form additional covalent bonds with hydrogen or oxygen atoms, and less often with nitrogen, phosphorus, sulfur, iron, or other elements.

A **carbohydrate** (kar-bō-Hī-drāt) is an organic molecule that contains carbon, hydrogen, and oxygen in a ratio near 1:2:1. Familiar carbohydrates include the sugars and starches that make up roughly half of the typical U.S. diet. Our tissues can break down most carbohydrates.

Carbohydrates are most important as sources of energy, although they sometimes have other functions. Despite their importance as an energy source, carbohydrates account for only about 1 percent of total body weight. The three major types of carbohydrates are *monosaccharides, disaccharides,* and *polysaccharides.*

Monosaccharides

A **simple sugar**, or **monosaccharide** (mon-ō-SAK-uh-rīd; *mono-*, single + *sakcharon*, sugar), is a carbohydrate containing from three to seven carbon atoms. This group includes **glucose** (GLOO-kōs), ($C_6H_{12}O_6$), the most important "fuel" in the body (**Figure 2-11**). Glucose and other monosaccharides dissolve readily in water. Blood and other body fluids rapidly distribute them throughout the body.

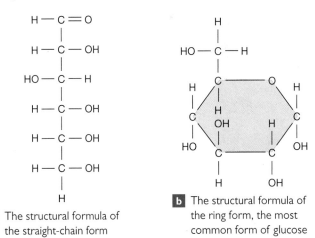

a The structural formula of the straight-chain form

b The structural formula of the ring form, the most common form of glucose

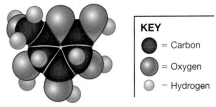

KEY
- = Carbon
- = Oxygen
- = Hydrogen

c A three-dimensional model that shows the organization of atoms in the ring form

Figure 2-11 The Structures of Glucose.

Figure 2-12 The Structure, Formation, and Breakdown of Complex Sugars.

a **Formation of the disaccharide sucrose through dehydration synthesis.** During dehydration synthesis, two molecules are joined by the removal of a water molecule.

b **Breakdown of sucrose into simple sugars by hydrolysis.** Hydrolysis reverses the steps of dehydration synthesis; a complex molecule is broken down by the addition of a water molecule.

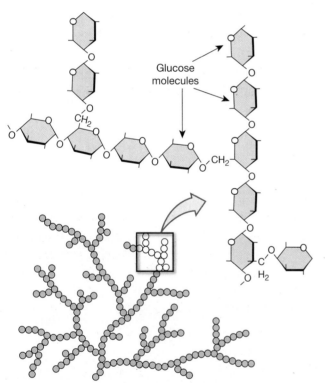

c **The structure of glycogen.** Liver and muscle cells store glucose as the polysaccharide glycogen, a long, branching chain of glucose molecules.

Disaccharides and Polysaccharides

Carbohydrates other than simple sugars are complex molecules made of monosaccharide building blocks. Two monosaccharides join together form a **disaccharide** (dī-SAK-uh-rīd; *di-*, two). Disaccharides such as *sucrose* (table sugar) have

a sweet taste. Like monosaccharides, they are quite soluble in water.

The formation of sucrose (**Figure 2-12a**) involves dehydration synthesis, a process introduced earlier in the chapter. ⟲ p. 33 Dehydration synthesis, or condensation, links molecules together by the removal of a water molecule. The breakdown of sucrose into simple sugars is an example of hydrolysis, the functional opposite of dehydration synthesis (**Figure 2-12b**).

All carbohydrates except monosaccharides must be disassembled through hydrolysis before they can provide useful energy. Many foods contain disaccharides. Most sweet junk foods, such as candy and soft drinks, abound in simple sugars (commonly fructose) and disaccharides (generally sucrose). Some people cannot tolerate table sugar (sucrose) for medical reasons. Others avoid it because they do not want to gain weight (excess sugars are stored as fat). Many of these people use artificial sweeteners in their foods and beverages. These compounds have a very sweet taste but either cannot be broken down in the body or are used in such small amounts that their breakdown does not affect the overall energy balance of the body.

Larger carbohydrate molecules are called **polysaccharides** (pol-ē-SAK-uh-rīdz; *poly-*, many). They form when repeated dehydration synthesis reactions add additional monosaccharides or disaccharides. *Starches* are glucose-based polysaccharides important in our diets. Most starches are manufactured by plants. Your digestive tract can break these molecules into simple sugars. Starches found in potatoes and grains are important energy sources. In contrast, *cellulose*, a component of the cell walls of plants, is a polysaccharide that our bodies cannot digest. The cellulose of foods such as

Table 2-4	Carbohydrates in the Body		
Structure	**Examples**	**Primary Functions**	**Remarks**
Monosaccharides (Simple Sugars)	Glucose, fructose	Energy source	Manufactured in the body and obtained from food; found in body fluids
Disaccharides	Sucrose, lactose, maltose	Energy source	Sucrose is table sugar, and lactose is present in milk; all must be broken down to monosaccharides before absorption
Polysaccharides	Glycogen	Storage of glucose molecules	Glycogen is in animal cells; other polysaccharides (starches and cellulose) are plant products

celery contributes to the bulk of digestive wastes but is useless as an energy source.

Glycogen (GLĪ-kō-jen), or *animal starch*, is a polysaccharide composed of interconnected glucose molecules (**Figure 2-12c**). Like most other large polysaccharides, glycogen will not dissolve in water or other body fluids. Liver and muscle tissues make and store glycogen. When these tissues have a high demand for energy, they break down glycogen molecules into glucose. When demands are low, the tissues absorb glucose from the bloodstream and rebuild glycogen reserves. **Table 2-4** summarizes information about the carbohydrates in the body.

CHECKPOINT

19. A food contains organic molecules with the elements C, H, and O in a ratio of 1:2:1. What class of compounds do these molecules represent, and what are their major functions in the body?

20. When two monosaccharides undergo a dehydration synthesis reaction, which type of molecule is formed?

See the blue Answers tab at the back of the book.

2-10 Lipids contain a carbon-to-hydrogen ratio of 1:2

Learning Objective Discuss the structures and functions of lipids.

Lipids (*lipos*, fat) also contain carbon, hydrogen, and oxygen, but the ratios do not approximate 1:2:1. The reason is because they have relatively less oxygen than do carbohydrates.

In addition, lipids may contain small quantities of other elements, including phosphorus, nitrogen, or sulfur. Familiar lipids include *fats, oils*, and *waxes*. Most lipids are insoluble in water. For this reason, special transport molecules carry them in the circulating blood.

Lipids form essential parts of the structure of all cells. In addition, lipid deposits are important as energy reserves. Based on equal weights, lipids provide roughly twice as much energy as carbohydrates when broken down in the body. When the supply of lipids exceeds the demand for energy, the excess is stored in fat deposits. For this reason, there has been great interest in developing *fat substitutes* that provide less energy but have the same taste and texture as lipids.

Lipids normally account for 12–18 percent of total body weight of adult men, and 18–24 percent of that of adult women. There are many kinds of lipids in the body. The major types are *fatty acids, fats, steroids*, and *phospholipids* (**Table 2-5**).

Fatty Acids

Fatty acids are long chains of carbon atoms with attached hydrogen atoms and end in a *carboxyl* (kar-BOK-sil) *group* (— COOH). The name *carboxyl* should help you remember that a carbon and a hydroxyl (— OH) group are the important structural features of fatty acids. When a fatty acid is in solution, only the carboxyl end dissolves in water. The carbon chain, known as the hydrocarbon *tail* of the fatty acid, is relatively insoluble. **Figure 2-13a** shows a representative fatty acid, *lauric acid*.

Table 2-5	Representative Lipids and Their Functions in the Body		
Lipid Type	**Examples**	**Primary Functions**	**Remarks**
Fatty Acids	Lauric acid	Energy sources	Absorbed from food or synthesized in cells; transported in the blood for use in many tissues
Fats	Monoglycerides, diglycerides, triglycerides	Energy source, energy storage, insulation, and physical protection	Stored in fat deposits; must be broken down to fatty acids and glycerol before they can be used as an energy source
Steroids	Cholesterol	Structural component of cell membranes, hormones, digestive secretions in bile	All have the same carbon-ring framework
Phospholipids	Lecithin	Structural components of cell membranes	Composed of fatty acids and nonlipid molecules

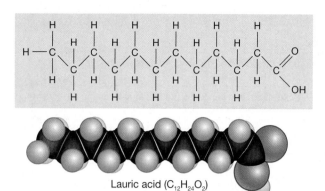

Lauric acid ($C_{12}H_{24}O_2$)

a Lauric acid shows the basic structure of a fatty acid: a long chain of carbon atoms and a carboxyl group (—COOH) at one end.

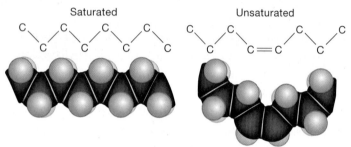

Saturated   Unsaturated

b A fatty acid is either saturated (has single covalent bonds only) or unsaturated (has one or more double covalent bonds). The presence of a double bond causes a sharp bend in the molecule.

Figure 2-13 Fatty Acids.

In a **saturated** fatty acid, such as lauric acid, the four single covalent bonds of each carbon atom permit each carbon to link to neighboring carbons on either side and to two hydrogen atoms. If any of the carbon-to-carbon bonds are double covalent bonds, then fewer hydrogen atoms are present and the fatty acid is **unsaturated**. The structures of saturated and unsaturated fatty acids are shown in **Figure 2-13b**. A *monounsaturated* fatty acid has a lone double bond in the hydrocarbon tail. A *polyunsaturated* fatty acid contains multiple double bonds.

Both saturated and unsaturated fatty acids can be broken down for energy, but a diet with large amounts of saturated fatty acids increases the risk of heart disease and other circulatory problems. Butter, fatty meat, and ice cream are popular dietary sources of saturated fatty acids. Vegetable oils such as olive oil or corn oil contain a mixture of unsaturated fatty acids.

Fats

Unlike simple sugars, individual fatty acids cannot be strung together in a chain by dehydration synthesis. But they can be attached to the compound **glycerol** (GLIS-er-ol) to make a **fat** through a similar reaction. In a **triglyceride** (trī-GLI-se-rīd), a glycerol molecule is attached to three fatty acids (**Figure 2-14**). Triglycerides are the most common fats in the body.

In addition to serving as an energy reserve, fat deposits under the skin serve as insulation. A mass of fat around a delicate organ, such as a kidney, provides a protective cushion. *Saturated fats*—triglycerides containing saturated fatty

CLINICAL NOTE

Fatty Acids and Health

Good news: The right fat can be good for you

Humans love fatty foods. Unfortunately, a diet containing large amounts of saturated fats has been shown to increase the risk of heart disease and other cardiovascular problems. Saturated fats contain only saturated fatty acids. These fats are found in such popular foods as fatty meat and dairy products (including such favorites as butter, cheese, and ice cream).

Vegetable oils contain a mixture of monounsaturated and polyunsaturated fatty acids. Recent studies indicate that monounsaturated fats may be more effective than polyunsaturated fats in lowering the risk of heart disease. According to current research, perhaps the healthiest choices are olive and canola oils. These oils contain an abundance of oleic acid, an 18-carbon monounsaturated fatty acid. Surprisingly, compounds

called *trans* fatty acids, produced from polyunsaturated oils during the manufacturing of some margarines and vegetable shortenings, appear to increase the risk of heart disease. U.S. Food and Drug Administration (FDA) guidelines now require that *trans* fatty acids be listed in the nutrition label of foods and dietary supplements.

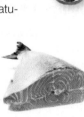

The Inuit people of the Arctic regions have lower rates of heart disease than do other populations, even though the typical Inuit diet is high in fats and cholesterol. Interestingly, the main fatty acids in their diet are omega-3s. These fatty acids have an unsaturated bond three carbons before the last (or omega) carbon, a position known as "omega minus 3." Fish flesh and fish oils, a large part of the Inuit diet, contain an abundance of omega-3 fatty acids. Why the presence of **omega-3 fatty acids** in the diet reduces the risks of heart disease, rheumatoid arthritis, and other inflammatory diseases is not yet apparent, but it is a research topic of great interest.

Figure 2-14 Triglyceride Formation. The formation of a triglyceride involves the attachment of three fatty acids to a glycerol molecule through dehydration synthesis. In this example, a triglyceride is formed by the attachment of one unsaturated and two saturated fatty acids to a glycerol molecule.

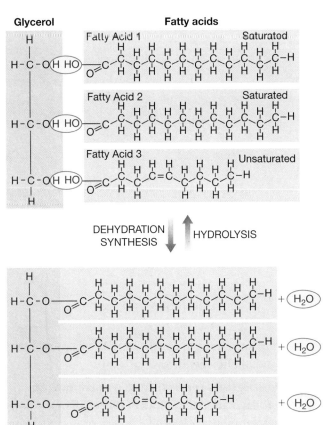

Figure 2-15 A Cholesterol Molecule. Like all steroids, cholesterol contains a complex four-ring structure.

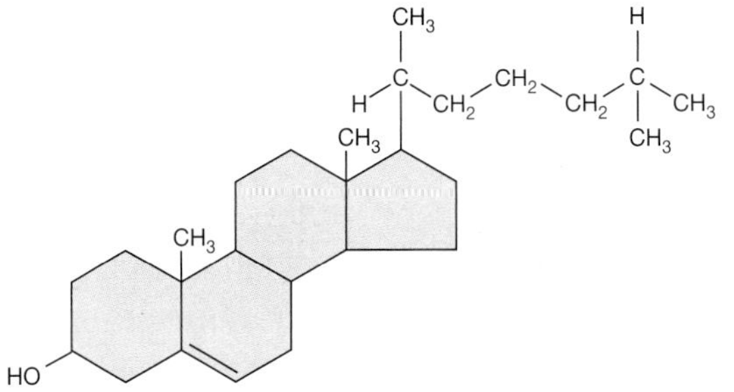

is the body itself. The liver can synthesize large amounts of cholesterol. The body's ability to synthesize this steroid can make it difficult to control blood cholesterol levels by dietary restriction alone. This difficulty can be a problem because a strong link exists between high blood cholesterol levels and heart disease. Current nutritional advice suggests limiting cholesterol intake to under 300 mg per day. This amount represents a 40 percent reduction for the average adult in the United States. (We will examine the connection between blood cholesterol levels and heart disease in Chapters 11 and 12.)

Phospholipids

Phospholipids (FOS-fō-lip-idz) consist of a glycerol and two fatty acids (a diglyceride) linked to a nonlipid group by a phosphate group (PO_4^{3-}) (**Figure 2-16**). The nonlipid portion of a phospholipid is soluble in water, but the fatty acid portion is relatively insoluble. Phospholipids are the most abundant lipid components of cell membranes.

> **CHECKPOINT**
>
> 21. Describe lipids.
> 22. Which kind of lipid would be found in a sample of fatty tissue taken from beneath the skin?
> 23. Which lipids would you find in human cell membranes?
>
> See the blue Answers tab at the back of the book.

acids—are usually solid at room temperature. *Unsaturated fats*, which are triglycerides containing unsaturated fatty acids, are usually liquid at room temperature. Such liquid fats are oils.

Steroids

Steroids are large lipid molecules composed of four connected rings of carbon atoms. They differ in the carbon chains that are attached to this basic structure. **Cholesterol** (koh-LES-ter-ol; *chole-*, bile + *stereos*, solid) is probably the best-known steroid (**Figure 2-15**). All our cells are surrounded by *cell membranes*, or *plasma membranes*, that contain cholesterol. Also, some chemical messengers, or *hormones*, are derived from cholesterol. Examples include the sex hormones testosterone and estrogen.

The cholesterol needed to maintain cell membranes and manufacture steroid hormones comes from two sources. One source is the diet. Animal products such as meat, cream, and egg yolks are especially rich in cholesterol. The second source

2-11 Proteins contain carbon, hydrogen, oxygen, and nitrogen and are formed from amino acids

Learning Objective Discuss the structures and functions of proteins.

Proteins are the most abundant organic molecules in the human body and in many ways the most important. The human body contains many different proteins, and they

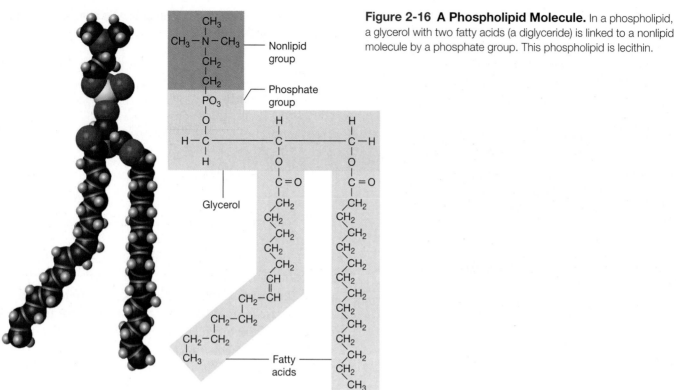

Figure 2-16 A Phospholipid Molecule. In a phospholipid, a glycerol with two fatty acids (a diglyceride) is linked to a nonlipid molecule by a phosphate group. This phospholipid is lecithin.

account for about 20 percent of total body weight. All proteins contain carbon, hydrogen, oxygen, and nitrogen. Smaller quantities of sulfur and phosphorus may also be present.

Protein Function

Proteins perform a variety of functions, which can be grouped into seven major categories:

1. **Support.** **Structural proteins** create a three-dimensional framework for the body, providing strength, organization, and support for cells, tissues, and organs.

2. **Movement.** **Contractile proteins** are responsible for muscular contraction. Related proteins are responsible for the movement of individual cells.

3. **Transport.** Insoluble lipids, respiratory gases, minerals such as iron, and several hormones are carried in the blood attached to **transport proteins**. Other specialized proteins transport materials between different parts of a cell.

4. **Buffering.** Proteins provide a buffering action, helping to prevent potentially dangerous changes in pH in body fluids.

5. **Metabolic regulation.** Many proteins are enzymes. Enzymes speed up chemical reactions in living cells. The sensitivity of enzymes to environmental factors is

extremely important in controlling the pace and direction of metabolic operations.

6. **Coordination and control.** Protein **hormones** can influence the metabolic activities of every cell in the body or affect the function of specific organs or organ systems.

7. **Defense.** The tough, waterproof proteins of the skin, hair, and nails protect the body from environmental hazards. In addition, proteins known as **antibodies** protect us from disease. Special **clotting proteins** restrict bleeding after an injury to the cardiovascular system.

Protein Structure

Proteins are long chains of organic molecules called **amino acids**. The human body contains significant quantities of the 20 different amino acids used in building proteins. Each amino acid consists of five parts: a central carbon atom, a hydrogen atom, an amino group ($—NH_2$), a carboxyl group ($—COOH$), and an R group (a variable *side chain* of one or more atoms) (**Figure 2-17a**). The name *amino acid* refers to the presence of the *amino* group and the acidic carboxyl group, which all amino acids have in common. (The carboxyl group is acidic because it can release a hydrogen ion.) The different R groups distinguish one amino acid from another, giving each its own chemical properties. For example, an R group may be polar, nonpolar, or electrically charged.

Figure 2-17 Amino Acids and the Formation of Peptide Bonds.

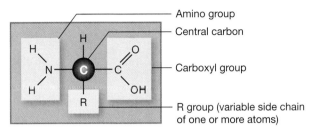

- Amino group
- Central carbon
- Carboxyl group
- R group (variable side chain of one or more atoms)

a **Structure of an Amino Acid.** Each amino acid consists of a central carbon atom to which four different groups are attached: a hydrogen atom, an amino group ($-NH_2$), a carboxyl group ($-COOH$), and a variable group generally designated R.

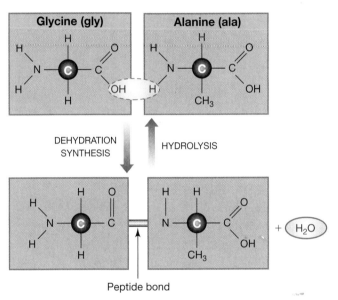

Glycine (gly)

Alanine (ala)

DEHYDRATION SYNTHESIS

HYDROLYSIS

$+ H_2O$

Peptide bond

b **Peptide Bond Formation.** Peptides form when a dehydration synthesis reaction creates a peptide bond between the carboxyl group of one amino acid and the amino group of another. In this example, glycine (for which R = H) and alanine (for which R = CH_3) are linked to form a dipeptide.

A typical protein contains 1000 amino acids. The largest protein complexes may have 100,000 or more. The individual amino acids are strung together like beads on a string, with the carboxyl group of one amino acid attached to the amino group of another. This connection is called a **peptide bond** (**Figure 2-17b**). **Peptides** are molecules made up of amino acids held together by peptide bonds. A molecule that consists of two amino acids is called a *dipeptide.* Tripeptides and larger chains of amino acids are called *polypeptides.* Polypeptides containing more than 100 amino acids are usually called proteins.

At its most basic level, the *structure* of a protein is established by the sequence of its amino acids (**Figure 2-18a**). The *characteristics* of a particular protein are determined in part by the R groups on its amino acids. But the properties of a protein are more than just the sum of the properties of its parts, for polypeptides can have highly complex shapes that are important to their function. Proteins can have four levels of structural complexity (**Figure 2-18**):

1. **Primary structure** is the sequence of amino acids linked by peptide bonds along the length of a single polypeptide chain (**Figure 2-18a**).

2. **Secondary structure** is the shape that results from hydrogen bonding between atoms at different parts of the polypeptide chain. Hydrogen bonding may create either an *alpha helix* (simple spiral) or *beta sheet* (a flat pleated sheet) (**Figure 2-18b**). A polypeptide chain may have both helical and pleated sections.

3. **Tertiary structure** is the complex coiling and folding that gives a protein its final three-dimensional shape (**Figure 2-18c**). Tertiary structure results mainly from interactions between the R groups of the polypeptide chain and the surrounding water molecules, and from interactions between the R groups of amino acids in different parts of the molecule.

4. **Quaternary structure** develops when individual polypeptide chains interact to form a protein complex (**Figure 2-18d**). Each of the polypeptide subunits has its own secondary and tertiary structures. For example, the protein *hemoglobin* contains four subunits. Hemoglobin is found within red blood cells, where it binds and transports oxygen. In *keratin* and *collagen*, two (keratin) or three (collagen) alpha-helical polypeptides are wound together like the strands of a rope. Keratin is the tough, water-resistant protein at the surface of the skin and in hair and nails. Collagen is the most abundant structural protein in the body. It is found in skin, bones, cartilages, and tendons. It forms the framework that supports cells in most tissues.

Proteins fall into two general structural classes based on their overall shape and properties:

- **Fibrous proteins** form extended sheets or strands. Fibrous proteins are tough, durable, and generally insoluble in water. They usually play structural roles in the body.

- **Globular proteins** are compact, generally rounded, and soluble in water. The unique shape of each globular protein comes from its tertiary structure. Many enzymes, hormones, and other molecules that circulate in the bloodstream are globular proteins. These proteins usually have active, functional roles in the body.

The shape of a protein determines its functional properties. The 20 common amino acids can be linked in an

Figure 2-18 Protein Structure.

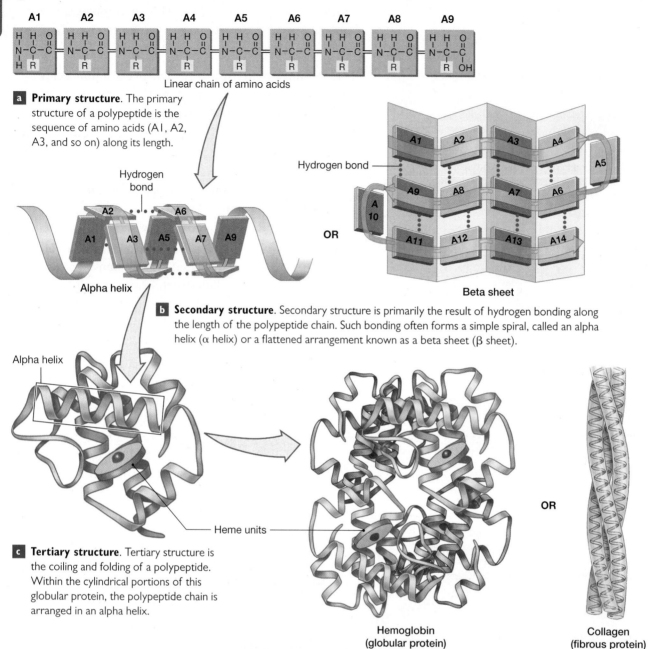

a **Primary structure**. The primary structure of a polypeptide is the sequence of amino acids (A1, A2, A3, and so on) along its length.

Linear chain of amino acids

b **Secondary structure**. Secondary structure is primarily the result of hydrogen bonding along the length of the polypeptide chain. Such bonding often forms a simple spiral, called an alpha helix (α helix) or a flattened arrangement known as a beta sheet (β sheet).

Alpha helix

Beta sheet

c **Tertiary structure**. Tertiary structure is the coiling and folding of a polypeptide. Within the cylindrical portions of this globular protein, the polypeptide chain is arranged in an alpha helix.

Hemoglobin (globular protein)

Collagen (fibrous protein)

d **Quaternary structure**. Quaternary structure develops when separate polypeptide subunits interact to form a larger molecule. A single hemoglobin molecule contains four globular subunits. Hemoglobin transports oxygen in the blood. In collagen, three helical polypeptide subunits intertwine. Collagen is the principal extracellular protein in most organs.

astonishing number of combinations, creating proteins of enormously varied shape and function. Small differences can have large effects. Changing one amino acid in a protein of 10,000 amino acids or more may make the protein incapable of performing its normal function. For example, several cancers and *sickle cell anemia*, a blood disorder, result from single changes in the amino acid sequences of complex proteins.

The shape of a protein—and thus its function—can be altered by small changes in the ionic composition, temperature, or pH of its surroundings. For example, very high body temperatures (over 43°C, or 110°F) cause death because at these temperatures proteins undergo **denaturation**, a change in their three-dimensional shape. Denatured proteins are nonfunctional, and the loss of structural proteins

Figure 2-19 A Simple Model of Enzyme Function. Each enzyme contains a specific active site somewhere on its exposed surface. Because the structure of the enzyme is not permanently affected, the entire process can be repeated.

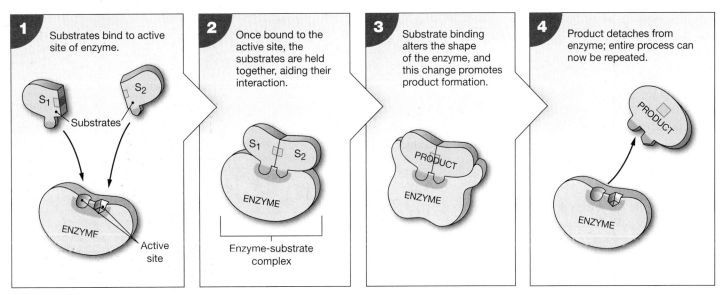

and enzymes causes irreparable damage to organs and organ systems. You see denaturation in progress each time you fry an egg. As the temperature rises, the structure of the abundant proteins dissolved in the clear egg white changes. Eventually the egg proteins form an insoluble white mass.

Enzyme Function

Enzymes are among the most important of all the body's proteins. ⟳ p. 34 These molecules catalyze the reactions that sustain life: Almost everything that happens inside the human body does so because a specific enzyme makes it possible.

Figure 2-19 shows a simple model of enzyme function. Recall that an enzyme functions as a catalyst—to speed up a chemical reaction without itself being permanently changed or consumed. The reactants in an enzymatic reaction are called **substrates**. They interact to form a specific **product**. For an enzyme to catalyze a reaction, the substrates must bind to a special region of the enzyme called the **active site**. This binding depends on the complementary shapes of the two molecules, much as a key fits into a lock. The shape of the active site is determined by the three-dimensional shape of the enzyme molecule. Substrate binding temporarily changes the shape of the enzyme. Once the reaction is completed and the products are released, the enzyme is free to catalyze another reaction. Enzymes work quickly. For example, an enzyme providing energy during a muscular contraction performs its reaction 100 times per second.

Each enzyme works best at an optimal temperature and pH. As temperatures rise or pH shifts outside normal limits,

bonds are broken and proteins change shape. Enzyme function deteriorates as a result.

Each enzyme catalyzes only one type of reaction. This *specificity* is due to the ability of its active sites to bind only to substrates with particular shapes and charges. The complex reactions that support life proceed in a series of interlocking steps, each step controlled by a different enzyme. Such a reaction sequence is called a *metabolic pathway.* (We will consider important metabolic pathways in later chapters.)

CHECKPOINT

24. Describe a protein.

25. How does boiling a protein affect its structural and functional properties?

See the blue Answers tab at the back of the book.

2-12 DNA and RNA are nucleic acids

Learning Objective Discuss the structures and functions of nucleic acids.

Nucleic (noo-KLĀ-ik) **acids** are large organic molecules made of carbon, hydrogen, oxygen, nitrogen, and phosphorus. Nucleic acids store and process information at the molecular level inside cells. The two classes of nucleic acid molecules are **deoxyribonucleic** (dē-oks-ē-rī-bō-noo-KLĀ-ik) **acid**, or **DNA**, and **ribonucleic** (rī-bō-noo-KLĀ-ik) **acid**, or **RNA**.

The DNA in our cells determines our inherited characteristics, including eye color, hair color, and blood type. DNA affects all aspects of body structure and function because DNA molecules encode the information needed to build proteins. By directing the synthesis of structural proteins, DNA controls the shape and physical characteristics of our bodies. By controlling the manufacture of enzymes, DNA regulates not only protein synthesis but also all aspects of cellular metabolism, including the creation and destruction of lipids, carbohydrates, and other vital molecules.

Several forms of RNA cooperate to manufacture specific proteins using the information provided by DNA. In Chapter 3, we will detail the ways DNA and RNA work together.

Structure of Nucleic Acids

A nucleic acid (**Figure 2-20**) is made up of subunits called **nucleotides**. Each nucleotide has three parts: a *sugar*, a *phosphate group* (PO_4^{3-}), and a *nitrogenous (nitrogen-containing) base* (**Figure 2-20a**). The sugar is always a five-carbon sugar, either **ribose** (in RNA) or **deoxyribose** (in DNA). There are five nitrogenous bases: **adenine (A)**, **guanine (G)**, **cytosine (C)**, **thymine (T)**, and **uracil (U)**. Both RNA and DNA contain adenine, guanine, and cytosine. Uracil is found only in RNA, and thymine only in DNA (**Figure 2-20b**).

Figure 2-20 The Structure of Nucleic Acids. Nucleic acids are long chains of nucleotides.

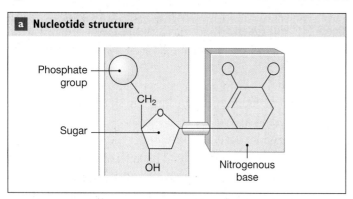

a Nucleotide structure

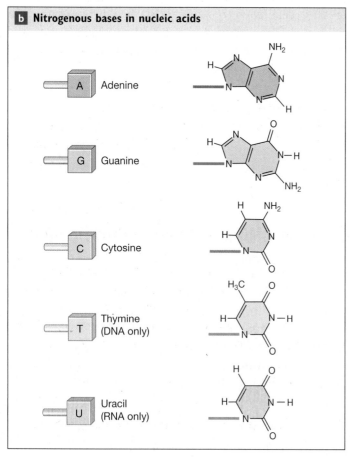

b Nitrogenous bases in nucleic acids

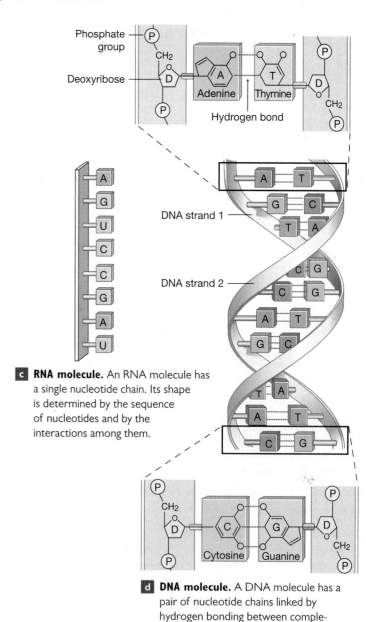

c **RNA molecule.** An RNA molecule has a single nucleotide chain. Its shape is determined by the sequence of nucleotides and by the interactions among them.

d **DNA molecule.** A DNA molecule has a pair of nucleotide chains linked by hydrogen bonding between complementary base pairs.

Table 2-6	A Comparison of RNA and DNA	
Characteristic	**RNA**	**DNA**
Sugar	Ribose	Deoxyribose
Nitrogenous Bases	Adenine	Adenine
	Guanine	Guanine
	Cytosine	Cytosine
	Uracil	Thymine
Number of Nucleotides in a Typical Molecule	Varies from fewer than 100 nucleotides to about 50,000	Always more than 45 million nucleotides
Shape of Molecule	Single strand	Paired strands coiled in a double helix
Function	Performs protein synthesis as directed by DNA	Stores genetic information that controls protein synthesis

Important structural differences between RNA and DNA are listed in **Table 2-6**. A molecule of RNA is a single chain of nucleotides (**Figure 2-20c**). A DNA molecule consists of two nucleotide chains. They are held together by weak hydrogen bonds between the opposing nitrogenous bases (**Figure 2-20d**). Because of their shapes, adenine can bond only with thymine, and cytosine only with guanine. For this reason, adenine–thymine and cytosine–guanine are known as **complementary base pairs**.

The two strands of DNA twist around one another in a **double helix**. This shape resembles a spiral staircase, with the stair steps corresponding to the nitrogenous base pairs.

CHECKPOINT

26. Describe a nucleic acid.

27. A large organic molecule composed of ribose sugars, nitrogenous bases, and phosphate groups is which kind of nucleic acid?

See the blue Answers tab at the back of the book.

2-13 ATP is a high-energy compound used by cells

Learning Objective Discuss the structures and functions of high-energy compounds.

The energy that powers a cell comes from the breakdown (catabolism) of organic molecules such as glucose. To get to where it is needed, that energy must be transferred from molecule to molecule or from one part of the cell to another.

The usual method of energy transfer involves the creation of high-energy bonds by enzymes within cells. A **high-energy bond** is a covalent bond that stores an unusually large amount of energy (as does a tightly twisted rubber band attached to the propeller of a model airplane). When that bond is later broken, the energy is released under controlled conditions (as when the propeller is turned by the untwisting rubber band).

In our cells, a high-energy bond usually connects a phosphate group (PO_4^{3-}) to an organic molecule, resulting in a **high-energy compound**. Most high-energy compounds are derived from nucleotides, the building blocks of nucleic acids. The most important high-energy compound in the body is **adenosine triphosphate**, or **ATP**. ATP is composed of the nucleotide *adenosine monophosphate* (*AMP*) and two phosphate groups (**Figure 2-21**). The addition of the two phosphate groups requires a significant amount of energy. When the first of these groups is added, AMP becomes *adenosine diphosphate* (*ADP*).

In ATP, a high-energy bond connects a phosphate group to **adenosine diphosphate (ADP)**. The conversion of ADP to ATP is the most important method of storing energy in our cells. The reverse reaction is the most important method of energy release. The two reactions can be diagrammed together as:

$$\text{ADP} + \text{phosphate group} + \text{energy} \rightleftharpoons \text{ATP} + \text{H}_2\text{O}$$

Throughout life, our cells continuously generate ATP from ADP and then use the energy stored in ATP to power vital functions, such as the synthesis of protein molecules or the contraction of muscles. **Figure 2-22** shows the recycling of ADP and ATP and its important role in cellular energy flow.

Figure 2-23 and **Table 2-7** review the major chemical compounds we have discussed in this chapter.

CHECKPOINT

28. Describe ATP.

29. What are the products of the hydrolysis of ATP?

See the blue Answers tab at the back of the book.

Figure 2-21 The Structure of ATP. A molecule of ATP is formed by attaching two phosphate groups to the nucleotide adenosine monophosphate (AMP). These two phosphate groups are connected by high-energy bonds.

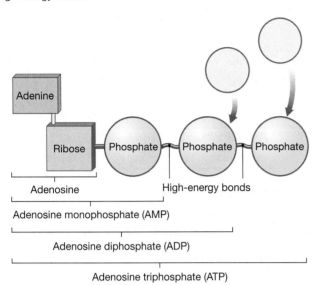

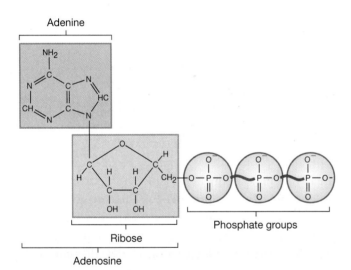

Figure 2-22 The Recycling of ADP and ATP and the Energy Flow within Cells.

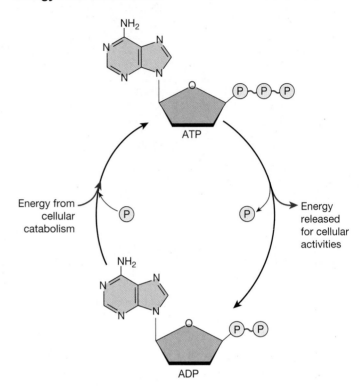

2-14 Chemicals form functional units called cells

Learning Objective Explain the relationship between chemicals and cells.

The human body is more than a random collection of chemicals. The biochemical building blocks discussed in this chapter are the components of *cells*. ⊃ p. 4 Each cell behaves like a miniature organism, responding to internal and external stimuli. A lipid membrane separates the cell from its environment, and internal membranes create compartments with specific functions. Proteins form an internal supporting framework and act as enzymes to accelerate and control the chemical reactions that maintain homeostasis. Nucleic acids direct the synthesis of all cellular proteins, including the enzymes that enable the cell to synthesize a wide variety of other substances. Carbohydrates provide energy for vital activities. They also form specialized compounds in combination with proteins or lipids. (In the next chapter, we consider the roles of such compounds within a living, functional cell.)

CHECKPOINT

30. Identify six elements common to organic compounds.

31. Identify the biochemical building blocks discussed in this chapter that are the components of cells.

See the blue Answers tab at the back of the book.

Figure 2-23 An Overview of the Structures of Organic Compounds in the Body. Each class of organic compounds is composed of simple structural subunits. Specific compounds within each class are depicted above the basic subunits. Fatty acids are the main subunits of all lipids except steroids. Only one type of lipid, a triglyceride, is represented here.

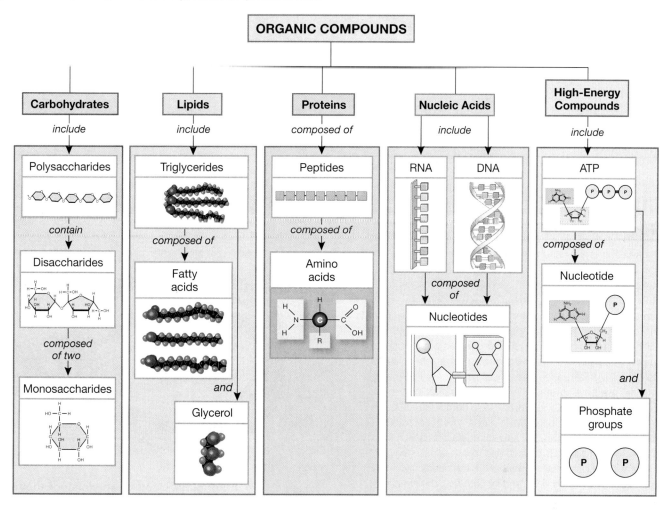

Table 2-7	The Structure and Function of Biologically Important Inorganic and Organic Compounds		
Class	**Building Blocks**	**Sources**	**Functions**
INORGANIC			
Water	Hydrogen and oxygen atoms	Absorbed as liquid water or generated by metabolism	Solvent; transport medium for dissolved materials and heat; cooling through evaporation; medium for chemical reactions; reactant in hydrolysis
Acids, bases, salts	H^+, OH^-, various anions and cations	Obtained from the diet or generated by metabolism	Structural components; buffers; sources of ions
Dissolved gases	Oxygen, carbon, nitrogen, and atoms of other elements	Atmosphere, metabolism	O_2: required for normal cellular metabolism

CO_2: generated by cells as a waste product |
ORGANIC			
Carbohydrates	C, H, and O; CHO in a 1:2:1 ratio	Obtained from the diet or manufactured in the body	Energy source; some structural role when attached to lipids or proteins; energy storage
Lipids	C, H, O, sometimes N or P; CHO not in 1:2:1 ratio	Obtained from the diet or manufactured in the body	Energy source; energy storage; insulation; structural components; chemical messengers; protection

(Continued)

Table 2-7	(Continued)		
Class	**Building Blocks**	**Sources**	**Functions**
Proteins	C, H, O, N, often S	20 common amino acids; roughly half can be manufactured in the body, others must be obtained from the diet	Catalysts for metabolic reactions; structural components; movement; transport; buffers; defense; control and coordination of activities
Nucleic acids	C, H, O, N, and P; nucleotides composed of phosphates, sugars, and nitrogenous bases	Obtained from the diet or manufactured in the body	Storage and processing of genetic information
High-energy compounds	Nucleotides joined to phosphates by high-energy bonds	Synthesized by all cells	Storage or transfer of energy

CLINICAL NOTE

Physical Properties of Emergency Medications

Many medications are used in prehospital care. Unlike in the hospital setting, medications used in the field are often exposed to environmental factors. In most cases, this rarely constitutes a problem. However, some medications are affected by environmental factors. Because of this, prehospital personnel must be familiar with the physical properties of the medications they use. Also, knowledge of the physical properties of prehospital medications helps in understanding their mechanism of action.

The three states of matter are *solid, liquid*, or *gas*. Two major factors affect the physical state of matter. The first factor is the intensity of the intermolecular forces that hold compounds together: solids have the strongest forces while gases have the weakest. The other factor is temperature. As the temperature rises, a substance will go from a solid to a liquid and then to a gaseous state.

As the material passes through these three phases from solid to liquid to gas, it absorbs heat, and its *enthalpy*, or heat content, increases.

Thus, the enthalpy of a liquid is greater than that of its solid, and the enthalpy of a gas is greater than that of its liquid, because heat is absorbed during melting and vaporization. The temperature at which a solid becomes a liquid is its *melting point*. The temperature at which a liquid becomes a gas is its *boiling point*. However, prior to reaching the boiling point, some liquids will begin to convert to the gaseous state through *evaporation*. Chemicals vary in their tendency to change physical states. The tendency to assume the gaseous state is *volatility*. Chemicals with high volatility rapidly evaporate and assume the gaseous state, while chemicals with low volatility tend to remain in the liquid state.

Most medications used in prehospital care are in a liquid state. This allows the medication to be administered into the body without having to be absorbed by the gastrointestinal tract. The boiling point and the freezing point of most emergency medicines will not be encountered in routine usage. However, some medications pose problems. For example, the medication mannitol is occasionally used in prehospital care to treat increased intracranial pressure, acute glaucoma, and blood transfusion reactions. Mannitol is a sugar and is used as an osmotic diuretic. It is supplied in liquid form in vials that contain a 20 percent solution. At temperatures less than 10°C (50°F), mannitol will begin

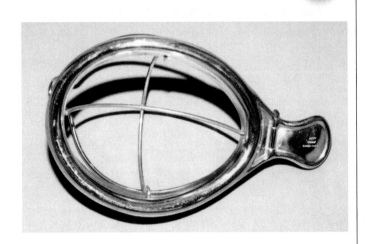

Figure 2-24 Ether Mask Used to Administer Ether as an Anesthetic. A cloth was placed in the frame and volatile ether was dripped onto the cloth for inhalation by the patient.

to crystallize. Initially, these crystals cannot be seen by the naked eye. If the temperature of the drug drops below 5°C (40°F), the entire vial will crystallize as the drug changes to the solid state. The higher the concentration of mannitol, the greater its tendency to crystallize. Because of this, mannitol should always be administered through a filter to prevent any crystals, including microscopic crystals, from entering the patient's circulation. Remelting mannitol with boiling water or in a microwave oven can potentially damage the drug and should not be attempted. Mannitol, like all EMS medications, should be maintained at the appropriate temperature.

The volatility of certain drugs is important in emergency care. For example, the general anesthetic agents are highly volatile, which allows their rapid delivery to patients. For example, the initial prototype anesthetic, ether, is highly volatile. In early anesthetic practice, it was dripped slowly into an ether mask and the patient inhaled the drug, which resulted in anesthesia (**Figure 2-24**). However, because ether is extremely flammable and hazardous to surgical personnel, it is rarely used in modern medicine.

(Continued)

An anesthetic agent occasionally used in modern medicine is *methoxyflurane* (Pentrane). In high doses, methoxyflurane is a general anesthetic, and in lower doses, it is an extremely effective analgesic agent. Although not approved for prehospital use in the United States, methoxyflurane is frequently used throughout Australian EMS as an analgesic agent. At room temperature, methoxyflurane is a liquid; however, it is highly volatile and rapidly evaporates. For analgesia, 3–6 milliliters of a 0.5 percent solution of methoxyflurane are placed on the absorbent wick of a methoxyflurane (Penthrane) inhaler. The inhaler is then handed to the patient, who breathes in and out through the mouthpiece. The onset of analgesia is rapid, and the effects of the drug quickly dissipate when removed. Because of this, it can be used in trauma, obstetrics, and other types of acute pain. A port on the methoxyflurane inhaler allows supplemental oxygen if required.

Nitrous oxide is another general anesthetic agent that has analgesic properties at lower concentrations. It is frequently used in the United States, Canada, and the United Kingdom for rapid analgesia. Because nitrous oxide can be an asphyxiant when used alone, it must always be administered with oxygen. Anesthesia is obtained when the level of nitrous oxide approaches 70 percent. Analgesia is obtained at a concentration of approximately 50 percent. In the United States, nitrous oxide and oxygen are administered from different cylinders. These gases are fed into a blender that mixes the correct 50 percent nitrous oxide/50 percent oxygen mixture. If the level of oxygen falls below 50 percent, then the unit shuts down. Unfortunately, requiring separate oxygen and nitrous oxide cylinders makes the unit much heavier, bulkier, and harder to use in emergency care. In the Commonwealth countries (former colonies of the United Kingdom), premixing nitrous oxide and oxygen into one cylinder is allowed (Entonox, Dolonox). This system is less bulky, less expensive, and easier to use in prehospital care.

One physical property of nitrous oxide affects its use in prehospital care. Nitrous oxide exists as a gas over liquid in pressurized steel containers at room temperature. However, at approximately −3.3°C (26°F), nitrous oxide returns to its liquid form. When this occurs, drug delivery ceases until the cylinder is warmed. Occasionally, inverting the cylinder two or three times may free enough gas to complete patient care. In the U.S. system (Nitronox), when nitrous oxide delivery ceases, the device allows the continued flow of pure oxygen. In the single-cylinder system, when the nitrous oxide liquefies, the mixture separates, and the gaseous oxygen occupies the top of the cylinder while the liquid nitrous oxide occupies the bottom of the cylinder. Administration of nitrous oxide through the single cylinder system in cold environments can cause decreased concentrations of the drug as it liquefies and leaves the mixture. Gentle rewarming of the cylinder at 20°C (68°F) and completely inverting the cylinder will restore the mixture.

RELATED CLINICAL TERMS

familial hypercholesterolemia: A genetic disorder resulting in high cholesterol levels in blood and cholesterol buildup in body tissues, especially the walls of blood vessels.

galactosemia: A metabolic disorder resulting from the lack of an enzyme that converts galactose, a monosaccharide in milk, to glucose within cells. Affected individuals have elevated galactose levels in the blood and urine. High levels of galactose during childhood can cause abnormalities in nervous system development and liver function, and cataracts.

nuclear imaging: A procedure in which an image is created on a photographic plate or video screen by the radiation emitted by injected radioisotopes.

phenylketonuria (PKU): A metabolic disorder resulting from a defect in the enzyme that normally converts the amino acid phenylalanine to tyrosine, another amino acid. If the resulting elevated phenylalanine levels are not detected in infancy, mental delay can result from damage to the developing nervous system. Treatment consists of controlling the amount of phenylalanine in the diet, especially during infancy and early childhood.

radiopharmaceuticals: Drugs that incorporate radioactive atoms; administered to expose specific target tissues to radiation.

tracer: A radioisotope-labeled compound that can be tracked in the body by the radiation it releases.

2 Chapter Review

Summary Outline

An Introduction to the Chemical Level of Organization *p. 26*

1. **Chemistry** is the study of *matter* and its interactions.

2-1 Atoms are the basic particles of matter *p. 26*

2. **Atoms** are the smallest units of matter. They consist of **protons, neutrons,** and **electrons** (*Figure 2-1*).

3. An **element** consists entirely of atoms with the same number of protons (**atomic number**). Within an atom, an **electron cloud** surrounds the nucleus (*Figure 2-2; Table 2-1*).

4. The **mass number** of an atom is equal to the total number of protons and neutrons in its nucleus. **Isotopes** are atoms of the same element whose nuclei contain different numbers of neutrons. The **atomic weight** of an element is its average mass because it takes into account the abundance of its various isotopes.

5. Electrons occupy a series of **electron shells** around the nucleus. The number of electrons in the outermost electron shell determines an element's chemical properties *(Figure 2-3)*.

2-2 Chemical bonds are forces formed by interactions among atoms *p. 28*

6. Atoms can combine through chemical reactions that create **chemical bonds**. A **molecule** is any chemical structure consisting of atoms held together by shared electrons. A **compound** is any chemical substance made up of atoms of two or more different elements in specific proportions.

7. An **ionic bond** results from the attraction between **ions**, which are atoms that have gained or lost electrons. **Cations** are positively charged ions, and **anions** are negatively charged ions *(Figure 2-4; Table 2-2)*.

8. Sharing one pair of electrons creates a single **covalent bond**; sharing two pairs forms a **double covalent bond**. An unequal sharing of electrons creates a **polar covalent bond** *(Figure 2-5)*.

9. A **hydrogen bond** is the attraction between a hydrogen atom with a slight positive charge and a negatively charged atom in another molecule or within the same molecule. Hydrogen bonds can affect the shapes and properties of molecules *(Figure 2-6)*.

2-3 Decomposition, synthesis, and exchange reactions are important chemical reactions in physiology *p. 31*

10. **Metabolism** refers to all the **chemical reactions** in the body. Our cells capture, store, and use energy to maintain homeostasis and support essential functions.

11. The rules of **chemical notation** are used to describe chemical compounds and reactions *(Spotlight Figure 2-7)*.

12. **Work** involves movement of an object or a change in its physical structure, and **energy** is the capacity to perform work. There are two major types of energy: kinetic and potential.

13. **Kinetic energy** is the energy of motion. **Potential energy** is stored energy that results from the position or structure of an object. Conversions from potential to kinetic energy are not 100 percent efficient; every energy exchange produces **heat**.

14. A chemical reaction may be classified as a **decomposition**, **synthesis**, or **exchange reaction**.

15. Cells gain energy to power their functions through **catabolism**, the breakdown of complex molecules. Much of this energy supports **anabolism**, the synthesis of new organic molecules.

16. Reversible reactions consist of simultaneous synthesis and decomposition reactions. At **equilibrium**, the rates of these two opposing reactions are in balance.

2-4 Enzymes catalyze specific biochemical reactions by lowering a reaction's activation energy *p. 34*

17. **Activation energy** is the amount of energy required to start a reaction. Molecules called **enzymes** control many chemical reactions within our bodies. Enzymes are **catalysts** that take part in reactions without themselves being permanently changed *(Figure 2-8)*.

18. **Exergonic** reactions release energy; **endergonic** reactions absorb energy.

2-5 Inorganic compounds usually lack carbon, and organic compounds always contain carbon *p. 34*

19. **Nutrients** and **metabolites** can be broadly classified as **organic** or **inorganic compounds**.

20. Living cells in the body consume oxygen and generate carbon dioxide.

2-6 Physiological systems depend on water *p. 35*

21. Water is the most important inorganic component of the body.

22. Water is an excellent solvent, has a high heat capacity, and participates in the metabolic reactions of the body.

23. Many inorganic compounds undergo **dissociation**, or **ionization**, in water to form ions *(Figure 2-9)*.

2-7 Body fluid pH is vital for homeostasis *p. 36*

24. The **pH** of a solution indicates the concentration of hydrogen ions it contains. Solutions are classified as neutral (pH = 7), acidic (pH < 7), or basic (alkaline) (pH > 7) on the basis of pH *(Figure 2-10)*.

25. **Buffers** maintain pH within normal limits (7.35−7.45 in most body fluids) by releasing or absorbing hydrogen ions.

2-8 Acids, bases, and salts have important physiological roles *p. 36*

26. An **acid** releases hydrogen ions into a solution, and a **base** removes hydrogen ions from a solution.

27. A **salt** is an ionic compound whose cation is not H^+ and whose anion is not OH^-. Acids, bases, and salts are **electrolytes**, compounds that dissociate in water and conduct an electrical current.

2-9 Carbohydrates contain carbon, hydrogen, and oxygen in a 1:2:1 ratio *p. 39*

28. Organic compounds always contain carbon and hydrogen.

29. **Carbohydrates** are most important as an energy source for metabolic processes. The three major types are **monosaccharides** (simple sugars), **disaccharides**, and **polysaccharides** *(Figures 2-11, 2-12; Table 2-3)*.

2-10 Lipids contain a carbon-to-hydrogen ratio of 1:2 *p. 41*

30. **Lipids** are water-insoluble molecules that include fats, oils, and waxes. There are four important classes of lipids: **fatty acids, fats, steroids**, and **phospholipids** (*Table 2-4*).

31. **Triglycerides (fats)** consist of three fatty acid molecules attached to a molecule of **glycerol** (*Figures 2-13, 2-14*).

32. Cholesterol is a building block of steroid hormones and is a component of cell membranes (*Figure 2-15*).

33. Phospholipids are the most abundant components of cell membranes (*Figure 2-16*).

2-11 Proteins contain carbon, hydrogen, oxygen, and nitrogen and are formed from amino acids *p. 43*

34. Proteins perform a great variety of functions in the body. Seven important types of proteins include **structural proteins, contractile proteins, transport proteins, buffering proteins, enzymes, hormones**, and **antibodies**.

35. Proteins are chains of **amino acids**. Each amino acid consists of an amino group, a carboxyl group, a hydrogen atom, and an R group (variable side chain) attached to a central carbon atom. Amino acids are linked by **peptide bonds**. The sequence of amino acids and the interactions of their R groups influence the final shape of a protein molecule (*Figures 2-17, 2-18*).

36. The four levels of protein structure are **primary structure** (amino acid sequence), **secondary structure** (amino acid interactions, such as hydrogen bonding), **tertiary structure** (complex folding and interaction with water molecules), and **quaternary structure** (formation of protein complexes from individual subunits). **Fibrous proteins** are tough,

durable, and generally insoluble in water. **Globular proteins** are generally rounded and soluble in water (*Figure 2-18*).

37. The shape of a protein determines its function. Each protein works best at an optimal combination of temperature and pH.

38. The reactants in an enzymatic reaction, called **substrates**, interact to form a **product** by binding to the enzyme at the **active site** (*Figure 2-19*).

2-12 DNA and RNA are nucleic acids *p. 47*

39. **Nucleic acids** store and process information at the molecular level. There are two kinds of nucleic acids: **deoxyribonucleic acid (DNA)** and **ribonucleic acid (RNA)** (*Figure 2-20; Table 2-5*).

40. Nucleic acids are chains of nucleotides. Each nucleotide contains a sugar, a **phosphate group**, and a **nitrogenous base**. The sugar is always **ribose** or **deoxyribose**. The nitrogenous bases found in DNA are **adenine, guanine, cytosine**, and **thymine**. In RNA, **uracil** replaces thymine.

2-13 ATP is a high-energy compound used by cells *p. 49*

41. Cells store energy in **high-energy compounds**. The most important high-energy compound is **ATP (adenosine triphosphate)**. When energy is available, cells make ATP by adding a phosphate group to ADP. When energy is needed, ATP is broken down to ADP and phosphate (*Figures 2-21, 2-22*).

42. Biologically important organic compounds are composed of simple structural subunits (*Figure 2-23; Table 2-6*).

2-14 Chemicals form functional units called cells *p. 50*

43. Biochemical building blocks form *cells*.

Review Questions
See the blue Answers tab at the back of the book.

Level 1 Reviewing Facts and Terms

Match each item in column A with the most closely related item in column B. Place the letters for answers in the spaces provided.

COLUMN A

_____ 1. Atomic number
_____ 2. Covalent bond
_____ 3. Ionic bond
_____ 4. Catabolism
_____ 5. Anabolism
_____ 6. Exchange reaction
_____ 7. Reversible reaction
_____ 8. Acid
_____ 9. Enzyme
_____ 10. Buffer
_____ 11. Organic compounds
_____ 12. Inorganic compounds

COLUMN B

a. Synthesis
b. Catalyst
c. Sharing of electrons
d. $A + B \rightleftharpoons AB$
e. Stabilizes pH
f. Number of protons
g. Decomposition
h. Carbohydrates, lipids, proteins
i. Electrical attraction
j. Water, NaCl
k. Donor
l. $AB + CD \longrightarrow AD + CB$

2

13. An oxygen atom has eight protons. **(a)** In the following diagram, sketch in the arrangement of electrons around the nucleus of the oxygen atom. **(b)** How many more electrons will it take to fill the outermost electron shell?

Oxygen atom

14. In atoms, protons and neutrons are found
   (a) only in the nucleus.
   (b) outside the nucleus.
   (c) inside and outside the nucleus.
   (d) in the electron cloud.

15. The number and arrangement of electrons in an atom's outer electron shell determine its element's
   (a) atomic weight.
   (b) atomic number.
   (c) electrical properties.
   (d) chemical properties.

16. The bond between sodium and chlorine in the compound sodium chloride (NaCl) is
   (a) an ionic bond.
   (b) a single covalent bond.
   (c) a nonpolar covalent bond.
   (d) a double covalent bond.

17. Explain how enzymes function in chemical reactions.

18. List the six most abundant elements in the body.

19. What four major classes of organic compounds are found in the body?

20. List seven major functions performed by proteins.

21. Identify the components of an amino acid in the following diagram.

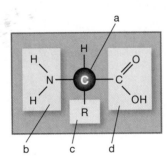

(a) _____   **(b)** _____
(c) _____   **(d)** _____

Level 2 Reviewing Concepts

22. Oxygen has eight protons, eight neutrons, and eight electrons. What is its atomic mass?
   (a) 8
   (b) 16
   (c) 24
   (d) 32

23. Which of the following groups contains only organic compounds?
   (a) Water, vitamins, oxygen, carbon dioxide
   (b) Oxygen, carbon dioxide, water, sugars
   (c) Water, fats, salts, nucleic acids
   (d) Carbohydrates, lipids, proteins, nucleic acids

24. Glucose and fructose are examples of
   (a) monosaccharides (simple sugars).
   (b) isotopes.
   (c) lipids.
   (d) a, b, and c are all correct.

25. Explain the differences among nonpolar covalent bonds, polar covalent bonds, and ionic bonds.

26. What does it mean to say a solution has a neutral pH?

27. How much more acidic or less acidic is a solution of pH 2 compared to one with a pH of 6?

28. An organic molecule contains the following elements: carbon, hydrogen, oxygen, nitrogen, and phosphorus. On the basis of this information, is the molecule a carbohydrate, a lipid, a protein, or a nucleic acid?

Level 3 Critical Thinking and Clinical Applications

29. The element sulfur has an atomic number of 16 and an atomic mass of 32. How many neutrons are in the nucleus of a sulfur atom? Assuming that sulfur forms covalent bonds with hydrogen, how many hydrogen atoms could bond to one sulfur atom?

30. An important buffer system in the human body involves carbon dioxide (CO_2) and bicarbonate ions (HCO_3^-) as shown:

$$CO_2 + H_2O \rightleftharpoons H_2CO_3 \rightleftharpoons H^+ + HCO_3^-$$

If a person becomes excited and exhales large amounts of CO_2, how will his or her body's pH be affected?

Cell Structure and Function

Learning Objectives

These objectives tell you what you should be able to do after completing the chapter. They correspond by number to this chapter's sections.

3-1 List the main points of the cell theory.

3-2 Describe the functions of the plasma membrane and the structures that enable it to perform those functions.

3-3 Describe the processes of cellular diffusion and osmosis, and explain their physiological roles.

3-4 Describe carrier-mediated transport and vesicular transport processes used by cells to absorb or remove specific substances.

3-5 Describe the organelles of a typical cell and indicate their specific functions.

3-6 Explain the functions of the cell nucleus.

3-7 Summarize the process of protein synthesis.

3-8 Describe the stages of the cell life cycle, including mitosis, interphase, and cytokinesis, and explain their significance.

3-9 Discuss the relationship between cell division and cancer.

3-10 Define differentiation and explain its importance.

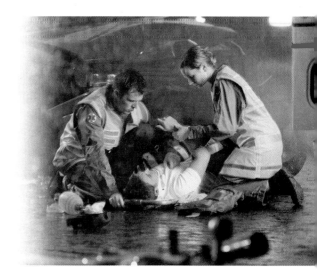

3

An Introduction to Cell Structure and Function

Cells are very small. A typical cell is only about 0.1 mm in diameter, similar to the thickness of a human hair. As a result, no one could actually examine the structure of a cell until effective microscopes were invented in the 17th century. In 1665, Robert Hooke inspected thin slices of cork and found that they were made up of millions of small, walled openings. Hooke used the term *cell* because the many, small bare spaces reminded him of the rooms, or cells, in a prison or monastery. Hooke saw only the outlines of cells, not the cells themselves, but he stimulated interest in the microscopic world and the nature of cellular life that continues to this day.

Build Your Knowledge

The Build Your Knowledge feature reminds you of what you already know and prepares you to learn new material. Be sure to read every Build Your Knowledge box or page so that you can build your knowledge—and confidence!

Recall that cells are the smallest living units that exhibit the basic functions of living things—responsiveness, growth, reproduction, movement, and metabolism (as you saw in **Chapter 1: An Introduction to Anatomy and Physiology**). Cells make up the cellular level of organization in the human body. ⊃ **p. 4**

3-1 The study of cells provides the foundation for understanding human physiology

Learning Objective List the main points of the cell theory.

Just as atoms are the building blocks of molecules, **cells** are the building blocks of the human body. Over the years, biologists have developed the **cell theory,** which includes the following four basic concepts:

1. Cells are the building blocks of all plants and animals.
2. Cells are the smallest functioning units of life.
3. Cells are produced through the division of preexisting cells.
4. Each cell maintains homeostasis.

An individual organism maintains homeostasis only through the combined and coordinated actions of many different types of cells. **Figure 3-1** shows some of the variety of cell shapes and sizes in the human body.

Numbering in the trillions, human body cells form anatomical structures and maintain them. Our cells allow us to perform activities as different as running and thinking. Thus, an understanding of how the human body functions requires a familiarity with the nature of cells.

The Study of Cells

The study of the structure and function of cells is called **cytology** (sī-TOL-ō-jē; *cyto-*, cell + *-logy*, the study of). What we have learned over the last 60 years has provided new insights into the physiology of cells and their means of homeostatic control. This knowledge resulted from improved equipment for viewing cells and new experimental techniques. It came not only from biology but also from chemistry and physics.

The two most common methods used to study cell and tissue structure are light microscopy and electron microscopy. Before the 1950s, cells were viewed through light microscopes. Using a series of glass lenses, *light microscopy* can magnify cellular structures about 1000 times. Light microscopy typically involves looking at thin sections sliced from a larger piece of tissue. A photograph taken through a light microscope is called a *light micrograph* (*LM*).

Many fine details of cell structure are too small to be seen with a light microscope. These details remained a mystery until cell biologists began using *electron microscopy*, a technique that replaced light with a focused beam of electrons. *Transmission electron micrographs* (*TEMs*) are photographs of very thin sections (slices), and they can reveal fine details of cell membranes and structures within

Figure 3-1 The Diversity of Cells in the Human Body. The cell types shown here have the dimensions they would have if magnified approximately 500 times.

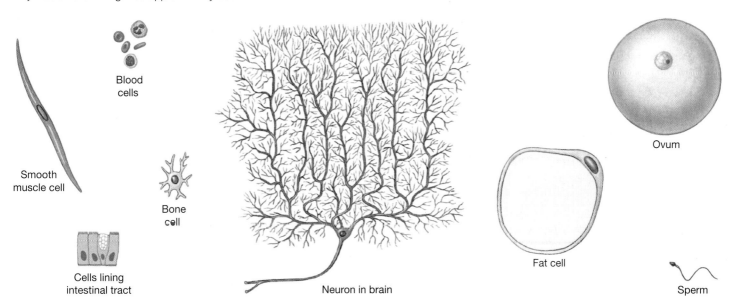

Blood cells

Smooth muscle cell

Bone cell

Cells lining intestinal tract

Neuron in brain

Ovum

Fat cell

Sperm

the cell. *Scanning electron micrographs* (*SEMs*) provide less magnification but reveal the three-dimensional nature of cell structures. An SEM provides a surface view of a cell, a portion of a cell, or structures outside the cell rather than a detailed sectional view.

You will see examples of light micrographs and both kinds of electron micrographs in figures throughout this text. The abbreviations LM, TEM, and SEM are followed by a number that tells you the total magnification of the image. For example, "LM × 160" indicates that the structures shown in a light micrograph have been magnified 160 times.

An Overview of Cell Anatomy

The "typical" cell is like the "average" person: Any such description masks enormous individual variations. Our representative, or model, cell shares features with most cells of the body without being identical to any specific one. **Spotlight Figure 3-2** summarizes the structures and functions of a model cell. We will refer to it during our discussion of the parts of a cell.

We begin our discussion of the cell with its **plasma membrane**, or **cell membrane**, which separates the cell contents, or **cytoplasm**, from its watery, surrounding environment. As noted in **Spotlight Figure 3-2**, this watery environment is called *extracellular fluid*. We then consider some of the ways cells interact with their external environment, as well as the activities of their specialized structures. We conclude with how typical body cells reproduce.

CHECKPOINT

1. The cell theory was developed over many years. What are its four basic concepts?
2. The study of cells is called _____.

See the blue Answers tab at the back of the book.

3-2 The plasma membrane separates the cell from its surrounding environment and performs various functions

Learning Objective Describe the functions of the plasma membrane and the structures that enable it to perform those functions.

We begin our look at cell structure with the plasma membrane. Its general functions include:

- ***Physical isolation.*** The plasma membrane is a physical barrier that separates the inside of the cell from the surrounding extracellular fluid. Conditions inside and outside the cell are very different. Those differences must be maintained to preserve homeostasis.

- ***Regulation of exchange with the environment.*** The plasma membrane controls the entry of ions and nutrients, the elimination of wastes, and the release of secretions.

- ***Sensitivity to the environment.*** The plasma membrane is the first part of the cell affected by changes in the extracellular fluid. It also contains a variety of molecules that act as receptors, enabling the cell to recognize and respond to specific molecules in its environment.

In our model cell, a *plasma membrane* separates the cell contents, called the *cytoplasm*, from its surroundings. The cytoplasm can be subdivided into the *cytosol*, or intracellular fluid, and intracellular structures collectively known as *organelles* (or-ga-NELZ). Organelles are structures suspended within the cytosol that perform specific functions within the cell and can be further subdivided into membranous and nonmembranous organelles. Cells are surrounded by a watery medium known as the **extracellular fluid.** The extracellular fluid in most tissues is called **interstitial** (in-ter-STISH-ul) **fluid.**

KEY

■	Plasma membrane
□	Nonmembranous organelles
□	Membranous organelles

Microvilli

Plasma membrane extensions containing microfilaments

Function
Increase surface area to aid absorption of extra-cellular materials

Centrioles

Cytoplasm contains two centrioles at right angles: each centriole is composed of 9 microtubule triplets in a 9 + 0 array

Functions
Essential for movement of chromosomes during cell division; organization of microtubules in cytoskeleton

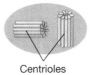

Centrioles

Cytoskeleton

Proteins organized in fine filaments or slender tubes

Microfilament

Functions
Strength and support; movement of cellular structures and materials

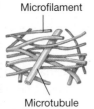

Microtubule

Plasma Membrane

Lipid bilayer containing phospholipids, steroids, proteins, and carbohydrates

Functions
Isolation; protection; sensitivity; support; controls entry and exit of materials

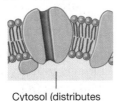

Cytosol (distributes materials by diffusion)

Secretory vesicles

CYTOSOL

NUCLEUS

Free ribosomes

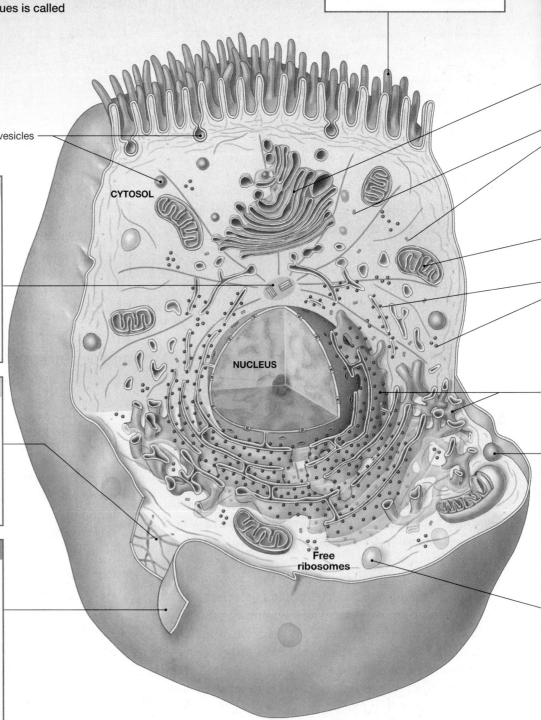

Cilia (not shown in model cell)

Cilia are long extensions of the plasma membrane containing microtubules. There are two types: motile and primary.

Function
Multiple motile cilia move materials over cell surfaces. A solitary primary cilium acts as a sensor.

Proteasomes

Hollow cylinders of proteolytic enzymes with regulatory proteins at their ends

Functions
Breakdown and recycling of damaged or abnormal intracellular proteins

Ribosomes

RNA + proteins; fixed ribosomes bound to rough endoplasmic reticulum, free ribosomes scattered in cytoplasm

Function
Protein synthesis

Peroxisomes

Vesicles containing degradative enzymes

Functions
Catabolism of fatty acids and other organic compounds, neutralization of toxic compounds generated in the process

Lysosomes

Vesicles containing digestive enzymes

Functions
Intracellular removal of damaged organelles or pathogens

Golgi apparatus

Stacks of flattened membranes (cisternae) containing chambers

Functions
Storage, alteration, and packaging of secretory products and lysosomal enzymes

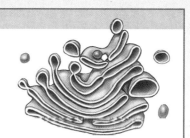

Mitochondria

Double membrane, with inner membrane folds (cristae) enclosing important metabolic enzymes

Functions
Produce 95 percent of the adenosine triphosphate (ATP) required by the cell

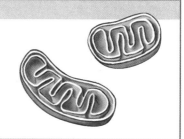

Endoplasmic reticulum (ER)

Network of membranous channels extending throughout the cytoplasm

Functions
Synthesis of secretory products; intracellular storage and transport

Rough ER modifies and packages newly synthesized proteins

Smooth ER synthesizes lipids and carbohydrates

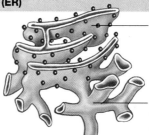

Chromatin

Nuclear envelope

Nucleolus (site of rRNA synthesis and assembly of ribosomal subunits)

NUCLEOPLASM

Nuclear pore

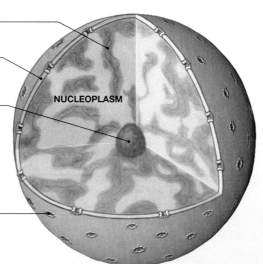

NUCLEUS

Nucleoplasm containing nucleotides, enzymes, nucleoproteins, and chromatin; surrounded by a double membrane, the nuclear envelope

Functions
Control of metabolism; storage and processing of genetic information; control of protein synthesis

3

- ***Structural support.*** Specialized connections between plasma membranes, or between membranes and materials outside the cell, give tissues a stable structure.

The plasma membrane is extremely thin, ranging from 6 to 10 nm in thickness. This membrane contains lipids, proteins, and carbohydrates (**Figure 3-3**).

Membrane Lipids

Phospholipids are a major component of plasma membranes. ⮌ p. 42 In a phospholipid, a phosphate group (PO_4^{3-}) serves as a link between a diglyceride (a glycerol molecule bonded to two fatty acid "tails") and a nonlipid "head."

The phospholipids in a plasma membrane lie in two distinct layers. For this reason, the plasma membrane is called a **phospholipid bilayer** (**Figure 3-3**). In each half of the bilayer, the phospholipids lie with their heads at the membrane surface and their tails on the inside. The heads are soluble in water, or **hydrophilic** (hī-drō-FI-lik; *hydro-*, water + *philos*, loving). The tails are insoluble in water, or **hydrophobic** (hī-drō-FŌB-ik; *hydro-*, + *phobos*, fear). In this arrangement, the hydrophilic heads of the two layers are in contact with watery environments on both sides of the membrane—the extracellular fluid on the outside of the cell and the *intracellular fluid* on the inside of the cell.

The hydrophobic lipid tails will not associate with water or charged molecules. This characteristic enables the plasma membrane to act as a selective physical barrier. Lipid-soluble molecules and compounds such as oxygen and carbon dioxide are able to cross the lipid portion of a plasma membrane, but ions and water-soluble compounds cannot pass. As a result, the plasma membrane isolates the cytoplasm from the surrounding extracellular fluid.

Mixed in with the fatty acid tails are cholesterol molecules and small quantities of other lipids. Cholesterol is present in a ratio of almost one cholesterol molecule for each phospholipid molecule. ⮌ p. 42 Cholesterol "stiffens" the plasma membrane, making it less fluid and less permeable.

Figure 3-3 The Plasma Membrane.

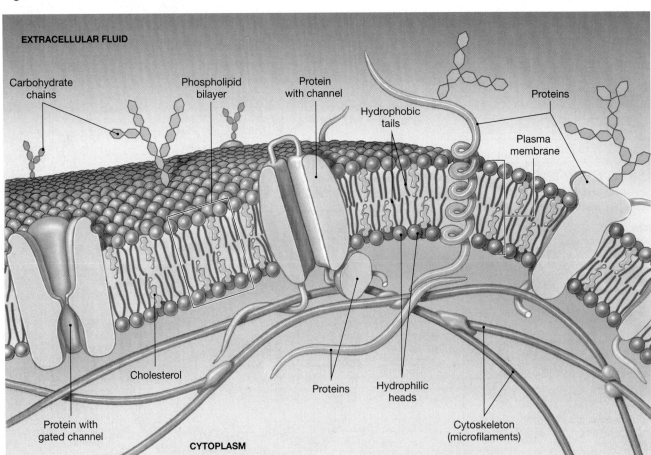

Table 3-1	Types of Membrane Proteins	
Class	Function	Example
Receptor proteins	Sensitive to specific extracellular materials that bind to them and trigger a change in a cell's activity.	Binding of the hormone insulin to membrane receptors increases the rate of glucose absorption by the cell.
Channel proteins	Form a central pore, or channel, that permits water, ions, and other solutes to bypass lipid portion of plasma membrane.	Calcium ion movement through channels is crucial to muscle contraction and the conduction of nerve impulses.
Carrier proteins	Bind and transport solutes across the plasma membrane. This process may or may not require ATP energy.	Carrier proteins bring glucose into the cytoplasm and also transport sodium, potassium, and calcium ions into and out of the cell.
Enzymes	Catalyze reactions in the extracellular fluid or cytosol (intracellular fluid).	Dipeptides are broken down into amino acids by enzymes on the exposed membranes of cells lining the intestinal tract.
Anchoring proteins	Attach the plasma membrane to other structures and stabilize its position.	Inside the cell, anchor proteins bind to the cytoskeleton (network of supporting filaments). Outside the cell, anchor proteins attach the cell to extracellular protein fibers or to another cell.
Recognition proteins (identifiers)	Identify a cell as self or nonself, normal or abnormal, to the immune system.	One group of such recognition proteins is the major histocompatibility complex (MHC) (discussed in Chapter 14: The Lymphatic System and Immunity).

Membrane Proteins

Several types of proteins are associated with the plasma membrane. The most common of these membrane proteins span the width of the membrane one or more times and are known as *transmembrane proteins*. Other membrane proteins are either partially embedded in the membrane's phospholipid bilayer or loosely bound to its inner or outer surface. Membrane proteins may function as *receptors, channels, carriers, enzymes, anchors*, or *identifiers*. **Table 3-1** provides a functional description and an example of each class of membrane protein.

Plasma membranes are not rigid, and their inner and outer surfaces differ in structure. Some embedded proteins always remain in specific areas of the membrane, but others drift from place to place along its surface like ice cubes in a punch bowl. In addition, the composition of the plasma membrane can change over time, as components of the membrane are added or removed.

Membrane Carbohydrates

Carbohydrates join with proteins and lipids to form complex molecules on the outer surface of the membrane. These complex molecules are known as *glycoproteins* and *glycolipids*. The carbohydrate portions function as cell lubricants and adhesives and act as receptors for compounds outside the cell. They also form part of a recognition system that keeps the immune system from attacking the body's own cells and tissues.

CHECKPOINT

3. List the general functions of the plasma membrane.

4. Which component of the plasma membrane is primarily responsible for forming a physical barrier between the cell's internal and external environments?

5. Which functional class of membrane proteins allows water and small ions to cross the plasma membrane?

See the blue Answers tab at the back of the book.

3-3 Diffusion is a passive transport process that assists membrane passage

Learning Objective Describe the processes of cellular diffusion and osmosis, and explain their physiological roles.

Permeability refers to the ease with which substances can cross a membrane. It is the property of the plasma membrane that determines precisely which substances can enter or leave the cytoplasm. If nothing can cross a membrane, it is described as **impermeable**. If any substance can cross without difficulty, the membrane is **freely permeable**. Plasma membranes are **selectively permeable**, permitting the free passage of some materials and restricting the passage of others. Whether or not a substance can cross the plasma membrane is based on the substance's size, electrical charge, molecular shape, lipid solubility, or some combination of these factors.

Movement across the membrane may be passive or active. **Passive processes** move ions or molecules across the plasma

3

membrane without any energy expenditure by the cell. **Active processes** require that the cell expend energy, generally from adenosine triphosphate (ATP). ⮌ p. 48

In this section, we consider the passive process of *diffusion*, including a special type of diffusion called *osmosis*. In the next section, we will examine some types of *carrier-mediated transport*, which includes both active and passive processes. We will consider *facilitated diffusion*, a passive carrier-mediated process, and *active transport*, an active carrier-mediated process. Finally, we will examine two active processes involving *vesicular transport*: endocytosis and exocytosis.

Diffusion

Ions and molecules are in constant motion, randomly colliding and bouncing off one another and off obstacles in their paths. Over time, one result of this motion is that the molecules in a given space tend to become evenly distributed, or spread out. **Diffusion** is the movement of molecules from an area of relatively high concentration (of many collisions) to an area of relatively low concentration (of fewer collisions). The difference between the high and low concentrations represents a **concentration gradient**. Diffusion is often described as proceeding "down a concentration gradient" or "downhill." As a result of diffusion, molecules eventually become uniformly distributed, and concentration gradients are eliminated.

Diffusion in air and water is slow. It is most important over very short distances. A simple, everyday example can give you a mental image of how diffusion works. Think about a colored sugar cube dropped into a beaker of water (**Figure 3-4**). As the cube dissolves, its sugar and dye molecules set up a steep concentration gradient with the surrounding clear water. Eventually, dissolved molecules of both types spread through the water until they are distributed evenly. (However, compared to a cell, a beaker of water is enormous. Additional factors—which we will ignore—account for dye and sugar distribution over distances of centimeters as opposed to micrometers.)

Diffusion is important in body fluids because it tends to eliminate local concentration gradients. For example, every cell in your body generates carbon dioxide, and its intracellular (within the cell) concentration is relatively high. Carbon dioxide concentrations are lower in the surrounding extracellular fluid, and lower still in the circulating blood. Plasma membranes are freely permeable to carbon dioxide. As a result, carbon dioxide diffuses down its concentration gradient, traveling from the cell's interior into the surrounding interstitial fluid, and then into the bloodstream, for delivery to the lungs.

Diffusion across Plasma Membranes

In extracellular fluids of the body, water and dissolved solutes diffuse freely. A plasma membrane, however, acts as a barrier that selectively restricts diffusion. Some substances

Figure 3-4 Diffusion.

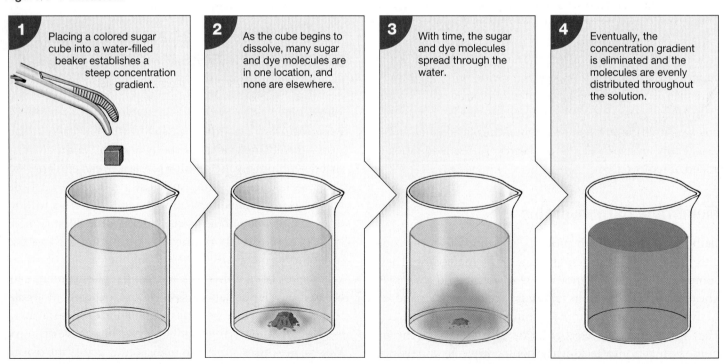

1 Placing a colored sugar cube into a water-filled beaker establishes a steep concentration gradient.

2 As the cube begins to dissolve, many sugar and dye molecules are in one location, and none are elsewhere.

3 With time, the sugar and dye molecules spread through the water.

4 Eventually, the concentration gradient is eliminated and the molecules are evenly distributed throughout the solution.

Figure 3-5 Diffusion across the Plasma Membrane. The way a substance crosses a plasma membrane depends on the substance's size and lipid solubility.

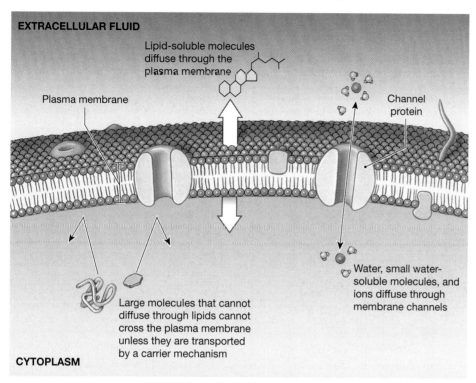

intracellular and extracellular fluids are solutions that contain a variety of dissolved materials, or **solutes**. ⊃ p. 35 Each solute tends to diffuse as if it were the only substance in solution. Thus, changes in the concentration of potassium ions, for example, have no effect on the rate or direction of sodium ion diffusion. Some ions and molecules (solutes) diffuse into the cytoplasm, others diffuse out, and a few, such as proteins, are unable to diffuse across a plasma membrane. Yet if we ignore the individual identities and simply count ions and molecules, we find that the total concentration of ions and molecules on either side of the plasma membrane stays the same.

Why does this state of solute equilibrium persist? The reason is because *the plasma membrane is freely permeable to water*. Whenever a solute concentration gradient exists across a plasma membrane, a concentration gradient for water exists also. Dissolved solute molecules occupy space that would otherwise be taken up by water molecules, so the higher the solute concentration, the lower the water concentration. As a result, *water molecules tend to flow across a membrane toward the solution containing the higher solute concentration*. This movement is down the concentration gradient for water molecules. Water will move until water concentrations—and thus, solute concentrations—are the same on either side of the membrane.

Three characteristics of osmosis are important to remember:

1. Osmosis is the diffusion of water molecules across a selectively permeable membrane.

2. Osmosis takes place across a selectively permeable membrane that is freely permeable to water but is not freely permeable to solutes.

3. In osmosis, water flows across a selectively permeable membrane toward the solution that has the higher concentration of solutes, because that is where the concentration of water is lower.

OSMOSIS AND OSMOTIC PRESSURE. **Figure 3-6** diagrams the process of osmosis: ❶ shows two solutions (A and B), with different solute concentrations, separated by a selectively permeable membrane. As osmosis takes place, water molecules cross the membrane until the solute concentrations in the two solutions are identical ❷. Thus, the volume of solution B increases

can pass through easily, but others cannot penetrate the membrane at all. An ion or molecule can independently diffuse across a plasma membrane only by (1) crossing the lipid portion of the membrane or (2) passing through a channel protein in the membrane. For this reason, the primary factors determining whether a substance can diffuse across a plasma membrane are its lipid solubility and its size relative to the sizes of membrane channels (**Figure 3-5**).

Alcohol, fatty acids, and steroids can enter cells easily because they can diffuse through the lipid portions of the membrane. Lipid-soluble drugs and dissolved gases such as oxygen and carbon dioxide also enter and leave cells by diffusing through the phospholipid bilayer.

Ions and most water-soluble compounds are not lipid soluble, so they must pass through membrane channels to enter the cytoplasm. These channels are very small, about 0.8 nm in diameter. Water molecules can enter or exit these channels freely, as can ions such as sodium and potassium. Water molecules may also enter or leave the cytoplasm through water channels called *aquaporins*. However, even a small organic molecule, such as glucose, is too big to fit through the channels.

Osmosis: A Special Case of Diffusion

The diffusion of water across a selectively permeable membrane is called **osmosis** (oz-M-sis; *osmos*, thrust). Both

Figure 3-6 Osmosis. The osmotic flow of water can create osmotic pressure across a selectively permeable membrane. The osmotic pressure of solution B is equal to the amount of hydrostatic pressure required to stop the osmotic flow.

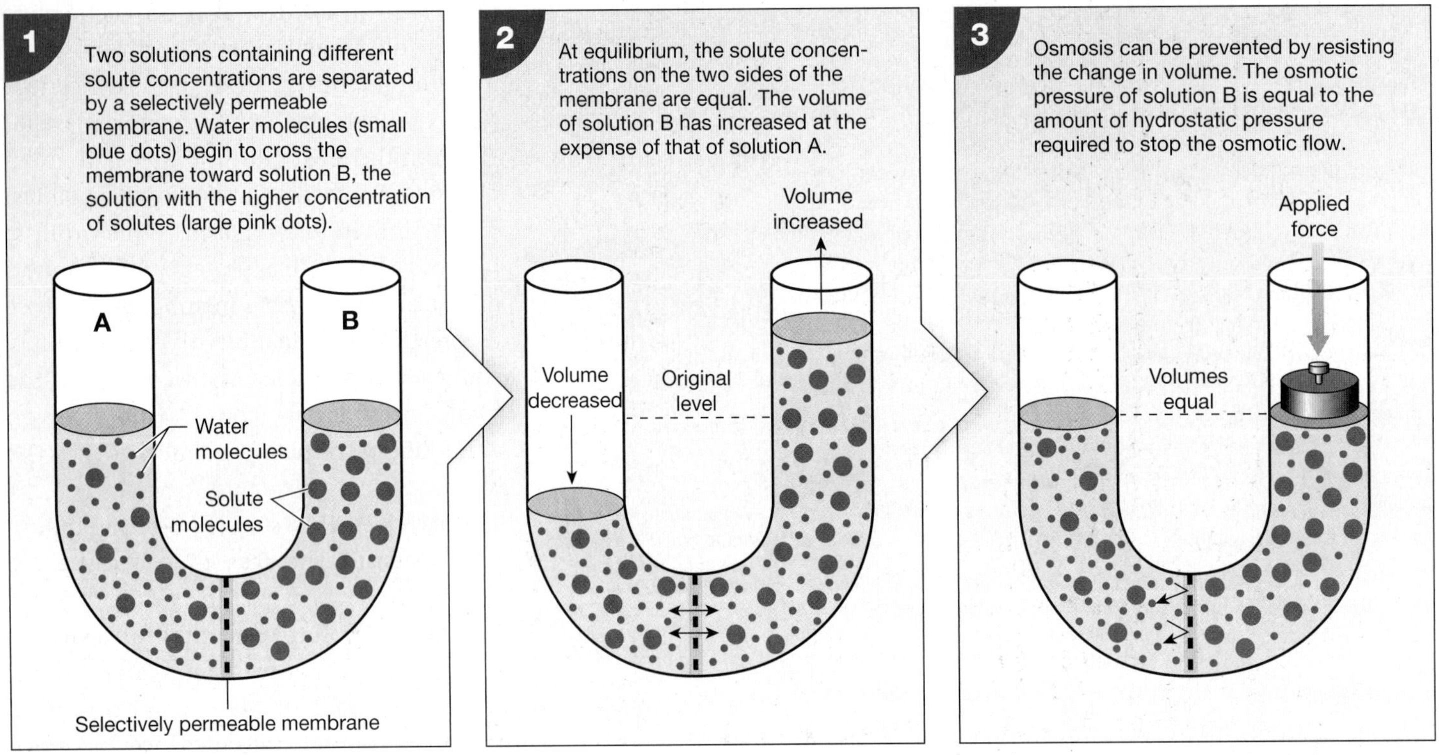
1
Two solutions containing different solute concentrations are separated by a selectively permeable membrane. Water molecules (small blue dots) begin to cross the membrane toward solution B, the solution with the higher concentration of solutes (large pink dots).
A
B
Water molecules
Solute molecules
Selectively permeable membrane
2
At equilibrium, the solute concentrations on the two sides of the membrane are equal. The volume of solution B has increased at the expense of that of solution A.
Volume increased
Volume decreased
Original level
3
Osmosis can be prevented by resisting the change in volume. The osmotic pressure of solution B is equal to the amount of hydrostatic pressure required to stop the osmotic flow.
Applied force
Volumes equal

while that of solution A decreases. The greater the initial difference in solute concentrations, the stronger is the osmotic flow.

The **osmotic pressure** of a solution is an indication of the force of water movement *into that solution* as a result of solute concentration. As the solute concentration of a solution increases, so does its osmotic pressure. Osmotic pressure can be measured in several ways. For example, an opposing pressure can prevent the entry of water molecules. Pushing against a fluid generates *hydrostatic pressure*. In 3, hydrostatic pressure opposes the osmotic pressure of solution B, so no net osmotic flow takes place.

Solutions of various solute concentrations are described as *isotonic, hypotonic*, or *hypertonic* with regard to their effects on the shape or tension of the plasma membrane of living cells. The effects of various osmotic solutions are difficult to see in most tissues, but they are readily seen in red blood cells (RBCs) (**Figure 3-7**).

In an **isotonic** (*iso-*, equal + *tonos*, tension) solution—one that does not cause a net movement of water into or out of the cell—RBCs retain their normal appearance (**Figure 3-7a**). In this case, an equilibrium exists: As one water molecule moves out of the cell, another moves in to replace it.

When an RBC is placed in a **hypotonic** (*hypo-*, below) solution, water will flow into the cell, causing it to swell up like a balloon (**Figure 3-7b**). Eventually the cell may burst, or *lyse*. In the case of RBCs, this event is known as **hemolysis** (*hemo-*, blood + *lysis*, a loosening).

RBCs in a **hypertonic** (*hyper-*, above) solution will lose water by osmosis. As they do, they shrivel and dehydrate. The shrinking of RBCs is called **crenation** (**Figure 3-7c**).

Build Your Knowledge

Recall that water is an excellent solvent (as you saw in **Chapter 2: The Chemical Level of Organization**). This property is due to the polar nature of water molecules. As a result of their polarity, water molecules can surround ions and keep them in solution by preventing ionic bonds from forming. Because of hydrogen bonding, water molecules can also link with many organic molecules containing polar covalent bonds and keep them in solution. ↺ **p. 30** As a solvent that can diffuse through selectively permeable membranes, water also affects the osmotic pressure of living cells. ↺ **p. 35**

CLINICAL NOTE

Fluid Movement

Prehospital personnel must have a good understanding of human cellular function. Many of the fluids and medications used in emergency medicine directly affect the cells. A major component of emergency medical care is monitoring and replacing the various fluids and electrolytes of the body. A decrease in the absolute volume of body fluids is referred to as *dehydration*. An increase in fluid volume is called *overhydration* and can result in edema and heart failure. In addition to fluids, the concentration of essential electrolytes can be disturbed in injury and illness. Optimal body function depends on a normal concentration of body fluids and electrolytes. Because of this, the fluid and electrolyte balance of the body must be maintained within fairly narrow limits. In critical situations, such as shock, the rapid replacement of lost fluids can be life-saving.

Water moves through the various membranes of the body by the process of osmosis (**Figure 3-7**). The rate at which the fluid moves depends upon the differences in the concentration of solutes in the fluid (also called *tonicity*). The total number of particles in a solution is measured in terms of *osmoles*. In general, the osmole is too large a unit for expressing osmotic activity of solutes in the body fluids. Instead, the term *milliOsmole (mOsm)*, which equals 1/1000 osmole, is commonly used. Normal body tonicity is approximately 280–310 milliOsmoles/liter. The terms *osmolality* and *osmolarity* are often used to describe the number of solute particles in a solution. *Osmolality* is the number of osmoles per kilogram of water. Osmolarity is the number of osmoles per liter of solution. In dilute solutions, such as body fluids, these two terms can be used almost synonymously because the differences are small. In practice, osmolarity is used more frequently than *osmolality*.

Sodium, the most abundant ion in the extracellular fluid, is responsible for the osmotic balance of the extracellular fluid compartment. Water follows sodium into the extracellular fluid. Potassium is the most abundant ion in the intracellular fluid compartment. Generally, the osmolarity of intracellular fluid does not change very rapidly. However, when there is a change in the osmolarity of extracellular fluid, water will move from the intracellular to the extracellular compartment, or vice versa, until osmotic equilibrium is regained.

Within the extracellular compartment, movement of water between the plasma in the intravascular space and fluid in the interstitial space is primarily a function of forces at play in the capillary beds. In general, the movement of water and solutes across a cell membrane is governed by *osmotic pressure*. Osmotic pressure is the pressure exerted by the concentration of solutes on one side of a semipermeable membrane, such as a cell membrane or the thin wall of a capillary. Osmotic pressure can be thought of as a "pull" rather than a "push" because a hypertonic concentration of solutes tends to pull water from the other side of the membrane.

Generally, there is a "two-way street" as solutes move out of a space while water moves into the space to balance the concentration of solutes on both sides of the membrane. However, a somewhat different osmotic mechanism operates between the plasma inside a capillary and the fluid in the interstitial space outside of the capillary. Blood plasma generates *oncotic force*, which is sometimes called *colloid osmotic pressure*. Plasma proteins are colloids, which are large particles that do not readily move across the capillary membrane. The most abundant of these is the plasma protein *albumin*. Because of their size, colloids tend to remain within the capillary. At the same time, there is usually very little water in the interstitial space. The small amount of water that does get into the interstitial space is usually taken up by the lymphatic system. Therefore, because there is little water outside the capillary and because plasma proteins do not readily move outside of the capillary, the forces governing water's movement between the capillary and the interstitial space are almost all on one side, governed by the plasma on the inside of the capillary.

Another force inside the capillaries is *hydrostatic pressure*, which is the blood pressure, or force against the vessel walls, created by contractions of the heart. Hydrostatic pressure tends to force some water out of the plasma and across the capillary wall into the interstitial space, a process that is called *filtration*. Hydrostatic pressure (a force that favors filtration, and pushes water out of the capillary) and *oncotic force* (a force that opposes filtration, and pulls water into the capillary) together are responsible for *net filtration*, which is described in *Starling's hypothesis*:

Net filtration = (forces that favor filtration)
          − (forces that oppose filtration)

Net filtration in a capillary is normally zero. It works this way: as plasma enters the capillary at the arterial end, hydrostatic pressure forces water to cross the capillary membrane into the interstitial space. This loss of water increases the relative concentration of plasma proteins and hence the colloid osmotic pressure. By the time the plasma reaches the venous end of the capillary, the oncotic force exerted by the increased concentration of plasma proteins is great enough to pull the water from the interstitial space back into the capillary. The outcome is that water is retained in the intravascular space and does not remain in the interstitial space.

In prehospital emergency care, the exact concentration of fluid and electrolytes is not known. Because of this, intravenous (IV) replacement fluids whose fluid and electrolyte concentrations are similar to those of the body are used initially. Later, when the patient's fluid and electrolyte status is known, IV fluids that will correct any detected underlying fluid and electrolyte problems are administered.

Figure 3-7 Osmotic Flow across a Plasma Membrane. The smaller paired arrows indicate an equilibrium and no net water movement. The larger arrows indicate the direction of osmotic water movement.

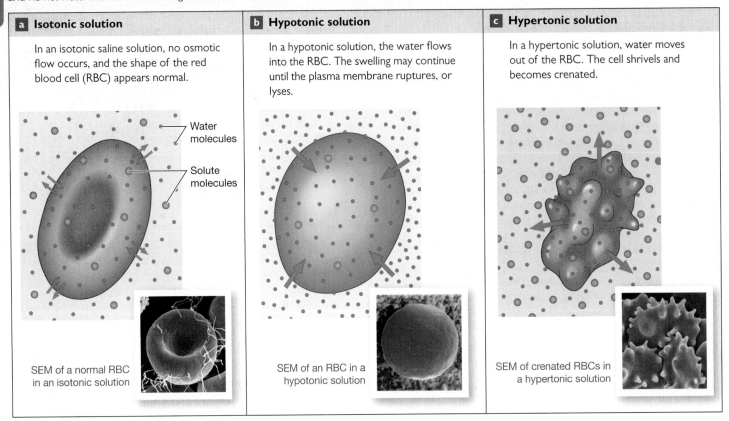

a Isotonic solution

In an isotonic saline solution, no osmotic flow occurs, and the shape of the red blood cell (RBC) appears normal.

Water molecules

Solute molecules

SEM of a normal RBC in an isotonic solution

b Hypotonic solution

In a hypotonic solution, the water flows into the RBC. The swelling may continue until the plasma membrane ruptures, or lyses.

SEM of an RBC in a hypotonic solution

c Hypertonic solution

In a hypertonic solution, water moves out of the RBC. The cell shrivels and becomes crenated.

SEM of crenated RBCs in a hypertonic solution

It is often necessary to give patients large volumes of fluid after severe blood loss or dehydration. One fluid frequently administered is a 0.9 percent (0.9 g/dL) solution of sodium chloride. This solution approximates the normal *osmotic concentration* (total solute concentration) of extracellular fluids and is called *normal saline*. It is used because sodium and chloride are the most abundant ions in the body's extracellular fluid. Little net movement of either type of ion occurs across plasma membranes, so normal saline is essentially isotonic with respect to body cells.

CHECKPOINT

6. What is meant by "selectively permeable," when referring to a plasma membrane?

7. Define diffusion.

8. How would a decrease in the concentration of oxygen in the lungs affect the diffusion of oxygen into the blood?

9. Define osmosis.

10. Relative to a surrounding hypertonic solution, the cytosol of a red blood cell is _____.

See the blue Answers tab at the back of the book.

3-4 Carrier-mediated and vesicular transport processes assist membrane passage

Learning Objective Describe carrier-mediated transport and vesicular transport processes used by cells to absorb or remove specific substances.

Besides diffusion, substances are brought into or removed from cells in two additional ways. *Carrier-mediated transport* uses specialized membrane proteins. It can be passive or active, depending on the substance being moved and the nature of the transport process. *Vesicular transport* involves the movement of materials within small membrane-enclosed sacs, or *vesicles*. Vesicular transport is always an active process.

Carrier-Mediated Transport

In **carrier-mediated transport**, membrane proteins bind specific ions or organic substrates and carry them across the plasma membrane. These proteins share several characteristics with enzymes. They may be used repeatedly, and they can only bind to specific substrates. For example, the carrier protein that transports glucose will not carry other simple sugars.

Carrier-mediated transport can be passive (no ATP required) or active (ATP dependent). In *passive transport*, solutes are typically carried from an area of high concentration to an area of low concentration. *Active transport* may follow or oppose an existing concentration gradient.

Many carrier proteins transport one ion or molecule at a time, but some move two solutes simultaneously. In *cotransport*, the carrier transports the two substances in the same direction, either into or out of the cell. In *countertransport*, one substance is moved into the cell while the other is moved out. Next, we discuss two major examples of carrier-mediated transport—*facilitated diffusion* and *active transport*.

Facilitated Diffusion

Many essential nutrients, including glucose and amino acids, are insoluble in lipids and too large to fit through membrane channels. However, these compounds can be passively transported across the membrane by carrier proteins in a process called **facilitated diffusion** (Figure 3-8). First, the molecule to be transported binds to a **receptor site** on the carrier protein. The shape of the protein then changes, moving the molecule across the plasma membrane and releasing it into the cytoplasm. This process takes place without ever creating a continuous open channel between the cell's exterior and interior.

Just as in the process of diffusion across a plasma membrane, no ATP is expended in facilitated diffusion. In each case, molecules move from an area of higher concentration to one of lower concentration. However, facilitated diffusion

Figure 3-8 Facilitated Diffusion. In this process, an extracellular molecule, such as glucose, binds to a specific receptor site on a carrier protein. This binding permits the molecule to diffuse across the plasma membrane.

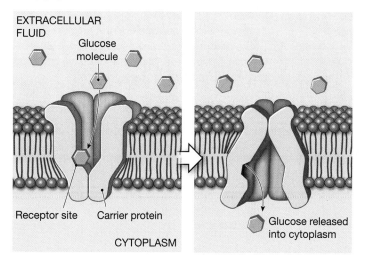

EXTRACELLULAR FLUID

Glucose molecule

Receptor site   Carrier protein

CYTOPLASM

Glucose released into cytoplasm

Build Your Knowledge

Recall that cations are atoms that have lost an electron and so have a positive electrical charge (as you saw in **Chapter 2: The Chemical Level of Organization**). Atoms that have gained electrons have a negative electrical charge and are called anions. ⮌ **p. 28**

also differs from simple diffusion. The rate of transport cannot increase indefinitely. The reason is that only a limited number of carrier proteins are available in the membrane. Once all of them are operating, any further increase in the solute concentration in the extracellular fluid will have no effect on the rate of movement into the cell.

Active Transport

In **active transport**, the high-energy bond in ATP provides the energy needed to move ions or molecules across the membrane. Despite the energy cost, active transport offers one great advantage: It is not dependent on a concentration gradient. This means that the cell can import or export specific materials *regardless of their intracellular or extracellular concentrations*.

All cells contain carrier proteins called **ion pumps** that actively transport the cations sodium (Na^+), potassium (K^+), calcium (Ca^{2+}), and magnesium (Mg^{2+}) across plasma membranes. Specialized cells have carrier proteins that can transport other ions, including iodide (I^-), chloride (Cl^-), and iron (Fe^{2+}). Many of these carrier proteins move a specific cation or anion in one direction only, either into or out of the cell. In a few cases, one carrier protein will move more than one ion at a time. The carrier protein is called an **exchange pump** if one kind of ion is moved in one direction and the other is moved in the opposite direction (countertransport).

A major function of exchange pumps is to maintain cell homeostasis. Sodium and potassium ions are the principal cations in body fluids. Sodium ion concentrations are high in the extracellular fluids but low in the cytoplasm. The distribution of potassium in the body is just the opposite—low in the extracellular fluids and high in the cytoplasm. Because of the presence of channel proteins in the membrane that are always open (so-called *leak channels*), sodium ions slowly diffuse into the cell, and potassium ions diffuse out.

Homeostasis within the cell depends on maintaining sodium and potassium ion concentration gradients with the extracellular fluid. The **sodium–potassium exchange pump** maintains these gradients by ejecting sodium ions

CLINICAL NOTE

IV Fluid Therapy

IV fluid therapy is the introduction of fluids and other substances into the venous side of the circulatory system. An important part of emergency care, it is used to replace blood lost through hemorrhage, to replace electrolytes or fluids, and to introduce medications directly into the vascular system.

Numerous types of IV fluids are available, each designed to treat a particular type of fluid and electrolyte imbalance. The two primary reasons for starting an IV in the emergency setting are (1) fluid volume replacement, and (2) IV access for drug administration. The following is a discussion of common IV fluids and their physiological actions after they enter the body.

IV Fluids

IV fluids are chemically prepared, sterile solutions tailored to the body's specific needs. They replace the body's lost fluids or aid in the delivery of IV medications. They also keep a vein patent when no fluid or drug therapy is required. IV fluids are supplied in four different forms: crystalloids, colloids, blood, and oxygen-carrying fluids.

Crystalloids

Crystalloids, the most commonly used IV fluid type in emergency medicine, contain water and electrolytes. They are classified based upon their tonicity and their relation to the tonicity of the body. **Table 3-2** illustrates the electrolyte concentration and tonicity of common IV crystalloids. Note that the tonicity of the fluids is measured in terms of osmolarity (reflected as milliOsmoles per liter). Classes of crystalloids include:

- *Isotonic solutions.* Isotonic solutions have a tonicity equal to that of blood plasma. In a normally hydrated patient, they will not cause any significant fluid or electrolyte shift.
- *Hypertonic solutions.* Hypertonic solutions have a higher solute concentration than do the body's cells. When administered to a normally hydrated patient, they cause a fluid shift from the intracellular compartment into the extracellular compartment. Later, solutes will diffuse in the opposite direction.
- *Hypotonic solutions.* Hypotonic solutions have a lower solute concentration than do the body's cells. When administered to a normally hydrated patient, they cause a fluid shift from the extracellular compartment into the intracellular compartment. Later, solutes will diffuse in the opposite direction.

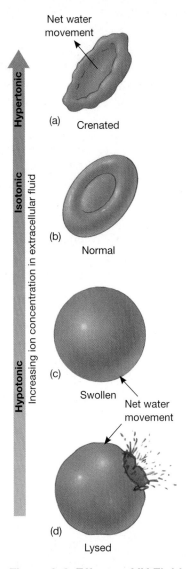

Figure 3-9 Effects of IV Fluids on Circulating Red Blood Cells (Erythrocytes). Hypertonic fluids cause cell shrinkage (crenation), while hypotonic fluids cause intracellular swelling that eventually leads to cell lysis.

The type of IV fluid used depends upon the patient's needs. In the prehospital setting, isotonic fluids are usually used, because the patient's underlying electrolyte and hydration status is unknown (**Figure 3-9**). However, once the patient arrives in the emergency department, blood electrolyte studies are used to guide fluid selection and administration. The IV fluids most frequently used in prehospital care include:

- *Lactated Ringer's.* Lactated Ringer's solution is an isotonic electrolyte solution that contains sodium chloride, potassium chloride, calcium chloride, and sodium lactate in water.
- *Normal saline.* Normal saline is an isotonic electrolyte solution that contains sodium chloride in water.
- *5 percent dextrose in water (D5W).* D_5W is a hypotonic glucose solution used to keep a vein patent and to dilute concentrated medications. While D_5W initially increases intravascular volume, glucose molecules rapidly diffuse across the vascular membrane and increase the amount of free water.

Both lactated Ringer's and normal saline are used for fluid replacement because of their immediate ability to expand the circulating fluid volume. However, due to the movement of electrolytes and water, two-thirds of either solution will be lost to the extravascular space within one hour.

Dextrose-Containing Solutions

Several IV fluids contain dextrose (d-glucose) in varying concentrations. The most commonly used of these are 50 percent dextrose ($D_{50}W$) and D_5W. Other dextrose solutions include 25 percent dextrose ($D_{25}W$) and 10 percent dextrose and water ($D_{10}W$). Some dextrose-containing solutions will also contain electrolytes, usually sodium and chloride. Examples of these include:

- 2.5 percent dextrose and 0.45 percent sodium chloride ($D_{2.5}NS$)
- 5 percent dextrose and 0.20 percent sodium chloride (D_5NS)
- 5 percent dextrose and 0.33 percent sodium chloride (D_5NS)
- 5 percent dextrose and 0.45 percent sodium chloride (D_5NS)
- 5 percent dextrose and 0.9 percent sodium chloride (D_5NS)
- 10 percent dextrose and 0.9 percent sodium chloride ($D_{10}NS$)
- 5 percent dextrose in lactated Ringer's (D_5LR)

Table 3-2	Contents and Characteristics of Common Emergency IV Fluids							
	Approximate Ionic Concentrations (mEq/L) and Calories per Liter							
	Ionic Concentrations (mEq/L)							
	Sodium	Potassium	Calcium	Chloride	Lactate	Calories Per Liter	Osmolarity[a] (mOsm/L)	pH Range[b]
Dextrose Injection, USP	0	0	0	0	0	170	252	3.5–6.5
10% Dextrose Injection, USP	0	0	0	0	0	340	505	3.5–6.5
0.9% Sodium Chloride Injection, USP	154	0	0	154	0	0	308	4.5–7.0
Sodium Lactate Injection, USP (M/6 Sodium Lactate)	167	0	0	0	167	54	334	6.0–7.3
2.5% Dextrose and 0.45% Sodium Chloride Injection, USP	77	0	0	77	0	85	280	3.5–6.0
5% Dextrose and 0.2% Sodium Chloride Injection, USP	34	0	0	34	0	170	321	3.5–6.0
5% Dextrose and 0.33% Sodium Chloride Injection, USP	56	0	0	56	0	170	365	3.5–6.0
5% Dextrose and 0.45% Sodium Chloride Injection, USP	77	0	0	77	0	170	406	3.5–6.0
5% Dextrose and 0.9% Sodium Chloride Injection, USP	154	0	0	154	0	170	560	3.5–6.0
10% Dextrose and 0.9% Sodium Chloride Injection, USP	154	0	0	154	0	340	813	3.5–6.0
Ringer's Injection, USP	147.5	4	4.5	156	0	0	309	5.0–7.5
Lactated Ringer's Injection	130	4	3	109	28	9	273	6.0–7.5
5% Dextrose in Ringer's Injection	147.5	4	4.5	156	0	170	561	3.5–6.5
Lactated Ringer's with 5% Dextrose	130	4	3	109	28	180	525	4.0–6.5

[a]Normal physiological isotonicity range is approximately 280–310 mOsm/L. Administration of substantially hypotonic solutions may cause hemolysis, and administration of substantially hypertonic solutions may cause vein damage.
[b]pH ranges are USP for applicable solution, corporate specification for non-USP solutions.

The high-concentration solutions, such as D$_{50}$W and D$_{25}$W, are used for glucose replacement in documented hypoglycemia. D$_{10}$W is used in patients such as chronic alcoholics who require calorie replacement in addition to water and electrolytes. D$_5$W and similar solutions are usually used for diluting IV medications and for conditions where an IV is started at a "to keep open" (TKO) or "keep vein open" (KVO) rate.

The solubility of dextrose is 1 gram per milliliter of water. Based on this property, dextrose-containing solutions are usually measured in weight-in-volume percentages. This system of measurement indicates the number of grams of dextrose in 100 mL of solution (water). A fully saturated solution contains 100 grams of dextrose per 100 mL of water and is considered a 100 percent solution (D$_{100}$W). D$_{50}$W, commonly used in prehospital care, contains 25 grams of glucose in 50 mL of water. Likewise, D$_{25}$W contains 12.5 grams of glucose in 50 mL of water. D$_{25}$W is preferred over D$_{50}$W when administering IV dextrose to infants and children. D$_{25}$W can be prepared by diluting 25 mL of D$_{50}$W with 25 mL of

sterile water for injection. This results in a solution that contains 12.5 grams of dextrose in 50 mL of water.

When considering glucose content, it is best to consider the amount of dextrose per milliliter of water. With a 50 percent dextrose solution, 1 mL of solution contains 0.5 grams of dextrose. Likewise, in a 25 percent dextrose solution, 1 mL of solution contains 0.25 grams of dextrose. A 100 percent dextrose solution would contain 1 g/mL. A solution of 5 percent dextrose in water contains 0.05 grams of dextrose per milliliter.

Most IV fluids contain 5 percent dextrose in water or an electrolyte solution. When administered at a TKO or KVO rate, the amount of dextrose delivered to the patient is negligible. However, if IV solutions that contain 5 percent dextrose are used for volume replacement, then the amount of dextrose administered can be potentially dangerous for the patient. A 1000 mL bag of D$_5$W contains 50 grams of dextrose. This is equivalent to two prefilled syringes of D$_{50}$W. In multiple trauma, it is not

(Continued)

uncommon to administer 2–3 liters of IV fluid in the prehospital setting. If D_5W were used, this would constitute a very high dextrose load. Infants and children are at increased risk of accidental overdose with dextrose. In documented hypoglycemia, the standard dose of dextrose is 0.5 grams per kilogram of body weight. A child who weighs 10 kilograms, for example, would receive 5 grams of dextrose for documented hypoglycemia (10 mL of $D_{50}W$ or 20 mL of $D_{25}W$). The amount of IV fluid administered to children who are dehydrated or in shock is 20 mL/kg of an isotonic crystalloid solution such as normal saline or lactated Ringer's. If D_5W were used by accident, 20 mL of fluid would provide 1 gram of dextrose per kilogram body weight. This is twice the recommended dose for documented hypoglycemia. Avoid using dextrose-containing solutions for any situation where volume replacement must be provided.

Colloids

Colloid solutions contain large proteins that cannot pass through the capillary membrane. Consequently, they remain in the intravascular compartment for a period of time. In addition, colloids have osmotic properties that attract water into the intravascular compartment. Thus, a small quantity of colloid can significantly increase intravascular volume. Common colloids include:

- *Plasma protein fraction (Plasmanate)*. Plasmanate is a protein-containing colloid solution. Its principle protein, albumin, is suspended in a saline solvent.

- *Salt-poor albumin*. Salt-poor albumin contains only human albumin. Each gram of albumin will retain approximately 18 mL of water in the intravascular space.

- *Dextran*. Dextran is not a protein but a large sugar molecule with osmotic properties similar to albumins. It is supplied in two molecular weights: 40,000 and 70,000 Daltons. Dextran 40 has from two to two and a half times the colloidal osmotic pressure of albumin.

- *Hetastarch (Hespan)*. Like dextran, hetastarch is a sugar molecule with osmotic properties similar to those of proteins such as albumin.

Although colloids help to maintain intravascular volume, their use in the field is impractical. Their high cost, short shelf life, and specific storage requirements make them better suited to the hospital setting.

Blood

The most desirable fluid for replacement is whole blood. Unlike colloids and crystalloids, the hemoglobin available in blood carries oxygen. Blood, however, is a precious commodity and must be conserved so that it can be of benefit to the most people. Its use in the field is usually limited to aeromedical operations or mass-casualty incidents. O-negative blood does not contain any antigenic proteins and is thus considered the "universal donor" type.

Figure 3-10 The Sodium–Potassium Exchange Pump. The operation of the sodium–potassium exchange pump is an example of active transport. For each ATP converted to ADP, this carrier protein pump carries three Na^+ out of the cell and two K^+ into the cell.

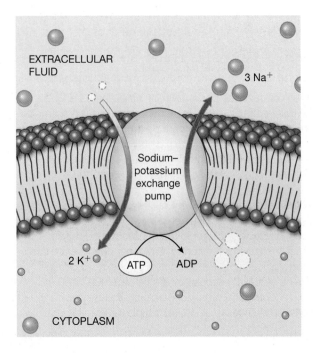

and recapturing lost potassium ions (**Figure 3-10**). For each ATP molecule consumed, the pump ejects three sodium ions and recaptures two potassium ions. The energy demands are impressive: The sodium–potassium exchange pump may use up to 40 percent of the ATP produced by a resting cell!

Vesicular Transport

In **vesicular transport**, materials move into or out of the cell in vesicles, small membrane-enclosed sacs that form at, or fuse with, the plasma membrane. The two major kinds of vesicular transport are *endocytosis* and *exocytosis*.

Endocytosis

The process called **endocytosis** (EN-dō-sī-TŌ-sis; *endo-*, inside + *cyte*, cell) is the packaging of extracellular materials in a vesicle at the cell surface for import *into* the cell. Relatively large volumes of extracellular material may be involved. There are three major types of endocytosis: *receptor-mediated endocytosis, pinocytosis*, and *phagocytosis*. All three are active processes that require ATP or other sources of energy.

- **Receptor-mediated endocytosis** produces vesicles containing a specific target molecule in high concentrations. Receptor-mediated endocytosis begins when molecules

Figure 3-11 Receptor-Mediated Endocytosis.

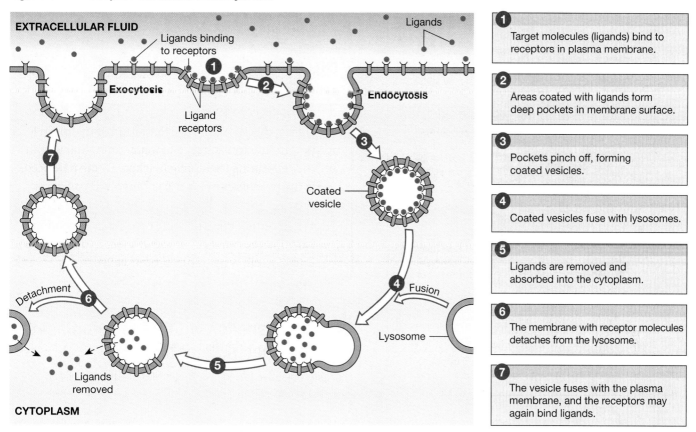

1 Target molecules (ligands) bind to receptors in plasma membrane.

2 Areas coated with ligands form deep pockets in membrane surface.

3 Pockets pinch off, forming coated vesicles.

4 Coated vesicles fuse with lysosomes.

5 Ligands are removed and absorbed into the cytoplasm.

6 The membrane with receptor molecules detaches from the lysosome.

7 The vesicle fuses with the plasma membrane, and the receptors may again bind ligands.

in the extracellular fluid bind to receptors on the plasma membrane surface (**Figure 3-11**). The receptors bind to specific target molecules, called **ligands** (LĪ-gandz), such as a transport protein (described below) or hormone, and then cluster together on the plasma membrane. The area of the membrane with the bound receptors pinches off to form a vesicle. This vesicle is surrounded by the cytoplasmic surface of the plasma membrane and is called a *coated vesicle*.

Many important substances, such as cholesterol and iron ions (Fe^{2+}), are carried throughout the body attached to special transport proteins. These transport proteins are too large to pass through membrane channels but can enter cells through receptor-mediated endocytosis.

- **Pinocytosis** (pi-nō-sī-TŌ-sis; *pinein*, to drink), or "cell drinking," is the formation of small vesicles filled with extracellular fluid. This process is common to most cells. A deep groove or pocket forms in the plasma membrane and then pinches off. No receptor proteins are involved. For this reason, pinocytosis is not as selective a process as receptor-mediated endocytosis.

- **Phagocytosis** (FAG-ō-sī-TŌ-sis; *phagein*, to eat), or "cell eating," produces vesicles containing solid objects that

may be as large as the cell itself (**Figure 3-12**). Cytoplasmic extensions called **pseudopodia** (soo-dō-PŌ-dē-ah; *pseudo-*, false + *podon*, foot) surround the object, and their membranes fuse to form a vesicle. This vesicle then fuses with many *lysosomes*. The vesicle contents are broken down by the lysosomal digestive enzymes.

Most cells carry out pinocytosis, but phagocytosis is performed only by specialized cells that protect tissues by engulfing bacteria, cell debris, and other abnormal materials. (We will consider phagocytic cells in chapters dealing with blood cells [Chapter 11] and the immune response [Chapter 14].)

Exocytosis

The process called **exocytosis** (ek-sō-sī-TŌ-sis; *exo-*, outside) is the functional reverse of endocytosis. In exocytosis, a vesicle created inside the cell fuses with the plasma membrane and discharges its contents into the extracellular environment. The ejected material may be secretory products such as a *hormone* (a compound that circulates in the blood and affects cells in other parts of the body) or mucus components, or waste products from the recycling of damaged organelles.

Figure 3-12 Phagocytosis.

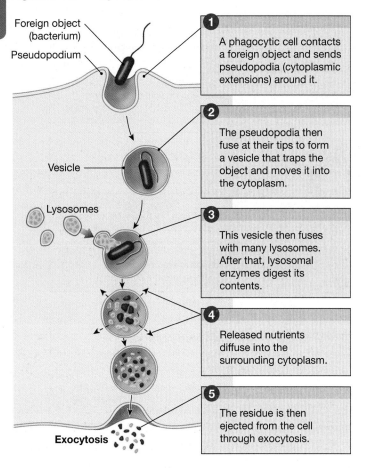

Foreign object (bacterium)

Pseudopodium

1 A phagocytic cell contacts a foreign object and sends pseudopodia (cytoplasmic extensions) around it.

2 The pseudopodia then fuse at their tips to form a vesicle that traps the object and moves it into the cytoplasm.

Vesicle

Lysosomes

3 This vesicle then fuses with many lysosomes. After that, lysosomal enzymes digest its contents.

4 Released nutrients diffuse into the surrounding cytoplasm.

5 The residue is then ejected from the cell through exocytosis.

Exocytosis

At any given moment, various transport processes are moving materials into and out of the cell. These processes are summarized in **Table 3-3**.

CHECKPOINT

11. What is the difference between active and passive transport processes?

12. During digestion, the concentration of hydrogen ions (H^+) in the stomach rises to many times that within the cells lining the stomach, where H^+ are produced. Is the type of transport process involved passive or active?

13. When certain types of white blood cells encounter bacteria, they are able to engulf them and bring them into the cell. What is this process called?

See the blue Answers tab at the back of the book.

3-5 Organelles within the cytoplasm perform specific functions

Learning Objective Describe the organelles of a typical cell and indicate their specific functions.

Cytoplasm is a general term for the material between the plasma membrane and the membrane that surrounds the nucleus. The cytoplasm contains cytosol and organelles.

Table 3-3	A Summary of Passive and Active Membrane Transport Processes		
Process	**Description**	**Factors Affecting Rate of Movement**	**Substances Involved**
Diffusion	Passive molecular movement of solutes; direction determined by relative concentrations	Steepness of concentration gradient, molecular size, electric charge, lipid solubility, temperature, and presence of channel proteins	Small inorganic ions: most gases and lipid-soluble materials (all cells)
Osmosis	Passive movement of water molecules toward solution containing a relatively higher solute concentration across a selectively permeable membrane	Concentration gradient, opposing osmotic or hydrostatic pressure	Water only (all cells)
Carrier-mediated Transport			
Facilitated diffusion	Passive: carrier proteins passively transport solutes down a concentration gradient	Steepness of gradient, temperature, and availability of carrier proteins	Glucose and amino acids (all cells)
Active transport	Active: carrier proteins actively transport solutes regardless of any concentration gradients	Availability of carrier proteins, substrate, and ATP	Na^+, K^+, Ca^{2+}, Mg^{2+} (all cells); other solutes by specialized cells
Vesicular Transport			
Endocytosis	Active: formation of vesicles containing extracellular fluid or solid material	Type depends on substance being moved into cell; requires ATP	Fluids, nutrients (all cells); debris, pathogens (specialized cells)
Exocytosis	Active: fusion of intracellular vesicles with plasma membrane to release fluids and/or solids from the cell	Type depends on substance being carried; requires ATP	Fluids, debris (all cells)

The Cytosol

The **cytosol**, or *intracellular fluid*, contains dissolved nutrients, ions, soluble and insoluble proteins, and waste products. The most important differences between the cytosol and the extracellular fluid that surrounds most of the cells in the body are as follows:

- **Potassium and sodium ions.** The concentration of potassium ions is higher in the cytosol than in the extracellular fluid. Conversely, the concentration of sodium ions is much lower in the cytosol than in the extracellular fluid.

- **Proteins.** The cytosol contains a higher concentration of suspended proteins than does the extracellular fluid. Many of the proteins are enzymes that regulate metabolic operations. Others are associated with various structures within the cell. These proteins give the cytosol a consistency that varies between that of thin maple syrup and almost-set gelatin.

- **Carbohydrates, amino acids, and lipids.** The cytosol usually contains small quantities of carbohydrates and small reserves of amino acids and lipids. The extracellular fluid is a transport medium only, and no amino acids or lipids are stored there. The carbohydrates are broken down to provide energy, and the amino acids are used to manufacture proteins. The lipids are used primarily as an energy source when carbohydrates are unavailable.

The cytosol may also contain insoluble materials known as **inclusions**. Examples include stored nutrients (such as glycogen granules in muscle and liver cells) and lipid droplets (in fat cells).

The Organelles

Organelles (or-gan-ELZ; "little organs") are internal structures that perform specific functions essential to normal cell structure, maintenance, and metabolism (see **Spotlight Figure 3-2** on pp. 58–59). Many organelles are membranous (membrane-enclosed). These organelles include the *nucleus, mitochondria, endoplasmic reticulum* (ER), *Golgi apparatus, lysosomes,* and *peroxisomes.* The membrane isolates the organelle from the cytosol, so that the organelle can manufacture or store secretions, enzymes, or toxins that might otherwise damage the cell. Nonmembranous organelles include the *cytoskeleton, microvilli, centrioles, cilia, flagella, ribosomes,* and *proteasomes.* Because they are not surrounded by membranes, their parts are in direct contact with the cytosol.

The Cytoskeleton

The **cytoskeleton** serves as the cell's skeleton. It is an internal protein framework of threadlike filaments and hollow tubules that gives the cytoplasm strength and flexibility (**Figure 3-11**). The cytoskeleton of all cells is made of microfilaments, intermediate filaments, and microtubules. Muscle cells contain these cytoskeletal parts plus thick filaments.

MICROFILAMENTS. The thinnest strands of the cytoskeleton are **microfilaments**, which are usually composed of the protein **actin**. In most cells, they form a dense layer just inside the plasma membrane. Microfilaments attach the plasma membrane to the underlying cytoplasm by forming connections with proteins of the plasma membrane. In muscle cells, actin microfilaments interact with **thick filaments**, made of the protein **myosin**, to produce powerful contractions.

INTERMEDIATE FILAMENTS. These cytoskeletal filaments are intermediate in size between microfilaments and the thick filaments of muscle cells. Their protein composition varies among cell types. Intermediate filaments strengthen the cell. They also stabilize its position with respect to surrounding cells through specialized attachments to the plasma membrane. Many cells contain intermediate filaments with unique functions. For example, keratin fibers in the superficial layers of the skin are intermediate filaments that make these layers strong and able to resist stretching.

MICROTUBULES. All body cells contain **microtubules**, hollow tubes built from the globular protein **tubulin**. Microtubules form the primary components of the cytoskeleton, giving the cell strength and rigidity, and anchoring the positions of major organelles. In size, they are the largest components of the cytoskeleton.

During cell division, microtubules form the *spindle apparatus,* which distributes the duplicated chromosomes to opposite ends of the dividing cell. We will consider this process in a later section.

Microvilli

Microvilli are small, finger-shaped projections of the plasma membrane on the exposed surfaces of many cells (**Spotlight Figure 3-2**). An internal core of microfilaments supports the microvilli and connects them to the cytoskeleton (**Figure 3-13**). Microvilli increase the surface area of the membrane. For this reason, they are common features of cells actively engaged in absorbing materials from the extracellular fluid. Examples include the cells of the digestive tract and kidneys.

Figure 3-13 The Cytoskeleton. The cytoskeleton provides strength and structural support for the cell and its organelles. Interactions between cytoskeletal components are also important in moving organelles and changing the shape of the cell.

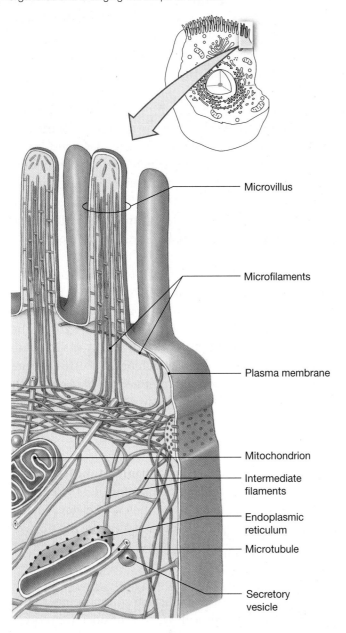

- Microvillus
- Microfilaments
- Plasma membrane
- Mitochondrion
- Intermediate filaments
- Endoplasmic reticulum
- Microtubule
- Secretory vesicle

Centrioles, Cilia, and Flagella

In addition to functioning individually in the cytoskeleton, microtubules also interact to form more complex structures known as *centrioles, cilia,* and *flagella*.

CENTRIOLES. A **centriole** is a cylindrical structure composed of triplets of microtubules (**Spotlight Figure 3-2**). All animal cells that are capable of dividing contain a pair of centrioles arranged perpendicular to each other. The centrioles produce the spindle fibers that move DNA strands during cell division. Mature RBCs, skeletal muscle cells, cardiac muscle cells, and typical neurons lack centrioles. As a result, these cells cannot divide.

CILIA. **Cilia** (SIL-ē-uh; singular *cilium*) are relatively long, slender extensions of the plasma membrane (**Spotlight Figure 3-2**). They are supported internally by a cylindrical array of pairs of microtubules surrounding a centrally located pair. Multiple *motile cilia* make coordinated active movements that require energy from ATP. Their coordinated actions move fluids or secretions across the cell surface. For example, motile cilia lining the respiratory passageways beat in a synchronized manner to move sticky mucus and trapped dust particles toward the throat and away from delicate respiratory surfaces. If these cilia are damaged or immobilized by heavy smoking or a metabolic problem, the cleansing action is lost, and the irritants will no longer be removed. As a result, a chronic cough and respiratory infections develop.

A single, nonmotile **primary cilium** is found on a wide variety of cells. It lacks the central pair of microtubules present in motile cilia. A primary cilium acts as a signal sensor, detecting extracellular stimuli.

FLAGELLA. Organelles called **flagella** (fla-JEL-uh; singular *flagellum,* whip) resemble cilia but are much longer. Flagella move a cell through the surrounding fluid, rather than moving the fluid past a stationary cell. Sperm cells are the only human cells that have a flagellum. If the flagella of sperm are paralyzed or otherwise abnormal, the individual will be sterile, because immobile sperm cannot carry out fertilization.

Ribosomes

Ribosomes are organelles that manufacture proteins, using information from the DNA of the nucleus. Each ribosome consists of a small and a large subunit composed of a form of RNA called *ribosomal RNA* and protein. Ribosomes are found in all cells, but their number varies depending on the type of cell and its activities. For example, liver cells, which manufacture blood proteins, have many more ribosomes than do fat cells, which synthesize triglycerides.

There are two major types of ribosomes. **Free ribosomes** are scattered throughout the cytoplasm. The proteins that they manufacture enter the cytosol. **Fixed ribosomes** are attached to the ER, a membranous organelle. Proteins manufactured by fixed ribosomes enter the ER, where they are modified and packaged for use within the cell or eventual secretion from the cell.

Proteasomes

Proteasomes are small organelles that remove proteins within the cytoplasm (**Spotlight Figure 3-2**). These organelles contain an assortment of protein-breaking, or proteolytic, enzymes called *proteases*. Proteasomes remove and recycle damaged or denatured proteins and break down abnormal proteins such as those produced within cells infected by viruses.

The Endoplasmic Reticulum

The **endoplasmic reticulum** (en-dō-PLAZ-mik re-TIK-ū-lum; *reticulum*, a network), or **ER**, is a network of intracellular membranes continuous with the membranous *nuclear envelope* surrounding the nucleus (**Spotlight Figure 3-2**). The ER forms hollow tubes, flattened sheets, and chambers called **cisternae** (sis-TUR-nē; singular, *cisterna*, a reservoir for water). The ER has four major functions:

1. **Synthesis.** Specialized regions of the ER manufacture proteins, carbohydrates, and lipids.
2. **Storage.** The ER can store synthesized molecules or materials absorbed from the cytosol without affecting other cellular operations.
3. **Transport.** Materials can travel from place to place in the ER.
4. **Detoxification.** The ER can absorb drugs or toxins and neutralize them with enzymes.

There are two types of ER: **smooth endoplasmic reticulum (SER)** and **rough endoplasmic reticulum (RER)** (**Figure 3-14**). The term *smooth* refers to the fact that no ribosomes are associated with the SER. The SER is where lipids and carbohydrates are produced. The membranes of the RER contain fixed ribosomes, giving the RER a beaded or rough appearance. The ribosomes take part in protein synthesis.

SER functions include (1) the synthesis of the phospholipids and cholesterol needed for maintenance and growth of the plasma membrane, ER, nuclear membrane, and Golgi apparatus in all cells; (2) the synthesis of steroid hormones, such as *testosterone* and *estrogen* (sex hormones) in cells of the reproductive organs; (3) the synthesis and storage of glycerides, especially triglycerides, in liver cells and fat cells; and (4) the synthesis and storage of glycogen in skeletal muscle and liver cells.

The RER functions as a combination workshop and shipping warehouse. The fixed ribosomes on its outer surface release newly synthesized proteins into the cisternae of the RER. Some proteins remain in the RER and function as enzymes. Others are chemically modified and packaged into

Figure 3-14 The Endoplasmic Reticulum. The three-dimensional relationships between the rough and smooth endoplasmic reticula are shown here.

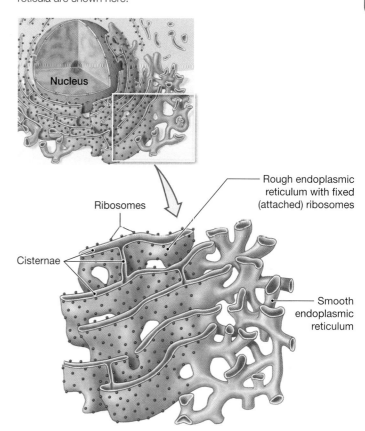

Nucleus

Ribosomes

Cisternae

Rough endoplasmic reticulum with fixed (attached) ribosomes

Smooth endoplasmic reticulum

small membrane-bound sacs that pinch off from the tips of the ER. The sacs, called *transport vesicles*, deliver the proteins to the Golgi apparatus, another membranous organelle. There the proteins are processed further (see **Spotlight Figure 3-16**).

The amount of ER and the ratio of RER to SER vary with the type of cell and its activities. For example, pancreatic cells that manufacture digestive enzymes contain an extensive RER, and their SER is relatively small. The proportions are just the reverse in reproductive system cells that synthesize steroid hormones.

The Golgi Apparatus

The **Golgi (GŌL-jē) apparatus** consists of a set of five or six flattened membranous discs called *cisternae*. A single cell may contain several of these organelles, each resembling a stack of dinner plates (**Figure 3-15**).

A Golgi apparatus has three major functions (**Spotlight Figure 3-17** on pp. 74–75). It

1. modifies and packages secretions, such as hormones or enzymes, for release from the cell;

Figure 3-15 The Golgi Apparatus.

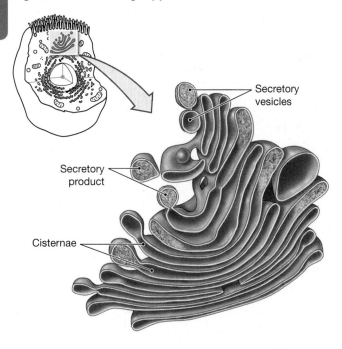

Secretory vesicles

Secretory product

Cisternae

2. renews or modifies the plasma membrane; and

3. packages special enzymes within vesicles (lysosomes) for use in the cytoplasm.

Lysosomes

Lysosomes (LĪ-sō-sōmz; *lyso-*, a loosening + *soma*, body) are vesicles filled with digestive enzymes. Lysosomes perform cleanup and recycling functions within the cell. One such function involves removing damaged organelles. Lysosomal enzymes are activated when lysosomes fuse with the membranes of damaged organelles, such as mitochondria or fragments of the ER. The activated enzymes break down the lysosomal contents. Nutrients re-enter the cytosol through passive or active transport processes. The remaining material is eliminated by exocytosis.

Lysosomes also function in defense against disease. Through endocytosis, immune system cells may engulf bacteria, fluids, and organic debris in their surroundings and isolate them within vesicles. ⊃ p. 68 Lysosomes fuse with vesicles created in this way. The digestive enzymes then break down the contents and free up usable substances such as sugars or amino acids.

Lysosomes also do essential recycling functions inside the cell. For example, when muscle cells are inactive, lysosomes gradually break down their contractile proteins. If the cells become active once again, this destruction ends. However, in damaged or dead cells, lysosome membranes disintegrate,

releasing active enzymes into the cytosol. These enzymes rapidly destroy the proteins and organelles of the cell, a process called **autolysis** (aw-TOL-i-sis; *auto-*, self). Because the breakdown of lysosomal membranes can destroy a cell, lysosomes have been called cellular "suicide packets." We do not know how to control lysosomal activities or why the enclosed enzymes do not digest the lysosomal membranes unless the cell is damaged.

Problems in producing lysosomal enzymes cause more than 30 serious inherited diseases affecting children. In these conditions, called *lysosomal storage disease*, the lack of a specific enzyme results in the buildup of waste products that lysosomes normally remove and recycle. Affected individuals may die when vital cells, such as those of the heart, can no longer function.

Peroxisomes

Peroxisomes are vesicles that are smaller than lysosomes and carry a different group of enzymes (**Spotlight Figure 3-2**). In contrast to lysosomes, which are produced at the Golgi apparatus, new peroxisomes arise from the growth and subdivision of existing peroxisomes. Peroxisomes absorb and break down fatty acids and other organic compounds. In the process, they generate hydrogen peroxide (H_2O_2), a potentially dangerous *free radical*. **Free radicals** are ions or molecules that contain unpaired electrons. They are highly reactive and enter additional reactions that can damage vital compounds such as proteins. Other enzymes in peroxisomes break down (H_2O_2) into oxygen and water, thus protecting the cell from the damaging effects of free radicals produced during catabolism. Found in all cells, peroxisomes are most abundant in metabolically active cells, such as liver cells.

Mitochondria

Mitochondria (mī-tō-KON-drē-uh; singular *mitochondrion*; *mitos*, thread + *chondrion*, granule) are small organelles that provide energy for the cell (**Spotlight Figure 3-2**). The number of mitochondria in a particular cell varies with the cell's energy demands. RBCs, for example, have no mitochondria, but these organelles may account for 30 percent of the volume of a heart muscle cell.

Mitochondria have an unusual double membrane (**Figure 3-17**, p. 76). Each membrane consists of a phospholipid bilayer. The outer membrane surrounds the entire organelle. The inner membrane contains numerous folds called **cristae**, which surround the fluid contents, or **matrix**.

Cristae increase the inner membrane surface area in contact with the matrix of the mitochondria. Metabolic enzymes in the matrix catalyze energy-producing reactions.

Most of the chemical reactions that release energy take place in the mitochondria, but most of the cellular activities that require energy occur in the surrounding cytoplasm. For this reason, cells must store energy in a form that can be moved from place to place. Energy is stored and transferred in the high-energy bond of ATP. ⟲ p. 48 Living cells break the high-energy phosphate bond under controlled conditions, reconverting ATP to ADP and releasing energy for the cell's use.

MITOCHONDRIAL ENERGY PRODUCTION. Most cells generate ATP and other high-energy compounds through the breakdown of carbohydrates, especially glucose. Most of the actual energy production occurs inside mitochondria, but the first steps take place in the cytosol. In this reaction sequence, called *glycolysis*, six-carbon glucose molecules are broken down into three-carbon *pyruvate* molecules. These molecules are then absorbed by the mitochondria. If glucose or other carbohydrates are not available, mitochondria can absorb and use small carbon chains produced by the breakdown of lipids or proteins. As long as oxygen is present, these molecules will be broken down to carbon dioxide, which diffuses out of the cell, and hydrogen atoms, which take part in a series of energy-releasing steps resulting in the enzymatic conversion of ADP to ATP.

Because the key reactions involved in mitochondrial activity consume oxygen, the process of mitochondrial energy production is known as **aerobic** (*aero-*, **air** + *bios*, **life**) **metabolism**, or *cellular respiration*. Aerobic metabolism in mitochondria produces about 95 percent of the energy a cell needs to stay alive. (We discuss aerobic metabolism in more detail in Chapters 7 and 17.)

CLINICAL NOTE

Inheritable Mitochondrial Disorders

Several inheritable disorders result from abnormal mitochondrial activity. Mitochondria have DNA and ribosomes to manufacture some of their own proteins. However, most of their proteins are coded by nuclear DNA and imported from the cytosol. For this reason, abnormal nuclear DNA or mtDNA may result in defective enzymes that reduce the efficiency of ATP production. A mitochondrial disorder may affect a single organ or involve many organ systems that affect cells throughout the body. Symptoms involving muscle cells, nerve cells, and the light receptor cells in the eye are most common. The reason is because these cells have especially high energy demands.

Mitochondria contain their own DNA (mtDNA) and ribosomes. The mtDNA codes for small numbers of RNA and polypeptide molecules. The polypeptides serve as enzymes in energy production. Although mitochondria contain their own DNA, their functions depend on imported proteins coded by nuclear DNA.

CHECKPOINT

14. Describe the difference between the cytoplasm and the cytosol.

15. Identify the membranous organelles and list their functions.

16. Cells lining the small intestine have numerous finger-like projections on their free surface. What are these structures, and what is their function?

17. How does the absence of centrioles affect a cell?

18. Explain why certain cells in the ovaries and testes contain large amounts of smooth endoplasmic reticulum (SER).

19. What does the presence of many mitochondria imply about a cell's energy requirements?

See the blue Answers tab at the back of the book.

3-6 The nucleus contains DNA and enzymes essential for controlling cellular activities

Learning Objective Explain the functions of the cell nucleus.

The **nucleus** is usually the largest and most conspicuous structure in a cell (**Spotlight Figure 3-2**). It is the control center for cellular operations. A single nucleus stores all the information needed to control the synthesis of the more than 100,000 different proteins in the human body. The nucleus determines the structure of the cell and the functions the cell can perform. The nucleus does so by controlling which proteins are synthesized, under what circumstances, and in what amounts.

Nuclear Structure and Contents

Most cells contain a single nucleus, but exceptions exist. For example, skeletal muscle cells have many nuclei, and mature RBCs have none. **Figure 3-18** shows the structure of a typical nucleus. A **nuclear envelope** consisting of a double membrane surrounds the nucleus and separates its fluid contents—called *nucleoplasm*—from the cytosol. The nucleoplasm contains ions, enzymes, RNA and DNA nucleotides, proteins, small amounts of RNA, and DNA.

The Golgi apparatus plays a major role in modifying and packaging newly synthesized proteins. Some proteins and glycoproteins synthesized in the rough endoplasmic reticulum (RER) are delivered to the Golgi apparatus by transport vesicles. Here's a summary of the process, beginning with DNA.

1 Protein synthesis begins when a gene on DNA produces messenger RNA (mRNA), the template for protein synthesis.

2 The mRNA leaves the nucleus and attaches to a free ribosome in the cytoplasm, or a fixed ribosome on the RER.

3a Proteins constructed on free ribosomes are released into the cytosol for use within the cell.

3b Protein synthesis on fixed ribosomes occurs at the RER. The newly synthesized protein folds into its three-dimensional shape.

4 The proteins are then modified within the ER. Regions of the ER then bud off, forming transport vesicles containing modified proteins and glycoproteins.

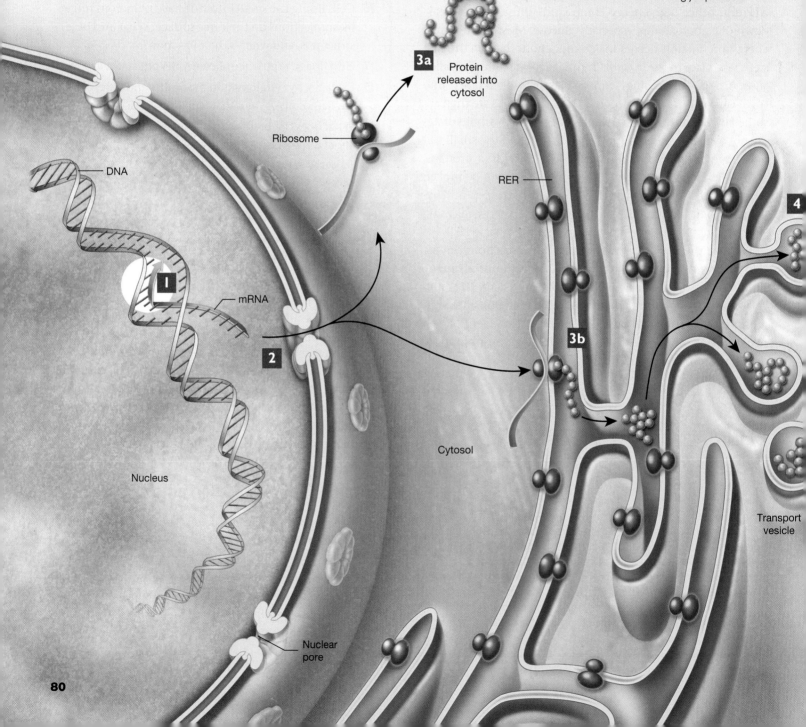

3a Protein released into cytosol

Ribosome

DNA

RER

mRNA

1

2

3b

4

Nucleus

Cytosol

Transport vesicle

Nuclear pore

5 The transport vesicles carry the proteins and glycoproteins generated in the ER toward the Golgi apparatus. The transport vesicles then fuse to create the forming face ("receiving side") of the Golgi apparatus.

6 Multiple transport vesicles combine to form cisternae on the forming face. Further protein and glycoprotein modification and packaging occur as the cisternae move toward the maturing face. Small transport vesicles return resident Golgi proteins to the forming face for reuse.

7 The maturing face ("shipping side") generates vesicles that carry modified proteins away from the Golgi apparatus. One type of vesicle becomes a lysosome, which contains digestive enzymes.

8 Two other types of vesicles proceed to the plasma membrane: secretory and membrane renewal. **Secretory vesicles** fuse with the plasma membrane and empty their products outside the cell by exocytosis. **Membrane renewal vesicles** add new lipids and proteins to the plasma membrane.

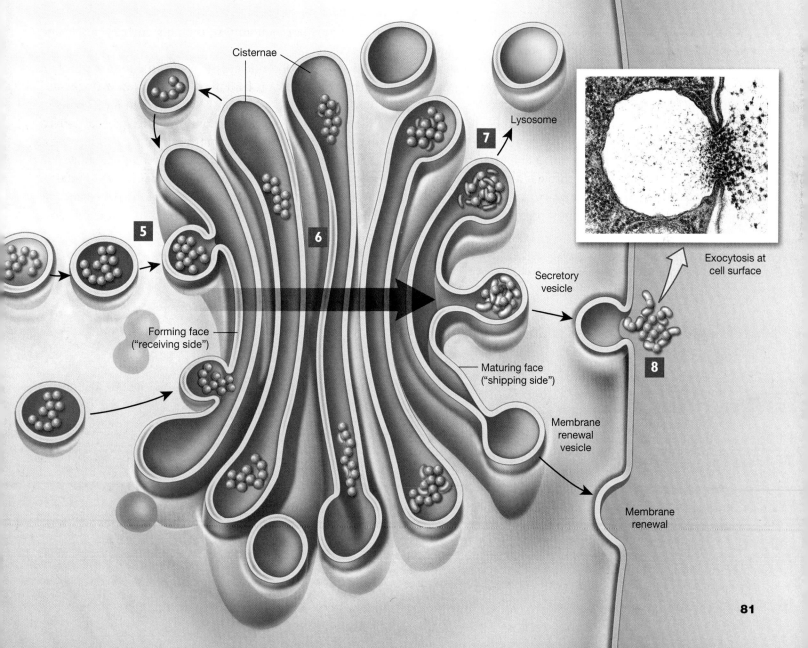

Cisternae

Lysosome

7

5

6

Forming face ("receiving side")

Secretory vesicle

Exocytosis at cell surface

Maturing face ("shipping side")

8

Membrane renewal vesicle

Membrane renewal

Figure 3-17 Mitochondria. Shown here is the three-dimensional organization of a typical mitochondrion and a color-enhanced TEM of a mitochondrion in section. Mitochondria absorb short carbon chains and oxygen, and generate carbon dioxide, ATP, and water.

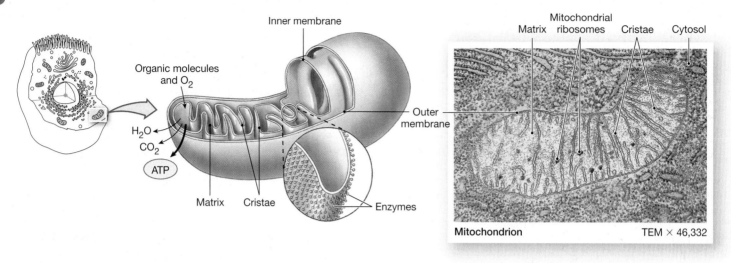

Chemical communication between the nucleus and the cytosol takes place through **nuclear pores**. These pores are large enough to allow the movement of ions and small molecules, yet small enough to regulate the transport of proteins and RNA.

Most nuclei have several **nucleoli** (noo-KLĒ-ō-lī; singular, *nucleolus*). Nucleoli are organelles that synthesize **ribosomal RNA (rRNA)**, and assemble the small and large ribosomal subunits. These subunits pass through the nuclear pores into the cytoplasm, where they will form functional ribosomes. For this reason, they are most prominent in cells that manufacture large amounts of proteins, such as muscle and liver cells.

The DNA in the nucleus stores instructions for protein synthesis. This DNA is contained in **chromosomes** (*chroma*, color). The nuclei of human body cells contain 23 pairs of chromosomes. One chromosome in each pair is derived from the mother and one from the father.

The structure of a typical chromosome is shown in **Figure 3-19**. Each chromosome contains DNA strands wrapped around proteins called *histones*. At intervals, the DNA and histones form a complex known as a *nucleosome*.

Figure 3-18 The Nucleus. The diagram and electron micrograph show important nuclear structures. The arrows on the TEM indicate the locations of nuclear pores.

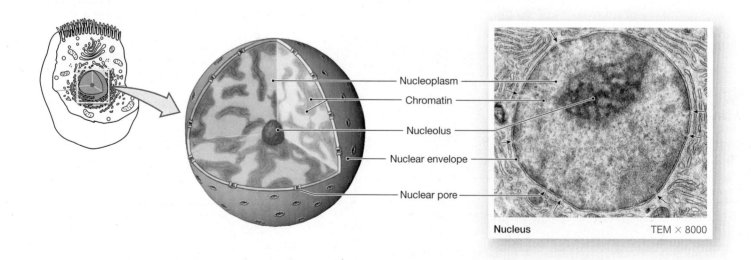

Figure 3-19 DNA Organization and Chromosome Structure.

DNA strands wound around histone proteins (at bottom) form coils that may be very tight or rather loose. In cells that are not dividing, the DNA is loosely coiled, forming a tangled network known as chromatin. When the coiling becomes tighter, as it does in preparation for cell division, the DNA becomes visible as distinct structures called chromosomes.

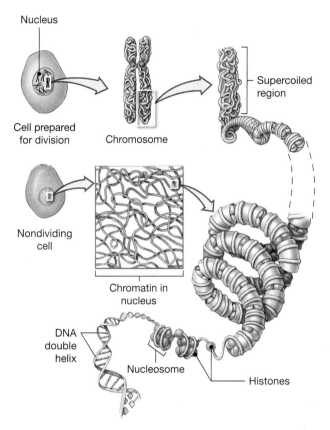

traits, such as hair color or blood type, are inherited from generation to generation.

How does the genetic code work? Recall the basic structure of nucleic acids described in Chapter 2. ⤴ p. 47 A single DNA molecule consists of a pair of DNA strands held together by hydrogen bonding between complementary nitrogenous bases. Information is stored in the sequence of nitrogenous bases (adenine, A; thymine, T; cytosine, C; and guanine, G) along the length of the DNA strands.

The genetic code is called a *triplet code* because a sequence of three nitrogenous bases represents a single amino acid. For example, the DNA triplet adenine–cytosine–adenine (ACA) codes for the amino acid cysteine.

A **gene** is the functional unit of heredity. Each protein-coding gene consists of all the triplets in the proper sequence needed to produce a specific protein. The number of triplets varies from gene to gene, depending on the size of the protein that will be produced. Each gene also contains special segments responsible for regulating its own activity. In effect these are triplets of nucleotides that say, "Do (or do not) read this message," "Message starts here," or "Message ends here." These "read me," "don't read me," and "start" signals form a special region of the DNA called the *promoter*, or control segment, at the start of each gene. Each gene ends with a "stop" signal.

The tightness of DNA coiling determines whether the chromosome is long and thin or short and fat. In cells that are not dividing, the nucleosomes are loosely coiled, forming a tangle of fine filaments known as **chromatin**. Chromosomes in a dividing cell contain very tightly coiled DNA. These chromosomes can be seen clearly as separate structures in light or electron micrographs.

Information Storage in the Nucleus

Each protein molecule consists of a unique sequence of amino acids. ⤴ p. 43 Any "recipe" for a protein, therefore, must specify the order of the amino acids it contains. This information is stored in the chemical structure of the DNA strands in the nucleus. The chemical "language" the cell uses is known as the **genetic code**. An understanding of the genetic code has enabled researchers to determine how cells build proteins and how various structural and functional

CLINICAL NOTE

DNA Fingerprinting

Every nucleated cell in the body carries a set of 46 chromosomes identical to the set formed at fertilization. Not all the DNA of these chromosomes codes for proteins. Within the DNA that does not code for proteins are regions called short tandem repeats (STRs), which contain the same nucleotide sequence repeated over and over. The number of STRs and the number of repetitions vary among individuals.

In the United States, 13 core STRs are used to identify individuals. The individual differences are reflected in the different lengths of these STRs. The chance that any two individuals, other than identical twins, will have the same length and pattern of repeating DNA segments in 13 STRs is approximately one in 575 trillion. For this reason, individuals can be identified on the basis of their DNA pattern, just as they can on the basis of a fingerprint. Skin scrapings, blood, semen, hair roots, or other tissues can serve as the DNA source. Information from **DNA fingerprinting** has been used to convict or acquit people accused of violent crimes, such as rape or murder. The U.S. Crime Act of 1994 mandates that DNA fingerprints of individuals convicted of certain crimes be kept in searchable criminal justice DNA databases. The science of molecular biology has become a useful addition to the crime-fighting toolbox.

Not all genes code for proteins. Some genes contain instructions for the synthesis of ribosomal RNA or another type, we will discuss shortly, *transfer RNA*. Some regulate other genes, and others have no apparent function.

CHECKPOINT

20. Describe the contents and structure of the nucleus.

21. What is a gene?

See the blue Answers tab at the back of the book.

3-7 DNA controls protein synthesis, cell structure, and cell function

Learning Objective Summarize the process of protein synthesis.

Each DNA molecule contains thousands of genes and, therefore, holds the information needed to synthesize thousands of proteins. Normally, the genes are tightly coiled, and bound histones keep the genes inactive, thus preventing the synthesis of proteins. Before a gene can be activated, enzymes must temporarily break the weak bonds between its nitrogenous bases and temporarily remove the histone that guards the *promoter* segment at the start of each gene.

The process of gene activation is only partially understood, but more is known about protein synthesis. The process of **protein synthesis** is divided into two main parts. *Transcription* is the production of RNA from a single strand of DNA. *Translation* is the assembly of a protein by ribosomes, using the information carried by the RNA molecule. Transcription takes place within the nucleus, and translation occurs in the cytoplasm.

Transcription

Ribosomes, the organelles of protein synthesis, are located in the cytoplasm, but the genes are confined to the nucleus. This problem of a separation between the protein manufacturing site and the DNA's protein blueprint is solved with a single strand of RNA known as **messenger RNA (mRNA)**. The process of mRNA formation is called **transcription** (**Figure 3-20**). Transcription means "copying" or "rewriting." This term makes sense because the newly formed mRNA is a transcript (a copy) of the information contained in the gene. The information that is "copied" is the sequence of nucleotides of the gene.

Transcription begins when an enzyme, *RNA polymerase*, binds to the promoter of a gene (❶ in **Figure 3-20**). This enzyme catalyzes the synthesis of an mRNA strand, using nucleotides

complementary to those in the gene (❷). The nucleotides involved are those typical of RNA, not those of DNA. RNA polymerase may use adenine, guanine, cytosine, or uracil (U), but never thymine. Thus, wherever an A occurs in the DNA strand, RNA polymerase attaches a U, not a T. The resulting mRNA strand contains a sequence of nucleotides that are complementary to those of the gene. A sequence of three nitrogenous bases along the new mRNA strand represents a **codon** (KŌ-don) that is complementary to the corresponding DNA triplet along the gene (❸). At the DNA "stop" signal, the enzyme and the mRNA strand detach, and the complementary DNA strands reattach.

The mRNA formed in this way may be altered, or edited, before it leaves the nucleus. For example, some regions (called *introns*) may be removed and the remaining segments (called *exons*) spliced together. This modification creates a shorter, functional mRNA strand that enters the cytoplasm through a nuclear pore. We now know that by removing different introns, a single gene can produce mRNAs that code for several different proteins. How this variable editing is regulated is unknown.

Translation

Translation is the synthesis of a protein using the information provided by the sequence of codons along the mRNA strand. Every amino acid has at least one unique and specific codon. **Table 3-4** includes several examples of DNA triplets and their corresponding mRNA codons and amino acids. During translation, the sequence of codons determines the sequence of amino acids in the protein. (For a complete table of mRNA codons, the amino acids, and the start or stop signals they represent, see the Appendix at the back of the book.)

Translation begins when the newly synthesized mRNA leaves the nucleus and binds with a ribosome in the cytoplasm. Molecules of a third form of RNA known as **transfer RNA (tRNA)** then deliver amino acids that will be used by the ribosome to assemble a protein. There are more than 20 different types of tRNA, at least one for each amino acid used in protein synthesis. Each tRNA molecule contains a triplet of nitrogenous bases, known as an **anticodon**, that is complementary to a specific codon on the mRNA and will bind to it.

Figure 3-21 illustrates the three phases of the translation process: *initiation, elongation, and termination*. During **initiation** (❶ and ❷), a functional ribosome forms as its two subunits (small and large) are joined, along with an mRNA strand and amino acid–carrying tRNA molecule. In **elongation** (❸ and ❹), amino acids are added one by one to the growing polypeptide chain. At **termination** (❺), the polypeptide

Figure 3-20 Transcription. In this figure, only a small portion of a single DNA molecule, containing a single gene, is undergoing transcription. **1** The two DNA strands separate, and RNA polymerase binds to the promoter of the gene. **2** The RNA polymerase moves from one nucleotide to the next along the length of the gene. At each site, complementary RNA nucleotides form hydrogen bonds with the DNA nucleotides of the gene. The RNA polymerase then bonds the arriving nucleotides together into a strand of mRNA. **3** On reaching the stop codon at the end of the gene, the RNA polymerase and the mRNA strand detach, and the two DNA strands reattach.

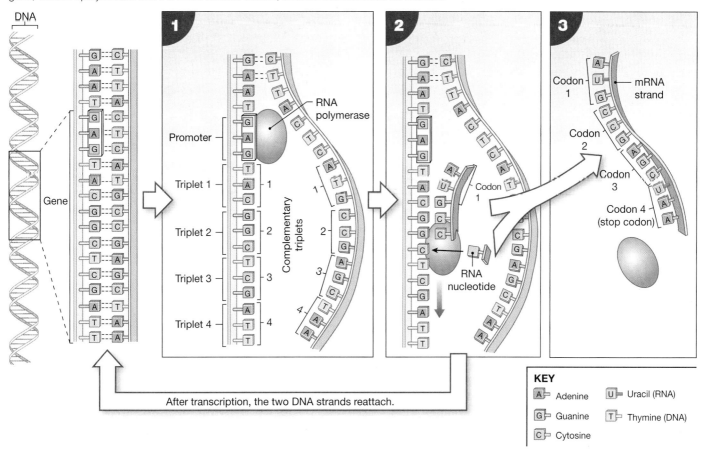

chain is released, and the ribosomal subunits separate, freeing an intact mRNA strand. The freed mRNA strand can interact with other ribosomes and create additional copies of the same polypeptide chain or protein.

A protein is a polypeptide containing 100 or more amino acids (as you may recall from Chapter 2). ⟳ p. 43 Translation proceeds swiftly, producing a typical protein (about 1000 amino acids) in around 20 seconds. The protein begins as a simple linear strand, but a more complex structure develops as it grows longer.

Table 3-4	Examples of the Genetic Code		
DNA Triplet	**mRNA Codon**	**tRNA Anticodon**	**Amino Acid (and/or Instruction)**
AAA	UUU	AAA	Phenylalanine
AAT	UUA	AAU	Leucine
ACA	UGU	ACA	Cysteine
CAA	GUU	CAA	Valine
GGG	CCC	GGG	Proline
CGA	GCU	CGA	Alanine
TAC	AUG	UAC	Methionine: start codon
ATT	UAA	[none]	Stop codon

CHECKPOINT

22. How does the nucleus control the cell's activities?

23. What process would be affected by the lack of the enzyme RNA polymerase?

24. During the process of transcription, a nucleotide was deleted from an mRNA sequence that coded for a protein. What effect would this deletion have on the amino acid sequence of the protein?

See the blue Answers tab at the back of the book.

Figure 3-21 Translation. Once transcription has been completed, the mRNA diffuses into the cytoplasm and interacts with a ribosome to assemble a protein or polypeptide.

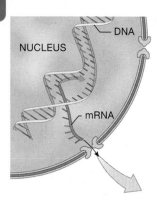

Initiation

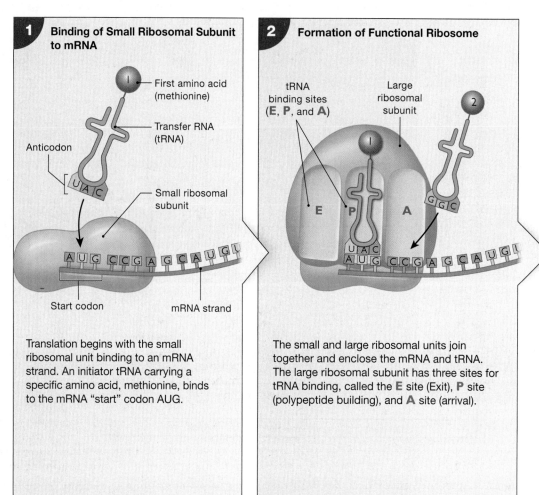

1 Binding of Small Ribosomal Subunit to mRNA

Translation begins with the small ribosomal unit binding to an mRNA strand. An initiator tRNA carrying a specific amino acid, methionine, binds to the mRNA "start" codon AUG.

2 Formation of Functional Ribosome

The small and large ribosomal units join together and enclose the mRNA and tRNA. The large ribosomal subunit has three sites for tRNA binding, called the **E** site (Exit), **P** site (polypeptide building), and **A** site (arrival).

KEY

 Adenine

 Guanine

 Cytosine

U Uracil

CLINICAL NOTE

Recombinant DNA Technology

Many important medications are derived from animals. For example, insulin, which is an important hormone in glucose metabolism, was initially derived from swine or cattle. However, there are slight differences in the structure of human insulin and the structure of pork or beef insulin. The amino acid sequence in the animal insulin molecules differs slightly from human insulin. While animal insulin works well in humans, the body eventually begins to produce anti-insulin antibodies against the foreign part of the insulin molecule. Over time, humans on animal insulin require more and more insulin as their immune systems destroy increasing quantities of the animal insulin. This insulin resistance becomes

a problem for long-term diabetics, as they require increasingly large doses of insulin.

However, scientists have developed a method of producing human insulin by a technique called *recombinant DNA technology*. With this technology, small fragments of human DNA that code for the production of insulin are inserted into specialized bacteria. These bacteria then begin producing insulin identical to human insulin. Diabetics can use this insulin without the risk of developing insulin resistance. Other medications produced by recombinant DNA technology include hepatitis B vaccines, "clot-busting" drugs (tPA) used in heart attacks, and others.

Elongation

Termination

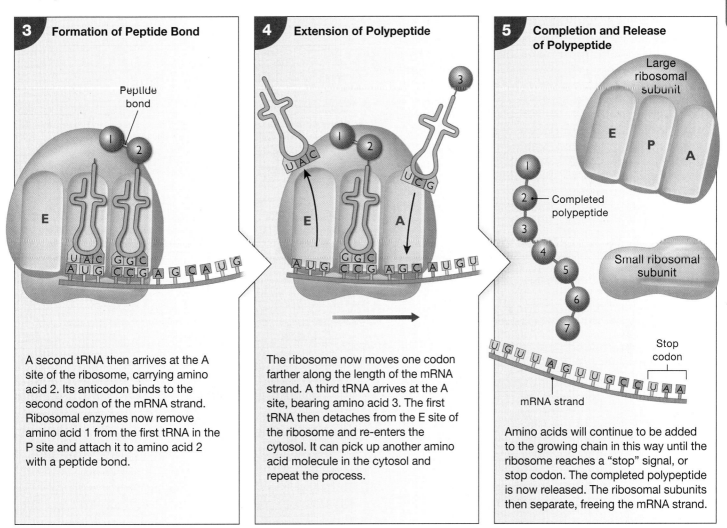

3 **Formation of Peptide Bond**

Peptide bond

E

UAC GGC
AUG CCGA GCAUG

A second tRNA then arrives at the A site of the ribosome, carrying amino acid 2. Its anticodon binds to the second codon of the mRNA strand. Ribosomal enzymes now remove amino acid 1 from the first tRNA in the P site and attach it to amino acid 2 with a peptide bond.

4 **Extension of Polypeptide**

UAC

UCG

E   A

GGC
AUG CCG AGCAUGU

The ribosome now moves one codon farther along the length of the mRNA strand. A third tRNA arrives at the A site, bearing amino acid 3. The first tRNA then detaches from the E site of the ribosome and re-enters the cytosol. It can pick up another amino acid molecule in the cytosol and repeat the process.

5 **Completion and Release of Polypeptide**

Large ribosomal subunit

E   P   A

Completed polypeptide

Small ribosomal subunit

mRNA strand

Stop codon

UGUUAGUUGCCUAA

Amino acids will continue to be added to the growing chain in this way until the ribosome reaches a "stop" signal, or stop codon. The completed polypeptide is now released. The ribosomal subunits then separate, freeing the mRNA strand.

3-8 Stages of a cell's life cycle include interphase, mitosis, and cytokinesis

Learning Objective Describe the stages of the cell life cycle, including mitosis, interphase, and cytokinesis, and explain their significance.

During the time between fertilization and physical maturity, the number of cells making up an individual increases from a single cell to roughly 75 trillion cells. This amazing increase in numbers takes place through a form of cellular reproduction called **cell division**. Even when development has been completed, cell division continues to be essential to survival because it replaces old and damaged cells.

For cell division to be successful, the genetic material in the nucleus must be duplicated accurately, and each daughter cell must receive a complete copy. The duplication of the cell's genetic material is called *DNA replication*. Nuclear division is called **mitosis** (mī-TŌ-sis). Mitosis takes place during the division of **somatic (*soma*, body) cells**, which include the vast majority of the cells in the body. The production of sex cells—sperm and oocytes (immature ova, or egg cells)— involves a different process, called **meiosis** (mī-Ō-sis), which we will describe in Chapter 19.

Figure 3-22 represents the life cycle of a typical cell. Most cells spend only a small part of their life cycle in cell division. For most of their lives, cells are in **interphase**, the period of time between cell divisions when they perform normal functions.

CLINICAL NOTE

Mutations and Mosaicism

Mutations are permanent changes in the nucleotide sequence of a cell's DNA. Mutations may involve changes in the number or structure of chromosomes and their long segments of DNA, or they may involve only single nucleotides. Chromosomal mutations can involve deletions, insertions, or inversions of DNA segments. Such changes may disrupt only the chromosome undergoing the change or may affect multiple chromosomes as one gains DNA and another loses DNA. The simplest mutation is called a *point mutation*, a change in a single nucleotide that affects one codon.

With roughly 3 billion pairs of nucleotides in the DNA of a human cell, a single mistake might seem relatively unimportant. Yet several hundred inherited disorders have been traced to abnormalities in enzyme or protein structure that reflect single changes in nucleotide sequence. In some disorders, a single change in the amino acid sequence of a structural protein or enzyme can prove fatal. For example, several cancers and two potentially lethal blood

disorders, *thalassemia* and *sickle cell anemia*, result from variations in a single nucleotide. Other mutations resulting from the addition or deletion of nucleotides can affect multiple codons in one gene, in several adjacent genes, or in the structure of one or more chromosomes.

Most mutations occur during DNA replication, when cells are preparing for cell division. A single cell or group of daughter cells may be affected. If the mutations take place early in development, however, subsets of cells or every cell in the body may be affected. **Mosaicism** occurs when a person's cells do not all have the same genetic makeup. Some amount of mosaicism is present in all of us.

If a mutation affects the DNA of an individual's sex cells, however, that mutation can be inherited by that individual's children. Our growing understanding of gene structure and genetic engineering is opening the possibility of diagnosing and correcting some of these problems.

Figure 3-22 Stages of a Cell's Life Cycle.

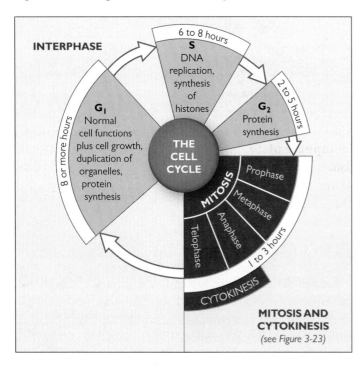

is called **apoptosis** (ap-op-TŌ-sis; *apo-*, off + *ptosis*, a falling). Apoptosis is a key process in homeostasis. During an immune response, for example, some types of white blood cells activate genes in abnormal or infected cells that tell the cell to die.

A cell ready to divide first enters the G_1 phase. In this phase, the cell makes enough organelles and cytosol for two functional cells. These preparations may take just eight hours in cells dividing at top speed, or days to weeks to complete, depending on the type of cell and the situation. For example, certain cells in the lining of the digestive tract divide every few days throughout life, but specialized cells in other tissues divide only under special circumstances, such as following an injury.

Once these preparations have been completed, the cell enters the S phase and replicates the DNA in its nucleus. This process takes six to eight hours. The goal of **DNA replication** is to copy the genetic information in the nucleus so that one set of chromosomes can be given to each of the two cells produced.

DNA replication starts when the complementary DNA strands begin to separate and unwind (**Figure 3-23**). Molecules of the enzyme *DNA polymerase* then bind to the exposed nitrogenous bases. As a result, complementary nucleotides present in the nucleoplasm attach to the exposed nitrogenous bases of the DNA strands and form a pair of identical DNA molecules.

Shortly after DNA replication is a brief G_2 phase for protein synthesis and for the completion of centriole replication. The cell then begins mitosis.

Interphase

Somatic cells differ in the length of time spent in interphase and their frequency of cell division. For example, unspecialized cells known as *stem cells* divide repeatedly with very brief interphase periods. In contrast, mature skeletal muscle cells and most nerve cells never undergo mitosis or cell division. Certain other cells appear to be programmed to self-destruct after a certain period of time because specific "suicide genes" in the nucleus are activated. The genetically controlled death of cells

Mitosis

Mitosis is a process that separates the duplicated chromosomes of the original cell into two identical nuclei. Division of the cytoplasm to form two distinct cells involves a separate,

Figure 3-23 DNA Replication. In replication, the DNA strands unwind, and DNA polymerase begins attaching complementary DNA nucleotides along each strand. The complementary copy of one original strand is produced as a continuous strand. The other copy is produced as short segments, which are then spliced together. The end result is that two identical copies of the original DNA molecule are produced.

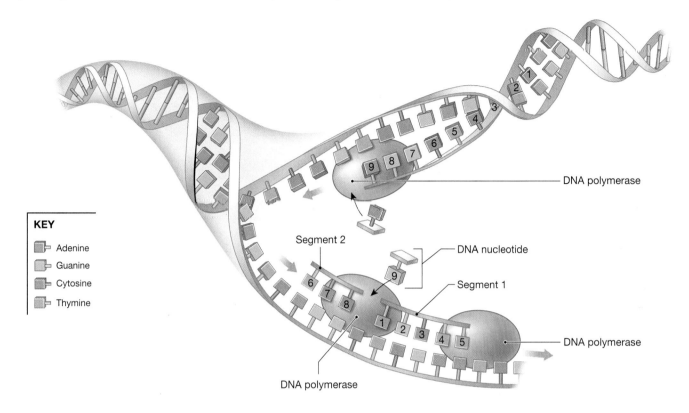

but related, process known as **cytokinesis** (sī-tō-ki-NĒ-sis; *cyto-*, cell + *kinesis*, motion). Mitosis is divided into four stages: *prophase, metaphase, anaphase,* and *telophase* (**Figure 3-22**).

Stage 1: Prophase

Prophase (PRŌ-fāz; *pro-*, before) begins when the DNA is coiled so tightly that the chromosomes become visible under a light microscope. As a result of DNA replication, there are now two copies of each chromosome. Each copy, called a **chromatid** (KRŌ-ma-tid), is connected to its duplicate copy at a single point, the **centromere** (SEN-trō-mēr).

As the chromosomes appear, the nucleoli disappear and the two pairs of centrioles begin moving toward opposite ends of the cell. An array of microtubules, called **spindle fibers**, extends between the centriole pairs. Late in prophase, the nuclear envelope disappears, and the chromatids become attached to the spindle fibers.

Stage 2: Metaphase

Metaphase (MET-a-fāz; *meta-*, after) begins as the chromosomes move to a narrow central zone called the **metaphase plate**. Metaphase ends when all the chromosomes are aligned in the plane of the metaphase plate. At this time, each chromosome still consists of a pair of chromatids.

Stage 3: Anaphase

Anaphase (AN-a-fāz; *ana-*, apart) begins when the centromere of each chromatid pair splits and the chromatids separate. The two resulting **daughter chromosomes** are now pulled toward opposite ends of the cell. Anaphase ends when the daughter chromosomes arrive near the centrioles at opposite ends of the cell.

Stage 4: Telophase

During **telophase** (TĒL-ō-fāz; *telos*, end), the cell prepares to return to interphase. The nuclear membranes re-form, the nuclei enlarge, and the chromosomes gradually uncoil. Once the fine filaments of chromatin become visible, nucleoli reappear and the nuclei resemble those of interphase cells. This stage marks the end of mitosis.

3

Figure 3-24 Interphase, Mitosis, and Cytokinesis.

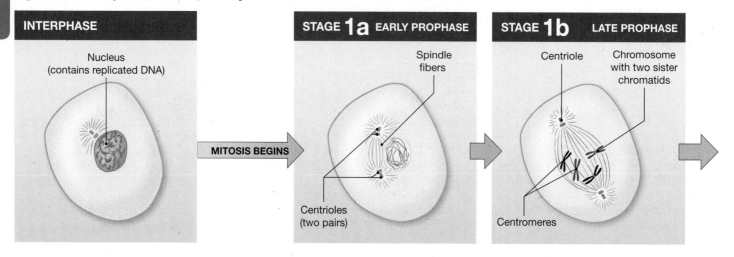

Cytokinesis

At the end of mitosis, the daughter cells have not yet completed their physical separation. **Cytokinesis** is the division of the cytoplasm into two daughter cells (**Figure 3-24**). It usually begins in late anaphase. As the daughter chromosomes near the ends of the spindle fibers, the cytoplasm constricts along the plane of the metaphase plate, forming a *cleavage furrow*. Cytokinesis continues throughout telophase, and is usually completed after a nuclear membrane has re-formed around each daughter nucleus. The completion of cytokinesis marks the end of cell division.

CHECKPOINT

25. Give the biological terms for (a) cellular reproduction and (b) cell death.

26. Describe interphase, and identify its stages.

27. Define mitosis, and list its four stages.

28. What would happen if spindle fibers failed to form in a cell during mitosis?

See the blue Answers tab at the back of the book.

3-9 Tumors and cancers are characterized by abnormal cell growth and division

Learning Objective Discuss the relationship between cell division and cancer.

Cancer cells result from mutations that disrupt the normal control processes that regulate cell division and growth. When the rates of cell division and growth exceed the rate of cell death, a tissue begins to enlarge. A **tumor**, or *neoplasm*, is a mass or swelling produced by abnormal cell growth and division. In a **benign tumor**, the cells usually remain in one place—within the epithelium (one of the four primary tissue types) or a connective tissue capsule. Such a tumor is seldom life threatening. It can usually be surgically removed if its size or position disturbs tissue function.

Cells in a **malignant tumor** no longer respond to normal controls. These cells do not remain within the epithelium or connective tissue capsule, but spread into surrounding tissues. The tumor of origin is called the *primary tumor* (or *primary neoplasm*). The spreading process is called **invasion**. Malignant cells may also travel to distant tissues and organs and produce *secondary tumors*. This migration, called **metastasis** (me-TAS-ta-sis; *meta-*, after + *stasis*, standing still), is difficult to control.

Cancer is an illness characterized by gene mutations leading to the formation of malignant cells and metastasis. Malignant cancer cells lose their resemblance to normal cells. The secondary tumors they form are extremely active metabolically. Their presence stimulates the growth of blood vessels into the area. The increased blood supply provides additional nutrients to the cancer cells, further accelerating tumor growth and metastasis.

As malignant tumors grow, organ function begins to deteriorate. The malignant cells may no longer perform their original functions, or they may perform normal functions in an abnormal way. Cancer cells do not use energy very efficiently. They grow and multiply at the expense of healthy tissues, competing for space and nutrients with normal cells. This competition accounts for the starved appearance of many patients in the late stages of cancer. Death may result from the compression of vital organs when nonfunctional

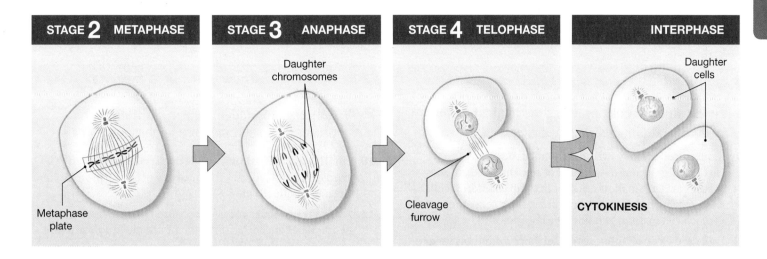

cancer cells have killed or replaced the healthy cells in those organs, or when the cancer cells have starved normal tissues of essential nutrients.

See the blue Answers tab at the back of the book.

CHECKPOINT

29. An illness characterized by mutations that disrupt normal control processes and produce potentially malignant cells is termed _____.

30. Define metastasis.

3-10 Differentiation is cellular specialization as a result of gene activation or repression

Learning Objective Define differentiation and explain its importance.

All the somatic cells that make up an individual have the same chromosomes and genes. Why then are liver cells, fat cells, and nerve cells quite different from each other in appearance and function? These differences exist because, in each case, a different set of genes has been repressed, or turned *off*. In other words, these cells differ because liver cells have one set of genes accessible for transcription, or activation, and fat cells have another. When a gene is functionally eliminated, the cell loses its ability to make a particular protein and to perform any functions involving that protein. As more genes are switched off, the cell's functions become more restricted or specialized. This development of specific cellular characteristics and functions that are different from the original cell is called **differentiation**.

Fertilization produces a single cell with all its genetic potential intact. A period of repeated cell divisions follows, and differentiation begins as the number of cells increases. Differentiation produces specialized cells with limited capabilities. These cells form organized collections known as *tissues*, each with different functional roles. (In the next chapter, we examine the structure and function of tissues, and the role of tissue interactions in the maintenance of homeostasis.)

CHECKPOINT

31. Define differentiation.

See the blue Answers tab at the back of the book.

RELATED CLINICAL TERMS

carcinogen (kar-SIN-ō-jen): A cancer-causing agent.

chemotherapy: The administration of drugs that either kill cancerous tissues or prevent mitotic divisions.

oncologists (on-KOL-o-jists): Physicians who specialize in identifying and treating cancers.

recombinant DNA: DNA created by inserting (splicing) a specific gene from one organism into the DNA strand of another organism.

remission: A stage in which a tumor stops growing or becomes smaller; a major goal of cancer treatment.

3

3 Chapter Review

Summary Outline

3-1 **The study of cells provides the foundation for understanding human physiology** *p. 58*

1. Modern **cell theory** includes several basic concepts: (1) **Cells** are the building blocks of all plants and animals; (2) cells are the smallest functioning units of life; (3) cells are produced by the division of preexisting cells; and (4) each cell maintains homeostasis *(Figure 3-1)*.

2. Light and electron microscopes are important tools used in **cytology**, the study of the structure and function of cells.

3. A cell is surrounded by **extracellular fluid**—specifically, **interstitial fluid**. The cell's outer boundary, the **plasma membrane (cell membrane)**, separates the **cytoplasm**, or cell contents, from the extracellular fluid *(Spotlight Figure 3-2)*.

3-2 **The plasma membrane separates the cell from its surrounding environment and performs various functions** *p. 59*

4. The functions of the plasma membrane include (1) physical isolation, (2) control of the exchange of materials with the cell's surroundings, (3) sensitivity, and (4) structural support.

5. The plasma membrane, or cell membrane, contains lipids, proteins, and carbohydrates. Its major components, lipid molecules, form a **phospholipid bilayer** *(Figure 3-3)*.

6. Membrane proteins may function as receptors, channels, carriers, enzymes, anchors, or identifiers *(Table 3-1)*.

3-3 **Diffusion is a passive transport process that assists membrane passage** *p. 63*

7. Plasma membranes are **selectively permeable**.

8. **Diffusion** is the movement of a substance from an area where its concentration is relatively high to an area where its concentration is lower. Diffusion occurs until the **concentration gradient** is eliminated *(Figures 3-4 and 3-5)*.

9. **Osmosis** is the diffusion of water across a selectively permeable membrane in response to differences in concentration. The force of movement is **osmotic pressure** *(Figures 3-6 and 3-7)*.

3-4 **Carrier-mediated and vesicular transport processes assist membrane passage** *p. 68*

10. **Facilitated diffusion** is a type of **carrier-mediated transport** and requires the presence of carrier proteins in the membrane *(Figure 3-8)*.

11. **Active transport** processes consume ATP and are independent of concentration gradients. Some **ion pumps** are **exchange pumps** *(Figure 3-9)*.

12. In **vesicular transport**, material moves into or out of a cell in membranous sacs. Movement into the cell occurs through **endocytosis**, an active process that includes **receptor-mediated endocytosis, pinocytosis** ("cell-drinking"), and **phagocytosis** ("cell-eating"). Movement of material out of the cell occurs through **exocytosis** *(Figures 3-10 and 3-11; Table 3-2)*.

3-5 **Organelles within the cytoplasm perform specific functions** *p. 74*

13. The *cytoplasm* surrounds the nucleus and contains a fluid cytosol and intracellular structures called organelles.

14. The **cytosol** *(intracellular fluid)* differs in composition from the extracellular fluid that surrounds most cells of the body.

15. Membrane-enclosed **organelles** are surrounded by phospholipid membranes that isolate them from the cytosol. Membranous organelles include the endoplasmic reticulum, the nucleus, the Golgi apparatus, lysosomes, and mitochondria *(Spotlight Figure 3-2)*.

16. Nonmembranous organelles are always in contact with the cytosol. They include the cytoskeleton, microvilli, centrioles, cilia, flagella, proteasomes, and ribosomes *(Spotlight Figure 3-2)*.

17. The **cytoskeleton** gives the cytoplasm strength and flexibility. Its main components are **microfilaments, intermediate filaments**, and **microtubules** *(Figure 3-12)*.

18. **Microvilli** are small projections of the plasma membrane that increase the surface area exposed to the extracellular environment *(Figure 3-12)*.

19. **Centrioles** direct the movement of chromosomes during cell division.

20. Multiple motile **cilia** move fluids or secretions across the cell surface by beating rhythmically. A single **primary cilium** is sensitive to environmental stimuli.

21. **Flagella** move a cell through surrounding fluid.

22. A **ribosome** manufactures proteins. **Free ribosomes** are in the cytoplasm, and **fixed ribosomes** are attached to the endoplasmic reticulum.

23. **Proteasomes** remove and break down damaged or abnormal proteins.

24. The **endoplasmic reticulum (ER)** is a network of intracellular membranes. **Rough endoplasmic reticulum (RER)** contains ribosomes and is involved in protein synthesis. **Smooth endoplasmic reticulum (SER)** does not contain ribosomes. It is involved in lipid and carbohydrate synthesis (*Figure 3-13; Spotlight Figure 3-17*).

25. The **Golgi apparatus** forms **secretory vesicles** and new membrane components, and it packages *lysosomes*. Secretions are discharged from the cell by exocytosis (*Spotlight Figure 3-2, Figure 3-14, Spotlight Figure 3-17*).

26. **Lysosomes** are vesicles filled with digestive enzymes. Their functions include ridding the cell of bacteria and debris.

27. **Mitochondria** are responsible for 95 percent of the ATP production within a typical cell. The **matrix**, or fluid contents of a mitochondrion, lies inside **cristae**, or folds of an inner mitochondrial membrane (*Figure 3-18*).

3-6 The nucleus contains DNA and enzymes essential for controlling cellular activities *p. 79*

28. The **nucleus** is the control center for cellular activities. It is surrounded by a **nuclear envelope,** through which it communicates with the cytosol by way of **nuclear pores** (*Figure 3-19*).

29. The nucleus controls the cell by directing the synthesis of specific proteins using information stored in the DNA of **chromosomes** (*Figure 3-20*).

30. The cell's information storage system, the **genetic code,** is called a *triplet code* because a sequence of three nitrogenous bases identifies a single amino acid. Each **gene** consists of all the DNA triplets needed to produce a specific protein (*Table 3-3*).

3-7 DNA controls protein synthesis, cell structure, and cell function *p. 84*

31. **Protein synthesis** includes both *transcription*, which occurs in the nucleus, and *translation,* which occurs in the cytoplasm.

32. During **transcription**, a strand of **messenger RNA (mRNA)** is formed and carries protein-making instructions from the nucleus to the cytoplasm (*Figure 3-21*).

33. During **translation**, a functional protein is constructed using the information contained in an mRNA strand. Each triplet of nitrogenous bases along the mRNA strand is a **codon**. The sequence of codons determines the sequence of amino acids in the protein.

34. During translation, complementary base pairing of **anticodons** and mRNA codons occurs, and **transfer RNA (tRNA)** molecules bring amino acids to the ribosome. Translation includes three phases: **initiation, elongation**, and **termination**.

3-8 Stages of a cell's life cycle include interphase, mitosis, and cytokinesis *p. 87*

35. **Cell division** is the reproduction of cells. **Apoptosis** is the genetically controlled death of cells. **Mitosis** is the nuclear division of **somatic** (body) **cells**.

36. Most somatic cells are in **interphase** most of the time. Cells preparing for mitosis undergo **DNA replication** in this phase (*Figures 3-23* and *3-24*).

37. Mitosis proceeds in four stages: **prophase, metaphase, anaphase,** and **telophase** (*Figure 3-24*).

38. During **cytokinesis,** the cytoplasm divides, producing two identical daughter cells.

3-9 Tumors and cancers are characterized by abnormal cell growth and division *p. 90*

39. Produced by abnormal cell growth and division, a **tumor**, or *neoplasm*, can be **benign** (non-cancerous) or **malignant** (able to invade other tissues). **Cancer** is a disease characterized by the presence of malignant tumors. Over time, cancer cells tend to spread to new areas of the body.

3-10 Differentiation is cellular specialization as a result of gene activation or repression *p. 91*

40. **Differentiation** is a process of specialization that produces cells with limited capabilities. These specialized cells form organized collections called *tissues*, each of which has specific functional roles.

Level 1 Reviewing Facts and Terms

Match each item in column A with the most closely related item in column B. Place letters for answers in the spaces provided.

COLUMN A

_____ **1.** Golgi apparatus
_____ **2.** Osmosis
_____ **3.** Hypotonic solution
_____ **4.** Hypertonic solution

_____ **5.** Isotonic solution
_____ **6.** Facilitated diffusion
_____ **7.** Carrier proteins
_____ **8.** Vesicular transport
_____ **9.** Cytosol
_____ **10.** Cytoskeleton
_____ **11.** Microvilli
_____ **12.** Ribosomes
_____ **13.** Mitochondria
_____ **14.** Lysosomes
_____ **15.** Nucleus
_____ **16.** Chromosomes
_____ **17.** Nucleolus

COLUMN B

a. Causes water to move out of a cell
b. Passive carrier-mediated transport
c. Endocytosis, exocytosis
d. Diffusion of water across a selectively permeable membrane
e. Cisternae
f. Normal saline is an example
g. Ion pump
h. Causes water to move into a cell
i. Manufacture proteins
j. Digestive enzymes
k. Internal protein framework
l. Control center for cellular operations
m. Intracellular fluid
n. DNA strands
o. Cristae
p. Synthesizes ribosome components
q. Increase cell surface area

18. The study of the structure and function of cells is called
 (a) histology.
 (b) cytology.
 (c) physiology.
 (d) biology.

19. The proteins in the plasma membranes may function as
 (a) receptors and channels.
 (b) carriers and enzymes.
 (c) anchors and identifiers.
 (d) a, b, and c are correct.

20. In the following diagram, identify the type of solution (hypertonic, hypotonic, or isotonic) in which each red blood cell is immersed.

Water molecules   Solute molecules

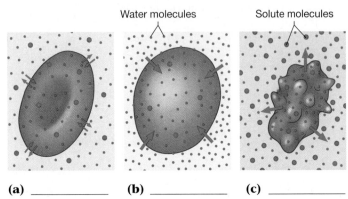

(a) _____   **(b)** _____   **(c)** _____

21. All of the following are passive membrane transport processes *except*
 (a) diffusion.
 (b) facilitated diffusion.
 (c) vesicular transport.
 (d) osmosis.

22. _____ ion concentrations are high in the extracellular fluids, and _____ ion concentrations are high in the cytoplasm.
 (a) Calcium, magnesium
 (b) Chloride, sodium
 (c) Potassium, sodium
 (d) Sodium, potassium

23. Structures that perform specific functions within the cell are
 (a) organs.
 (b) organisms.
 (c) organelles.
 (d) chromosomes.

24. The assembly of a functional protein using the information provided by an mRNA strand is
 (a) translation.
 (b) transcription.
 (c) replication.
 (d) gene activation.

25. The term *differentiation* refers to
   (a) the loss of genes from cells.
   (b) the acquisition of new functional capabilities by cells.
   (c) the production of functionally specialized cells.
   (d) the division of genes among different types of cells.

26. What are the four general functions of the plasma membrane?

27. By what three major transport processes do substances get into and out of cells?

28. What are the four major functions of the endoplasmic reticulum?

Level 2 Reviewing Concepts

29. Diffusion is important in body fluids because this process tends to
   (a) increase local concentration gradients.
   (b) eliminate local concentration gradients.
   (c) move substances against their concentration gradients.
   (d) create concentration gradients.

30. When placed in a _____ solution, a cell will lose water through osmosis. The process results in the _____ of red blood cells.
   (a) hypotonic, crenation
   (b) hypertonic, crenation
   (c) isotonic, hemolysis
   (d) hypotonic, hemolysis

31. Suppose that a DNA segment has the following nucleotide sequence: CTC ATA CGA TTC AAG TTA. Which of the following nucleotide sequences would be found in a complementary mRNA strand?
   (a) GAG UAU GAU AAC UUG AAU
   (b) GAG TAT GCT AAG TTC AAT
   (c) GAG UAU GCU AAG UUC AAU
   (d) GUG UAU GGA UUG AAC GGU

32. How many amino acids are coded in the DNA segment in the previous question?
   (a) 18
   (b) 9
   (c) 6
   (d) 3

33. Construct a simple table indicating the similarities of and differences between facilitated diffusion and active transport.

34. How does the cytosol, or intracellular fluid, differ in composition from the extracellular fluid?

35. What are the products of transcription and translation?

36. List the stages of mitosis, and briefly describe the events that occur in each.

37. What is cytokinesis, and what role does it play in the cell cycle?

Level 3 Critical Thinking and Clinical Applications

38. The transport of a certain molecule exhibits the following characteristics: (1) The molecule moves down its concentration gradient; (2) at concentrations above a given level, there is no increase in the rate of transport; and (3) cellular energy is not required for transport to occur. Which type of transport process is at work?

39. Solutions A and B are separated by a selectively permeable membrane. Over time, the level of fluid on side A increases. Which solution initially had the higher concentration of solute?

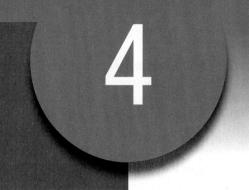

The Tissue Level of Organization

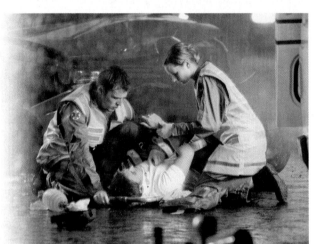

Learning Objectives

These objectives tell you what you should be able to do after completing the chapter. They correspond by number to this chapter's sections.

4-1 Identify the body's four basic types of tissues and describe their roles.

4-2 Describe the characteristics and functions of epithelial cells.

4-3 Describe the relationship between form and function for each type of epithelium.

4-4 Compare the structures and functions of the various types of connective tissues.

4-5 Explain how epithelial and connective tissues combine to form four types of tissue membranes, and specify the functions of each.

4-6 Describe the three types of muscle tissue and the special structural features of each.

4-7 Discuss the basic structure and role of neural tissue.

4-8 Describe how injuries affect the tissues of the body.

4-9 Describe how aging affects the tissues of the body.

An Introduction to the Tissue Level of Organization

In this chapter, we discuss how a variety of cell types arranged in various combinations form tissues, which are structures with distinct structural and functional properties. Tissues in combination form organs, such as the heart and liver, and in turn organs can be grouped into 11 organ systems.

Build Your Knowledge

The Build Your Knowledge feature reminds you of what you already know and prepares you to learn new material. Be sure to read every Build Your Knowledge box or page so that you can build your knowledge—and confidence!

Recall that a tissue is made up of similar cells working together to perform a specific function (as you saw in **Chapter 1: An Introduction to Anatomy and Physiology**). Our example there was cardiac muscle tissue. This tissue combines with other tissues to form the heart. The heart, blood, and blood vessels are the components of the cardiovascular system. ↺ **p. 4**

4-1 The four tissue types are epithelial, connective, muscle, and neural

Learning Objective Identify the body's four basic types of tissues and describe their roles.

No single cell is able to perform the many functions of the human body. Instead, through differentiation, each cell specializes to perform a relatively restricted range of functions. There are trillions of individual cells in the human body, but only about 200 different types of cells. These cell types combine to form **tissues**, collections of specialized cells and cell products that perform a limited number of functions.

Build Your Knowledge

Recall that differentiation is the development of specific cellular characteristics and functions that are different from the original cell. This cellular specialization occurs as different genes are activated or repressed (as you saw in **Chapter 3: The Cellular Level of Organization**). This process underlies why cells such as liver cells, fat cells, and nerve cells differ in appearance and function. ↺ **p. 85**

Histology (*histos*, tissue) is the study of tissues. Histologists recognize four basic *types* of tissues: *epithelial tissue, connective tissue, muscle tissue*, and *neural tissue* (**Figure 4-1**).

CHECKPOINT

1. Define histology.

2. List the four basic types of tissues in the body.

See the blue Answers tab at the back of the book.

4-2 Epithelial tissue covers body surfaces, lines cavities and tubular structures, and serves essential functions

Learning Objective Describe the characteristics and functions of epithelial cells.

Our discussion begins with *epithelial tissue*, because it includes a familiar feature—the surface of your skin. **Epithelial tissue** includes epithelia and *glands*. **Epithelia** (ep-i-THĒ-lē-a; singular, *epithelium*) are layers of cells that cover internal or external surfaces. **Glands** are composed of fluid-secreting cells derived from epithelia.

Epithelia have the following important characteristics:

- Cells that are bound closely together. In other tissue types, the cells are often widely separated by extracellular materials.

4

Figure 4-1 An Orientation to the Tissues of the Body.

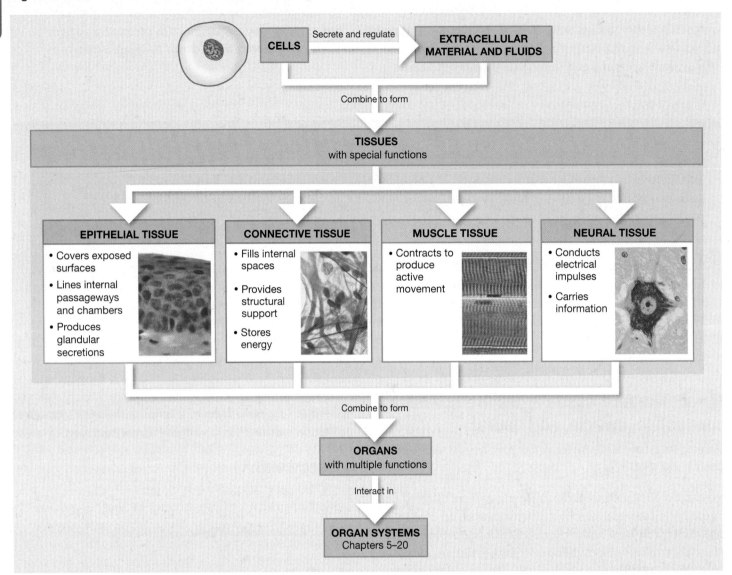

- A free (apical) surface exposed to the environment or to an internal chamber or passageway.

- Attachment to underlying connective tissue by a *basement membrane*.

- The absence of blood vessels. Because of this **avascular** (ā-VAS-kū-lar; *a-*, without + *vas,* vessel) condition, epithelial cells must obtain nutrients across their attached surface from deeper tissues or across their exposed surfaces.

- Continual replacement or regeneration of epithelial cells that are damaged or lost at the exposed surface.

Epithelia cover both external and internal body surfaces. In addition to covering the skin, epithelia line internal passageways that open to the outside world, such as the digestive, respiratory, reproductive, and urinary tracts. These epithelia form selective barriers that separate the deep tissues of the body from the external environment.

Epithelia also line internal cavities and passageways, such as the body cavities surrounding the lungs and heart; the fluid-filled chambers in the brain, eye, and internal ear; and the inner surfaces of the heart and blood vessels. These epithelia prevent friction, regulate the fluid composition of internal cavities, and restrict communication between the blood and tissue fluids.

Functions of Epithelia

Epithelia perform four essential functions. They:

1. ***Provide physical protection.*** Epithelia protect exposed and internal surfaces from abrasion, dehydration, and destruction by chemical or biological agents. For

example, as long as it remains intact, the epithelium of your skin resists impacts and scrapes, restricts water loss, and prevents bacteria from invading underlying structures.

2. ***Control permeability.*** Any substance that enters or leaves the body must cross an epithelium. Some epithelia are relatively impermeable; others are easily crossed by compounds as large as proteins.

3. ***Provide sensation.*** Specialized epithelial cells can detect changes in the environment and relay information about such changes to the nervous system. For example, touch receptors in the deepest layers of the epithelium of the skin respond to touch by stimulating neighboring sensory nerves.

4. ***Produce specialized secretions.*** Epithelial cells that produce secretions are called **gland cells**. Individual gland cells are typically scattered among other cell types in an epithelium. In a **glandular epithelium**, most or all of the cells actively produce secretions. These secretions are classified according to where they are discharged:

- **Exocrine** (*exo-*, outside + *krinein*, to secrete) secretions are discharged onto the surface of the epithelium. Examples include enzymes entering the digestive tract, perspiration on the skin, and milk produced by mammary glands.

- **Endocrine** (*endo-*, inside) secretions are released into the surrounding tissue (interstitial) fluid and blood. These secretions, called *hormones*, act as chemical messengers and regulate or coordinate the activities of other tissues, organs, and organ systems. (We discuss hormones further in Chapter 10.) Endocrine secretions are produced in organs such as the pancreas, and thyroid and pituitary glands.

Intercellular Connections

To be effective in protecting other tissues, epithelial cells must remain firmly attached to the basement membrane and to one another to form a complete cover or lining. If an epithelium is damaged or the connections are broken, it is no longer an effective barrier. For example, when the epithelium of the skin is damaged by a burn or an abrasion, bacteria can enter underlying tissues and cause an infection.

Undamaged epithelia form effective barriers because of intercellular connections that involve either large areas of opposing plasma membranes or specialized attachment sites. The large areas of opposing plasma membranes are interconnected by transmembrane proteins called *cell adhesion*

molecules (CAMs). These proteins bind to each other and extracellular materials by a thin layer of *proteoglycans* (a protein–polysaccharide mixture).

More specialized attachment sites that attach a cell to another cell or to extracellular materials are known as **cell junctions**. Three common cell junctions are *tight junctions, gap junctions*, and *desmosomes* (**Figure 4-2**).

At a **tight junction**, the lipid layers of adjacent plasma membranes are tightly bound together by interlocking membrane proteins (**Figure 4-2a,c**). Inferior to the tight junctions, a continuous *adhesion belt* forms a band that encircles cells and binds them to their neighbors. The bands are connected to a network of actin filaments in the cytoskeleton.

Tight junctions prevent the passage of water and solutes between cells. These junctions are common between epithelial cells exposed to harsh chemicals or powerful enzymes. For example, tight junctions between epithelial cells lining the digestive tract keep digestive enzymes, stomach acids, or waste products from damaging underlying tissues.

Some epithelial functions require rapid intercellular communication. At a **gap junction**, two cells are held together by embedded membrane proteins called *connexons* (**Figure 4-2b**). Together, the connexons form a narrow passageway that lets small molecules and ions pass from cell to cell. Gap junctions are most abundant in cardiac muscle and smooth muscle tissue, where they are essential to the coordination of muscle contractions. They also interconnect cells in ciliated epithelia (discussed shortly).

Most epithelial cells are subject to mechanical stresses such as stretching, bending, twisting, or compression. For this reason, they must have durable interconnections. At a **desmosome** (DEZ-mō-sōm; *desmos*, ligament + *soma*, body), the plasma membranes of two cells are locked together by CAMs and proteoglycans between the opposite dense areas of each cell. Each *dense area* is linked to the cytoskeleton by a network of intermediate filaments (**Figure 4-2d**).

Desmosomes that form a small disc are called *spot desmosomes. Hemidesmosomes* resemble half of a spot desmosome and attach a cell to the basement membrane (**Figure 4-2e**). Desmosomes are abundant between cells in the superficial layers of the skin. As a result, damaged skin cells are usually lost in sheets rather than as individual cells. (That is why your skin peels after a sunburn, rather than coming off as a powder.)

The Epithelial Surface

The *apical surface* of epithelial cells is exposed to an internal or external environment. The surfaces of these cells often have specialized structures unlike other body cells (**Figure 4-3**).

Figure 4-2 Cell Junctions.

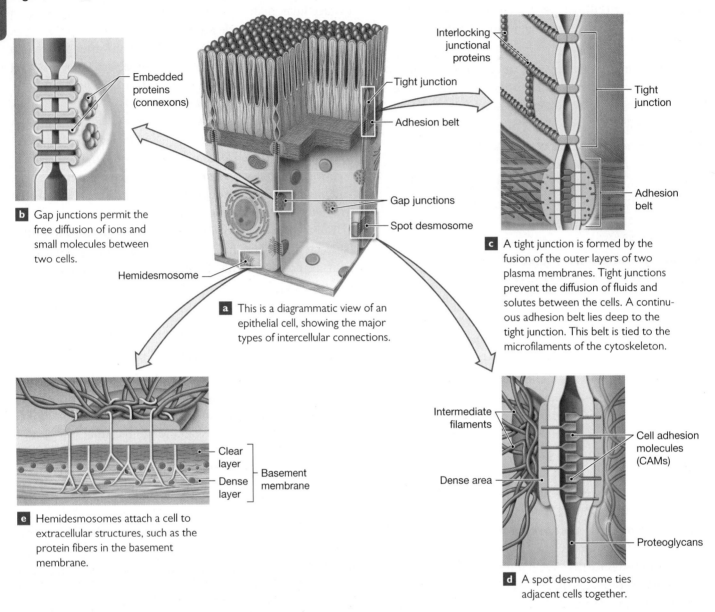

b Gap junctions permit the free diffusion of ions and small molecules between two cells.

Embedded proteins (connexons)

Hemidesmosome

Tight junction

Adhesion belt

Gap junctions

Spot desmosome

a This is a diagrammatic view of an epithelial cell, showing the major types of intercellular connections.

Interlocking junctional proteins

Tight junction

Adhesion belt

c A tight junction is formed by the fusion of the outer layers of two plasma membranes. Tight junctions prevent the diffusion of fluids and solutes between the cells. A continuous adhesion belt lies deep to the tight junction. This belt is tied to the microfilaments of the cytoskeleton.

Clear layer

Dense layer

Basement membrane

e Hemidesmosomes attach a cell to extracellular structures, such as the protein fibers in the basement membrane.

Intermediate filaments

Dense area

Cell adhesion molecules (CAMs)

Proteoglycans

d A spot desmosome ties adjacent cells together.

Many epithelia that line internal passageways have microvilli on their exposed surfaces. ⤴ p. 70 Microvilli may vary in number from just a few to so many that they carpet the entire surface. They are especially abundant on epithelial surfaces where absorption and secretion take place, such as portions of the digestive system and kidneys. The epithelial cells in these locations are transport specialists. A cell with microvilli has at least 20 times the surface area of a cell without them. The greater the surface area of the plasma membrane, the more transport proteins are exposed to the extracellular environment.

Some epithelia contain cilia on their exposed surfaces. ⤴ p. 71 A typical cell within a *ciliated epithelium* has roughly 250 cilia that beat in a coordinated manner to move materials across the epithelial surface. For example, the ciliated epithelium that lines the respiratory tract moves mucus-trapped irritants away from the lungs and toward the throat.

The Basement Membrane

Epithelial cells not only must adhere to one another but also must remain firmly connected to the rest of the body. This function is performed by the **basement membrane**, which lies between the epithelium and underlying connective tissues (**Figure 4-3**). There are no cells within the basement

Figure 4-3 The Surfaces of Epithelial Cells. The surfaces of most epithelia are specialized for specific functions. In this diagram of a generalized epithelium, the free (apical) surfaces of different cells bear microvilli or cilia. Mitochondria are shown concentrated near the basal surface of the cells, where they likely provide energy for the cell's transport activities.

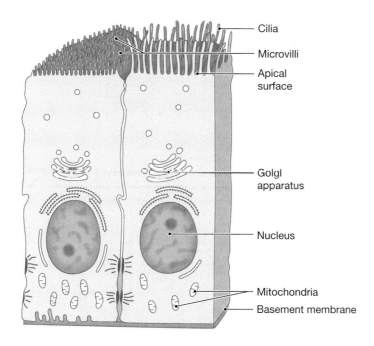

Cilia
Microvilli
Apical surface
Golgi apparatus
Nucleus
Mitochondria
Basement membrane

Build Your Knowledge

Epithelial cells of certain body surfaces are transport specialists. Recall that the transport of materials across plasma membranes involves passive and active processes (as you saw in **Chapter 3: The Cellular Level of Organization**). Active processes require the cell to expend energy. The three main transport processes involved in getting substances into and out of cells are (1) diffusion, (2) carrier-mediated transport, and (3) vesicular transport. Diffusion is a passive process. Carrier-mediated transport includes both passive and active processes. Vesicular transport is an active process. ⟳ **p. 69**

membrane, which consists of a network of protein fibers. The epithelial cells adjacent to the basement membrane are firmly attached to these protein fibers by hemidesmosomes. In addition to providing strength and resisting distortion, the basement membrane also acts as a barrier. It restricts proteins and other large molecules from moving from the underlying connective tissue into the epithelium.

Epithelial Renewal and Repair

An epithelium must continually repair and renew itself. Epithelial cells may survive for just a day or two, because they are lost or destroyed by exposure to disruptive enzymes, toxic chemicals, pathogenic microorganisms, or mechanical abrasion. The only way the epithelium can maintain its structure over time is through the continuous division of unspecialized cells known as **stem cells,** or *germinative cells*. These cells are found in the deepest layers of the epithelium, near the basement membrane.

CHECKPOINT

3. List five important characteristics of epithelial tissue.

4. Identify four essential functions of epithelial tissue.

5. Identify the three main types of epithelial cell junctions.

6. What physiological functions are enhanced by the presence of microvilli or cilia on epithelial cells?

See the blue Answers tab at the back of the book.

4-3 Cell shape and number of layers determine the classification of epithelia

Learning Objective Describe the relationship between form and function for each type of epithelium.

There are many different specialized types of epithelia. They can easily be classified according to the number of cell layers and the shape of the exposed cells. This classification scheme recognizes two types of layering—*simple* and *stratified*—and three cell shapes—*squamous, cuboidal,* and *columnar* (**Table 4-1**).

Cell Layers

A **simple epithelium** consists of a single layer of cells covering the basement membrane. Simple epithelia are thin. A single layer of cells is fragile and cannot provide much mechanical protection. For this reason, simple epithelia are found only in protected areas inside the body. They line internal compartments and passageways, including the pleural, pericardial, and peritoneal cavities, the heart chambers, and blood vessels.

Simple epithelia are also characteristic of regions where secretion or absorption occurs. Examples are the lining of the intestines and the gas-exchange surfaces of the lungs. In these places, thinness is an advantage. It reduces the time for materials to cross the epithelial barrier.

Table 4-1	Classifying Epithelia		
	Squamous	**Cuboidal**	**Columnar**
Simple	Simple squamous epithelium	Simple cuboidal epithelium	Simple columnar epithelium
Stratified	Stratified squamous epithelium	Stratified cuboidal epithelium	Stratified columnar epithelium

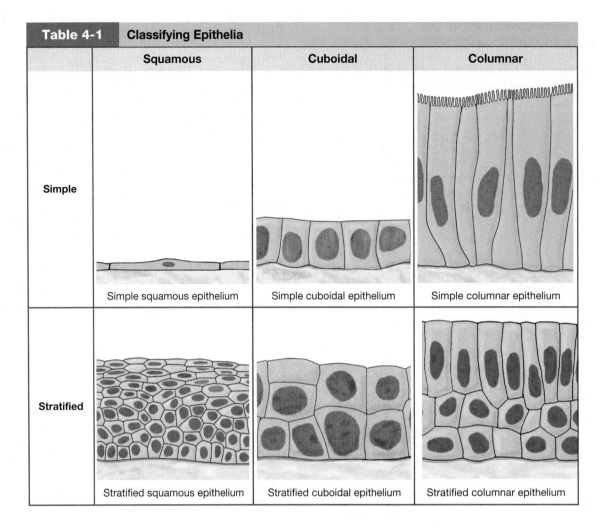

A **stratified epithelium** provides greater protection because it has several layers of cells above the basement membrane. Stratified epithelia are usually found in areas exposed to mechanical or chemical stresses. Examples include the surface of the skin and the lining of the mouth.

Cell Shapes

In sectional view (perpendicular to the exposed surface and basement membrane), cells at the surface of the epithelium usually have one of three basic shapes.

1. *Squamous.* In a **squamous epithelium** (SKWĀ-mus; *squama,* plate or scale), the cells are thin and flat. The nucleus occupies the thickest portion of each cell. Viewed from the surface, the cells look like fried eggs laid side by side.

2. *Cuboidal.* The cells of a **cuboidal epithelium** resemble little hexagonal (six-sided) boxes when seen from their free, apical surfaces. In typical sectional view, they appear square. The round nuclei lie near the center of each cell, and the distance between neighboring nuclei is about equal to the height of the epithelium.

3. *Columnar.* In a **columnar epithelium**, the cells are also hexagonal but taller and more slender, resembling rectangles in sectional view. The nuclei are crowded into a narrow band close to the basement membrane. The height of the epithelium is several times the distance between two nuclei.

Classification of Epithelia

The two basic epithelial arrangements (simple and stratified) and the three possible cell shapes (squamous, cuboidal, and columnar) enable us to describe almost every epithelium in the body. We will focus here on only a few major types of epithelia.

Simple Squamous Epithelia

A **simple squamous epithelium** is found in protected regions where absorption takes place or where a slippery surface reduces friction (**Figure 4-4a**). Examples are portions of the kidney tubules, the exchange surfaces of the lungs, the linings of the pericardial, pleural, and peritoneal cavities, blood vessels, and the inner surfaces of the heart.

Figure 4-4 Simple Epithelia.

Simple Squamous Epithelium

LOCATIONS: Epithelia lining pleural, pericardial, and peritoneal cavities; lining heart and blood vessels; portions of kidney tubules (thin sections of nephron loops); inner lining of cornea; alveoli (air sacs) of lungs

FUNCTIONS: Reduces friction; controls vessel permeability; performs absorption and secretion

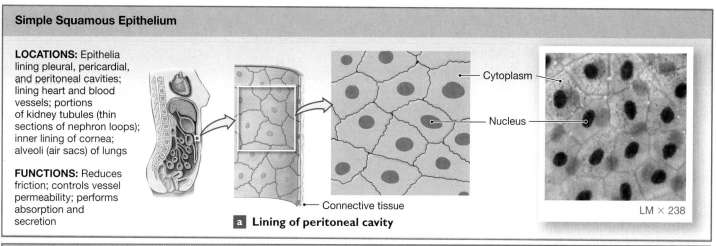

Cytoplasm

Nucleus

Connective tissue

a **Lining of peritoneal cavity**

LM × 238

Simple Cuboidal Epithelium

LOCATIONS: Glands; ducts; portions of kidney tubules; thyroid gland

FUNCTIONS: Limited protection, secretion, absorption

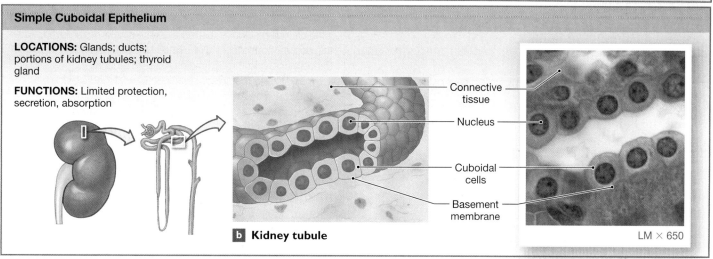

Connective tissue

Nucleus

Cuboidal cells

Basement membrane

b **Kidney tubule**

LM × 650

Simple Columnar Epithelium

LOCATIONS: Lining of stomach, intestine, gallbladder, uterine tubes, and collecting ducts of kidneys

FUNCTIONS: Protection, secretion, absorption

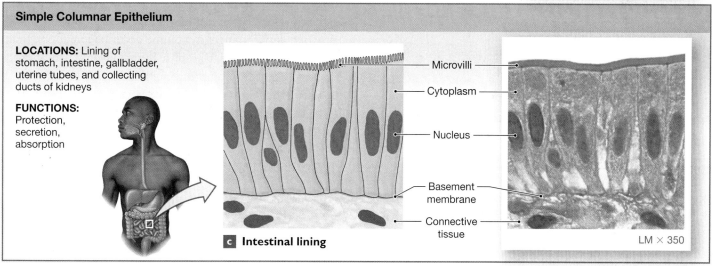

Microvilli

Cytoplasm

Nucleus

Basement membrane

Connective tissue

c **Intestinal lining**

LM × 350

4

Simple Cuboidal Epithelia

A **simple cuboidal epithelium** provides limited protection and occurs where secretion or absorption takes place (**Figure 4-4b**). These functions are enhanced by larger cells, which have more room for the necessary organelles. Simple cuboidal epithelia in the pancreas and salivary glands secrete enzymes and buffers and line the ducts that discharge these secretions. Simple cuboidal epithelia also line portions of the kidney tubules involved in producing urine.

Simple Columnar Epithelia

A **simple columnar epithelium** provides some protection and may also occur in areas of absorption or secretion (**Figure 4-4c**). This type of epithelium lines the stomach, the intestinal tract, and many excretory ducts.

Stratified Squamous Epithelia

A **stratified squamous epithelium** is found where mechanical stresses are severe. Examples include the surface of the skin and the lining of the mouth, tongue, esophagus, and anus (**Figure 4-5a**).

Stratified Cuboidal Epithelia

Stratified cuboidal epithelium is relatively rare. It occurs along the ducts of sweat glands and in the larger ducts of the mammary glands. (It is not shown with the other stratified epithelia.)

Stratified Columnar Epithelia

Stratified columnar epithelium is also relatively rare. It is found along portions of the pharynx, epiglottis, anus, urethra, and a few, large excretory ducts. If more than two layers are present, only the superficial cells are columnar. (It is also not shown with the other stratified epithelia.)

Pseudostratified Epithelia

Portions of the respiratory tract contain **pseudostratified columnar epithelium**, a columnar epithelium that includes a mixture of cell types. The distances between the cell nuclei and the exposed surface vary, so the epithelium appears layered, or stratified (**Figure 4-5b**). It is not truly stratified, though, because all the cells contact the basement membrane.

Epithelial cells of this tissue typically possess cilia. A pseudostratified ciliated columnar epithelium lines most of the nasal cavity, the trachea (windpipe) and bronchi, and portions of the male reproductive tract.

CLINICAL NOTE

Cellular Adaptation

Cells can change or adapt to their environment in order to protect themselves from injury. This process, called *cellular adaptation*, is a common and central aspect of many disease states. Cells can adapt by decreasing their size (*atrophy*), increasing their size (*hypertrophy*), increasing their numbers (*hyperplasia*), or by reversibly replacing one mature cell type with another, less mature type (*metaplasia*).

A good example of metaplasia is the response of bronchial (airway) tissues to prolonged exposure to cigarette smoke. In this process, normal columnar ciliated epithelial cells of the bronchial lining are replaced with stratified squamous epithelial cells. The newly formed replacement cells do not have cilia and do not secrete mucus. This results in a loss of two important pulmonary protective mechanisms. Bronchial metaplasia can often be reversed if the offending stimulus, usually cigarette smoke, is removed. When this occurs, normal columnar ciliated epithelial cells begin replacing the cells changed through the metaplastic process.

In addition to metaplasia, continued, prolonged exposure to cigarette smoke can result in the cancerous transformation of bronchial epithelial cells (*dysplasia*). Bronchogenic (lung) cancers are a major health problem in industrialized countries. The mortality rate is high: lung cancers represent 32 percent of all cancer deaths.

Transitional Epithelia

A **transitional epithelium** is a stratified epithelium that tolerates repeated cycles of stretching and recoiling. It is called transitional because the appearance of the epithelium changes as stretching takes place. It lines the ureters and urinary bladder, where large changes in volume occur (**Figure 4-5c**). In an empty urinary bladder, the epithelium is layered, and the outermost cells appear plump and cuboidal. In a full urinary bladder, when the volume of urine has stretched the lining to its limits, the epithelium appears flattened. It looks more like a stratified squamous epithelium.

Glandular Epithelia

Many epithelia contain gland cells that produce exocrine or endocrine secretions. Exocrine secretions are produced by exocrine glands, which discharge their products through a *duct*, or tube, onto some external or internal surface. Endocrine secretions (*hormones*) are produced by ductless endocrine glands and released into blood or tissue fluids.

Based on their structure, exocrine glands can be categorized as unicellular glands (called *mucous* or *goblet cells*) or as multicellular glands. The simplest multicellular exocrine gland is a *secretory sheet*, such as the epithelium of mucin-secreting

Figure 4-5 Stratified Epithelia.

Stratified Squamous Epithelium

LOCATIONS: Surface of skin; lining of mouth, throat, oeophague, rectum, anue, and vagina

FUNCTIONS: Provides physical protection against abrasion, pathogens, and chemical attack

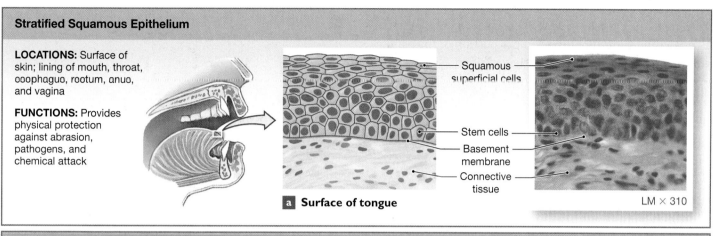

Squamous superficial cells

Stem cells

Basement membrane

Connective tissue

LM × 310

a **Surface of tongue**

Pseudostratified Ciliated Columnar Epithelium

LOCATIONS: Lining of nasal cavity, trachea, and bronchi; portions of male reproductive tract

FUNCTIONS: Protection, secretion, moves mucus with cilia

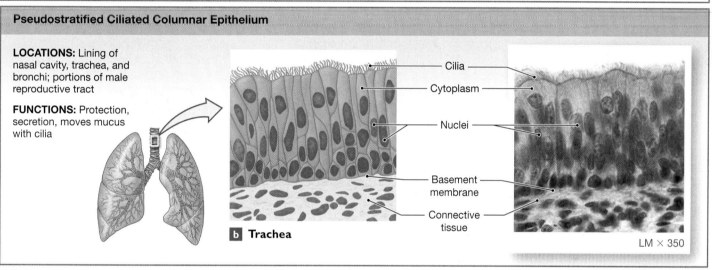

Cilia

Cytoplasm

Nuclei

Basement membrane

Connective tissue

b **Trachea**

LM × 350

Transitional Epithelium

LOCATIONS: Urinary bladder, renal pelvis, ureters

FUNCTIONS: Permits expansion and recoil after stretching

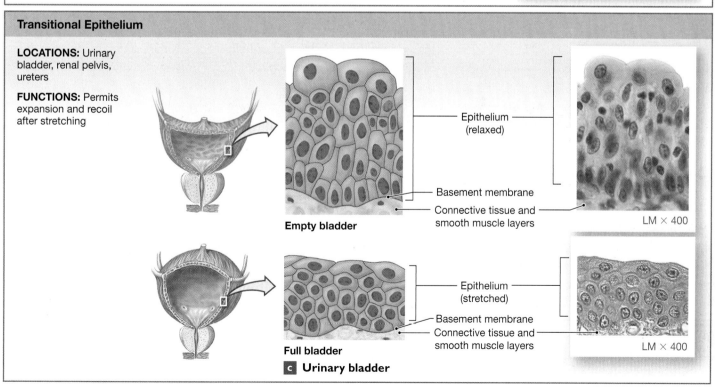

Epithelium (relaxed)

Basement membrane

Connective tissue and smooth muscle layers

LM × 400

Empty bladder

Epithelium (stretched)

Basement membrane

Connective tissue and smooth muscle layers

LM × 400

Full bladder

c **Urinary bladder**

cells that lines the stomach and protects it from its own acids and enzymes. Multicellular glands are further classified according to the branching pattern of the duct and the shape and branching pattern of the secretory portion of the gland. Additionally, exocrine glands can be classified according to their *mode of secretion* or *type of secretion*.

Mode of Secretion

A glandular epithelial cell releases its secretions by (1) *merocrine secretion*, (2) *apocrine secretion*, or (3) *holocrine secretion* (**Figure 4-6**).

Figure 4-6 Modes of Glandular Secretion.

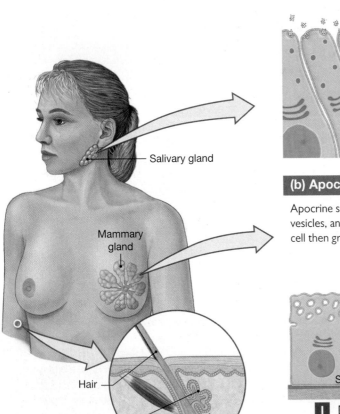

(a) Merocrine secretion

In merocrine secretion, the product is released from secretory vesicles at the apical surface of the gland cell by exocytosis.

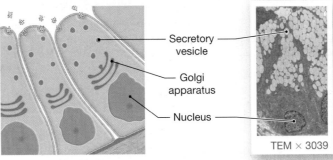

Secretory vesicle

Golgi apparatus

Nucleus

TEM × 3039

(b) Apocrine secretion

Apocrine secretion involves the loss of apical cytoplasm. Inclusions, secretory vesicles, and other cytoplasmic components are shed in the process. The gland cell then grows and repairs itself before it releases additional secretions.

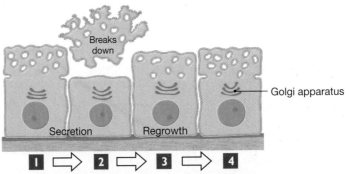

Breaks down

Golgi apparatus

Secretion   Regrowth

1   2   3   4

(c) Holocrine secretion

Holocrine secretion occurs as superficial gland cells burst. Continued secretion involves the replacement of these cells through the divisions of underlying stem cells.

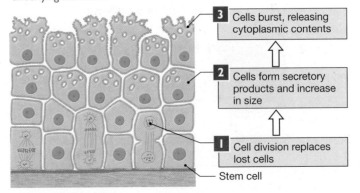

3 Cells burst, releasing cytoplasmic contents

2 Cells form secretory products and increase in size

1 Cell division replaces lost cells

Stem cell

Salivary gland

Mammary gland

Hair

Sebaceous gland

Hair follicle

Table 4-2	A Classification of Exocrine Glands	
Feature	**Description**	**Examples**
MODE OF SECRETION		
Merocrine	Secretion occurs through exocytosis.	Saliva from salivary glands; mucus in digestive and respiratory tracts; perspiration on the skin; milk in breasts
Apocrine	Secretion occurs through loss of cytoplasm containing secretory product.	Milk in breasts; viscous underarm perspiration
Holocrine	Secretion occurs through loss of entire cell containing secretory product.	Skin oils and waxy coating of hair (produced by sebaceous glands of the skin)
TYPE OF SECRETION		
Serous	Watery solution containing enzymes	Secretions of parotid salivary gland
Mucous	Thick, slippery mucus	Secretions of sublingual salivary gland
Mixed	Contains more than one type of secretion	Secretions of submandibular salivary gland (serous and mucous)

In **merocrine secretion** (MER-u-krin; *meros*, part + *krinein*, to secrete), the product is released from secretory vesicles by exocytosis (**Figure 4-6a**). ↻ p. 68 This is the most common mode of exocrine secretion. One product of merocrine secretion, *mucin*, mixes with water to form **mucus**. Mucus is an effective lubricant, a protective barrier, and a sticky trap for foreign particles and microorganisms.

Apocrine secretion (AP-ō-krin; *apo-*, off) involves the loss of both cytoplasm and the secretory product (**Figure 4-6b**). The outermost portion of the cytoplasm becomes packed with secretory vesicles before it is shed. Milk production in the mammary glands involves both merocrine and apocrine secretions. Merocrine and apocrine secretions leave a cell intact and able to continue secreting.

Holocrine secretion (HOL-ō-krin; *holos*, entire) does not leave a cell intact. Instead, the entire cell becomes packed with secretory vesicles and then bursts, releasing the secretion, but killing the cell (**Figure 4-6c**). Sebaceous glands, associated with hair follicles, produce an oily hair coating by holocrine secretion.

Type of Secretion

There are many kinds of exocrine secretions, all performing a variety of functions. Examples are enzymes entering the digestive tract, perspiration on the skin, and the milk produced by mammary glands.

Based on the type or types of secretions produced, exocrine glands can also be categorized as serous, mucous, or mixed. The secretions can have a variety of functions. *Serous glands* secrete a watery solution containing enzymes. *Mucous glands* secrete mucins that form a thick, slippery mucus. *Mixed glands* contain more than one type of gland cell. They may produce two different exocrine secretions, one serous and the other mucous.

Table 4-2 summarizes the classification of exocrine glands according to their mode of secretion and type of secretion.

CLINICAL NOTE

Exfoliative Cytology

Exfoliative cytology (eks-FŌ-lē-a-tiv; *ex-*, from ō + *folium*, leaf) is the study of cells shed or removed from epithelial surfaces. The cells are examined for a variety of reasons—for example, to check for cellular changes that indicate cancer or to do genetic screening of a fetus. The cells are collected by sampling the fluids that cover the epithelia lining the respiratory, digestive, urinary, or reproductive tracts; by removing fluid from the pericardial, peritoneal, or pleural cavities; or by removing cells from an epithelial surface.

A common example of exfoliative cytology is a *Pap test*, named after Dr. George Papanicolaou, who pioneered its use. The most familiar Pap test is that for cervical cancer. The test involves scraping a small number of cells from the tip of the *cervix*, the portion of the uterus that projects into the vagina.

Amniocentesis is another important test involving exfoliative cytology. In this procedure, epithelial cells that have been shed are collected from a sample of *amniotic fluid*, the fluid that surrounds and protects a developing fetus. Examination of these cells can determine whether the fetus has a genetic abnormality, such as *Down's syndrome*, that affects the number or structure of chromosomes.

CHECKPOINT

7. Identify the three cell shapes characteristic of epithelial cells.

8. Using a light microscope, a tissue appears as a simple squamous epithelium. Can this be a sample of the skin surface? Why or why not?

9. Name the two primary types of glandular epithelia.

10. The secretory cells of sebaceous glands fill with secretions and then rupture, releasing their contents. Which mode of secretion occurs in sebaceous glands?

11. Which type of gland releases its secretions directly into the extracellular fluid?

See the blue Answers tab at the back of the book.

4-4 Connective tissue provides a protective structural framework for other tissue types

Learning Objective Compare the structures and functions of the various types of connective tissues.

Connective tissue is the most diverse tissue of the body. Bone, blood, and fat are familiar connective tissues with very different functions and characteristics. All connective tissues have three basic components: (1) specialized cells, (2) extracellular protein fibers, and (3) a fluid known as **ground substance**. The extracellular fibers and ground substance form the **matrix** that surrounds the cells. This extracellular matrix accounts for most of the volume of connective tissues. Connective tissue differs in this way from epithelial tissues, which consist almost entirely of cells.

Connective tissues occur throughout the body but are never exposed to the outside environment. Many connective tissues are highly vascular (that is, they have many blood vessels). They also contain sensory receptors that detect pain, pressure, temperature, and other stimuli. Connective tissue functions include:

- *Support and protection.* The minerals and fibers produced by connective tissue cells form a strong structural framework for the body, protect delicate organs, and surround and interconnect other tissue types.

- *Transportation of materials.* Fluid connective tissues move dissolved materials efficiently from one region of the body to another.

- *Storage of energy reserves.* Fats are stored in connective tissue cells called *adipose cells* until needed.

- *Defense of the body.* Specialized connective tissue cells respond to invasions by microorganisms through cell-to-cell interactions and the production of *antibodies.*

Based on their physical properties, connective tissues are classified into three major types (**Figure 4-7**):

Figure 4-7 Major Types of Connective Tissue.

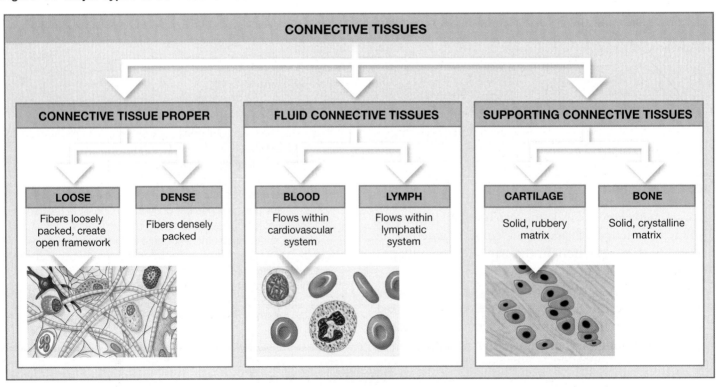

1. **Connective tissue proper** consists of many cell types within a matrix containing extracellular fibers and a syrupy ground substance. Examples are the tissue that underlies the skin, fatty tissue, and *tendons* and *ligaments*.

2. **Fluid connective tissues** have a distinctive population of cells suspended in a matrix of watery ground substance containing dissolved proteins. The two fluid connective tissues are *blood* and *lymph*.

3. **Supporting connective tissues** have a less diverse cell population than connective tissue proper, and a matrix of dense ground substance and closely packed fibers. The body contains two supporting connective tissues: *cartilage* and *bone*. The fibrous matrix of bone is said to be calcified because it contains mineral deposits (primarily calcium salts) that give the bone strength and rigidity.

Connective Tissue Proper

Connective tissue proper contains a varied cell population, extracellular fibers, and a syrupy ground substance (**Figure 4-8**). Some cells of connective tissue proper are "permanent residents." Others are not always present because they leave to defend and repair areas of injured tissue.

Cells of Connective Tissue Proper

Connective tissue proper includes these four major cell types:

* **Fibroblasts** (FĪ-brō-blasts) are the only cells that are always present in connective tissue proper. They are also the most abundant permanent, or fixed, cells in connective tissue proper. Fibroblasts produce connective tissue fibers and ground substance. **Fibrocytes** (FĪ-brō-sīts) are next in abundance and differentiate from fibroblasts. Fibrocytes maintain the connective tissue fibers of connective tissue proper.

* **Macrophages** (MAK-rō-fā-jez; *phagein*, to eat) are large phagocytic cells (*phagocytes*) scattered throughout the matrix. These "big eater" cells engulf, or *phagocytize*, damaged cells or pathogens that enter the tissue. They also release chemicals that mobilize the immune system, attracting additional macrophages and other cells involved in tissue defense. ⟳ p. 68 Macrophages that spend long periods of time in connective tissue are known as *fixed macrophages*. When an infection occurs, migrating macrophages (called *free macrophages*) are drawn to the affected area.

* **Fat cells**, also known as adipose cells or **adipocytes** (AD-i-pō-sīts), are permanent residents. A typical fat cell contains a large lipid droplet that squeezes the nucleus and other organelles to one side of the cell. The number of fat cells varies from one connective tissue to another, from one region of the body to another, and among individuals.

* **Mast cells** are small, mobile connective tissue cells often found near blood vessels. The cytoplasm of a mast cell is packed with granules filled with *histamine* and *heparin*. These chemicals are released to begin the body's defensive activities after an injury or infection (as we will discuss later in the chapter).

Figure 4-8 Cells and Fibers of Connective Tissue Proper. This diagrammatic view shows the common cell types and fibers of connective tissue proper.

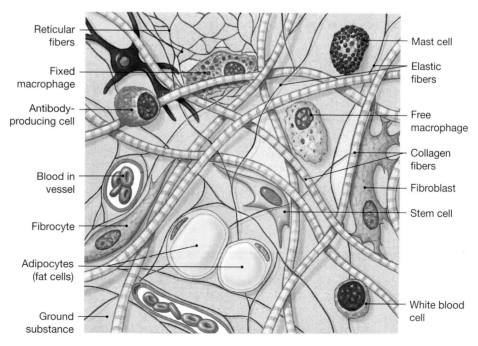

Reticular fibers
Fixed macrophage
Antibody-producing cell
Blood in vessel
Fibrocyte
Adipocytes (fat cells)
Ground substance

Mast cell
Elastic fibers
Free macrophage
Collagen fibers
Fibroblast
Stem cell
White blood cell

4

In addition to mast cells and free macrophages, both phagocytic and antibody-producing white blood cells may move through connective tissue proper. Their numbers increase markedly if the tissue is damaged, as does the production of **antibodies**, proteins that destroy invading microorganisms or foreign substances. *Stem cells* also respond to local injury by dividing to produce daughter cells that differentiate into fibroblasts, macrophages, or other connective tissue cells.

Connective Tissue Fibers

The three basic types of fibers—*collagen, elastic*, and *reticular*—are formed from protein subunits secreted by fibroblasts (**Figure 4-8**):

1. **Collagen fibers** are long, straight, and unbranched. These strong but flexible fibers are the most common fibers in connective tissue proper.

2. **Elastic fibers** contain the protein *elastin*. Elastic fibers are branched and wavy. After stretching, they return to their original length.

3. **Reticular fibers** (*reticulum*, a network) are made up of the same protein subunits as collagen fibers, but arranged differently. The least common of the three fibers, they are thinner than collagen fibers. Reticular fibers form a branching, interwoven framework in various organs.

Ground Substance

Ground substance fills the spaces between cells and surrounds connective tissue fibers (**Figure 4-8**). In normal connective tissue proper, it is clear, colorless, and similar in consistency to maple syrup. This dense consistency slows the movement of bacteria and other pathogens, making them easier for phagocytes to catch.

Types of Connective Tissue Proper

Connective tissue proper is categorized as either *loose connective tissues* or *dense connective tissues* on the basis of the relative proportions of cells, fibers, and ground substance. Loose connective tissues are the "packing materials" of the body. They fill spaces between organs, provide cushioning, and support epithelia. They also anchor blood vessels and nerves, store lipids, and provide a route for the diffusion of materials. Dense connective tissues are tough, strong, and durable. They resist tension and distortion and interconnect bones and muscles.

CLINICAL NOTE

Marfan's Syndrome

Marfan's syndrome is an inherited condition caused by the production of an abnormally weak form of *fibrillin*, a carbohydrate–protein complex important to normal connective tissue strength and elasticity. The effects of this defect are widespread because most organs contain connective tissues. The most visible sign of Marfan's syndrome involves the skeleton. Most individuals with this condition are tall and have abnormally long arms, legs, and fingers. The most serious consequences, affecting roughly 90 percent of individuals with Marfan's syndrome, are structural abnormalities in their cardiovascular systems. The most dangerous possibility is that the weakened connective tissues in the walls of major arteries, such as the aorta, may burst, causing a sudden, fatal loss of blood. Worldwide, the incidence of Marfan's syndrome is about 1 in 5000. Most cases have a family history of the disorder, but about one-fourth of the cases do not, and these result from a new mutation in the fibrillin gene.

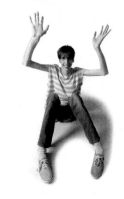

Loose Connective Tissues

Areolar tissue (*areola,* little space) is the least specialized connective tissue in adults (**Figure 4-9a**). It contains all the cells and fibers found in any connective tissue proper, as well as an extensive blood supply.

CLINICAL NOTE

Blunt Chest Trauma

The heart and great vessels are supported within the chest by strong connective tissues. These tissues allow limited movement of the heart and great vessels within the chest. The aortic arch is somewhat mobile, while the descending aorta is virtually immobile, particularly at the attachment of the fibrous *ligamentum arteriosum*. Vehicular trauma often involves a sudden and rapid deceleration, during which the heart continues to travel forward within the chest. This can place the aorta under great stress, and often results in tearing and rupture, typically at the point where the *ligamentum arteriosum* attaches. Traumatic thoracic aortic rupture has a very high mortality rate; 80–90 percent of victims die at the scene.

Figure 4-9 Loose Connective Tissues.

Areolar Tissue

LOCATIONS: Within and deep to the dermis of skin, and covered by the epithelial lining of the digestive, respiratory, and urinary tracts; between muscles; around joints, blood vessels, and nerves

FUNCTIONS: Cushions organs; provides support but permits independent movement; phagocytic cells provide defense against pathogens

Areolar tissue from pleura

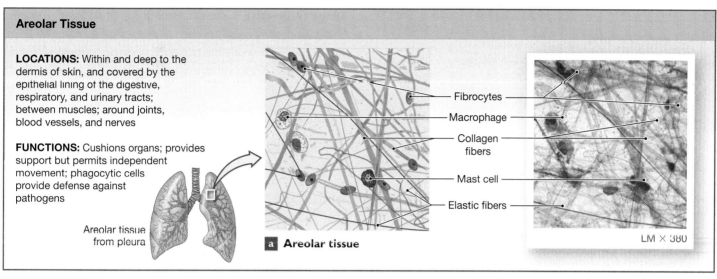

Fibrocytes
Macrophage
Collagen fibers
Mast cell
Elastic fibers

LM × 380

a **Areolar tissue**

Adipose Tissue

LOCATIONS: Deep to the skin, especially at sides, buttocks, and breasts; padding around eyes and kidneys

FUNCTIONS: Provides padding and cushions shocks; insulates (reduces heat loss); stores energy

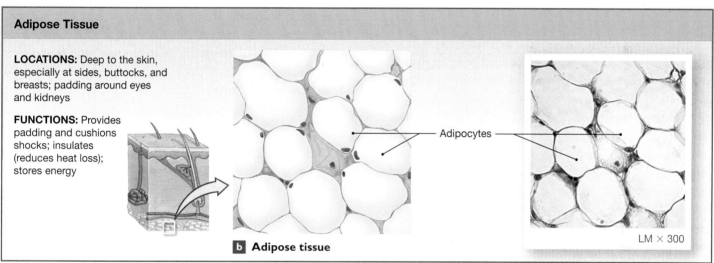

Adipocytes

LM × 300

b **Adipose tissue**

Reticular Tissue

LOCATIONS: Liver, kidney, spleen, lymph nodes, and bone marrow

FUNCTIONS: Provides supporting framework

Reticular tissue from liver

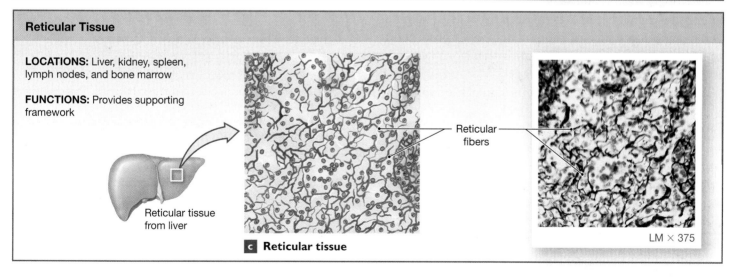

Reticular fibers

LM × 375

c **Reticular tissue**

4

EMS and Obesity

Emergency Medical Services (EMS) is thought of as an intense, exciting, and physically challenging profession. In actuality, EMS is a fairly sedentary job punctuated by short periods of intense activity. Because of this, EMS providers are at risk for gaining weight. In addition, they also run the risk of physical injury if they do not remain physically fit.

As an EMS provider, you should carefully monitor your weight and maintain a healthy lifestyle. This should include some form of regular physical exercise, rational eating, and adequate rest and relaxation. You cannot depend on the job alone to provide the exercise required to maintain optimal fitness. If your agency does not have an ongoing fitness program, encourage them to start one. The result is a healthier, safer, and more satisfying career.

Areolar tissue forms a layer that separates the skin from deeper structures. In addition to providing padding, its elastic properties allow a considerable amount of independent movement. Pinching the skin of your arm, for example, does not distort the underlying muscle. Conversely, a contracting muscle does not pull against the skin. As the muscle bulges, the areolar tissue stretches. The ample blood supply in this tissue carries wandering cells to and from the tissue and provides for the metabolic needs (oxygen and nutrients) of nearby epithelial tissue.

Adipose tissue, or fat, is a loose connective tissue containing large numbers of fat cells, or adipocytes (**Figure 4-9b**). The difference between loose connective tissue and adipose tissue is one of degree. A loose connective tissue is called adipose tissue when it becomes dominated by fat cells. Adipose tissue is another source of padding and shock absorption for the body. It also serves as insulation that slows heat loss through the skin, and it stores energy.

Adipose tissue is common under the skin of the flanks (between the last rib and the hips), buttocks, and breasts. It fills the bony sockets behind the eyes and surrounds the kidneys. It is also common beneath the epithelial lining of the pericardial and peritoneal cavities.

Reticular tissue is a loose connective tissue whose reticular fibers form a complex three-dimensional network (**Figure 4-9c**). They stabilize the positions of functional cells in lymph nodes and bone marrow and in organs such as the spleen and liver. Fixed macrophages, fibroblasts, and fibrocytes are associated with the reticular fibers. These cells are seldom visible, however, because specialized cells with other functions dominate the organs.

Dense Connective Tissues

Dense connective tissues consist mostly of collagen fibers. For this reason, they are also called *fibrous*, or *collagenous* (ko-LAJ-e-nus), tissues. The body has two types of dense connective tissues.

In **dense regular connective tissue**, the collagen fibers are parallel to each other, packed tightly, and aligned with the forces applied to the tissue. **Tendons** are cords of dense regular connective tissue that attach skeletal muscles to bones (**Figure 4-10a**). Their collagen fibers run along the length of the tendon and transfer the pull of the contracting muscle to the bone. **Ligaments** (LIG-a-ments) resemble tendons but connect one bone to another. Ligaments often contain elastic fibers as well as collagen fibers and thus can tolerate a modest amount of stretching.

In contrast, the fibers of **dense irregular connective tissue** (**Figure 4-10b**) form an interwoven meshwork in no consistent pattern. This tissue strengthens and supports areas subjected to stresses from many directions. Dense irregular connective tissue gives skin its strength and covers bone and cartilage (except at joints). It also forms a thick fibrous layer, or **capsule**, which surrounds internal organs such as the liver, kidneys, and spleen and encloses joint cavities.

Fluid Connective Tissues

Blood and **lymph** are connective tissues that contain distinctive collections of cells in a fluid matrix. Under normal conditions, the proteins dissolved in this watery matrix do

Adipose Tissue and Weight Control

Adipocytes are metabolically active cells. Their lipids are continually being broken down and replaced. When nutrients are scarce, adipocytes deflate like collapsing balloons. This deflation occurs during a weight-loss program. Because the cells are not killed but merely reduced in size, the lost weight can easily be regained in the same areas of the body.

In adults, adipocytes cannot divide. However, an excess of circulating lipids can stimulate connective tissue stem cells to divide. These cells then differentiate into additional fat cells. As a result, areas of areolar tissue can become adipose tissue after chronic overeating. In the procedure known as *liposuction*, unwanted adipose tissue is surgically removed. Because adipose tissue can regenerate through differentiation of stem cells, liposuction provides only a temporary and potentially risky solution to the problem of excess weight.

Figure 4-10 Dense Connective Tissues.

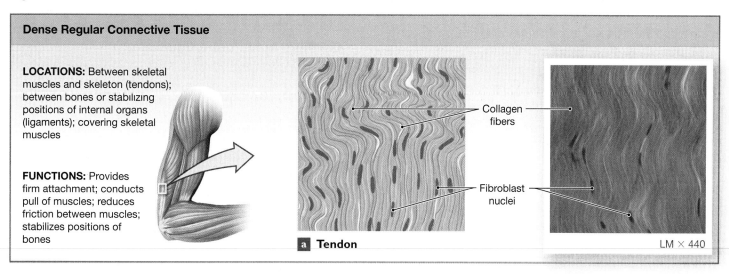

Dense Regular Connective Tissue

LOCATIONS: Between skeletal muscles and skeleton (tendons); between bones or stabilizing positions of internal organs (ligaments); covering skeletal muscles

FUNCTIONS: Provides firm attachment; conducts pull of muscles; reduces friction between muscles; stabilizes positions of bones

Collagen fibers

Fibroblast nuclei

a **Tendon**

LM × 440

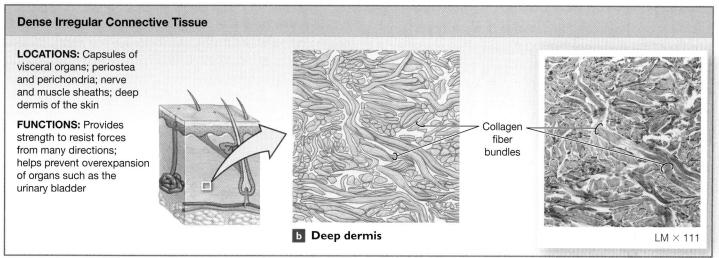

Dense Irregular Connective Tissue

LOCATIONS: Capsules of visceral organs; periostea and perichondria; nerve and muscle sheaths; deep dermis of the skin

FUNCTIONS: Provides strength to resist forces from many directions; helps prevent overexpansion of organs such as the urinary bladder

Collagen fiber bundles

b **Deep dermis**

LM × 111

not form large insoluble fibers. In blood, the watery matrix is called **plasma**.

A single cell type, the **red blood cell**, accounts for almost half the volume of blood. Red blood cells transport oxygen in the blood. Blood also contains small numbers of **white blood cells**, important cells of the immune system, and **platelets**, cell fragments that play a role in blood clotting.

Together, plasma, lymph, and interstitial fluid make up most of the extracellular fluid of the body. Plasma is confined to the blood vessels of the cardiovascular system and is kept in constant motion by contractions of the heart. As blood flows through body tissues within thin-walled vessels called *capillaries*, water and small solutes move from the plasma into the interstitial fluid surrounding the body's cells. Lymph forms as interstitial fluid drains into small passageways, or *lymphatic vessels*, that eventually return it to the cardiovascular system. Along the way, cells of the immune system monitor the composition of the lymph and respond to signs of injury and infection. This recirculation of fluid is essential for homeostasis.

Supporting Connective Tissues

Cartilage and bone are called supporting connective tissues because they provide a strong framework that supports the rest of the body. In these connective tissues, the matrix contains numerous fibers and, in some cases, deposits of solid calcium salts.

Cartilage

The matrix of **cartilage** is a firm gel containing embedded fibers. **Chondrocytes** (KON-drō-sīts) are the only cells found within the cartilage matrix. They occupy small pockets known as *lacunae* (la-KOO-nē; *lacus,* pool). Unlike other connective tissues, cartilage is avascular, so chondrocytes must obtain nutrients and eliminate waste products by diffusion through the matrix. This lack of a blood supply also limits the repair capabilities of cartilage. Structures of cartilage are covered and set apart from surrounding tissues by a **perichondrium** (per-i-KON-drē-um; *peri-,* around + *chondros,* cartilage) made up of an inner cellular layer and an outer fibrous layer.

The three major types of cartilage are *hyaline cartilage, elastic cartilage,* and *fibrocartilage* (**Figure 4-11**):

1. **Hyaline cartilage** (HĪ-uh-lin; *hyalos,* glass) is the most common type of cartilage (**Figure 4-11a**). The matrix contains closely packed collagen fibers, making hyaline cartilage tough but somewhat flexible. This type of cartilage connects the ribs to the sternum (breastbone), supports the conducting passageways of the respiratory tract, and covers opposing bone surfaces within joints.

2. **Elastic cartilage** contains numerous elastic fibers that make it extremely resilient and flexible (**Figure 4-11b**). Elastic cartilage forms the external flap (the *auricle,* or *pinna*) of the external ear, the epiglottis, an airway to the middle ear (the *auditory tube*), and small cartilages in the larynx (voice box).

3. **Fibrocartilage** has little ground substance, and its matrix is dominated by collagen fibers (**Figure 4-11c**). These fibers are densely interwoven, making this tissue extremely durable and tough. Pads of fibrocartilage lie between the spinal vertebrae, between the pubic bones of the pelvis, around tendons, and around or within a few joints. In these positions, the pads resist compression, absorb shocks, and prevent damaging bone-to-bone contact. Cartilages heal poorly, and damaged fibrocartilage in joints such as the knee can interfere with normal movements.

Bone

Here we focus on significant differences between cartilage and bone. We will examine the detailed histology of **bone**, or *osseous* (OS-ē-us; *os,* bone) *tissue* in Chapter 6. The volume of ground substance in bone is very small. The matrix of bone consists mainly of hard calcium compounds and flexible collagen fibers. This combination gives bone truly remarkable properties, making it both strong and resistant to shattering. In its overall properties, bone can compete with the best steel-reinforced concrete.

The general organization of bone is shown in **Figure 4-12**. Lacunae in the matrix contain bone cells, or **osteocytes**

CLINICAL NOTE

Cartilages and Joint Injuries

Several complex joints, including the knee, contain both hyaline cartilage and fibrocartilage. The hyaline cartilage covers bony surfaces. Fibrocartilage pads in the joint prevent bone-to-bone contact when movements are under way. Injuries to these joints can produce tears in the fibrocartilage pads that do not heal. This loss of cushioning places more strain on the cartilages within joints and leads to further joint damage. Eventually, joint mobility is severely reduced. Cartilages heal poorly because they are avascular. Joint cartilages heal even more slowly than other cartilages. Surgery to repair cartilage usually results in only a temporary or incomplete repair.

(OS-tē-ō-sīts; *os,* bone + *cyte,* cell). The lacunae surround the blood vessels that branch through the bony matrix. Diffusion cannot take place through the bony matrix, but osteocytes obtain nutrients through cytoplasmic extensions that reach blood vessels and other osteocytes. These extensions run through a branching network within the matrix called **canaliculi** (kan-a-LIK-ū-lē; little canals).

Except in joint cavities, where a layer of hyaline cartilage covers bone, all other bone surfaces are surrounded by a **periosteum** (per-ē-OS-tē-um), a covering made up of fibrous (outer) and cellular (inner) layers. Unlike cartilage, bone is constantly being remodeled throughout life. Complete repairs can be made even after severe damage. **Table 4-3** summarizes the similarities and differences between cartilage and bone.

CHECKPOINT

12. Identify several functions of connective tissues.

13. List the three types of connective tissues.

14. Which type of connective tissue contains primarily triglycerides?

15. Lack of vitamin C in the diet interferes with the ability of fibroblasts to produce collagen. What effect might this interference have on connective tissue?

16. Which two types of connective tissue have a fluid matrix?

17. Identify the two types of supporting connective tissue.

18. Why does cartilage heal more slowly than bone?

See the blue Answers tab at the back of the book.

Figure 4-11 Types of Cartilage.

Hyaline Cartilage

LOCATIONS: Between tips of ribs and bones of sternum; covering bone surfaces at freely movable (synovial) joints; supporting larynx (voice box), trachea, and bronchi; forming part of nasal septum

FUNCTIONS: Provides stiff but somewhat flexible support; reduces friction between bony surfaces

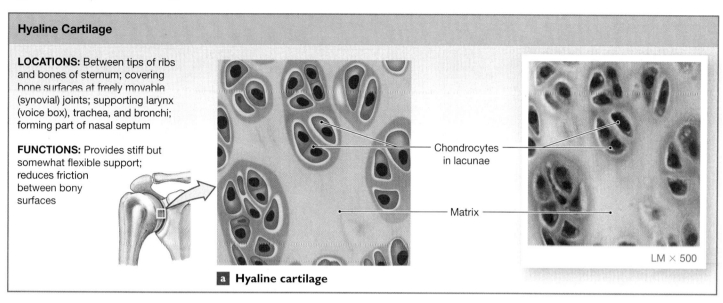

Chondrocytes in lacunae

Matrix

LM × 500

a **Hyaline cartilage**

Elastic Cartilage

LOCATIONS: Auricle of external ear; epiglottis; auditory tube; cuneiform cartilages of larynx

FUNCTIONS: Provides support, but tolerates distortion without damage and returns to original shape

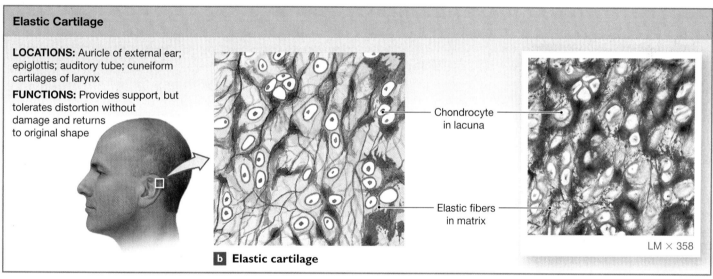

Chondrocyte in lacuna

Elastic fibers in matrix

LM × 358

b **Elastic cartilage**

Fibrocartilage

LOCATIONS: Pads within knee joint; between pubic bones of pelvis; intervertebral discs

FUNCTIONS: Resists compression; prevents bone-to-bone contact; limits movement

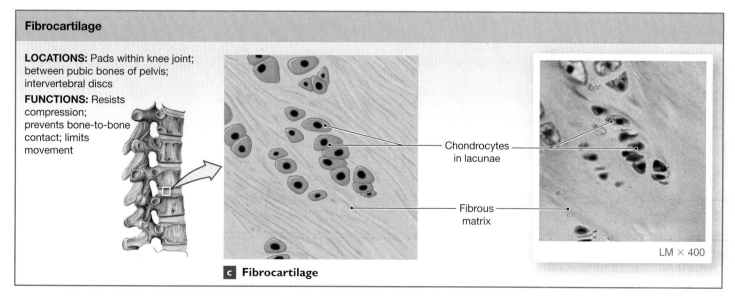

Chondrocytes in lacunae

Fibrous matrix

LM × 400

c **Fibrocartilage**

Figure 4-12 Bone. The osteocytes in bone are usually organized in groups around a central space that contains blood vessels. In the micrograph, bone dust produced during preparation of the bone section fills the lacunae and the central canal, making them appear dark.

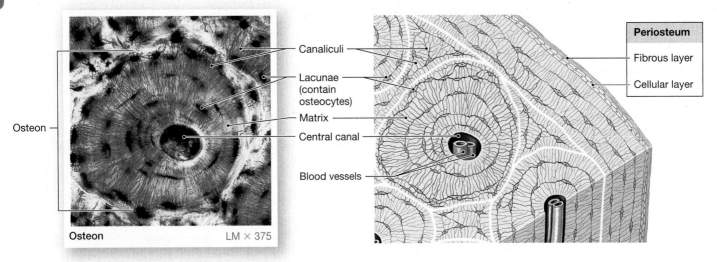

4-5 Tissue membranes are physical barriers of four types: mucous, serous, cutaneous, and synovial

Learning Objective Explain how epithelial and connective tissues combine to form four types of tissue membranes, and specify the functions of each.

Some anatomical terms have more than one meaning, depending on the context. One such term is *membrane*. For example, at the cellular level, plasma membranes are lipid bilayers that restrict the passage of ions and other solutes. ⤶ p. 60 A tissue membrane is a physical barrier. Tissue membranes line or cover body surfaces. Each consists of an epithelium supported by connective tissue. The body has four such membranes: *mucous membranes, serous membranes, the cutaneous membrane*, and *synovial membranes* (**Figure 4-13**).

Mucous Membranes

Mucous membranes, or **mucosae** (mū-KŌ-sē), line passageways and chambers that open to the exterior, including those in the digestive, respiratory, reproductive, and urinary tracts (**Figure 4-13a**). The epithelial surfaces are kept moist at all times, typically by mucous secretions from mucous cells or multicellular glands, or by fluids such as urine or semen.

Table 4-3	A Comparison of Cartilage and Bone	
Characteristic	**Cartilage**	**Bone**
STRUCTURAL FEATURES		
Cells	Chondrocytes in lacunae	Osteocytes in lacunae
Ground substance	Protein–polysaccharide gel and water	A small volume of liquid surrounding insoluble crystals of calcium salts (calcium phosphate and calcium carbonate)
Fibers	Collagen, elastic, reticular fibers (proportions vary)	Collagen fibers predominate
Vascularity (blood supply)	None (avascular)	Extensive
Covering	Perichondrium	Periosteum
Strength	Limited: bends easily but difficult to break	Strong: resists distortion until breaking point is reached
METABOLIC FEATURES		
Oxygen demands	Low	High
Nutrient delivery	By diffusion through matrix	By diffusion through cytoplasm and fluid in canaliculi
Repair capabilities	Limited	Extensive

Figure 4-13 Tissue Membranes.

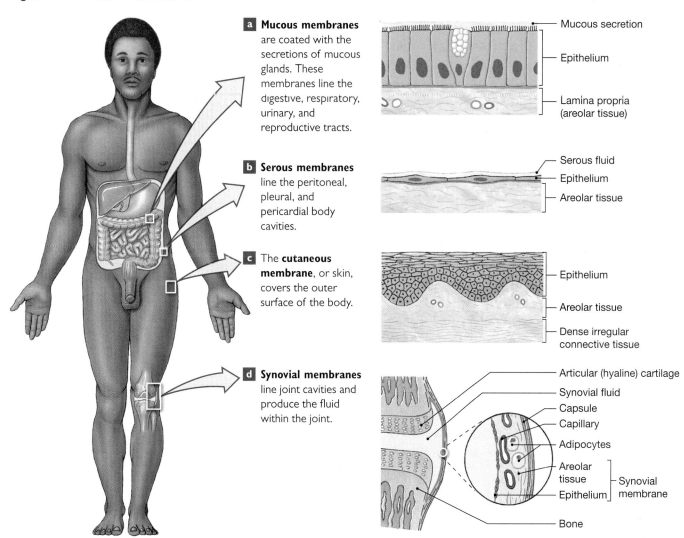

a **Mucous membranes** are coated with the secretions of mucous glands. These membranes line the digestive, respiratory, urinary, and reproductive tracts.

- Mucous secretion
- Epithelium
- Lamina propria (areolar tissue)

b **Serous membranes** line the peritoneal, pleural, and pericardial body cavities.

- Serous fluid
- Epithelium
- Areolar tissue

c The **cutaneous membrane**, or skin, covers the outer surface of the body.

- Epithelium
- Areolar tissue
- Dense irregular connective tissue

d **Synovial membranes** line joint cavities and produce the fluid within the joint.

- Articular (hyaline) cartilage
- Synovial fluid
- Capsule
- Capillary
- Adipocytes
- Areolar tissue — Synovial membrane
- Epithelium
- Bone

The areolar tissue portion of a mucous membrane is called the *lamina propria* (PRŌ-prē-uh).

Many mucous membranes contain simple epithelia with absorptive or secretory functions, such as the simple columnar epithelium of the digestive tract. However, other types of epithelia may be involved. For example, a stratified squamous epithelium is part of the mucous membrane of the mouth. Also, the mucous membrane along most of the urinary tract has a transitional epithelium.

Serous Membranes

A **serous membrane** consists of a simple epithelium supported by areolar tissue (**Figure 4-13b**). Serous membranes line the sealed, internal cavities of the trunk, which are not open to the exterior. There are three serous membranes. The **pleura** (PLOO-ra; *pleura*, rib) lines the pleural cavities and covers the lungs. The **peritoneum** (per-i-tō-NĒ-um; *peri*, around + *teinein*, to stretch) lines the peritoneal cavity and covers the surfaces of enclosed organs such as the liver and stomach. The **pericardium** (per-i-KAR-dē-um) lines the pericardial cavity and covers the heart.

A serous membrane has *parietal* and *visceral* portions that are in close contact at all times. ↺ p. 17 The parietal portion lines the inner surface of the cavity. The visceral portion, or *serosa*, covers the outer surface of organs projecting into the body cavity. For example, the visceral pericardium covers the heart, and the parietal pericardium lines the inner surfaces of the pericardial sac that surrounds the pericardial cavity. The primary function of any serous membrane is to reduce friction between the opposing parietal and visceral surfaces when an organ moves or changes shape. Friction is reduced by a watery, *serous fluid* formed by fluids diffusing from underlying tissues.

4

The Cutaneous Membrane

The **cutaneous membrane** is the skin that covers the surface of your body (**Figure 4-13c**). It consists of a stratified squamous epithelium and a layer of areolar tissue reinforced by underlying dense irregular connective tissue. In contrast to serous or mucous membranes, the cutaneous membrane is thick, relatively waterproof, and usually dry. (We discuss the skin in detail in Chapter 5.)

Synovial Membranes

Bones contact one another at joints, or **articulations** (ar-tik-ū-LĀ-shuns). Joints that allow free movement are surrounded by a fibrous capsule and contain a joint cavity lined by a **synovial (si-NŌ-vē-ul) membrane** (**Figure 4-13d**). Unlike the other three membranes, the synovial membrane consists primarily of areolar tissue and an incomplete layer of epithelial tissue.

In freely movable joints, the bony surfaces do not come into direct contact with one another. If they did, impacts and abrasion would damage the opposing surfaces, and smooth movement would become almost impossible. Instead, the ends of the bones are covered with hyaline cartilage and separated by a viscous *synovial fluid* produced by fibroblasts in the connective tissue of the synovial membrane. The synovial fluid helps lubricate the joint and permits smooth movement.

CHECKPOINT

19. Identify the four types of tissue membranes found in the body.

20. How does a plasma (cell) membrane differ from a tissue membrane?

21. What is the function of fluids produced by serous membranes?

22. The lining of the nasal cavity is normally moist, contains numerous mucous cells, and rests on a layer of areolar tissue. Which type of membrane is this?

See the blue Answers tab at the back of the book.

4-6 The three types of muscle tissue are skeletal, cardiac, and smooth

Learning Objective Describe the three types of muscle tissue and the special structural features of each.

Muscle tissue is specialized for contraction. Muscle cells contract due to interaction between filaments of the proteins *myosin* and *actin*. ↺ p. 70 These two proteins are found in the cytoskeletons of many cells, but in muscle cells, the filaments are more numerous and arranged so that their interaction produces a contraction of the entire cell.

There are three types of muscle tissue in the body—*skeletal, cardiac,* and *smooth muscle tissues* (**Figure 4-14**). The contraction process is the same in all of them, but the organization of their actin and myosin filaments differs. In this discussion, we will focus on general characteristics rather than specific details (which we will examine in Chapter 7).

Skeletal Muscle Tissue

Skeletal muscle tissue contains very large, multinucleated cells (**Figure 4-14a**). A skeletal muscle cell may be 100 micrometers (μm; 1 μm = 0.001 mm = 1/25,000 in.) in diameter and up to 0.3 m (1 ft) long. The individual muscle cells are usually called *muscle fibers* because they are relatively long and slender. Skeletal muscle fibers are incapable of dividing, but new muscle fibers are produced through the divisions of stem cells in adult skeletal muscle tissue. As a result, at least partial repairs can take place after an injury.

In skeletal muscle fibers, actin and myosin filaments are organized into repeating patterns that give the cells a *striated*, or banded, appearance. The *striations*, or bands, are easy to see in light micrographs. Skeletal muscle fibers will not usually contract unless stimulated by nerves. Because the nervous system provides voluntary control over its activities, skeletal muscle is described as *striated voluntary muscle*.

Cardiac Muscle Tissue

Cardiac muscle tissue is found in the heart. Like skeletal muscle tissue, cardiac muscle tissue is striated. A typical cardiac muscle cell, or *cardiocyte*, is much smaller than a skeletal muscle fiber and usually has only a single nucleus (**Figure 4-14b**). Cardiac muscle cells branch and form extensive connections with one another. These cells are interconnected at **intercalated** (in-TER-ka-lā-ted) **discs**, specialized attachment sites containing gap junctions and desmosomes. Cardiac muscle cells thus form a network that efficiently conducts the stimulus and force for contraction from one area of the heart to another. Cardiac muscle tissue has a very limited ability to repair itself. Stem cells are lacking. Some cardiac muscle cells do divide after an injury to the heart, but the repairs are incomplete.

Figure 4-14 Muscle Tissue.

Skeletal Muscle Tissue

Cells are long, cylindrical, striated, and multinucleate.

LOCATIONS. Combined with connective tissues and neural tissue in skeletal muscles

FUNCTIONS: Moves or stabilizes the position of the skeleton; guards entrances and exits to the digestive, respiratory, and urinary tracts; generates heat; protects internal organs

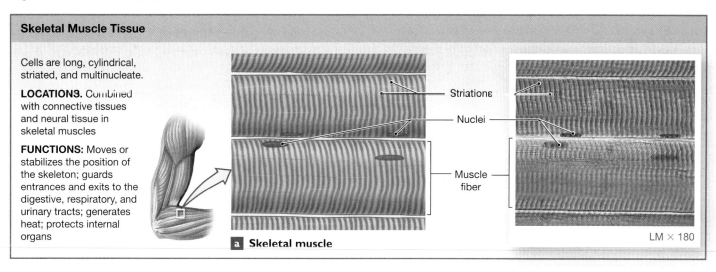

a **Skeletal muscle**

Striations

Nuclei

Muscle fiber

LM × 180

Cardiac Muscle Tissue

Cells are short, branched, and striated, usually with a single nucleus; cells are interconnected by intercalated discs.

LOCATION: Heart

FUNCTIONS: Circulates blood; maintains blood pressure

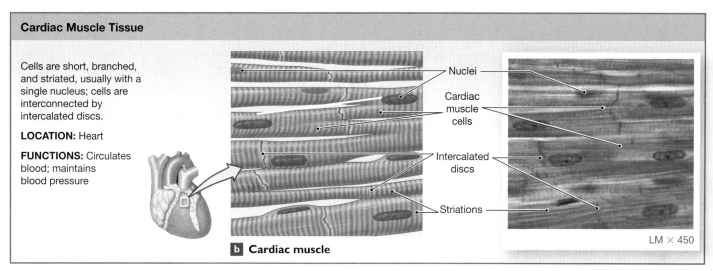

b **Cardiac muscle**

Nuclei

Cardiac muscle cells

Intercalated discs

Striations

LM × 450

Smooth Muscle Tissue

Cells are short, spindle-shaped, and nonstriated, with a single, central nucleus.

LOCATIONS: Found in the walls of blood vessels and in digestive, respiratory, urinary, and reproductive organs

FUNCTIONS: Moves food, urine, and reproductive tract secretions; controls diameter of respiratory passageways; regulates diameter of blood vessels

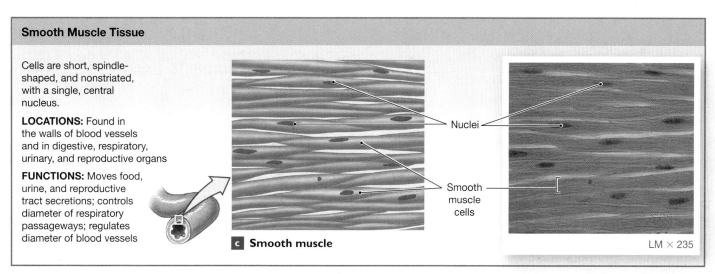

c **Smooth muscle**

Nuclei

Smooth muscle cells

LM × 235

4

Cardiac muscle cells do not rely on nerve activity to start a contraction. Instead, specialized *pacemaker cells* establish a regular rate of contraction. The nervous system can alter the rate of pacemaker activity, but it does not provide voluntary control over individual cardiac muscle cells. For this reason, cardiac muscle is called *striated involuntary muscle.*

Smooth Muscle Tissue

Smooth muscle tissue is found in the walls of blood vessels; around hollow organs such as the urinary bladder; and in layers around the respiratory, circulatory, digestive, and reproductive tracts.

A smooth muscle cell is small and slender. It tapers to a point at each end and contains a single nucleus (**Figure 4-14c**). Unlike skeletal and cardiac muscle, smooth muscle cells have no striations. The reason is because their actin and myosin filaments are scattered throughout the cytoplasm. Smooth muscle cells can divide, so smooth muscle tissue can regenerate after injury.

Smooth muscle cells may contract on their own, or their contractions may be triggered by neural activity. The nervous system usually does not provide voluntary control over smooth muscle contractions, so smooth muscle is known as *nonstriated involuntary muscle.*

CHECKPOINT

23. Identify the three types of muscle tissue in the body.

24. Voluntary control of muscle contractions is restricted to which type of muscle tissue?

25. Which type of muscle tissue has small, tapering cells with single nuclei and no obvious striations?

See the blue Answers tab at the back of the book.

4-7 Neural tissue responds to stimuli and propagates electrical impulses throughout the body

Learning Objective Discuss the basic structure and role of neural tissue.

Neural tissue, also known as *nervous tissue* or *nerve tissue*, is specialized for propagating (transmitting) electrical impulses from one region of the body to another. Most neural tissue (98 percent) is concentrated in the brain and spinal cord, the control centers for the nervous system.

Neural tissue contains two basic types of cells: (1) neurons (NOO-ronz; *neuro-*, nerve) and (2) several different kinds of supporting cells, or **neuroglia** (noo-ROG-lē-uh; *glia*, glue). Our conscious and unconscious thought processes are due to communication among neurons in the brain. Neurons communicate through electrical events that affect their plasma membranes. The neuroglia provide physical support for neural tissue, maintain the chemical composition of the neural tissue fluids, supply nutrients to neurons, and defend the tissue from infection.

The longest cells in your body are neurons. Many reach up to a meter (39 in.) long. Most neurons cannot divide under normal circumstances, so they have a very limited ability to repair themselves after injury.

A typical neuron has three main parts: (1) a **cell body** containing a large nucleus, (2) numerous branching projections called **dendrites** (DEN-drīts; *dendron,* tree), and (3) one projection called an **axon** (**Figure 4-15**). Dendrites receive information, typically from other neurons, and axons carry that information to other cells. Axons are also called *nerve fibers* because they tend to be very long and slender. Each axon ends at *axon terminals,* where the neuron communicates with other cells. (In Chapter 8, we consider the properties of neural tissue.)

CHECKPOINT

26. A tissue contains irregularly shaped cells with many projections, including some several centimeters long. These are probably which type of cell?

27. Why are both skeletal muscle cells and axons also called fibers?

See the blue Answers tab at the back of the book.

4-8 The response to tissue injury involves inflammation and regeneration

Learning Objective Describe how injuries affect the tissues of the body.

The different tissues in the body are not isolated from each other. They combine to form organs with diverse functions. Any injury will affect several tissue types at the same time. The repair process depends on the coordinated response of these tissues to restore homeostasis.

Restoring homeostasis after a tissue injury involves two related processes: *inflammation* and *regeneration*. First, the area is isolated from neighboring healthy tissue while damaged cells, tissue components, and any dangerous microorganisms are cleaned up. This phase, which coordinates the

Figure 4-15 Neural Tissue.

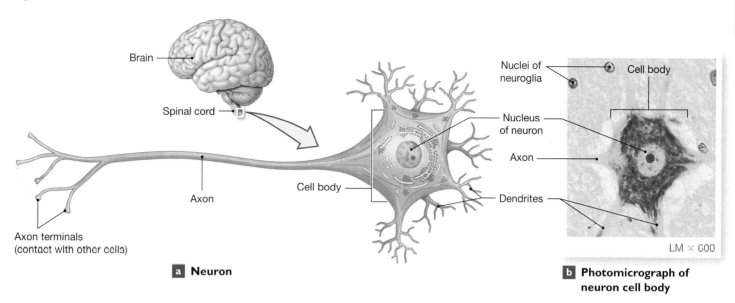

Brain

Spinal cord

Axon

Axon terminals
(contact with other cells)

Cell body

Nuclei of
neuroglia

Cell body

Nucleus
of neuron

Axon

Dendrites

LM × 600

a **Neuron**

b **Photomicrograph of
neuron cell body**

activities of several different tissues, is called **inflammation**, or the *inflammatory response*. It produces several familiar signs and symptoms, including swelling, heat (warmth), redness, and pain.

Many stimuli can produce inflammation. They include impact, abrasion, chemical irritation, *infection* (invasion and presence of pathogens, such as harmful bacteria or viruses), and extreme temperatures (hot or cold). When any of these stimuli either kill cells, damage fibers, or injure tissues, they trigger the inflammatory response by stimulating mast cells. ↻ p. 103 The mast cells release chemicals (*histamine* and *heparin*) that cause local blood vessels to *dilate* (enlarge in diameter) and become more permeable. As a result, increased blood flow to the injured region makes it red and warm to the touch, and the diffusion of blood plasma causes the injured area to swell. The abnormal tissue conditions and chemicals released by the mast cells also stimulate sensory nerve endings that produce sensations of pain. These local circulatory changes increase the delivery of nutrients, oxygen, phagocytic white blood cells, and blood-clotting proteins. They also speed up the removal of waste products and toxins. Over a period of hours to days, this coordinated response generally succeeds in eliminating the inflammatory stimulus. (We will examine inflammation further in Chapter 14.)

In the second phase following injury, damaged tissues are replaced or repaired to restore normal function. This repair process is called **regeneration**. During regeneration, fibroblasts produce a dense network of collagen fibers known as *scar tissue* or *fibrous tissue*. Over time, scar tissue gradually assumes a more normal appearance.

Each organ has a different tissue organization, and this organization affects its ability to regenerate after injury. Epithelia, connective tissues (except cartilage), and smooth muscle tissue usually regenerate well. Other muscle tissues and neural tissue regenerate relatively poorly, if at all.

Your skin, which is made up mostly of epithelia and connective tissues, regenerates rapidly. (We will examine the regeneration of skin in Chapter 5.) In contrast, damage to the heart is more serious. Although its connective tissue can be repaired, most of the damaged cardiac muscle cells are replaced only by fibrous connective tissue. Such permanent replacement of normal tissues is called **fibrosis** (fī-BRŌ-sis). Fibrosis may occur in muscle and other tissues in response to injury, disease, or aging. **Spotlight Figure 4-16** shows the tissue response to injury and the process of tissue regeneration.

CHECKPOINT

28. Identify the two phases in the response to tissue injury.

29. What signs and symptoms are associated with inflammation?

30. What is fibrosis?

See the blue Answers tab at the back of the book.

Tissues are not isolated, and they combine to form organs with diverse functions. Therefore, any injury affects several types of tissue at the same time. To preserve homeostasis, the tissues must respond in a coordinated way. Restoring homeostasis involves two related processes: inflammation and regeneration.

stimulates

Mast Cell Activation

When an injury damages connective tissue, mast cells release a variety of chemicals. This process, called **mast cell activation**, stimulates inflammation.

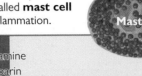

Mast cell

Histamine
Heparin

Exposure to Pathogens and Toxins

Injured tissue contains an abnormal concentration of pathogens, toxins, wastes, and the chemicals from injured cells.

INFLAMMATION

Inflammation produces several familiar indications of injury, including swelling, redness, heat (warmth), pain, and sometimes loss of function. Inflammation may also result from the presence of pathogens, such as harmful bacteria, within the tissues. The invasion and presence of these pathogens is an **infection**.

When a tissue is injured, a general defense mechanism is activated.

Increased Blood Flow	Increased Vessel Permeability	Pain
In response to the released chemicals, blood vessels dilate, increasing blood flow through the damaged tissue. 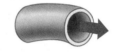	Vessel dilation is accompanied by an increase in the permeability of the capillary walls. Plasma now diffuses into the injured tissue, so the area becomes swollen. 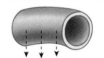	The abnormal conditions within the tissue and the chemicals released by mast cells stimulate nerve endings that produce the sensation of pain. 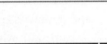 PAIN

Increased Local Temperature	Increased Oxygen and Nutrients	Increased Phagocytosis	Removal of Toxins and Wastes
The increased blood flow and permeability causes the tissue to become warm and red.	Vessel dilation, increased blood flow, and increased vessel permeability result in enhanced delivery of oxygen and nutrients.  O₂	Phagocytes in the tissue are activated, and they begin engulfing tissue debris and pathogens. 	Enhanced circulation carries away toxins and wastes, distributing them to the kidneys for excretion, or to the liver for inactivation. Toxins and wastes

Normal tissue conditions restored

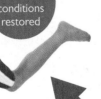

Regeneration

Regeneration is the repair that occurs after the damaged tissue has been stabilized and the inflammation has subsided. Fibroblasts move into the area, laying down a collagenous framework known as **scar tissue**. Over time, scar tissue is usually "remodeled" and gradually assumes a more normal appearance.

Inflammation Subsides

Over a period of hours to days, the cleanup process generally succeeds in eliminating the inflammatory stimuli.

Inhibits mast cell activation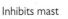

4-9 With advancing age, tissue repair declines and cancer rates increase

Learning Objective Describe how aging affects the tissues of the body.

Aging has two important effects on tissues. The body's ability to repair damage to tissues decreases, and cancer is more likely to occur.

Aging and Tissue Structure

Tissues change with age. The speed and effectiveness of tissue repairs decrease. Maintenance and repair activities throughout the body slow down, and energy consumption generally declines. These changes reflect various hormonal alterations that take place with age, often coupled with reduced physical activity and a more sedentary lifestyle. These factors combine to alter the structure and chemical composition of many tissues. Epithelia get thinner and connective tissues more fragile. Individuals bruise more easily and bones become brittle. Joint pain and broken bones are common in the elderly. Cardiac muscle fibers and neurons cannot be replaced, and cumulative losses from relatively minor damage can contribute to major health problems, such as cardiovascular disease or deterioration in mental functioning.

Some of the effects of aging are genetically programmed. For example, as people age, their chondrocytes produce a slightly different form of the gelatinous compound making up the cartilage matrix. This difference probably accounts for the thinner and less resilient cartilage of older people.

Other age-related changes in tissue structure have multiple causes. The age-related reduction in bone strength in women is a condition called *osteoporosis*. It is often caused by a combination of inactivity, low dietary calcium intake, and a reduction in circulating estrogens (sex hormones). A program of exercise, calcium supplements, and in some cases medication can generally maintain normal bone structure for many years.

Aging and Cancer Rates

Cancer rates increase with age, and roughly 25 percent of all people in the United States develop cancer at some point in their lives. It has been estimated that 70–80 percent of cancer cases result from mutations due to chemical exposure, environmental factors, or some combination of the two, and 40 percent of these cancers are caused by cigarette smoke. Each year in the United States, over 500,000 individuals die of cancer. It is second only to heart disease as a cause of death.

Build Your Knowledge

Recall that cancer is an illness characterized by gene mutations leading to the formation of malignant cells and metastasis (as you saw in **Chapter 3: The Cellular Level of Organization**). Cancer cells result when these mutations lead to disruptions in the control of normal cycles of cell division and growth. ⊃ p. 84

CHECKPOINT

31. Identify some age-related factors that affect tissue repair and structure.

See the blue Answers tab at the back of the book.

RELATED CLINICAL TERMS

adhesions: Restrictive fibrous connections that can result from surgery, infection, or other injuries to serous membranes.

anaplasia (a-nuh-PLĀ-zē-uh)**:** An irreversible change in the size and shape of tissue cells.

dysplasia (dis-PLĀ-zē-uh)**:** A change in the normal shape, size, and organization of tissue cells.

metaplasia (me-tuh-PLĀ-zē-uh)**:** A structural change in cells that alters the character of a tissue.

necrosis (ne-KRŌ-sis)**:** Tissue destruction that occurs after cells have been injured or killed.

pericarditis: An inflammation of the pericardial lining that may lead to the accumulation of pericardial fluid (*pericardial effusion*).

peritonitis: An inflammation of the peritoneum after infection or injury.

pleural effusion: The accumulation of fluid within the pleural cavities as a result of chronic infection or inflammation of the pleura.

pleuritis (*pleurisy*)**:** An inflammation of the pleural cavities.

4 Chapter Review

Summary Outline

4-1 The four tissue types are epithelial, connective, muscle, and neural *p. 97*

1. **Tissues** are collections of specialized cells and cell products that are organized to perform a relatively limited number of functions. The four **tissue types** are epithelial tissue, connective tissues, muscle tissue, and neural tissue. **Histology** is the study of tissues *(Figure 4-1)*.

4-2 Epithelial tissue covers body surfaces, lines cavities and tubular structures, and serves essential functions *p. 97*

2. An **epithelium** is an **avascular** layer of cells that forms a barrier that covers internal or external surfaces. **Glands** are secretory structures derived from epithelia.

3. Epithelia provide physical protection, control permeability, provide sensations, and produce specialized secretions.

4. **Gland cells** are epithelial cells that produce secretions. **Exocrine** secretions are released onto body surfaces; **endocrine** secretions, known as hormones, are released by gland cells into the surrounding tissue fluid.

5. The individual cells that make up tissues connect to one another or to extracellular protein fibers by means of *cell adhesion molecules (CAMs)* and/or proteoglycans, or at specialized attachment sites called **cell junctions.** The three major types of cell junctions are **tight junctions, gap junctions**, and **desmosomes** *(Figure 4-2)*.

6. Many epithelial cells have microvilli that increase absorptive surface area. The coordinated beating of the cilia on a ciliated epithelium moves materials across the epithelial surface *(Figure 4-3)*.

7. The basal surface of each epithelium is connected to a non-cellular **basement membrane.**

8. Divisions by **stem cells**, or *germinative cells*, continually replace the short-lived epithelial cells.

4-3 Cell shape and number of layers determine the classification of epithelia *p. 101*

9. Epithelia are classified on the basis of the number of cell layers and the shape of the exposed cells *(Table 4-1)*.

10. A **simple epithelium** has a single layer of cells covering the basement membrane: a **stratified epithelium** has several layers. In a **squamous epithelium**, the cells are thin and flat. Cells in a **cuboidal epithelium** resemble little boxes;

those in a **columnar epithelium** are taller and more slender *(Figures 4-4 and 4-5)*.

11. A glandular epithelial cell may release its secretions by *merocrine, apocrine,* or *holocrine* secretory modes *(Figure 4-6)*.

12. In **merocrine secretion** (the most common method of secretion), the product is released through exocytosis. **Apocrine secretion** involves the loss of both secretory product and cytoplasm. **Holocrine secretion** destroys the cell, which becomes packed with secretions before it finally bursts.

13. Exocrine secretions may be serous (watery, usually containing enzymes), mucous (thick and slippery), or mixed (containing enzymes and lubricants) *(Table 4-2)*.

4-4 Connective tissue provides a protective structural framework for other tissue types *p. 108*

14. All **connective** tissues have specialized cells and a **matrix**, composed of extracellular protein fibers and a **ground substance**.

15. Connective tissues are internal tissues with many important functions: establishing a structural framework; transporting fluids and dissolved materials; protecting delicate organs; supporting, surrounding, and interconnecting tissues; storing energy reserves; and defending the body from microorganisms.

16. **Connective tissue proper** refers to connective tissues that contain varied cell populations and fiber types surrounded by a syrupy ground substance *(Figure 4-7)*.

17. **Fluid connective tissues** have a distinctive population of cells suspended in a watery ground substance containing dissolved proteins. The two types are *blood* and *lymph* *(Figure 4-7)*.

18. **Supporting connective tissues** have a less diverse cell population than connective tissue proper and a dense matrix that contains closely packed fibers. The two types of supporting connective tissues are cartilage and bone *(Figure 4-7)*.

19. Connective tissue proper contains fibers, a viscous ground substance, and a varied cell population, including **fibroblasts, fibrocytes, macrophages, fat cells, mast cells**, and various white blood cells *(Figure 4-8)*.

20. There are three types of fibers in connective tissue: **collagen fibers, elastic fibers**, and **reticular fibers**.

21. Connective tissue proper is classified as **loose** or **dense connective tissue**. Loose connective tissues include **areolar tissue, adipose tissue**, and **reticular tissue** *(Figure 4-9)*.

22. Most of the volume in dense connective tissue consists of fibers. **Dense regular connective tissue** forms **tendons** and **ligaments. Dense irregular connective tissue** forms organ capsules, bone and cartilage sheaths, and the deep dermis of the skin *(Figure 4-10)*.

23. **Blood** and **lymph** are connective tissues that contain distinctive collections of cells in a fluid matrix.

24. Blood contains **red blood cells, white blood cells**, and **platelets**: the watery ground substance is called **plasma**.

25. Lymph forms as *interstitial fluid* enters the *lymphatic vessels*, which return lymph to the cardiovascular system.

26. Cartilage and bone are called supporting connective tissues because they support the rest of the body.

27. The matrix of **cartilage** consists of a firm gel and cells called **chondrocytes**. A fibrous **perichondrium** separates cartilage from surrounding tissues. The three types of cartilage are **hyaline cartilage, elastic cartilage**, and **fibrocartilage** *(Figure 4-11)*.

28. Chondrocytes obtain nutrients by diffusion through the avascular matrix.

29. **Bone**, or *osseous tissue*, has a matrix consisting primarily of collagen fibers and calcium salts, which give it unique properties *(Figure 4-12; Table 4-3)*.

30. **Osteocytes** depend on diffusion through **canaliculi** for nutrient intake.

31. Each bone is surrounded by a **periosteum** with fibrous and cellular layers.

4-5 Tissue membranes are physical barriers of four types: mucous, serous, cutaneous, and synovial *p. 116*

32. Membranes form a barrier or interface. Epithelia and connective tissues combine to form membranes that cover and protect other structures and tissues *(Figure 4-13)*.

33. **Mucous membranes** line passageways and chambers that communicate with the exterior. Their surfaces are normally moistened by mucous secretions.

34. **Serous membranes** line the body's sealed internal cavities of the trunk. They form a fluid that prevents friction between the inner surface of the cavity and the surfaces of visceral organs projecting into the cavity.

35. The **cutaneous membrane**, or skin, covers the body surface. Unlike serous and mucous membranes, it is relatively thick, waterproof, and usually dry.

36. **Synovial membranes**, located at joints (articulations), produce *synovial fluid* in joint cavities. Synovial fluid helps lubricate the joint and promotes smooth movement.

4-6 The three types of muscle tissue are skeletal, cardiac, and smooth *p. 118*

37. **Muscle tissue** is specialized for contraction *(Figure 4-14)*.

38. **Skeletal muscle tissue** contains large cells, or *muscle fibers*, that are multinucleate and have a banded (striated) appearance. Because we can control the contraction of skeletal muscle fibers through the nervous system, skeletal muscle is considered *striated voluntary muscle*.

39. **Cardiac muscle tissue** is found only in the heart. The nervous system does not provide voluntary control over cardiac muscle cells. Thus, cardiac muscle is *striated involuntary muscle*.

40. **Smooth muscle tissue** is found in the walls of blood vessels, around hollow organs, and in layers around various tracts (respiratory, circulatory, digestive, and reproductive). It is classified as *nonstriated involuntary muscle*.

4-7 Neural tissue responds to stimuli and propagates electrical impulses throughout the body *p. 120*

41. **Neural tissue** is specialized to propagate, or transmit, electrical impulses that convey information from one area of the body to another.

42. Cells in neural tissue are either neurons or neuroglia. **Neurons** transmit information as electrical impulses in their plasma membranes. Several kinds of **neuroglia** serve both supporting and defense functions *(Figure 4-15)*.

43. A typical neuron has a **cell body, dendrites**, and an **axon**, which ends at *axon terminals*.

4-8 The response to tissue injury involves inflammation and regeneration *p. 120*

44. Any injury affects several tissue types at the same time, and they respond in a coordinated manner. Homeostasis is restored through two processes: *inflammation* and *regeneration*.

45. **Inflammation**, or the *inflammatory response*, isolates the injured area while damaged cells, tissue components, and any dangerous microorganisms are cleaned up *(Spotlight Figure 4-16)*.

46. **Regeneration** is the repair process that restores normal function *(Spotlight Figure 4-16)*.

4-9 With advancing age, tissue repair declines and cancer rates increase *p. 122*

47. Tissues change with age. Repair and maintenance grow less efficient, and the structure and chemical composition of many tissues are altered.

48. Cancer rates increase with age; roughly three-quarters of all cases are due to mutations caused by exposure to chemicals or by other environmental factors, such as cigarette smoke.

Level 1 Reviewing Facts and Terms

Match each item in column A with the most closely related item in column B. Place letters for answers in the spaces provided.

COLUMN A

_____ 1. Histology
_____ 2. Microvilli
_____ 3. Gap junction
_____ 4. Tight junction
_____ 5. Stem cells
_____ 6. Destroys gland cell
_____ 7. Hormones
_____ 8. Adipocytes
_____ 9. Bone-to-bone attachment
_____ 10. Muscle-to-bone attachment
_____ 11. Skeletal muscle tissue
_____ 12. Cardiac muscle tissue

COLUMN B

a. Repair and renewal
b. Ligament
c. Endocrine secretion
d. Enhance absorption and secretion
e. Fat cells
f. Holocrine secretion
g. Study of tissues
h. Tendon
i. Prevents the passage of water and solutes between cells
j. Permits ions to pass from cell to cell
k. Intercalated discs
l. Striated, voluntary

13. Identify the six categories of epithelial tissue shown in the drawing below.

(a) _____   (b) _____
(c) _____   (d) _____
(e) _____   (f) _____

14. The four basic tissue types found in the body are
   (a) epithelial, connective, muscle, neural.
   (b) simple, cuboidal, squamous, stratified.
   (c) fibroblasts, adipocytes, melanocytes, mesenchymal.
   (d) lymphocytes, macrophages, microphages, adipocytes.

15. The most abundant connections between cells in the superficial layers of the skin are
   (a) intermediate junctions.   (b) gap junctions.
   (c) desmosomes.   (d) tight junctions.

16. The three cell shapes making up epithelial tissue are
   (a) simple, stratified, transitional.
   (b) simple, stratified, pseudostratified.
   (c) hexagonal, cuboidal, spherical.
   (d) cuboidal, squamous, columnar.

17. Mucous secretions that coat the passageways of the digestive and respiratory tracts result from secretion.
   (a) Apocrine   (b) Merocrine
   (c) Holocrine   (d) Endocrine

18. Matrix is characteristic of which type of tissue?
   (a) Epithelial   (b) Neural
   (c) Muscle   (d) Connective

19. The three major types of cartilage in the body are
   (a) collagen, reticular, elastic.
   (b) areolar, adipose, reticular.
   (c) hyaline, elastic, fibrocartilage.
   (d) keratin, reticular, elastic.

20. The primary function of serous membranes in the body is
   (a) to minimize friction between opposing surfaces.
   (b) to line cavities that are open to the exterior.
   (c) to perform absorptive and secretory functions.
   (d) to cover the surface of the body.

21. Large muscle fibers that are multinucleated, striated, and voluntary are found in
   (a) cardiac muscle tissue.   (b) skeletal muscle tissue.
   (c) smooth muscle tissue.   (d) a, b, and c are correct.

22. Intercalated discs and pacemaker cells are characteristic of
   (a) smooth muscle tissue.   (b) cardiac muscle tissue.
   (c) skeletal muscle tissue.   (d) All of the above

23. Dendrites, an axon, and a cell body are characteristics of cells found in
    (a) neural tissue.   **(b)** muscle tissue.
    (c) connective tissue.   **(d)** epithelial tissue.

24. Identify the four kinds of tissue membranes shown in the drawing below.

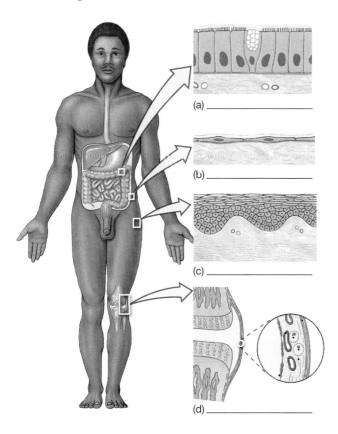

(a) _____

(b) _____

(c) _____

(d) _____

25. What two types of layering make epithelial tissue recognizable?

26. What three basic components are found in connective tissues?

27. Which fluid connective tissues and supporting connective tissues are found in the human body?

28. What two cell populations make up neural tissue? What is the function of each?

Level 2 Reviewing Concepts

29. In body surfaces where mechanical stresses are severe, the dominant epithelium is
    (a) stratified squamous epithelium.
    (b) simple cuboidal epithelium.
    (c) simple columnar epithelium.
    (d) stratified cuboidal epithelium.

30. Why does holocrine secretion require continuous cell division?

31. What is the difference between an exocrine secretion and an endocrine secretion?

32. A significant structural feature in the digestive system is the presence of tight junctions located near the exposed surfaces of cells lining the digestive tract. Why are these junctions so important?

33. Why are infections always a serious threat after a severe burn or an abrasion?

34. What characteristics make the cutaneous membrane different from serous and mucous membranes?

Level 3 Critical Thinking and Clinical Applications

35. Your lab partner in a biology class loses the labels of two prepared slides—one of an animal's intestine, the other an animal's esophagus. How could you help her tell which slide is which?

36. You are asked to develop a scheme that can be used to identify the three types of muscle tissue in just two steps. What would the two steps be?

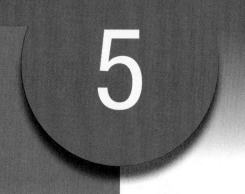

The Integumentary System

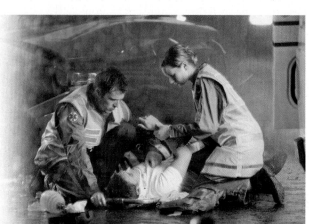

Learning Objectives

These objectives tell you what you should be able to do after completing the chapter. They correspond by number to this chapter's sections.

5-1 Describe the main structural features of the epidermis, and explain the functional significance of each.

5-2 Explain what accounts for individual differences in skin color, and discuss the response of melanocytes to sunlight exposure.

5-3 Describe the interaction between sunlight and vitamin D_3 production.

5-4 Describe the structure and functions of the dermis.

5-5 Describe the structure and functions of the hypodermis.

5-6 Describe the processes that produce hair and the structural basis for hair texture and color.

5-7 Discuss the various kinds of glands in the skin, and list the secretions of those glands.

5-8 Describe the anatomical structure of nails, and explain how they are formed.

5-9 Explain how the skin responds to injury and repairs itself.

5-10 Summarize the effects of aging on the skin.

An Introduction to the Integumentary System

The integumentary system consists of the skin, hair, nails, and various glands. It is the most visible organ system of the body. We devote a lot of time to improving its appearance. Washing your face and hands, brushing or trimming your hair, clipping your nails, showering, and applying deodorant—all these activities modify the appearance or properties of the skin. And when something goes wrong with your skin, the effects are immediately apparent. You may notice a minor skin condition or blemish at once, yet ignore more serious problems in other organ systems. Physicians also pay attention to the skin because changes in its color, flexibility, or sensitivity can be important clues about a disorder in another body system.

The **integumentary system**, or simply the **integument** (in-TEG-ū-ment), has two major parts: the cutaneous membrane and accessory structures (**Figure 5-1**). The **cutaneous membrane**, or *skin*, is an organ composed of the superficial epithelium, or **epidermis** (*epi-*, above), and the underlying connective tissues of the **dermis**. The **accessory structures** include hair, exocrine glands, and nails. They are located primarily in the dermis and protrude through the epidermis to the skin surface.

Beneath the dermis, the loose connective tissue of the **hypodermis**, or *subcutaneous layer*, separates the integument from deeper tissues and organs. It is often not considered to be part of the integumentary system, but we include it here because its connective tissue fibers are interwoven with those of the dermis.

The integument has five major functions:

1. ***Protection.*** The skin covers and protects underlying tissues and organs from impacts, chemicals, and infections. It also prevents the loss of body fluids.

2. ***Temperature maintenance.*** The skin maintains normal body temperature by regulating heat exchange with the environment.

3. ***Synthesis and storage of nutrients.*** The epidermis synthesizes vitamin D_3, a steroid building block for a hormone that aids calcium uptake. The dermis stores large reserves of lipids in adipose tissue.

4. ***Sensory reception.*** Receptors in the integument detect touch, pressure, pain, and temperature stimuli and relay that information to the nervous system.

5. ***Excretion and secretion.*** Integumentary glands excrete salts, water, and organic wastes. Also, specialized integumentary glands of the breasts secrete milk.

Figure 5-1 The General Structure of the Integumentary System. This diagrammatic section of the skin shows the relationships among the major parts of the integumentary system (with the exception of nails, shown in **Figure 5-8**).

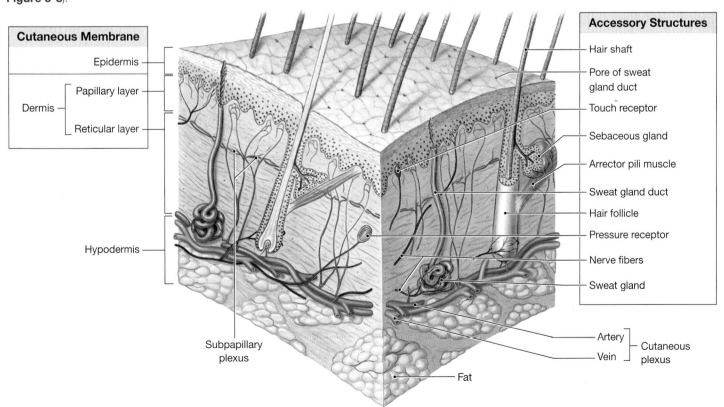

Cutaneous Membrane
- Epidermis
- Dermis
  - Papillary layer
  - Reticular layer

Hypodermis

Subpapillary plexus

Fat

Accessory Structures
- Hair shaft
- Pore of sweat gland duct
- Touch receptor
- Sebaceous gland
- Arrector pili muscle
- Sweat gland duct
- Hair follicle
- Pressure receptor
- Nerve fibers
- Sweat gland
- Artery ⎱ Cutaneous
- Vein ⎰ plexus

Build Your Knowledge

The Build Your Knowledge feature reminds you of what you already know and prepares you to learn new material. Be sure to read every Build Your Knowledge box or page so that you can build your knowledge—and confidence!

Recall that the epidermis is a stratified squamous epithelium and is found where mechanical stresses are severe (as you saw in **Chapter 4: The Tissue Level of Organization**). Such an epithelium provides physical protection against abrasion and chemical attack, and helps keep microorganisms outside the body. ⊃ **p. 99**

We will explore these functions more fully as we discuss the individual components of the integument. We begin with the superficial layer of the skin: the epidermis.

CHECKPOINT

1. List five major functions of the integumentary system.

See the blue Answers tab at the back of the book.

5-1 The epidermis is composed of strata (layers) with various functions

Learning Objective Describe the main structural features of the epidermis, and explain the functional significance of each.

Like all other epithelia, the epidermis is avascular and contains no blood vessels. For this reason, epidermal cells must rely on the diffusion of nutrients and oxygen from capillaries within the underlying dermis. As a result, the epidermal cells with the highest metabolic demands lie closest to the basement membrane, where diffusion distance is short. The outer, superficial cells far removed from the source of nutrients are dead.

Keratinocytes (ke-RAT-i-nō-sīts) are the body's most abundant epithelial cells. They dominate the epidermis. They form several layers of cells and contain the protein keratin (discussed shortly). **Thick skin**, found on the palms of the hands and soles of the feet, contains five layers of cells. Only four layers make up **thin skin**, which covers the rest of the body. The words *thin* and *thick* refer to the relative thickness of the epidermis only, not to that of the integument as a whole.

Spotlight Figure 5-4 shows the five cell layers, or **strata** (singular *stratum*), in a section of thick skin. In order, from the basement membrane toward the free surface, they are the *stratum basale*, three intermediate layers (the *stratum spinosum*, the *stratum granulosum*, and the *stratum lucidum*), and the *stratum corneum*.

CLINICAL NOTE

Dermatology

The integumentary system consists of the skin, hair, nails, and various glands. The largest and one of the most versatile organs of the body, it plays a major role in the maintenance of homeostasis. The study and treatment of diseases of the skin, hair, and nails is called *dermatology*, and physicians who specialize in the medical and surgical treatment of these disorders are called *dermatologists*. Dermatologists diagnose and treat skin, hair, and nail conditions and perform minor skin surgeries such as lesion removal. Physicians who perform major skin surgery are referred to as *plastic surgeons*. There are two general categories of plastic surgery: reconstructive and cosmetic (esthetic). Reconstructive surgery corrects defects due to trauma, tumors, and disease, whereas cosmetic surgery is elective surgery that changes the physical appearance of a part of the body.

The integumentary system is essential to the body's continued maintenance of homeostasis. Its functions include:

- **Protection.** The skin is a barrier that prevents the entry of microorganisms and other harmful substances. It also prevents the loss of water from the body to the environment.
- **Temperature maintenance.** The integument plays a major role in temperature balance by regulating heat gain or heat loss to the environment.
- **Nutrient storage.** The subcutaneous tissues contain a large reserve of lipids for use in metabolism and hormone production.
- **Sensory reception.** The skin contains a vast network of sensory fibers and nerves that detect touch, pressure, pain, and temperature.
- **Excretion and secretion.** The skin secretes water, salt, and organic wastes as the body strives to maintain homeostasis. The skin is important in the synthesis of important chemicals and hormones including the production of vitamin D.

The skin consists of the epidermis, the dermis, and the subcutaneous tissues. It is thickest on the lower back and thinnest on the genitalia. Various tensions on the skin cause it to be oriented into patterns called *cleavage lines* or *Langer's lines* (**Figures 5–2** and **5–3**). Incisions and wounds perpendicular to cleavage lines tend to gape open, while incisions and wounds parallel to the cleavage lines tend to heal with a thin, less noticeable scar.

Figure 5–2 Cleavage Lines or Langer's Lines. These lines represent natural tension patterns in the skin. If possible, surgeons try to make their incisions parallel to the cleavage lines so that the tension on the wound edges is kept to a minimum.

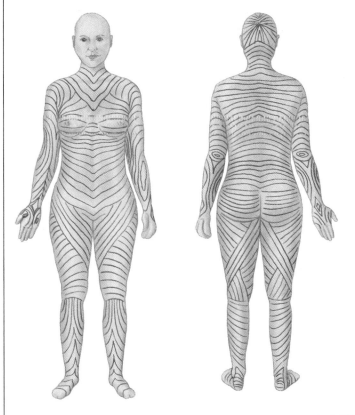

Figure 5–3 Cleavage Lines of the Face.

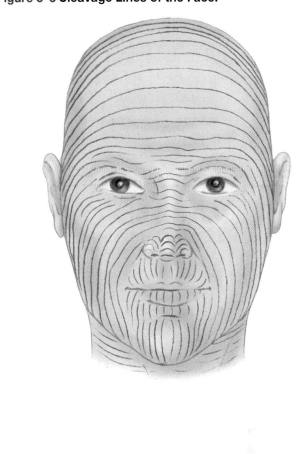

Stratum Basale

The deepest epidermal layer is called the **stratum basale** (STRA-tum buh-SAHL-āy; *basis,* base), or *stratum germinativum* (STRA-tum jer-mi-na-TĒ-vum; *stratum,* layer + *germinare,* to start growing). Hemidesmosomes attach the cells of this layer firmly to the basement membrane. ⊃ p. 93 The basement membrane separates the epidermis from the areolar connective tissue of the adjacent dermis.

The stratum basale forms **epidermal ridges**, which extend into the dermis. Between the ridges, dermal projections called *dermal papillae* (singular *papilla;* a nippleshaped mound) extend upward into the epidermis (**Spotlight Figure 5-4**). The combination of ridges and papillae increases the area of contact between the two regions and strengthens the bond between them. It also increases the available surface area for diffusion of nutrients between the dermis and epidermis.

The contours of the skin surface follow the ridge patterns, which vary from small cone-shaped pegs (in thin skin) to the complex whorls on the thick skin of the palms and soles. The superficial ridges on the palms and soles (which overlie the dermal papillae) increase the surface area of the skin and increase friction, ensuring a secure grip. The ridge patterns on the tips of the fingers are also the basis of fingerprints. These ridge shapes are determined partly by genes and partly by the environment inside the uterus. That is, during fetal development, contact with amniotic fluid, another fetus (in the case of twins), or the uterine wall will affect the fingerprint pattern of a fetus. For this reason, identical twins do not have identical fingerprints. The pattern of your epidermal ridges is unique and does not change over the course of a lifetime.

BASIC ORGANIZATION OF THE EPIDERMIS

The epidermis consists of stratified squamous epithelium. It is separated from the dermis by a basement membrane. The stratum basale and the underlying dermis interlock, strengthening the bond between the two. The epidermis forms epidermal ridges, which extend into the dermis and are adjacent to dermal papillae that project into the epidermis.

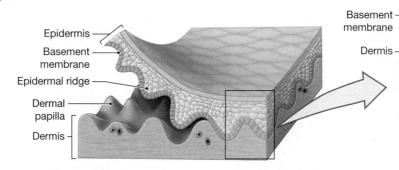

Epidermis
Basement membrane
Epidermal ridge
Dermal papilla
Dermis

Stratum corneum
Basement membrane
Dermis

Thin skin   LM × 200

Thin skin contains four layers of keratinocytes and is about as thick as the wall of a plastic sandwich bag (about 0.08 mm).

LAYERS OF THE EPIDERMIS

The layers of the epidermis are best shown in a sectional view of thick skin. **Thick skin** contains a fifth layer, the *stratum lucidum*. Because thick skin also has a much thicker superficial layer (the *stratum corneum*), it is about as thick as a standard paper towel (about 0.5 mm).

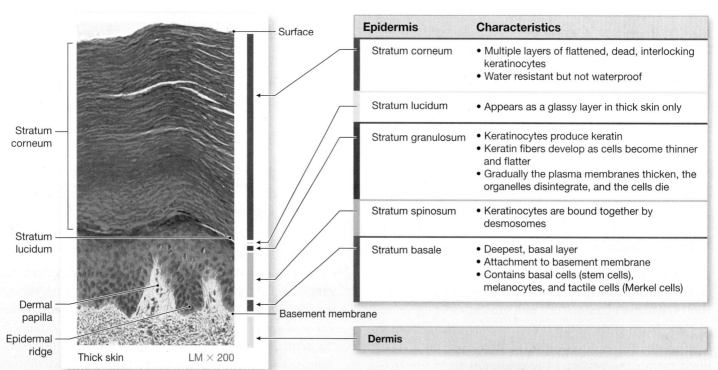

Stratum corneum
Stratum lucidum
Dermal papilla
Epidermal ridge

Thick skin   LM × 200

Surface

Basement membrane

Dermis

Epidermis	Characteristics
Stratum corneum	• Multiple layers of flattened, dead, interlocking keratinocytes • Water resistant but not waterproof
Stratum lucidum	• Appears as a glassy layer in thick skin only
Stratum granulosum	• Keratinocytes produce keratin • Keratin fibers develop as cells become thinner and flatter • Gradually the plasma membranes thicken, the organelles disintegrate, and the cells die
Stratum spinosum	• Keratinocytes are bound together by desmosomes
Stratum basale	• Deepest, basal layer • Attachment to basement membrane • Contains basal cells (stem cells), melanocytes, and tactile cells (Merkel cells)

EPIDERMAL RIDGES OF THICK SKIN

Fingerprints reveal the pattern of epidermal ridges. The scanning electron micrograph to the right shows the ridges on a fingertip.

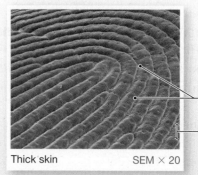

Pores of sweat gland ducts
Epidermal ridge

Thick skin   SEM × 20

melanin, a red-yellow to brown-black pigment that colors the epidermis.

Intermediate Strata

The cells in the three layers of the intermediate strata are progressively displaced from the basal layer as they become specialized to form the outer protective barrier of the skin. Each time a stem cell divides, one of the resulting daughter cells enters the next layer, the **stratum spinosum** (spiny layer). There it may continue to divide and add to the thickness of the epithelium. This stratum consists of keratinocytes held together by desmosomes. It also contains branched *dendritic cells* that take part in the immune response.

The **stratum granulosum** (grainy layer) consists of cells displaced from the stratum spinosum. They have stopped dividing and have begun making large amounts of the protein **keratin** (KER-a-tin; *keros,* horn). ⟲ p. 44 Keratin is extremely durable and water-resistant. In humans, keratin not only coats the surface of the skin but also forms the basic structure of hair, calluses, and nails. In various other animals, it forms structures such as horns and hooves, feathers, and baleen plates (in the mouths of filter-feeding whales).

In the thick skin of the palms and soles, a glassy **stratum lucidum** (clear layer) covers the stratum granulosum. The cells in this layer are flattened, densely packed, and filled with keratin.

Stratum Corneum

At the exposed surface of the skin is the **stratum corneum** (KOR-nē-um; *cornu,* horn). It normally contains 15–30 layers of flattened and dead epithelial cells packed with filaments of keratin. Such cells are said to be **keratinized** (ker-A-tin-īzed), or **cornified** (KOR-ni-f īd; *cornu,* horn + *facere,* to make). The dead cells in each layer of the stratum corneum remain tightly connected by desmosomes. As a result, these cells are generally shed in large groups or sheets rather than individually.

It takes 7–10 days for a cell to move from the stratum basale to the stratum corneum. During this time, the cell is displaced from its oxygen and nutrient supply, becomes filled with keratin, and finally dies. The dead cells usually remain in the stratum corneum for two more weeks before they are shed or washed away. As superficial layers are lost, new layers arrive from the underlying strata. Thus, the deeper layers of the epithelium and underlying tissues remain protected by a barrier of dead, durable, and expendable cells. Normally, the surface of the stratum corneum is relatively dry, so it is unsuitable for the growth of many microorganisms.

CLINICAL NOTE

Drug Administration through the Skin

Drugs dissolved in oils or other lipid-soluble solvents can be carried across the plasma membranes of the epidermal cells. The movement is slow, particularly through the stratum corneum, but 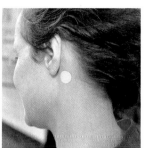 once a drug reaches the underlying tissues, it will be absorbed into the circulation.

A useful technique for long-term drug administration involves putting a sticky, drug-containing patch over an area of thin skin. To overcome the slow rate of diffusion, the patch must contain an extremely high concentration of the drug. This technique, called *transdermal administration*, has the advantage that a single patch may work for several days, making daily pills unnecessary. Two drugs routinely administered transdermally are:

- Nitroglycerin which can be used to treat angina pectoris.
- Nicotine, the addictive compound in tobacco, for suppressing the craving for a cigarette. The transdermal dosage of nicotine can gradually be reduced in small controlled steps.

Other transdermal procedures include so-called "active" patches containing sharp microneedles and procedures using a brief pulse of electricity to the skin.

Large stem cells, called **basal cells** or *germinative cells*, dominate the stratum basale. Their continuous division replaces cells that are lost or shed at the epithelial surface. The stratum basale also contains *Merkel cells* (specialized epithelial cells sensitive to touch) and *melanocytes*, squeezed between or deep to the cells in this layer. Melanocytes synthesize

Build Your Knowledge

To form an effective barrier that protects underlying tissues, the epithelial cells of the skin must hold onto one another and also be connected to the rest of the body. They do this with specialized cell junctions known as desmosomes and hemidesmosomes (as you saw in **Chapter 4: The Tissue Level of Organization**). Desmosomes lock together the plasma membranes of epithelial cells forming the different strata of the epidermis. Hemidesmosomes firmly attach the deepest cells of the stratum basale to the extracellular basement membrane. ⟲ **p. 93**

CLINICAL NOTE

Disorders of Keratin Production

The excessive production of keratin is called hyperkeratosis (hī-per-ker-a-TŌ-sis). Calluses and corns are easily observed examples. Calluses are thickened areas that appear on already thick-skinned areas, such as the palms of the hands or the soles or heels of the feet. They form in response to chronic abrasion and distortion. Corns are more lo-

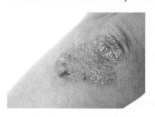

calized areas of excessive keratin production that form in areas of thin skin on or between the toes.

In psoriasis (so-RĪ-a-sis), basal cells (stem cells) in the stratum basale are unusually ac-tive, causing hyperkeratosis in specific areas, such as the scalp, elbows, palms, soles, groin, or nails. Normally, an individual stem cell divides once about every 20 days, but in psoriasis it may divide every day and a half. Keratinization is abnormal and typically incomplete by the time the outer layers are shed. The affected areas have red bases covered with vast numbers of small, silvery scales that continu-ously flake off. Psoriasis develops in 20–30 percent of individuals with an inherited tendency for the condition. Roughly 5 percent of the U.S. population has psoriasis to some degree. It is fre-quently aggravated by stress and anxiety. Most cases are pain-less and controllable, but not curable.

CHECKPOINT

2. Identify the five layers of the epidermis.

3. Dandruff is caused by excessive shedding of cells from the outer layer of skin in the scalp. Thus, dandruff is composed of cells from which epidermal layer?

4. Some criminals sand their fingertips to avoid leaving recognizable fingerprints. Would this practice perma-nently remove fingerprints? Why or why not?

See the blue Answers tab at the back of the book.

5-2 Factors influencing skin color are epidermal pigmentation and dermal circulation

Learning Objective Explain what accounts for individual differences in skin color, and discuss the response of melanocytes to sunlight exposure.

One of the most obvious differences among humans is skin color. What gives skin its various colors? Here we examine how pigments in the epidermis and blood flow in the dermis influence skin color.

The Role of Pigmentation

The epidermis contains variable amounts of two pigments, carotene and melanin. **Carotene** (KAR-uh-tēn) is an orange-yellow pigment that normally accumulates in epidermal cells. It is found in a variety of orange-colored vegetables, such as carrots and squashes. Eating lots of carrots can actu-ally cause the skin of light-skinned individuals to turn or-ange. The color change is less striking in the skin of darker individuals. Carotene can be converted to vitamin A, which is required for the normal maintenance of epithelial tissues and the synthesis of photoreceptor pigments in the eye.

Melanin is a pigment made by pigment-producing cells called **melanocytes** (me-LAN-ō-sīts). There are two types of melanin, a red-yellow form and a brown-black form. Melanocytes manufacture and store melanin within intracel-lular vesicles called *melanosomes* (**Figure 5-5**). These vesicles are transferred to the epithelial cells of the stratum basale, coloring the entire epidermis. Melanocyte activity slowly increases in re-sponse to sunlight exposure, peaking around 10 days after the initial exposure. *Freckles* are small pigmented spots that appear on the skin of pale-skinned individuals. Freckles represent areas of greater-than-average melanin production. They tend to be most abundant on surfaces exposed to the sun, such as the face.

The ratio of melanocytes to basal cells ranges between 1:4 and 1:20, depending on the region of the body. The skin cov-ering most areas of the body has about 1000 melanocytes per square millimeter. The cheeks and forehead, the nipples, and the genital region (the scrotum in males and labia majora in females) have about twice that density.

People of all skin colors produce both types of melanin. The differences in skin pigmentation among individuals are due to the amount of each type produced. A deficiency or ab-sence of melanin production leads to a disorder known as *al-binism*. Individuals with albinism have a normal abundance and distribution of melanocytes, but these cells are not able to produce melanin.

Sunlight contains significant amounts of **ultraviolet (UV) radiation**. A small amount of UV radiation is benefi-cial because it stimulates the synthesis of vitamin D_3 in the epidermis. (We discuss this process in a later section.) Too much ultraviolet radiation, however, produces immediate effects of mild or even serious burns. Melanin helps prevent skin damage by absorbing UV radiation before it reaches the deep layers of the epidermis and dermis. Within epi-dermal cells, melanin concentrates around the nuclear en-velope. There it absorbs UV radiation before it can damage nuclear DNA.

Figure 5-5 Melanocytes. These views show the location and orientation of melanocytes in the deepest layer of the epidermis (stratum basale) of a dark-skinned person.

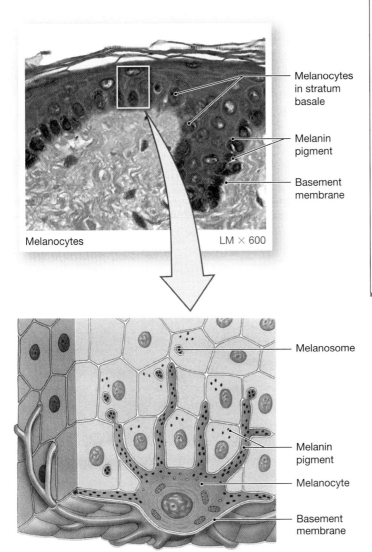

Melanocytes in stratum basale

Melanin pigment

Basement membrane

Melanocytes LM × 600

Melanosome

Melanin pigment

Melanocyte

Basement membrane

CLINICAL NOTE

Skin Color

Skin color is an important indicator of body function and varies from person to person. Changes in skin color are often evidence of a systemic disease. Normal skin color in light-skinned people is pink, which indicates adequate cardiorespiratory function and vascular integrity. In dark-skinned people, inspect the mucous membranes (such as the lips) to detect skin color changes. Paleness indicates decreased blood flow through the skin and results from anemia or conditions such as hypothermia or hypovolemia. A bluish discoloration of the skin is called *cyanosis* and is due to increased amounts of unoxygenated hemoglobin. The presence of cyanosis should alert care providers to an underlying problem that adversely affects oxygenation or perfusion. A yellowish discoloration of the skin, called *jaundice*, is due to the accumulation of bilirubin in the skin tissues. This is seen in liver diseases such as hepatitis and liver failure. A red coloration to the skin may be due to carbon monoxide poisoning. As carbon monoxide replaces oxygen on the hemoglobin molecules, the red color of the blood is enhanced, and this is evident in the skin.

The Role of Dermal Circulation

Blood with abundant oxygen is bright red, so blood vessels in the dermis normally give the skin a reddish tint that is most apparent in lightly pigmented individuals. If those vessels dilate (widen), the red tones become much more pronounced. For example, skin becomes flushed and red when body temperature rises because the superficial blood vessels dilate so that the skin can act like a radiator and lose heat. ↰ p. 11 When the vessels are temporarily constricted, as when you are frightened, the skin becomes relatively pale.

During a sustained reduction in circulatory supply, the blood in the skin loses oxygen to surrounding tissues and takes on a darker red tone. Seen from the surface, the skin then takes on a bluish coloration called **cyanosis** (sī-uh-NŌ-sis; *kyanos*, blue). In individuals of any skin color, cyanosis is most apparent in areas of thin skin, such as the lips, ears, or beneath the nails. It can be a response to extreme cold or a result of circulatory or respiratory disorders, such as heart failure or severe asthma.

Despite the presence of melanin, long-term damage can result from repeated exposure to sunlight, even in dark-skinned individuals. Over time, cumulative UV damage to the skin can harm fibroblasts, impairing maintenance of the dermis. The result is premature wrinkling. In addition, skin cancers can result from chromosomal damage in stem cells of the stratum basale or in melanocytes. One of the major consequences of the global depletion of the ozone layer in the upper atmosphere is likely to be a sharp increase in the rate of skin cancers (such as *malignant melanoma*). For this reason, it makes sense to limit your UV exposure by wearing protective clothing and sunscreens during outdoor activities.

CHECKPOINT

5. Name the two pigments in the epidermis.

6. Why does exposure to sunlight or sunlamps darken skin?

7. Why does the skin of a light-skinned person appear red during exercise in hot weather?

See the blue Answers tab at the back of the book.

5-3 Sunlight has beneficial and detrimental effects on the skin

Learning Objective Describe the interaction between sunlight and vitamin D_3 production.

In this section, we briefly consider how interactions between sunlight and skin cells regularly produce an important vitamin, and can sometimes result in skin cancers.

The Epidermis and Vitamin D_3

Too much sunlight can damage epithelial cells and deeper tissues, but limited exposure to sunlight is beneficial. When exposed to UV radiation, epidermal cells in the stratum spinosum and stratum basale convert a cholesterol-related steroid into **vitamin D_3**. The liver then converts vitamin D_3 into an intermediary product used by the kidneys to synthesize the hormone *calcitriol*. Calcitriol is essential for the absorption of calcium and phosphorus in the small intestine. An inadequate supply of vitamin D_3 can lead to abnormally weak and flexible bones.

Skin Cancers

Almost everyone has several benign tumors of the skin. Moles and warts are common examples. Skin cancers, however, are more dangerous. They are the most common form of cancer. Any cancer of epithelial tissue is called a **carcinoma** (kar-si-NŌ-mah). The most common *skin* cancer is **basal cell carcinoma**, which often looks like a waxy bump (**Figure 5-6a**). This cancer originates in the stratum basale. Less common are **squamous cell carcinomas**, which involve more superficial layers of epidermal cells. Metastasis seldom occurs in either cancer, and most people survive these cancers. The usual treatment involves surgical removal of the tumor.

Figure 5-6 Skin Cancers.

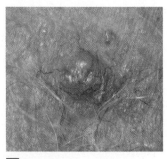
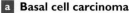
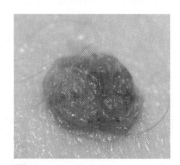

a Basal cell carcinoma   **b** Melanoma

Compared with these common and seldom life-threatening cancers, **malignant melanomas** (mel-a-NŌ-maz) are extremely dangerous (**Figure 5-6b**). In this condition, cancerous melanocytes grow rapidly and metastasize through the lymphatic system. A melanoma usually begins from a mole but may appear anywhere in the body. The outlook for long-term survival depends on when the condition is detected and treated. Avoiding exposure to UV radiation in sunlight (especially during the middle of the day) and using a sunblock (not a tanning oil) would largely prevent all three forms of cancer.

> **CHECKPOINT**
>
> 8. Explain the relationship between sunlight exposure and vitamin D_3 synthesis.
>
> 9. What is the most common skin cancer?
>
> See the blue Answers tab at the back of the book.

5-4 The dermis is the tissue layer that supports the epidermis

Learning Objective Describe the structure and functions of the dermis.

The dermis lies between the epidermis and the hypodermis. It has two major layers: a superficial *papillary layer* and a deeper *reticular layer* (**Figure 5-1**).

The **papillary layer**, named after the dermal papillae, consists of areolar tissue that supports and nourishes the epidermis. This region contains the capillaries, lymphatic vessels, and sensory neurons that supply the surface of the skin.

The deeper **reticular layer** consists of an interwoven meshwork of dense irregular connective tissue containing both *elastic fibers* and *collagen fibers*. The elastic fibers provide flexibility, and the collagen fibers limit that flexibility to prevent damage to the tissue. Bundles of collagen fibers blend into those of the papillary layer above, blurring the boundary between these layers. Collagen fibers of the reticular layer also extend into the deeper hypodermis.

In addition to protein-based elastic and collagen fibers, the dermis contains the mixed cell populations of connective tissue proper. The dominant cell type of the dermis is the fibroblast. ↺ p. 103 Accessory organs derived from the epidermis, such as hair follicles and sweat glands, extend into the dermis (**Figure 5-1**).

Other organ systems interact with the skin through their connections to the dermis. For example, both dermal layers contain a network of blood vessels (cardiovascular system), lymphatic vessels (lymphatic system), and nerve fibers (nervous system).

CLINICAL NOTE

Dermatitis

Inflammation is a complex process that helps defend the body against pathogens and injury. ⟲ p. 114 Skin inflammation can be very painful because skin contains an abundance of sensory receptors.

Dermatitis (der-muh-TĪ-tis) is an inflammation of the skin that mainly involves the papillary layer of the dermis. The inflammation typically begins in an area of the skin exposed to infection or irritated by chemicals, radiation, or mechanical stimuli, such as scratching. Dermatitis may cause no discomfort, or it may produce an annoying itch. Sometimes the condition can be quite painful, and the inflammation can spread rapidly across the entire integument.

Dermatitis has many forms. Some of them are common:

- Contact dermatitis generally occurs in response to strong chemical irritants. It produces an itchy rash that may spread to other areas. One example is poison ivy.
- Eczema (EK-se-muh) can be triggered by temperature changes, fungi, chemical irritants, greases, detergents, or stress. Hereditary factors, environmental factors, or both can promote its development.
- Diaper rash is a localized dermatitis caused by a combination of moisture, irritating chemicals from fecal or urinary wastes, and microorganisms, frequently the yeast Candida, which is a fungus.
- Urticaria (ur-ti-KAR-ē-uh), also called hives, is an extensive allergic response to a food, drug, insect bite, infection, stress, or some other stimulus.

Arteries supplying the skin lie deep in the hypodermis. Branches of the arteries form two networks, or *plexuses*, in the dermis. The deeper network lies along the border of the hypodermis with the reticular layer of the dermis. This network is called the *cutaneous plexus* (**Figure 5-1**). Branches of these arteries supply both the adipose tissue in the hypodermis and the tissues of the integument. As small arteries travel toward the epidermis, branches supply the hair follicles, sweat glands, and other structures in the dermis.

On reaching the papillary layer, the small arteries form another network called the *subpapillary plexus* (**Figure 5-1**). It provides blood to capillary loops that follow the contours of the epidermis–dermis boundary. (Capillaries are the smallest blood vessels. They are where nutrients and oxygen are exchanged for carbon dioxide and waste products. ⟲ p. 107) The capillaries empty into small veins of the subpapillary plexus. These small veins, in turn, drain into veins accompanying arteries of the cutaneous plexus. This network connects to larger veins in the deep hypodermis.

Both the blood vessels and the lymphatic vessels in the dermis help local tissues defend and repair themselves after injury or infection. The nerve fibers control blood flow, adjust gland secretion rates, and monitor sensory receptors in the dermis and the deeper layers of the epidermis. These receptors provide sensations of touch, pain, pressure, and temperature. (We will describe them in Chapter 9.)

CHECKPOINT

10. Describe the location of the dermis.

11. Where are the capillaries that supply the epidermis located?

See the blue Answers tab at the back of the book.

5-5 The hypodermis connects the dermis to underlying tissues

Learning Objective Describe the structure and functions of the hypodermis.

The **hypodermis**, or subcutaneous layer, lies deep to the dermis (**Figure 5-1**). The boundary between the two is generally indistinct because the connective tissue fibers of the reticular layer are extensively interwoven with those of the hypodermis. The hypodermis is not a part of the integument, but it is important in stabilizing the position of the skin relative to underlying tissues, such as skeletal muscles or other organs, while permitting them to move independently.

The hypodermis consists of areolar tissue with many fat cells. These adipose cells provide infants and small children with a layer of "baby fat," which helps to reduce heat loss. Subcutaneous fat also serves as an energy reserve and a shock absorber for the rough-and-tumble activities of our early years.

As we grow and mature, the distribution of subcutaneous fat changes. The greatest change takes place in response to circulating sex hormones. Beginning at puberty, men accumulate subcutaneous fat at the neck, upper arms, along the lower back, and over the buttocks. Women do so in the breasts, buttocks, hips, and thighs. Both women and men, however, may accumulate distressing amounts of adipose tissue in the abdominal region, producing a prominent "potbelly." An excessive amount of such abdominal fat is strongly correlated with cardiovascular disease.

The hypodermis is quite elastic. Its superficial region contains the large blood vessels of the cutaneous plexus. Below this region, the hypodermis contains few capillaries and no vital organs. The lack of vital organs makes *subcutaneous injection* a useful method for administering drugs using a *hypodermic needle*.

5

CLINICAL NOTE

Medical Conditions of the Skin

Many diseases affect the skin. These can be localized to the skin or can involve other body organs and systems. Often, skin lesions are due to infections or problems elsewhere in the body.

Exanthems

Many of the viruses that infect humans cause characteristic skin rashes during the course of the infection. An exanthem is an acute, generalized skin eruption that can be caused by drugs, viruses, or certain bacteria. Usually, the eruption causes macules or papules, although some will have vesicles. Most of the childhood viral infections are characterized by recognizable viral exanthems (**Figure 5–7**). These include: rubella (three-day, or German measles), rubeola (red measles), roseola, and varicella (chicken pox). Certain bacterial infections also result in the development of an exanthem. The most common of these, scarlet fever (scarletina), is caused by group A beta-hemolytic streptococcus infection, usually pharyngitis. The rash of scarlet fever feels like sandpaper, and the face is flushed with an obvious pallor around the mouth.

Many of the viral exanthems are asymptomatic. Some, however, can cause itching and pain. Varicella causes vesicles that can actually shed the virus. Exanthems do not require specific treatment. Instead, treatment is directed at the underlying cause or at the symptoms that make the patient uncomfortable.

Herpes Zoster

Herpes zoster (shingles) is a disease characterized by the eruption of groups of vesicles along the dermatome of a sensory nerve. The virus that causes varicella (chicken pox) and herpes zoster is the varicella-zoster virus (VZV). After the initial infection

Figure 5-7 Examples of Viral Exanthems Associated with Childhood Illness. (a) varicella or chicken pox; (b) rubeola or red measles.

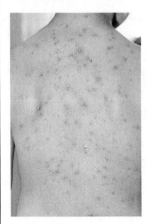
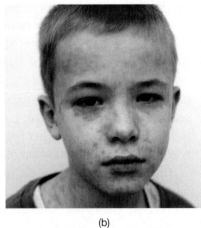

(a)   (b)

with VZV, the patient will develop varicella. This usually occurs during childhood. During the course of the varicella infection, the VZV enters the ganglia for the sensory nerve and remains there for life. Later in life, the virus becomes reactivated and spreads along the sensory nerve that it infected. Stress, disease, and immunosuppression appear to be causes of virus reactivation, although in most cases the cause is idiopathic (cannot be determined). Initially, zoster causes pain that is often severe, followed by redness of the affected area. The redness and rash are limited to the dermatome of the affected nerve, and the rash does not cross the midline of the body. Zoster infections can also affect the cranial nerves or involve the eye. Eventually, the vesicles will break out. Although antiviral drugs do not eradicate the virus, they are effective to decrease the severity of the infection and the length of the outbreak, which may last for several weeks.

Staphylococcal Scalded Skin Syndrome

Staphylococcal scalded skin syndrome (SSSS) is most frequently seen in children less than 5 years of age. It is caused by infection with group II staphylococci, which produces a toxin that causes separation of the skin just below the granular layer of the epidermis. This results in sloughing of the skin in the affected areas. The toxin, an epidermolysin, is usually produced at a site other than the skin and is delivered to the skin via the circulatory system.

SSSS begins with fever, malaise, irritability, and runny nose, followed by generalized erythema (redness) with exquisite tenderness. The erythema spreads from the face and trunk to cover the entire body with the exception of the palms of the hands, soles of the feet, and mucous membranes. Within 48 hours, blisters and bullae may form and the pain becomes severe. As the blisters rupture, fluid is lost, which results in dehydration. In severe cases, the skin of the entire body may slough. Treatment of SSSS includes antibiotics to eradicate the underlying infection and replacement fluids if needed. The skin should be treated the same as with a severe burn. Children with a large area of skin involvement are best treated in a burn center.

Toxic Epidermal Necrolysis

Toxic epidermal necrolysis (TEN) is a serious and sometimes fatal drug reaction that is similar to staphylococcal scalded skin syndrome. It primarily affects adults. Antibiotics of the sulfonamide class, nonsteroidal anti-inflammatory drugs, and anticonvulsants seem to be the cause of most cases of TEN. The skin eruption is preceded by fever, malaise, anorexia, and inflammation of the eyelids and mucous membranes. The skin becomes reddened and is very tender, first in the axillae and groin, then extends over the body surface. Blisters and bullae form, and the entire epidermis may be shed. TEN causes full-thickness necrosis (death) of the epidermis with subepidermal blister formations. Treatment is identical as for burns, and severe cases are best managed in a burn unit.

CHECKPOINT

12. List the two terms for the tissue that connects the dermis to underlying tissues.

13. Describe the hypodermis.

See the blue Answers tab at the back of the book.

5-6 Hair is composed of dead, keratinized cells that have been pushed to the skin surface

Learning Objective Describe the processes that produce hair and the structural basis for hair texture and color.

Hair and several other structures—hair follicles, sebaceous and sweat glands, and nails—are considered accessory structures of the integument. During embryonic development, these structures originate from the epidermis.

Hairs are nonliving, keratinized structures produced in organs called **hair follicles** (**Figure 5-8a**). Hairs project above the surface of the skin almost everywhere. We do not have hairs on the sides and soles of the feet, the palms of the hands, the sides of the fingers and toes, the lips, and portions of the external genital organs.

The Structure of Hair and Hair Follicles

Hair follicles project deep into the dermis and usually into the underlying hypodermis (**Figure 5-8b**). The walls of each follicle contain all the cell layers found in the epidermis. The epithelium at the base of a follicle forms a cap over the **hair papilla**, a peg of connective tissue containing capillaries and nerves. Hair is formed by the repeated divisions of epithelial stem cells in the **hair matrix** surrounding the hair papilla. As the daughter cells are pushed toward the

Figure 5-8 Hair Follicles and Hairs.

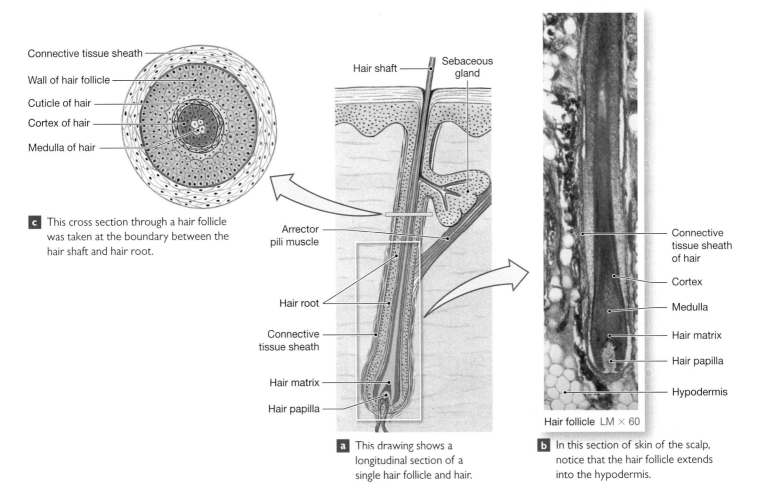

Connective tissue sheath

Wall of hair follicle

Cuticle of hair

Cortex of hair

Medulla of hair

c This cross section through a hair follicle was taken at the boundary between the hair shaft and hair root.

Hair shaft

Sebaceous gland

Arrector pili muscle

Hair root

Connective tissue sheath

Hair matrix

Hair papilla

a This drawing shows a longitudinal section of a single hair follicle and hair.

Connective tissue sheath of hair

Cortex

Medulla

Hair matrix

Hair papilla

Hypodermis

Hair follicle LM × 60

b In this section of skin of the scalp, notice that the hair follicle extends into the hypodermis.

5

CLNICAL NOTE

Hair Loss

Some people feel anxious when they find hairs clinging to their hairbrush instead of to their heads. On the average, we lose about 50 hairs from the head each day, but several factors may affect this rate. Sustained losses of over 100 hairs per day generally indicate a net loss of hair. The absence or loss of hair is called *alopecia* (al-ō-PĒ-shē-uh). Temporary increases in hair loss can result from drugs (including chemotherapeutic agents), radiation, dietary factors, high fever, stress, or hormonal factors related to pregnancy.

In males, changes in the level of circulating sex hormones can affect the scalp, causing a shift in production from normal hair to fine "peach fuzz" hairs, beginning at the temples and the crown of the head. This alteration is called *male pattern baldness*. Some cases of male pattern baldness respond to drug therapies, such as topical application of *minoxidil (Rogaine)*.

Chemotherapy and radiation therapy for cancer treatment can cause hair loss because both cancer cells and normal cells,

notably hair matrix stem cells, are affected. Such hair loss is generally not permanent, but may affect all the hair on the body. In treatment with radiation, only the hair in the area receiving the radiation is affected. Radiation therapy to the head often causes hair loss from the scalp.

Not all drugs administered during chemotherapy cause hair loss. However, when hair loss does occur, it most often begins within a few weeks and generally increases up to two months into treatment. Hair usually begins to regrow a few months after treatment ends, with complete regrowth within a year. The color, thickness, and texture of the new hair may be different from the original hair.

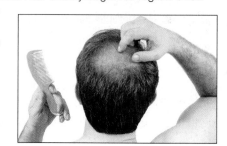

surface, the hair lengthens, and the cells undergo keratinization and die. The point at which this occurs is about halfway to the skin surface and marks the boundary between the **hair root** (the portion that anchors the hair into the skin) and the **hair shaft** (the part we see on the surface) (**Figure 5-8a**).

Each hair shaft consists of three layers of dead, keratinized cells (**Figure 5-8c**). The surface layer, or **cuticle**, is made up of an overlapping shingle-like layer of cells. The underlying layer is called the **cortex**, and the **medulla** makes up the core of the hair. The medulla contains a flexible *soft keratin*. The cortex and cuticle contain thick layers of *hard keratin*, which give the hair its stiffness.

Hairs grow and are shed according to a *hair growth cycle* based on the activity level of hair follicles. In general, a hair in the scalp grows for two to five years, at a rate of about 0.3 mm per day. Then its follicle may become inactive for a similar period of time. When another growth cycle begins, the follicle produces a new hair, and the old hair gets pushed toward the surface to be shed. Variations in growth rate and in the length of the hair growth cycle account for individual differences in the length of uncut hair.

What makes hair curly or straight? These differences result from the cross-sectional shape of the hair shaft and its hair follicle. A curly hair and its follicle are oval or flattened. A straight hair and its follicle are round.

Functions of Hair

The 2.5 million hairs on the human body have important functions. The roughly 500,000 hairs on the head protect the scalp from UV light, help cushion a light blow to the head, and provide insulation for the skull. The hairs guarding the entrances to the nostrils and external ear canals help keep out foreign particles. The eyelashes perform a similar function for the surface of the eye.

A sensory nerve fiber is associated with the base of each hair follicle. As a result, you can even feel the movement of a single hair shaft. This sensitivity provides an early-warning system that may help prevent injury. For example, you may be able to swat a mosquito before it reaches the surface of your skin.

A bundle of smooth muscle cells forms the **arrector pili** (a-REK-tor PI-lē) muscle. It extends from the papillary dermis to the connective tissue sheath around each hair follicle (**Figure 5-8a**). When stimulated, the arrector pili pulls on the follicle, forcing the hair to stand up. Contraction may be caused by emotional states (such as fear or rage) or a response to cold, producing "goose bumps."

Hair Color

Hair color reflects differences in the type and amount of pigment produced by melanocytes at the hair papilla. The two different forms of melanin produce hair colors that can range from black to blond. These pigment differences are

5

CLNICAL NOTE

The Hair in Disease

The hair is a tactile sensory organ that covers the entire body, with the exception of the palms, soles, and parts of the genitalia. Like other body organs, the hair can be affected by disease. Changes in hair growth or distribution can be an aid in the diagnostic process.

Loss of hair occurs with aging. Normally, about 50 hairs are lost each day. Loss of more than 100 hairs per day (*alopecia*) may indicate underlying disease. Severe malnutrition and chemotherapy can cause hair loss. Chemotherapy, often used to treat cancer, inhibits cell growth. This is especially apparent in cells that are rapidly dividing. Cells in the hair follicle divide more rapidly than other body cells. Thus, hair loss often results from chemotherapy.

Hair growth and distribution are primarily controlled by masculine hormones (*androgens*). Diseases that cause an increase in androgens often result in excessive hair growth (*hirsutism*). These include certain tumors, polycystic ovarian disease, and hyperplasia of the adrenal glands. Both hair loss and excessive hair growth should be investigated to determine the underlying cause.

genetically determined, but hormonal and environmental factors also influence the condition of your hair.

What about gray hair? As pigment production decreases with age, hair color lightens. White hair results from both a lack of pigment and the presence of air bubbles within the hair shaft. As the proportion of white hairs increases, the individual's hair color is described as gray. Because each hair is dead and inert, changes in color are gradual. Unless bleach is used, it is not possible for hair to "turn white overnight," as some horror stories would have made us believe.

CHECKPOINT

14. Describe a typical strand of hair.
15. What happens when the arrector pili muscle contracts?
16. If a burn on the forearm destroys the epidermis and the deep dermis and then heals, will hair grow again in the affected area?

See the blue Answers tab at the back of the book.

5-7 Sebaceous glands and sweat glands are exocrine glands found in the skin

Learning Objective Discuss the various kinds of glands in the skin, and list the secretions of those glands.

The integument contains two types of exocrine glands: *sebaceous glands* and *sweat glands*.

Sebaceous (Oil) Glands

Sebaceous (se-BĀ-shus) glands, or *oil glands*, discharge an oily lipid secretion into hair follicles or, in some cases, onto the skin (**Figure 5-9**). The gland cells produce large quantities of lipids as they mature. The lipid is released through holocrine secretion, a process that involves the rupture and death of the cells. ⤴ p. 100 The contraction of the arrector pili muscle that elevates a hair also squeezes the sebaceous gland, forcing the oily secretions into the hair follicle and onto the surrounding skin. This secretion, called **sebum** (SĒ-bum), inhibits the growth of bacteria, lubricates the hair,

Figure 5-9 Sebaceous Glands and Their Relationship to Hair Follicles.

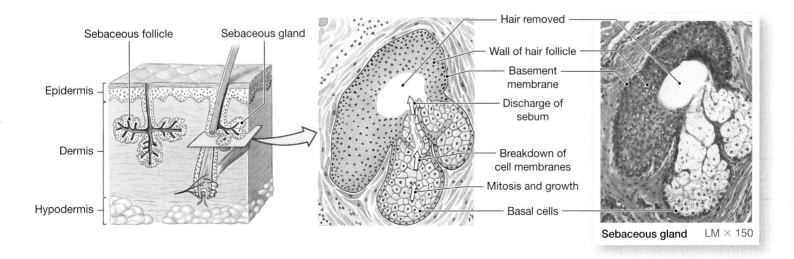

5

and conditions the surrounding skin. **Sebaceous follicles** are large sebaceous glands that discharge sebum directly onto the skin. They are located on the face, back, chest, nipples, and external genitalia.

Sebaceous glands are sensitive to changes in the concentrations of sex hormones. Their secretions accelerate at puberty. For this reason, individuals with large sebaceous glands may be especially prone to develop **acne** during adolescence. In acne, sebaceous ducts become blocked and secretions accumulate, causing inflammation and a raised "pimple." The trapped secretions provide a fertile environment for bacterial infection.

Sweat Glands

The skin contains two types of sweat glands, or *sudoriferous glands*: *apocrine sweat glands* and *merocrine sweat glands* (**Figure 5-10**).

Apocrine Sweat Glands

Apocrine sweat glands secrete their products into hair follicles in the armpits, around the nipples, and in the pubic region. The name *apocrine* was originally chosen because it was thought these gland cells use an apocrine method of

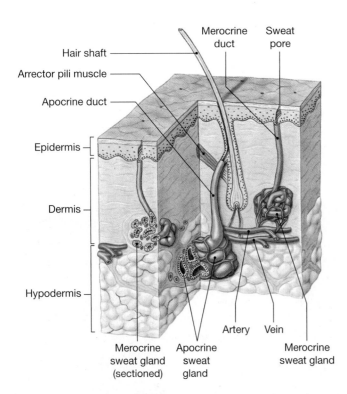

Merocrine duct

Sweat pore

Hair shaft

Arrector pili muscle

Apocrine duct

Epidermis

Dermis

Hypodermis

Merocrine sweat gland (sectioned)

Apocrine sweat gland

Artery

Vein

Merocrine sweat gland

Figure 5-10 Sweat Glands. Merocrine sweat glands secrete directly onto the skin. Apocrine sweat glands secrete into hair follicles.

secretion. ↺ p. 98 We now know that they rely on merocrine secretion, but the name has not changed.

At puberty, these glands begin discharging a sticky, cloudy, and potentially odorous secretion. The sweat is a food source for bacteria, which intensify its odor. In other mammals, this odor is an important form of communication. In our culture, whatever function it might have is masked by products such as deodorants. Other products, such as antiperspirants, contain astringent compounds that contract the skin and its sweat gland openings, thereby decreasing the quantity of both apocrine and merocrine secretions.

Merocrine Sweat Glands

Merocrine sweat glands, or *eccrine* (EK-rin) *sweat glands*, are coiled tubular glands that discharge their secretions directly onto the surface of the skin. They are far more numerous and widely distributed than apocrine glands. The skin of an adult contains 2–5 million eccrine glands. Palms and soles have the highest numbers. It has been estimated that the palm of the hand has about 500 glands per square centimeter (3000 per square inch).

The perspiration, or sweat, produced by merocrine glands is 99 percent water. Sweat also contains a mixture of electrolytes (chiefly sodium chloride), organic nutrients, and waste products such as urea. Sodium chloride gives sweat its salty taste.

The primary function of merocrine gland activity and perspiration is to cool the surface of the skin and lower body temperature. When a person is sweating in the hot sun, all the merocrine glands are working together. The blood vessels beneath the epidermis are dilated and flushed with blood, the skin reddens in light-colored individuals, and the skin surface becomes warm and wet. As the moisture evaporates, the skin cools. If body temperature then falls below normal, perspiration ceases, and blood flow to the skin is reduced. The skin surface then cools and dries, releasing little heat into the environment. (We considered the roles of the skin and negative feedback in thermoregulation, or temperature control, in Chapter 1 on p. 10. In Chapter 17 we will examine this process in greater detail.)

Perspiration results in the loss of water and electrolytes from the body. For this reason, excessive perspiration to maintain normal body temperature can lead to problems. For example, when all the merocrine sweat glands are working at maximum, perspiration may exceed a gallon (about 4 liters) per hour, and dangerous fluid and electrolyte losses can occur. For this reason, marathoners and other endurance athletes must drink fluids at regular intervals.

Build Your Knowledge

Recall that exocrine glands secrete their products onto an epithelial surface (as you saw in **Chapter 4: The Tissue Level of Organization**). These secretions reach the surface either directly (mucous cells) or through tubular ducts that open onto the surface of the skin or onto an epithelium lining an internal passageway that connects to the exterior. ⤴ **p. 98**

Sweat also provides protection from environmental hazards. Sweat dilutes harmful chemicals in contact with the skin and flushes microorganisms from its surface. The presence of *dermicidin*, a small peptide molecule with antibiotic properties, provides additional protection from microorganisms.

The skin also contains other types of modified sweat glands with specialized secretions. For example, the mammary glands of the breasts are structurally related to apocrine sweat glands but secrete milk. Another example is the *ceruminous glands* in the passageway of the external ear. Their secretions combine with those of nearby sebaceous glands to form a mixture called *cerumen*, or earwax.

CHECKPOINT

17. Identify two types of exocrine glands found in the skin.

18. What are the functions of sebaceous secretions?

19. Deodorants are used to mask the effects of secretions from which type of skin gland?

See the blue Answers tab at the back of the book.

5-8 Nails are keratinized epidermal cells that protect the tips of fingers and toes

Learning Objective Describe the anatomical structure of nails, and explain how they are formed.

Nails protect the dorsal surfaces of the tips of the fingers and toes (**Figure 5-11a**). They also help limit distortion of the digits when they are subjected to mechanical stress—for example, when you run or grasp objects. The **nail body** is the visible portion of the nail. It consists of a dense mass of dead, keratinized cells. The nail body covers an area of epidermis called the **nail bed** (**Figure 5-11b**). The nail body is recessed

Figure 5-11 The Structure of a Nail.

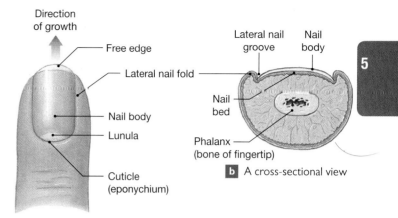

a   A superficial view

b   A cross-sectional view

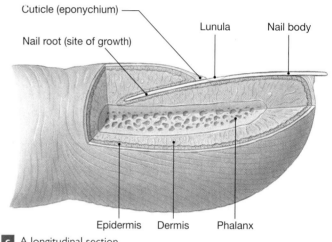

c   A longitudinal section

beneath the level of the surrounding epithelium and is bordered by **lateral nail folds**.

The nail is produced at the **nail root**, an epithelial fold not visible from the surface. The deepest portion of the nail root lies very close to the bone of the fingertip. A portion of the stratum corneum of the fold extends over the exposed nail nearest the root, forming the **cuticle**, or *eponychium* (ep-ō-NIK-ē-um; *epi-*, over + *onyx*, nail) (**Figure 5-11c**). Underlying blood vessels give the nail its pink appearance. Near the root these vessels may be obscured, leaving a pale crescent known as the **lunula** (LOO-nū-la; *luna*, moon).

CHECKPOINT

20. What substance makes nails hard?

21. Where does nail growth take place?

See the blue Answers tab at the back of the book.

5-9 Several steps are involved in repairing the integument following an injury

Learning Objective Explain how the skin responds to injury and repairs itself.

The integumentary system can respond directly and independently to many local influences or stimuli, without involving the nervous or endocrine systems. For example, when the skin is subjected to mechanical stresses, stem cells in the stratum basale divide more rapidly, and the thickness of the epithelium increases. That is why calluses form on your palms when you perform manual labor. After an injury to the skin, you can see a more dramatic example of a local response.

Repair of Skin Injuries

The skin can regenerate effectively even after considerable damage because stem cells are present in both its epithelial and connective tissues. Division of stem cells of the stratum basale replaces epithelial cells. Connective tissue stem cells divide to replace cells lost from the dermis. This process can be slow. When large surface areas are involved, infection and fluid loss complicate the repair process.

The relative speed and effectiveness of skin repair vary, depending on the type of wound. A slender, straight cut, or *incision*, may heal relatively quickly. A scrape, or *abrasion*, which involves a much greater area, may heal more slowly.

The skin regenerates in four phases after an injury: an inflammatory phase, a migratory phase, a proliferation phase, and a scarring phase (**Figure 5-12**).

When damage extends through the epidermis and into the dermis, bleeding generally takes place. Mast cells in the dermis trigger an *inflammatory response* that results in enhanced blood flow to the surrounding region and attraction of phagocytes ❶.

A blood clot, or **scab**, forms at the surface as part of the *migratory phase*. The scab temporarily restores the integrity of the epidermis and restricts the entry of additional microorganisms ❷. Most of the clot consists of an insoluble network of *fibrin*, a fibrous protein that forms from blood proteins during the clotting response. Cells of the stratum basale rapidly divide and

Figure 5-12 Repair of Injury to the Skin.

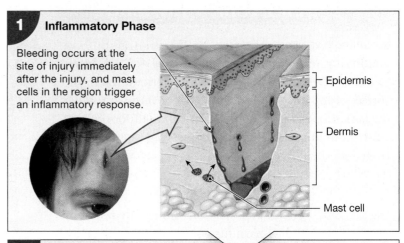

1 Inflammatory Phase

Bleeding occurs at the site of injury immediately after the injury, and mast cells in the region trigger an inflammatory response.

- Epidermis
- Dermis
- Mast cell

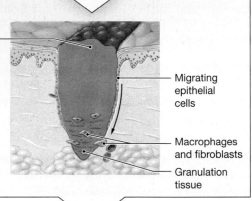

2 Migratory Phase

After several hours, a scab has formed and cells of the stratum basale are migrating along the edges of the wound. Phagocytic cells are removing debris, and more of these cells are arriving with the enhanced circulation in the area. Clotting around the edges of the affected area partially isolates the region.

- Migrating epithelial cells
- Macrophages and fibroblasts
- Granulation tissue

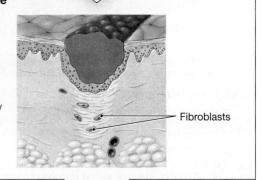

3 Proliferation Phase

About a week after the injury, the scab has been undermined by epidermal cells migrating over the collagen fiber meshwork produced by fibroblast activity. Phagocytic activity around the site has almost ended, and the fibrin clot is dissolving.

- Fibroblasts

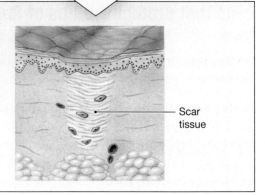

4 Scarring Phase

After several weeks, the scab has been shed, and the epidermis is complete. A shallow depression marks the injury site, but fibroblasts in the dermis continue to create scar tissue that will gradually elevate the overlying epidermis.

- Scar tissue

begin to migrate along the sides of the wound to replace the missing epidermal cells. Meanwhile, fixed macrophages and newly arriving phagocytes patrol the damaged area of the dermis and clear away debris and pathogens.

If the wound covers an extensive area or involves a region covered by thin skin, dermal repairs must be under way before epithelial cells can cover the surface. Fibroblasts and connective tissue stem cells divide to produce mobile cells that invade the deeper areas of injury. Epithelial cells lining damaged blood vessels also begin to divide, and capillaries follow the fibroblasts, enhancing circulation. The combination of blood clot, fibroblasts, and an extensive capillary network is called **granulation tissue**.

Over time, deeper portions of the clot dissolve and the number of capillaries declines in the *proliferation phase* ❸. Fibroblast activity has formed an extensive meshwork of collagen fibers in the dermis. These repairs do not restore the integument to its original condition, however, because the dermis now contains an abnormally large number of collagen fibers and relatively few blood vessels. Severely damaged hair follicles, sebaceous or sweat glands, muscle cells, and nerves are seldom repaired. Instead, they are replaced by fibrous tissue.

In the *scarring phase*, the formation of rather inflexible, fibrous, noncellular **scar tissue** completes the repair process, but without restoring the tissue to its original condition. ❹. The process of scar tissue formation is highly variable. For example, surgical procedures performed on a fetus do not leave scars. In some adults, most often those with dark skin, scar tissue formation may continue beyond what is needed for tissue repair. The result is a flattened mass of scar tissue that begins at the injury site and grows into the surrounding dermis. This thickened area of scar tissue, called a **keloid** (KĒ-loyd), is covered by a shiny, smooth epidermal

CLNICAL NOTE

Traumatic Conditions of the Skin

Traumatic disruption of the layers of the skin exposes the tissues underneath. This increases the likelihood of infection, loss of body fluids, and pain. Skin trauma can result from direct trauma (either sharp or blunt) or burns (either thermal or chemical).

Soft-Tissue Wounds

Trauma that results in the disruption of the layers of the skin is called a wound. There are several classifications of wounds. These include:

- *Abrasion*—is a simple scrape or scratch where the outer layer of skin is damaged but not all of the layers are penetrated (**Figure 5–13**).
- *Laceration*—commonly called a cut, a laceration may be smooth or jagged (**Figure 5–14**). Smooth wounds are usually caused by a sharp edge such as a razor blade or glass. Jagged wounds can be due to injury from duller objects such as jagged metal. They can also occur as a result of blunt trauma such as a blow or fall.
- *Puncture*—occurs when a sharp, pointed object penetrates the skin or other tissues (**Figure 5–15**). Common causes include such items as nails, ice picks, splinters, or knives. There are two types of puncture wounds, penetrating and perforating. *Penetrating puncture wounds* can be shallow or deep and can injure underlying tissues and blood vessels. Penetrating puncture wounds carry an increased incidence of infection as foreign material may be carried into the wound during injury and remain there due to sealing of the surface. *Perforating puncture wounds* have both an entrance wound and an exit wound. Often, the exit wound is more serious than the entrance wound. An example of a penetrating puncture wound is a gunshot wound.
- *Avulsion*—is an injury where a flap of skin and tissues are torn loose or pulled completely off (**Figure 5–16**). Avulsions can cause serious tissue defects and subsequent scarring. A special type of avulsion is the *degloving avulsion*. This is a potentially devastating wound where the skin, usually of the hand, is stripped off like a glove (**Figure 5–17**).
- *Amputation*—occurs when an extremity, or part of an extremity is completely cut through or torn off (**Figure 5–18**). Amputations often are caused by machinery and can be life-threatening. Today, using microsurgical techniques, amputated body parts can be replanted if the condition of the tissues is satisfactory.
- *Crush injury*—results when a body part, usually an extremity, becomes caught between heavy items such as parts of machinery. There is often massive damage to underlying blood vessels, nerves, and bone.

Figure 5-13 An Abrasion of the Left Side of the Face.

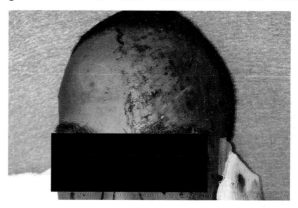

(Continued)

5

Figure 5-14 Jagged Laceration of the Forehead.

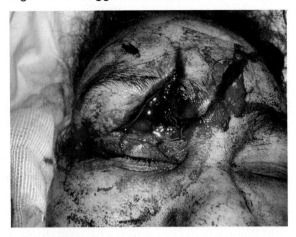

Figure 5-15 Examples of Puncture Wounds.
(a) Nail gun injury with embedded carpet fibers. **(b)** Gun shot wound of the left thigh—the entry wound is on the left and the exit wound is on the right.

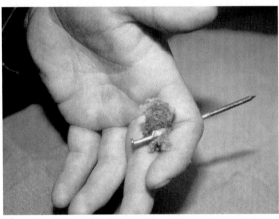

(a)

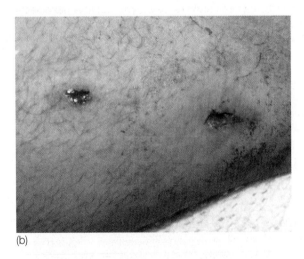

(b)

Figure 5-16 Avulsion.

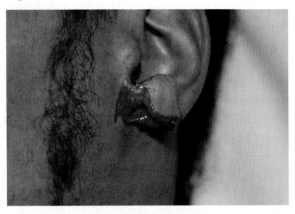

Figure 5-17 Degloving Injury.

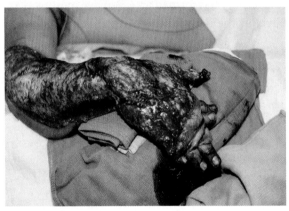

Figure 5-18 Partial Amputation of the Right Hand.

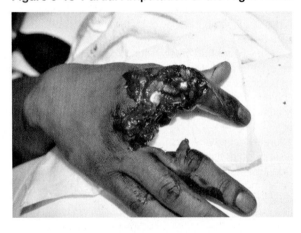

Soft-tissue injuries are commonly encountered in emergency care. They are often grotesque and can distract from other patient care activities. Fortunately, they are rarely life-threatening. In the pre-hospital setting, they are usually dressed to prevent further contamination, and definitive care, such as wound repair or surgery, is carried out at the hospital.

Limb Replantation

With the advent of microsurgical techniques, many body parts can be surgically reattached, or replanted, following amputation (**Figure 5–19**). Amputated body parts should be located

Figure 5-19 Amputation and Replantation. (a) Complete amputation of the left forearm caused by tractor power takeoff device—contraction of the forearm muscles exposes the radius and ulna. **(b)** The amputated hand was found and retrieved by EMS personnel.

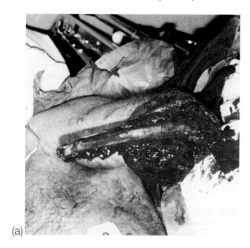

(a)

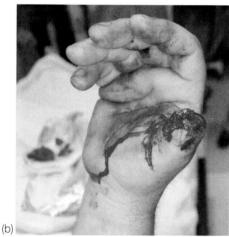

(b)

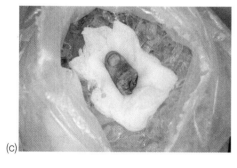

(c)

at the emergency scene and should accompany the patient to the hospital if at all possible. Even if an amputated part is too damaged for replantation, the tissues can be used to help repair the wound.

The separated body part should be cleaned of any gross debris, exposed areas covered with a lightly moistened gauze, and then placed into a sealed plastic bag. The bag should be immersed into saline with a few pieces of ice added. Packing the body part in ice, as was the old practice, caused tissue damage at a cellular level, and adversely impacted limb survival. Many body parts have been successfully replanted including arms, hands, feet, legs, ears, the nose, and the penis. Patients with amputations where replantation is a possibility should be transported to medical centers with microsurgical replant capabilities.

The material placed directly on a wound is called a *dressing*. These are sterile and designed to control bleeding and protect the wound from contamination. A dressing is held in place by a *bandage*. Bandages can be made from gauze, elastic material, cloth, and many other materials. Sometimes, wounds require splinting. This is especially true in cases where there may be an associated fracture or where movement might cause the wound to open.

Injury and Repair

The skin is an amazingly resilient organ. It can regenerate effectively, even after considerable damage. This is due to stem cells in the epithelial and connective tissues. The rate of wound repair is related to several factors such as wound size, infection, fluid loss, vascular supply, and overall patient condition. Small lacerations may heal quickly while large avulsions and burns can take considerably more time.

Regeneration of a wound following injury involves several distinct stages. If the wound extends through the epidermis and into the dermis or connective tissue, bleeding usually occurs. The blood at the site of the wound will collect and clot, and eventually form a *scab*. This serves to temporarily restore the integrity of the epidermis and limits the entry of additional organisms. Next, the cells of the stratum germinativum, which is the deepest layer of the epidermis, begin to undergo rapid division. As this occurs, they migrate along the sides of the wound, and attempt to replace the lost epidermal cells. Scavenger, phagocytic cells remove debris from the wound. Additional phagocytic cells are transported to the injury site via the circulatory system.

If the wound is extensive or deep, repairs to the dermis must be under way before epithelial cells can be laid down. Fibroblast and mesenchymal cells begin to divide, producing mobile cells that penetrate the deeper areas of the wound. Damaged blood vessels begin to repair themselves through division of endothelial cells. These cells follow the fibroblasts into the deeper areas of the wound, providing a blood supply. Together, fibroblasts, the blood clot, and the developing capillary network are called *granulation tissue*. Ultimately, the clot dissolves and the number of capillaries declines as the needs of the healing tissue decrease. Fibroblast activity leads to the formation of collagen fibers and *ground substance*.

The repaired wound is different from the original tissues. There is an increased number of collagen fibers and a decreased number of blood vessels that result in scar tissue. This scar tissue varies based upon the type of wound and the age and health of the patient.

Burns

Skin injury caused by heat, chemicals, electricity, and radiation is called a *burn*. Although burns usually affect the skin, they can also affect underlying tissues such as the subcutaneous tissues, muscle, blood vessels, nerves, and even bone (**Figure 5–20**).

Burns are classified by depth and include the following:

- *First-degree burns*—also called superficial burns, first-degree burns involve only the epidermis. They can be quite painful, as nerve fibers are uninjured. Example: sunburn (**Figure 5–21**).

(Continued)

Figure 5-20 Burn Classification System.

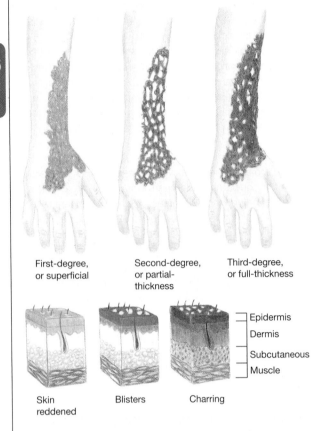

First-degree, or superficial

Second-degree, or partial-thickness

Third-degree, or full-thickness

- Epidermis
- Dermis
- Subcutaneous
- Muscle

Skin reddened

Blisters

Charring

Figure 5-21 First-Degree Burn.
(Note that some areas of second-degree burn are also present.)

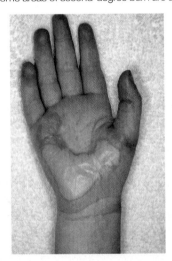

- *Second-degree burns*—also called partial-thickness burns, the epidermis is burned through and the dermis is damaged (**Figure 5–22**). There is usually intense pain and blistering. The blisters develop as plasma and interstitial fluids are released into the skin and elevate the top layer. Example: scald injury.
- *Third-degree burns*—also called full-thickness burns, third-degree burns are characterized by damage to all layers of the skin (**Figure 5–23**). The patient may not suffer as much pain as would be expected, because pain fibers in the skin may be

Figure 5-22 Second-Degree Burn.

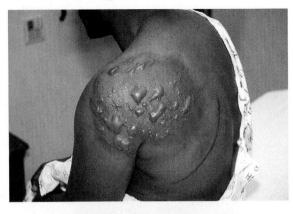

Figure 5-23 Third-Degree Burn of the Left Hand.

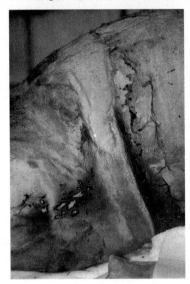

destroyed by the injury. Third-degree burns are almost always accompanied by partial-thickness burns and some degree of pain is usually present. Third-degree burns usually require skin grafting and are very disfiguring.

Deep burns are sometimes seen with prolonged exposure to heat and with electrical and lightning injuries. In some cases, muscle tissue and bone will be involved. Although these are technically considered full-thickness burns, they are occasionally called fourth-degree burns to separate them from less severe injuries.

The severity of a burn is determined by consideration of the following factors:

- Body regions burned
- Depth of the burn
- Extent of the burn
- Agent or source of the burn
- Age of the patient
- Other associated illnesses and injuries

The agent or source of the burn can be significant. For example, electrical burns may cause only a small area of skin injury but cause massive injury to underlying tissues. Chemical burns are of special concern, because the chemical can remain on the skin and continue to burn for hours or even days.

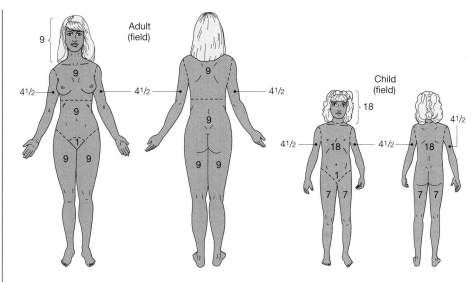

Figure 5-24 Rule of Nines, a System for Approximating the Severity of a Burn Injury.

The extent of a burn is important to determine. The amount of body surface area (BSA) involved can be quickly estimated by using the *rule of nines* (**Figure 5–24**). In an adult, each of the following areas represents 9 percent of the BSA: head and neck, each upper extremity, chest, abdomen, upper back, lower back, the front of each lower extremity, and the back of each lower extremity. Together, these total 99 percent. The remaining 1 percent of BSA is assigned to the genital region. In children, the head is proportionally large compared to the body, and the body regions are adjusted accordingly. Another system of estimating the amount of BSA burned is the palmar method. The patient's palm equals about 1 percent of the patient's BSA. Considering this, the percentage of BSA burned can be quickly approximated. This system is particularly useful for smaller burns.

surface (**Figure 5-25**). Keloids most commonly develop on the upper back, shoulders, anterior chest, and earlobes. They are harmless. Some aboriginal cultures intentionally produce keloids as a form of body decoration.

Effects of Burns

Burns are relatively common injuries. They result from exposure of the skin to heat, radiation, electrical shock, or strong chemical agents. The severity of a burn depends on the depth of penetration and the total area affected, as detailed in *Clinical Note: Burns* on p. 136.

The most common classification of burns is based on the depth of penetration. The larger the area affected, the greater the impact on integumentary function.

Figure 5-25 A Keloid. A keloid is an area of raised fibrous scar tissue.

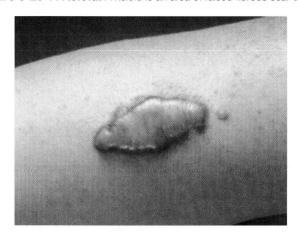

CHECKPOINT

22. What term describes the combination of fibrin clots, fibroblasts, and the extensive network of capillaries in healing tissue?

23. Why can skin regenerate effectively even after considerable damage?

See the blue Answers tab at the back of the book.

5-10 Effects of aging include dermal thinning, wrinkling, and reduced melanocyte activity

Learning Objective Summarize the effects of aging on the skin.

Aging affects all parts of the integumentary system. Major age-related changes include the following:

- ***Skin injuries and infections become more common.*** Such problems are more likely because the epidermis thins as stem cell activity declines, and connections between the epidermis and dermis weaken.

- ***The sensitivity of the immune system is reduced.*** The number of macrophages and dendritic cells in the skin decreases to about one-half the levels seen at maturity (roughly, at the age of 21 years). This loss further encourages skin damage and infection.

- ***Muscles become weaker, and bone strength decreases.*** Such changes are related to reduced calcium and phosphate absorption due to a decline in vitamin D_3 production of around 75 percent.

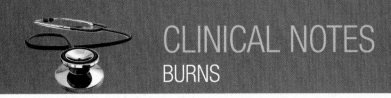

CLINICAL NOTES
BURNS

Burns are relatively common injuries that result from skin exposure to heat, friction, radiation, electrical shock, or strong chemical agents. Each year in the United States, roughly 4000 people die from fires and burns. In evaluating burns in a clinical setting, two key factors must be determined: the depth of the burn and the percentage of skin surface area that has been burned.

Classification by Depth of Burn

Partial-Thickness Burns

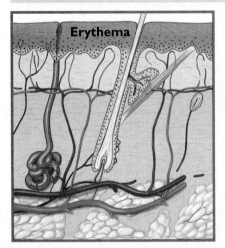 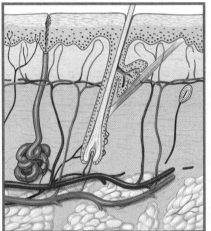

In a **first-degree burn**, only the surface of the epidermis is affected. In this type of burn, which includes most sunburns, the skin reddens and can be painful. The redness, a sign called **erythema** (er-i-THĒ-muh), results from inflammation of the sun-damaged tissues.

In a **second-degree burn**, the entire epidermis and perhaps some of the dermis are damaged. Accessory structures such as hair follicles and glands are generally not affected, but blistering, pain, and swelling occur. If the blisters rupture at the surface, infection can easily develop. Healing typically takes one to two weeks, and some scar tissue may form.

Full-Thickness Burns

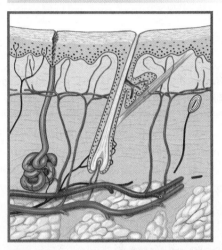

Third-degree burns, or full-thickness burns, destroy the epidermis and dermis, extending into the hypodermis. Despite swelling, these burns are less painful than second-degree burns, because sensory nerves are destroyed. Extensive third-degree burns cannot repair themselves, because granulation tissue cannot form and epithelial cells are unable to cover the injury. Skin grafting is usually necessary.

Estimation of Surface Burn Area

A simple method for estimating burn area is the **rule of nines**. The surface area in adults is divided into multiples of 9 and then the damaged regions are totaled. This rule is modified for children because their body proportions are different.

The depth of the burn can be quickly assessed with a pin. Because loss of sensation is characteristic of a full-thickness burn, the absence of a reaction to a pin prick indicates the presence of third-degree damage.

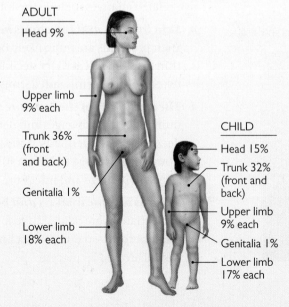

ADULT
Head 9%
Upper limb 9% each
Trunk 36% (front and back)
Genitalia 1%
Lower limb 18% each

CHILD
Head 15%
Trunk 32% (front and back)
Upper limb 9% each
Genitalia 1%
Lower limb 17% each

Burns and Skin Function

Burns that cover more than 20 percent of the skin surface threaten critical homeostatic functions of the skin.

Skin Functions Affected by Burns

- **Fluid and Electrolyte Balance**. Burns cause the skin to lose its effectiveness as a barrier to fluid and electrolyte loss. In full-thickness burns, the rate of fluid loss through the skin may reach five times the normal level.

- **Thermoregulation**. Increased fluid loss means increased evaporative cooling. As a result, more energy must be expended to keep body temperature within acceptable limits.

- **Protection from Infection**. Widespread bacterial infection, or **sepsis** (sepsis, rotting), is the leading cause of death in burn victims.

- *Sensitivity to sun exposure increases.* Less melanin is produced because melanocyte activity declines. The skin of light-skinned individuals becomes very pale, and sunburn is more likely.

- *The skin becomes dry and often scaly.* Glandular activity declines, reducing sebum production and perspiration.

- *Hair thins and changes color.* Follicles stop functioning or produce finer hairs. With decreased melanocyte activity, these hairs are gray or white.

- *Sagging and wrinkling of the skin occur.* The dermis becomes thinner, and the elastic fiber network decreases in size. The integument therefore becomes weaker and less resilient. Sagging and wrinkling are most noticeable in areas exposed to the sun.

- *The ability to lose heat decreases.* The blood supply to the dermis is reduced just as the sweat glands become less active. This combination makes elderly people less able than younger people to lose body heat. As a result, overexertion or overexposure to high temperatures (as in a sauna or hot tub) can cause dangerously high body temperatures.

- *Skin repairs take place more slowly.* For example, it takes three to four weeks to repair an uninfected blister site in a young adult. The same repairs could take six to eight weeks at ages 65–75 years. Recurrent infections may result because repairs are slow.

The Build Your Knowledge figure on p. 138 reviews the integumentary system. Such reviews appear after each body system to gradually build your understanding of the interconnections among all body systems. Because we have covered only one body system so far, references to body systems to be discussed in upcoming chapters are not included.

CHECKPOINT

24. Older individuals do not tolerate summer heat as well as they did when they were young, and they are more prone to heat-related illnesses. What accounts for these changes?

25. Why does hair turn gray or white with age?

See the blue Answers tab at the back of the book.

RELATED CLINICAL TERMS

biopsy (BĪ-op-sē): The removal and examination of tissue from the body for the diagnosis of disease.

cavernous hemangioma (strawberry nevus): A mass of large blood vessels that can occur in the skin or other organs in the body; a "port wine stain" birthmark generally lasts a lifetime.

lesions (LĒ-zhuns): Changes in tissue structure caused by injury or disease.

pruritus (proo-RĪ-tus): An irritating itching sensation, common in skin conditions such as psoriasis or dermatitis.

ulcer: A localized shedding of an epithelium.

xerosis (ze-RŌ-sis): "Dry skin," a common complaint of older persons and almost anyone living in an arid climate.

Build Your Knowledge
How the INTEGUMENTARY SYSTEM integrates with the other body systems presented so far

5

Integumentary System

The integumentary system performs five major functions for the human body. It:

- covers and protects underlying tissues and organs from impacts, chemicals, and infections, and it prevents the loss of body fluids

- maintains normal body temperature by regulating heat exchange with the environment

- synthesizes vitamin D_3 in the epidermis, which aids calcium uptake, and stores large reserves of lipids in the dermis

- detects touch, pressure, pain, and temperature stimuli

- excretes salts, water, and organic wastes

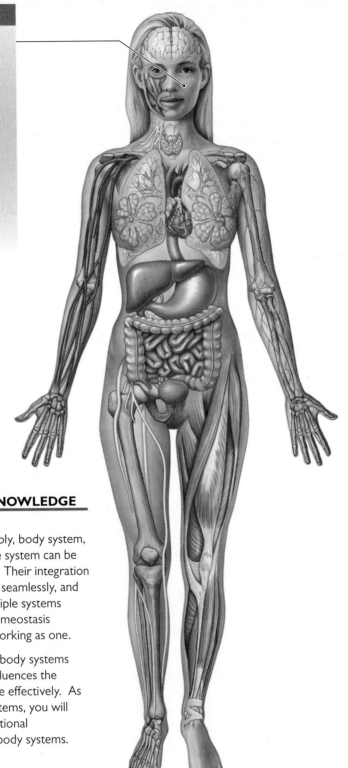

ABOUT THE BUILD YOUR KNOWLEDGE FIGURES

Because each organ system, or simply, body system, interacts with all the others, no one system can be completely understood in isolation. Their integration allows the human body to function seamlessly, and when disease or injury strikes, multiple systems must respond to heal the body. Homeostasis depends on all the body systems working as one.

These figures will introduce the body systems one by one and show how each influences the others to make them function more effectively. As we progress through the organ systems, you will *build your knowledge* about the functional relationships between the various body systems.

5 Chapter Review

Summary Outline

An Introduction to the Integumentary System *p. 129*

1. The **integumentary system**, or **integument**, consists of the **cutaneous membrane**, which includes the **epidermis** and **dermis**, and the **accessory structures**. Beneath it lies the **hypodermis** (or *subcutaneous layer*) *(Figure 5-1)*.

2. Major functions of the integument include *protection, temperature maintenance, synthesis and storage of nutrients, sensory reception*, and *excretion and secretion*.

5-1 The epidermis is composed of strata (layers) with various functions *p. 130*

3. **Thin skin**, made up of four layers of **keratinocytes**, covers most of the body. Heavily abraded body surfaces may be covered by **thick skin** *(Spotlight Figure 5-4)*.

4. Cell divisions by **basal cells** (stem cells) that make up most of the **stratum basale** replace more superficial cells. As epidermal cells age, they move up through the **stratum spinosum**, the **stratum granulosum,** the **stratum lucidum** (in thick skin), and the **stratum corneum.** In the process, they accumulate large amounts of **keratin.** Ultimately, the cells are shed or lost *(Spotlight Figure 5-4)*.

5. **Epidermal ridges** interlock with the **dermal papillae** of the dermis. Together, they form superficial ridges on the palms and soles that improve the gripping ability of the hands and feet and are the basis of fingerprints *(Spotlight Figure 5-4)*.

5-2 Factors influencing skin color are epidermal pigmentation and dermal circulation *p. 134*

6. The color of the epidermis depends on two factors: blood supply and the concentrations of the pigments **melanin** and **carotene. Melanocytes** protect stem cells from **ultraviolet (UV) radiation** *(Figure 5-5)*.

5-3 Sunlight has beneficial and detrimental effects on the skin *p. 136*

7. Epidermal cells synthesize **vitamin D$_3$** when exposed to sunlight.

8. Skin cancer is the most common form of cancer. **Basal cell carcinoma** and **squamous cell carcinoma** are not as dangerous as **melanoma** *(Figure 5-6)*.

5-4 The dermis is the tissue layer that supports the epidermis *p. 136*

9. The dermis consists of the **papillary layer** and the deeper **reticular layer.**

10. The papillary layer of the dermis contains blood vessels, lymphatic vessels, and sensory nerves. This layer supports and nourishes the overlying epidermis. The reticular layer consists of a meshwork of collagen and elastic fibers oriented to resist tension in the skin.

11. Components of other organ systems (cardiovascular, lymphatic, and nervous) that communicate with the skin are in the dermis. Arteries to the skin form the *cutaneous plexus* within the superficial region of the hypodermis. The *subpapillary plexus* is at the base of the papillary layer of the dermis.

5-5 The hypodermis connects the dermis to underlying tissues *p. 137*

12. The **hypodermis,** or subcutaneous layer, stabilizes the skin's position against underlying organs and tissues.

5-6 Hair is composed of dead, keratinized cells that have been pushed to the skin surface *p. 139*

13. **Hairs** originate in complex organs called **hair follicles.** Each hair has a **shaft** composed of dead, keratinized cells. Hairs have a central **medulla** of soft keratin surrounded by a **cortex** and an outer **cuticle** of hard keratin *(Figure 5-8)*.

14. Each **arrector pili** muscle can raise a single hair.

15. Hairs grow and are shed according to the *hair growth cycle*. A single hair grows for 2–5 years and is then shed after a period of inactivity in the hair follicle.

5-7 Sebaceous glands and sweat glands are exocrine glands found in the skin *p. 141*

16. Typical **sebaceous glands** discharge waxy **sebum** into hair follicles. *Sebaceous follicles* are sebaceous glands that empty directly onto the skin *(Figure 5-9)*.

17. **Apocrine sweat glands** produce an odorous secretion; the more numerous **merocrine sweat glands** produce perspiration, a watery secretion *(Figure 5-10)*.

5-8 Nails are keratinized epidermal cells that protect the tips of fingers and toes *p. 143*

18. The **nail body** of a **nail** covers the **nail bed**. Nail production occurs at the **nail root**, which is covered by the **cuticle** *(Figure 5-11)*.

5-9 Several steps are involved in repairing the integument following an injury *p. 144*

19. The skin can regenerate effectively even after considerable damage *(Figure 5-12)*.

20. Burns are relatively common injuries characterized by damage to layers of the epidermis and perhaps the dermis.

5-10 Effects of aging include dermal thinning, wrinkling, and reduced melanocyte activity *p. 149*

21. With aging, the integument thins, blood flow decreases, cellular activity decreases, and repairs occur more slowly.

Review Questions

See the blue Answers tab at the back of the book.

Level 1 Reviewing Facts and Terms

Match each item in column A with the most closely related item in column B. Place letters for answers in the spaces provided.

COLUMN A

_____ 1. Cutaneous membrane
_____ 2. Carotene
_____ 3. Melanocytes
_____ 4. Stratum basale
_____ 5. Merocrine (eccrine)_glands
_____ 6. Stratum corneum
_____ 7. Bluish skin
_____ 8. Sebaceous glands
_____ 9. Smooth muscle
_____ 10. Vitamin D$_3$

COLUMN B

a. Arrector pili
b. Cyanosis
c. Perspiration
d. Sebum
e. Epidermal layer of flattened and dead cells
f. Skin
g. Orange-yellow pigment
h. Bone growth
i. Pigment cells
j. Epidermal layer containing stem cells

11. The two major components of the integument are
 (a) the cutaneous membrane and the accessory structures.
 (b) the epidermis and the hypodermis.
 (c) the hair and the nails.
 (d) the dermis and the subcutaneous layer.

12. The fibrous protein that forms the basic structural component of hair and nails is
 (a) collagen.
 (b) melanin.
 (c) elastin.
 (d) keratin.

13. Identify the different portions (a–d) of the cutaneous membrane and the underlying layer of loose connective tissue (e) in the following diagram.

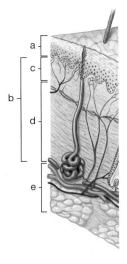

 (a) _____
 (b) _____
 (c) _____
 (d) _____
 (e) _____

14. The two types of exocrine glands in the skin are
 (a) merocrine and sweat glands.
 (b) sebaceous and sweat glands.
 (c) apocrine and sweat glands.
 (d) eccrine and sweat glands.

15. All of the following are accessory structures of the integumentary system *except*
 (a) nails.
 (b) hair.
 (c) dermal papillae.
 (d) sweat glands.

16. Sweat glands that communicate with hair follicles in the armpits and produce an odorous secretion are
  (a) apocrine glands.
  (b) merocrine glands.
  (c) sebaceous glands.
  (d) a, b, and c are correct.

17. The reason elderly people are more sensitive to sun exposure and more likely to get sunburned is that with age
  (a) melanocyte activity declines.
  (b) vitamin D_3 production declines.
  (c) glandular activity declines.
  (d) skin thickness decreases.

18. Identify the different portions (a–e) of a hair and hair follicle.

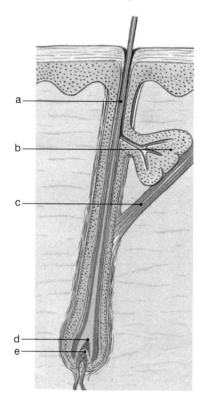

  (a) _____   **(b)** _____
  (c) _____   **(d)** _____
  (e) _____

19. Which two skin pigments are found in the epidermis?

20. Which two major layers constitute the dermis, and what components are found in each layer?

21. Which two groups of sweat glands occur in the skin?

Level 2 Reviewing Concepts

22. In elderly people, blood supply to the dermis is reduced and sweat glands are less active. This combination of factors would most affect the
  (a) ability to thermoregulate.
  (b) ability to heal injured skin.
  (c) ease with which the skin is injured.
  (d) physical characteristics of the skin.
  (e) ability to grow hair.

23. In clinical practice, drugs can be delivered by diffusion across the skin. This delivery method is called transdermal administration. Why are fat-soluble drugs more desirable for transdermal administration than drugs that are water soluble?

24. In our society, a tanned body is associated with good health. However, medical research constantly warns about the dangers of excessive exposure to the sun. What are the benefits of a tan?

25. In some cultures, women must be covered completely, except for their eyes, when they go outside. These women exhibit a high incidence of bone problems. Why?

26. Why is a subcutaneous injection with a hypodermic needle a useful method for administering drugs?

27. Why does skin sag and wrinkle as a person ages?

Level 3 Critical Thinking and Clinical Applications

28. A new mother notices that her 6-month-old son has a yellow-orange complexion. Fearful that the child may have jaundice (a condition caused by bilirubin, a toxic yellow-orange pigment produced during the destruction of red blood cells), she takes him to her pediatrician. After examining the child, the pediatrician declares him perfectly healthy and advises the mother to watch the child's diet. Why?

29. Vanessa notices that even though her 80-year-old grandmother keeps her thermostat set at 80°F, she still wears a sweater in her house. When Vanessa asks her grandmother why, her grandmother says she is cold. Vanessa can't understand this. How would you explain it to her?

30. A 32-year-old woman is admitted to the hospital with third-degree burns on her entire right leg, entire right arm, and the back of her trunk. Estimate the percentage of her body surface area affected by these burns.

6

The Skeletal System

Learning Objectives

These objectives tell you what you should be able to do after completing the chapter. They correspond by number to this chapter's sections.

6-1 Describe the primary functions of the skeletal system.

6-2 Classify bones according to shape, and compare the structures and functions of compact and spongy bone.

6-3 Compare the processes of intramembranous ossification and endochondral ossification.

6-4 Describe the remodeling and homeostatic processes of the skeletal system.

6-5 Summarize the effects of aging on the skeletal system.

6-6 Define a bone marking and name the components and functions of the axial and appendicular skeletons.

6-7 Identify the bones of the skull, discuss the differences in structure and function of the various vertebrae, and describe the roles of the thoracic cage.

6-8 Identify the bones of the pectoral and pelvic girdles and the upper and lower limbs, and describe their various functions.

6-9 Contrast the major categories of joints, and link their structural features to joint functions.

6-10 Describe how the structure and functions of synovial joints permit the movements of the skeleton.

6-11 Explain the relationship between joint structure and mobility of representative axial and appendicular articulations.

6-12 Describe the interactions between the skeletal system and other body systems.

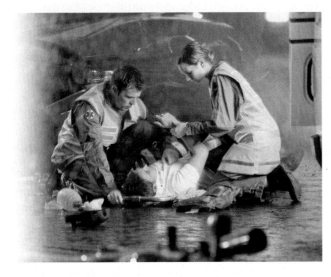

An Introduction to the Skeletal System

The skeleton has many functions. The most obvious is supporting the weight of the body. This support is provided by bones, structures as strong as reinforced concrete but considerably lighter. Unlike concrete, bones can be remodeled and reshaped to meet changing metabolic demands and patterns of activity. Bones work with muscles to maintain body position and to produce controlled, precise movements. With the skeleton to pull against, contracting muscles can make us sit, stand, walk, or run.

Build Your Knowledge

Recall that bone is a supporting connective tissue (as you saw in **Chapter 4: The Tissue Level of Organization**). All of the features and properties of the skeletal system ultimately depend on the unique and constantly changing properties of bone. ⊃ **p. 102**

6-1 The skeletal system has five primary functions

Learning Objective Describe the primary functions of the skeletal system.

The skeletal system includes the bones of the skeleton and the cartilages, joints, ligaments, and other connective tissues that stabilize or connect the bones. This system has five primary functions:

1. **Support.** The skeletal system provides structural support for the entire body. Individual bones or groups of bones provide a framework for the attachment of soft tissues and organs.

2. **Storage of minerals and lipids.** The calcium salts of bone serve as a valuable mineral reserve that maintains normal concentrations of calcium and phosphate ions in body fluids. In addition, bones store lipids as energy reserves in areas filled with *yellow bone marrow.*

3. **Blood cell production.** Red blood cells, white blood cells, and other blood elements are produced within the *red bone marrow,* which fills the internal cavities of many bones.

4. **Protection.** Skeletal structures surround many soft tissues and organs. The ribs protect the heart and lungs, the skull encloses the brain, the vertebrae shield the spinal cord, and the pelvis cradles delicate digestive and reproductive organs.

5. **Leverage.** Many bones function as levers that change the magnitude (size) and direction of the forces generated by skeletal muscles. The resulting movements range from the delicate motion of a fingertip to powerful changes in the position of the entire body.

CHECKPOINT

1. Name the five primary functions of the skeletal system.

See the blue Answers tab at the back of the book.

6-2 Bones are classified according to shape and structure

Learning Objective Classify bones according to shape, and compare the structures and functions of compact and spongy bone.

Bone, or **osseous tissue,** is a supporting connective tissue that contains specialized cells and a matrix consisting of extracellular protein fibers and a ground substance. ⊃ p. 107 The distinctive texture of bone results from the calcium salts deposited within the matrix. Calcium phosphate, $Ca_3(PO_4)_2$, accounts for almost two-thirds of the weight of bone. The remaining third is dominated by collagen fibers. Osteocytes and other cell types make up only around 2 percent of the mass of a bone.

Build Your Knowledge

Recall that a salt is an ionic compound made up of any cation except a hydrogen ion (H^+) and any anion except a hydroxide ion (OH^-) (as you saw in **Chapter 2: The Chemical Level of Organization**). Calcium phosphate, $Ca_3(PO_4)_2$, is a calcium salt. The cation is a calcium ion (Ca^{2+}), and the anion is a phosphate ion (PO_4^{3-}). ⊃ **p. 37**

Figure 6-1 A Classification of Bones by Shape.

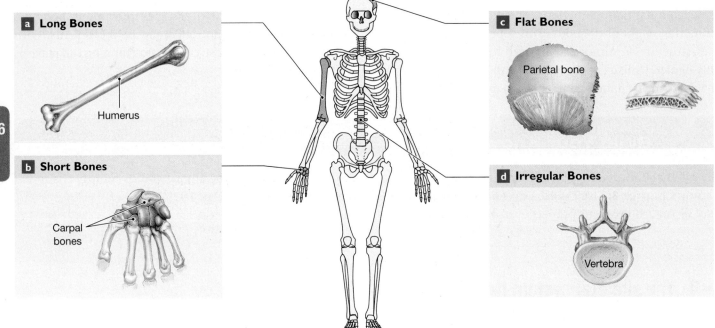

a Long Bones

Humerus

b Short Bones

Carpal bones

c Flat Bones

Parietal bone

d Irregular Bones

Vertebra

Macroscopic Features of Bone

The typical human skeleton contains 206 major bones. They have four general shapes: long, short, flat, and irregular (**Figure 6-1**). **Long bones** are longer than they are wide. In **short bones** these dimensions are roughly equal. Examples of long bones are bones of the limbs, such as the bones of the arm (*humerus*) and thigh (*femur*). Short bones include the bones of the wrist (*carpal bones*) and ankles (*tarsal bones*). **Flat bones** are thin and relatively broad, such as the *parietal bones* of the skull, the ribs, and the shoulder blades (*scapulae*). **Irregular bones** have complex shapes that do not fit easily into any other category. Examples include the vertebrae of the spinal column and several bones of the skull.

Figure 6-2 shows the typical features of a long bone on the humerus. A long bone has a central shaft, or **diaphysis** (dī-AF-i-sis), that surrounds a central space called the **marrow cavity**, or *medullary cavity* (*medulla*, innermost part). This space contains **bone marrow**, a soft, fatty tissue. The expanded portions at each end are called **epiphyses** (ē-PIF-i-sēz). They are covered by *articular cartilages*. Each epiphysis (ē-PIF-i-sis) of a long bone articulates with an adjacent bone at a joint.

Two types of bone tissue are shown in **Figure 6-2**. **Compact bone** is relatively dense and solid. **Spongy bone**, or *trabecular* (tra-bek-YŪ-lar) *bone*, consists of an interlacing network of bony rods or struts separated by spaces. Compact bone forms the wall of the diaphysis, and spongy bone fills the epiphyses

Figure 6-2 The Structure of a Long Bone.

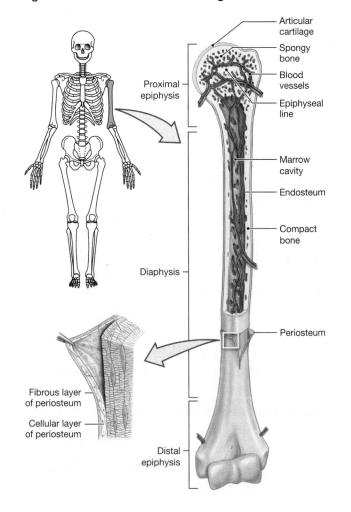

Proximal epiphysis

Diaphysis

Distal epiphysis

Articular cartilage

Spongy bone

Blood vessels

Epiphyseal line

Marrow cavity

Endosteum

Compact bone

Periosteum

Fibrous layer of periosteum

Cellular layer of periosteum

CLINICAL NOTE

Intraosseous Needle Placement

The bones are highly vascular, living tissues. By taking advantage of this characteristic, we can place a needle into the medullary cavity of the bone in order to provide emergency fluids and medications. Recent literature has shown that the intraosseous (IO) route of medication administration in cardiac arrest is equal to intravenous administration. The IO route should be considered for life-threatening cases, particularly cardiac arrest, when an IV cannot be placed.

The concept of placing a needle into the bone marrow was described as early as 1922. However, the technique was all but abandoned until the mid-1980s when it was reintroduced as an alternative fluid administration route in pediatric patients who needed fluids or medications emergently. Since then, the technique has become widespread and is now used in adults as well as children.

Large bones, such as the tibia and humerus, are extremely vascular and can accept large volumes of fluids and transfer them to the central circulation. The sternum is also used for IO administration in certain situations. The bone receives most of

its blood supply through a nutrient artery, which enters the cortex of the bone and divides into ascending and descending branches. These branches further divide into arterioles and then capillaries. The capillaries drain into the medullary venous sinusoids throughout the medullary space of the bone (**Figure 6-3**). Specially designed IO needles are available to pierce the cortex of the bone (**Figures 6-4** through **6-7**). Fluids and medications administered through a properly

Figure 6-3 Intraosseous Needle Properly Placed in Marrow Cavity and Medullary Sinusoids. Fluid primarily drains from the sinusoids and exits via the emissary vein or nutrient vein and enters the central venous circulation.

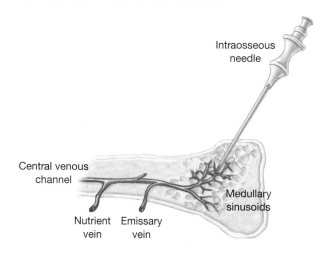

Figure 6-4 Special Intraosseous Needle for Emergency Intraosseous Access.

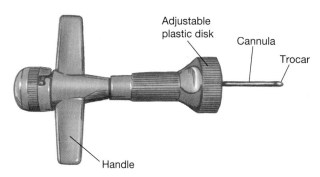

Figure 6-5 Bone Injection Gun (BIG) IO Device.
(a) Adult; **(b)** pediatric.

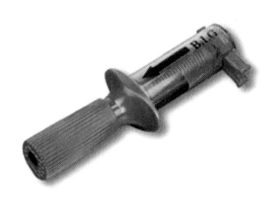

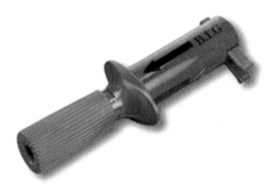

Figure 6-6 F.A.S.T.1 Sternal IO.

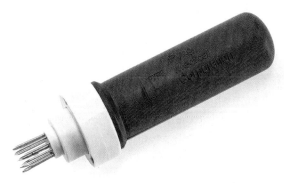

(Continued)

Figure 6-7 EZ-IO Device.

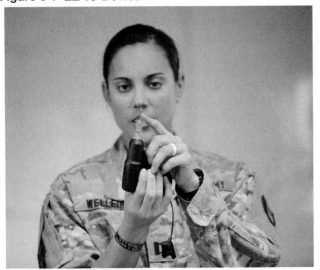

placed IO needle enter the medullary sinusoids. The medullary cavity functions as a rigid, non-collapsible vein, even in the setting of cardiac arrest or shock. The medullary sinusoids act as a central venous channel that exits the bone as either nutrient veins or emissary veins. Fluids and medications administered through an IO needle enter the central circulation promptly, nearly as fast as through an intravenous line. Virtually all fluids and medications used in the prehospital setting can be administered by the IO route.

The IO route provides a viable alternative for critically ill or critically injured patients when medications or fluids are required. Current trauma practices call for limited fluid administration in trauma, so the expanding role of IO therapy appears to be in cardiac arrest when an IV cannot be placed.

and lines the marrow cavity. A thin layer of compact bone covers the spongy bone of each epiphysis.

The outer surface of a bone is covered by a **periosteum** (**Figure 6-2**). The periosteum consists of an outer fibrous layer and an inner cellular layer. The fibers of *tendons* and *ligaments* intermingle with those of the fibrous layer of the periosteum. Tendons attach skeletal muscles to bones, and ligaments attach one bone to another. The periosteum isolates the bone from surrounding tissues, provides a route for blood vessels and nerves, and takes part in bone growth and repair.

Within the bone, a cellular **endosteum** covers the spongy bone of the marrow cavity and other inner surfaces. The endosteum is active during bone growth and during repair or remodeling.

Microscopic Features of Bone

Bone is a supporting connective tissue. We introduced its general histology in Chapter 4. **Figure 6-8** presents further details of the microscopic structure of bone. Both compact bone and spongy bone contain bone cells, or **osteocytes** (OS-tē-ō-sīts; *osteon*, bone), in small pockets called **lacunae** (la-KOO-nē) (**Figure 6-8a,b**). Lacunae are found between narrow sheets of calcified matrix that are known as **lamellae** (lah-MEL-lē; *lamella*, thin plate). Small channels, called **canaliculi** (ka-na-LIK-ū-lē), radiate through the matrix. They interconnect lacunae and link them to nearby blood vessels. The canaliculi contain cytoplasmic extensions of the osteocytes. Nutrients from the blood and waste products from osteocytes diffuse through the extracellular fluid that surrounds these cells, as well as through their cytoplasmic extensions.

Compact and Spongy Bones

The basic functional unit of compact bone is the **osteon** (OS-tē-on), or *Haversian system* (**Figure 6-8a,b**). Within an osteon, the osteocytes are arranged in concentric layers around a **central canal**, or *Haversian canal*, that contains one or more blood vessels. The lamellae of each osteon form a series of nested cylinders around the central canal. The central canals generally run parallel to the surface of the bone. **Perforating canals** provide passageways that link the blood vessels of the central canals with those of the periosteum and the marrow cavity.

Spongy bone has no osteons and a different arrangement of lamellae. Its lamellae form rods or plates called **trabeculae** (tra-BEK-ū-lē; *trabecula,* wall). Frequent branchings of the thin trabeculae create an open network. Canaliculi radiating from the lacunae of spongy bone end at the exposed surfaces of the trabeculae, where nutrients and wastes diffuse between the marrow and osteocytes.

A layer of compact bone covers bone surfaces everywhere except inside *joint capsules,* where articular cartilages protect opposing surfaces. Compact bone is usually found where stresses come from a limited range of directions. The limb bones, for example, are built to withstand forces applied at either end. Because osteons are parallel to the long axis of the shaft, a limb bone does not bend when a force (even a large one) is applied to either end. However, a much smaller force applied to the side of the shaft can break the bone.

In contrast, spongy bone is found where bones are not heavily stressed or where stresses arrive from many directions. For example, spongy bone is present in the epiphyses of long bones, where stresses are transferred across joints. It is

Figure 6-8 The Microscopic Structure of a Typical Bone.

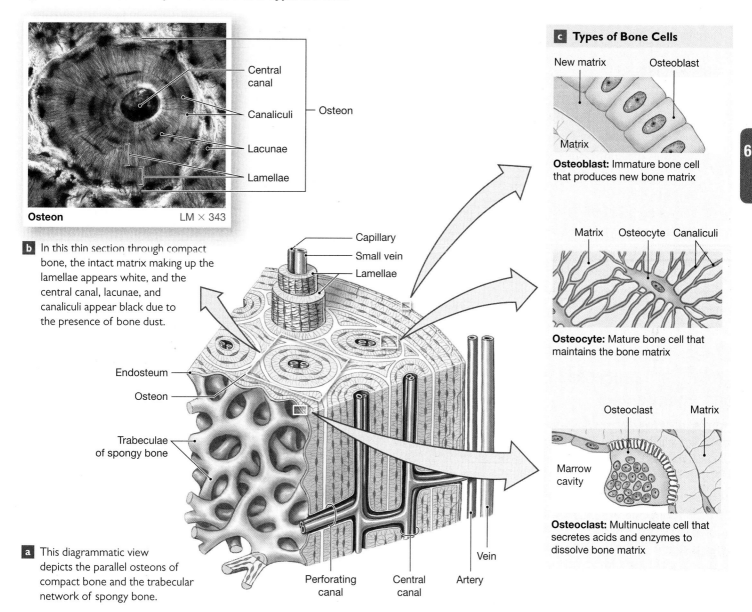

Osteon LM × 343

b In this thin section through compact bone, the intact matrix making up the lamellae appears white, and the central canal, lacunae, and canaliculi appear black due to the presence of bone dust.

a This diagrammatic view depicts the parallel osteons of compact bone and the trabecular network of spongy bone.

c Types of Bone Cells

Osteoblast: Immature bone cell that produces new bone matrix

Osteocyte: Mature bone cell that maintains the bone matrix

Osteoclast: Multinucleate cell that secretes acids and enzymes to dissolve bone matrix

also much lighter than compact bone. Spongy bone reduces the weight of the skeleton, making it easier for muscles to move the bones. Finally, the trabecular network of spongy bone supports and protects the cells of red bone marrow, where blood cells form.

Cells in Bone

Osteocytes are the most abundant cells in bone, but other cells types are also present (**Figure 6-8c**). These cells, called *osteoblasts* and *osteoclasts*, are associated with the endosteum that lines the inner cavities of both compact and spongy bones, and with the cellular layer of the periosteum. The three primary cell types are:

1. **Osteoblasts** (OS-tē-ō-blasts; *blast,* precursor) produce new bone, in a process called **ossification**. They produce new bone matrix and promote the deposition of calcium salts in the organic matrix. When an osteoblast becomes completely surrounded by calcified matrix, it differentiates into an osteocyte.

2. **Osteocytes** are mature bone cells. They maintain normal bone structure by recycling the calcium salts in the bony matrix and by assisting in repairs.

3. **Osteoclasts** (OS-tē-ō-clasts; *clast,* break) are giant cells with 50 or more nuclei. They secrete acids and enzymes that dissolve the bony matrix and release the stored minerals through *osteolysis* (os-tē-OL-i-sis), or *resorption.* This

process helps regulate calcium and phosphate concentrations in body fluids. At any given moment, osteoclasts are removing matrix and osteoblasts are adding to it.

CHECKPOINT

2. Identify the four general shapes of bones.

3. How would a bone's strength be affected if the ratio of collagen to calcium increased?

4. A sample of a long bone shows concentric layers surrounding a central canal. Is it from the shaft or the end of the bone?

5. Mature bone cells are known as _____, bone-building cells are called _____, and _____ are bone-resorbing cells.

6. If the activity of osteoclasts exceeds that of osteoblasts in a bone, how will the mass of the bone be affected?

See the blue Answers tab at the back of the book.

6-3 Ossification and appositional growth are processes of bone formation and enlargement

Learning Objective Compare the processes of intramembranous ossification and endochondral ossification.

The growth of your skeleton determines the size and proportions of your body. The bony skeleton begins to form about six weeks after fertilization, when an embryo is about 12 mm (0.5 in.) long. (At this time, all skeletal elements are made of cartilage.) Bone growth continues through adolescence, and portions of the skeleton generally do not stop growing until about age 25.

During development, bone replaces cartilage or other connective tissues. The process of replacing other tissues with bone is called **ossification.** (**Calcification** is the deposition of calcium salts. It occurs during ossification, but it can also take place in tissues other than bone.) There are two forms of ossification. In *intramembranous ossification*, bone develops within sheets or membranes of connective tissue. In *endochondral ossification*, bone replaces existing cartilage. **Figure 6-9** shows some of the bones formed by these two processes in a 16-week-old fetus.

Intramembranous Ossification

Intramembranous (in-tra-MEM-bra-nus) ossification begins when osteoblasts differentiate within embryonic or fetal fibrous connective tissue. This type of ossification takes

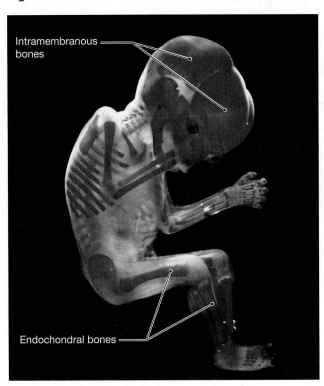

Figure 6-9 Bone Formation in a 16-Week-Old Fetus.

Intramembranous bones

Endochondral bones

place in the deeper layers of the dermis. The osteoblasts differentiate from connective tissue stem cells after the organic components of the matrix secreted by the stem cells become calcified. Ossification first occurs in an **ossification center**. As ossification proceeds and new bone branches outward, some osteoblasts become trapped inside bony pockets and change into osteocytes.

Bone growth is an active process, and osteoblasts require oxygen and a supply of nutrients. Blood vessels begin to grow into the area to meet these demands and over time become trapped within the developing bone. At first, the intramembranous bone resembles spongy bone. Further remodeling around the trapped blood vessels can produce osteons typical of compact bone. The flat bones of the skull, the lower jaw (*mandible*), and the collarbones (*clavicles*) form this way.

Endochondral Ossification

Most bones of the skeleton form through **endochondral (en-dō-KON-drul;** *endo,* **inside** + *chondros,* **cartilage) ossification** of existing hyaline cartilage. The cartilages develop first, serving as miniature models of the future bone (**Figure 6-9**). By the time an embryo is 6 weeks old, these cartilage models begin to be replaced by true bone. Steps in the

Figure 6-10 Endochondral Ossification.

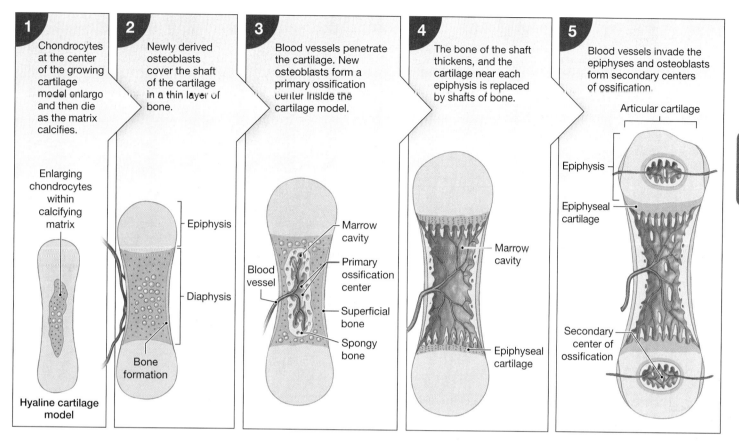

1 Chondrocytes at the center of the growing cartilage model enlarge and then die as the matrix calcifies.

Enlarging chondrocytes within calcifying matrix

Hyaline cartilage model

2 Newly derived osteoblasts cover the shaft of the cartilage in a thin layer of bone.

Epiphysis

Diaphysis

Bone formation

3 Blood vessels penetrate the cartilage. New osteoblasts form a primary ossification center inside the cartilage model.

Marrow cavity

Blood vessel

Primary ossification center

Superficial bone

Spongy bone

4 The bone of the shaft thickens, and the cartilage near each epiphysis is replaced by shafts of bone.

Marrow cavity

Epiphyseal cartilage

5 Blood vessels invade the epiphyses and osteoblasts form secondary centers of ossification.

Articular cartilage

Epiphysis

Epiphyseal cartilage

Secondary center of ossification

---

growth and ossification of a limb bone are diagrammed in **Figure 6-10**:

1 Endochondral ossification starts as chondrocytes within the growing cartilage model enlarge and their surrounding matrix begins to calcify. The chondrocytes die because the calcified matrix slows the diffusion of nutrients.

2 Bone formation first occurs at the shaft surface. Blood vessels grow around the edges of the cartilage, and the cells of the perichondrium differentiate into osteoblasts. The osteoblasts begin producing a superficial layer of bone around the shaft surface. ↰ p. 145

3 Blood vessels invade the inner region of the cartilage, along with migrating fibroblasts that differentiate into osteoblasts. The new osteoblasts form spongy bone within the center of the shaft at a *primary ossification center*. Bone development proceeds toward either end, filling the shaft with spongy bone.

4 As the bone enlarges, osteoclasts break down some of the spongy bone and create a marrow cavity. The **epiphyseal cartilages**, or *epiphyseal plates*, on the ends

continue to enlarge, increasing the length of the developing bone. Osteoblasts from the shaft continuously invade the epiphyseal cartilages, but the bone grows longer because new cartilage is continuously added in front of the advancing osteoblasts. This situation is like a pair of joggers, one in front of the other: As long as they run at the same speed, the one in back will never catch the one in front.

5 The centers of the epiphyses begin to calcify. As blood vessels and osteoblasts enter these areas, *secondary ossification centers* form. The epiphyses eventually become filled with spongy bone. A thin cap of the original cartilage model remains exposed to the joint cavity as the **articular cartilage**. At this stage, the bone of the shaft and the bone of each epiphysis are still separated by epiphyseal cartilage. As long as the rate of cartilage growth keeps pace with the rate of osteoblast invasion, the epiphyseal cartilage persists, and the bone continues to grow longer.

When sex hormone production increases at puberty, bone growth speeds up. The osteoblasts begin to produce bone faster than the epiphyseal cartilages expand. As a result, the

Figure 6-11 Appositional Bone Growth.

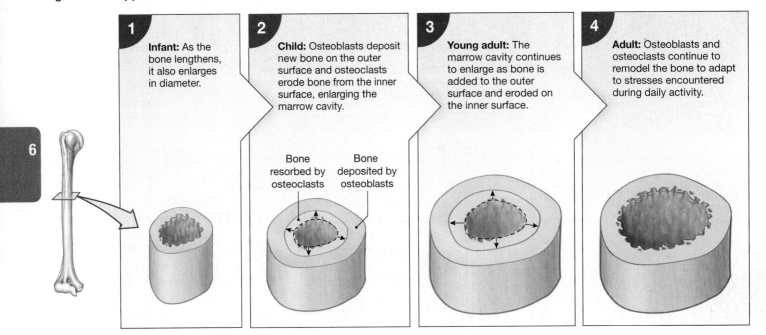

1 **Infant:** As the bone lengthens, it also enlarges in diameter.

2 **Child:** Osteoblasts deposit new bone on the outer surface and osteoclasts erode bone from the inner surface, enlarging the marrow cavity.

Bone resorbed by osteoclasts

Bone deposited by osteoblasts

3 **Young adult:** The marrow cavity continues to enlarge as bone is added to the outer surface and eroded on the inner surface.

4 **Adult:** Osteoblasts and osteoclasts continue to remodel the bone to adapt to stresses encountered during daily activity.

epiphyseal cartilages at each end of the bone get increasingly narrow, until they disappear. In adults, the former location of the epiphyseal cartilage is marked by a distinct **epiphyseal line** (**Figure 6-10**) that can be seen in X-rays. The end of epiphyseal growth is called *epiphyseal closure*.

While the bone lengthens, its diameter also enlarges. This enlargement process, called **appositional growth**, occurs as cells of the periosteum develop into osteoblasts and produce additional bony matrix (**Figure 6-11**). As new bone is deposited on the outer surface of the shaft, the inner surface is eroded by osteoclasts, and the marrow cavity gradually enlarges.

Bone Growth and Body Proportions

The timing of epiphyseal closure varies from bone to bone and individual to individual. Ossification of the toes may be complete by age 11, but portions of the pelvis or the wrist may enlarge until age 25. The epiphyseal cartilages in the arms and legs usually close by age 18 (women) or 20 (men). Differences in sex hormones account for variations in body size and proportions between men and women.

Requirements for Normal Bone Growth

Normal bone growth and maintenance depend on a reliable source of minerals, especially calcium salts. During prenatal development, these minerals are absorbed from the mother's bloodstream. The demands are so great that the maternal skeleton often loses bone mass during pregnancy. From infancy to adulthood, the diet must provide adequate amounts of calcium and phosphate. The body must also be able to absorb and transport these minerals to sites of bone formation.

Vitamin D₃ plays an important role in normal calcium metabolism. This vitamin can be manufactured by epidermal cells exposed to UV radiation or obtained from dietary supplements. ⤴ p. 127 After vitamin D_3 is processed in the liver, the kidneys convert a derivative of this vitamin into *calcitriol*, a hormone that stimulates the absorption of calcium and phosphate ions in the digestive tract. A deficiency of vitamin D_3 can lead to softening of bones as a result of poor mineralization. This disorder is called *osteomalacia* in adults and *rickets* in children. In growing children, affected individuals develop a bowlegged appearance as the leg bones bend laterally under the weight of the body.

Vitamin A and *vitamin C* are also essential for normal bone growth and maintenance. For example, a deficiency of vitamin C can cause *scurvy*. In this condition, a reduction in osteoblast activity leads to weak and brittle bones. Various hormones are also essential to normal skeletal growth and development. They include growth hormone, thyroid hormones, sex hormones, and hormones involved in calcium metabolism.

CHECKPOINT

7. During intramembranous ossification, which type of tissue is replaced by bone?

8. How could X-rays of the femur be used to determine if a person had reached full height?

9. A child who enters puberty several years later than the average age is generally taller than average as an adult. Why?

10. Why are pregnant women given calcium supplements and encouraged to drink milk even though their skeletons are fully formed?

See the blue Answers tab at the back of the book.

6-4 Bone growth and development depend on a balance between bone formation and resorption, and on calcium availability

Learning Objective Describe the remodeling and homeostatic processes of the skeletal system.

The process of **remodeling** continuously recycles and renews the organic and mineral components of the bone matrix. Two of the five major functions of the skeleton, support and storage of minerals, depend on this dynamic nature of bone. In adults, osteocytes maintain the matrix surrounding their lacunae, continually removing and replacing calcium salts. But osteoclasts and osteoblasts also remain active, even after the epiphyseal cartilages have closed. Normally, their activities are balanced. As one osteon forms through the activity of osteoblasts, another is destroyed by osteoclasts.

The turnover rate for bone is quite high. In young adults almost one-fifth of the skeleton is recycled and replaced, or remodeled, each year. Not every part of every bone is affected. For example, the spongy bone in the head of the femur may be replaced two or three times each year, yet the compact bone along the shaft remains largely untouched.

The Role of Remodeling in Support

Regular mineral turnover gives each bone the ability to adapt to new stresses. Heavily stressed bones become thicker and stronger and develop more pronounced surface ridges. Bones not subjected to ordinary stresses become thin and brittle. For this reason, regular exercise is an important stimulus in maintaining normal bone structure.

Degenerative changes take place in the skeleton after even brief periods of inactivity. For example, using a crutch while wearing a cast takes the weight off the injured leg. After a few weeks, the unstressed leg will lose up to about a third of its bone mass. However, the bones rebuild just as quickly once they again carry their normal weight.

The Skeleton as a Calcium Reserve

The bones of the skeleton are important mineral reserves—especially for calcium, the most abundant mineral in the human body. A typical human body contains 1–2 kg (2.2–4.4 lb) of calcium, with 99 percent deposited in the skeleton.

CHECKPOINT

11. Describe bone remodeling.

12. Why would you expect the arm bones of a weight lifter to be thicker and heavier than those of a jogger?

13. What general effects do the hormones PTH, calcitriol, and calcitonin have on blood calcium levels?

14. What is the difference between a closed fracture and an open fracture?

See the blue Answers tab at the back of the book.

6-5 Osteopenia has a widespread effect on aging skeletal tissue

Learning Objective Summarize the effects of aging on the skeletal system.

Bones become thinner and relatively weaker as a normal part of aging. Inadequate ossification is called **osteopenia** (os-t–PĒ-n-uh; *penia,* lacking). All of us become slightly osteopenic as we age.

The reduction in bone mass begins between ages 30 and 40. Osteoblast activity begins to decline, while osteoclast activity continues at previous levels. Once the reduction begins, women lose roughly 8 percent of their skeletal mass every decade. Men lose less—about 3 percent per decade. Not all parts of the skeleton are equally affected. Epiphyses, vertebrae, and the jaws lose more than their fair share. The result is fragile limbs, a reduction in height, and the loss of teeth.

CHECKPOINT

15. Define osteopenia.

16. Why is osteoporosis more common in older women than in older men?

See the blue Answers tab at the back of the book.

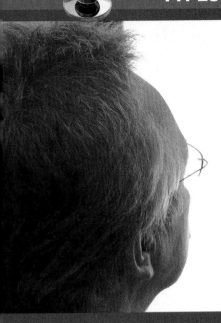
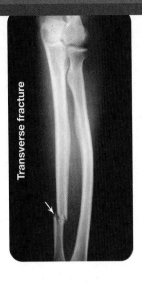
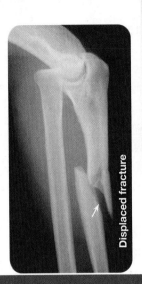
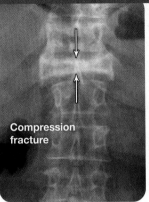
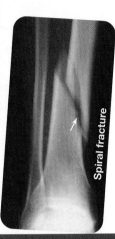

Transverse fracture

Displaced fracture

Compression fracture

Spiral fracture

TYPES OF FRACTURES

Fractures are named according to their external appearance, their location, and the nature of the crack or break in the bone. Important types of fractures are shown here by representative x-rays. The broadest general categories are closed fractures and open fractures. **Closed**, or *simple*, fractures are completely internal. They can be seen only on x-rays, because they do not involve a break in the skin. **Open**, or *compound*, fractures project through the skin. These fractures, which are obvious on inspection, are more dangerous than closed fractures, due to the possibility of infection or uncontrolled bleeding. Many fractures fall into more than one category, because the terms overlap.

Transverse fractures, such as this fracture of the ulna, break a bone shaft across its long axis.

Displaced fractures produce new and abnormal bone arrangements. **Nondisplaced fractures** retain the normal alignment of the bones or fragments.

Compression fractures occur in vertebrae subjected to extreme stresses, such as those produced by the forces that arise when you land on your seat in a fall. Compression fractures are often associated with osteoporosis.

Spiral fractures, such as this fracture of the tibia, are produced by twisting stresses that spread along the length of the bone.

REPAIR OF A FRACTURE

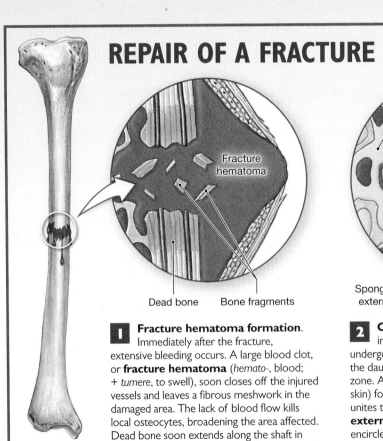
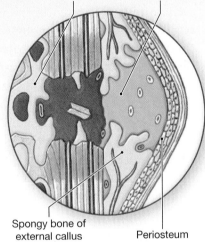

Fracture hematoma

Spongy bone of internal callus

Cartilage of external callus

Dead bone   Bone fragments

Spongy bone of external callus

Periosteum

1 **Fracture hematoma formation.** Immediately after the fracture, extensive bleeding occurs. A large blood clot, or **fracture hematoma** (*hemato-*, blood; + *tumere*, to swell), soon closes off the injured vessels and leaves a fibrous meshwork in the damaged area. The lack of blood flow kills local osteocytes, broadening the area affected. Dead bone soon extends along the shaft in either direction.

2 **Callus formation.** The cells of the intact endosteum and periosteum undergo rapid cycles of cell division, and the daughter cells migrate into the fracture zone. An **internal callus** (*callum*, hard skin) forms as a network of spongy bone unites the inner edges of the fracture. An **external callus** of cartilage and bone encircles and stabilizes the outer edges of the fracture.

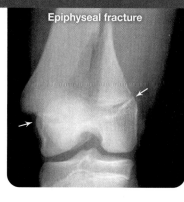

Epiphyseal fracture

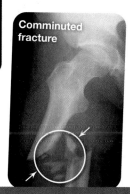

Comminuted fracture

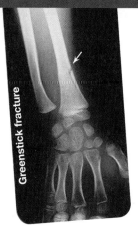

Greenstick fracture

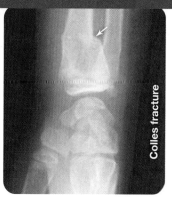

Colles fracture

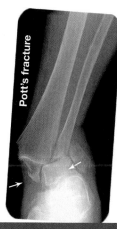

Pott's fracture

Epiphyseal fractures, such as this fracture of the femur, tend to occur where the bone matrix is undergoing calcification and chondrocytes are dying. A clean transverse fracture along this line generally heals well. Unless carefully treated, fractures between the epiphysis and the epiphyseal cartilage can permanently stop growth at this site.

Comminuted fractures, such as this fracture of the femur, shatter the affected area into a multitude of bony fragments.

In a **greenstick fracture,** such as this fracture of the radius, only one side of the shaft is broken, and the other is bent. This type of fracture generally occurs in children, whose long bones have yet to ossify fully.

A **Colles fracture,** a break in the distal portion of the radius, is typically the result of reaching out to cushion a fall.

A **Pott's fracture,** also called a bimalleolar fracture, occurs at the ankle and affects both the medial malleolus of the distal tibia and the lateral malleolus of the distal fibula.

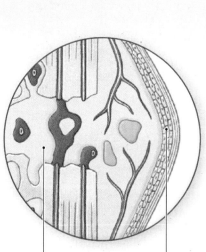

Internal callus   External callus

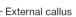

— External callus

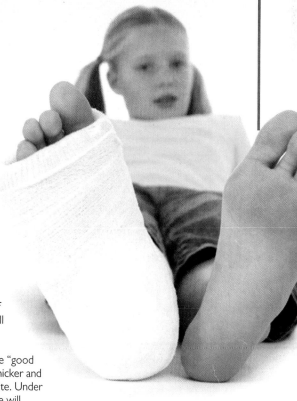

3 **Spongy bone formation.**
Osteoblasts replace the central cartilage of the external callus with spongy bone, which then unites the broken ends. Fragments of dead bone and the areas of bone closest to the break are resorbed and replaced. The ends of the fracture are now held firmly in place and can withstand normal stresses from muscle contractions.

4 **Compact bone formation.**
A swelling marks the location of the fracture. Over time, this region will be remodeled by osteoblasts and osteoclasts, and little evidence of the fracture will remain. The repair may be "good as new" or the bone may be slightly thicker and stronger than normal at the fracture site. Under comparable stresses, a second fracture will generally occur at a different site.

CLINICAL NOTE

Skeletal Injuries

There are four general types of skeletal and joint injuries: sprains, subluxations, dislocations, and fractures.

Sprains

The *sprain* is an injury that stretches or tears one or more ligaments within a joint. This tearing of ligaments weakens the joint. Stresses to a joint can extend the joint beyond its normal range of motion, which causes ligamentous injury (**Figure 6-12**). The injury results in acute pain at the site, followed shortly by inflammation and swelling. Sprains are classified, or graded, according to their severity, using the following criteria:

- *Grade I.* Minor and incomplete tear. The ligament is painful and tender, but there is no laxity. Swelling and ecchymosis are usually minimal. The joint is stable.

Figure 6-12 Grade II Ankle Sprain Following Common Inversion Injury. The anterior talofibular ligament appears completely torn, while the posterior talofibular ligament is only partially torn. The vast majority of ankle sprains involve the lateral ligaments.

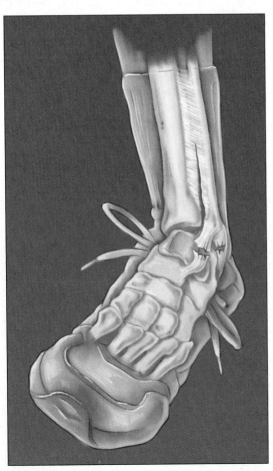

- *Grade II.* Significant but incomplete tear. There is laxity, but also an endpoint beyond which no further opening of the joint occurs. Swelling and ecchymosis may be moderate to severe, and pain may range from moderate to severe. The joint is unstable but intact.
- *Grade III.* Complete tear and total failure of the ligament or ligaments involved. No endpoint is felt when stress is applied to the ligament during examination of the joint. Pain and muscle spasm can often mask a grade III sprain, so the diagnosis is easily missed. Due to severe pain and spasm, the injury may be mistaken for a fracture. A repeat examination several days later can help confirm the diagnosis. The joint is unstable.

Subluxation

A *subluxation*, also called a *partial dislocation*, is a partial displacement of a bone end from its position within a joint capsule. It occurs as the joint separates under stress, which stretches the ligaments. A subluxation differs from a sprain in that it more significantly reduces the joint's integrity.

Dislocation

A *dislocation* is a complete displacement of bone ends from their normal position within a joint. The joint often fixes in an abnormal position with noticeable deformity (**Figure 6-13**).

Figure 6-13 Anterior Dislocation of the Knee. This rare injury poses a significant threat to blood vessels and nerves that transverse the knee. Immediate reduction is indicated.

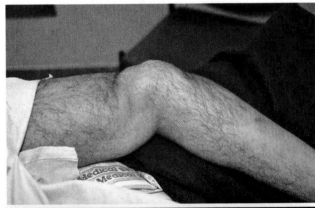

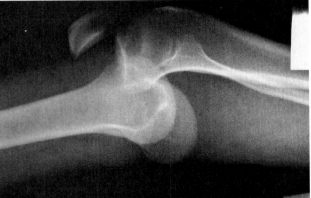

This injury occurs when the bones of the joint move beyond their normal range of motion, usually with great force. It carries with it the danger of entrapping, compressing, or tearing nearby blood vessels and nerves. A dislocation should be suspected whenever a joint is deformed or does not move in a normal fashion.

Fracture

A *fracture* is an injury that interrupts the structural integrity of a bone. Most fractures are the result of significant trauma to a healthy bone. The bony cortex may be disrupted by many different forces including a direct blow, angular (bending) forces, axial loading, twisting (torque) stress, or any combination of these.

Fractures also can occur in a bone that is diseased or otherwise abnormal. These pathological processes weaken the bone, making it susceptible to fracture by forces that would, under normal circumstances, not typically disrupt the cortex. These fractures are called pathological fractures and can result from relatively minor trauma. Examples of pathological fractures include fractures through lytic metastatic (cancerous) lesions, fractures through benign bone cysts, and vertebral compression fractures in patients with advanced osteoporosis. Vertebral compression fractures are the most common type of pathological fracture.

Growth-plate Injuries

Fractures can involve the epiphyseal growth plate in children. The cartilaginous epiphyseal plate, also called the physis, is readily injured because it is weaker than ossified bone or ligaments (**Figure 6-14**). Damage to the epiphyseal plate during a child's growth may destroy all or part of the bone's ability to produce new bone, which results in stunted or deformed growth thereafter. The potential for a growth disturbance from a growth-plate injury is related to the number of years the child has yet to grow. Thus, the older the child, the less time remains for a deformity to develop. The *Salter-Harris system* is often used to classify growth-plate injuries. The potential for growth disturbance increases as the classification number increases. The prognosis is best for

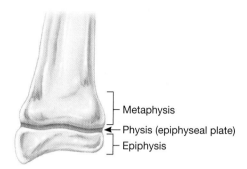

Figure 6-14 Growth Plate in a Child's Long Bone. This growth plate is also called the physis or epiphyseal plate. The portion of bone proximal to the physis is the metaphysics; the segment distal to the physis is the epiphysis.

— Metaphysis
— Physis (epiphyseal plate)
— Epiphysis

type I fractures and worst for type V fractures. The Salter-Harris classifications for growth-plate injuries are as follows (**Figure 6-15**):

- *Salter-Harris Type I.* The fracture line runs through the physis. There is usually little, if any, separation of the epiphysis from the rest of the bone. It is often difficult to see the fracture line on an X-ray, as the line is hidden within the growth plate. A type I injury is the least severe epiphyseal fracture type.
- *Salter-Harris Type II.* The entire epiphysis and a portion of the metaphysis are broken off. The fracture line runs through the physis and into the metaphysis.
- *Salter-Harris Type III.* A portion of the epiphysis is broken off. The fracture line runs through the physis, into the epiphysis, and into the joint.
- *Salter-Harris Type IV.* A portion of the epiphysis and a portion of the metaphysis are broken off. The fracture line runs through the metaphysis, the physis, the epiphysis, and into the joint.
- *Salter-Harris Type V.* The epiphyseal plate is compressed, usually through an axial loading type force. These injuries are difficult to diagnose and are sometimes only evident retrospectively when a growth disturbance develops.

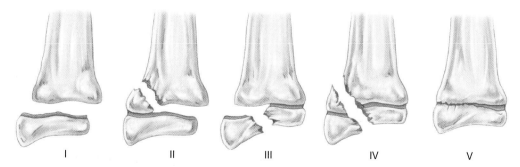

| I | II | III | IV | V |

Figure 6-15 Salter-Harris System of Classifying Growth Plate Injuries. The likelihood of a permanent growth plate deformity increases as the classification number increases.

(Continued)

Figure 6-16 Open and Closed Fractures. Open fractures, also called compound fractures, have a direct communication with the environment. Closed fractures, also called simple fractures, do not have any communication with the environment.

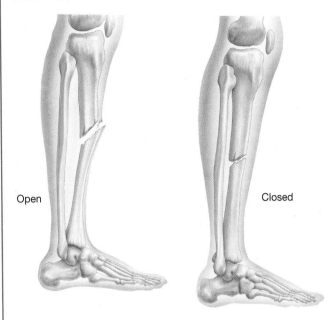

Open   Closed

Types of Fractures

There are many systems for classifying fractures. Generally, fractures are classified as either closed or open. In a *closed fracture*, the skin is not broken and there is no communication between the fracture site and the environment. In an

open fracture, the skin is broken and a communication exists between the fracture site and the environment. The difference in these two classifications has significant emergency care considerations. Open fractures are usually taken to the operating room, where the fracture site is exposed, cleansed, and irrigated to prevent infection. Closed fractures can be splinted, placed in a cast, or otherwise immobilized (**Figure 6-16**).

Fractures are also classified based upon the orientation of the fracture line as seen in radiographic (X-ray) studies (**Figure 6-17**).

- *Greenstick fracture.* Greenstick fractures are seen almost exclusively in children. In a greenstick fracture, one side of the bone is broken and the other side bent. This occurs due to the large amount of cartilage in the bones of children.
- *Torus fracture.* Torus fractures occur almost exclusively in children. In a torus fracture, there is localized buckling or swelling (or torus) of the cortex, with little or no displacement of the bone itself.
- *Transverse fracture.* A transverse fracture is a fracture line perpendicular to the long axis of the bone.
- *Oblique fracture.* In an oblique fracture, the break extends obliquely to the long axis of the bone.
- *Spiral fracture.* A spiral fracture, also called a torsion fracture, occurs when a twisting force is applied to a long bone.
- *Comminuted fracture.* Comminuted fractures are those where the bone at the fracture site has multiple bone fragments.
- *Segmental fracture.* A segmental fracture is an injury where there are multiple fracture sites along the axis of the bone, which leaves a free-floating segment of bone between the

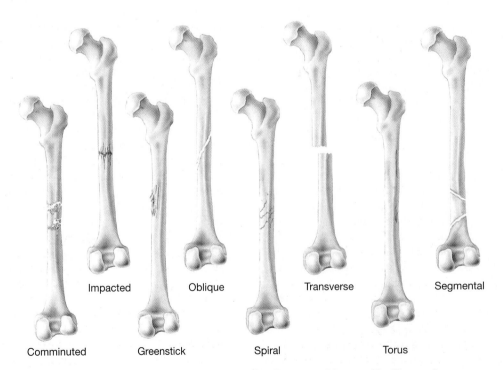

Impacted   Oblique   Transverse   Segmental

Comminuted   Greenstick   Spiral   Torus

Figure 6-17 Types of Fracture Based on the Appearance of the Fracture Line on Radiographs.

Figure 6-18 Colles' Fracture. In these common forearm fractures, the shape of the wrist after the injury often resembles a dinner fork.

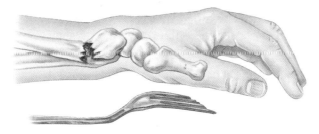

two fracture sites. Segmental fractures are often mistakenly called comminuted fractures.

- *Impacted fracture.* An impacted fracture is an injury where an axial loading force is applied to the bone, which drives the bone ends at the fracture site together.

Specific Fractures

Several specific types of fractures are important to emergency medical care.

Upper Extremity Fractures

Upper extremity fractures are common. Falls on an outstretched arm can result in fractures of the wrist, elbow, humerus, and clavicle. In fact, the clavicle is the most frequently fractured bone in the body. A common forearm fracture is the *Colles' fracture* (**Figure 6-18**). It usually results from a fall on an outstretched arm. The deformity resembles that of a dinner fork. Supracondylar fractures are fractures of the distal humerus, just above the elbow. Fractures that result from extension-type injuries usually cause posterior displacement of the distal segment. With flexion-type injuries, the distal fracture segment is usually displaced anteriorly. Flexion-type injuries occur much less frequently than extension-type injuries. Most supracondylar fractures occur in children and are associated with a number of complications, including nerve and vascular injuries due to the close proximity of these structures to the fracture site (**Figure 6-19**). Supracondylar fractures that involve a growth plate can cause growth abnormalities that often result in permanent deformity. Because of the high complication rate, supracondylar fractures should be promptly evaluated and treated by an orthopaedic surgeon.

Hip Fractures

Although the femur is the largest bone in the body, fractures of the proximal femur, or hip, are frequently seen, especially in the elderly. The hip is a ball-and-socket joint that consists of the acetabulum and the proximal femur, two to three inches below the lesser trochanter. The incidence of hip fracture increases with age and doubles for every decade past the age of 50. The incidence is two to three times higher in women than men, primarily due to decreased bone density secondary to osteoporosis. Hip fractures are usually classified as either intracapsular or extracapsular, depending on their location. With intracapsular fractures, the blood vessels that supply the femoral head are often compromised, which can lead to necrosis of the femoral head. The four types of intracapsular hip fractures are capital, subcapital,

Figure 6-19 Supracondylar Fracture. Supracondylar fractures have a high incidence of associated nervous and vascular tissue injury. In children, some supracondylar fractures can involve the growth plate, and possibly lead to permanent deformity or disability.

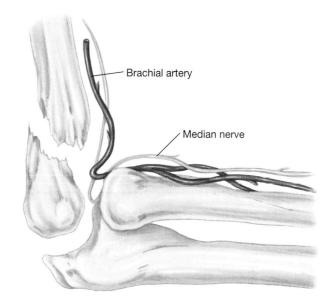

Brachial artery

Median nerve

transcervical, or basicervical (**Figure 6-20**). Subcapital fractures are by far the most common type of intracapsular hip fracture. There are three types of extracapsular hip fractures: trochanteric, intertrochanteric, and subtrochanteric. Of these, intertrochanteric fractures are the most common. All hip fractures in ambulatory patients require open reduction and internal fixation in the operating room. Intracapsular fractures usually require replacement of the entire hip joint with a prosthetic hip and acetabulum. Most extracapsular fractures can be stabilized by placement of a surgical pin or nail to hold the bone segments together while healing. As a rule, early fixation of hip fractures (less than 72 hours) in the elderly reduces morbidity and mortality.

Facial Fractures

Fractures of the maxilla usually result from high-energy injuries. As a result, patients with facial fractures may also sustain other associated injuries such as spinal, chest, and abdominal injuries. There are several identifiable facial fracture patterns that were first described by LeFort. He developed a facial fracture classification system that bears his name (**Figure 6-21**). A LeFort I fracture is limited to the maxilla at the level of the nares. In a LeFort I fracture, only the hard palate and upper teeth move with gentle palpation and mobilization. With a LeFort II injury, the triangular fracture line extends across the ridge of the cheeks and into the orbits. Mobilization of the fracture segment will move the nose but not the eyes. In a LeFort III fracture, the facial skeleton is separated from the skull. The entire face, including both orbits, shifts with palpation and gentle mobilization. This injury is also called a *cranial-facial disjunction.* Although not identified by LeFort, a LeFort IV facial fracture has been described. It is similar to a LeFort III fracture, but the fracture line extends upward into the frontal bones.

(Continued)

Figure 6-20 Types of Hip Fractures. Subcapital and intertrochanteric are the most common.

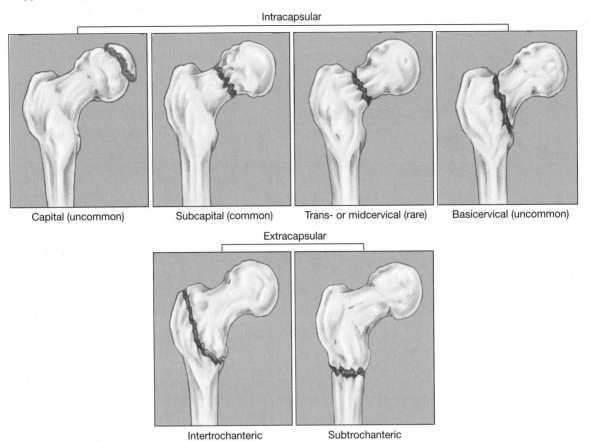

Intracapsular

Capital (uncommon)   Subcapital (common)   Trans- or midcervical (rare)   Basicervical (uncommon)

Extracapsular

Intertrochanteric   Subtrochanteric

Figure 6-21 LeFort System of Classifying Facial Fractures.

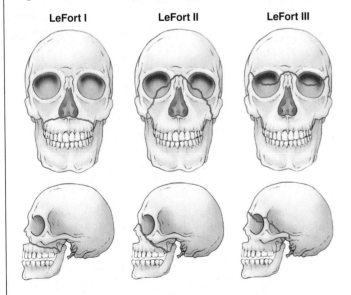

LeFort I   LeFort II   LeFort III

Fracture Healing

A fracture heals in three phases: inflammatory, reparative, and remodeling. Each phase of healing gradually blends into the next.

Immediately following a fracture, microscopic blood vessels that cross the fracture line are severed, which interrupts blood supply to the injured bone ends. In the following days, these blood-deprived bone ends become necrotic. This triggers a classic inflammatory response and essential inflammatory cells migrate to the fracture site. Soon, granulation tissue begins to fill the affected area. Within the inflammatory response are cells capable of forming cartilage, collagen, and bone. Together, these three components form the bone callus that gradually surrounds the fractured bone ends and stabilizes them. There are both internal and external calluses. Over time, the external callus becomes harder as minerals, especially calcium, are laid down. Underneath the callus, the necrotic edges of bone at the fracture site are removed by osteoclasts, which are cells whose function is to resorb bone. Finally, following the reparative phase, the remodeling phase begins. Remodeling is the tendency of the bone to regain its original shape and contour. During this phase, the excess parts of the callus are removed and new bone is laid down along natural lines of stress. Remodeling can continue for years and is affected by such factors as the patient's age and health and the magnitude of the original fracture. Typically, within a year or so, all evidence that a fracture occurred has disappeared and the bone appears completely normal. Fractures heal most rapidly in young children and slowest in the elderly. A 5-year-old child with an uncomplicated wrist fracture may only need to be in a cast for three weeks while an elderly patient with the same injury can expect to be in a cast for six weeks or more.

Calcium ions play an important role in many physiological processes, so calcium ion concentrations must be closely controlled. Even small variations from the normal concentration affect cellular operations. Larger changes can cause a clinical crisis.

Parathyroid hormone (PTH) from the parathyroid glands and *calcitriol* from the kidneys work together to increase calcium levels in body fluids. Their actions are opposed by *calcitonin*, a hormone from the thyroid gland that decreases calcium levels in body fluids. (We discuss these hormones and their regulation in Chapter 10.)

By providing a calcium reserve, the skeleton helps maintain calcium homeostasis in body fluids. This function can directly affect the shape and strength of the bones in the skeleton. When large numbers of calcium ions are released from the bones, the bones become weaker. When calcium salts are deposited, the bones become denser and stronger.

Repair of Fractures

Despite its strength, bone will crack or even break if subjected to extreme loads, sudden impacts, or stresses from unusual directions. Such bone damage is called a **fracture**. Most fractures heal even after severe damage, as long as the blood supply remains and the cellular components of the endosteum and periosteum survive. Steps in the repair process may take from four months to well over a year. The different types of fractures and the repair process are described in the Clinical Note: Types of Fractures and Steps in Repair on pp 166-167.

CLINICAL NOTE

Osteoporosis

Osteoporosis (os-tē-ō-po-RŌ-sis; *porosus*, porous) is a condition that reduces bone mass so much that normal function is compromised. The difference between the "normal" osteopenia of aging and osteoporosis is a matter of degree.

Sex hormones are important in maintaining normal rates of bone deposition. Over age 45, an estimated 29 percent of women and 18 percent of men have osteoporosis. In women, the condition accelerates after menopause because circulating estrogens (female sex hormones) decline. Severe osteoporosis is less common in men under age 60 than in women under 60 because men continue to produce androgens (male sex hormones) until late in life.

Osteoporotic bones break easily and do not repair well. Fractures frequently occur in the hip, wrist, and spine. Vertebrae may collapse and create pressure on spinal nerves.

6-6 The bones of the skeleton are distinguished by bone markings and grouped into two skeletal divisions

Learning Objective Define a bone marking and name the components and functions of the axial and appendicular skeletons.

Bone Markings (Surface Features)

The surfaces of each bone in your body have characteristic features related to specific functions. Projections form where muscles, tendons, or ligaments attach, and where adjacent bones form at joints. *Depressions, grooves, and openings* indicate sites where blood vessels and nerves run alongside or penetrate the bone. These landmarks are called **bone markings**, or *surface features*. **Figure 6-22** lists and illustrates the most common terms used to describe bone markings.

Skeletal Divisions

The skeletal system consists of 206 separate bones and associated cartilages (**Figure 6-23**). It is divided into axial and appendicular divisions (**Figure 6-24**).

The **axial skeleton** forms the longitudinal axis of the body. This division has 80 bones. They can be subdivided into four groups:

1. The 22 bones of the **skull** (8 *cranial bones* and 14 *facial bones*).

2. The seven bones associated with the skull (six **auditory ossicles** [*ear bones*] and the **hyoid bone**).

3. The 25 bones of the **thoracic cage** (24 *ribs* and the *sternum*).

4. The 26 bones of the **vertebral column**.

The **appendicular skeleton** includes the bones of the limbs and those of the **pectoral** and **pelvic girdles**, which attach the limbs to the trunk. All together there are 126 appendicular bones. Of these, 32 are associated with each upper limb, and 31 with each lower limb.

CHECKPOINT

17. Define a bone marking.

18. Identify the bones of the axial skeleton.

See the blue Answers tab at the back of the book.

6-7 The bones of the skull, vertebral column, and thoracic cage make up the axial skeleton

Learning Objective Identify the bones of the skull, discuss the differences in structure and function of the various vertebrae, and describe the roles of the thoracic cage.

The **axial skeleton** creates a framework that supports and protects the brain, the spinal cord, and the thoracic and abdominal organs. It also provides an extensive surface area for

Figure 6-22 An Introduction to Bone Markings.

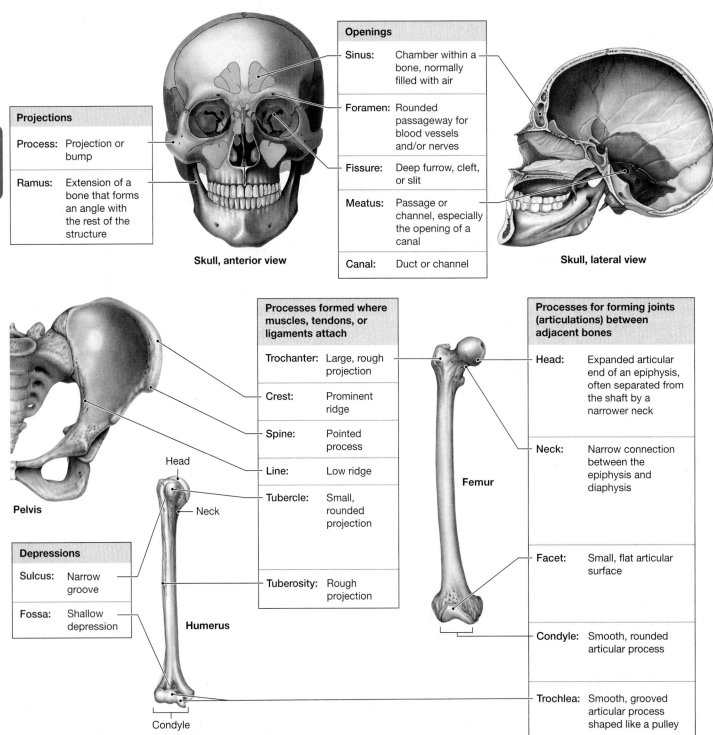

Projections

Process:	Projection or bump
Ramus:	Extension of a bone that forms an angle with the rest of the structure

Skull, anterior view

Openings

Sinus:	Chamber within a bone, normally filled with air
Foramen:	Rounded passageway for blood vessels and/or nerves
Fissure:	Deep furrow, cleft, or slit
Meatus:	Passage or channel, especially the opening of a canal
Canal:	Duct or channel

Skull, lateral view

Pelvis

Processes formed where muscles, tendons, or ligaments attach

Trochanter:	Large, rough projection
Crest:	Prominent ridge
Spine:	Pointed process
Line:	Low ridge
Tubercle:	Small, rounded projection
Tuberosity:	Rough projection

Head

Neck

Depressions

Sulcus:	Narrow groove
Fossa:	Shallow depression

Humerus

Condyle

Femur

Processes for forming joints (articulations) between adjacent bones

Head:	Expanded articular end of an epiphysis, often separated from the shaft by a narrower neck
Neck:	Narrow connection between the epiphysis and diaphysis
Facet:	Small, flat articular surface
Condyle:	Smooth, rounded articular process
Trochlea:	Smooth, grooved articular process shaped like a pulley

the attachment of muscles that (1) adjust the positions of the head, neck, and trunk; (2) perform respiratory movements; and (3) stabilize or position elements of the appendicular skeleton.

The Skull

The bones of the skull protect the brain and guard the entrances to the digestive and respiratory systems. The skull also houses

special sense organs for smell, taste, hearing, balance, and sight. The skull is made up of 22 bones: 8 form the **cranium**, and 14 are associated with the face. Seven additional bones are associated with the skull: six *auditory ossicles,* tiny bones involved in sound detection, are encased by the *temporal bones* of the cranium; and the *hyoid bone* is connected to the inferior surface of the skull by a pair of ligaments.

Figure 6-23 The Skeleton.

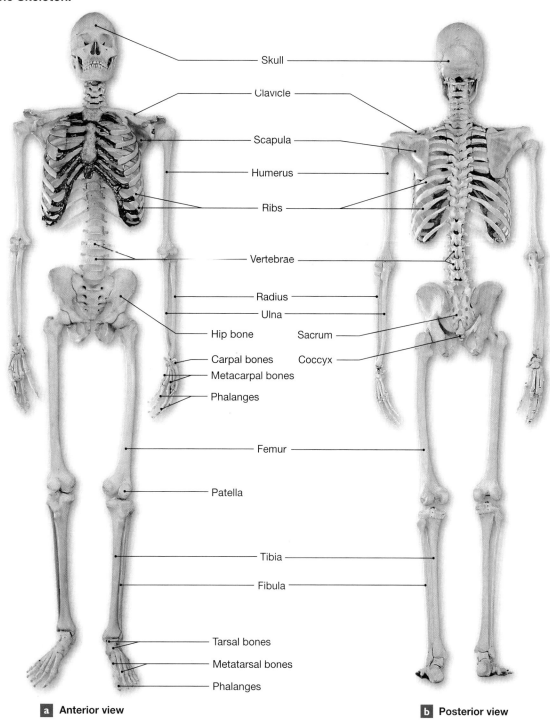

Skull

Clavicle

Scapula

Humerus

Ribs

Vertebrae

Radius

Ulna

Hip bone   Sacrum

Carpal bones   Coccyx

Metacarpal bones

Phalanges

Femur

Patella

Tibia

Fibula

Tarsal bones

Metatarsal bones

Phalanges

a **Anterior view**   **b** **Posterior view**

The cranium encloses the **cranial cavity**, a chamber that supports the brain. Membranes that stabilize the position of the brain are attached to the inner surface of the cranium. The outer surface of the cranium provides an extensive area for the attachment of muscles that move the eyes, jaws, and head.

The Bones of the Cranium

THE FRONTAL BONE. The **frontal bone** of the cranium forms the forehead and the roof of the **orbits**, or eye sockets (**Figures 6-25** and **6-26a**). A **supra-orbital foramen** pierces the bony ridge above each orbit, forming a passageway for

6

Figure 6-24 The Axial and Appendicular Divisions of the Skeleton.

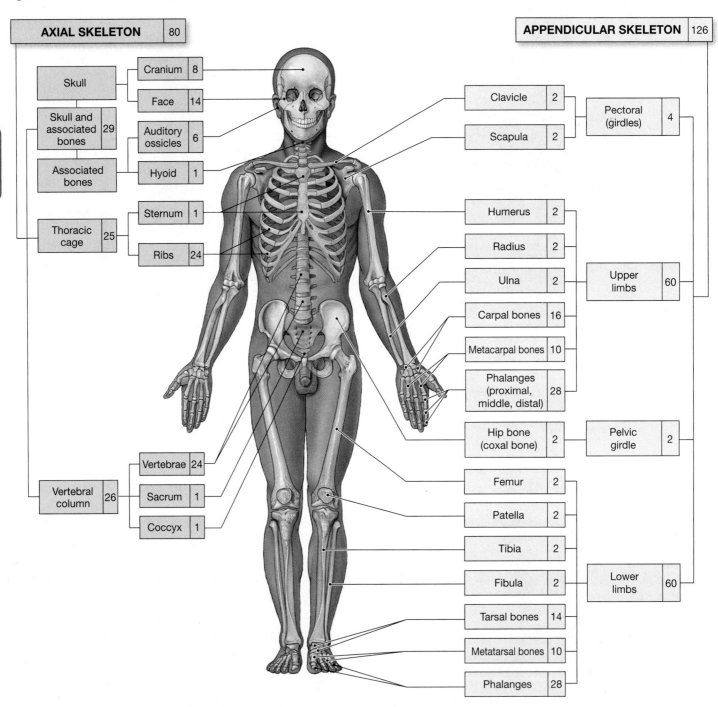

blood vessels and nerves passing to or from the eyebrows and eyelids (**Figure 6-25**). (Sometimes the foramen is incomplete, and the vessels then cross the rim of the orbit in a deep groove, called the *supra-orbital notch.*)

Above the orbit, the frontal bone contains air-filled chambers that connect with the nasal cavity. These **frontal sinuses** make the bone lighter and produce mucus that cleans and moistens the nasal cavities (**Figure 6-27b**).

THE PARIETAL BONES. On either side of the skull, a **parietal (pa-RĪ-e-tal) bone** is posterior to the frontal bone (**Figures 6-26a** and **6-27**). Together the parietal bones form the roof and the superior walls of the cranium. The parietal bones interlock along the **sagittal suture**, which extends along the midline of the cranium (**Figure 6-26a**). Anteriorly, the two parietal bones articulate with the frontal bone along the **coronal suture** (**Figure 6-25**).

Figure 6-25 The Adult Skull, Part I. The adult skull is shown in lateral view.

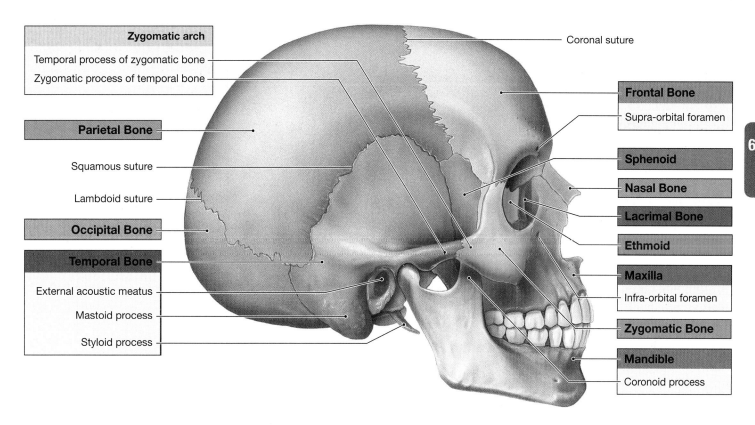

THE OCCIPITAL BONE. The **occipital bone** forms the posterior and inferior portions of the cranium (**Figures 6-26** and **6-26b**). Along its superior margin, the occipital bone contacts the two parietal bones at the **lambdoid (LAM-doyd) suture**. The **foramen magnum** connects the cranial cavity with the vertebral canal, which is enclosed by the vertebral column. This passageway surrounds the connection between the brain and spinal cord. On either side of the foramen magnum are the **occipital condyles**, the sites of articulation between the skull and the first vertebra of the neck.

THE TEMPORAL BONES. The **temporal bones** form part of both the sides of the cranium and the zygomatic arches. The temporal bones contact the parietal bones along the **squamous (SKWĀ-mus) suture** on each side (**Figure 6-25**).

The temporal bones have a number of distinctive surface features. One of them, the **external acoustic meatus**, leads to the *tympanic membrane,* or eardrum. The eardrum separates the external acoustic meatus from the *middle ear,* an air-filled chamber which contains the *auditory ossicles,* or *ear bones*. (We will consider structures of the ear in Chapter 9.)

Anterior to the external acoustic meatus is a transverse depression, the **mandibular fossa**, which marks the point of articulation with the lower jaw (mandible) (**Figure 6-26b**). The prominent bulge just posterior and inferior to the entrance to the external acoustic meatus is the **mastoid process**. It is a site of the attachment of muscles that rotate or extend the head. Next to the base of the mastoid process is the long, sharp **styloid (STĪ-loyd; *stylos,* pillar) process**. Ligaments that support the hyoid bone are attached to the styloid process. It also anchors muscles associated with the tongue and pharynx.

THE SPHENOID BONE. The **sphenoid (SFĒ-noyd) bone** forms part of the floor of the cranium (**Figure 6-27b**). It also acts like a bridge, uniting the cranial and facial bones, and it braces the sides of the skull. The general shape of the sphenoid is like a giant bat with wings extended (**Figure 6-27a**). Viewed anteriorly (**Figure 6-26a**) or laterally (**Figure 6-25**), the sphenoid is covered by other bones. Like the frontal bone, the sphenoid bone also contains a pair of sinuses, called **sphenoidal sinuses (Figure 6-27b,c)**.

Figure 6-26 The Adult Skull, Part II.

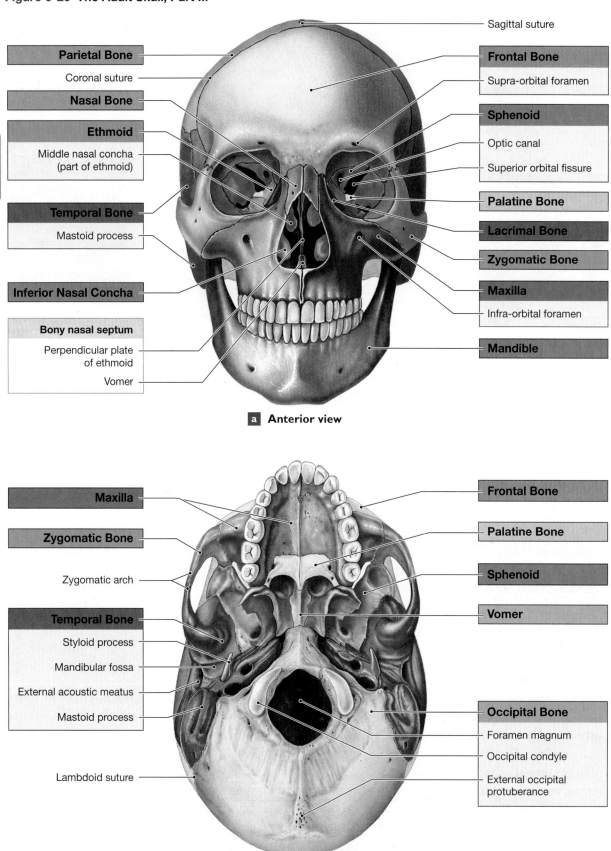

Sagittal suture

Parietal Bone

Coronal suture

Nasal Bone

Ethmoid

Middle nasal concha
(part of ethmoid)

Temporal Bone

Mastoid process

Inferior Nasal Concha

Bony nasal septum

Perpendicular plate
of ethmoid

Vomer

Frontal Bone

Supra-orbital foramen

Sphenoid

Optic canal

Superior orbital fissure

Palatine Bone

Lacrimal Bone

Zygomatic Bone

Maxilla

Infra-orbital foramen

Mandible

a **Anterior view**

Maxilla

Zygomatic Bone

Zygomatic arch

Temporal Bone

Styloid process

Mandibular fossa

External acoustic meatus

Mastoid process

Lambdoid suture

Frontal Bone

Palatine Bone

Sphenoid

Vomer

Occipital Bone

Foramen magnum

Occipital condyle

External occipital
protuberance

b **Inferior view**

Figure 6-27 Sectional Anatomy of the Skull.

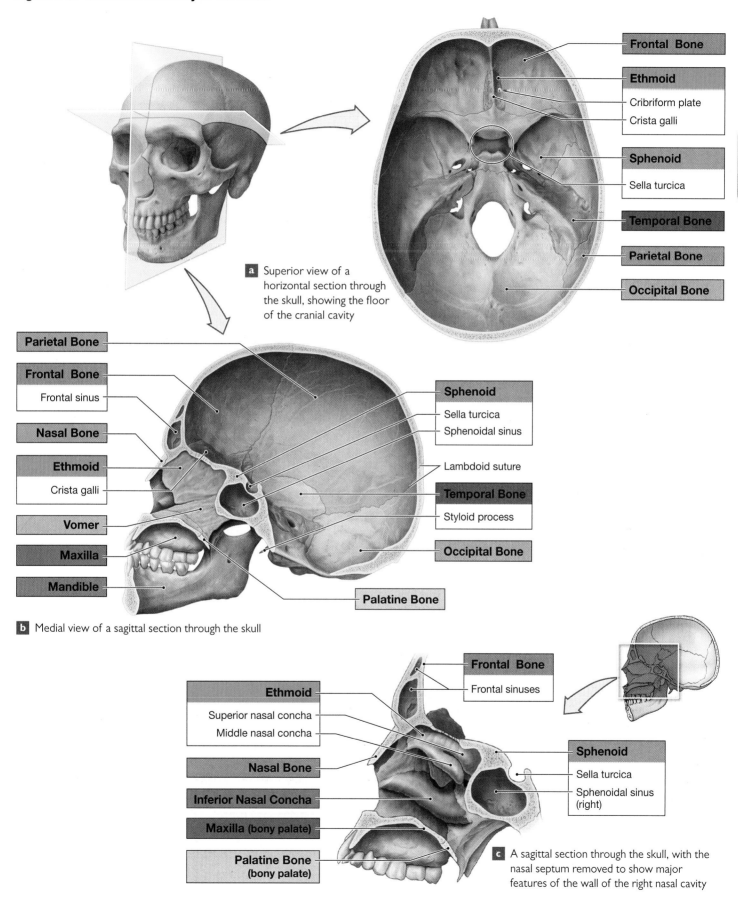

Frontal Bone

Ethmoid
Cribriform plate
Crista galli

Sphenoid
Sella turcica

Temporal Bone

Parietal Bone

Occipital Bone

a Superior view of a horizontal section through the skull, showing the floor of the cranial cavity

Parietal Bone

Frontal Bone
Frontal sinus

Nasal Bone

Ethmoid
Crista galli

Vomer

Maxilla

Mandible

Sphenoid
Sella turcica
Sphenoidal sinus

Lambdoid suture

Temporal Bone
Styloid process

Occipital Bone

Palatine Bone

b Medial view of a sagittal section through the skull

Frontal Bone
Frontal sinuses

Ethmoid
Superior nasal concha
Middle nasal concha

Nasal Bone

Inferior Nasal Concha

Maxilla (bony palate)

Palatine Bone
(bony palate)

Sphenoid
Sella turcica
Sphenoidal sinus
(right)

c A sagittal section through the skull, with the nasal septum removed to show major features of the wall of the right nasal cavity

The lateral "wings" of the sphenoid extend to either side from a central depression called the **sella turcica** (TUR-si-kuh) (Turk's saddle) (**Figure 6-27a,b**). It encloses the pituitary gland, which is connected to the inferior surface of the brain by a narrow stalk of neural tissue.

THE ETHMOID BONE. The **ethmoid bone** is anterior to the sphenoid bone. The ethmoid consists of two honeycombed masses of bone. It forms part of the cranial floor, contributes to the medial surfaces of the orbit of each eye, and forms the roof and sides of the nasal cavity (**Figures 6-26a and 6-27b**). A prominent ridge, the **crista galli**, or "cock's comb," projects above the superior surface of the ethmoid (**Figure 6-27a,b**). Holes in the **cribriform plate** (*cribrum*, sieve) permit passage of the olfactory nerves, which provide the sense of smell.

The lateral portions of the ethmoid bone contain the **ethmoidal sinuses**, which drain into the nasal cavity. Projections called the **superior** and **middle nasal conchae** (KONG-k; singular *concha*, shell) extend into the nasal cavity toward the *nasal septum* (*septum*, wall), which divides the nasal cavity into left and right portions (**Figures 6-26a and 6-27b,c**). The superior and middle nasal conchae, along with the inferior nasal conchae bones (discussed shortly), slow and break up the airflow through the nasal cavity. This allows time for the air to be cleaned, moistened, and warmed before it reaches the delicate portions of the respiratory tract. These bones also direct air into contact with olfactory (smell) receptors in the superior portions of the nasal cavity. The **perpendicular plate** of the ethmoid bone extends inferiorly from the crista galli, passing between the conchae to contribute to the nasal septum (**Figure 6-26a**).

The Bones of the Face

The facial bones protect and support the entrances to the digestive and respiratory tracts. They are sites for the attachment of muscles that control our facial expressions and help us manipulate food. Of the 14 facial bones, only the lower jaw, or mandible, is movable.

THE MAXILLAE. The **maxillae**, or *maxillary* (MAK-si-ler-ē) *bones*, articulate with all other facial bones except the mandible. The maxillae are the largest facial bones. The maxillary bones form (1) the floor and medial portion of the rim of the orbit (**Figure 6-26a**); (2) the walls of the nasal cavity; and (3) the anterior roof of the mouth, or *bony palate* (**Figure 6-27c**). The **maxillary sinuses** in these bones

produce mucus that flushes the inferior surfaces of the nasal cavities. These sinuses lighten the portion of the maxillae above the embedded teeth. Infections of the gums or teeth can sometimes spread into the maxillary sinuses, increasing pain and making treatment more complicated. The **infra-orbital foramen** is an opening for a major sensory nerve from the face (**Figures 6-25 and 6-26a**).

THE PALATINE BONES. The paired **palatine bones** form the posterior surface of the *bony palate*, or *hard palate*—the "roof of the mouth" (**Figures 6-26b and 6-27b,c**). The superior surfaces of the horizontal portion of each palatine bone contribute to the floor of the nasal cavity. The superior tip of the vertical portion of each palatine bone forms part of the floor of each orbit.

THE VOMER. The inferior margin of the **vomer** articulates with the paired palatine bones (**Figures 6-26b and 6-27b**). The vomer supports a prominent partition that forms part of the *nasal septum*, along with the ethmoid bone (**Figures 6-26a and 6-27b**).

THE ZYGOMATIC BONES. On each side of the skull, a **zygomatic** (zī-gō-MA-tik) **bone** articulates with the frontal bone and the maxilla to complete the lateral wall of the orbit (**Figures 6-25 and 6-26a**). Along its lateral margin, each zygomatic bone gives rise to a slender *temporal process* that curves laterally and posteriorly to meet the *zygomatic process* of the temporal bone. Together these processes form the **zygomatic arch**, or *cheekbone* (**Figure 6-25**).

THE NASAL BONES. The **nasal bones** form the bridge of the nose midway between the orbits. They articulate with the frontal bone and the maxillary bones (**Figures 6-25 and 6-26a**).

THE LACRIMAL BONES. The **lacrimal** (*lacrimae*, tears) **bones** are located within the orbit on its medial surface. They articulate with the frontal, ethmoid, and maxillary bones (**Figures 6-25 and 6-26a**).

THE INFERIOR NASAL CONCHAE. The paired **inferior nasal conchae** project from the lateral walls of the nasal cavity (**Figures 6-26a and 6-27c**). They slow airflow and deflect inhaled air toward the olfactory (smell) receptors located near the upper portions of the nasal cavity.

THE NASAL COMPLEX. The **nasal complex** includes the bones that form the superior and lateral walls of the nasal cavities and the sinuses that drain into them.

The ethmoid bone and vomer form the bony portion of the **nasal septum**, which separates the left and right portions of the nasal cavity (**Figure 6-26a**).

The air-filled chambers of the frontal, sphenoid, ethmoid, palatine, and maxillary bones are collectively known as the **paranasal sinuses** (**Figure 6-28**). (The tiny palatine sinuses, not shown, open into the sphenoidal sinuses.) These sinuses lighten the skull and provide an extensive area of mucous epithelium. Their mucous secretions are released into the nasal cavities, where the ciliated epithelium passes the mucus back toward the throat. There it is swallowed or expelled by coughing. Incoming air is humidified and warmed as it flows across this carpet of mucus. Dust and bacteria become trapped in the sticky mucus and are swallowed or expelled. This mechanism helps protect delicate portions of the respiratory tract.

THE MANDIBLE. The broad **mandible** is the bone of the lower jaw. It forms a broad, horizontal curve with vertical processes at either side. Each vertical process, or **ramus**, bears two processes. The more posterior **condylar process** ends at the *mandibular condyle*, a curved surface that articulates with the mandibular fossa of the temporal bone on that side. This joint is quite mobile. A disadvantage of such mobility is that the jaw is easily dislocated. The anterior **coronoid (kor-Ō-noyd) process** (**Figure 6-25**) is the attachment point for the *temporalis muscle*, a powerful muscle that closes the jaws.

The Hyoid Bone

The small, U-shaped **hyoid bone** is suspended below the skull (**Figure 6-29**). Ligaments extend from the styloid processes of the temporal bones to the *lesser horns*. The hyoid (1) serves as a base for muscles associated with the *larynx* (voicebox), tongue, and pharynx. It also (2) supports and stabilizes the larynx.

The Skulls of Infants and Children

Many different centers of ossification are involved in forming the skull. During development, the centers fuse into a smaller number of composite bones. For example, the sphenoid begins as 14 separate ossification centers. At birth, there are two frontal bones, four occipital bones, and several sphenoid and temporal elements.

The skull organizes around the developing brain. The brain enlarges rapidly prior to birth, but the bones of the skull fail to keep pace. At birth the cranial bones are connected

Figure 6-28 The Paranasal Sinuses.

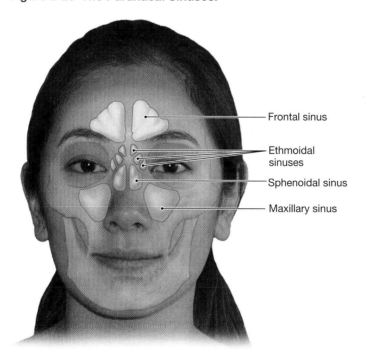

- Frontal sinus
- Ethmoidal sinuses
- Sphenoidal sinus
- Maxillary sinus

Figure 6-29 The Hyoid Bone.

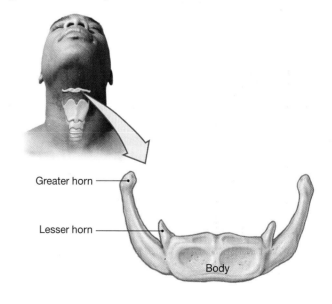

Greater horn

Lesser horn

Body

by areas of fibrous connective tissue (**Figure 6-30**). The connections are quite flexible, so the skull can be distorted without damage. During delivery, changes in head shape ease the passage of the infant along the birth canal. The largest fibrous areas between the cranial bones are known as **fontanelles** (fon-tah-NELZ; sometimes spelled *fontanels*). The anterior fontanelle is the "soft spot" on newborns. By about age 4, these areas disappear and skull growth is completed.

Figure 6-30 The Skull of an Infant.

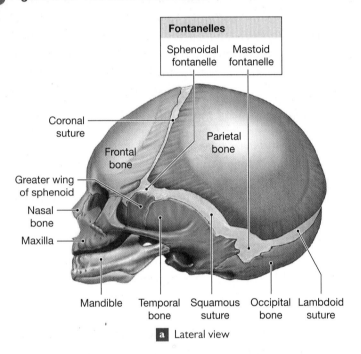

a Lateral view

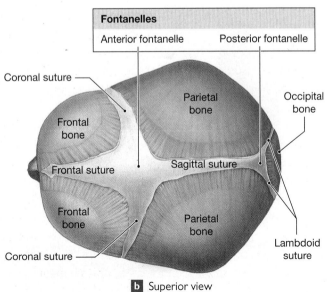

b Superior view

The Vertebral Column and Thoracic Cage

The rest of the axial skeleton consists of the vertebral column and the thoracic cage. The **vertebral column**, or **spine**, consists of 26 bones: the 24 **vertebrae**, the *sacrum* (SĀ-krum), and the *coccyx* (KOK-siks) or *tailbone*. The vertebrae provide a column of support. They bear the weight of the head, neck, and trunk, and ultimately transfer the weight to the appendicular skeleton of the lower limbs. The vertebrae also protect the spinal cord and help maintain an upright body position when sitting or standing.

The vertebral column is subdivided on the basis of vertebral structure (**Figure 6-31**). The **cervical region** of the vertebral column consists of the seven **cervical vertebrae** of the neck (abbreviated as C_1 to C_7). The cervical region begins at the articulation of C_1 with the occipital condyles of the skull. This region extends inferiorly to the articulation of C_7 with the first thoracic vertebra. The **thoracic region** consists of the 12 **thoracic vertebrae** (T_1 to T_{12}). Each articulates with one or more pairs of ribs. The **lumbar region** contains the five **lumbar vertebrae** (L_1 to L_5). The first lumbar vertebra articulates with T_{12}, and the fifth lumbar vertebra articulates with the **sacrum**. The sacrum is a single bone formed by the fusion of the five embryonic vertebrae of the **sacral region**. The **coccygeal region** is made up of the small **coccyx**, which also consists of fused vertebrae. The total length of the adult vertebral column averages 71 cm (28 in.).

Spinal Curvature

Even when we stand up straight, the vertebral column is not straight and rigid. A lateral view shows four **spinal curves** (**Figure 6-31**). The *thoracic* and *sacral curves* are called **primary curves** because they are present at birth. The C-shape of an infant's body axis results from these primary curves. The *cervical* and *lumbar curves*, known as **secondary curves**, develop several months after birth. All four spinal curves are fully developed by age 10.

Several abnormal distortions of spinal curvature may appear before adulthood. Three examples are (1) **kyphosis** (kī-FŌ-sis; *kyphos*, humpbacked, bent), caused by an exaggerated thoracic curvature; (2) **lordosis** (lor-DŌ-sis; *lordosis*, a bending backward), an exaggerated lumbar curvature; and (3) **scoliosis** (skō-lē-Ō-sis; *scoliosis*, crookedness), an abnormal lateral curvature.

Figure 6-31 The Vertebral Column. The major regions of the vertebral column and the four spinal curves are shown in this lateral view.

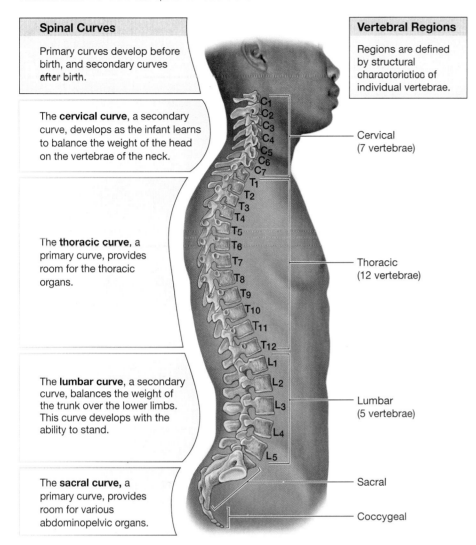

Spinal Curves

Primary curves develop before birth, and secondary curves after birth.

The **cervical curve**, a secondary curve, develops as the infant learns to balance the weight of the head on the vertebrae of the neck.

The **thoracic curve**, a primary curve, provides room for the thoracic organs.

The **lumbar curve**, a secondary curve, balances the weight of the trunk over the lower limbs. This curve develops with the ability to stand.

The **sacral curve,** a primary curve, provides room for various abdominopelvic organs.

Vertebral Regions

Regions are defined by structural characteristics of individual vertebrae.

Cervical (7 vertebrae)

Thoracic (12 vertebrae)

Lumbar (5 vertebrae)

Sacral

Coccygeal

Vertebral Anatomy

Figure 6-32 shows representative vertebrae from three different regions of the vertebral column. All vertebrae have a *vertebral body*, a *vertebral arch*, and *articular processes*. The **vertebral body** is the more massive, weight-bearing portion. An **intervertebral disc** of fibrocartilage lies between the bony faces of the vertebral bodies, preventing contact. Intervertebral discs are not found in the sacrum and coccyx, where the vertebrae have fused, or between the first and second cervical vertebrae.

The **vertebral arch** forms the posterior margin of each **vertebral foramen** (plural, *foramina*). Together, the vertebral foramina of successive vertebrae form the **vertebral canal**, which encloses the spinal cord. The vertebral arch has walls, called *pedicles* (PED-i-kulz), and a roof formed by flat layers called *laminae* (LAM-i-nē; singular, *lamina,* a thin plate). *Transverse processes* project laterally or dorsolaterally from the pedicles and are sites for muscle attachment. A *spinous process*, or spinal process, projects posteriorly from where the laminae fuse together. The spinous processes form the bumps that can be felt along the midline of your back.

The **articular processes** arise at the junction between the pedicles and laminae. Each side of a vertebra has a *superior* and *inferior articular process*. The articular processes of successive vertebrae contact one another at the **articular facets**. Gaps between the pedicles of successive vertebrae—the *intervertebral foramina*—permit the passage of nerves running to or from the enclosed spinal cord.

Some structural differences among vertebrae reflect differences in function, as we discuss next.

The Cervical Vertebrae

The seven cervical vertebrae extend from the head to the thorax. A typical cervical vertebra is shown in **Figure 6-33**. Notice that the body of the vertebra is not much larger than the vertebral foramen.

Distinctive features of a typical cervical vertebra include (1) an oval, concave vertebral body; (2) a relatively large vertebral foramen; (3) a stumpy spinous process, usually with a notched tip; and (4) round **transverse foramina** within the transverse processes. These foramina protect blood vessels supplying the brain.

The first two cervical vertebrae have unique characteristics that allow for specialized movements. The **atlas** (C_1) holds up the head, articulating with the occipital condyles of the skull. It is named after Atlas, who, according to Greek myth, holds the world on his shoulders. The articulation between the occipital condyles and the atlas permits you to nod (as when indicating "yes"). The atlas forms a pivot joint with the **axis** (C_2) through a projection on the axis called the **dens** (*denz;* tooth), or *odontoid process*. This articulation permits rotation (as when shaking your head "no") (**Figure 6-33**).

Figure 6-32 Typical Vertebrae of the Cervical, Thoracic, and Lumbar Regions.

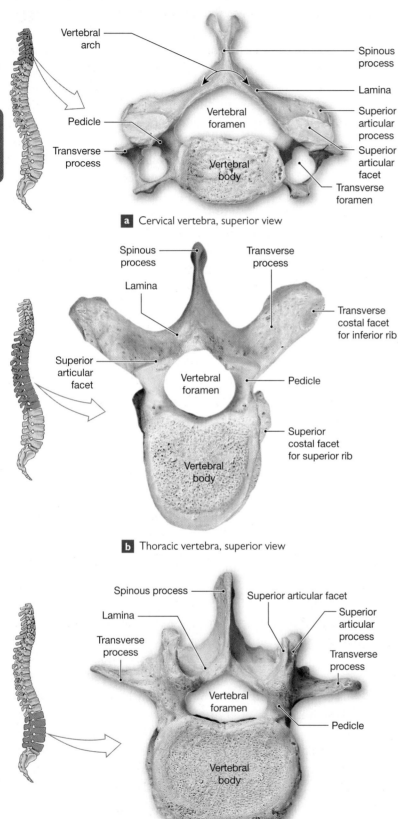

a Cervical vertebra, superior view

b Thoracic vertebra, superior view

c Lumbar vertebra, superior view

Figure 6-33 The Atlas and Axis. The arrows indicate the direction of rotation at the articulation between the atlas (C_1) and the axis (C_2).

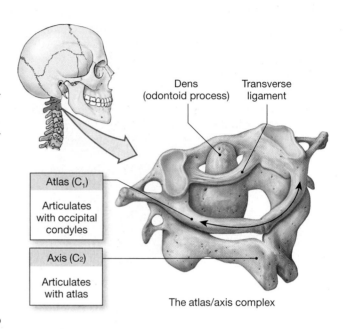

| Atlas (C_1) |
| Articulates with occipital condyles |

| Axis (C_2) |
| Articulates with atlas |

The atlas/axis complex

The Thoracic Vertebrae

There are 12 thoracic vertebrae (**Figure 6-31b**). From the first thoracic vertebra to the sacrum, the diameter of the spinal cord decreases, and so does the size of the vertebral foramen. At the same time, the vertebral bodies gradually enlarge, because they must bear more weight. Distinctive features of a thoracic vertebra include (1) a characteristic heart-shaped body that is more massive than that of a cervical vertebra; (2) a large, slender spinous process that points inferiorly; and (3) *costal facets* on the body (and, in most cases, on the transverse processes) for articulating with the head of one or two pairs of ribs.

The Lumbar Vertebrae

The five lumbar vertebrae are the largest vertebrae (**Figure 6-32c**). Their distinctive features include (1) a vertebral body that is thicker and more oval than that of a thoracic vertebra; (2) a relatively massive, stumpy spinous process that projects posteriorly, providing a surface for the attachment of the lower back muscles; and (3) blade-like transverse processes that lack articulations for ribs.

These vertebrae support most of the body weight. With increasing weight, the intervertebral discs become increasingly important as shock absorbers. The lumbar discs, which are subjected to the most pressure, are the thickest of all.

CLINICAL NOTE

Compression Fractures

Aging affects virtually every body system, and the skeletal system is no exception. Bone mass is normally lost with age in a process called *osteopenia*. However, some people will lose significantly more bone in a process called *osteoporosis*. In severe osteoporosis, over 50 percent of the bone mass can be lost. This is a particular problem in women following menopause where decreasing levels of female hormones (*estrogens*) result in loss of bone mass. This causes the bones to become weak and subject to fracture.

The weight-bearing parts of the spinal bones (*vertebral bodies*) are particularly vulnerable to osteoporosis. With advanced osteoporosis, relatively minor trauma, even as simple as rolling over in bed, can cause compression fractures. *Compression fractures* cause the vertebral body to collapse (much like crushing a soft drink can), which results in pain, limited movement, and a loss in body height. Elderly patients with multiple compression fractures may actually lose several inches of body height.

The Sacrum and Coccyx

The sacrum consists of the fused parts of five sacral vertebrae. It protects the reproductive, digestive, and excretory organs. Through paired articulations, it attaches the axial skeleton to the pelvic girdle of the appendicular skeleton. The broad surface area of the sacrum provides an extensive area for the attachment of muscles, especially those used for leg movement (**Figure 6-34**).

Notice that the sacrum resembles a triangle. The narrow caudal portion is called the **apex**. The broad superior surface is the **base**. The superior articular processes of the first sacral vertebra articulate with the last lumbar vertebra. The **sacral canal** is a passageway that begins between those processes and extends the length of the sacrum. Nerves and the membranes that line the vertebral canal in the spinal cord continue into the sacral canal. Its inferior end, the *sacral hiatus* (hī–tus), is covered by connective tissues. A prominent bulge at the anterior tip of the base is the **sacral promontory**. It is an important landmark in females during pelvic examinations and during labor and delivery.

The sacral vertebrae begin fusing shortly after puberty. They are typically completely fused at ages 25–30. Their fused spinal processes form a series of elevations along the *median sacral crest*. Four pairs of **sacral foramina** open on either side of the median sacral crest.

The coccyx provides an attachment site for a muscle that closes the anal opening. The fusion of the three to five (most often four) coccygeal vertebrae is not complete until late in adulthood. In elderly people, the coccyx may also fuse with the sacrum.

Figure 6-34 The Sacrum and Coccyx.

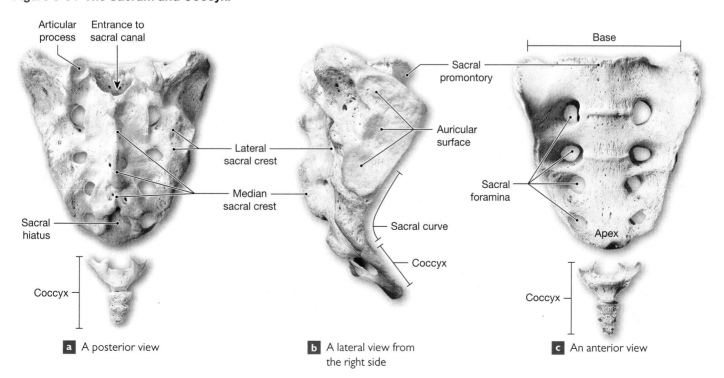

a A posterior view

b A lateral view from the right side

c An anterior view

6

The Thoracic Cage

The skeleton of the chest, or **thoracic cage**, consists of the thoracic vertebrae, the ribs, and the sternum (**Figure 6-35**). It provides bony support for the walls of the thoracic cavity. The ribs and the sternum form the *rib cage*. The thoracic cage protects the heart, lungs, and other internal organs. It also serves as a base for muscles involved in respiration.

Ribs, or *costal bones*, are long, curved, flattened bones that originate on or between the thoracic vertebrae and end in the wall of the thoracic cavity. Each of us, regardless of sex, has 12 pairs of ribs. The first seven pairs are called **true ribs**, or *vertebrosternal ribs*. These ribs reach the anterior body wall and are connected to the sternum by separate cartilaginous extensions, the **costal cartilages**. Ribs 8–12 are called the **false ribs** because they do not attach directly to the sternum. The costal cartilages of ribs 8–10, the *vertebrochondral ribs*, fuse together and merge with the cartilages of rib pair 7 before they reach the sternum. The last two pairs of ribs (11 and 12) are called **floating ribs** because they have no connection with the sternum.

The ribs provide attachment sites for muscles of the pectoral girdle and trunk, and between individual ribs. With their complex musculature, dual articulations at the vertebrae (ribs 2–9), and flexible connection to the sternum, the ribs are quite mobile. Because they are curved, their movements affect both the width and the depth of the thoracic cage, increasing or decreasing its volume.

The adult **sternum**, or breastbone, has three parts. The broad, triangular **manubrium** (ma-NOO-brē-um) articulates with the *clavicles* of the appendicular skeleton and with the cartilages of the first pair of ribs. The *jugular notch* is the shallow indentation on the superior surface of the manubrium. The elongated **body** ends at the slender **xiphoid (ZI-foyd) process**.

Ossification of the sternum begins at 6–10 different centers. Fusion is not complete until at least age 25. The xiphoid process is usually the last part to ossify and fuse. Its connection to the body of the sternum can be broken by impact or strong pressure, creating a spear of bone that can severely damage the liver. Cardiopulmonary resuscitation (CPR) training strongly emphasizes the proper positioning of the hand to avoid breaking ribs or the xiphoid process.

Figure 6-35 The Thoracic Cage.

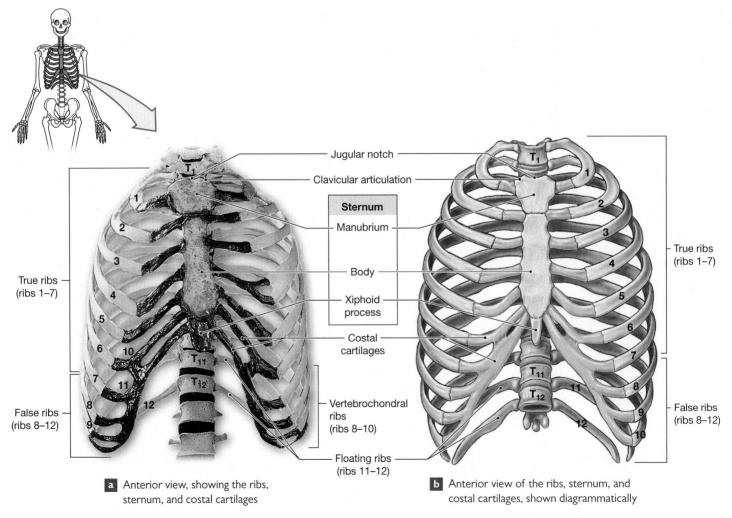

Sternum
Manubrium
Body
Xiphoid process

Jugular notch

Clavicular articulation

Costal cartilages

Vertebrochondral ribs (ribs 8–10)

Floating ribs (ribs 11–12)

True ribs (ribs 1–7)

False ribs (ribs 8–12)

True ribs (ribs 1–7)

False ribs (ribs 8–12)

a Anterior view, showing the ribs, sternum, and costal cartilages

b Anterior view of the ribs, sternum, and costal cartilages, shown diagrammatically

CHECKPOINT

19. The mastoid and styloid processes are found on which skull bones?

20. What bone contains the depression called the sella turcica? What is located in this depression?

21. Which bone of the cranium articulates directly with the vertebral column?

22. During baseball practice, a ball hits Casey in the eye, fracturing the bones directly above and below the orbit. Which bones were broken?

23. What are the functions of the paranasal sinuses?

24. Why would a fracture of the coronoid process of the mandible make it difficult to close the mouth?

25. What signs would you expect to see in a person suffering from a fractured hyoid bone?

26. Joe suffered a hairline fracture at the base of the dens. Which bone is fractured, and where would you find it?

27. In adults, five large vertebrae fuse to form what single structure?

28. Why are the bodies of lumbar vertebrae so large?

29. What are the differences between true ribs and false ribs?

30. Improper administration of CPR (cardiopulmonary resuscitation) could result in a fracture of which bone(s)?

See the blue Answers tab at the back of the book.

6-8 The pectoral girdles and upper limb bones, and the pelvic girdle and lower limb bones, make up the appendicular skeleton

Learning Objective Identify the bones of the pectoral and pelvic girdles and the upper and lower limbs, and describe their various functions.

The appendicular skeleton includes the bones of the upper and lower limbs, and the supporting bones of the pectoral and pelvic girdles that connect the limbs to the trunk.

The Pectoral Girdles

Each upper limb articulates with the trunk at a **pectoral girdle**, or *shoulder girdle*. The pectoral girdles consist of two broad, flat **scapulae** (SKAP-ū-lē; singular, *scapula,* SKAP-ū-luh) or shoulder blades and two slender, curved **clavicles** (KLAV-i-kulz; collarbones) (**Figure 6-36**). Each clavicle articulates with the manubrium of the sternum. These joints are the only direct connections between the pectoral girdles and the axial skeleton. Skeletal muscles support and position each scapula, which has no bony or ligamentous connections to the thoracic cage.

Movements of the clavicle and scapula position the shoulder joint and provide a base for arm movement. Once the shoulder joint is in position, muscles that originate on the pectoral girdle help to move the arm. The surfaces of the scapulae and clavicles are, therefore, extremely important as sites for muscle attachment.

The Clavicles

Each S-shaped clavicle articulates with the manubrium of the sternum at its *sternal end* and with a process of the scapula, the *acromion* (a-KRŌ-mē-on), at its *acromial end* (**Figure 6-36**). The smooth superior surface of the clavicle lies just beneath the skin. The rough inferior surface of the acromial end has prominent lines and tubercles, attachment sites for muscles and ligaments.

The clavicles are relatively small and fragile, so fractures are fairly common. For example, you can fracture a clavicle in a simple fall if you land on your hand with your arm outstretched. Fortunately, most fractures of the clavicle heal rapidly without a cast.

The Scapulae

The anterior surface of the *body* of each scapula forms a broad triangle bounded by **superior**, **medial**, and **lateral borders** (**Figure 6-37**). Muscles that position the scapula attach along

Figure 6-36 The Clavicle. The right clavicle is shown in a superior view.

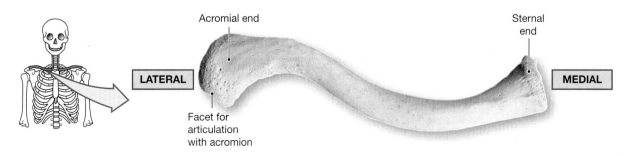

Acromial end

Sternal end

LATERAL

MEDIAL

Facet for articulation with acromion

Figure 6-37 The Scapula. These photographs show the major landmarks on the right scapula.

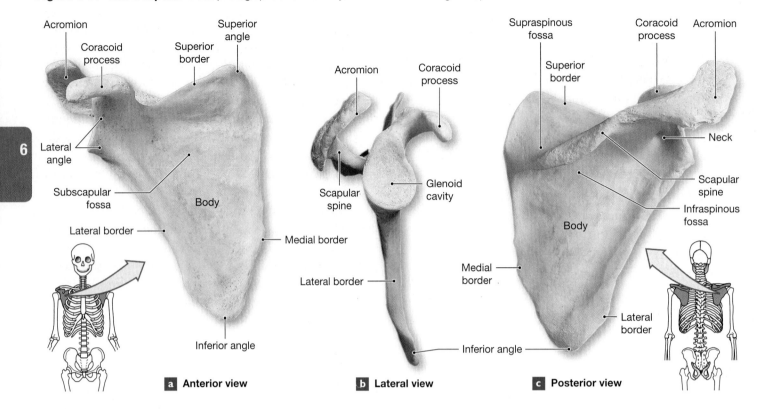

a Anterior view

b Lateral view

c Posterior view

these edges. The three tips are called the *superior angle, inferior angle,* and *lateral angle.* The lateral angle, or *head,* of the scapula forms a broad process that supports the shallow, cup-shaped **glenoid cavity**, or *glenoid fossa* (FOS-sah). ⟲ p. 153 At the glenoid cavity, the scapula forms the *shoulder joint* with the humerus, the proximal bone of the upper limb. The depression in the anterior surface of the body of the scapula is called the **subscapular fossa**. The *subscapularis muscle* attaches here and to the humerus.

Figure 6-37b shows a lateral view of the scapula and the two large processes that extend over the glenoid cavity. The smaller, anterior projection is the **coracoid (KOR-uh-koyd) process**. The **acromion** is the larger, posterior process. If you run your fingers along the superior surface of the shoulder joint, you will feel this process. The acromion articulates with the distal end of the clavicle.

The **scapular spine** divides the posterior surface of the scapula into two regions (**Figure 6-37c**). The area superior to the spine is the **supraspinous fossa** (*supra-*, above); the *supraspinatus muscle* attaches here. The region below the spine is the **infraspinous fossa** (*infra-*, beneath), where the *infraspinatus muscle* attaches. Both muscles are also attached to the humerus.

The Upper Limb

The skeleton of each upper limb consists of the bones of the arm, forearm, wrist, and hand. Anatomically, the term *arm* refers only to the proximal portion of the upper limb (from shoulder to elbow), not to the entire limb. ⟲ p. 14 The arm, or *brachium*, contains a single bone, the **humerus**, which extends from the scapula to the elbow.

The Humerus

At its proximal end, the round **head** of the humerus articulates with the scapula. The prominent **greater tubercle** of the humerus is a rounded projection near the lateral surface of the head (**Figure 6-38**). It establishes the lateral contour of the shoulder. The **lesser tubercle** lies more anteriorly, separated from the greater tubercle by a deep *intertubercular groove*. Muscles are attached to both tubercles, and a large tendon runs along the groove. The *anatomical neck* lies between the tubercles and below the surface of the head. Distal to the tubercles, the narrow *surgical neck* corresponds to the region of growing bone, the *epiphyseal cartilage.* ⟲ p. 147 The surgical neck earned its name because it is a common fracture site.

Figure 6-38 **The Humerus.** Major landmarks on the right humerus are labeled.

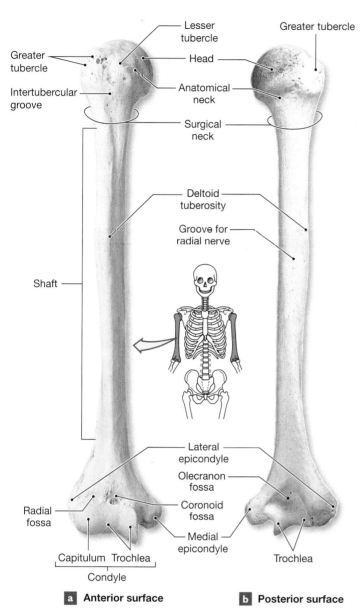

Lesser tubercle

Greater tubercle

Greater tubercle

Head

Anatomical neck

Intertubercular groove

Surgical neck

Deltoid tuberosity

Groove for radial nerve

Shaft

Lateral epicondyle

Olecranon fossa

Coronoid fossa

Medial epicondyle

Radial fossa

Capitulum Trochlea

Condyle

Trochlea

a **Anterior surface**

b **Posterior surface**

The proximal shaft of the humerus is round in section. The elevated **deltoid tuberosity** that runs along the lateral border of the shaft is named after the *deltoid muscle,* which attaches to it.

Distally, the posterior surface of the shaft flattens, and the humerus expands to either side, forming a broad triangle. **Medial** and **lateral epicondyles** project to either side, providing additional surface area for muscle attachment. The smooth **condyle** dominates the inferior surface of the humerus. At the condyle, the humerus articulates with the bones of the forearm, the *radius* and *ulna.*

A low ridge crosses the condyle, dividing it into two distinct regions. The **trochlea** is the large medial portion shaped like a spool or pulley (*trochlea,* a pulley). The trochlea extends from the base of the **coronoid** (*corona,* crown) **fossa** on the anterior surface to the **olecranon** (ō-LEK-ruh-non) **fossa** on the posterior surface. These depressions accept projections from the ulna as the elbow reaches its limits of motion. The **capitulum** forms the lateral region of the condyle. A shallow **radial fossa** proximal to the capitulum accommodates a small projection on the radius.

The Radius and Ulna

The **radius** and **ulna** are the bones of the forearm (**Figure 6-39**). In the anatomical position, the radius lies along the lateral (thumb) side of the forearm while the ulna provides medial support of the forearm (**Figure 6-39a**).

The **olecranon** of the ulna is the point of the elbow. On its anterior surface, the **trochlear notch** articulates with the trochlea of the humerus at the elbow joint. **Figure 6-39b** shows the trochlear notch in a lateral view. The olecranon forms the superior lip of the notch, and the **coronoid process** forms its inferior lip. At the limit of *extension,* when the arm and forearm form a straight line, the olecranon swings into the olecranon fossa on the posterior surface of the humerus. At the limit of *flexion,* when the arm and forearm form a V, the coronoid process projects into the coronoid fossa on the anterior surface of the humerus.

A fibrous sheet, or *interosseus membrane,* connects the lateral margin of the ulna to the radius along its length. Near the wrist, the ulnar shaft ends at a disc-shaped head whose posterior margin bears a short **styloid process**. The distal end of the ulna is separated from the wrist joint by a pad of cartilage, and only the large distal portion of the radius participates in the wrist joint. The styloid process of the radius stabilizes the joint by preventing lateral movement of the bones of the wrist (*carpal bones*). The lateral surface of the ulnar head articulates with the distal end of the radius at the *distal radio-ulnar joint.*

A narrow *neck* extends from the head of the radius to the **radial tuberosity,** which marks the attachment site of the *biceps brachii,* a large muscle on the anterior surface of the arm. The disc-shaped head of the radius articulates with the capitulum of the humerus at the elbow joint and with the ulna at the **radial notch**. This articulation with the ulna, the *proximal radio-ulnar joint,* allows the radius to roll across the ulna, rotating the palm in a movement known as *pronation.* The reverse movement, which returns the forearm to the anatomical position, is called *supination.*

6

Figure 6-39 The Right Radius and Ulna.

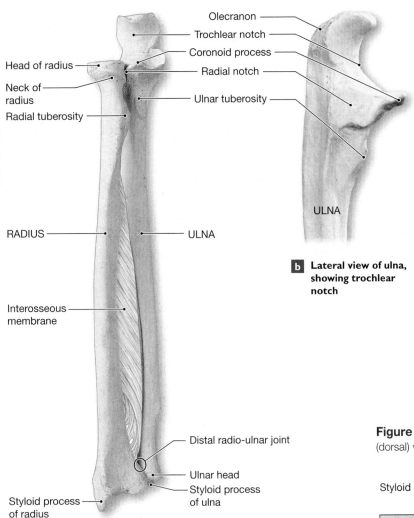

Olecranon
Trochlear notch
Coronoid process
Head of radius
Radial notch
Neck of radius
Ulnar tuberosity
Radial tuberosity

RADIUS
ULNA

Interosseous membrane

Distal radio-ulnar joint

Ulnar head
Styloid process of ulna

Styloid process of radius

a Anterior view

ULNA

b Lateral view of ulna, showing trochlear notch

Bones of the Wrist and Hand

The wrist, palm, and fingers are supported by 27 bones (**Figure 6-40**). The eight **carpal bones** of the wrist, or *carpus*, form two rows. There are four proximal carpal bones: (1) the *scaphoid bone*; (2) the *lunate bone*; (3) the *triquetrum bone*; and (4) the *pisiform* (PIS-i-form) *bone*. There are also four distal carpal bones: (1) the *trapezium*; (2) the *trapezoid bone*; (3) the *capitate bone*; and (4) the *hamate bone*. Joints between the carpal bones permit a limited degree of sliding and twisting.

Five **metacarpal (met-uh-KAR-pul) bones** articulate with the distal carpal bones and form the palm of the hand. The metacarpal bones in turn articulate with the finger bones, or **phalanges** (fa-LAN-jēz; singular, *phalanx*). Each

hand has 14 phalangeal bones. Four of the fingers contain three phalanges each (proximal, middle, and distal). The thumb, or **pollex** (POL-eks), has only two phalanges (proximal and distal).

The Pelvic Girdle

The **pelvic girdle** articulates with the thigh bones (**Figure 6-41**). Because of the stresses involved in weight bearing and locomotion, the bones of the pelvic girdle and lower limbs are more massive than those of the pectoral girdles and upper limbs. The pelvic girdle is also much more firmly attached to the axial skeleton.

The pelvic girdle consists of two large **hip bones**, or **coxal bones**. Each hip bone forms by the fusion of three bones: an **ilium** (IL-ē-um), an **ischium** (IS-kē-um), and a **pubis** (PŪ-bis) (**Figure 6-41a,c,d**). Posteriorly, the hip bones articulate with the sacrum at the **sacroiliac joints** (**Figure 6-41d**). Anteriorly, the hip bones are connected by a pad of fibrocartilage at a joint called the *pubic symphysis*. At the hip joint on either

Figure 6-40 The Bones of the Wrist and Hand. A posterior (dorsal) view of the right hand is shown.

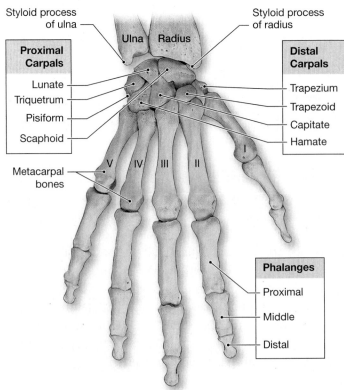

Styloid process of ulna
Styloid process of radius
Ulna   Radius

Proximal Carpals
Lunate
Triquetrum
Pisiform
Scaphoid

Distal Carpals
Trapezium
Trapezoid
Capitate
Hamate

Metacarpal bones

V   IV   III   II   I

Phalanges
Proximal
Middle
Distal

Figure 6-41 The Hip Bones and the Pelvis.

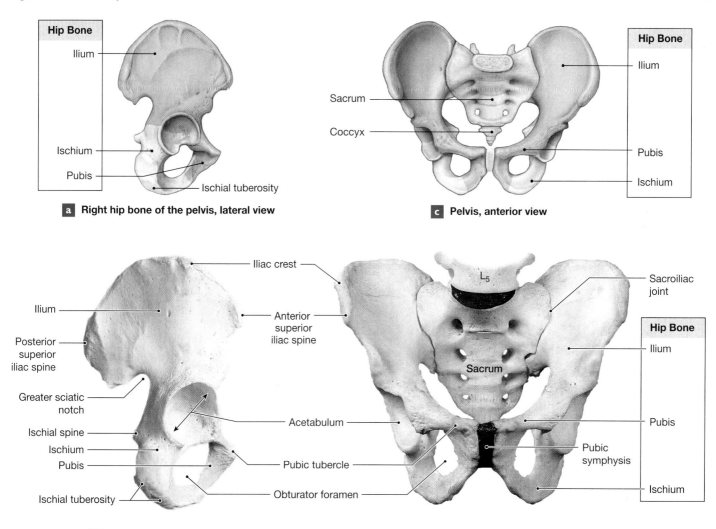

a Right hip bone of the pelvis, lateral view

c Pelvis, anterior view

b Right hip bone, lateral view

d Adult male pelvis, anterior view

side, the head of the femur (thigh bone) articulates with the curved surface of the **acetabulum** (as-e-TAB-ū-lum; *acetabulum*, a vinegar cup).

The Hip Bone (Coxal Bone)

The ilium is the most superior and largest component of the hip bone (**Figure 6-41**). Above the acetabulum, the ilium forms a broad, curved surface that provides an extensive area for the attachment of muscles, tendons, and ligaments. The superior margin of the ilium, the **iliac crest**, marks the sites of attachments of both ligaments and muscles (**Figure 6-41b,d**). Near the superior and posterior margin of the acetabulum, the ilium fuses with the ischium. A roughened projection at the posterior and lateral edge of the ischium, called the *ischial tuberosity*, supports the body's weight when sitting.

The fusion of a narrow branch of the ischium with a branch of the pubis completes the encirclement of the **obturator (OB-tū-rā-tor) foramen**. This space is closed by a sheet of collagen fibers whose inner and outer surfaces provide a base for the attachment of muscles of the hip.

The anterior and medial surface of the pubis contains a roughened area that marks the **pubic symphysis**, an articulation with the pubis of the opposite side. This joint limits movement between the two pubic bones.

The Pelvis

The **pelvis** consists of the two hip bones, the sacrum and the coccyx (**Figure 6-41c,d**). It includes portions of both the appendicular and axial skeletons. An extensive network of ligaments connects the sacrum with the iliac crests, the ischia, and the pubic bones. Other ligaments tie the ilia to the

Figure 6-42 Differences in the Anatomy of the Pelvis in Males and Females.

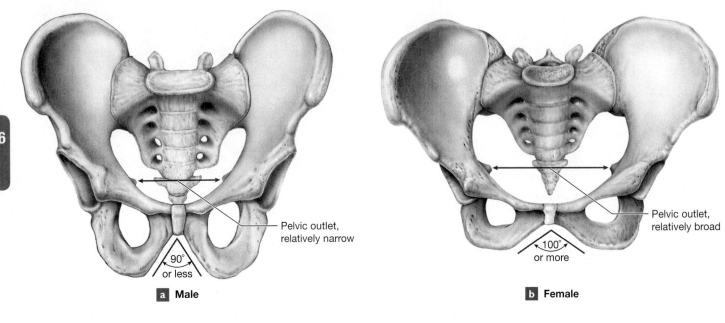

a Male

b Female

posterior lumbar vertebrae. These interconnections increase the structural stability of the pelvis.

The shape of the pelvis of a female is somewhat different from that of a male (**Figure 6-42**). Some differences result from variations in body size and muscle mass. For example, in females the pelvis is generally smoother, lighter in weight, and has less prominent markings. Other differences are adaptations for childbearing. They help to support the weight of the developing fetus and to ease its passage through the pelvic outlet during delivery. The *pelvic outlet* is the inferior opening of the pelvis. Compared to males, females have a relatively broad, low pelvis; a larger pelvic outlet; and a broader *pubic angle* (the angle between the pubic bones).

The Lower Limb

The skeleton of each lower limb consists of a *femur* (thigh bone), a *patella* (kneecap), a *tibia* and a *fibula* (leg), and the bones of the ankle and foot.

The Femur

The **femur** is the longest and heaviest bone in the body (**Figure 6-43**). The rounded epiphysis, or head, of the femur articulates with the pelvis at the acetabulum. The **greater** and **lesser trochanters** are large, rough projections that extend laterally from the juncture of the neck and the shaft. Both trochanters develop where large tendons attach to the

femur. On the posterior surface of the femur is a prominent ridge, the **linea aspera**. It marks the attachment of powerful muscles that pull the shaft of the femur toward the midline, a movement called *adduction* (*ad-*, toward + *duco*, to lead).

The proximal shaft of the femur is round in cross section. More distally, the shaft becomes more flattened and ends in two large **epicondyles** (**lateral** and **medial**). The inferior surfaces of the epicondyles form the **lateral** and **medial condyles**. They form part of the knee joint.

The **patella** (*kneecap*) glides over the smooth anterior surface, or *patellar surface*, between the lateral and medial condyles. ⟲ p. 155 The patella forms within the tendon of the *quadriceps femoris*, a group of muscles that straighten the knee.

CLINICAL NOTE

Hip Fractures

In the aged, simple falls can cause a *fractured* (broken) hip. These injuries are devastating; most patients require ambulance transport to the hospital. Most hip fractures require surgical repair. Fractures that occur low on the femoral neck can often be treated with a specialized nail that retains the native ball-and-socket joint. Fractures higher up the femoral neck usually require a prosthesis that replaces the native ball-and-socket joint. Hip fractures can be extremely debilitating and are one of the most common reasons for nursing home placement.

Figure 6-43 The Femur. The labels indicate the various bone markings on the right femur.

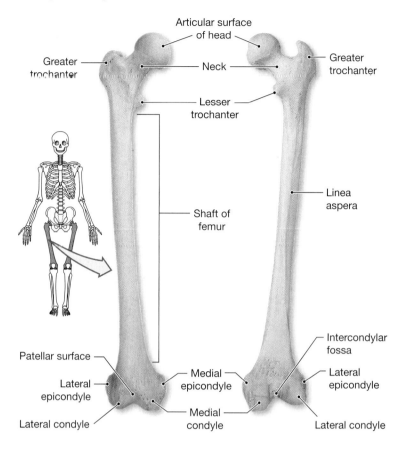

Figure 6-44 The Right Tibia and Fibula. These bones are shown in an anterior view.

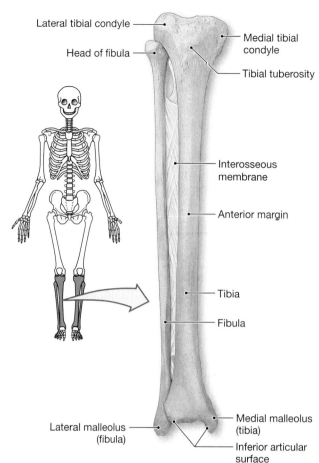

The Tibia and Fibula

The **tibia** (TIB-ē-uh), or *shinbone*, is the large medial bone of the leg (**Figure 6-44**). The lateral and medial condyles of the femur articulate with the *lateral* and *medial condyles* of the tibia. The *patellar ligament* connects the patella to the **tibial tuberosity** just below the knee joint.

A projecting **anterior margin** extends almost the entire length of the anterior tibial surface. The tibia broadens at its distal end into a large process, the **medial malleolus** (ma-LĒ-o-lus; *malleolus,* hammer), which provides medial support for the ankle. The inferior surface of the tibia forms a joint with the proximal bone of the ankle.

The slender **fibula** (FIB-ū-luh) parallels the lateral border of the tibia. The fibula articulates with the tibia inferior to the lateral condyle of the tibia. The fibula does not articulate with the femur or help transfer weight to the ankle and foot. However, it is an important surface for muscle attachment, and the distal **lateral malleolus**

provides lateral stability to the ankle. An interosseus membrane between the two bones stabilizes their relative positions and provides additional surface area for muscle attachment.

Bones of the Ankle and Foot

The ankle, or *tarsus*, includes seven separate **tarsal bones** (**Figure 6-45a**): (1) the *talus,* (2) the *calcaneus,* (3) the *navicular bone,* (4) the *cuboid bone,* and (5–7) the *medial, intermediate,* and *lateral cuneiform bones.* Only the **talus** articulates with the tibia and fibula. It passes the body's weight from the tibia toward the toes.

When you stand normally, most of your weight is transmitted to the ground through the talus to the large **calcaneus** (kal-KĀ-nē-us), or *heel bone* (**Figure 6-45b,c**). The posterior projection of the calcaneus is the attachment site for the *calcaneal tendon,* or *Achilles tendon,* which arises from the calf muscles. These muscles raise the heel and depress the sole,

Figure 6-45 The Bones of the Ankle and Foot.

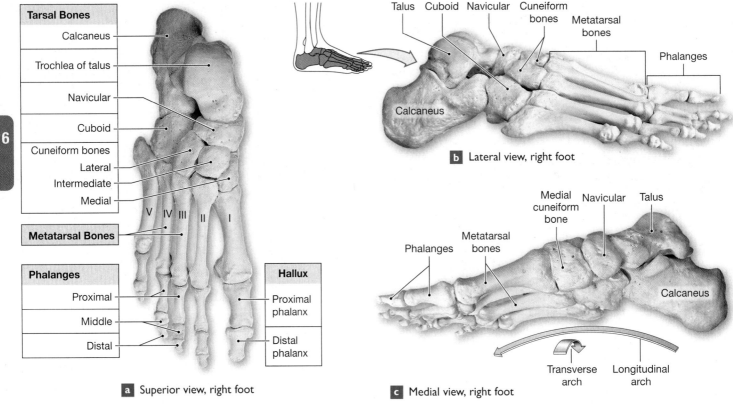

Tarsal Bones
Calcaneus
Trochlea of talus
Navicular
Cuboid
Cuneiform bones
Lateral
Intermediate
Medial

Metatarsal Bones

Phalanges
Proximal
Middle
Distal

Hallux
Proximal phalanx
Distal phalanx

a Superior view, right foot

Talus Cuboid Navicular Cuneiform bones Metatarsal bones Phalanges Calcaneus

b Lateral view, right foot

Medial cuneiform bone Navicular Talus Metatarsal bones Phalanges Calcaneus Transverse arch Longitudinal arch

c Medial view, right foot

---

as when you stand on tiptoes. The rest of the body weight is passed through the cuboid bone and cuneiform bones to the **metatarsal bones**, which support the sole of the foot.

The basic organization of the metatarsals and phalanges of the foot resembles that of the hand. The metatarsals are numbered by Roman numerals I to V from medial to lateral, and their distal ends form the ball of the foot. Like the thumb, the great toe (or **hallux**) has two phalanges. Like the fingers, the other toes have three.

Weight is transferred along the *longitudinal arch* of the foot (**Figure 6-45c**). Ligaments and tendons maintain this arch by tying the calcaneus to the distal portions of the metatarsal bones. However, the lateral portion of this arch has less curvature than the medial portion. Part of the reason is that there is more elasticity in the medial portion. As a result, the medial plantar surface of the foot remains elevated and the muscles, nerves, and blood vessels that supply the inferior surface are not squeezed between the metatarsal bones and the ground. In the condition known as *flatfeet*, normal arches are "lost" or never form.

The *transverse arch* describes the degree of curvature change from the medial to lateral borders of the foot.

CHECKPOINT

31. How would a broken clavicle affect the mobility of the scapula?

32. The rounded projections on either side of the elbow are parts of which bone?

33. Which of the two bones of the forearm is lateral in the anatomical position?

34. Which three bones make up a hip bone?

35. The fibula neither participates in the knee joint nor bears weight. When it is fractured, however, walking becomes difficult. Why?

36. While jumping off the back steps at his house, 10-year-old Cesar lands on his right heel and breaks his foot. Which bone is most likely broken?

See the blue Answers tab at the back of the book.

6-9 Joints are categorized according to their range of motion or anatomical organization

Learning Objective Contrast the major categories of joints, and link their structural features to joint functions.

Joints, or **articulations**, exist wherever two bones meet. The structure of a joint determines the type of movement that may take place. Each joint reflects a compromise between the need for strength and stability and the need for movement. When movement is not required or could be dangerous, joints can be very strong. For example, the sutures of the skull lock the bones together as if they were a single bone. At other joints, movement is more important than strength. For example, the shoulder joint permits a range of arm movement that is limited more by the surrounding muscles than by joint structure. The joint itself is relatively weak, so shoulder injuries are rather common.

Joints can be classified according to their structure or function. The structural classification is based on their anatomy. Joints are described as **fibrous**, **cartilaginous**, or **synovial** (si-NŌ-vē-ul). The first two reflect the type of connective tissue binding them together. Such joints permit either no movement or only slight movements. Synovial joints permit free movement. They are surrounded by fibrous tissue, and the ends of bones are covered by cartilage that prevents bone-to-bone contact.

In a functional classification—one we will emphasize—joints are classified according to *range of motion*, the amount of movement possible. An immovable joint is a **synarthrosis** (sin-ar-THRŌ-sis; *syn-*, together + *arthros*, joint). A slightly movable joint is an **amphiarthrosis** (am-fē-ar-THRŌ-sis;

Build Your Knowledge

Recall that a synovial membrane lines the cavity of a freely movable joint (as you in saw **Chapter 4: The Tissue Level of Organization**). The synovial fluid it secretes lubricates the joint and permits smooth movement ⮌ **p. 111**

amphi-, on both sides). A freely movable joint is a **diarthrosis** (dī-ar-THRŌ-sis; *dia-*, through), or *synovial joint*. **Table 6-1** presents a functional classification, relates it to the structural classification scheme, and provides examples.

Immovable Joints (Synarthroses)

At a synarthrosis, the bony edges are quite close together and may even interlock. A synarthrosis can be fibrous or cartilaginous. Two examples of fibrous immovable joints can be found in the skull. In a **suture** (*sutura,* a sewing together), the bones of the skull are interlocked and bound together by dense connective tissue. In a **gomphosis** (gom-FŌ-sis; *gomphosis,* a bolting together), a ligament binds each tooth in the mouth within a bony socket (*alveolus*).

A rigid, cartilaginous connection is called a **synchondrosis** (sin-kon-DRŌ-sis; *syn,* together + *chondros,* cartilage). The connection between the first pair of ribs and the sternum is a synchondrosis. Another example is the epiphyseal cartilage that connects the diaphysis and epiphysis in a growing long bone. ⮌ p. 147

Table 6-1	A Functional and Structural Classification of Joints			
Functional Category	**Structural Category and Type**		**Description**	**Example**
SYNARTHROSIS (NO MOVEMENT)				
	Fibrous	Suture	Fibrous connections plus interlocked surfaces	Between the bones of the skull
	Fibrous	Gomphosis	Fibrous connections plus insertion in bony socket (alveolus)	Between the teeth and bony sockets in the maxillae and mandible
	Cartilaginous	Synchondrosis	Interposition of cartilage bridge or plate	Between the first pair of ribs and the sternum; epiphyseal cartilages
AMPHIARTHROSIS (LITTLE MOVEMENT)				
	Fibrous	Syndesmosis	Ligamentous connection	Between the tibia and fibula
	Cartilaginous	Symphysis	Connection by a fibrocartilage pad	Between the two pubic bones; between adjacent vertebrae of spinal column
DIARTHROSIS (FREE MOVEMENT)				
	Synovial		Complex joint bounded by joint capsule and containing synovial fluid	Numerous; subdivided by range of motion (**Spotlight Figure 6-50**)

Slightly Movable Joints (Amphiarthroses)

An amphiarthrosis permits very limited movement. The bones are usually farther apart than in a synarthrosis. Structurally, an amphiarthrosis can be fibrous or cartilaginous.

A **syndesmosis** (sin-dez-MŌ-sis; *desmos*, a band or ligament) is a fibrous joint connected by a ligament. The distal articulation between the two bones of the leg, the tibia and fibula, is an example. A **symphysis** is a cartilaginous joint between bones separated by a broad disc or pad of fibrocartilage. The articulations between the spinal vertebrae (at an *intervertebral disc*) and the joint between the two pubic bones are examples of a symphysis.

Freely Movable Joints (Diarthroses)

Diarthroses, or **synovial joints**, permit a wide range of motion (**Figure 6-46a**).

Synovial joints are typically found at the ends of long bones, such as those of the arms and legs. Under normal conditions the bony surfaces are not in contact, for they are covered with special **articular cartilages**. Although they resemble hyaline cartilage, articular cartilages have no

perichondrium and their matrix contains more water than other cartilages. The joint is surrounded by a fibrous **joint capsule**, or *articular capsule*. A synovial membrane lines the joint cavity. **Synovial fluid** in the joint cavity lubricates moving surfaces in the joint and reduces friction.

Some complex joints have additional padding between the opposing surfaces. An example of such shock-absorbing, fibrocartilage pads are the **menisci** (me-NIS-kē; singular *meniscus*, crescent) in the knee (**Figure 6-46b**). Such joints also have **fat pads** which protect the articular cartilages and act as packing material. When the bones move, the fat pads fill in the spaces created as the joint cavity changes shape.

The joint capsule surrounding the entire joint is continuous with the periostea of the articulating bones. In addition, **ligaments** join bone to bone outside or inside the joint capsule. **Bursae** (BUR-sē; singular *bursa,* a pouch) are small packets of connective tissue containing synovial fluid. They form where a tendon or ligament rubs against other tissues. They reduce friction and act as shock absorbers. Bursae are characteristic of many synovial joints. They may also be found surrounding a tendon, covering a bone, or within other connective tissues exposed to friction or pressure.

Figure 6-46 The Structure of a Synovial Joint.

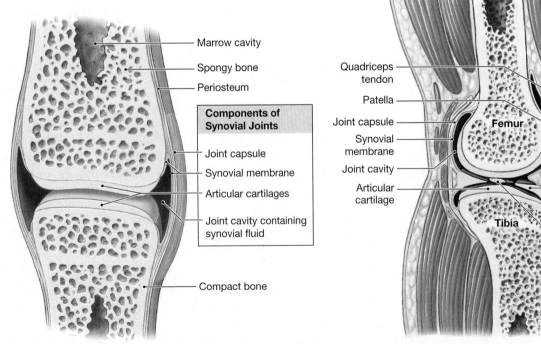

Components of Synovial Joints

- Marrow cavity
- Spongy bone
- Periosteum
- Joint capsule
- Synovial membrane
- Articular cartilages
- Joint cavity containing synovial fluid
- Compact bone

a Synovial joint, sagittal section

- Quadriceps tendon
- Patella
- Joint capsule
- Synovial membrane
- Joint cavity
- Articular cartilage
- Femur
- Tibia

Accessory Structures of a Knee Joint

- Bursa
- Fat pad
- Meniscus

Ligaments

- Extracapsular ligament (patellar)
- Intracapsular ligament (cruciate)

b Knee joint, sagittal section

CLINICAL NOTE

Rheumatism and Arthritis

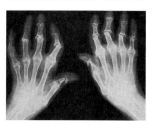

Problems with joints are relatively common, especially in older people. Rheumatism (ROO-muh-tiz-um) is a general term for pain and stiffness in the skeletal or muscular systems, or both. Arthritis (ar-THRĪ-tis) includes all the rheumatic diseases that affect synovial joints. It always involves damage to the articular cartilages. Causes can be bacterial or viral infection, injury to the joint, metabolic problems, or severe physical stresses.

Osteoarthritis (os-tē-ō-ar-THRĪ-tis), or *degenerative arthritis* or *degenerative joint disease*, is the most common form of arthritis. It generally affects individuals of age 60 or older. It can result from wear and tear at the joint surfaces or from genetic factors affecting collagen formation. In the United States, 25 percent of women and 15 percent of men over age 60 show signs of this disease.

Rheumatoid arthritis is an inflammatory condition that affects about 0.5–1 percent of the adult population. At least some cases result when the immune response mistakenly attacks the joint tissues. Allergies, bacteria, viruses, and genetic factors have all been proposed as contributing to or triggering the destructive inflammation.

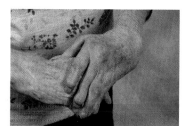

CHECKPOINT

37. Name and describe the three types of joints as classified by their range of motion.

38. In a newborn, the large bones of the skull are joined by fibrous connective tissue but later form immovable joints. Structurally, which type of joints are these?

See the blue Answers tab at the back of the book.

6-10 The structure and functions of synovial joints enable various skeletal movements

Learning Objective Describe how the structure and functions of synovial joints permit the movements of the skeleton.

Synovial joints are involved in all of our day-to-day movements. In everyday speech we use phrases such as "bend the leg" or "raise the arm," but anatomists use more precise language to describe types of movement and types of synovial joints.

Types of Movements at Synovial Joints

Gliding

In **gliding**, two opposing surfaces slide past each other. Gliding occurs between articulating carpal bones and articulating tarsal bones, and between the clavicles and sternum. The movement is slight but can take place in almost any direction. The joint capsule and ligaments usually prevent rotation.

Angular Movement

Angular movements include *flexion, extension, adduction, abduction*, and *circumduction*. The description of each movement refers to an individual in the anatomical position.

Flexion (FLEK-shun) is movement in the anterior-posterior, or sagittal, plane that decreases the angle between articulating bones (**Figure 6-47a**). **Extension** occurs in the same plane, but it increases the angle between articulating bones. Flexion at the shoulder joint or hip joint moves the limbs forward (*anteriorly*). Extension moves them back (*posteriorly*). Flexion of the wrist joint moves the hand forward, and extension moves it back.

Flexion and extension usually describe movements of the long bones, but they are also used for movements of the axial skeleton. For example, when you bring your head toward your chest, you flex the intervertebral joints of the neck. When you bend at the waist to touch your toes, you flex the entire vertebral column. Extension reverses these movements. In these examples, extension can continue past the anatomical position. In these cases, **hyperextension** occurs. When you gaze at the ceiling, you hyperextend the neck. Ligaments, bony processes, or soft tissues prevent hyperextension of other joints.

Abduction (*ab-*, from) is movement *away* from the longitudinal axis of the body in the frontal plane. For example,

Figure 6-47 Angular Movements. The red dots mark the locations of the joints involved in the movements illustrated.

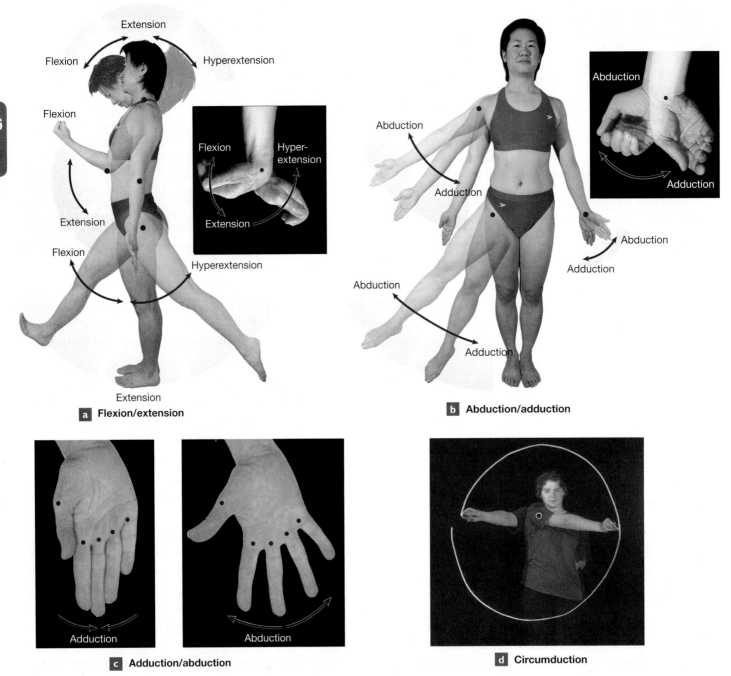

a **Flexion/extension**

b **Abduction/adduction**

c **Adduction/abduction**

d **Circumduction**

swinging the upper limb to the side is abduction of the limb (**Figure 6-47b**). Moving it back to the anatomical position is **adduction** (*ad,* to). Adduction of the wrist moves the heel of the hand toward the body, and abduction moves it farther away. Spreading the fingers or toes apart abducts them, because they move *away* from a central digit (finger or toe), as in **Figure 6-47c**. Bringing fingers or toes together

is adduction. Abduction and adduction always refer to movements of the appendicular skeleton, not to those of the axial skeleton.

Circumduction (*circum,* around) is another type of angular movement. An example is moving your arm in a loop, as when drawing a large circle on a chalkboard (**Figure 6-47d**).

Rotation

Rotation involves turning around the longitudinal axis of the body or a limb (**Figure 6-48**). For example, you may rotate your head to look to one side or rotate your arm to screw in a lightbulb.

The articulations between the radius and ulna permit the rotation of the distal end of the radius across the anterior

Figure 6-48 Rotational Movements.

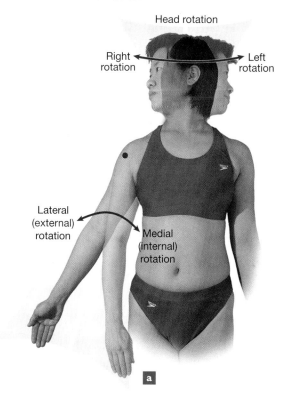

Head rotation

Right rotation — Left rotation

Lateral (external) rotation

Medial (internal) rotation

a

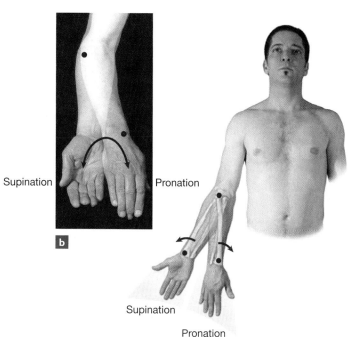

Supination — Pronation

b

Supination

Pronation

surface of the ulna. This rotation moves the wrist and hand from palm-facing-front to palm-facing-back. This motion is called **pronation** (prō-NĀ-shun) (**Figure 6-48b**). The opposing movement, in which the palm is turned forward, is called **supination** (soo-pi-NĀ-shun).

Special Movements

Some specific terms describe unusual or special types of movement (**Figure 6-49**).

- **Inversion** (*in-*, into + *vertere*, to turn) is a twisting motion of the foot that turns the sole inward, elevating the medial edge of the sole. The opposite movement is called **eversion** (ē-VER-zhun; *e-*, out).

- **Dorsiflexion** is flexion at the ankle joint and elevation of the sole, as when you dig in your heel. **Plantar flexion** (*planta*, sole) is extension at the ankle joint and elevation of the heel, as when you stand on tiptoe.

- **Opposition** is the movement of the thumb toward the palm or fingertips. It enables you to grasp and hold an object. **Reposition** returns the thumb from opposition.

- **Protraction** occurs when you move a part of the body anteriorly in the horizontal plane. **Retraction** is the reverse movement. You protract your jaw when you grasp your upper lip with your lower teeth, and you protract your clavicles when you cross your arms.

- **Elevation** and **depression** take place when a structure moves in a superior or inferior direction, respectively. You depress your mandible when you open your mouth and elevate it as you close it.

- **Lateral flexion** occurs when your vertebral column bends to the side.

Types of Synovial Joints

Based on the shapes of the articulating surfaces, anatomists describe synovial joints as *gliding, hinge, condylar, saddle, pivot,* or *ball-and-socket joints.* Each type of joint permits a different type and range of motion. **Spotlight Figure 6-50** lists the categories and the types of movement each joint permits.

CHECKPOINT

39. Give the proper term for each of the following types of motion: (a) moving the humerus away from the longitudinal axis of the body, (b) turning the palms so that they face forward, and (c) bending the elbow.

40. Which movements are associated with hinge joints?

See the blue Answers tab at the back of the book.

Figure 6-49 Special Movements.

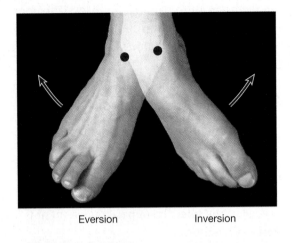

Eversion   Inversion

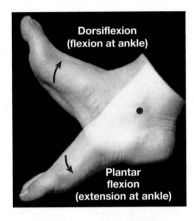

Dorsiflexion (flexion at ankle)

Plantar flexion (extension at ankle)

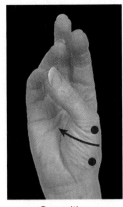

Opposition

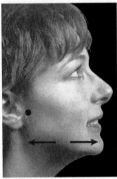
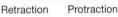

Retraction   Protraction

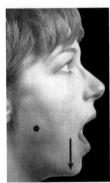

Depression

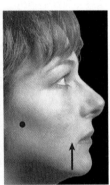

Elevation

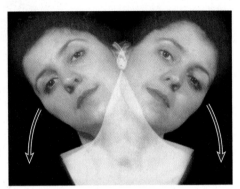

Lateral flexion

6-11 Intervertebral articulations and appendicular articulations demonstrate functional differences in support and mobility

Learning Objective Explain the relationship between joint structure and mobility of representative axial and appendicular articulations.

In this section, we describe examples of joints that demonstrate important functional principles.

Intervertebral Articulations

From the axis to the sacrum, the vertebrae articulate with one another in two ways: (1) at gliding joints (diarthroses) between the *superior* and *inferior articular processes*, and (2) at *symphyseal joints* (amphiarthroses) between the vertebral bodies (**Figure 6-51**). Articulations between the superior and inferior articular processes of adjacent vertebrae permit small movements during flexion and rotation of the vertebral column. Little gliding occurs between adjacent vertebral bodies.

Except for the first cervical vertebra, the vertebrae are separated and cushioned by pads called **intervertebral discs**. Each intervertebral disc has a tough outer layer of fibrocartilage. The collagen fibers of that layer attach the discs to adjacent vertebrae. The fibrocartilage surrounds a soft, elastic, and gelatinous core. The core gives intervertebral discs resiliency and enables them to act as shock absorbers, compressing and distorting when stressed. This resiliency prevents bone-to-bone contact that might damage the vertebrae or jolt the spinal cord and brain.

Shortly after physical maturity, the gelatinous mass within each disc begins to degenerate, and the "cushion" becomes less effective. Over the same period, the outer fibrocartilage loses its elasticity. If the stresses are great enough, the inner mass may break through the surrounding fibrocartilage and protrude beyond the intervertebral space. This condition, called a *herniated disc*, further reduces disc function. The term *slipped disc* is often used to describe this problem, although the disc does not actually slip.

The discs make a significant contribution to an individual's height. They account for about one-quarter of the length of the spinal column above the sacrum. As we grow older,

SPOTLIGHT Figure 6-50
SYNOVIAL JOINTS

Synovial joints are described as gliding, hinge, condylar, saddle, pivot, or ball-and-socket on the basis of the shapes of the articulating surfaces. Each type permits a different range and type of motion.

Gliding joint

Gliding joints have flattened or slightly curved surfaces that slide across one another, but the amount of movement is very slight.

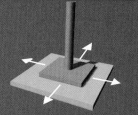

Movement: multidirectional in a single plane

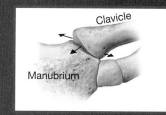

Clavicle

Manubrium

Examples:
- Joints at both ends of the clavicles
- Joints between the carpal bones, the tarsal bones, and the articular facets of adjacent vertebrae
- Joints at the sacrum and hip bones

Hinge joint

Hinge joints permit angular motion in a single plane, like the opening and closing of a door.

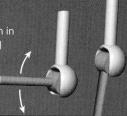

Movement: angular in a single plane

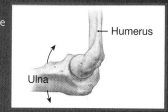

Humerus

Ulna

Examples:
- Joints at the elbow, knee and ankle, and between the phalanges

Condylar joint

Condylar joints, or ellipsoidal joints, have an oval articular face nestled within a depression on the opposing surface.

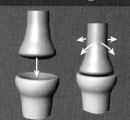

Movement: angular in two planes

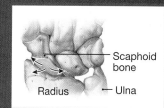

Scaphoid bone

Radius   Ulna

Examples:
- Joint between the radius and the proximal carpal bones
- Joints between the phalanges of the fingers with the metacarpal bones
- Joints between the phalanges of the toes with the metatarsal bones

Saddle joint

Saddle joints have articular faces that fit together like a rider in a saddle. Each face is concave along one axis and convex along the other.

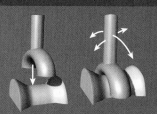

Movement: angular in two planes, and circumduction

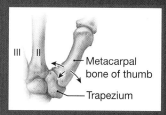

III II

Metacarpal bone of thumb

Trapezium

Examples:
- Carpometacarpal joint at the base of the thumb

Pivot joint

Pivot joints only permit rotation.

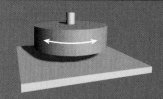

Movement: rotation in a single plane

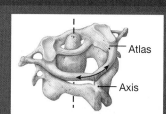

Atlas

Axis

Examples:
- Joint between the atlas and the axis
- Joint between the head of the radius and the proximal shaft of the ulna

Ball-and-socket joint

In a ball-and-socket joint, the round head of one bone rests within a cup-shaped depression in another.

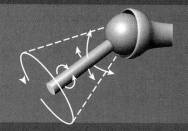

Movement: angular, rotation, and circumduction

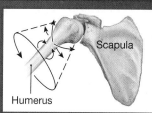

Scapula

Humerus

Examples:
- Joints at the shoulders and hips

201

6

Figure 6-51 Intervertebral Articulations.

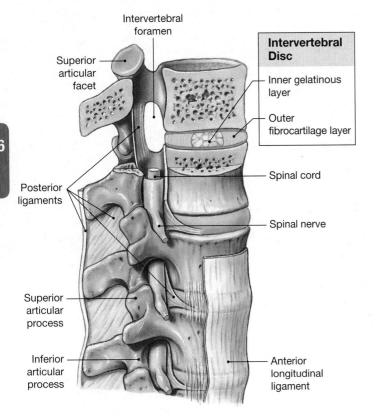

Intervertebral foramen

Superior articular facet

Posterior ligaments

Superior articular process

Inferior articular process

Intervertebral Disc

Inner gelatinous layer

Outer fibrocartilage layer

Spinal cord

Spinal nerve

Anterior longitudinal ligament

Figure 6-52 The Shoulder Joint. The structure of the right shoulder joint is visible in this anterior view of a frontal section.

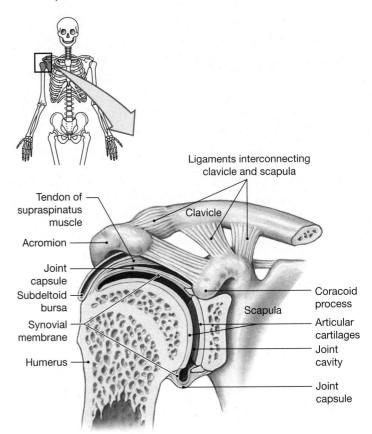

Tendon of supraspinatus muscle

Acromion

Joint capsule

Subdeltoid bursa

Synovial membrane

Humerus

Ligaments interconnecting clavicle and scapula

Clavicle

Coracoid process

Scapula

Articular cartilages

Joint cavity

Joint capsule

the water content of each disc decreases. This loss causes the vertebral column to shorten, accounting for the characteristic decrease in height with advancing age.

Articulations of the Upper Limb

The shoulder, elbow, and wrist work together to position the hand, which performs precise and controlled movements. The shoulder has great mobility, the elbow has great strength, and the wrist makes fine adjustments in the orientation of the palm and fingers.

The Shoulder Joint

The shoulder joint permits the greatest range of motion of any joint in the body. Because it is also the most frequently dislocated joint, it demonstrates the principle that stability must be sacrificed to obtain mobility.

The shoulder joint is a ball-and-socket joint (**Figure 6-52**). The relatively loose joint capsule extends from the scapular neck to the humerus. This oversized capsule permits an extensive range of motion.

Bursae at the shoulder, like those at other joints, reduce friction where large muscles and tendons pass across the joint capsule. The bursae of the shoulder are especially

large and numerous. Several bursae are associated with the capsule, the processes of the scapula, and large shoulder muscles. Inflammation of any of these bursae—a condition called *bursitis*—can restrict motion and produce pain.

CLINICAL NOTE

Dislocations

The disruption or displacement of a joint due to trauma is a *dislocation*. In order for a joint to dislocate, the soft tissue of the joint capsule and ligaments must be stretched beyond the normal range of motion. Oftentimes, the ligaments are torn, which allows the bones of the joint to separate. Because of the associated soft-tissue damage, dislocations can cause paralysis of the affected limb as the nerves and arteries that lead to the extremity pass quite close to the joint and may be compressed or torn.

Dislocations are common in fingers, elbows, shoulders, hips, knees, and toes. Often, in addition to the dislocation, a fracture (broken bone) occurs at the time of injury.

The joints of the spine are at risk for dislocation, especially in high-energy accidents such as auto and motorcycle collisions, skiing injuries, and diving injuries. Spinal dislocations can be catastrophic as the spinal cord can be damaged when the dislocation occurs.

Figure 6-53 The Elbow Joint.
This longitudinal section reveals the anatomy of the right elbow joint.

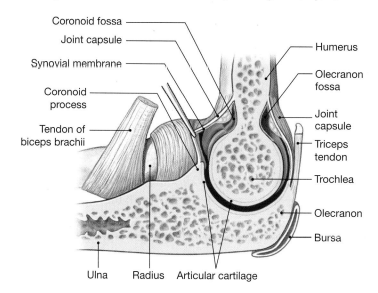

Figure 6-54 The Hip Joint.

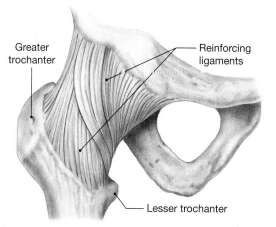

a The hip joint is extremely strong and stable, in part because of the massive joint capsule and surrounding ligaments.

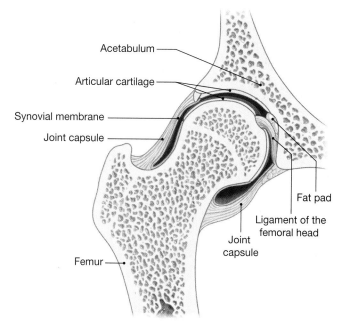

b This sectional view of the right hip shows the structure of the joint and the position of the ligament of the femoral head.

The muscles that move the humerus do more to stabilize the shoulder joint than all its ligaments and capsular fibers combined. Powerful muscles originating on the trunk, shoulder girdle, and humerus cover the anterior, superior, and posterior surfaces of the capsule. These muscles form the *rotator cuff*, a group of muscles that swing the arm through an impressive range of motion.

The Elbow Joint

The elbow joint consists of two articulations: between the humerus and ulna and between the humerus and radius (**Figure 6-53**). The larger and stronger articulation is between the humerus and the ulna. This hinge joint provides stability and limits movement at the elbow joint.

The elbow joint is extremely stable because (1) the bony surfaces of the humerus and ulna interlock, (2) the joint capsule is very thick, and (3) the capsule is reinforced by strong ligaments. Nevertheless, severe impacts or unusual stresses can damage the joint. If you fall on your hand with a partially flexed elbow, contractions of the muscles that extend the elbow may break the ulna at the center of the trochlear notch.

Articulations of the Lower Limb

The joints of the hip, ankle, and foot are sturdier than those at corresponding locations in the upper limb, and they have smaller ranges of motion. The knee has a range of motion comparable to that of the elbow, but the knee is subjected to much greater forces. For this reason, it is less stable.

The Hip Joint

The hip joint is a ball-and-socket diarthrosis (**Figure 6-54**). The articulating surface of the acetabulum has a fibrocartilage pad along its edges, a fat pad covered by synovial membrane in its central portion, and a central, intracapsular ligament. This structural combination resists compression, absorbs shocks, and stretches and distorts without damage.

The joint capsule of the hip joint is denser and stronger than that of the shoulder. It extends from the lateral and inferior surfaces of the pelvic girdle to the femur and encloses both the femoral head and neck. This arrangement helps keep the head from moving away from the acetabulum. Three broad ligaments reinforce the joint capsule, while a fourth, the *ligament of the femoral head* (the *ligamentum teres*), is inside the acetabulum and attaches to the center of the femoral head. Additional stabilization comes from the bulk of the surrounding muscles.

The combination of an almost complete bony socket, a strong joint capsule, supporting ligaments, and muscular padding makes this an extremely stable joint. However, this ball-and-socket joint is not directly aligned with the weight distribution along the shaft. As a result, *hip fractures* (fractures of the femoral neck or between the trochanters) are actually more common than *hip dislocations* (articulating surfaces are forced out of position). Flexion, extension, adduction, abduction, and rotation are permitted, but the total range of motion is considerably less than that of the shoulder. Flexion is the most important normal hip movement, and range of flexion is primarily limited by the surrounding muscles. Other directions of movement are restricted by ligaments and the joint capsule.

The Knee Joint

The hip joint passes weight to the femur, and at the knee joint the femur transfers the weight to the tibia. The knee functions as a hinge joint, but the articulation is far more complex than that of the elbow or even the ankle. The rounded condyles of the femur roll across the top of the tibia, so the points of contact are constantly changing.

Structurally, the knee combines three separate articulations. There are two between the femur and tibia (medial condyle to medial condyle, and lateral condyle to lateral condyle), and one between the patella and the femur. There is no single unified joint capsule, nor is there a common synovial cavity. A pair of fibrocartilage pads, the **medial** and **lateral menisci**, lies between the femoral and tibial surfaces (**Figure 6-55b**). The pads act as cushions and conform to the shape of the articulating surfaces as the femur changes position. Fat pads provide padding around the margins of the joint and assist the bursae in reducing friction between the patella and other tissues.

Ligaments stabilize the anterior, posterior, medial, and lateral surfaces of this joint. A complete dislocation of the knee is an extremely rare event. The tendon from the muscles responsible for extending the knee passes over the anterior surface of the joint. The patella lies within this tendon, and the **patellar ligament** continues its attachment on the anterior surface of the tibia (**Figure 6-55**). This ligament provides support to the front of the knee joint. Posterior ligaments

Figure 6-55 The Knee Joint.

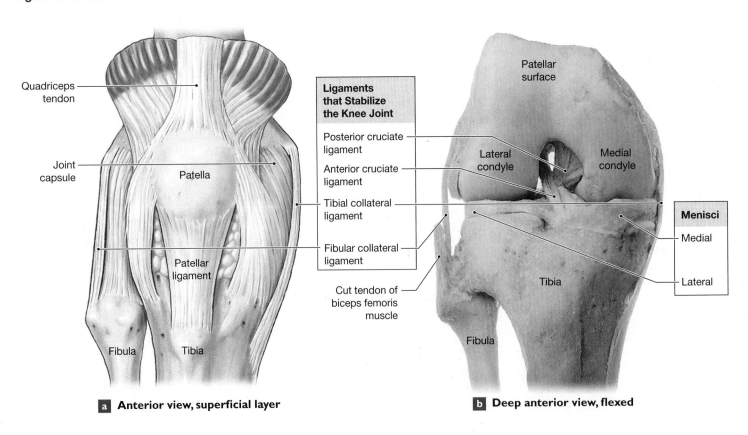

Ligaments that Stabilize the Knee Joint

- Posterior cruciate ligament
- Anterior cruciate ligament
- Tibial collateral ligament
- Fibular collateral ligament

Quadriceps tendon

Joint capsule

Patella

Patellar ligament

Fibula

Tibia

Cut tendon of biceps femoris muscle

Patellar surface

Lateral condyle

Medial condyle

Menisci
- Medial
- Lateral

Tibia

Fibula

a Anterior view, superficial layer

b Deep anterior view, flexed

between the femur and the heads of the tibia and fibula reinforce the back of the knee joint. The *fibular collateral ligament*, also called the *lateral collateral ligament*, reinforces the lateral surface of the knee joint. The *tibial collateral ligament*, also called the *medial collateral ligament (MCL)*, reinforces the medial surface of the knee joint. Together, they stabilize the joint at full extension.

Additional ligaments are found inside the joint capsule (**Figure 6-55b**). Inside the joint, the *anterior cruciate ligament (ACL)* and *posterior cruciate ligament* cross each other as they attach the tibia to the femur. (The term *cruciate* is derived from the Latin word *crucialis*, meaning a cross.) These ligaments limit the anterior and posterior movement of the femur. Rupture of the ACL is a common sports injury. It affects women two to five times more often than men. ACL injuries are frequently caused by twisting an extended weight-bearing knee. This movement is common in football, basketball, and skiing. A strong hit or force to the lateral surface of the knee, as in a football tackle or a flying hockey puck, may damage both the ACL and the MCL.

CHECKPOINT

41. Would a tennis player or a jogger be more likely to develop inflammation of the subdeltoid bursa? Why?

42. Daphne falls on her hands with her elbows slightly flexed. After the fall, she can't move her left arm at the elbow. If a fracture exists, which bone is most likely broken?

43. Why is a complete dislocation of the knee joint an infrequent event?

See the blue Answers tab at the back of the book.

6-12 The Skeletal System Supports and Stores Energy and Minerals for Other Body Systems

Learning Objective Describe the interactions between the skeletal system and other body systems.

Bones may seem inert, but by now you know they are quite dynamic. They undergo continuous remodeling. The balance between bone formation and bone recycling involves interactions between the skeletal system and other organ systems. Bones provide attachment sites for muscles. Bones are extensively interconnected with the cardiovascular and lymphatic systems. They are largely under the physiological control of the endocrine system. The digestive and urinary systems provide calcium and phosphate minerals for bone growth.

CHECKPOINT

44. Describe the functional relationship between the skeletal system and the integumentary system.

See the blue Answers tab at the back of the book.

Build Your Knowledge

How the SKELETAL SYSTEM integrates with the other body systems presented so far on **p. 185** reviews the major functional relationships between the skeletal and integumentary systems.

RELATED CLINICAL TERMS

ankylosis (ang-ki-LŌ-sis): An abnormal fusion between articulating bones in response to trauma and friction within a joint.

arthroscopy: Insertion of a narrow tube containing optical fibers and a tiny camera (arthroscope) directly into the joint for visual examination.

gigantism: A condition of extreme height resulting from an overproduction of growth hormone before puberty.

luxation (luks-Ā-shun): A dislocation; a condition in which the articulating surfaces are forced out of position.

orthopedics (or-tho-PĒ-diks): A branch of surgery concerned with disorders of the bones and joints and their associated muscles, tendons, and ligaments.

osteomyelitis (os-tē-ō-mī-e-LĪ-tis): A painful infection in a bone, generally caused by bacteria.

spina bifida (SPĪ-nuh BI-fi-duh): A birth defect resulting from the failure of the vertebral laminae to unite during development; commonly associated with developmental abnormalities of the brain and spinal cord.

sprain: A condition in which a ligament is stretched to the point at which some of the collagen fibers are torn. The ligament remains functional, and the structure of the joint is not affected.

whiplash: An injury resulting when a sudden change in body position injures the cervical vertebrae.

Build Your Knowledge:
How the SKELETAL SYSTEM integrates with the other body systems presented so far

6

Integumentary System

- The Integumentary System removes excess body heat, synthesizes vitamin D_3 for calcium and phosphate ion absorption, and protects underlying bones and joints

- The skeletal system provides structural support for the skin

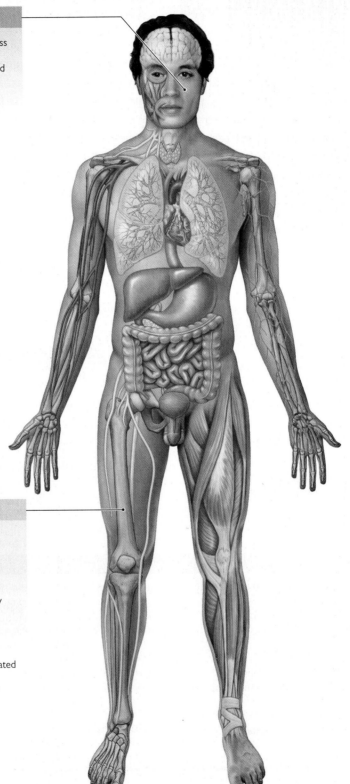

Skeletal System

The skeletal system performs five primary functions for the human body. It
- provides structural support for the body
- stores calcium, phosphate, and other minerals necessary for many functions in other organ systems, and lipids as energy reserves
- produces blood cells and other blood elements in red bone marrow
- protects many soft tissues and organs
- provides leverage for movements generated by skeletal muscles

6 Chapter Review

Summary Outline

An Introduction to the Skeletal System *p. 157*

1. The components of the skeletal system have a variety of purposes, such as providing a framework for body posture and allowing for precise movements.

6-1 The Skeletal System Has Five Primary Functions *p. 157*

2. The skeletal system includes the bones of the skeleton and the cartilages, ligaments, and other connective tissues that stabilize or interconnect bones. Its functions include structural support, storage of minerals and lipids, blood cell production, protection, and leverage.

6-2 Bones Are Classified According to Shape and Structure *p. 157*

3. **Bone**, or **osseous tissue**, is a supporting connective tissue with a solid *matrix*.

4. General categories of bones are **long bones, short bones, flat bones**, and **irregular bones** *(Figure 6-1)*.

5. The features of a long bone include a **diaphysis**, two **epiphyses**, and a central *marrow cavity (Figure 6-2)*.

6. The two types of bone tissue are **compact bone** and **spongy** *(trabecular)* **bone**.

7. A bone is covered by a **periosteum** and lined with an **endosteum**.

8. Both types of bone tissue contain **osteocytes** in **lacunae**. Layers of calcified matrix are **lamellae**, interconnected by **canaliculi** *(Figure 6-8a,b)*.

9. The basic functional unit of compact bone is the **osteon**, containing osteocytes arranged around a **central canal**.

10. Spongy bone contains **trabeculae**, often in an open network.

11. Compact bone is located where stresses come from a limited range of directions. Spongy bone is located where stresses are few or come from many different directions.

12. Cells other than osteocytes are also present in bone. **Osteoblasts** synthesize the matrix in the process of *ossification*. **Osteoclasts** dissolve the bony matrix through the process of *osteolysis* or *resorption (Figure 6-8c)*.

6-3 Ossification and Appositional Growth Are Processes of Bone Formation and Enlargement *p. 162*

13. **Ossification** is the process of converting other tissues to bone.

14. **Intramembranous ossification** begins when stem cells in connective tissue differentiate into osteoblasts and produce spongy or compact bone *(Figure 6-10)*.

15. **Endochondral ossification** begins with the formation of a cartilage model of a bone that is gradually replaced by bone. In this process, bone length also increases *(Figure 6-9)*.

16. Bone diameter increases through **appositional growth** *(Figure 6-11)*.

17. The timing of epiphyseal closure differs among bones and among individuals.

18. Normal ossification requires a reliable source of minerals, vitamins, and hormones.

6-4 Bone Growth and Development Depend on a Balance between Bone Formation and Resorption, and on Calcium Availability *p. 165*

19. The organic and mineral components of bone are continuously recycled and renewed through the process of **remodeling**.

20. The shapes and thicknesses of bones reflect the stresses applied to them. Mineral turnover enables bone to adapt to new stresses.

21. Calcium is the most abundant mineral in the human body, with roughly 99 percent of it located in the skeleton. The skeleton acts as a calcium reserve.

22. A **fracture** is a crack or break in a bone. **Closed** fractures are internal. **Open** fractures project through the skin. Repair of a fracture involves the formation of a **fracture hematoma**, an **external callus**, and an **internal callus** *(Clinical Note: Types of Fractures and Steps in Repair)*.

6-5 Osteopenia Has a Widespread Effect on Aging Skeletal Tissue *p. 165*

23. The effects of aging on the skeleton can include **osteopenia** and **osteoporosis**.

6-6 The Bones of the Skeleton Are Distinguished by Bone Markings and Grouped into Two Skeletal Divisions *p. 173*

24. A **bone marking** (surface feature) is an area on the surface of a bone with a specific function. Bone markings can be used to describe and identify specific bones *(Figure 6-22)*.

25. The **axial skeleton** can be subdivided into the **skull** and associated bones (including the **auditory ossicles**, or ear bones, and the **hyoid**); the **thoracic cage**, composed of the **ribs** and **sternum** *(rib cage)* and thoracic vertebrae; and the **vertebral column** *(Figures 6-23 and 6-24)*.

26. The **appendicular skeleton** includes the bones of the upper and lower limbs and the **pectoral** and **pelvic girdles**.

6

6-7 The Bones of the Skull, Vertebral Column, and Thoracic Cage Make Up the Axial Skeleton *p. 173*

27. The **cranium** encloses the **cranial cavity**, which encloses the brain.

28. The **frontal bone** forms the forehead and superior surface of each **orbit** *(Figures 6-25 to 6-27)*.

29. The **parietal bones** form the upper sides and roof of the cranium *(Figures 6-25 and 6-26)*.

30. The **occipital bone** surrounds the **foramen magnum** and articulates with the sphenoid, temporal, and parietal bones to form the back of the cranium *(Figures 6-25 to 6-27)*.

31. The **temporal bones** help form the sides and base of the cranium and fuse with the parietal bones along the **squamous suture** *(Figures 6-25 to 6-27)*.

32. The **sphenoid bone** acts like a bridge that unites the cranial and facial bones *(Figures 6-25 to 6-27)*.

33. The **ethmoid bone** stabilizes the brain and forms the roof and sides of the nasal cavity. Its **cribriform plate** contains perforations for olfactory nerves, and the **perpendicular plate** forms part of the bony *nasal septum (Figures 6-25 to 6-27)*.

34. The left and right **maxillae**, or *maxillary bones*, articulate with all the other facial bones except the *mandible (Figures 6-25 to 6-27)*.

35. The **palatine bones** form the posterior portions of the hard palate and contribute to the walls of the nasal cavity and to the floor of each orbit *(Figures 6-25 to 6-27)*.

36. The **vomer** forms the inferior portion of the bony nasal septum *(Figures 6-25 to 6-27)*.

37. The **zygomatic bones** help complete the orbit and together with the temporal bones form the **zygomatic arch** *(cheekbone) (Figures 6-25 to 6-27)*.

38. The **nasal bones** articulate with the frontal bone and the maxillary bones *(Figures 6-25 to 6-27)*.

39. The **lacrimal bones** are within the orbit on its medial surface *(Figures 6-25 to 6-27)*.

40. The **inferior nasal conchae** inside the nasal cavity aid the **superior** and **middle nasal conchae** of the ethmoid bone in slowing incoming air *(Figures 6-25 to 6-27)*.

41. The **nasal complex** includes the bones that form the superior and lateral walls of the nasal cavity and the sinuses that drain into them. The **nasal septum** divides the nasal cavities. Together, the **frontal, sphenoidal, ethmoidal, palatine,** and **maxillary sinuses** make up the **paranasal sinuses** *(Figures 6-26 to 6-28)*.

42. The **mandible** is the bone of the lower jaw *(Figures 6-25 to 6-27)*.

43. The **hyoid bone** is suspended below the skull by ligaments from the styloid processes of the temporal bones *(Figure 6-29)*.

44. Fibrous tissue connections called **fontanelles** permit the skulls of infants and children to continue growing *(Figure 6-30)*.

45. The **vertebral column** consists of the vertebrae, sacrum, and coccyx. We have 7 **cervical vertebrae**, 12 **thoracic vertebrae**, and 5 **lumbar vertebrae**. The **sacrum** and **coccyx** consist of fused vertebrae *(Figure 6-31)*.

46. The spinal column has four **spinal curves,** which accommodate the unequal distribution of body weight and keep it in line with the body axis *(Figure 6-31)*.

47. A typical vertebra has a **body** and a **vertebral arch**; it articulates with other vertebrae at the **articular processes**. Adjacent vertebrae are separated by an **intervertebral disc** *(Figure 6-32)*.

48. Cervical vertebrae are distinguished by the oval body and **transverse foramina** on either side *(Figures 6-32 and 6-33)*.

49. Thoracic vertebrae have distinctive heart-shaped bodies and articulate with the ribs *(Figure 6-32)*.

50. The lumbar vertebrae are the most massive, least mobile, and are subjected to the greatest strains *(Figure 6-32)*.

51. The sacrum protects reproductive, digestive, and excretory organs. At its **apex**, the sacrum articulates with the coccyx. At its **base**, the sacrum articulates with the last lumbar vertebra *(Figure 6-34)*.

52. The skeleton of the chest, or **thoracic cage**, consists of the thoracic vertebrae, the ribs, and the sternum. The **ribs** and **sternum** form the *rib cage (Figure 6-35)*.

53. Ribs 1 to 7 are **true ribs**. Ribs 8 to 12 lack direct connections to the sternum and are called **false ribs**; they include two pairs of **floating ribs**. The medial end of each rib articulates with a thoracic vertebra *(Figure 6-35)*.

54. The sternum consists of a **manubrium**, a **body**, and a **xiphoid process** *(Figure 6-35)*.

6-8 The Pectoral Girdles and Upper Limb Bones, and the Pelvic Girdle and Lower Limb Bones, Make Up the Appendicular Skeleton *p. 187*

55. Each arm articulates with the trunk at a **pectoral girdle**, or *shoulder girdle*, which consists of a **scapula** and a **clavicle** *(Figures 6-8, 6-9, 6-35, 6-36)*.

56. The clavicle and scapula position the shoulder joint, help move the arm, and provide a base for arm movement and muscle attachment *(Figures 6-35 and 6-36)*.

57. Both the **coracoid process** and the **acromion** are attached to ligaments and tendons. The **scapular spine** crosses the posterior surface of the scapular body *(Figure 6-36)*.

58. The **humerus** articulates with the scapula at the shoulder joint. The **greater tubercle** and **lesser tubercle** of the humerus are important sites for muscle attachment. Other prominent landmarks include the **deltoid tuberosity**, the **medial** and **lateral epicondyles**, and the articular **condyle** *(Figure 6-37)*.

59. Distally, the humerus articulates with the radius and ulna. The medial **trochlea** extends from the **coronoid fossa** to the **olecranon fossa** *(Figure 6-37)*.

60. The **radius** and **ulna** are the bones of the forearm. The olecranon fossa accommodates the **olecranon process** during extension of the arm. The coronoid and radial fossae accommodate the **coronoid process** of the ulna (*Figure 6-38*).

61. The bones of the wrist form two rows of **carpal bones**. The distal carpal bones articulate with the **metacarpal bones** of the palm. The metacarpal bones articulate with the proximal **phalanges**, or finger bones. Four of the fingers contain three phalanges; the **pollex**, or thumb, has only two (*Figure 6-40*).

62. The **pelvic girdle** consists of two **hip bones**, or **coxal bones** (*Figures 6-8, 6-9 and 6-41*).

63. The largest part of the hip bone, the **ilium**, fuses with the **ischium**, which in turn fuses with the **pubis**. The **pubic symphysis** limits movement between the pubic bones of the left and right hip bones (*Figure 6-41*).

64. The **pelvis** consists of the hip bones, the sacrum, and the coccyx (*Figures 6-41 and 6-42*).

65. The **femur**, or *thigh bone*, is the longest bone in the body. It articulates with the **tibia** at the knee joint. The patellar ligament from the **patella** (the *kneecap*) attaches at the **tibial tuberosity** (*Figures 6-43 and 6-44*).

66. Other tibial landmarks include the **anterior margin** and the **medial malleolus**. The **head** of the **fibula** articulates with the tibia below the knee, and the **lateral malleolus** stabilizes the ankle (*Figure 6-44*).

67. The ankle includes seven **tarsal bones**; only the **talus** articulates with the tibia and fibula. When we stand normally, most of our weight is transferred to the **calcaneus**, or *heel bone*, and the rest is passed on to the **metatarsal bones** (*Figure 6-45*).

68. The basic organizational pattern of the metatarsals and phalanges of the foot resembles that of the hand.

6-9 Joints Are Categorized According to Their Range of Motion or Anatomical Organization *p. 195*

69. **Articulations** (joints) exist wherever two bones interact. Immovable joints are **synarthroses**, slightly movable joints are **amphiarthroses**, and those that are freely movable are called **diarthroses** (*Table 6-1*).

70. Examples of synarthroses are a **suture**, a **gomphosis**, and a **synchondrosis**.

71. Examples of amphiarthroses are a **syndesmosis** and a **symphysis**.

72. The bony surfaces at diarthroses, or **synovial joints**, are covered by **articular cartilages**, lubricated by **synovial fluid**, and enclosed within a **joint capsule**. Other synovial structures include **menisci, fat pads, bursae**, and various **ligaments** (*Figure 6-45*).

6-10 The Structure and Functions of Synovial Joints Enable Various Skeletal Movements *p. 197*

73. Important terms that describe movements at synovial joints are **flexion, extension, hyperextension, abduction, adduction, circumduction**, and **rotation** (*Figures 6-46 and 6-47*).

74. The bones in the forearm permit **pronation** and **supination** (*Figure 6-47*).

75. Movements of the foot include **inversion** and **eversion**. The ankle undergoes flexion and extension, also known as **dorsiflexion** and **plantar flexion**, respectively. **Opposition** is the thumb movement that enables us to grasp and hold objects. **Reposition** is the opposite of opposition (*Figure 6-48*).

76. **Protraction** involves moving a part of the body forward; **retraction** involves moving it back. **Depression** and **elevation** occur when we move a structure inferiorly and superiorly, respectively (*Figure 6-48*).

77. Major types of synovial joints include gliding joints, hinge joints, pivot joints, condylar joints, saddle joints, and ball-and-socket joints (*Spotlight Figure 6-50*).

6-11 Intervertebral Articulations and Appendicular Articulations Demonstrate Functional Differences in Support and Mobility *p. 200*

78. The articular processes of adjacent vertebrae form gliding joints. *Symphyseal joints* connect adjacent vertebral bodies and are separated by pads called **intervertebral discs** (*Figure 6-50*).

79. The shoulder joint is formed by the **glenoid cavity** and the head of the humerus. This ball-and-socket joint is extremely mobile and, for that reason, it is also unstable and easily dislocated (*Figure 6-50*).

80. Bursae at the shoulder joint reduce friction from muscles and tendons during movement (*Figure 6-50*).

81. The elbow joint permits only flexion and extension. It is extremely stable because of extensive ligaments and the shapes of the articulating bones (*Figure 6-51*).

82. The hip joint is formed by the union of the **acetabulum** with the head of the femur. This ball-and-socket joint permits flexion and extension, adduction and abduction, circumduction, and rotation (*Figure 6-52*).

83. The knee joint is a complicated hinge joint. The joint permits flexion–extension and limited rotation (*Figure 6-53*).

6-12 The Skeletal System Supports and Stores Energy and Minerals for Other Body Systems *p. 205*

84. Growth and maintenance of the skeletal system is supported by the integumentary system. The skeletal system also interacts with the muscular, cardiovascular, lymphatic, digestive, urinary, and endocrine systems.

Review Questions

See the blue Answers tab at the back of the book.

Level 1 Reviewing Facts and Terms

Match each item in column A with the most closely related item in column B. Place letters for answers in the spaces provided.

6–2 COLUMN A

_____ 1. Osteocytes
_____ 2. Diaphysis
_____ 3. Auditory ossicles
_____ 4. Cribriform plate
_____ 5. Osteoblasts
_____ 6. C_1
_____ 7. C_2
_____ 8. Hip and shoulder
_____ 9. Patella
_____ 10. Calcaneus
_____ 11. Synarthrosis
_____ 12. Moving the hand into a palm-front position
_____ 13. Osteoclasts
_____ 14. Raising the arm laterally
_____ 15. Elbow and knee

COLUMN B

a. Abduction
b. Heel bone
c. Ball-and-socket joints
d. Bone-resorbing cells
e. Hinge joints
f. Axis
g. Immovable joint
h. Bone shaft
i. Mature bone cells
j. Bone-producing cells
k. Atlas
l. Olfactory nerves
m. Ear bones
n. Supination
o. Kneecap

16. Skeletal bones store lipids as energy reserves in areas of
    (a) red marrow.
    (b) yellow marrow.
    (c) the matrix of bone tissue.
    (d) the ground substance.

17. The two types of osseous tissue are
    (a) compact bone and spongy bone.
    (b) dense bone and compact bone.
    (c) spongy bone and cancellous bone.
    (d) a, b, and c are correct

18. The basic functional units of mature compact bone are
    (a) lacunae.   (b) osteocytes.
    (c) osteons.   (d) canaliculi.

19. The axial skeleton consists of the bones of the
    (a) pectoral and pelvic girdles.
    (b) skull, thorax, and vertebral column.
    (c) arm, legs, hand, and feet.
    (d) limbs, pectoral girdle, and pelvic girdle.

20. The appendicular skeleton consists of the bones of the
    (a) pectoral and pelvic girdles.
    (b) skull, thorax, and vertebral column.
    (c) arm, legs, hand, and feet.
    (d) limbs, pectoral girdles, and pelvic girdle.

21. Identify the cranial and facial bones in the diagrams below.

Cranial bones   **Facial bones**

(a) _____   (b) _____
(c) _____   (d) _____
(e) _____   (f) _____
(g) _____   (h) _____
(i) _____   (j) _____
(k) _____   (l) _____

22. Which of the following lists contains only bones of the cranium?
    (a) Frontal, parietal, occipital, sphenoid
    (b) Frontal, occipital, zygomatic, parietal
    (c) Occipital, sphenoid, temporal, palatine
    (d) Mandible, maxilla, nasal, zygomatic

23. Of the following bones, which one is unpaired?
    (a) Vomer   (b) Maxilla
    (c) Palatine   (d) Nasal

24. At the glenoid cavity, the scapula articulates with the proximal end of the
    (a) humerus.   (b) radius.
    (c) ulna.   (d) femur.

25. While an individual is in the anatomical position, the ulna lies
    (a) medial to the radius.   (b) lateral to the radius.
    (c) inferior to the radius.   (d) superior to the radius.

26. Each hip bone of the pelvic girdle consists of three fused bones: the
    (a) ulna, radius, humerus.
    (b) ilium, ischium, pubis.
    (c) femur, tibia, fibula.
    (d) hamate, capitate, trapezium.

27. Joints that are typically located at the end of long bones are
    (a) synarthroses.   (b) amphiarthroses.
    (c) diarthroses.   (d) sutures.

28. Label the structures in the following illustration of a synovial joint.

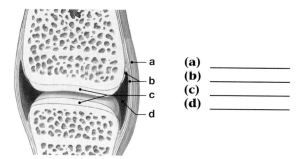

(a) _____
(b) _____
(c) _____
(d) _____

29. The function of synovial fluid is
(a) to nourish chondrocytes.
(b) to provide lubrication.
(c) to absorb shock.
(d) a, b, and c are correct.

30. Abduction and adduction always refer to movements of the
(a) axial skeleton. **(b)** appendicular skeleton.
(c) skull. **(d)** vertebral column.

31. Standing on tiptoe is an example of a movement called
(a) elevation. **(b)** dorsiflexion.
(c) plantar flexion. **(d)** retraction.

32. What is the primary difference between intramembranous ossification and endochondral ossification?

33. What unique characteristic of the hyoid bone makes it different from all the other bones in the body?

34. What two primary functions are performed by the thoracic cage?

35. Which two large scapular processes are associated with the shoulder joint?

Level 2 Reviewing Concepts

36. Why are stresses or impacts to the side of the shaft of a long bone more dangerous than stress applied along the long axis of the shaft?

37. During the growth of a long bone, how is the epiphysis forced farther from the shaft?

38. Why are ruptured intervertebral discs more common in lumbar vertebrae, and dislocations and fractures more common in cervical vertebrae?

39. Why are clavicular injuries common?

40. What is the difference in skeletal structure between the pelvic girdle and the pelvis?

41. How do articular cartilages differ from other cartilages in the body?

42. What is the significance of the fact that the pubic symphysis is a slightly movable joint?

Level 3 Critical Thinking and Clinical Applications

43. While playing on her swing set, 10-year-old Yasmin falls and breaks her right leg. At the emergency room, the physician tells Yasmin's parents that the proximal end of the tibia, where the epiphysis meets the diaphysis, is fractured. The fracture is properly set and eventually heals. During a routine physical when she is 18, Yasmin learns that her right leg is 2 cm shorter than her left, probably because of her accident. What might account for this difference?

44. Tess is diagnosed with a disease that affects the membranes surrounding the brain. The physician tells Tess's family that the disease is caused by an airborne virus. Explain how this virus could have entered the cranium.

45. While working at an excavation, an archaeologist finds several small skull bones. She examines the frontal, parietal, and occipital bones and concludes that the skulls are those of children not yet 1 year old. How can she tell their ages from examining these bones?

46. Firefighter Frank is fighting a fire in a building when part of the ceiling collapses and a beam strikes him on his left shoulder. He is rescued by his friends, but he has a great deal of pain in his shoulder and cannot move his arm properly, especially anteriorly. His clavicle is not broken, and his humerus is intact. What is the probable nature of Frank's injury?

47. Ed "turns over" his ankle while playing tennis. He experiences swelling and pain, but after examination he is told that there are no torn ligaments and that the structure of the ankle is not affected. On the basis of the signs and symptoms and the examination results, what do you think happened to Ed's ankle?

The Muscular System

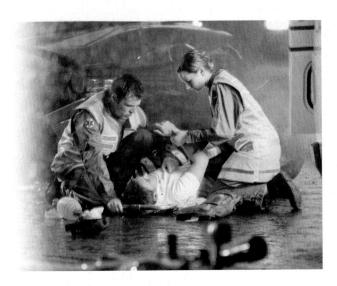

Learning Objectives

These Learning Objectives tell you what you should be able to do after completing the chapter. They correspond by number to this chapter's sections.

7-1 Specify the functions of skeletal muscle tissue.

7-2 Describe the organization of muscle at the tissue level.

7-3 Identify the structural components of a sarcomere.

7-4 Explain the key steps in the contraction of a skeletal muscle fiber beginning at the neuromuscular junction.

7-5 Compare the different types of muscle contractions.

7-6 Describe the processes by which muscles obtain the energy to power contractions.

7-7 Relate the types of muscle fibers to muscle performance, and distinguish between aerobic and anaerobic endurance.

7-8 Contrast the structures and functions of skeletal, cardiac, and smooth muscle tissues.

7-9 Explain how the name of a muscle can help identify its location, appearance, or function.

7-10 Identify the main axial muscles of the body and their origins, insertions, and actions.

7-11 Identify the main appendicular muscles of the body and their origins, insertions, and actions.

7-12 Describe the effects of aging on muscle tissue.

7-13 Discuss the interactions between the muscular system and other body systems when the body is at rest, and explain the homeostatic responses to exercise by the muscular system and various other body systems.

An Introduction to Muscle Tissue

Muscle tissue is one of the four primary tissue types. It consists of elongated muscle cells that are highly specialized for contraction. We introduced the three types of muscle tissue—*skeletal muscle, cardiac muscle,* and *smooth muscle*—in Chapter 4. ↻ p. 111 Without these muscle tissues, nothing in the body would move, and the body itself could not move. We would not be able to sit, stand, walk, speak, or grasp objects. Our blood would not circulate, because we would have no heartbeat to propel it through the vessels. Our lungs could not empty and fill, nor could food move through the digestive tract.

We begin this chapter by discussing skeletal muscle tissue, the most abundant muscle tissue in the body. We then give an overview of the differences among skeletal, cardiac, and smooth muscle tissue. Finally, we describe the gross anatomy of the muscular system and look at the working relationships between the muscles and bones of the body.

Build Your Knowledge

Recall that skeletal muscle tissue is described as striated voluntary muscle tissue (as you saw in **Chapter 4: The Tissue Level of Organization**). This description is based on the presence of regularly repeating groups of actin and myosin filaments within skeletal muscle cells. It also refers to the fact that the nervous system provides voluntary control over this tissue. ↻ **p. 113**

7-1 Skeletal muscle performs five primary functions

Learning Objective Specify the functions of skeletal muscle tissue.

Skeletal muscles are organs composed primarily of skeletal muscle tissue, but they also contain connective tissues, nerves, and blood vessels. These muscles are directly or indirectly attached to the bones of the skeleton. The muscular system includes approximately 700 skeletal muscles that perform the following functions:

1. ***Move the skeleton.*** When skeletal muscles contract, they pull on tendons and thereby move the bones. These contractions may produce a simple motion, such as extending the arm, or the highly coordinated movements of swimming, skiing, or typing.

2. ***Maintain posture and body position.*** Continuous muscle contractions maintain body posture. Without this constant action, you could not sit upright without collapsing, or stand without toppling over.

3. ***Support soft tissues.*** The abdominal wall and the floor of the pelvic cavity consist of layers of skeletal muscle. These muscles support the weight of our visceral organs and shield our internal tissues from injury.

4. ***Guard entrances and exits.*** Skeletal muscles encircle openings of the digestive and urinary tracts. These muscles give us voluntary control over swallowing, defecating, and urinating.

5. ***Maintain body temperature.*** Muscle contractions use energy, and whenever energy is used in the body, some of it is converted to heat. The heat from working muscles keeps body temperature in the range required for normal functioning.

To understand how skeletal muscle contracts, we must study the structure of skeletal muscle. We begin with the organ-level structure of skeletal muscle and then describe its cellular-level structure. In the following discussions, you will often see the Greek words *sarkos* (flesh) and *mys* (muscle) as word roots in the names of the structural features of muscles and their components.

CHECKPOINT

1. What are the five primary functions of skeletal muscle?

See the blue Answers tab at the back of the book.

7-2 A skeletal muscle contains muscle tissue, connective tissues, blood vessels, and nerves

Learning Objective Describe the organization of muscle at the tissue level.

Figure 7-1 illustrates the organization of a typical skeletal muscle. A skeletal muscle contains skeletal muscle tissue as well as connective tissues, blood vessels, and nerves. Each cell in skeletal muscle tissue is a single muscle *fiber*.

Figure 7-1 The Organization of Skeletal Muscles.

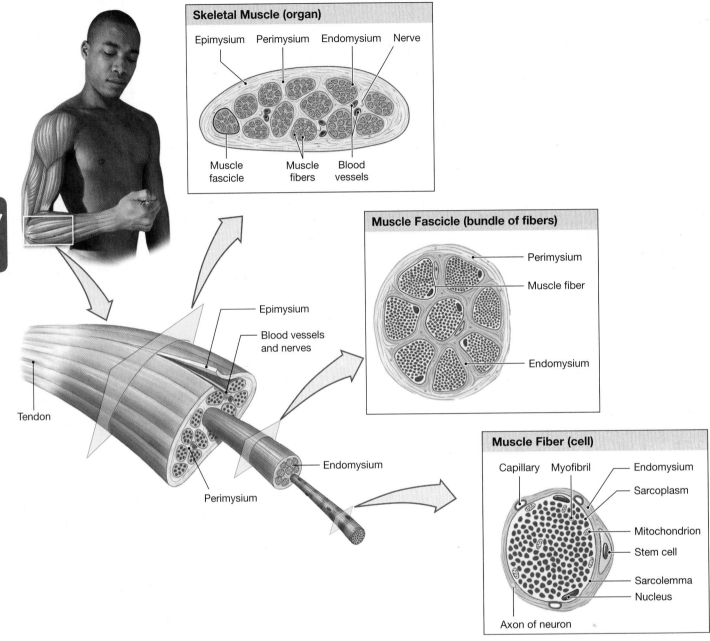

Skeletal Muscle (organ)

Epimysium   Perimysium   Endomysium   Nerve

Muscle fascicle   Muscle fibers   Blood vessels

Muscle Fascicle (bundle of fibers)

Perimysium

Muscle fiber

Endomysium

Epimysium

Blood vessels and nerves

Tendon

Endomysium

Perimysium

Muscle Fiber (cell)

Capillary   Myofibril   Endomysium

Sarcoplasm

Mitochondrion

Stem cell

Sarcolemma

Nucleus

Axon of neuron

Connective Tissue Organization

Three layers of connective tissue are part of each muscle: the epimysium, the perimysium, and the endomysium (**Figure 7-1**).

The **epimysium** (ep-i-MIZ-ē-um; *epi-*, on + *mys*, muscle) is a layer of collagen fibers that surrounds the entire muscle. It separates the muscle from surrounding tissues and organs.

The connective tissue fibers of the **perimysium** (per-i-MIZ-ē-um; *peri-*, around) divide the skeletal muscle into compartments. Each compartment contains a bundle of muscle fibers called a **fascicle** (FAS-i-kl; *fasciculus,* a

bundle). In addition to collagen and elastic fibers, the perimysium contains blood vessels and nerves that supply the fascicles.

Within a fascicle, the **endomysium** (en-dō-MIZ-ē-um; *endo-*, inside) surrounds each skeletal muscle fiber (cell) and ties adjacent muscle fibers together. Stem cells scattered among the fibers help repair damaged muscle tissue. The endomysium also contains capillaries that supply blood to the muscle fibers, and nerve fibers (axons) that control the muscle.

At each end of the muscle, the collagen fibers of all three layers come together to form either a bundle known as a

tendon, or a broad sheet called an **aponeurosis** (ap-ō-noo-RŌ-sis). Tendons are bands of collagen fibers that attach skeletal muscles to bones, and aponeuroses connect different skeletal muscles. ⟲ p. 104 The tendon fibers are interwoven into the periosteum of the bone, providing a firm attachment. Any contraction of the muscle exerts a pull on its tendon and in turn on the attached bone.

Blood Vessels and Nerves

The connective tissues of the epimysium and perimysium provide a passageway for the blood vessels and nerves that are necessary for muscle fibers to function. Muscle contraction uses tremendous amounts of energy. An extensive network of blood vessels delivers the necessary oxygen. It also carries away the metabolic wastes generated by active skeletal muscles.

Skeletal muscles contract only when they are stimulated by the central nervous system. *Axons* (nerve fibers) penetrate the epimysium, branch through the perimysium, and enter the endomysium to control individual muscle fibers. Skeletal muscles are often called *voluntary muscles* because we have voluntary control over their contractions. Many skeletal muscles may also be controlled at a subconscious level. For example, skeletal muscles involved with breathing, such as the *diaphragm*, usually work outside our conscious awareness.

CHECKPOINT

2. Describe the connective tissue layers associated with a skeletal muscle.

3. How would severing the tendon attached to a muscle affect the muscle's ability to move a body part?

See the blue Answers tab at the back of the book.

7-3 Skeletal muscle fibers have distinctive features

Learning Objective Identify the structural components of a sarcomere.

Skeletal muscle fibers are quite different from the "typical" cell we described in Chapter 3. ⟲ p. 57 One major difference is size. A skeletal muscle fiber from a leg muscle, for example, could have a diameter of 100 μm and a length equal to that of the entire muscle (up to 60 cm, or 24 in.). In addition, each skeletal muscle fiber contains hundreds of nuclei just beneath the plasma membrane. For this reason, it is said to be *multinucleate*. In the next sections, we examine the components of a typical skeletal muscle fiber.

The Sarcolemma and Transverse Tubules

The basic structure of a muscle fiber is shown in **Figure 7-2a**. The plasma membrane, or **sarcolemma** (sar-kō-LEM-uh; *sarkos,* flesh + *lemma*, husk), of a muscle fiber surrounds the cytoplasm, or **sarcoplasm** (SAR kō plazm). Openings scattered across the surface of the sarcolemma lead into a network of narrow tubules called **transverse tubules**, or **T tubules**. Filled with extracellular fluid, the T tubules form passageways through the muscle fiber, like a series of tunnels through a mountain.

The T tubules play a major role in making all regions of the muscle fiber contract at the same time. A muscle fiber contraction takes place through the orderly interaction of both electrical and chemical events. Electrical impulses conducted by the sarcolemma trigger a contraction by altering the chemical environment everywhere inside the muscle fiber. These electrical impulses reach the cell's interior by traveling along the transverse tubules that extend deep into the sarcoplasm of the muscle fiber.

Myofibrils

Inside each muscle fiber, branches of T tubules encircle cylinder-shaped structures called **myofibrils (Figure 7-2a)**. A myofibril is 1–2 μm in diameter and as long as the entire muscle fiber. Each muscle fiber contains hundreds to thousands of myofibrils. Myofibrils are bundles of **myofilaments**, protein filaments made primarily of the proteins *actin* and *myosin* (**Figure 7-2a**). Actin molecules are found in **thin filaments**, and myosin molecules in **thick filaments**. ⟲ p. 70

Myofibrils can actively shorten. As they do so, they create muscle fiber contraction. Because they are attached to the sarcolemma at each end of the cell, their contraction shortens the entire cell. Scattered among the myofibrils are mitochondria and granules of glycogen, a source of glucose. The breakdown of glucose and the activity of mitochondria provide the ATP that powers muscular contractions.

The Sarcoplasmic Reticulum

The **sarcoplasmic reticulum (SR)** is a specialized form of smooth endoplasmic reticulum (**Figure 7-2a**). The SR forms a tubular network around each myofibril and is tightly bound to T tubules. Expanded chambers of the SR called *terminal cisternae* (singular: *cisterna*) lie on either side of T tubules that encircle a myofibril, forming a *triad*.

The terminal cisternae contain high concentrations of calcium ions. The calcium ion concentration in the cytosol

Figure 7-2 The Organization of a Skeletal Muscle Fiber.

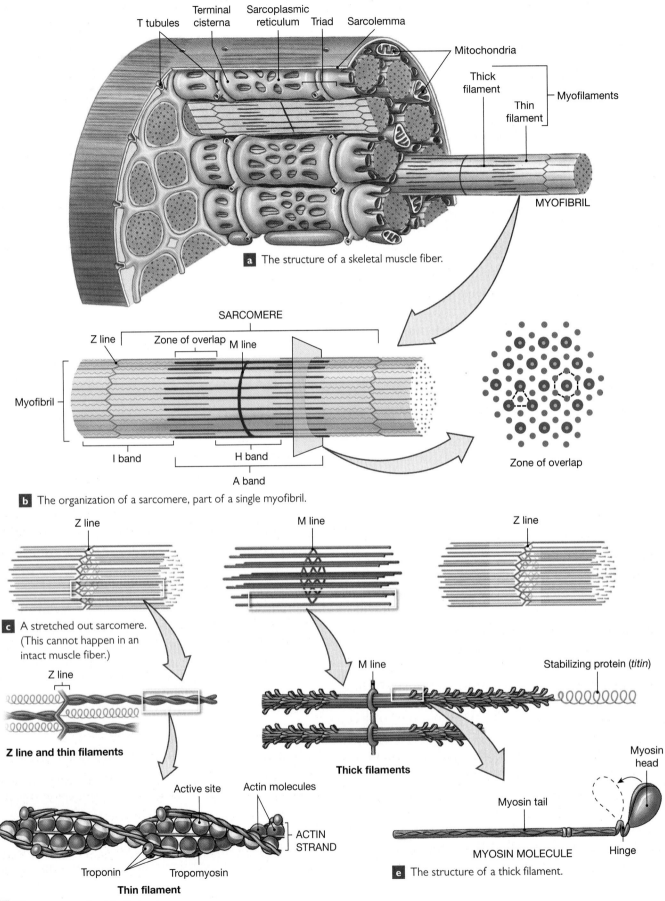

T tubules Terminal cisterna Sarcoplasmic reticulum Triad Sarcolemma

Mitochondria

Thick filament Thin filament Myofilaments

MYOFIBRIL

a The structure of a skeletal muscle fiber.

SARCOMERE

Z line Zone of overlap M line

Myofibril

I band H band

A band

Zone of overlap

b The organization of a sarcomere, part of a single myofibril.

Z line M line Z line

c A stretched out sarcomere. (This cannot happen in an intact muscle fiber.)

Z line

Z line and thin filaments

M line

Thick filaments

Stabilizing protein (*titin*)

Myosin head

Myosin tail

Hinge

MYOSIN MOLECULE

e The structure of a thick filament.

Active site Actin molecules

ACTIN STRAND

Troponin Tropomyosin

Thin filament

d The structure of a thin filament.

Build Your Knowledge

Calcium is the most abundant mineral in the human body. Calcium ions (Ca^{2+}) are important in many physiological processes, not the least of which is muscle contraction. Recall that the skin plays an important role in calcium metabolism by synthesizing vitamin D_3 (as you saw in **Chapter 5: The Integumentary System**). This vitamin is modified by the liver and converted by the kidneys into calcitriol, the hormone essential for calcium and phosphate absorption by the small intestine. ↺ **p. 127** Our bones also have a role in calcium metabolism (as you saw in **Chapter 6: The Skeletal System**). They provide a mineral reserve for maintaining normal concentrations of calcium (and phosphate) ions in body fluids. ↺ **p. 143**

of all cells is kept very low. Most cells, including skeletal muscle fibers, pump calcium ions across their plasma membranes and into the extracellular fluid. Skeletal muscle fibers, however, also actively transport calcium ions into the terminal cisternae of the SR. A muscle contraction begins when these stored calcium ions are released into the cytosol of the sarcoplasm.

Sarcomeres

The myofilaments (thin and thick filaments) that make up myofibrils are organized into repeating functional units called **sarcomeres** (SAR-kō-mērz; *sarkos*, flesh + *meros*, part) (**Figure 7-2b**). Each myofibril consists of approximately 10,000 sarcomeres arranged end to end. The sarcomere is the smallest functional unit of the muscle fiber. Interactions between the thick and thin filaments of sarcomeres are responsible for muscle contraction.

The arrangement of thick and thin filaments within a sarcomere produces a banded appearance. All the myofibrils lie parallel to the long axis of the cell, with their sarcomeres lying side by side. As a result, the entire muscle fiber has a banded, or *striated*, appearance corresponding to the bands of the individual sarcomeres (**Figure 7-2a**).

Figure 7-2b diagrams the external and internal structure of a single sarcomere. Each sarcomere has a resting length of about 2 μm. Neither type of filament spans the entire length of a sarcomere. The thick filaments (purple) lie in the center of the sarcomere. Thin filaments (red) at either end of

the sarcomere are attached to interconnecting proteins that make up the **Z lines**, the boundaries of each sarcomere.

Differences in the sizes and densities of thick and thin filaments account for the banded appearance of the sarcomere. The dark **A band** is the area containing thick filaments. The light region between two successive A bands—including the Z line—is the **I band**. (It may help you to remember that in a light micrograph, the A band appears d**A**rk and the I band is l**I**ght.)

From the Z lines, the thin filaments extend toward the center of the sarcomere, passing among the thick filaments in the *zone of overlap*. Strands of another protein (*titin*) extend from the Z lines to the ends of the thick filaments and keep both types of filaments aligned. The **M line** is made up of proteins that connect the central portions of each thick filament to its neighbors. An **H band** includes the M line and light regions on either side of the M line. It contains only thick filaments. The relationships of Z lines and M lines are shown in **Figure 7-2c**.

Thin and Thick Filaments

Each thin filament consists of a twisted strand of actin molecules (**Figure 7-2d**). Each actin molecule has an **active site** that can interact with myosin. In a resting muscle, the active sites along the thin filaments are covered by strands of the protein **tropomyosin** (trō-pō-MĪ-ō-sin; *trope*, turning). The tropomyosin strands are held in position by molecules of **troponin** (TRŌ-pō-nin) that are bound to the actin strand.

Thick filaments are composed of myosin molecules, each with a *tail* and a globular *head* (**Figure 7-2c,e**). The myosin molecules are oriented away from the center of the sarcomere, with the heads projecting outward. During a contraction, the myosin heads attach to actin molecules. This interaction takes place only when the troponin changes position, moving the tropomyosin and uncovering the active sites on actin.

Calcium is the "key" that "unlocks" the active sites and starts a contraction. When calcium ions bind to troponin, the protein changes shape, swinging the tropomyosin away from the active sites. Myosin–actin binding can then occur, and a contraction begins. The source of the calcium is the terminal cisternae of the SR.

Sliding Filaments and Cross-Bridges

When a sarcomere contracts, the I bands get smaller, the Z lines move closer together, the H bands decrease, and the zones of overlap get larger, but the length of the A bands does not change (**Figure 7-3**). These observations make sense only if the thin filaments slide toward the center of the sarcomere, alongside the stationary thick filaments. This explanation for sarcomere contraction is called the *sliding filament theory*.

Figure 7-3 Changes in the Appearance of a Sarcomere during Contraction of a Skeletal Muscle Fiber.

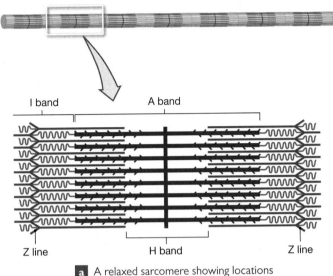

| I band | A band |
| Z line | H band | Z line |

a A relaxed sarcomere showing locations of the A band, Z lines, and I band.

| I band | A band |
| Z line | H band | Z line |

b During a contraction, the A band stays the same width, but the Z lines move closer together and the I band gets smaller.

The mechanism responsible for sliding filaments involves the binding of the myosin heads of thick filaments to active sites on the thin filaments. When the myosin heads interact with thin filaments during a contraction, they are called **cross-bridges**. When a cross-bridge binds to an active site, it pivots toward the center of the sarcomere (**Figure 7-2e**), pulling the thin filament in that direction. The cross-bridge then detaches and returns to its original position, ready to repeat a cycle of "attach, pivot, detach, and return," like a person pulling in a rope one-handed.

CHECKPOINT

4. Describe the basic structure of a sarcomere.

5. Why do skeletal muscle fibers appear striated when viewed through a light microscope?

6. Where would you expect the greatest concentration of calcium ions to be in a resting skeletal muscle fiber?

See the blue Answers tab at the back of the book.

7-4 The nervous system and skeletal muscles communicate at neuromuscular junctions

Learning Objective Explain the key steps in the contraction of a skeletal muscle fiber beginning at the neuromuscular junction.

Skeletal muscle fibers contract only under nervous system control. The nervous system and a skeletal muscle fiber communicate at a specialized intercellular connection known as a **neuromuscular junction (NMJ)**.

The Neuromuscular Junction

Each skeletal muscle fiber is controlled by a nerve cell called a *motor neuron*. A single axon of this neuron branches within the perimysium to form a number of fine branches. Each branch ends at an expanded **axon terminal**. ↪ p. 113 The axon terminal becomes part of a NMJ midway along the fiber's length.

The cytoplasm of the axon terminal contains mitochondria and vesicles filled with molecules of **acetylcholine** (as-ē-til-KŌ-lēn), or **ACh**. Acetylcholine is a *neurotransmitter*, a chemical released by a neuron to communicate with other cells. The release of ACh from the axon terminal results in changes in the sarcolemma that trigger the contraction of the muscle fiber.

A narrow space, the **synaptic cleft**, separates the axon terminal from the sarcolemma. This portion of the sarcolemma, known as the **motor end plate**, contains receptors that bind ACh. Both the synaptic cleft and the motor end plate contain the enzyme **acetylcholinesterase** (**AChE**, or *cholinesterase*), which breaks down molecules of ACh.

Neurons control skeletal muscle fibers by stimulating the production of an **action potential**, or electrical impulse, in the sarcolemma. The steps in this process are shown in **Spotlight Figure 7-4**.

CLINICAL NOTE

Neuromuscular Blockade

Certain emergency situations require chemically paralyzing a patient so that an endotracheal tube can be placed to assist or manage breathing. This procedure, referred to as *rapid sequence intubation (or induction) (RSI)*, involves the use of medications that act on the neuromuscular junction, the connection between the peripheral nerves and the skeletal muscle. Nerve impulses travel down the nerve and release a chemical neurotransmitter that stimulates (depolarizes) the associated skeletal muscle fibers, which results in contraction. Acetylcholine is the principle neurotransmitter in the neuromuscular junction. Blocking its action results in relaxation of skeletal (voluntary) muscles.

There are two ways to block the neuromuscular junction. One is by the administration of depolarizing agents that substitute for acetylcholine. Unlike acetylcholine, these depolarizing agents act over a prolonged time, which results in continued muscle depolarization and muscle paralysis. Because they have a stimulating effect, they often produce fasiculations (generalized, involuntary muscle twitching), especially in children, immediately after administration. The prototypical depolarizing neuromuscular blocker is succinylcholine (Anectine). It is the most commonly used neuromuscular blocker for RSI.

The other way to block the neuromuscular junction is to administer a drug that blocks the reuptake of acetylcholine into the nerve terminal. This produces an excess of acetylcholine in the neuromuscular junction, and inhibits the stimulation of the muscle. Because these drugs do not depolarize the affected muscle fibers, they are referred to as *nondepolarizing blockers*. They do not cause muscle fasiculations. Drugs in this class are similar in action to curare and include vecuronium, rocuronium, atracurium, and pancuronium.

Chemically paralyzing a patient causes complete voluntary muscle relaxation, including the muscles of respiration. This allows caregivers to take control of the airway and provide unimpeded mechanical ventilation. Esophageal and stomach muscles, and therefore sphincter tone, also relax, which increases the risk of vomiting and aspiration. Because neuromuscular blocking agents do not affect mental status or pain sensation, patients should be sedated or put to sleep before administration of neuromuscular blockers. If pain is present or expected, an analgesic should be administered.

Build Your Knowledge

Recall that neurons communicate through electrical events that affect their plasma membranes (as you saw in **Chapter 4: The Tissue Level of Organization**). ⤴ p. 113 These events also occur in the sarcolemma of skeletal muscle fibers. (We discuss these electrical events in detail in Chapter 8: The Nervous System.)

CLINICAL NOTE

Interference at the NMJ and Muscular Paralysis

Any condition that interferes with the generation of an action potential in the sarcolemma will cause muscular paralysis. Two examples are worth noting.

Botulism is a disease that results from the consumption of foods (often canned or smoked) contaminated with a bacterial toxin. The toxin prevents the release of ACh at the axon terminals, leading to a severe, potentially fatal muscular paralysis.

The progressive muscular paralysis seen in the autoimmune disease myasthenia gravis (mī-as-THĒ-nē-uh GRA-vis) results from the loss of ACh receptors at the motor end plate. The primary cause is a misguided attack on ACh receptors by the immune system. Genetic factors play a role in predisposing individuals to develop this condition. Estimates of the incidence of myasthenia gravis in the United States range from 2 to 10 cases per 100,000 population.

CLINICAL NOTE

Myasthenia Gravis

Myasthenia gravis is an autoimmune disease characterized by muscle weakness and fatigue. It is particularly evident with repetitive use of voluntary muscles. Antibodies against acetylcholine receptors impair the function of the acetylcholine receptor at the neuromuscular junction, which causes varying degrees of motor weakness. The muscle weakness is most pronounced in the proximal muscles and is generally relieved by rest.

The signs and symptoms of myasthenia gravis can be quite varied. The first symptom is usually weakness of the eye muscles and drooping eyelids. The facial muscles are also often weak and can result in a peculiar smile known as the myasthenic snarl. As the illness progresses, the patient develops trouble swallowing and has difficulty holding his head upright. The weakness then spreads to the muscles of the trunk.

The diagnosis of myasthenia gravis can usually be made by performing a Tensilon test. Prior to administering Tensilon, a patient is given an apple to bite and chew. Then, a dose of the cholinesterase inhibitor *edrophonium chloride (Tensilon)* is administered. The patient is then asked to bite and chew the apple. A marked increase in muscle strength and the ability to eat the apple after administration of Tensilon helps establish the diagnosis. In myasthenia gravis, edrophonium causes a dramatic difference in the patient's ability to eat the apple. Cholinesterase inhibitors, such as edrophonium or neostigmine, inhibit the enzyme cholinesterase. Cholinesterase breaks down acetylcholine at the neuromuscular junction. Inhibition of cholinesterase allows acetylcholine to accumulate in the neuromuscular junction and overcome the effects of the acetylcholine receptor antibodies. For chronic treatment of myasthenia gravis, long-acting cholinesterase agents can be used to prevent skeletal muscle weakness.

SPOTLIGHT Figure 7-4
EVENTS AT THE NEUROMUSCULAR JUNCTION

A single axon may branch to control more than one skeletal muscle fiber, but each muscle fiber has only one neuromuscular junction (NMJ). At the NMJ, the axon terminal of the neuron lies near the motor end plate of the muscle fiber.

Motor neuron

Path of electrical impulse (action potential)

Axon

Neuromuscular junction

Axon terminal

SEE BELOW

Sarcoplasmic reticulum

Motor end plate

Myofibril

Motor end plate

1 The cytoplasm of the axon terminal contains vesicles filled with molecules of acetylcholine, or ACh. ACh is a neurotransmiter, a chemical released by a neuron to change the permeability or other properties of another cell's plasma membrane. The synaptic cleft and the motor end plate contain molecules of the enzyme acetylcholinesterase (AChE), which breaks down ACh.

2 The stimulus for ACh release is the arrival of an electrical impulse, or action potential, at the axon terminal. The action potential arrives at the NMJ after traveling along the length of the axon.

Arriving action potential

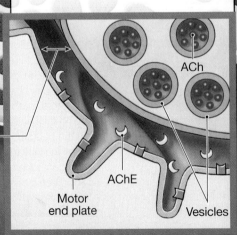

The synaptic cleft, a narrow space, separates the axon terminal of the neuron from the opposing motor end plate.

ACh

AChE

Motor end plate

Vesicles

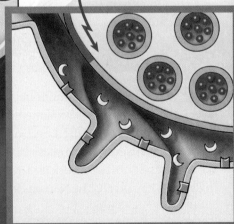

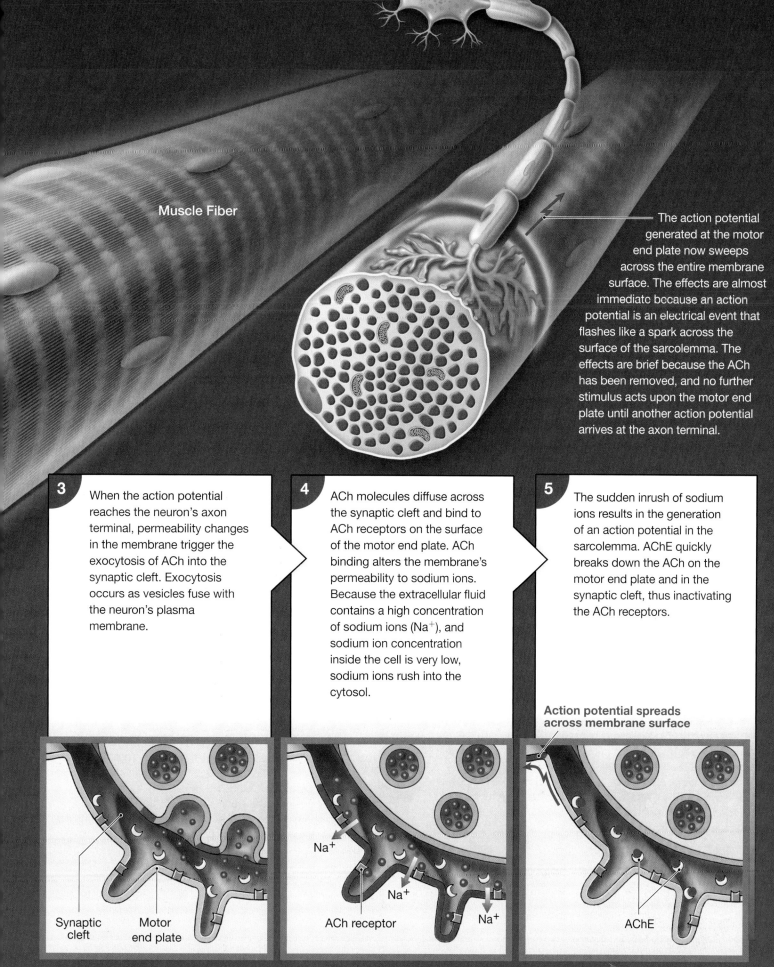

Muscle Fiber

The action potential generated at the motor end plate now sweeps across the entire membrane surface. The effects are almost immediate because an action potential is an electrical event that flashes like a spark across the surface of the sarcolemma. The effects are brief because the ACh has been removed, and no further stimulus acts upon the motor end plate until another action potential arrives at the axon terminal.

3 When the action potential reaches the neuron's axon terminal, permeability changes in the membrane trigger the exocytosis of ACh into the synaptic cleft. Exocytosis occurs as vesicles fuse with the neuron's plasma membrane.

4 ACh molecules diffuse across the synaptic cleft and bind to ACh receptors on the surface of the motor end plate. ACh binding alters the membrane's permeability to sodium ions. Because the extracellular fluid contains a high concentration of sodium ions (Na$^+$), and sodium ion concentration inside the cell is very low, sodium ions rush into the cytosol.

5 The sudden inrush of sodium ions results in the generation of an action potential in the sarcolemma. AChE quickly breaks down the ACh on the motor end plate and in the synaptic cleft, thus inactivating the ACh receptors.

Action potential spreads across membrane surface

Synaptic cleft   Motor end plate

Na$^+$

Na$^+$

ACh receptor

Na$^+$

AChE

CLINICAL NOTE

Rigor Mortis

Upon death, circulation ceases, depriving skeletal muscles of nutrients and oxygen. Within a few hours, skeletal muscle fibers run out of ATP. The sarcoplasmic reticulum then can no longer remove calcium ions from the cytosol. Calcium ions diffusing into the cytosol from the extracellular fluid or leaking out of the sarcoplasmic reticulum trigger a sustained contraction. Without ATP, the cross-bridges cannot detach from the active sites, and the muscle locks in the contracted position. All of the body's skeletal muscles are involved, and the individual becomes "stiff as a board." This physical state—called rigor mortis—lasts until the lysosomal enzymes released by autolysis break down the myofilaments. Rigor mortis begins two to seven hours after death and ends after one to six days or when decomposition begins. The timing is dependent on environmental factors, such as temperature.

The Contraction Cycle

The link between the generation of an action potential in the sarcolemma and the start of a muscle contraction occurs at the triads. There, the passage of the action potential along the T tubules triggers a massive release of calcium ions from the terminal cisternae. The presence of the calcium ions begins muscle contraction. The interlocking steps of the contraction cycle are shown in **Spotlight Figure 7-5** (pp. 224–225).

Figure 7-6 (p. 226) provides a summary of the contraction process, beginning with ACh release and ending with relaxation.

CHECKPOINT

7. Describe the neuromuscular junction.

8. How would a drug that blocks acetylcholine release affect muscle contraction?

9. What would you expect to happen to a resting skeletal muscle if the sarcolemma suddenly became very permeable to calcium ions?

See the blue Answers tab at the back of the book.

7-5 Sarcomere shortening and muscle fiber stimulation produce tension

Learning Objective Compare the different types of muscle contractions.

Now that you are familiar with the contraction of individual muscle fibers, let's examine the performance of skeletal muscles. In this section, we consider the coordinated contractions of an entire population of muscle fibers.

The individual muscle cells in muscle tissue are surrounded and tied together by connective tissue. When muscle cells contract, they pull on collagen fibers, producing an active force called **tension**. Tension applied to

CLINICAL NOTE

Tetanus

Children are often told to be careful around rusty nails. Parents should worry most not about the rust or the nail, but about infection with a very common bacterium, *Clostridium tetani*. This bacterium can cause the disease called tetanus. Although they share a name, the disease tetanus has no relation to the normal muscle response to neural stimulation. The *Clostridium* bacteria are found virtually everywhere but thrive only in tissues that contain abnormally low amounts of oxygen. For this reason, a deep puncture wound, such as that from a nail, carries a much greater risk than a shallow, open cut that bleeds freely.

When active in body tissues, these bacteria release a powerful toxin that affects the central nervous system. Motor neurons, which control skeletal muscles throughout the body, are particularly sensitive to it. The toxin suppresses the mechanism that inhibits motor neuron activity. The result is a sustained, powerful contraction of skeletal muscles throughout the body.

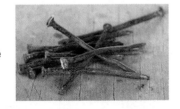

The incubation period (the time between exposure and the onset of symptoms) is usually less than two weeks. The most common early complaints are headache, muscle stiffness, and difficulty swallowing. Because it soon becomes difficult to open the mouth, this disease is also called *lockjaw*. Widespread muscle spasms usually develop within two to three days of the initial symptoms and continue for a week before subsiding. After two to four weeks, surviving patients recover with no aftereffects.

Severe tetanus has a 40–60 percent mortality rate, but immunization is effective in preventing the disease. Of the approximately 500,000 cases of tetanus worldwide each year, only about 100 occur in the United States, thanks to an effective immunization program. ("Tetanus shots," with booster shots every 10 years, are recommended.) Severe symptoms in unimmunized patients can be prevented by early administration of an antitoxin, usually *human tetanus immune globulin*. However, this treatment does not reduce symptoms that have already appeared.

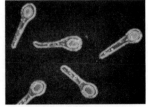

Clostridium tetani

an object tends to pull the object toward the source of the tension. However, before movement can take place, the applied tension must overcome the object's **resistance**, a passive force that opposes movement. The amount of resistance can depend on an object's weight and shape, friction, and other factors. In contrast, **compression**—a push applied to an object—tends to force the object away from the source of compression. Muscle cells can only contract (that is, shorten and generate tension). They cannot actively lengthen and generate compression.

The amount of tension produced by an individual muscle fiber depends solely on the number of pivoting cross-bridges it contains. All the sarcomeres of the fiber are involved. There is no way to regulate the amount of tension produced in that contraction by changing the number of contracting sarcomeres. The muscle fiber is either "on" (producing tension) or "off" (relaxed).

Tension does vary, however. It depends on

1. the muscle fiber's resting length at the time of stimulation, which determines the degree of overlap between thick and thin filaments, and

2. the frequency of stimulation, which affects the internal concentration of calcium ions and thus the amount bound to troponin molecules.

An entire skeletal muscle contracts when its component muscle fibers are stimulated. The amount of tension produced in the skeletal muscle *as a whole* is determined by

1. the frequency of muscle fiber stimulation, and

2. the number of muscle fibers activated.

Frequency of Muscle Fiber Stimulation

A **twitch** is a single stimulus–contraction–relaxation sequence in a muscle fiber. Its duration can be as brief as 7.5 ms, as in an eye muscle fiber, or up to 100 ms in fibers of the *soleus*, a small calf muscle. A *myogram* is a graph of tension development in a muscle fiber during a twitch. **Figure 7-7** is a myogram of the phases of a 40-ms twitch in a fiber from the *gastrocnemius muscle*, a prominent calf muscle:

- The **latent period** begins at stimulation and typically lasts about 2 ms. Over this period, the action potential sweeps across the sarcolemma, and calcium ions are released by the SR. No tension is produced by the muscle fiber because contraction has yet to begin.

- In the **contraction phase**, tension rises to a peak. Throughout this period, the cross-bridges are

interacting with the active sites on the actin filaments. Maximum tension is reached roughly 15 ms after stimulation.

- During the **relaxation phase**, muscle tension falls to resting levels as calcium levels drop, active sites are being covered, and the number of cross-bridges declines. This phase lasts about 25 ms.

A single stimulation produces a single twitch, but twitches in a skeletal muscle do not accomplish anything useful. All normal activities involve sustained muscle contractions. Such contractions result from repeated stimulations.

Summation and Incomplete Tetanus

If a second stimulus arrives before the relaxation phase has ended, a second, more powerful contraction occurs. The addition of one twitch to another in this way is called **summation** (**Figure 7-8a**). If the muscle is stimulated repeatedly and is never allowed to relax completely, the tension rises and peaks (**Figure 7-8b**). A muscle producing almost peak tension during rapid cycles of contraction and relaxation is said to be in **incomplete tetanus** (*tetanos*, convulsive tension). Virtually all normal muscular contractions involve incomplete tetanus of the participating muscle fibers.

Complete Tetanus

Complete tetanus occurs when the rate of stimulation is increased until the relaxation phase is completely eliminated, producing maximum tension (**Figure 7-8c**). In complete tetanus, the action potentials are arriving so fast that the SR does not have time to reclaim calcium ions. The high calcium ion concentration in the cytosol prolongs the contraction, making it continuous.

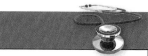

THE MUSCULAR DYSTROPHIES NOTE

The Muscular Dystrophies

Abnormalities in the genes that code for structural and functional proteins in muscle fibers are responsible for a number of inherited diseases collectively known as the *muscular dystrophies* (DIS-trō-fēz). These conditions, which cause progressive muscular weakness and deterioration, are the result of abnormalities in the sarcolemma or in the structure of internal proteins. The best-known example is *Duchenne's muscular dystrophy*, which typically develops in males ages 3–7 years.

THE CONTRACTION CYCLE

1 Contraction Cycle Begins

The contraction cycle, which involves a series of interrelated steps, begins with the arrival of calcium ions within the zone of overlap.

2 Active-Site Exposure

Calcium ions bind to troponin, weakening the bond between actin and the troponin–tropomyosin complex. This reaction leads to the exposure of the active sites on the actin molecules of the thin filaments.

3 Cross-Bridge Formation

Once the active sites are exposed, the energized myosin heads bind to them, forming cross-bridges.

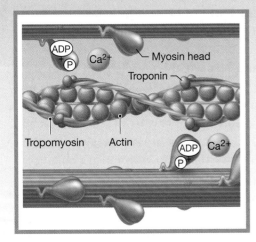

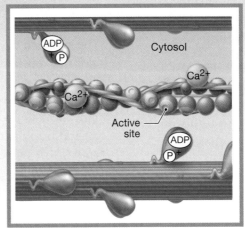

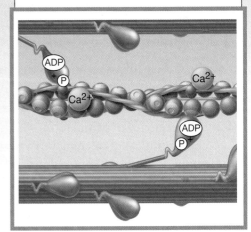

Resting Sarcomere

In the resting sarcomere, each myosin head is already "energized"—charged with the energy that will be used to power a contraction. Each myosin head points away from the M line. In this position, the myosin head is "cocked" like the spring in a mousetrap. Cocking the myosin head requires energy, which is obtained by breaking down ATP. At the start of the contraction cycle, the breakdown products, ADP and phosphate (often represented as P), remain bound to the myosin head.

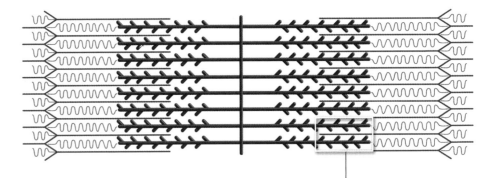

Zone of Overlap
(shown in sequence above)

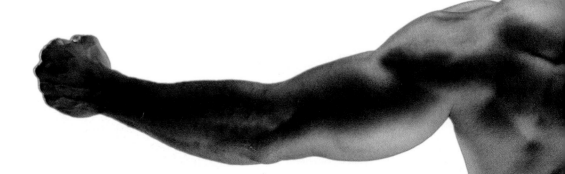

4. Myosin Head Pivoting

After cross-bridge formation, the stored energy is used to pivot the myosin head toward the M line. This action is called the power stroke; when it occurs, the bound ADP and phosphate group are released.

5. Cross-Bridge Detachment

When another ATP binds to the myosin head, the link between the myosin head and the active site on the actin molecule is broken. The active site is now exposed and able to form another cross-bridge.

6. Myosin Reactivation

Myosin reactivation occurs when the free myosin head splits ATP into ADP and P. The energy released is used to recock the myosin head.

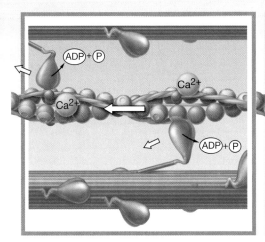

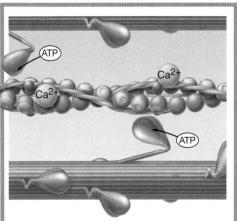

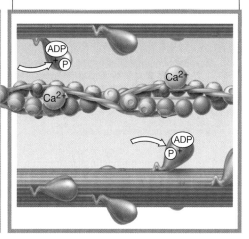

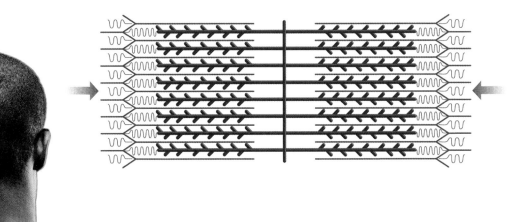

Contracted Sarcomere

The entire cycle is repeated several times each second, as long as Ca^{2+} concentrations remain elevated and ATP reserves are sufficient. Calcium ion levels will remain elevated only as long as action potentials continue to pass along the T tubules and stimulate the terminal cisternae. Once that stimulus is removed, calcium ion pumps pull Ca^{2+} from the cytosol and store it within the terminal cisternae. Troponin molecules then shift position, swinging the tropomyosin strands over the active sites and preventing further cross-bridge formation.

Figure 7-6 Steps Involved in Skeletal Muscle Contraction and Relaxation.

Steps that Initiate a Muscle Contraction

1 ACh released

ACh is released at the neuromuscular junction and binds to ACh receptors on the sarcolemma.

2 Action potential reaches T tubule

An action potential is generated and spreads across the membrane surface of the muscle fiber and along the T tubules.

3 Sarcoplasmic reticulum releases Ca²⁺ ions

The sarcoplasmic reticulum releases stored calcium ions.

4 Active site exposure and cross-bridge formation

Calcium ions bind to troponin, exposing the active sites on the thin filaments. Cross-bridges form when myosin heads bind to those active sites.

5 Contraction cycle begins

The contraction cycle begins as repeated cycles of cross-bridge binding, pivoting, and detachment occur, all powered by ATP.

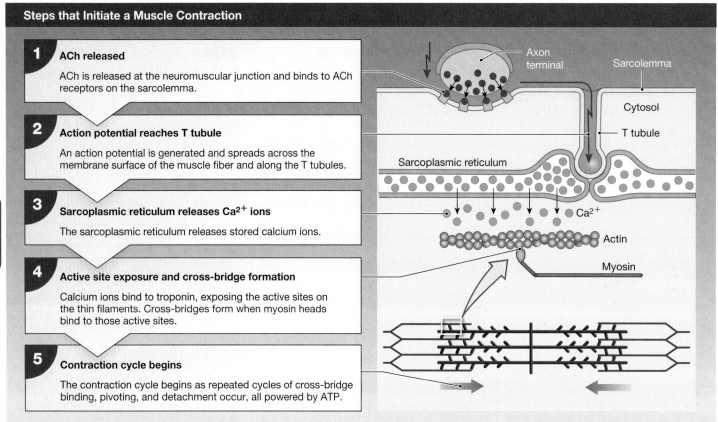

Steps that End a Muscle Contraction

6 ACh is broken down

ACh is broken down by acetylcholinesterase (AChE), ending action potential generation.

7 Sarcoplasmic reticulum reabsorbs Ca²⁺ ions

As the calcium ions are reabsorbed, their concentration in the cytosol declines.

8 Active sites covered, and cross-bridge formation ends

Without calcium ions, the tropomyosin returns to its normal position and the active sites are covered again.

9 Contraction ends

Without cross-bridge formation, contraction ends.

10 Muscle relaxation occurs

The muscle returns passively to its resting length.

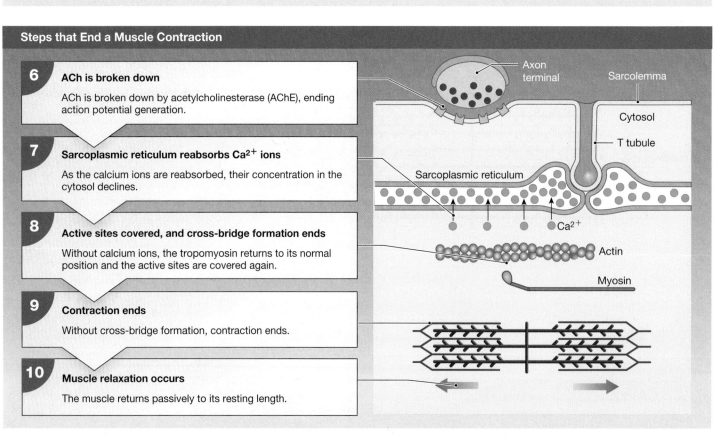

Figure 7-7 The Development of Tension in a Twitch.

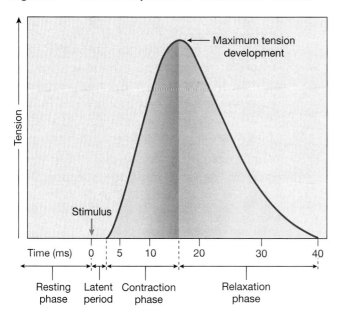

Number of Muscle Fibers Activated

We have a remarkable ability to control the amount of tension exerted by our skeletal muscles so that our muscles contract smoothly during a normal movement, not jerkily. Such control is accomplished by controlling the number of stimulated muscle fibers in the skeletal muscle.

A typical skeletal muscle contains thousands of muscle fibers. Some motor neurons control a single muscle fiber, but most control hundreds or thousands of muscle fibers through multiple axon terminals. A **motor unit** is a single motor neuron and all the muscle fibers it controls.

The size of a motor unit indicates how fine the control of movement can be. In the muscles of the eye, where precise control is extremely important, a motor neuron may control two or three muscle fibers. We have much less precise control over our leg muscles, where up to 2000 muscle fibers may respond to stimulation by a single motor neuron.

The muscle fibers of each motor unit are intermingled with those of other motor units (**Figure 7-9**). This mixing ensures that the direction of pull on a tendon does not change when the number of activated motor units varies. When you decide to perform a specific arm movement, specific groups of motor neurons within the spinal cord are stimulated. The contraction begins with the activation of the smallest motor units in the stimulated muscle. Over time, the number of activated motor units gradually increases. The activation of more and more motor units is called **recruitment**, and the result is a smooth, steady increase in muscular tension.

Peak tension production occurs when all the motor units in the muscle are contracting in complete tetanus. Such contractions do not last long, however, because the muscle fibers soon use up their available energy supplies. During a sustained contraction, motor units are activated on a rotating basis, so that some are resting while others are contracting. As a result, when your muscles contract for sustained periods, they produce slightly less than maximal tension.

Muscle Tone

Some of the motor units within any particular muscle are always active, even when the entire muscle is not contracting. Their contractions do not produce enough tension to cause

Figure 7-8 Effects of Repeated Stimulations.

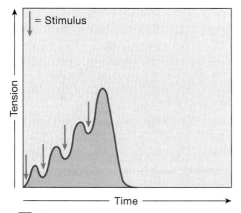

a **Summation**. Summation of twitches occurs when successive stimuli arrive before the relaxation phase has been completed.

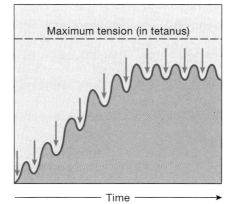

b **Incomplete tetanus**. Incomplete tetanus occurs if the stimulus frequency increases further. Tension production rises to a peak, and the periods of relaxation are very brief.

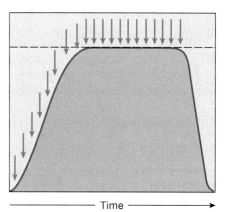

c **Complete tetanus**. During complete tetanus, the stimulus frequency is so high that the relaxation phase is eliminated; tension plateaus at maximal levels.

Figure 7-9 The Arrangement of Motor Units in a Skeletal Muscle. Each motor unit is a single motor neuron and all the muscle fibers it innervates. Muscle fibers of different motor units are intermingled, so the forces applied to the tendon remain roughly balanced regardless of which muscle groups are stimulated.

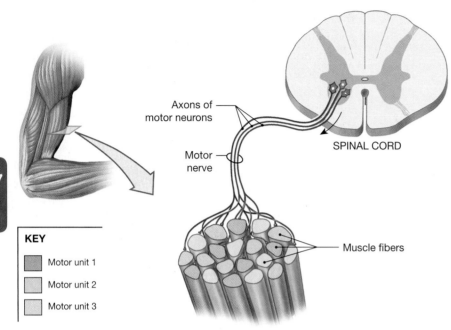

Axons of
motor neurons

SPINAL CORD

Motor
nerve

Muscle fibers

KEY

- Motor unit 1
- Motor unit 2
- Motor unit 3

movement, but they do tense and firm the muscle. This resting tension in a skeletal muscle is called **muscle tone**. A muscle with little muscle tone is limp and flaccid, but one with moderate muscle tone is quite firm and solid. Resting muscle tone stabilizes the positions of bones and joints. For example, in muscles involved with balance and posture, enough motor units are stimulated to produce the tension needed to maintain body position.

A skeletal muscle that is not regularly stimulated by a motor neuron will **atrophy** (AT-rō-fē; *a,* without + *-trophy,* nourishing): Its muscle fibers will become smaller and weaker. Individuals paralyzed by spinal injuries or other damage to the nervous system gradually lose muscle size and tone in the areas affected. Even a temporary reduction in muscle use can lead to muscular atrophy. Compare, for example, arm muscles after a cast has been worn to the same muscles in the other arm. Muscle atrophy is reversible at first, but dying muscle fibers are not replaced. In extreme atrophy, the functional losses are permanent. That is why physical therapy is so important for patients who are temporarily unable to move normally.

Isotonic and Isometric Contractions

We can classify muscle contractions on the basis of their pattern of tension production. In an **isotonic** (*iso-,* **equal** + *tonos,* **tension) contraction**, tension rises and the skeletal muscle's length changes. Tension in the muscle remains at

a constant level until relaxation takes place. Lifting an object off a desk, walking, and running involve isotonic contractions.

In an **isometric** (*metron,* **measure) contraction**, the muscle as a whole does not change length, and the tension produced never exceeds the load. Examples of isometric contractions are pushing against a closed door and trying to pick up a car. These examples are rather unusual, but many of the everyday reflexive muscle contractions that keep your body upright when you stand or sit involve isometric contractions of muscles that oppose the force of gravity.

Normal daily activities involve a combination of isotonic and isometric muscular contractions. As you sit reading this text, isometric contractions of postural muscles stabilize your vertebrae and maintain your upright position. When you turn a page, isotonic contractions move your arm, forearm, hand, and fingers.

Muscle Elongation Following Contraction

Recall that no active mechanism for muscle fiber elongation exists. ⤴ p. 200 Contraction is active, but elongation is passive. After a contraction, a muscle fiber usually returns to its original length through a combination of *elastic forces,* the *movements of opposing muscles,* and *gravity.*

Elastic forces are generated when a muscle fiber contracts and tugs on the flexible extracellular fibers of the endomysium, perimysium, epimysium, and tendons. These fibers are also somewhat elastic, and their recoil gradually helps return the muscle fiber to its original resting length.

Much more rapid returns to resting length result from the contraction of opposing muscles. For example, contraction of the *biceps brachii* muscle on the anterior part of your arm flexes your elbow, and contraction of the *triceps brachii* muscle on the posterior surface of your arm extends your elbow. When the biceps brachii contracts, the triceps brachii is stretched. When the biceps brachii relaxes, contraction of the triceps brachii extends the elbow and stretches the muscle fibers of the biceps brachii to their original length.

Gravity may also help lengthen a muscle after a contraction. For example, imagine your biceps brachii muscle fully contracted with your elbow pointing at the ground. When the muscle relaxes, gravity will pull your forearm down and stretch the muscle.

CLINICAL NOTE

Interference with Neural Control Mechanisms

Any condition that interferes with the generation of an action potential in the sarcolemma will cause muscular paralysis. Two examples are worth noting.

Botulism results from the consumption of foods (often canned or smoked) contaminated with a toxin. The toxin, produced by the bacteria *Clostridium botulinum*, prevents the release of ACh at the synaptic terminals, which leads to a potentially fatal muscular paralysis.

The progressive muscular paralysis seen in *myasthenia gravis* results from the loss of ACh receptors at the motor end plate. The primary cause is a misguided attack on the ACh receptors by the immune system. Genetic factors play a role in predisposing individuals to develop this condition.

CHECKPOINT

10. What factors are responsible for the amount of tension a skeletal muscle develops?

11. A motor unit from a skeletal muscle contains 1500 muscle fibers. Would this muscle be involved in fine, delicate movements or in powerful, gross movements? Explain.

12. Can a skeletal muscle contract without shortening? Explain.

See the blue Answers tab at the back of the book.

7-6 ATP is the energy source for muscle contraction

Learning Objective Describe the processes by which muscles obtain the energy to power contractions.

Muscle contraction requires large amounts of energy. For example, an active skeletal muscle fiber may require some 600 trillion molecules of ATP each second, not including the energy needed to pump the calcium ions back into the SR. This enormous amount of energy is not available before a contraction begins in a resting muscle fiber. Instead, a resting muscle fiber contains only enough energy reserves to sustain a contraction until additional ATP can be generated. Throughout the rest of the contraction, the muscle fiber will generate ATP at roughly the same rate as it is used. This section discusses how muscle fibers meet the demand for ATP.

Build Your Knowledge

Recall that the most important high-energy compound in the body is adenosine triphosphate, or ATP (as you saw in **Chapter 2: The Chemical Level of Organization**). ATP is made up of the nucleotide adenosine monophosphate (AMP) connected with two phosphate groups by high energy bonds. Cells most often obtain energy by removing one phosphate group from ATP, forming adenosine diphosphate, or ADP. ADP can be converted back to ATP by attaching another phospahate group. ↻ **p. 48**

ATP and CP Reserves

The primary function of ATP is the transfer of energy from one location to another, not the long-term storage of energy. At rest, a skeletal muscle fiber produces more ATP than it needs. Under these conditions, ATP transfers energy to *creatine* (KRĒ-uh-tēn), a small molecule that muscle cells assemble from fragments of amino acids. As **Figure 7-10a** shows, the energy transfer creates another high-energy compound, **creatine phosphate (CP)**:

$$\text{ATP} + \text{creatine} \rightarrow \text{ADP} + \text{creatine phosphate}$$

During a contraction, each cross-bridge breaks down ATP, producing ADP and a phosphate group. Then the energy stored in CP is used to "recharge" the ADP back to ATP through the reverse reaction:

$$\text{ADP} + \text{creatine phosphate} \rightarrow \text{ATP} + \text{creatine}$$

The enzyme that regulates this reaction is **creatine phosphokinase (CPK or CK)**. When muscle cells are damaged, CPK leaks into the bloodstream. For this reason, a high blood level of CPK usually indicates serious muscle damage.

A resting skeletal muscle fiber contains about six times as much CP as ATP. But when a muscle fiber is undergoing a sustained contraction, these energy reserves are exhausted in about 15 seconds. The muscle fiber must then rely on other processes to convert ADP to ATP.

ATP Generation

Cells in the body generate ATP through *aerobic* (oxygen-requiring) *metabolism* in mitochondria and through *glycolysis* in the cytoplasm. ↻ p. 73 Glycolysis is an **anaerobic** (non-oxygen-requiring) process.

Figure 7-10 Muscle Metabolism.

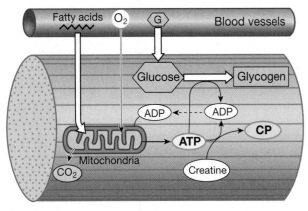

7 **a** **Resting:** Fatty acids are broken down; the ATP produced is used to build energy reserves of ATP, CP, and glycogen.

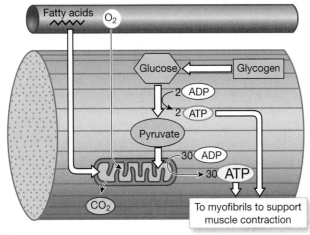

b **Moderate activity:** Glucose and fatty acids are broken down; the ATP produced is used to power contraction.

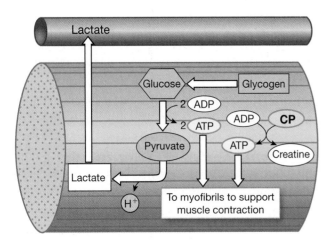

c **Peak activity:** Most ATP is produced through glycolysis, with lactate and hydrogen ions as by-products. Mitochondrial activity (not shown) now provides only about one-third of the ATP consumed.

Aerobic Metabolism

Aerobic metabolism normally provides 95 percent of the ATP needed by a resting cell. In this process, mitochondria absorb oxygen, ADP, phosphate ions, and organic substrate molecules from the surrounding cytoplasm. The organic substrates are carbon chains produced by the breakdown of carbohydrates, lipids, or proteins. The molecules enter the *citric acid cycle* (also known as the *tricarboxylic acid cycle* or the *Krebs cycle*) and are then completely disassembled by a series of chemical reactions. In brief, the carbon atoms and oxygen atoms are released as carbon dioxide (CO_2). The hydrogen atoms are shuttled to *respiratory enzymes* in the inner mitochondrial membrane, where their electrons are removed. The protons and electrons thus produced ultimately recombine with oxygen to form water (H_2O). Along the way, large amounts of energy are released and used to make ATP. The aerobic metabolism of a common carbohydrate substrate, pyruvate, is quite efficient: For each pyruvate molecule that enters the citric acid cycle, the cell gains 15 ATP molecules.

Resting skeletal muscle fibers rely primarily on the aerobic metabolism of fatty acids to make ATP (**Figure 7-10a**). These fatty acids are absorbed from the circulation. When the muscle starts contracting, the mitochondria begin breaking down molecules of pyruvate instead of fatty acids. The pyruvate is provided through the process of glycolysis (discussed shortly).

The maximum rate of ATP generation within mitochondria is limited by the availability of oxygen. A sufficient supply of oxygen becomes a problem as the energy demands of the muscle fiber increase. Oxygen consumption and energy production by mitochondria can increase to 40 times resting levels, but the energy demands of the muscle fiber may increase by 120 times. Thus, at peak levels of exertion, mitochondrial activity provides only around one-third of the required ATP.

Glycolysis

Glycolysis is the anaerobic breakdown of glucose to pyruvate in the cytoplasm of the cell. The ATP yield of glycolysis is much lower than that of aerobic metabolism. However, glycolysis can proceed without oxygen. For this reason, *glycolysis can continue to provide ATP when the availability of oxygen limits the rate of mitochondrial ATP production.*

The glucose broken down under these conditions comes from glycogen reserves in the sarcoplasm. Glycogen is a polysaccharide chain of glucose molecules. ⟲ p. 39 Typical skeletal muscle fibers contain large glycogen reserves in the form of insoluble granules. When the muscle fiber begins to run short of ATP and CP, enzymes break the glycogen molecules apart, releasing glucose that can be used to generate more ATP.

Energy Use and the Level of Muscle Activity

The demand for ATP is low in a resting skeletal muscle cell. More than enough oxygen is available for mitochondria to meet this demand and produce a surplus of ATP. The extra ATP is used to build up reserves of CP and glycogen (**Figure 7-10a**).

At moderate levels of activity, the demand for ATP increases (**Figure 7-10b**). As the rate of mitochondrial ATP production rises, so does the rate of oxygen consumption. So long as sufficient oxygen is available, the mitochondria can meet the demand for ATP. The amount of ATP provided by glycolysis remains relatively minor.

At peak levels of activity, oxygen cannot diffuse into the muscle fiber fast enough to enable the mitochondria to produce the required ATP. Mitochondrial activity can provide only about one-third the ATP needed, and glycolysis becomes the primary source of ATP (**Figure 7-10c**). The anaerobic process of glycolysis enables the cell to continue generating ATP when mitochondrial activity alone cannot meet the demand.

This pathway has its drawbacks. For example, when glycolysis produces pyruvate faster than it can be used by the mitochondria, pyruvate levels rise in the sarcoplasm. Under these conditions, the pyruvate is converted to **lactic acid**, a related three-carbon molecule. This conversion poses a problem because lactic acid dissociates into a hydrogen ion and a *lactate ion* in body fluids. The accumulation of hydrogen ions can lower the pH within the cell and alter the normal functioning of key enzymes. The muscle fiber then cannot continue to contract.

Glycolysis is also an inefficient way to generate ATP. Under anaerobic conditions, each glucose generates two pyruvate molecules, which are converted to lactic acid. In return, the cell gains two ATP molecules. If those two pyruvate molecules had been broken down aerobically in a mitochondrion, the cell would have gained an additional 30 ATP molecules.

Muscle Fatigue

A skeletal muscle fiber is said to be fatigued when it can no longer perform at the required level of activity despite continued neural stimulation. **Muscle fatigue** is caused by the depletion of energy reserves or the decline in pH due to the production and dissociation of lactic acid.

If the muscle contractions use ATP at or below the maximum rate of mitochondrial ATP generation, the muscle fiber can function aerobically. Under these conditions, fatigue does not occur until glycogen and other reserves such as lipids and amino acids are depleted. This type of fatigue affects the muscles of endurance athletes, such as marathon runners, after hours of exertion.

When a muscle produces a sudden, intense burst of activity, the ATP is provided by glycolysis. After a relatively short time (seconds to minutes), the rising lactic acid levels lower the tissue pH, and the muscle can no longer function normally. Athletes running sprints, such as the 100-yard dash, suffer from this type of muscle fatigue.

The Recovery Period

When a muscle fiber contracts, conditions in the sarcoplasm change: Energy reserves are consumed, heat is released, and lactic acid may be produced. During the **recovery period**, conditions within the muscle return to normal pre-exertion levels. The muscle's metabolic activity removes lactic acid and replaces intracellular energy reserves. The body as a whole loses the heat generated during intense muscular contraction.

Lactic Acid Recycling

The reaction that converts pyruvate to lactate is freely reversible. During the recovery period, when oxygen is available, lactate can be recycled by converting it back to pyruvate. This pyruvate can then be used as a building block to synthesize glucose or be used by mitochondria to generate ATP. The ATP is used to convert creatine to CP and to store the newly synthesized glucose as glycogen.

During the recovery period, the body's oxygen demand remains elevated above normal resting levels. The **oxygen debt** is the additional oxygen required during the recovery period to restore normal pre-exertion conditions in muscle tissue. Liver cells and muscle cells consume most of the extra oxygen. The liver cells produce ATP for converting lactate absorbed from the blood back to glucose, and muscle cells restore their reserves of ATP, CP and glycogen. Other cells, including sweat gland cells, also increase their rate of oxygen use and ATP generation. While the oxygen debt is being repaid, breathing rate and depth are increased. That is why you continue to breathe heavily for a time after you stop exercising.

CLINICAL NOTE

Rhabdomyolysis

Patients who are unconscious or immobile for a prolonged time are at risk for developing rhabdomyolysis, which is a breakdown of muscle tissue where the patient has been lying. When this occurs, numerous substances, most notably myoglobin, muscle enzymes, and electrolytes, are released from the damaged muscle. Myoglobin concentrates in the urine (myoglobinuria), turning it dark reddish brown. In severe cases, the patient can develop kidney failure.

Heat Loss

Muscular activity generates substantial amounts of heat that warms the sarcoplasm, interstitial fluid, and circulating blood. Muscle contractions play an important role in maintaining normal body temperature because muscle makes up a large portion of total body mass. Shivering, for example, can help keep you warm in a cold environment. But when skeletal muscles are contracting at peak levels, body temperature soon begins to climb. In response, blood flow to the skin increases, promoting heat loss through processes described in Chapters 1 and 5. ↪ pp. 10, 133

CHECKPOINT

13. How do muscle cells continuously synthesize ATP?

14. What is muscle fatigue?

15. Define oxygen debt.

See the blue Answers tab at the back of the book.

Build Your Knowledge

A primary function of the integumentary system is to help maintain normal body temperature by regulating heat exchange with the environment (as you saw in **Chapter 5: The Integumentary System**). Excess body heat may be lost from the skin when superficial blood vessels dilate (widen) and merocrine sweat glands secrete perspiration. The heat released by the superficial blood flow warms and evaporates the sweat on the skin, cooling the skin and lowering body temperature. ↪ **pp. 127, 133**

7-7 Muscle performance depends on muscle fiber type and physical conditioning

Learning Objective Relate the types of muscle fibers to muscle performance, and distinguish between aerobic and anaerobic endurance.

We can consider muscle performance in terms of **force**, the maximum amount of tension produced by a particular muscle or muscle group, and **endurance**, the amount of time over which the individual can perform a particular activity. Two major factors determine the performance capabilities of a particular skeletal muscle: the types of muscle fibers within the muscle, and physical conditioning or training.

Types of Skeletal Muscle Fibers

The human body contains two contrasting types of skeletal muscle fibers: fast (or fast-twitch) fibers and slow (or slow-twitch) fibers.

Fast Fibers

Most of the skeletal muscle fibers in the body are called **fast fibers** because they can reach peak twitch tension in 0.01 second or less after stimulation. Fast fibers are large in diameter and contain densely packed myofibrils, large glycogen reserves, and relatively few mitochondria. The tension produced by a muscle fiber is directly proportional to the number of myofibrils, so fast-fiber muscles produce powerful contractions. However, fast fibers fatigue rapidly because their contractions use ATP very quickly and they have few mitochondria to produce ATP. As a result, their activity is primarily supported by glycolysis.

Slow Fibers

Slow fibers are only about half the diameter of fast fibers, and they take three times as long to reach peak tension after stimulation. These fibers are specialized to contract for extended periods, long after a fast muscle would have become fatigued. Three specializations make this possible. They are related to the availability and use of oxygen:

1. ***Oxygen supply.*** Slow muscle tissue contains a more extensive network of capillaries than does typical fast muscle tissue, so oxygen supply is dramatically increased.

2. ***Oxygen storage.*** Slow muscle fibers contain the red pigment **myoglobin** (MĪ-ō-glō-bin). This globular protein

is structurally related to hemoglobin, the oxygen-carrying pigment found in blood, and also binds oxygen molecules. ⤴ p. 44 For this reason, resting slow muscle fibers contain oxygen reserves that can be mobilized during a contraction.

3. *Oxygen use.* Slow muscle fibers contain a relatively larger number of mitochondria than do fast muscle fibers.

The Distribution of Muscle Fibers and Muscle Performance

The percentages of fast and slow muscle fibers can vary considerably among skeletal muscles. Muscles dominated by fast fibers appear pale, and they are often called **white muscles**. Chicken breasts contain "white meat" because chickens use their wings only briefly, as when fleeing a predator. The power for their flight comes from the anaerobic process of glycolysis in the fast fibers of their breast muscles. In contrast, slow muscle fibers have a reddish color due to extensive blood vessels and myoglobin, and muscles dominated by slow fibers are known as **red muscles**. Chickens walk around all day, and these movements are powered by aerobic metabolism in the slow muscle fibers of the "dark meat" of their legs.

What about human muscles? Most contain a mixture of fiber types and so appear pink. However, there are no slow fibers in muscles of the eye and hand, where swift, but brief, contractions are required. Many back and calf muscles are dominated by slow fibers. These muscles contract almost continuously to keep us upright. The percentage of fast versus slow fibers in each muscle is genetically determined, but athletic training can increase the fatigue resistance of fast muscle fibers.

Physical Conditioning

Physical conditioning and training schedules enable athletes to improve both power and endurance. In practice, the training schedule varies depending on whether the activity is primarily supported by aerobic or anaerobic energy production.

Anaerobic endurance is the length of time muscle contractions can be supported by glycolysis and existing energy reserves of ATP and CP. Examples of activities that require anaerobic endurance are a 50-yard dash or swim, a pole vault, and a weight-lifting competition. Such activities involve contractions of fast muscle fibers. Athletes training to develop anaerobic endurance do frequent, brief, intense workouts. The net effect is an enlargement, or **hypertrophy** (hī-PER-trō-fē), of the stimulated muscles, as seen in champion weight lifters or bodybuilders. The number of muscle fibers does not change, but the muscle as a whole gets larger because each muscle fiber increases in diameter.

Aerobic endurance is the length of time a muscle can continue to contract while supported by mitochondrial activities. Aerobic endurance is determined by the availability of substrates for aerobic metabolism from the breakdown of carbohydrates, lipids, or amino acids. Aerobic activities do not promote muscle hypertrophy. Training to improve aerobic endurance usually involves sustained low levels of muscular activity. Examples are jogging, distance swimming, and other exercises that do not require peak tension production. Because glucose is a preferred energy source, endurance athletes often "load up" on carbohydrates ("carboload") for the three days before an event. They may also consume glucose-rich "sports drinks" during a competition.

CHECKPOINT

16. Why would a sprinter experience muscle fatigue before a marathon runner would?

17. Which activity would be more likely to create an oxygen debt in an individual who regularly exercises: swimming laps or lifting weights?

18. Which type of muscle fibers would you expect to dominate in the large leg muscles of someone who excels at endurance activities such as cycling or long-distance running?

See the blue Answers tab at the back of the book.

7-8 Cardiac and smooth muscle tissues differ in structure and function from skeletal muscle tissue

Learning Objective Contrast the structures and functions of skeletal, cardiac, and smooth muscle tissues.

We introduced cardiac muscle tissue and smooth muscle tissue previously (Chapter 4). Here we consider their structural and functional properties in greater detail.

Cardiac Muscle Tissue

Cardiac muscle tissue is found only in the heart. Cardiac muscle cells are relatively small and usually have a single, centrally placed nucleus.

Build Your Knowledge

Cardiac muscle is described as striated involuntary muscle because of its regular arrangement of actin and myosin filaments forming striations and the lack of voluntary nervous control over its contraction (as you saw in **Chapter 4: The Tissue Level of Organization**). Smooth muscle is known as nonstriated involuntary muscle because it lacks striations and the nervous system does not provide voluntary control over its contractions. ⊃ **p. 113**

Like skeletal muscle fibers, cardiac muscle cells contain an orderly arrangement of myofibrils and are striated, but significant differences exist in their structures and functions. The most obvious structural difference is that cardiac muscle cells are branched, and each cardiac cell contacts several others at specialized sites called **intercalated** (in-TER-ka-lā-ted) **discs** (**Figure 7-11a**). These cellular connections contain gap junctions that allow the movement of ions and small molecules and the rapid passage of action potentials from cell to cell, resulting in their simultaneous contraction. The cells "pull together" quite efficiently because the myofibrils are also attached to the intercalated discs.

Cardiac muscle and skeletal muscle also have these important functional differences:

- **Automaticity.** Cardiac muscle tissue contracts without neural stimulation, a property called *automaticity.* Specialized cardiac muscle cells called **pacemaker cells** normally determine the timing of contractions.

- **Longer contractions.** Cardiac muscle cell contractions last roughly 10 times longer than those of skeletal muscle fibers.

- **No tetanus.** The properties of cardiac muscle plasma membranes differ from those of skeletal muscle fibers. As a result, cardiac muscle tissue cannot undergo tetanus (sustained contraction). This property is important because a heart in tetany could not pump blood.

- **Extracellular calcium ions.** An action potential not only triggers the release of calcium from the SR but also increases the permeability of the plasma membrane to extracellular calcium ions.

Figure 7-11 Cardiac and Smooth Muscle Tissues.

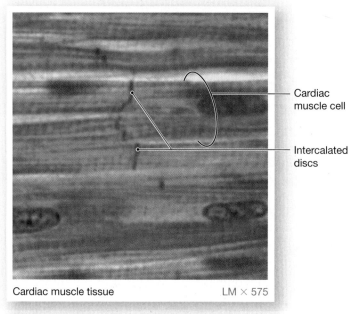

Cardiac muscle tissue   LM × 575

— Cardiac muscle cell

— Intercalated discs

a A light micrograph of cardiac muscle tissue.

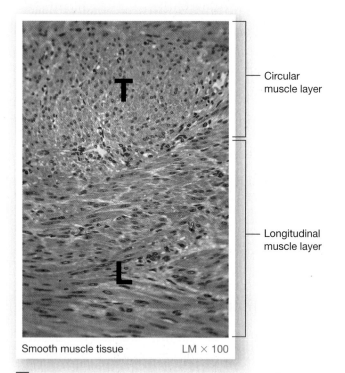

Smooth muscle tissue   LM × 100

— Circular muscle layer

— Longitudinal muscle layer

b Many visceral organs contain several layers of smooth muscle tissue oriented in different directions. Here, a single sectional view shows smooth muscle cells in both longitudinal (L) and transverse (T) sections.

- **Reliance on aerobic metabolism.** Cardiac muscle cells rely on aerobic metabolism for the energy needed to continue contracting. The sarcoplasm contains large numbers of mitochondria and abundant reserves of myoglobin that store oxygen.

Smooth Muscle Tissue

Smooth muscle cells are similar in size to cardiac muscle cells. They also contain a single, centrally located nucleus within each spindle-shaped cell (**Figure 7-11b**). Smooth muscle tissue is found within almost every organ, forming sheets, bundles, or sheaths around other tissues. Smooth muscles around blood vessels regulate blood flow through vital organs in the skeletal, muscular, nervous, and endocrine systems. Rings of smooth muscles, called *sphincters*, regulate movement of materials along internal passageways in the digestive and urinary systems.

Actin and myosin are present in all three muscle types. However, the internal organization of a smooth muscle cell differs from that of skeletal or cardiac muscle cells in these ways:

- **No sarcomeres.** Smooth muscle tissue lacks myofibrils, sarcomeres, or striations.

- **Scattered thick filaments.** In smooth muscle cells, the thick filaments are scattered throughout the sarcoplasm. The thin filaments are anchored within the cytoplasm and to the sarcolemma. The anchoring sites on the sarcolemma are not arranged in straight lines. As a result, when a contraction takes place, the muscle cell twists like a corkscrew.

- **Cells bound together.** Adjacent smooth muscle cells are bound together at these anchoring sites, thereby transmitting the contractile forces throughout the tissue.

Functionally, smooth muscle tissue differs from other muscle types in several major ways:

- **Contractions triggered differently.** Calcium ions trigger contractions through a different mechanism than that found in other muscle types. Also, most of the calcium ions that trigger contractions enter the cell from the extracellular fluid.

- **Contraction over a greater range of lengths.** Smooth muscle cells are able to contract over a greater range of lengths than skeletal or cardiac muscle because the actin and myosin filaments are not rigidly organized. This property is important because layers of smooth muscle are found in the walls of organs that undergo large changes in volume, such as the urinary bladder and stomach. Like skeletal muscle fibers, smooth muscle fibers can undergo sustained contractions.

- **Automaticity or neural or hormonal stimulation.** Many smooth muscle cells are not innervated by motor neurons. Instead, these muscle cells contract either automatically (in response to *pacesetter cells*) or in response to environmental or hormonal stimulation. When smooth muscle fibers are innervated by motor neurons, the neurons involved are not under voluntary control.

Table 7-1 summarizes the structural and functional properties of skeletal, cardiac, and smooth muscle tissue.

When myocardial ischemia is suspected, patients are usually admitted to the hospital and serial lab tests are performed, usually over a 24-hour period. The chance of detecting myocardial ischemia with a single sampling of CK-MB is only 34 percent. However, repeated sampling over 24 hours increases the accuracy to 90 percent or better.

Table 7-1	A Comparison of Skeletal, Cardiac, and Smooth Muscle Tissues		
Property	**Skeletal Muscle Fiber**	**Cardiac Muscle Cell**	**Smooth Muscle Cell**
Fiber dimensions (diameter × length)	100 μm × up to 60 cm	10–20 μm × 50–100 μm	5–10 μm × 30–200 μm
Nuclei	Multiple, near sarcolemma	Usually single, centrally located	Single, centrally located
Filament organization	In sarcomeres along myofibrils	In sarcomeres along myofibrils	Scattered throughout sarcoplasm
Control mechanism	Neural, at single neuromuscular junction	Automaticity (pacemaker cells)	Automaticity (pacesetter cells), neural or hormonal control
Ca²⁺ Source	Release from SR	Extracellular fluid and release from SR	Extracellular fluid and release from SR
Contraction	Rapid onset; tetanus can occur; rapid fatigue	Slower onset; tetanus cannot occur; resistant to fatigue	Slow onset; tetanus can occur; resistant to fatigue
Energy source	Aerobic metabolism at moderate levels of activity; glycolysis (anaerobic during peak activity)	Aerobic metabolism, usually lipid or carbohydrate substrates	Primarily aerobic metabolism

CLINICAL NOTE

Laboratory Testing in Heart Attack

Diagnosing a heart attack is often difficult. A heart attack (*acute myocardial infarction*) occurs when an artery that supplies blood to the heart muscle is blocked. Initially, the area of heart muscle supplied by the artery will become injured (*myocardial ischemia*). If this continues, the affected area of heart muscle will die (*myocardial infarction*). Because of this, it is important for emergency personnel to recognize heart attacks, now referred to as *acute coronary syndrome*, so that treatment can be provided and blood flow restored before a significant mass of the heart muscle is permanently damaged.

Several diagnostic tools are routinely used to determine whether a heart attack has occurred. These include the electrocardiogram (ECG), X-rays, laboratory tests, and others. Following injury to the heart muscle, its chemical components are released into the circulation. Laboratory assays of these chemicals can aid in the diagnosis of heart attack. Commonly assayed chemicals include:

* *Creatine kinase (CK).* CK is an enzyme found in muscle and brain tissues. There are subtle differences in CK structure (*isoenzymes*), depending on the source. CK-MM comes from skeletal muscle, CK-BB comes from brain tissue, and CH-MB comes from heart tissue. The amount of CK-MB in the blood does not normally exceed 2–4 percent of total CK values. Any elevation in the percentage of CK-MB indicates myocardial injury. The CK-MB level begins to increase within four to six hours of injury, peaks at 18–24 hours, and remains elevated for three to four days.
* *Lactic dehydrogenase (LD or LDH).* LDH is found in heart muscle, skeletal muscle, liver, erythrocytes, kidney, and some types of tumors. It is increased in over 90 percent of myocardial infarctions. However, it can be increased in diseases of any of the above organs or hemolysis. There are five LDH isoenzymes:

  * LDH1: heart, erythrocytes, renal cortex
  * LDH2: reticuloendothelial system
  * LDH3: lung tissue
  * LDH4: placenta, kidney, pancreas
  * LDH5: skeletal muscle, liver

  Reversal of LDH1/LDH2 ratio is characteristic of an acute myocardial infarction; with an 80–85 percent sensitivity. LDH begins to rise within 24 hours of myocardial infarction, peaks in three days and returns to normal in eight to nine days.

* *Myoglobin.* Myoglobin is found in striated muscle and contains iron. It stores oxygen and gives muscle its red color. Damage to skeletal or cardiac muscle releases myoglobin into circulation. Myoglobin rapid assay kits are available that allow testing in the prehospital setting. Myoglobin rises fast (two hours) after myocardial infarction, peaks at six to eight hours and returns to normal in 20–36 hours.
* *Troponin I, T, and C.* The troponins are the contractile proteins of the myofibril. The cardiac isoforms are very specific for cardiac injury and are not present in serum from healthy people. Troponin I is the form frequently assessed. There is a new form (Troponin L) which may be detected earlier. Troponin rapid assay kits are available that allow testing in the prehospital setting. The troponins rise four to six hours after injury, peak in 12–16 hours, and remain elevated for up to 10 days. High-sensitivity troponin testing is rapidly becoming available that will shorten the diagnostic time for cardiac enzyme testing.
* *B-natriuretic peptide (BNP).* BNP is a peptide found in the ventricles of the heart and increases when ventricular filling pressures are high. It can be used to detect congestive heart failure.

CHECKPOINT

19. How do intercalated discs enhance the functioning of cardiac muscle tissue?
20. Extracellular calcium ions are important for the contraction of what type(s) of muscle tissue?
21. Why can smooth muscle contract over a wider range of resting lengths than skeletal muscle?

See the blue Answers tab at the back of the book.

7-9 Descriptive terms are used to name skeletal muscles

Learning Objective Explain how the name of a muscle can help identify its location, appearance, or function.

The **muscular system** includes all the skeletal muscles (**Figure 7-12**). The general appearance of each of the nearly 700 skeletal muscles provides clues to its primary function. Muscles involved with locomotion and posture work across joints, producing movement of the skeleton. Those that support soft tissue form slings or sheets between relatively stable bony parts. Muscles that guard an entrance or an exit completely encircle the opening.

The separation of the skeletal system into axial and appendicular divisions provides a useful guideline for subdividing the muscular system as well:

* The **axial muscles** arise on the axial skeleton. They position the head and spinal column and also move the rib cage, assisting in the movements that make breathing possible. They do not play a role in movement or support of the pectoral or pelvic girdles or the limbs. This category includes roughly 60 percent of the skeletal muscles in the body.

* The **appendicular muscles** stabilize or move components of the appendicular skeleton.

Figure 7-12 An Overview of the Major Skeletal Muscles.

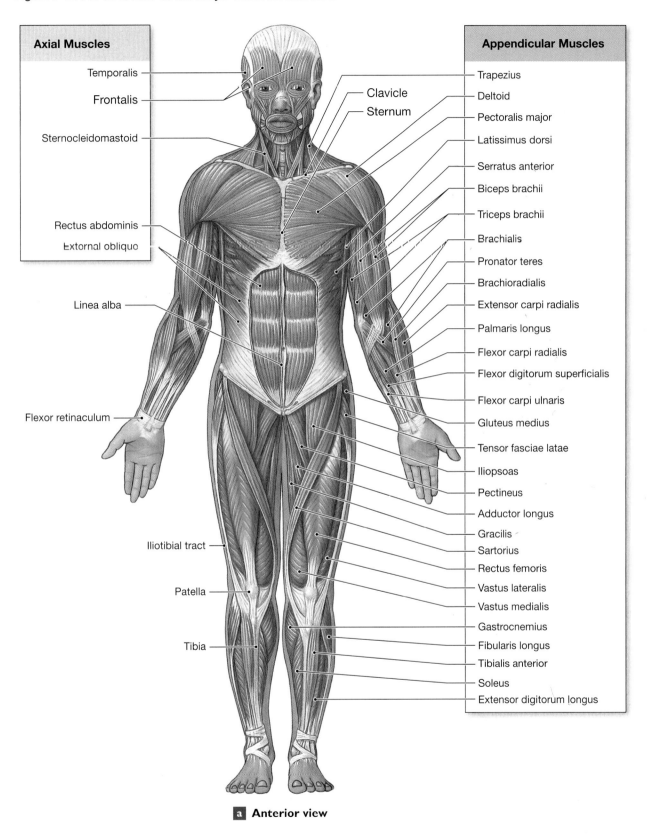

Axial Muscles

Temporalis
Frontalis
Sternocleidomastoid
Rectus abdominis
External oblique
Linea alba
Flexor retinaculum
Iliotibial tract
Patella
Tibia

Clavicle
Sternum

Appendicular Muscles

Trapezius
Deltoid
Pectoralis major
Latissimus dorsi
Serratus anterior
Biceps brachii
Triceps brachii
Brachialis
Pronator teres
Brachioradialis
Extensor carpi radialis
Palmaris longus
Flexor carpi radialis
Flexor digitorum superficialis
Flexor carpi ulnaris
Gluteus medius
Tensor fasciae latae
Iliopsoas
Pectineus
Adductor longus
Gracilis
Sartorius
Rectus femoris
Vastus lateralis
Vastus medialis
Gastrocnemius
Fibularis longus
Tibialis anterior
Soleus
Extensor digitorum longus

a **Anterior view**

7

(*continued*)

Figure 7-12 An Overview of the Major Skeletal Muscles. (*continued*)

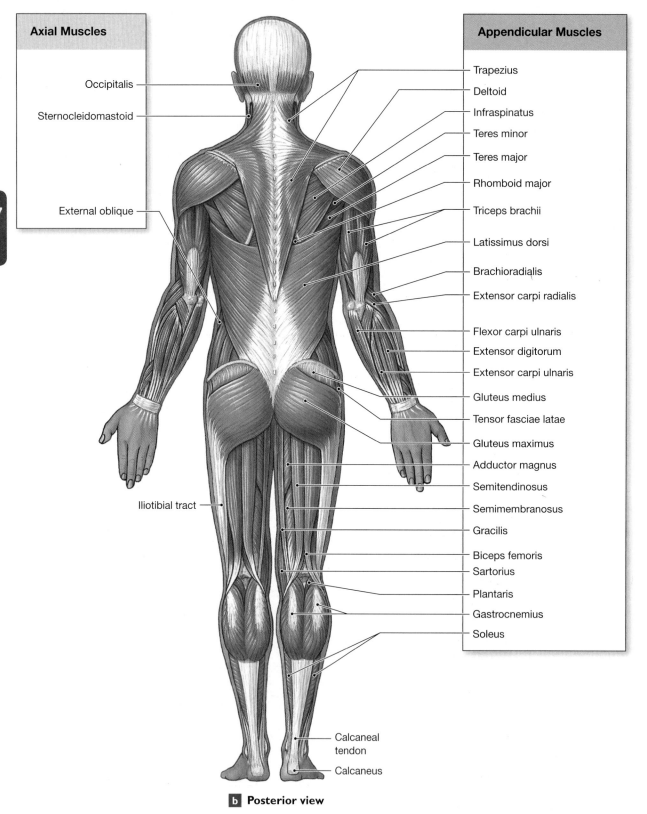

Axial Muscles

Occipitalis

Sternocleidomastoid

External oblique

Appendicular Muscles

Trapezius

Deltoid

Infraspinatus

Teres minor

Teres major

Rhomboid major

Triceps brachii

Latissimus dorsi

Brachioradialis

Extensor carpi radialis

Flexor carpi ulnaris

Extensor digitorum

Extensor carpi ulnaris

Gluteus medius

Tensor fasciae latae

Gluteus maximus

Adductor magnus

Semitendinosus

Semimembranosus

Gracilis

Biceps femoris

Sartorius

Plantaris

Gastrocnemius

Soleus

Iliotibial tract

Calcaneal tendon

Calcaneus

b Posterior view

7

Here we consider several features of muscles that are used to name them: their attachment sites, known as origins and insertions, and their actions.

Origins, Insertions, and Actions

Each muscle begins at an **origin**, ends at an **insertion**, and contracts to produce a specific **action**. In general, a muscle's origin remains stationary while the insertion moves. For example, the *gastrocnemius* muscle (in the calf) has its origin on the distal portion of the femur and inserts on the calcaneus. Its contraction pulls the insertion closer to the origin, resulting in the action called *plantar flexion*. The determinations of origin and insertion are usually based on movement from the anatomical position.

Almost all skeletal muscles either originate or insert on the skeleton. When they contract, they may produce *flexion, extension, adduction, abduction, protraction, retraction, elevation, depression, rotation, circumduction, pronation, supination, inversion,* or *eversion.* (You may wish to review Figures 6-32 to 6-34, pp. 177–179.)

We can describe actions of muscles in two ways. The first describes muscle actions in terms of the bone affected. Accordingly, we say the *biceps brachii* muscle performs "flexion of the forearm." The second way, which is increasingly used by specialists of human motion *(kinesiologists),* describes muscle action in terms of the joint involved. Thus, we say the biceps brachii muscle performs "flexion at (or of) the elbow." We will primarily use the second way.

We can also describe muscles by their **primary actions**:

- A **prime mover, or agonist** (AG-o-nist), is a muscle whose contraction is chiefly responsible for producing a particular movement. The *biceps brachii* muscle is a prime mover that flexes the elbow.

- An **antagonist** (an-TAG-o-nist) is a muscle whose action opposes the movement produced by another muscle. An antagonist may also be a prime mover. For example, the *triceps brachii* muscle is a prime mover that extends the elbow. It is, therefore, an antagonist of the biceps brachii, and the biceps brachii is an antagonist of the triceps brachii. Agonists and antagonists are functional opposites—if one produces flexion, the other's primary action is extension.

- A **synergist** (*syn-,* together + *ergon,* work) is a muscle that helps a prime mover work efficiently. Synergists may either provide additional pull near the insertion or stabilize the point of origin. For example, the *deltoid muscle* acts to

lift the arm away from the body (abduction). A smaller muscle, the *supraspinatus muscle,* assists the deltoid in starting this movement. **Fixators** are synergists that stabilize the origin of a prime mover by preventing movement at another joint.

Names of Skeletal Muscles

You need not learn the name of every skeletal muscle, but you should become familiar with the most important ones. Fortunately, the names of muscles provide clues to their identification. **Table 7-2** summarizes muscle terminology and can be a useful reference as you go through the rest of this chapter. (With the exception of the platysma and the diaphragm, the complete name of every muscle includes the word *muscle.* For simplicity, we have not included the word *muscle* in figures and tables.)

Some names, often those with Greek or Latin roots, refer to the orientation of the muscle fascicles. For example, *rectus* means "straight," and *rectus muscles* are parallel muscles whose fascicles run parallel to the long axis of the muscle, as in the *rectus abdominis muscle.* In a few cases, a muscle is such a prominent feature that the regional name alone can identify it, such as the *temporalis muscle* of the head.

Other muscles are named after structural features. For example, a biceps muscle has two tendons of origin (*bi-,* two + *caput,* head), and the *triceps* has three. **Table 7-2** also lists names reflecting shape, length, or size, or whether a muscle is visible at the body surface (*externus, superficialis*) or lies beneath (*internus, profundus*). Superficial muscles that position or stabilize an organ are called *extrinsic muscles.* Those that operate within an organ are called *intrinsic muscles.*

The first part of many names indicates the muscle's origin, and the second part its insertion. The *sternohyoid muscle,* for example, originates at the sternum and inserts on the hyoid bone. Other names may also indicate the primary function of the muscle. For example, the *extensor carpi radialis muscle* is found along the radial (lateral) border of the forearm, and its contraction produces extension at the wrist (carpal) joint.

CHECKPOINT

22. Identify the kinds of descriptive information used to name skeletal muscles.

23. Which muscle is the antagonist of the biceps brachii?

24. What does the name *flexor carpi radialis longus* tell you about this muscle?

See the blue Answers tab at the back of the book.

Table 7-2	Muscle Terminology		
Terms Indicating Position, Direction, or Muscle Fiber Orientation	**Terms Indicating Specific Regions of the Body***	**Terms Indicating Structural Characteristics of the Muscle**	**Terms Indicating Actions**
Anterior (front)	Abdominis (abdomen)	**Origin**	**General**
Externus (superficial)	Anconeus (elbow)	Biceps (two heads)	Abductor (movement away)
Extrinsic (outside)	Auricularis (auricle of ear)	Triceps (three heads)	Adductor (movement toward)
Inferioris (inferior)	Brachialis (brachium)	Quadriceps (four heads)	Depressor (lowering movement)
Internus (deep, internal)	Capitis (head)	**Shape**	Extensor (straightening movement)
Intrinsic (inside)	Carpi (wrist)	Deltoid (triangle)	Flexor (bending movement)
Lateralis (lateral)	Cervicis (neck)	Orbicularis (circle)	Levator (raising movement)
Medialis/medius (medial, middle)	Cleido-/-clavius (clavicle)	Pectinate (comblike)	Pronator (turning into prone position)
Obliquus (oblique)	Coccygeus (coccyx)	Piriformis (pear-shaped)	Supinator (turning into supine position)
Posterior (back)	Costalis (ribs)	Platy- (flat)	Tensor (tensing movement)
Profundus (deep)	Cutaneous (skin)	Pyramidal (pyramid)	**Specific**
Rectus (straight)	Femoris (femur)	Rhomboid (parallelogram)	Buccinator (trumpeter)
Superficialis (superficial)	Genio- (chin)	Serratus (serrated)	Risorius (laugher)
Superioris (superior)	Glosso-/-glossal (tongue)	Splenius (bandage)	Sartorius (like a tailor)
Transversus (transverse)	Hallucis (great toe)	Teres (long and round)	
	Ilio- (ilium)	Trapezius (trapezoid)	
	Inguinal (groin)	**Other Striking Features**	
	Lumborum (lumbar region)	Alba (white)	
	Nasalis (nose)	Brevis (short)	
	Nuchal (back of neck)	Gracilis (slender)	
	Oculo- (eye)	Lata (wide)	
	Oris (mouth)	Latissimus (widest)	
	Palpebrae (eyelid)	Longissimus (longest)	
	Pollicis (thumb)	Longus (long)	
	Popliteus (behind knee)	Magnus (large)	
	Psoas (loin)	Major (larger)	
	Radialis (radius)	Maximus (largest)	
	Scapularis (scapula)	Minimus (smallest)	
	Temporalis (temples)	Minor (smaller)	
	Thoracis (thoracic region)	Vastus (great)	
	Tibialis (tibia)		
	Ulnaris (ulna)		
	Uro- (urinary)		

*For other regional terms, refer to Figure 1-6, p. 14, which shows anatomical landmarks.

7-10 Axial muscles are muscles of the head and neck, vertebral column, trunk, and pelvic floor

Learning Objective Identify the main axial muscles of the body and their origins, insertions, and actions.

The axial muscles fall into four logical groups based on location, function, or both:

1. *Muscles of the head and neck.* These muscles include those responsible for facial expression, chewing, and swallowing.

2. *Muscles of the spine.* This group includes flexors and extensors of the head, neck, and spinal column.

3. *Muscles of the trunk.* The *oblique* and *rectus* muscles form the muscular walls of the thoracic and abdomino-pelvic cavities.

4. *Muscles of the pelvic floor.* These muscles extend between the sacrum and pelvic girdle and form the muscular *perineum*, which closes the pelvic outlet.

Muscles of the Head and Neck

The muscles of the head and neck are shown in **Figures 7-13** and **7-14** (pp. 241–242) and detailed in **Table 7-3**. The

Figure 7-13 Muscles of the Head and Neck.

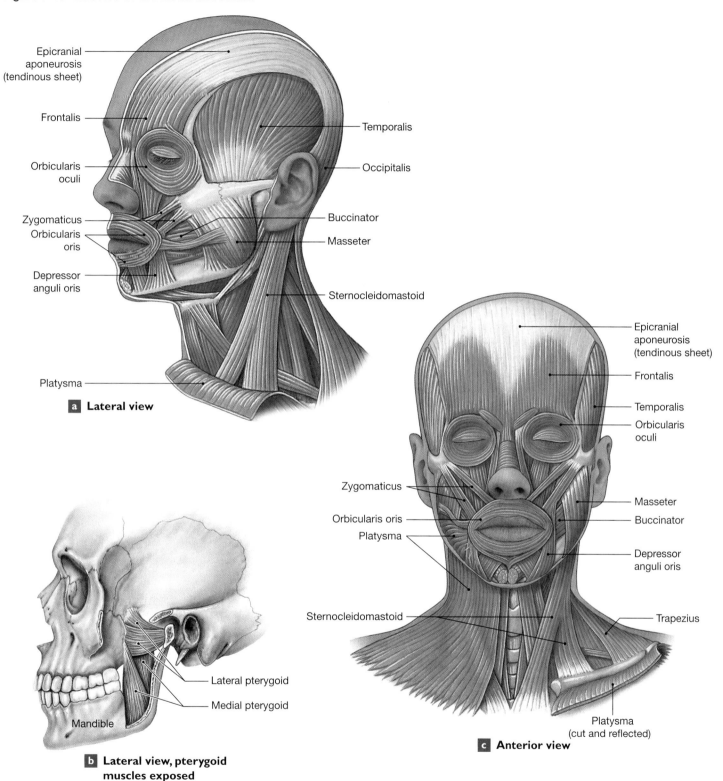

a **Lateral view**

b **Lateral view, pterygoid muscles exposed**

c **Anterior view**

muscles of the face originate on the surface of the skull and insert into the dermis of the skin. When they contract, the skin moves.

The largest group of facial muscles is associated with the mouth. The **orbicularis oris** constricts the opening,

and other muscles move the lips or the corners of the mouth. The **buccinator** (BUK-si-nā-tor) muscle compresses the cheeks, as when pursing the lips and blowing forcefully. (*Buccinator* translates as "trumpeter.") During chewing, contraction and relaxation of the buccinators

Figure 7-14 Muscles of the Anterior Neck.

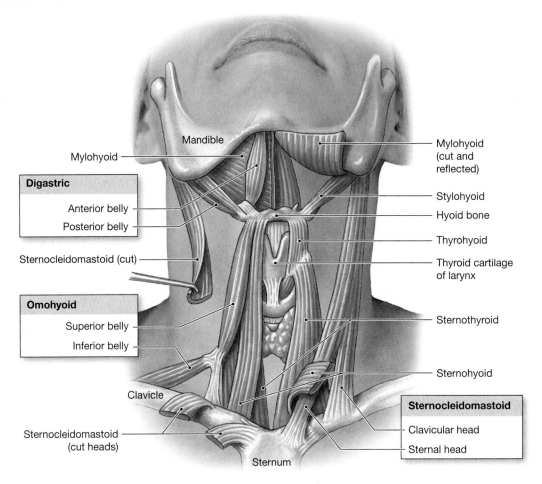

move food back across the teeth from the space inside the cheeks. In infants, the buccinator produces suction for suckling at the breast. The chewing motions are primarily produced by contractions of the **masseter**, assisted by the **temporalis** and the **pterygoid** muscles used in various combinations.

Smaller groups of muscles control movements of the eyebrows and eyelids, the scalp, the nose, and the external ear. The **epicranium** (ep-i-KRĀ-nē-um), or *scalp*, contains a two-part muscle, the *occipitofrontalis*. The anterior **frontalis** muscle and the posterior **occipitalis** muscle of the occipitofrontalis are separated by an *aponeurosis,* or tendinous sheet, called the **epicranial aponeurosis**. The **platysma** (pla-TIZ-muh; *platys*, flat) covers the ventral surface of the neck, extending from the base of the neck to the mandible and the corners of the mouth.

The muscles of the neck control the position of the larynx, depress the mandible, tense the floor of the mouth, and provide a stable foundation for muscles of the tongue

and pharynx (**Figure 7-14**). These muscles include the following:

- The **digastric**, which has two bellies (*di-,* two + *gaster*, stomach), opens the mouth by depressing the mandible.

- The broad, flat **mylohyoid** provides a muscular floor to the mouth and supports the tongue.

- The **stylohyoid** forms a muscular connection between the hyoid bone and the styloid process of the skull.

- The **sternocleidomastoid** (ster-nō-klī-dō-MAS-toyd) extends from the clavicle and the sternum to the mastoid region of the skull. It can rotate the head or flex the neck.

- The **omohyoid** attaches to the scapula, the clavicle and first rib, and the hyoid bone. Its superior and inferior bellies join at a central tendon anchored to the clavicle and first rib.

Table 7-3	Muscles of the Head and Neck		
Region/Muscle	**Origin**	**Insertion**	**Action**
MOUTH			
Buccinator	Maxillary bone and mandible	Blends into fibers of orbicularis oris	Compresses cheeks
Orbicularis oris	Maxillary bone and mandible	Lips	Compresses, purses lips
Depressor anguli oris	Anterolateral surface of mandible	Skin at angle of mouth	Depresses corner of mouth
Zygomaticus	Zygomatic bone	Angle of mouth; upper lip	Draws corner of mouth back and up
EYE			
Orbicularis oculi	Medial margin of orbit	Skin around eyelids	Closes eye
SCALP			
Frontalis	Epicranial aponeurosis	Skin of eyebrow and bridge of nose	Raises eyebrows, wrinkles forehead
Occipitalis	Occipital bone	Epicranial aponeurosis	Tenses and retracts scalp
LOWER JAW			
Masseter	Zygomatic arch	Lateral surface of mandible	Elevates mandible
Temporalis	Along temporal lines of skull	Coronoid process of mandible	Elevates mandible
Pterygoids	Inferior processes of sphenoid	Medial surface of mandible	Elevate, protract, and/or move mandible to either side
NECK			
Platysma	From cartilage of second rib to acromion of scapula	Mandible and skin of cheek	Tenses skin of neck, depresses mandible
Digastric	Mastoid region of temporal bone and inferior surface of mandible	Hyoid bone	Depresses mandible and/or elevates larynx
Mylohyoid	Medial surface of mandible	Median connective tissue band that runs to hyoid bone	Elevates floor of mouth and hyoid, and/or depresses mandible
Omohyoid	Superior border of scapula	Hyoid bone	Depresses hyoid bone and larynx
Sternohyoid	Clavicle and sternum	Hyoid bone	Depresses hyoid bone and larynx
Sternothyroid	Dorsal surface of sternum and 1st rib	Thyroid cartilage of larynx	Depresses hyoid bone and larynx
Stylohyoid	Styloid process of temporal bone	Hyoid bone	Elevates larynx
Sternocleidomastoid	Superior margins of sternum and clavicle	Mastoid region of skull	Both sides together flex the neck; one side alone bends head toward shoulder and turns face to opposite side

CLINICAL NOTE

Spasmodic Torticollis

Spasmodic torticollis is an intermittent or continuous spasm of the muscles of the neck, most commonly the *sternocleidomastoid* and *trapezius* muscles. It is usually more pronounced on one side, which results in turning or tipping of the head toward the affected muscles. Torticollis is involuntary and cannot be inhibited. It tends to be worse when the patient sits, stands, or walks. Torticollis affects women twice as often as men.

Torticollis should not be confused with a cervical muscle strain or spasm. Torticollis belongs to a class of diseases referred to as focal dystonias. Dystonias are an abnormal state of muscle tone. Focal dystonias affect a single area of the body. They occur more frequently in adults than in children, remain stable, and rarely spread to other body parts. Spasmodic torticollis is the most common focal dystonia. It is always important to exclude an extrapyramidal system reaction as a cause of spasmodic torticollis. Many of the antipsychotic drugs can cause focal dystonias, including torticollis, especially when administered in higher doses.

A simple neck muscle spasm, generally referred to as a "crick in the neck," often results from overuse, awkward positioning, or sleeping in an unusual position. The spasm can be quite intense and painful and can last for several days. The initial "injury" can slightly tear or stretch the affected muscle and cause pain and spasm. Most cases respond to local ice or heat, immobilization, and anti-inflammatory drugs. In severe cases, narcotics may be required for pain control, and intravenous diazepam (Valium) may be needed to help alleviate the muscle spasm.

Muscles of the Spine

The muscles of the spine are covered by more superficial back muscles, such as the trapezius and latissimus dorsi (**Figure 7-12b**). The most superior of the spinal muscles are the posterior neck muscles: the superficial **splenius capitis** and the deeper **semispinalis capitis** (**Figure 7-15** and **Table 7-4**). When the left and right pairs of these muscles contract together, they assist each other in extending the head. When both contract on one side, they assist in tilting the head. Due to its more lateral insertion, contraction of the splenius capitis also acts to rotate the head.

The *spinal extensors*, or **erector spinae**, act to maintain an erect spinal column and head. Moving laterally from the spine, these muscles can be subdivided into **spinalis**, **longissimus**, and **iliocostalis** divisions. In the lower lumbar and sacral regions, the border between the longissimus and iliocostalis muscles is indistinct, and they are sometimes known as the *sacrospinalis* muscles. When contracting together, these muscles extend the spinal column. When only the muscles on one side contract, the spine is bent laterally (lateral flexion). Deep to the spinalis muscles, smaller muscles interconnect and stabilize the vertebrae. In the lumbar region, the large **quadratus lumborum** muscles flex the spinal column and depress the ribs.

The extensor muscles of the vertebral column outnumber its flexor muscles. Fewer flexor muscles are needed because many large trunk muscles flex the vertebral column. Also, most of the body weight lies anterior to the vertebral column, so gravity tends to flex the spine.

Figure 7-15 Muscles of the Spine.

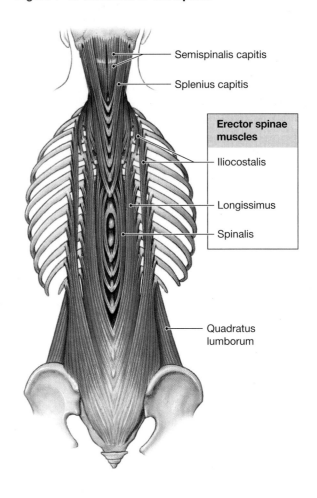

Semispinalis capitis

Splenius capitis

Erector spinae muscles

Iliocostalis

Longissimus

Spinalis

Quadratus lumborum

Table 7-4	Muscles of the Spine		
Region/Muscle	**Origin**	**Insertion**	**Action**
SPINAL EXTENSORS			
Splenius capitis	Spinous processes of lower cervical and upper thoracic vertebrae	Mastoid process, base of the skull, and upper cervical vertebrae	The two sides act together to extend the neck; either alone rotates and laterally flexes head to that side
Semispinalis capitis	Spinous processes of lower cervical and upper thoracic vertebrae	Base of skull, upper cervical vertebrae	The two sides act together to extend the neck; either alone laterally flexes head to that side
Spinalis group	Spinous processes and transverse processes of cervical, thoracic, and upper lumbar vertebrae	Base of skull and spinous processes of cervical and upper thoracic vertebrae	The two sides act together to extend vertebral column; either alone extends neck and laterally flexes head or rotates vertebral column to that side
Longissimus group	Processes of lower cervical, thoracic, and upper lumbar vertebrae	Mastoid process of temporal bone, transverse process of cervical vertebrae, and inferior surfaces of ribs	The two sides act together to extend vertebral column; either alone rotates and laterally flexes head or vertebral column to that side
Iliocostalis group	Superior borders of ribs and iliac crest	Transverse processes of cervical vertebrae and inferior surfaces of ribs	Extends vertebral column or moves laterally to that side; moves ribs
SPINAL FLEXOR			
Quadratus lumborum	Iliac crest	Last rib and transverse processes of lumbar vertebrae	Together they depress ribs, flex vertebral column; one side acting alone produces lateral flexion

CLINICAL NOTE

Hernias

Contraction of the abdominal muscles can significantly increase the pressure within the abdominal cavity. During forceful exercise or lifting, the pressures within the abdominopelvic cavity can increase even more. If a weakness exists in the wall of the abdominal cavity, this increased pressure can force a portion of a visceral organ into the weakened area. The presence of a visceral organ in a weakened area of the abdominal wall is referred to as a *hernia.* Hernias can develop virtually anywhere in the abdominal wall. However, the inguinal region is particularly vulnerable to hernia development.

During development of the male, the testes descend from the abdominal cavity into the scrotum. They pass through the abdominal wall at the inguinal canals and carry remnants of the abdominal wall and membranes with them. In the adult male, the spermatic ducts and associated blood vessels penetrate the abdominal wall at the inguinal canals on their way to the testicles. The inguinal canal is weaker than other portions of the muscular abdominal wall. With age and increased intra-abdominal pressure, the inguinal canal slowly enlarges. On occasion, the inguinal canal enlarges and allows some of the abdominal contents, usually a portion of the small intestine, to enter. The presence of abdominal viscera in the inguinal canal is referred to as an *inguinal hernia.* Usually, the affected small intestine is forced into the canal when pressure within the abdomen increases; it returns to the abdomen when pressure is relieved. If the affected portion of the hernial site becomes trapped, and cannot return to the abdominal cavity, the hernia is said to be *incarcerated.* If blood supply to the hernia is compromised, the hernia is said to be *strangulated.* Emergency surgery is necessary to remove the hernia sac from the inguinal canal before bowel ischemia and necrosis occurs (**Figure 7-16**).

In addition to inguinal hernias, several other types of hernias can occur. Patients who have had abdominal surgery may have a weakness in the abdominal wall along the scar of the incision. When intra-abdominal pressure increases, a visceral organ can be forced through this weakness to form an *incisional hernia.* This situation is more common in obese patients. Often, a piece of surgical mesh must be placed in the abdominal wall in order to prevent hernia formation. Females tend to develop *femoral hernias,* which develop in the femoral ring underneath the inguinal ligament. The incidence of femoral hernias is much lower than that of inguinal hernias.

A weakness in the diaphragm can result in some of the abdominal contents being forced into the chest cavity. A *hiatal hernia* is common. In these, the proximal portion of the stomach is forced upward through the esophageal hiatus (the point where the esophagus enters the abdomen). Hiatal hernias are usually managed with diet, weight loss, and medication. Surgery is rarely indicated.

Figure 7-16 Inguinal Hernia. An inguinal hernia occurs when a loop of abdominal viscera, usually the small intestine, enters a weakened and dilated inguinal canal. In severe cases, the loop of small intestine can be entrapped within the canal, often cutting off the blood supply. This situation, referred to as a strangulated inguinal hernia, is a surgical emergency.

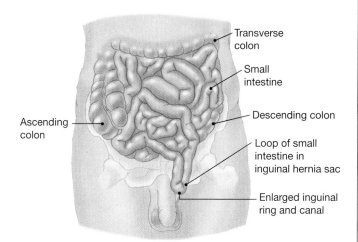

Transverse colon

Small intestine

Descending colon

Loop of small intestine in inguinal hernia sac

Enlarged inguinal ring and canal

Ascending colon

CLINICAL NOTE

Musculoskeletal Back Disorders

Back pain is one of the most common complaints encountered in modern emergency medical practice. In fact, low back pain is secondary only to the common cold as a cause of missed time from work. It is also the primary cause of reduced work capacity. Between 60 and 90 percent of the population will experience back pain in their lifetime. Emergency medical services (EMS) is a physically demanding occupation (**Figure 7-17**). EMS personnel are particularly vulnerable to back injury and should take precautions to minimize the chances of injury. This includes proper lifting techniques and requesting assistance when needed (**Figures 7-17** to **7-19**).

There are numerous causes of back pain, which range from a simple muscle strain to a ruptured aortic aneurysm. Back strains usually occur when an abnormal or exaggerated movement stretches or tears a muscle or group of muscles in the back (**Figure 7-18**). Carrying heavy loads can also stress or tear back muscles and result in a strain. Back strains, especially those that involve a group of muscles, initially causes localized bleeding at the injury site. This is followed by the formation of a hematoma. Hematoma formation is often accompanied by pain. Often, the

(*Continued*)

Figure 7-17 Physical Demands of EMS. Lifting and moving patients and equipment can cause low back injury if not performed correctly.

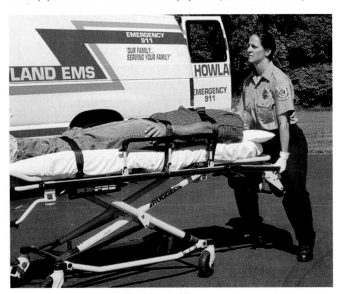

Figure 7-18 Proper Lifting Technique. By lifting with the legs, the large paraspinous muscles of the back are not overstressed.

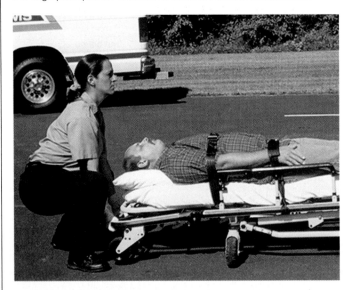

affected muscles, and other muscles in the area, will spasm. This causes increased irritation of the previously injured muscle and increased pain. Occasionally, the spasm can be so severe that

Figure 7-19 Lifting in Unison. Back strains in EMS personnel usually occur when a team member moves awkwardly during a lift. Twisting, turning, or other movements can place stress on the large back muscles and result in back strain.

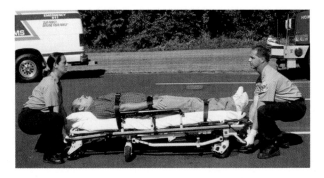

pressure is placed on nerve roots that exit the spine at each level. Irritation of the nerve roots can cause pain along the distribution of the affected spinal nerve.

There are three layers of muscles along the spine, collectively referred to as the *paraspinous muscles*. The superficial layer, which consists of the *spinalis*, the *longissimus*, and the *iliocostalis*, is palpable during physical examination. Tenderness or spasm can usually be palpated. Occasionally, spasm is limited to one side and an obvious lateral curvature of the spine can be seen.

A lumbar muscle strain can be quite painful. It is not uncommon for these patients to be in such severe pain that they must be medicated before they can lie down on the ambulance stretcher for transport. The definitive treatment of a lumbar strain is to rest the affected muscles and minimize inflammation. Initially, this should include the application of ice and rest. Later, moist heat can be applied to the affected muscles. Anti-inflammatory medications are also helpful. Moderate to severe pain may require a short course of narcotic pain medicine. Muscle relaxant medications are somewhat controversial. Their effectiveness in the treatment of lumbar muscle strains varies significantly from patient to patient. Most of the muscle relaxants have sedating side effects that may help a patient to sleep. The application of physical therapy modalities, osteopathic manipulation, or chiropractic adjustment can sometimes help to alleviate acute pain and shorten the recovery period.

The Axial Muscles of the Trunk

The *oblique muscles* and the *rectus muscles* form the muscular walls of the thoracic and abdominopelvic cavities between the first thoracic vertebra and the pelvis. In the thoracic area, these muscles are partitioned by the ribs, but over the abdominal surface they form broad muscular sheets (**Figure 7-20** and **Table 7-5**). The oblique muscles can compress underlying structures or rotate the spinal column,

depending on whether one or both sides are contracting. The rectus muscles are important flexors of the spinal column; they oppose the erector spinae.

The axial muscles of the trunk include (1) the **external** and **internal intercostals**, (2) the muscular **diaphragm** that separates the thoracic and abdominopelvic cavities, (3) the **external** and **internal obliques**, (4) the **transversus abdominis**, (5) the **rectus abdominis**, and (6) the muscles that form the floor of the pelvic cavity.

Figure 7-20 Oblique and Rectus Muscles and the Diaphragm.

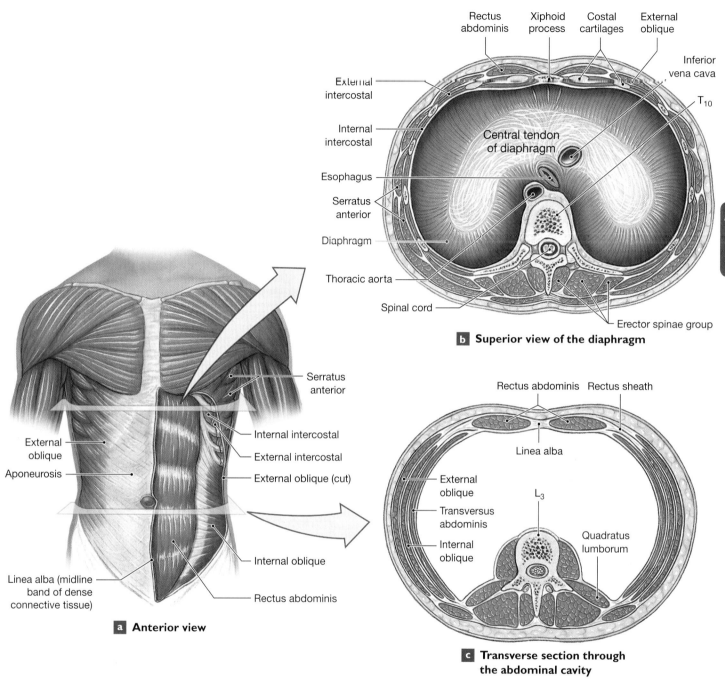

b **Superior view of the diaphragm**

a **Anterior view**

c **Transverse section through the abdominal cavity**

Build Your Knowledge

The pelvic cavity lies inferior to the abdominal cavity (as you saw in **Chapter 1: An Introduction to Anatomy and Physiology**). It contains the urinary bladder, various reproductive organs, and the distal portion of the large intestine. ⮌ **p. 18**

Muscles of the Pelvic Floor

The floor of the pelvic cavity is called the **perineum** (**Figure 7-21** and **Table 7-6**). It is formed by a broad sheet of muscles that connects the sacrum and coccyx to the ischium and pubis. These muscles support the organs of the pelvic cavity, flex the coccyx, and control the movement of materials through the urethra and anus.

Table 7-5	Axial Muscles of the Trunk		
Region/Muscle	Origin	Insertion	Action
THORACIC REGION			
External intercostals	Inferior border of each rib	Superior border of next rib	Elevate ribs
Internal intercostals	Superior border of each rib	Inferior border of the preceding rib	Depress ribs
Diaphragm	Xiphoid process, cartilages of ribs 4–10, and anterior surfaces of lumbar vertebrae	Central tendinous sheet	Contraction expands thoracic cavity, compresses abdominopelvic cavity
ABDOMINAL REGION			
External oblique	Lower eight ribs	Linea alba and iliac crest	Compresses abdomen, depresses ribs, flexes or laterally flexes vertebral column
Internal oblique	Iliac crest and adjacent connective tissues	Lower ribs, xiphoid of sternum, and linea alba	Compresses abdomen, depresses ribs, flexes or laterally flexes vertebral column
Transversus abdominis	Cartilages of lower ribs, iliac crest, and adjacent connective tissues	Linea alba and pubis	Compresses abdomen
Rectus abdominis	Superior surface of pubis around symphysis	Inferior surfaces of costal cartilages (ribs 5–7) and xiphoid process	Depresses ribs, flexes vertebral column

CHECKPOINT

25. If you were contracting and relaxing your masseter muscle, what would you probably be doing?

26. Which facial muscle would you expect to be well developed in a trumpet player?

27. Damage to the external intercostal muscles would interfere with what important process?

28. If someone were to hit you in your rectus abdominis muscle, how would your body position change?

See the blue Answers tab at the back of the book.

Table 7-6	Muscles of the Pelvic Floor		
Muscle	Origin	Insertion	Action
SUPERFICIAL MUSCLES			
Bulbospongiosus			
Males	Base of penis; fibers cross over urethra	Midline and central tendon of perineum	Compresses base and stiffens penis; ejects urine or semen
Females	Base of clitoris; fibers run on either side of urethral and vaginal openings	Central tendon of perineum	Compresses and stiffens clitoris; narrows vaginal opening
Ischiocavernosus	Inferior medial surface of ischium	Symphysis pubis anterior to base of penis or clitoris	Compresses and stiffens penis or clitoris
Transverse perineal	Inferior medial surface of ischium	Central tendon of perineum	Stabilizes central tendon of perineum
DEEP MUSCLES			
External Urethral Sphincter			
Males	Inferior medial surfaces of ischium and pubis	Midline at base of penis; inner fibers encircle urethra	Closes urethra, compresses prostate and bulbo-urethral glands
Females	Inferior medial surfaces of ischium and pubis	Midline; inner fibers encircle urethra	Closes urethra, compresses vagina and greater vestibular glands
External anal sphincter	By tendon from coccyx	Encircles anal opening	Closes anal opening
Levator ani	Ischial spine, pubis	Coccyx	Tenses floor of pelvis, supports pelvic organs, flexes coccyx, elevates and retracts anus

Figure 7-21 Muscles of the Pelvic Floor.

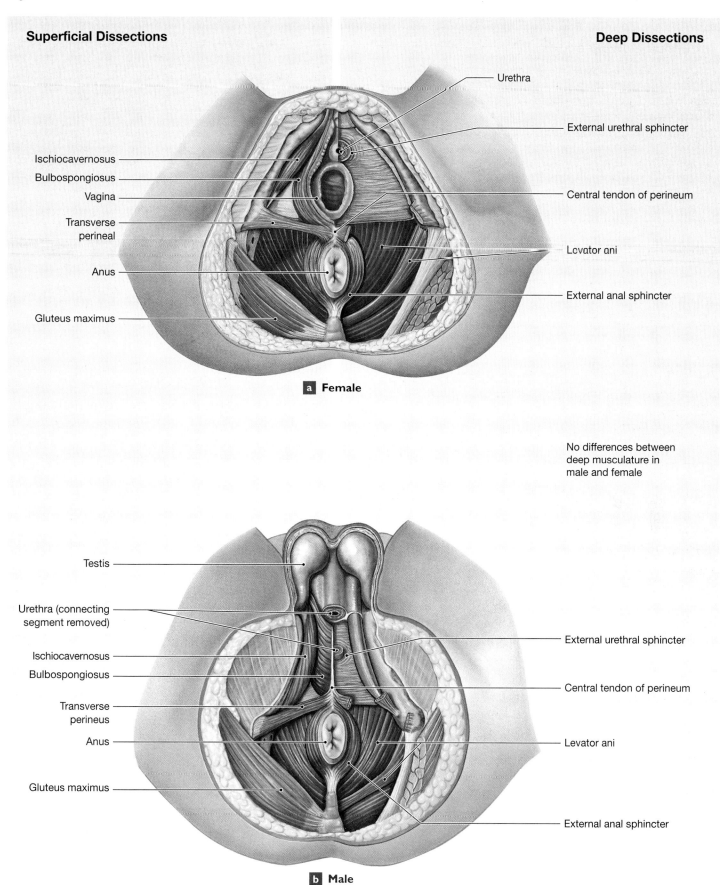

Superficial Dissections — Deep Dissections

a Female

No differences between deep musculature in male and female

b Male

CLINICAL NOTE

Intramuscular Injections

Drugs are commonly injected into tissues rather than directly into the bloodstream. This method makes it possible to introduce a large amount of a drug at one treatment, yet have it enter the circulation gradually. An intramuscular (IM) injection introduces the drug into the mass of a large skeletal muscle. Uptake is usually faster and accompanied by less tissue irritation than when drugs are administered *intradermally* or *subcutaneously* (injected into the dermis or subcutaneous layer, respectively). ↻ p. 129 Up to 5 mL of fluid may be injected at one time, and multiple injections are possible.

The most common complications involve accidental injection into a blood vessel or the piercing of a nerve. The sudden entry of massive quantities of a drug into the bloodstream can have unpleasant or even fatal effects. Damage to a nerve can cause motor paralysis or sensory loss. For these reasons, the injection site must be selected with care.

Bulky muscles that contain few large vessels or nerves make ideal injection sites. The gluteus medius or the posterior, lateral, superior portion of the gluteus maximus is often selected. The deltoid muscle of the arm, about 2.5 cm (1 in.) distal to the acromion, is another common site.

Probably the most satisfactory site from a technical point of view is the vastus lateralis of the thigh. An injection into this thick muscle will not encounter vessels or nerves. This injection site is preferred in infants and young children, who have relatively small gluteal and deltoid muscles. This site is also used in elderly patients or others with atrophied gluteal and deltoid muscles.

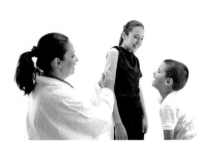

7-11 Appendicular muscles are muscles of the shoulders, upper limbs, pelvic girdle, and lower limbs

Learning Objective Identify the main appendicular muscles of the body and their origins, insertions, and actions.

The appendicular musculature includes (1) the muscles of the shoulders and upper limbs and (2) the muscles of the pelvic girdle and lower limbs. The two groups have very different functions and ranges of motion. The muscular connections between the pectoral girdle and the axial skeleton increase the mobility of the upper limb and must also act as shock absorbers. For example, people can still perform delicate hand movements while jogging. The reason is that the muscular connections between the axial and appendicular skeleton smooth out the bounces in their stride. In contrast, the pelvic girdle has evolved to transfer weight from the axial to the appendicular skeleton. A muscular connection would reduce the efficiency of the transfer, and the emphasis is on sheer power rather than mobility.

Muscles of the Shoulders and Upper Limbs

Muscles that Position the Pectoral Girdle

The large, superficial **trapezius** muscles cover the back and portions of the neck, reaching to the base of the skull. These muscles form a broad diamond (**Figure 7-22a** and **Table 7-7**). Its actions are quite varied because specific regions can be made to contract independently. The **rhomboid** muscles

and the **levator scapulae** are covered by the trapezius. Both originate on vertebrae and insert on the scapula. Contraction of the rhomboids adducts (retracts) the scapula, pulling it toward the center of the back. The levator scapulae elevates the scapula, as when you shrug your shoulders.

On the chest, the **serratus anterior** originates along the anterior surfaces of several ribs (**Figure 7-22b**) and inserts along the vertebral border of the scapula. When the serratus anterior contracts, it abducts (protracts) the scapula and swings the shoulder anteriorly. The **pectoralis minor** attaches to the coracoid process of the scapula. The **subclavius** (sub-KLĀ-vē-us; *sub*, below + *clavius*, clavicle) inserts on the inferior border of the clavicle. The contraction of each of these muscles depresses and protracts the scapula.

Muscles that Move the Arm

The muscles that move the arm (**Figure 7-23** and **Table 7-8**) are easiest to remember when grouped by primary actions:

- The **deltoid** is the major abductor of the arm, and the **supraspinatus** assists at the start of this movement.

- The **subscapularis**, **teres major**, **infraspinatus**, and **teres minor** rotate the arm.

- The **pectoralis major**, which extends between the chest and the greater tubercle of the humerus, produces flexion at the shoulder joint. The **latissimus dorsi**, which extends between the thoracic vertebrae and the intertubercular groove of the humerus, produces extension. The two muscles also work together to produce adduction and rotation of the humerus.

Figure 7-22 **Muscles that Position the Pectoral Girdle.**

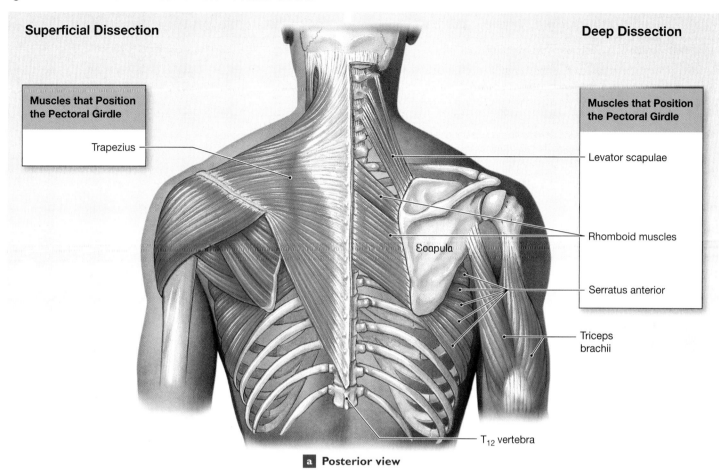

Superficial Dissection

Deep Dissection

Muscles that Position the Pectoral Girdle

Trapezius

Muscles that Position the Pectoral Girdle

Levator scapulae

Rhomboid muscles

Scapula

Serratus anterior

Triceps brachii

T$_{12}$ vertebra

a **Posterior view**

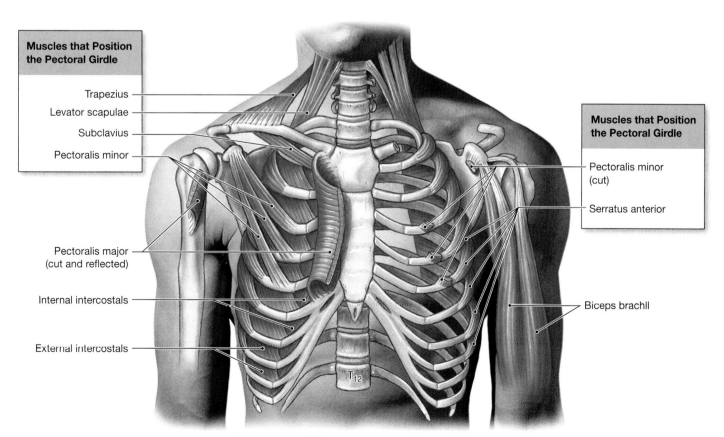

Muscles that Position the Pectoral Girdle

Trapezius

Levator scapulae

Subclavius

Pectoralis minor

Pectoralis major (cut and reflected)

Internal intercostals

External intercostals

T$_{12}$

Muscles that Position the Pectoral Girdle

Pectoralis minor (cut)

Serratus anterior

Biceps brachii

b **Anterior view**

Table 7-7	Muscles that Position the Pectoral Girdle		
Muscle	**Origin**	**Insertion**	**Action**
Levator scapulae	Transverse processes of first 4 cervical vertebrae	Vertebral border of scapula	Elevates scapula
Pectoralis minor	Anterior surfaces of ribs 3–5	Coracoid process of scapula	Depresses and abducts (protracts) shoulder; rotates scapula laterally (downward); elevates ribs if scapula is stationary
Rhomboid muscles	Spinous processes of lower cervical and upper thoracic vertebrae	Vertebral border of scapula	Adducts (retracts) and rotates scapula laterally (downward)
Serratus anterior	Anterior and superior margins of ribs 1–9	Anterior surface of vertebral border of scapula	Protracts shoulder, abducts and medially rotates scapula (upward)
Subclavius	First rib	Clavicle	Depresses and protracts shoulder
Trapezius	Occipital bone and spinous processes of thoracic vertebrae	Clavicle and scapula (acromion and scapular spine)	Depends on active region and state of other muscles; may elevate, adduct, depress, or rotate scapula and/or elevate clavicle; can also extend or hyperextend neck

These muscles provide substantial support for the shoulder joint. The tendons of the supraspinatus, infraspinatus, teres minor, and subscapularis blend with and support the capsular fibers that enclose the shoulder joint. They are the muscles of the *rotator cuff*, a common site of sports injuries. Sports that involve throwing a ball, such as a baseball or football, place considerable strain on the muscles of the rotator cuff. A **muscle strain** (a tear or break in the muscle), *bursitis*, and other painful injuries can result.

Muscles that Move the Forearm and Wrist

Most of the muscles that insert on the forearm and wrist (**Figure 7-24** and **Table 7-9**) originate on the humerus, but there are two notable exceptions. The **biceps brachii** and the *long head* tendon of the **triceps brachii** originate on the scapula and insert on the bones of the forearm. Their primary actions are at the elbow, although their contractions can have a secondary effect on the shoulder. The triceps brachii

Table 7-8	Muscles that Move the Arm		
Muscle	**Origin**	**Insertion**	**Action**
Coracobrachialis	Coracoid process of scapula	Medial margin of shaft of humerus	Adduction and flexion at shoulder
Deltoid	Clavicle and scapula (acromion and adjacent scapular spine)	Deltoid tuberosity of humerus	Abduction at shoulder
Latissimus dorsi	Spinous processes of lower thoracic vertebrae, ribs, and lumbar vertebrae	Intertubercular groove of humerus	Extension, adduction, and medial rotation at shoulder
Pectoralis major	Cartilages of ribs 2–6, body of sternum, and clavicle	Greater tubercle of humerus	Flexion, adduction, and medial rotation at shoulder
Supraspinatus*	Supraspinous fossa of scapula	Greater tubercle of humerus	Abduction at shoulder
Infraspinatus*	Infraspinous fossa of scapula	Greater tubercle of humerus	Lateral rotation at shoulder
Subscapularis*	Subscapular fossa of scapula	Lesser tubercle of humerus	Medial rotation at shoulder
Teres minor*	Lateral border of scapula	Greater tubercle of humerus	Lateral rotation at shoulder
Teres major	Inferior angle of scapula	Intertubercular groove of humerus	Adduction and medial rotation at shoulder

*Rotator cuff muscles

Figure 7-23 Muscles that Move the Arm. The four muscles of the rotator cuff are marked by an asterisk (*).

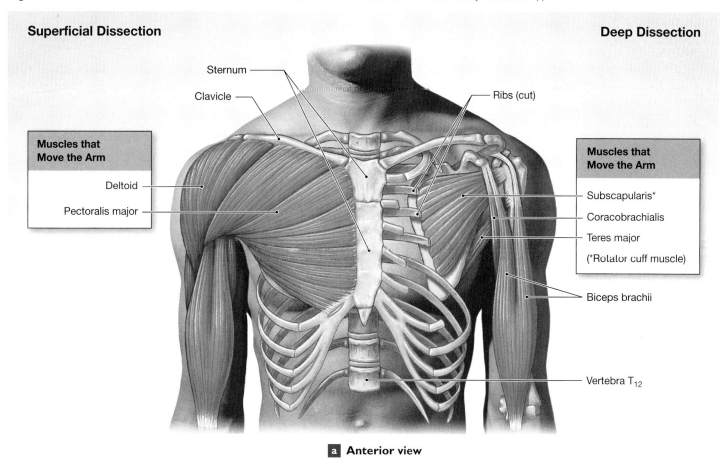

Superficial Dissection

Deep Dissection

Sternum
Clavicle
Ribs (cut)

Muscles that Move the Arm

Deltoid
Pectoralis major

Muscles that Move the Arm

Subscapularis*
Coracobrachialis
Teres major
(*Rotator cuff muscle)

Biceps brachii

Vertebra T_{12}

a **Anterior view**

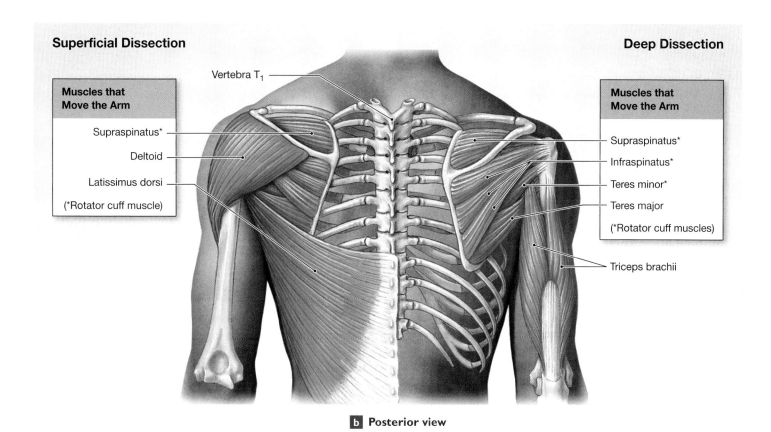

Superficial Dissection

Deep Dissection

Vertebra T_1

Muscles that Move the Arm

Supraspinatus*
Deltoid
Latissimus dorsi
(*Rotator cuff muscle)

Muscles that Move the Arm

Supraspinatus*
Infraspinatus*
Teres minor*
Teres major
(*Rotator cuff muscles)

Triceps brachii

b **Posterior view**

Figure 7-24 Muscles that Move the Forearm and Wrist.

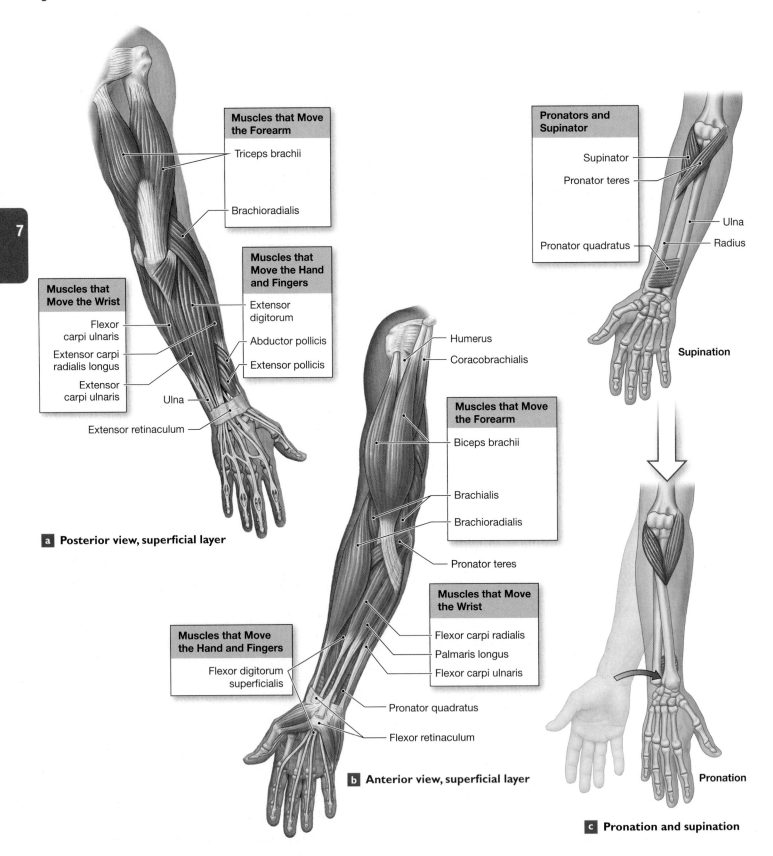

Muscles that Move the Forearm

Triceps brachii

Brachioradialis

Muscles that Move the Wrist

Flexor carpi ulnaris

Extensor carpi radialis longus

Extensor carpi ulnaris

Ulna

Extensor retinaculum

Muscles that Move the Hand and Fingers

Extensor digitorum

Abductor pollicis

Extensor pollicis

a **Posterior view, superficial layer**

Humerus

Coracobrachialis

Muscles that Move the Forearm

Biceps brachii

Brachialis

Brachioradialis

Pronator teres

Muscles that Move the Wrist

Flexor carpi radialis

Palmaris longus

Flexor carpi ulnaris

Muscles that Move the Hand and Fingers

Flexor digitorum superficialis

Pronator quadratus

Flexor retinaculum

b **Anterior view, superficial layer**

Pronators and Supinator

Supinator

Pronator teres

Pronator quadratus

Ulna

Radius

Supination

Pronation

c **Pronation and supination**

Table 7-9	Muscles that Move the Forearm, Wrist, and Hand		
Muscle	**Origin**	**Insertion**	**Action**
ACTION AT THE ELBOW			
Flexors			
Biceps brachii	*Short head* from the coracoid process and *long head* from the supraglenoid tubercle (both on the scapula)	Tuberosity of radius	Flexion at shoulder and elbow; supination
Brachialis	Anterior, distal surface of humerus	Tuberosity of ulna	Flexion at elbow
Brachioradialis	Lateral epicondyle of humerus	Styloid process of radius	Flexion at elbow
Extensors			
Triceps brachii	Superior, posterior, and lateral margins of humerus, and the scapula	Olecranon of ulna	Extension at elbow
PRONATORS/SUPINATOR			
Pronator quadratus	Medial surface of distal portion of ulna	Anterior and lateral surface of distal portion of radius	Pronation
Pronator teres	Medial epicondyle of humerus and coronoid process of ulna	Distal lateral surface of radius	Pronation
Supinator	Lateral epicondyle of humerus and ulna	Anterior and lateral surface of radius distal to the radial tuberosity	Supination
ACTION AT THE WRIST			
Flexors			
Flexor carpi radialis	Medial epicondyle of humerus	Bases of second and third metacarpal bones	Flexion and abduction at wrist
Flexor carpi ulnaris	Medial epicondyle of humerus and adjacent surfaces of ulna	Pisiform bone, hamate bone, and base of fifth metacarpal bone	Flexion and adduction at wrist
Palmaris longus	Medial epicondyle of humerus	A tendinous sheet on the palm	Flexion at wrist
Extensors			
Extensor carpi radialis	Distal lateral surface and lateral epicondyle of humerus	Bases of second and third metacarpal bones	Extension and abduction at wrist
Extensor carpi ulnaris	Lateral epicondyle of humerus and adjacent surface of ulna	Base of fifth metacarpal bone	Extension and adduction at wrist
ACTION AT THE HAND			
Extensor digitorum	Lateral epicondyle of humerus	Posterior surfaces of the phalanges, fingers 2–5	Extension at finger joints and wrist
Flexor digitorum	Medial epicondyle of humerus; anterior surfaces of ulna and radius; medial and posterior surfaces of ulna	Distal phalanges of fingers 2–5	Flexion at finger joints and wrist
Abductor pollicis	Proximal dorsal surfaces of ulna and radius	Lateral margin of 1st metacarpal bone	Abduction at thumb joints and wrist
Extensor pollicis	Distal shaft of radius and the interosseus membrane	Base of phalanges of the thumb	Extension at thumb joints; abduction at wrist

extends the elbow when, for example, you do pushups. The biceps brachii both flexes the elbow and supinates the forearm. With the forearm pronated (palm facing back), the biceps brachii cannot function effectively. As a result, you are strongest when you flex your elbow with a supinated forearm. You will see that the biceps brachii then makes a prominent bulge.

Other important muscles include the following:

- The **brachialis** and **brachioradialis** also flex the elbow, opposed by the triceps brachii.
- The **flexor carpi radialis**, the **flexor carpi ulnaris**, and the **palmaris longus** are superficial muscles that

work together to produce flexion of the wrist. Because they originate on opposite sides of the humerus, the flexor carpi radialis flexes and abducts the wrist, whereas the flexor carpi ulnaris flexes and adducts the wrist.

- The **extensor carpi radialis** muscles and the **extensor carpi ulnaris** have a similar relationship. The former produces extension and abduction at the wrist. The latter produces extension and adduction.

- The **pronators** and the **supinator** rotate the radius at its proximal and distal articulations with the ulna. They do not flex or extend the elbow.

Muscles that Move the Hand and Fingers

The muscles of the forearm flex and extend the finger joints (**Table 7-9**). These muscles end before reaching the hand, and only their tendons cross the wrist. These are relatively large muscles, and keeping them clear of the joints ensures maximum mobility at both the wrist and hand. Wide bands of connective tissue cross the posterior and anterior surfaces of the wrist. The *extensor retinaculum* (ret-i-NAK-ū-lum; plural, *retinacula*) holds the tendons of the extensor muscles in place. The *flexor retinaculum* does the same for the flexor muscles. Both groups of tendons pass through *synovial tendon sheaths*, wide tubular bursae that reduce friction. ↪ p. 175

Inflammation of the retinacula and synovial tendon sheaths can restrict movement and irritate the *median nerve*, a nerve that innervates the palm of the hand. Chronic pain, often associated with weakness in the hand muscles, is the result. This condition is known as **carpal tunnel syndrome**. A common cause is repetitive hand or wrist movements. Fine control of the hand involves small *intrinsic muscles*, which originate on the carpal and metacarpal bones. No muscles originate on the phalanges, and only tendons extend across the distal joints of the fingers.

CHECKPOINT

29. Which muscle do you use to shrug your shoulders?

30. Sometimes baseball pitchers suffer rotator cuff injuries. Which muscles are involved in this type of injury?

31. Injury to the flexor carpi ulnaris would impair which two movements?

See the blue Answers tab at the back of the book.

Muscles of the Pelvis and Lower Limbs

The muscles of the pelvis and the lower limb can be divided into three functional groups: (1) muscles that work across the hip joint to move the thigh; (2) muscles that work across the knee joint to move the leg; and (3) muscles that work across the various joints of the foot to move the ankles, feet, and toes.

Muscles that Move the Thigh

The muscles that move the thigh are detailed in **Figure 7-25** and **Table 7-10**.

- **Gluteal muscles** cover the lateral surfaces of the ilia (**Figure 7-25a,b**). The **gluteus maximus** is the largest and most posterior of the gluteal muscles. They produce extension, rotation, and abduction at the hip joint.

- The adductors of the thigh include the **adductor magnus**, the **adductor brevis**, the **adductor longus**, the **pectineus** (pek-ti-NĒ-us), and the **gracilis** (GRAS-i-lis) (**Figure 7-25c**). When an athlete suffers a *pulled groin*, the problem is a *strain*—a muscle tear—in one of these adductor muscles.

- The largest hip flexor is the **iliopsoas** (il-ē-ō-SŌ-us) muscle (**Figure 7-25c**). The iliopsoas is really two muscles, the **psoas major** and the **iliacus** (il-Ī-ah-kus). They share a common insertion at the lesser trochanter of the femur.

Muscles that Move the Leg

The pattern of muscle distribution in the lower limb is like that in the upper limb: Extensors are found along the anterior and lateral surfaces of the limb, and flexors lie along the posterior and medial surfaces (**Figure 7-26**).

- The flexors of the knee include three muscles collectively known as the *hamstrings*. They are the **biceps femoris** (FEM-or-is), the **semimembranosus** (sem-ē-mem-bra-NŌ-sus), and the **semitendinosus** (sem-ē-ten-di-NŌ-sus)—and the **sartorius** (sar-TŌR-ē-us) (**Figure 7-26a**). The sartorius muscle crosses both the hip and knee joints. It produces flexion at the knee and lateral rotation at the hip when you cross your legs. A *pulled hamstring* is a relatively common sports injury caused by a strain affecting one of the hamstring muscles.

- Collectively the *knee extensors* are known as the **quadriceps femoris**. The three **vastus** muscles and

Figure 7-25 Muscles that Move the Thigh.

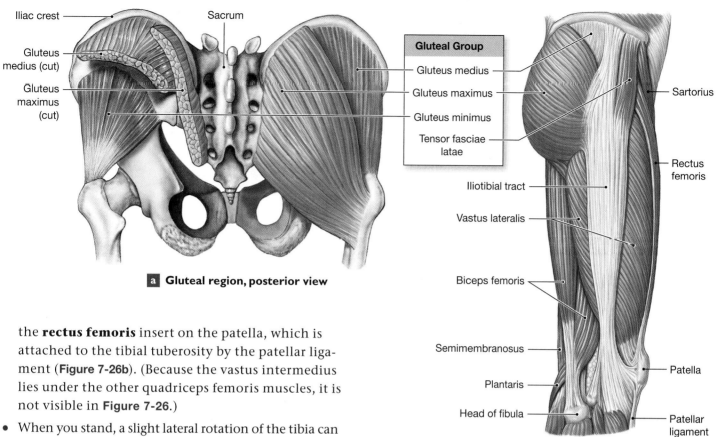

Iliac crest

Sacrum

Gluteus medius (cut)

Gluteus maximus (cut)

Gluteal Group
- Gluteus medius
- Gluteus maximus
- Gluteus minimus
- Tensor fasciae latae

Sartorius

Rectus femoris

Iliotibial tract

Vastus lateralis

Biceps femoris

Semimembranosus

Plantaris

Head of fibula

Patella

Patellar ligament

a **Gluteal region, posterior view**

b **Lateral view**

the **rectus femoris** insert on the patella, which is attached to the tibial tuberosity by the patellar ligament (**Figure 7-26b**). (Because the vastus intermedius lies under the other quadriceps femoris muscles, it is not visible in **Figure 7-26**.)

- When you stand, a slight lateral rotation of the tibia can lock the knee joint in the extended position. This enables you to stand for long periods with minimal muscular effort, but the locked knee cannot be flexed. The small **popliteus** (pop-LI-tē-us) muscle unlocks the joint by medially rotating the tibia back into its normal position (**Figure 7-26a**).

The muscles that move the leg are detailed in **Table 7-11**.

Muscles that Move the Foot and Toes

Muscles that move the foot and toes are shown in **Figure 7-27** (p. 260) and detailed in **Table 7-12** (p. 261). Most of the muscles that move the ankle produce the plantar flexion involved with walking and running movements.

- The large **gastrocnemius** (gas-trok-NĒ-mē-us; *gaster,* stomach + *kneme,* knee) of the calf is assisted by the underlying **soleus** (SŌ-lē-us) muscle. These muscles share a common tendon, the **calcaneal tendon,** or *Achilles tendon.*

- A pair of deep **fibularis** muscles, or *peroneus* muscles, produces eversion of the foot as well as extension (plantar flexion) at the ankle. A third fibularis muscle also everts the foot but produces flexion (dorsiflexion) at the ankle.

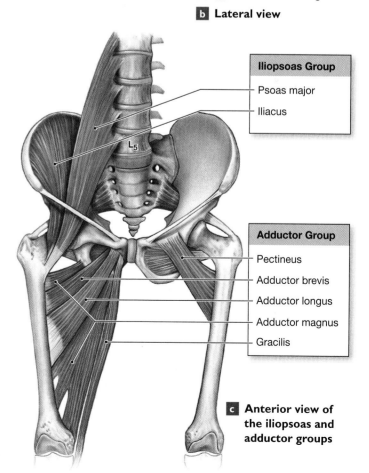

Iliopsoas Group
- Psoas major
- Iliacus

L$_5$

Adductor Group
- Pectineus
- Adductor brevis
- Adductor longus
- Adductor magnus
- Gracilis

c **Anterior view of the iliopsoas and adductor groups**

Table 7-10	Muscles that Move the Thigh		
Group/Muscle	**Origin**	**Insertion**	**Action**
GLUTEAL GROUP			
Gluteus maximus	Iliac crest of ilium, sacrum, and coccyx	Iliotibial tract and gluteal tuberosity of femur	Extension and lateral rotation at hip
Gluteus medius	Anterior iliac crest and lateral surface of ilium	Greater trochanter of femur	Abduction and medial rotation at hip
Gluteus minimus	Lateral surface of ilium	Greater trochanter of femur	Abduction and medial rotation at hip
Tensor fasciae latae	Iliac crest and surface of ilium between anterior iliac spines	Iliotibial tract	Flexion and medial rotation at hip; tenses fasciae latae, which laterally supports the knee
ADDUCTOR GROUP			
Adductor brevis	Inferior ramus of pubis	Linea aspera of femur	Adduction, flexion, and medial rotation at hip
Adductor longus	Inferior ramus of pubis anterior to adductor brevis	Linea aspera of femur	Adduction, flexion, and medial rotation at hip
Adductor magnus	Inferior ramus of pubis posterior to adductor brevis	Linea aspera of femur	Adduction at hip joint; superior portion produces flexion; inferior portion produces extension
Pectineus	Superior ramus of pubis	Inferior to lesser trochanter of femur	Adduction, flexion, and medial rotation at hip joint
Gracilis	Inferior ramus of pubis	Medial surface of tibia inferior to medial condyle	Flexion at knee; adduction and medial rotation at hip
ILIOPSOAS GROUP			
Iliacus	Medial surface of ilium	Femur distal to lesser trochanter; tendon fused with that of psoas major	Flexion at hip
Psoas major	Anterior surfaces and transverse processes of T_{12} and lumbar vertebrae	Lesser trochanter in company with iliacus	Flexion at hip or lumbar intervertebral joints

Table 7-11	Muscles that Move the Leg		
Muscle	**Origin**	**Insertion**	**Action**
FLEXORS			
Biceps femoris*	Ischial tuberosity and linea aspera of femur	Head of fibula, lateral condyle of tibia	Flexion at knee, extension and lateral rotation at hip
Semimembranosus*	Ischial tuberosity	Posterior surface of medial condyle of tibia	Flexion at knee; extension and medial rotation at hip
Semitendinosus*	Ischial tuberosity	Proximal medial surface of tibia	Flexion at knee; extension and medial rotation at hip
Sartorius	Anterior superior spine of ilium	Medial surface of tibia near tibial tuberosity	Flexion at knee; flexion and lateral rotation at hip
Popliteus	Lateral condyle of femur	Posterior surface of proximal tibial shaft	Rotates tibia medially (or rotates femur laterally); flexion at knee
EXTENSORS			
Rectus femoris	Anterior inferior iliac spine and superior acetabular rim of ilium	Tibial tuberosity by way of patellar ligament	Extension at knee, flexion at hip
Vastus intermedius	Anterior and lateral surface of femur along linea aspera	Tibial tuberosity by way of patellar ligament	Extension at knee
Vastus lateralis	Anterior and inferior to greater trochanter of femur and along linea aspera	Tibial tuberosity by way of patellar ligament	Extension at knee
Vastus medialis	Entire length of linea aspera of femur	Tibial tuberosity by way of patellar ligament	Extension at knee

*Hamstring muscles

Figure 7-26 Muscles that Move the Leg. The three muscles collectively referred to as the hamstrings are marked by an asterisk (*).

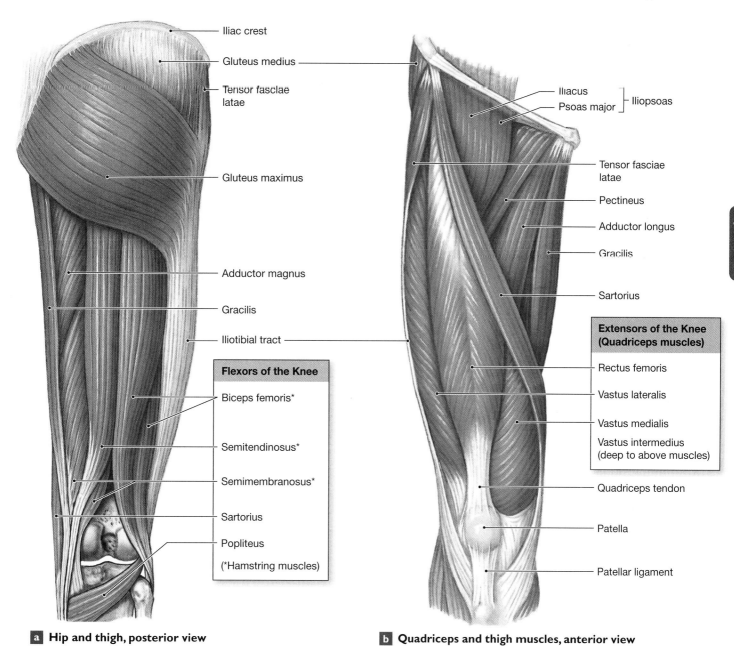

Flexors of the Knee

Biceps femoris*

Semitendinosus*

Semimembranosus*

Sartorius

Popliteus

(*Hamstring muscles)

Extensors of the Knee (Quadriceps muscles)

Rectus femoris

Vastus lateralis

Vastus medialis

Vastus intermedius (deep to above muscles)

a **Hip and thigh, posterior view**

b **Quadriceps and thigh muscles, anterior view**

- Inversion of the foot is caused by contraction of the **tibialis** (tib-ē-A-lis) muscles. The large **tibialis anterior** dorsiflexes the ankle and opposes the gastrocnemius.

Important digital muscles originate on the surface of the tibia, the fibula, or both. Their tendons are surrounded by synovial tendon sheaths at the ankle joint. The positions of these sheaths are stabilized by *retinacula*. Several smaller intrinsic muscles originate on the tarsal and metatarsal bones. Their contractions move the toes.

CHECKPOINT

32. You often hear of athletes suffering a "pulled hamstring." To what does this phrase refer?

33. How would a torn calcaneal tendon to affect movement of the foot?

34. Which three functional groups make up the muscles of the lower limbs?

35. Which muscle of the leg crosses both the hip and knee joints?

See the blue Answers tab at the back of the book.

Figure 7-27 Muscles that Move the Foot and Toes.

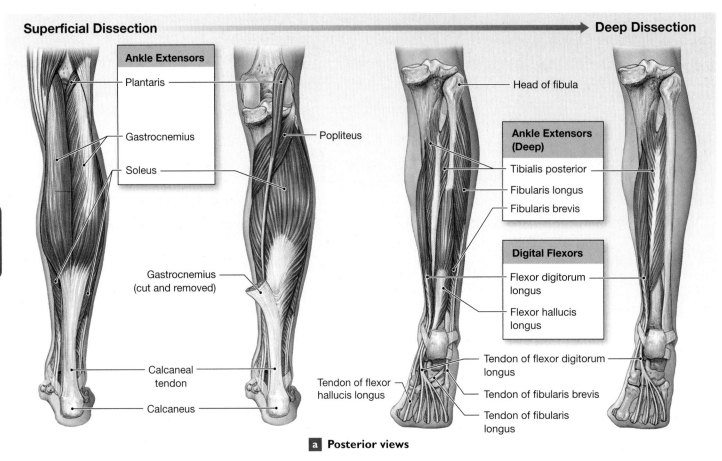

Superficial Dissection → **Deep Dissection**

Ankle Extensors
- Plantaris
- Gastrocnemius
- Soleus

Popliteus

Head of fibula

Ankle Extensors (Deep)
- Tibialis posterior
- Fibularis longus
- Fibularis brevis

Digital Flexors
- Flexor digitorum longus
- Flexor hallucis longus

Gastrocnemius (cut and removed)

Calcaneal tendon

Calcaneus

Tendon of flexor hallucis longus

Tendon of flexor digitorum longus

Tendon of fibularis brevis

Tendon of fibularis longus

a Posterior views

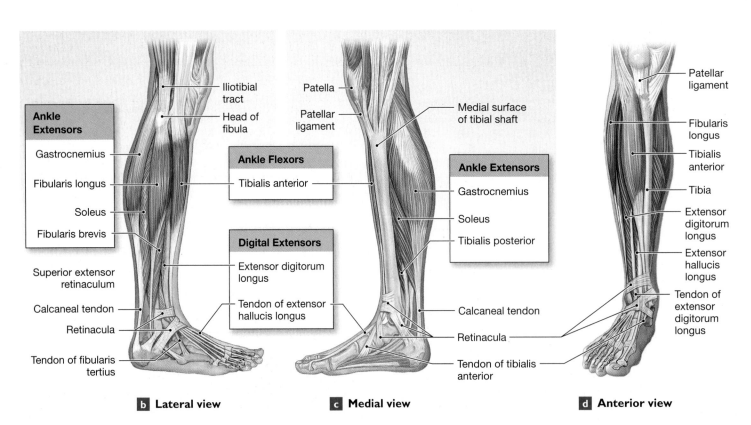

Ankle Extensors
- Gastrocnemius
- Fibularis longus
- Soleus
- Fibularis brevis

Superior extensor retinaculum

Calcaneal tendon

Retinacula

Tendon of fibularis tertius

Iliotibial tract

Head of fibula

Ankle Flexors
- Tibialis anterior

Digital Extensors
- Extensor digitorum longus
- Tendon of extensor hallucis longus

Patella

Patellar ligament

Medial surface of tibial shaft

Ankle Extensors
- Gastrocnemius
- Soleus
- Tibialis posterior

Calcaneal tendon

Retinacula

Tendon of tibialis anterior

Patellar ligament

Fibularis longus

Tibialis anterior

Tibia

Extensor digitorum longus

Extensor hallucis longus

Tendon of extensor digitorum longus

b Lateral view   **c** Medial view   **d** Anterior view

Table 7-12	Muscles that Move the Foot and Toes			
Muscle	**Origin**	**Insertion**		**Action**
ACTION AT THE ANKLE				
Flexors (Dorsiflexors)				
Tibialis anterior	Lateral condyle and proximal shaft of tibia	Base of first metatarsal bone		Flexion (dorsiflexion) at ankle, inversion of foot
Fibularis tertius	Distal anterior surface of fibula and interosseus membrane	Dorsal surface of fifth metatarsal bone		Flexion (dorsiflexion) at ankle; eversion of foot
Extensors (Plantar flexors)				
Gastrocnemius	Femoral condyles	Calcaneus by way of calcaneal tendon		Extension (plantar flexion) at ankle; inversion and adduction of foot; flexion at knee
Fibularis brevis	Midlateral margin of fibula	Base of fifth metatarsal bone		Eversion of foot and extension (plantar flexion) at ankle
Fibularis longus	Lateral condyle of tibia, head and proximal shaft of fibula	Base of first metatarsal bone and medial cuneiform bone		Eversion of foot and extension (plantar flexion) at ankle
Plantaris	Lateral supracondylar ridge of femur	Posterior calcaneus		Extension (plantar flexion) at ankle; flexion at knee
Soleus	Head and proximal shaft of fibula, and adjacent shaft of tibia	Calcaneus by way of calcaneal tendon		Extension (plantar flexion) at ankle; adduction of foot
Tibialis posterior	Interosseus membrane and adjacent shafts of tibia and fibula	Tarsal and metatarsal bones		Adduction and inversion of foot; extension (plantar flexion) at ankle
ACTION AT THE TOES				
Flexors				
Flexor digitorum longus	Posterior and medial surface of tibia	Inferior surface of phalanges, toes 2–5		Flexion at joints of toes 2–5
Flexor hallucis longus	Posterior surface of fibula	Inferior surface, distal phalanx of great toe		Flexion at joints of great toe; assists in extension (plantar flexion) at ankle
Extensors				
Extensor digitorum longus	Lateral condyle of tibia, anterior surface of fibula	Superior surfaces of phalanges, toes 2–5		Extension at joints of toes 2–5
Extensor hallucis longus	Anterior surface of fibula	Superior surface, distal phalanx of great toe		Extension at joints of great toe

CLINICAL NOTE

Fibromyalgia

Fibromyalgia is a chronic inflammatory disorder of the muscular system. It is classified by the American Academy of Rheumatology as the presence of 11 of 18 specific tender points, nonrestorative sleep, muscle stiffness, and generalized aching pain, with symptoms present for more than three months' duration. Furthermore, the pains and stiffness cannot be explained by other mechanisms. Fibromyalgia can be quite debilitating. It commonly affects women under 40 years of age and is almost always associated with chronic fatigue. Many of the problems associated with fibromyalgia can be attributed to other conditions, such as depression. However, the presence of the tender points is the diagnostic key to fibromyalgia.

7-12 The size and power of muscle tissue decrease with advancing age

Learning Objective Describe the effects of aging on muscle tissue.

The effects of aging on the muscular system can be summarized as follows:

1. ***Skeletal muscle fibers become smaller in diameter.*** The reduction in size reflects a decrease in the number of myofibrils. In addition, muscle fibers contain smaller ATP, CP, and glycogen reserves and less myoglobin. Overall, muscle strength and endurance are reduced, and muscles tend to fatigue rapidly. Also, blood flow to active muscles does not increase with

exercise as rapidly as it does in younger people because cardiovascular performance decreases with age.

2. *Skeletal muscles become less elastic.* Aging skeletal muscles develop increasing amounts of fibrous connective tissue, a process called *fibrosis.* Fibrosis makes the muscle less flexible, and the collagen fibers can restrict movement and circulation.

3. *Tolerance for exercise decreases.* A lower tolerance for exercise as age increases results in part from the tendency to tire quickly and in part from reduced thermoregulation (described in Chapters 1 and 5). ↺ pp. 10, 127 Individuals over age 65 years cannot eliminate heat generated by muscles as effectively as younger people, which leads to overheating.

4. *The ability to recover from muscular injuries decreases.* When an injury occurs, repair capabilities are limited. As a result, scar tissue usually forms.

The *rate* of decline in muscular performance is the same in all people, regardless of their exercise patterns or lifestyle. For this reason, to be in good shape late in life, an individual must be in *very* good shape early in life. Regular exercise helps control body weight, strengthens bones, and generally improves the quality of life at all ages. Extremely demanding exercise is not as important as regular exercise. In fact, extreme exercise in the elderly can damage tendons, bones, and joints.

CHECKPOINT

36. Describe general age-related effects on skeletal muscle tissue.

See the blue Answers tab at the back of the book.

7-13 Exercise produces responses in multiple body systems

Learning Objective Discuss the interactions between the muscular system and other body systems when the body is at rest, and explain the homeostatic responses to exercise by the muscular system and various other body systems.

Even when the body is at rest, the muscular system is interacting with other body systems.

To work at maximum efficiency and maintain homeostasis, the muscular system must be supported by many other

Build Your Knowledge

How the MUSCULAR SYSTEM integrates with the other body systems presented so far on **p. 238** summarizes the major functional relationships between it and the integumentary and skeletal systems.

systems. The changes that take place during exercise are a good example of such interactions. Responses of the muscular system and other organ systems to exercise include the following:

- *Muscular system.* Active muscles consume oxygen and generate carbon dioxide and heat.

- *Cardiovascular system.* Blood vessels in active muscles and in the skin dilate, and heart rate increases. These adjustments speed delivery of oxygen and removal of carbon dioxide at the muscle. They also bring heat to the skin where it can pass into the environment.

- *Respiratory system.* The rate and depth of respiration increase during exercise. Air moves into and out of the lungs more quickly, keeping pace with the increased rate of blood flow through the lungs.

- *Integumentary system.* Blood vessels dilate, and sweat gland secretion increases. This combination promotes evaporation at the skin surface and removes the excess heat generated by muscular activity.

- *Nervous and endocrine systems.* These systems direct the responses of other organ systems by controlling heart rate, respiratory rate, sweat gland activity, and the release of stored energy reserves.

CHECKPOINT

37. What major function does the muscular system perform for the body as a whole?

38. Identify the physiological effects of exercise on the cardiovascular, respiratory, and integumentary systems. What is the relationship between these physiological effects and the nervous and endocrine systems?

See the blue Answers tab at the back of the book.

Build Your Knowledge
How the MUSCULAR SYSTEM integrates with the other body systems presented so far

Integumentary System

• The Integumentary System removes excess body heat; synthesizes vitamin D₃ for calcium and phosphate absorption; protects underlying muscles

• The muscular system includes facial muscles that pull on the skin of the face to produce facial expressions

Skeletal System

• The Skeletal System provides mineral reserves for maintaining normal calcium and phosphate levels in body fluids; supports skeletal muscles; and provides sites of muscle attachment

• The muscular system provides skeletal movement and support; stabilizes bones and joints; stresses exerted by tendons of contracting skeletal muscles help to maintain normal bone structure and mass

Muscular System

The muscular system performs five primary functions for the human body. It
• produces skeletal movement
• helps maintain posture and body position
• supports soft tissues
• guards entrances and exits to the body
• helps maintain body temperature

7

RELATED CLINICAL TERMS

compartment syndrome: Ischemia (defined shortly) resulting from accumulated blood and fluid trapped within limb muscle compartments formed by partitions of dense connective tissue.

ischemia (is-KĒ-mē-uh): A deficiency of blood ("blood starvation") in a body part, sometimes due to compression of regional blood vessels.

muscle cramps: Prolonged, involuntary, painful muscular contractions.

muscular dystrophies (DIS-trō-fēz): A varied collection of inherited diseases that produce progressive muscle weakness and deterioration. The most familiar is *Duchenne muscular dystrophy*, which typically develops in males ages 3–7 years.

myalgia (mī-AL-jē-uh): Muscular pain; a common symptom of a wide variety of conditions and infections.

myoma: A benign tumor of muscle tissue.

myositis (mī-ō-SĪ-tis): Inflammation of muscle tissue.

polio: A viral disease in which the destruction of motor neurons produces paralysis and atrophy of motor units.

sarcoma: A malignant tumor of mesoderm-derived tissue (muscle, bone, or other connective tissue).

tendinitis: Inflammation of the connective tissue surrounding a tendon.

7 Chapter Review

Summary Outline

An Introduction to Muscle Tissue *p. 213*

1. The three types of muscle tissue are *skeletal muscle, cardiac muscle,* and *smooth muscle*. The muscular system includes all of the body's skeletal muscles, which can be controlled voluntarily.

7-1 Skeletal muscle performs five primary functions *p. 213*

2. **Skeletal muscles** attach to bones directly or indirectly. They (1) produce movement of the skeleton, (2) maintain posture and body position, (3) support soft tissues, (4) guard entrances and exits, and (5) maintain body temperature.

7-2 A skeletal muscle contains muscle tissue, connective tissues, blood vessels, and nerves *p. 213*

3. Each muscle fiber is surrounded by an **endomysium**. Bundles of muscle fibers are sheathed by a **perimysium,** and the entire muscle is covered by an **epimysium**. At the ends of the muscle is a **tendon** or **aponeurosis** *(Figure 7-1)*.

7-3 Skeletal muscle fibers have distinctive features *p. 215*

4. A muscle cell has a **sarcolemma** (plasma membrane), **sarcoplasm** (cytoplasm), and a **sarcoplasmic reticulum,** similar to the smooth endoplasmic reticulum of other cells. **Transverse tubules (T tubules)** and **myofibrils** have roles in contraction. Filaments in a myofibril are organized into repeating functional units called **sarcomeres** *(Figure 7-2a–c)*.

5. **Myofilaments** consist of **thin filaments** *(actin)* and **thick filaments** *(myo sin) (Figure 7-2d,e)*.

6. As a myofilament contracts and shortens, the **Z lines** of adjacent sarcomeres move closer together as the thin filaments slide past the thick filaments *(Figure 7-3)*.

7. The explanation for sarcomere contraction is the *sliding filament theory*. The process involves **active sites** on thin filaments and **cross-bridges** of the thick filaments. At rest, the necessary interactions are prevented by **tropomyosin** and **troponin** proteins on the thin filaments.

7-4 The nervous system and skeletal muscles communicate at neuromuscular junctions *p. 218*

8. Neural control of muscle function links electrical activity in the sarcolemma with the initiation of a contraction.

9. A neuron controls the activity of a muscle fiber at a **neuromuscular junction (NMJ)** *(Spotlight Figure 7-4)*.

10. When an **action potential** arrives at the axon terminal, acetylcholine is released into the synaptic cleft. The binding of ACh to receptors on the motor end plate leads to the generation of an action potential in the sarcolemma. The passage of an action potential along a transverse tubule triggers the release of calcium ions from the *terminal cisternae* of the sarcoplasmic reticulum *(Spotlight Figure 7-4)*.

11. A contraction involves a repeated cycle of "attach, pivot, detach, and return." It begins when calcium ions are released by the sarcoplasmic reticulum. The calcium ions bind to troponin, which changes position and moves tropomyosin away from the active sites of actin. Cross-bridge binding of

myosin heads to actin can then occur. After binding, each myosin head pivots at its base, pulling the actin filament toward the center of the sarcomere *(Spotlight Figure 7-5).*

12. A summary of the contraction process, from ACh release to the end of the contraction and relaxation, is shown in *Figure 7-6.*

7-5 Sarcomere shortening and muscle fiber stimulation produce tension *p. 222*

13. The amount of tension produced by a muscle fiber depends on the number of cross-bridges formed.

14. Both the number of activated muscle fibers and their rate of stimulation control the tension of a skeletal muscle.

15. A muscle fiber **twitch** is a cycle of contraction and relaxation produced by a single stimulus *(Figure 7-7).*

16. Repeated stimulation before the relaxation phase ends can result in the addition of twitches (known as **summation**). The result can be either **incomplete tetanus** (in which tension peaks because the muscle is never allowed to relax completely) or **complete tetanus** (in which the relaxation phase is completely eliminated) *(Figure 7-8).*

17. The number and size of a muscle's **motor units** indicate how precisely the muscle's movements are controlled *(Figure 7-9).*

18. Muscle tension is increased by increasing the number of motor units involved—a process called **recruitment**.

19. Resting **muscle tone** stabilizes bones and joints. Inadequate stimulation causes muscles to **atrophy**.

20. Normal activities usually include both **isotonic contractions** (a muscle's tension remains constant as it shortens) and **isometric contractions** (a muscle's tension rises but its length remains constant).

21. Elongation of a muscle fiber is passive. Elongation can result from elastic forces, the contraction of opposing muscles, or the effects of gravity.

7-6 ATP is the energy source for muscle contraction *p. 229*

22. Muscle contractions require large amounts of energy from ATP.

23. ATP is an energy-transfer molecule, not an energy-storage molecule. **Creatine phosphate (CP)** can release stored energy to convert ADP to ATP. A resting muscle cell contains many times more CP than ATP *(Figure 7-10a).*

24. At rest or moderate levels of activity, aerobic metabolism in mitochondria can provide most of the ATP required to support muscle contractions.

25. When a muscle fiber runs short of ATP and CP, enzymes can break down glycogen molecules to release glucose that can be broken down by **glycolysis** *(Figure 7-10b).*

26. At peak levels of activity, the cell relies heavily on the **anaerobic** process of glycolysis to generate ATP, because the mitochondria cannot obtain enough oxygen to meet the existing ATP demands *(Figure 7-10c).*

27. **Muscle fatigue** occurs when a muscle can no longer contract, because of a drop in the pH due to the buildup and dissociation of **lactic acid**, a lack of energy resources, or other factors.

28. The **recovery period** begins after a period of muscle activity and continues until conditions inside the muscle have returned to pre-exertion levels. The *oxygen debt* is the amount of oxygen used to restore normal conditions.

7-7 Muscle performance depends on muscle fiber type and physical conditioning *p. 232*

29. Muscle performance can be considered in terms of **force** (the maximum amount of tension produced by a particular muscle or muscle group) and **endurance** (the duration of muscular activity).

30. The two types of human skeletal muscle fibers are **fast fibers** and **slow fibers.**

31. Fast fibers are large in diameter, contain densely packed myofibrils, large reserves of glycogen, and few mitochondria. They produce rapid and powerful contractions of relatively short duration.

32. Slow fibers are smaller in diameter and take three times as long to contract after stimulation. An extensive capillary supply, abundant mitochondria, and high concentrations of **myoglobin** enable them to contract for long periods of time.

33. **Anaerobic endurance** is the time over which a muscle can support sustained, powerful contractions anaerobically. Training to develop anaerobic endurance can lead to **hypertrophy** (enlargement) of the stimulated muscles.

34. **Aerobic endurance** is the time over which a muscle can continue to contract while supported by mitochondrial activities.

7-8 Cardiac and smooth muscle tissues differ in structure and function from skeletal muscle tissue *p. 233*

35. Cardiac muscle cells differ from skeletal muscle fibers in that they are smaller, typically have a single central nucleus, rely more greatly on aerobic metabolism when contracting at peak levels, and have **intercalated discs** *(Figure 7-11a; Table 7-1).*

36. Cardiac muscle cells have *automaticity* and do not require neural stimulation to contract. Their contractions last longer than those of skeletal muscles, and cardiac muscle cannot undergo tetanus.

37. Smooth muscle is nonstriated, involuntary muscle tissue that can contract over a greater range of lengths than skeletal muscle cells *(Figure 7-11b; Table 7-1)*.

38. Many smooth muscle cells lack direct connections to motor neurons. If innervated, they are not under voluntary control.

7-9 Descriptive terms are used to name skeletal muscles *p. 236*

39. The **muscular system** includes approximately 700 skeletal muscles, which can be voluntarily controlled *(Figure 7-12)*.

40. The **axial muscles** arise on the axial skeleton; they position the head and spinal column and move the rib cage. The **appendicular muscles** stabilize or move components of the appendicular skeleton.

41. Each muscle can be identified by its **origin, insertion,** and **primary action.** A muscle can be classified by its primary action as a **prime mover,** or **agonist;** as a **synergist;** or as an **antagonist.**

42. The names of muscles often provide clues to their location, fascicle orientation, or function *(Table 7-2)*.

7-10 Axial muscles are muscles of the head and neck, vertebral column, trunk, and pelvic floor *p. 240*

43. The axial muscles fall into four groups based on location and/or function: muscles of (a) the head and neck, (b) the spine, (c) the trunk, and (d) the pelvic floor.

44. The muscles of the head include the **frontalis, orbicularis oris, buccinator, masseter, temporalis,** and **pterygoids** *(Figure 7-13; Table 7-3)*.

45. The muscles of the neck include the **platysma, digastric, mylohyoid, stylohyoid, omohyoid,** and **sternocleidomastoid** *(Figures 7-13, 7-14; Table 7-3)*.

46. The **splenius capitis** and **semispinalis capitis** are the most superior muscles of the spine. The extensor muscles of the spine, or **erector spinae,** can be classified into the **spinalis, longissimus,** and **iliocostalis** groups. In the lower lumbar and sacral regions, the longissimus and iliocostalis are sometimes called the *sacrospinalis* muscles *(Figure 7-16; Table 7-4)*.

47. The muscles of the trunk include the **oblique** and **rectus** muscles. The thoracic region muscles include the **intercostal** and **transversus** muscles. Also important to respiration is the **diaphragm** *(Figure 7-20; Table 7-5)*.

48. The muscular floor of the pelvic cavity is called the **perineum.** These muscles support the organs of the pelvic cavity and control the movement of materials through the urethra and anus *(Figure 7-21; Table 7-6)*.

7-11 Appendicular muscles are muscles of the shoulders, upper limbs, pelvic girdle, and lower limbs *p. 250*

49. Together, the **trapezius** and the sternocleidomastoid affect the position of the shoulder, head, and neck. Other muscles inserting on the scapula include the **rhomboids,** the **levator scapulae,** the **serratus anterior,** and the **pectoralis minor** *(Figure 7-22; Table 7-7)*.

50. The **deltoid** and the **supraspinatus** produce abduction of the arm at the shoulder. The **subscapularis, teres major, infraspinatus,** and **teres minor** rotate the arm at the shoulder *(Figure 7-23; Table 7-8)*.

51. The **pectoralis major** flexes the shoulder joint, and the **latissimus dorsi** extends it. Both of these muscles adduct and rotate the arm at the shoulder joint *(Figure 7-23; Table 7-8)*.

52. The primary actions of the **biceps brachii** and the **triceps brachii** affect the elbow. The **brachialis** and **brachioradialis** flex the elbow. The **flexor carpi radialis,** the **flexor carpi ulnaris,** and the **palmaris longus** cooperate to flex the wrist. They are opposed by the **extensor carpi radialis** and the **extensor carpi ulnaris.** The **pronator** muscles pronate the forearm, opposed by the **supinator** and the biceps brachii *(Figure 7-24; Table 7-9)*.

53. *Gluteal muscles* cover the lateral surfaces of the ilia. They produce extension, abduction, and rotation at the hip *(Figure 7-25a,b; Table 7-10)*.

54. Adductors of the thigh work across the hip joint. These muscles include the **adductor magnus, adductor brevis, adductor longus, pectineus,** and **gracilis** *(Figure 7-25c; Table 7-10)*.

55. The **psoas major** and the **iliacus** merge to form the **iliopsoas** muscle, a powerful flexor of the hip *(Figure 7-25c; Table 7-10)*.

56. The flexors of the knee include the hamstrings (**biceps femoris, semimembranosus,** and **semitendinosus**) and **sartorius.** The **popliteus** aids flexion by unlocking the knee *(Figure 7-26; Table 7-11)*.

57. The *knee extensors* are known as the **quadriceps femoris.** This group includes the three **vastus** muscles and the **rectus femoris** *(Figure 7-26; Table 7-11)*.

58. The **gastrocnemius** and **soleus** muscles produce plantar flexion (ankle extension). A pair of **fibularis** muscles produces eversion as well as plantar flexion and a third also produces dorsiflexion (ankle flexion). The **tibialis anterior** performs dorsiflexion *(Figure 7-27; Table 7-12)*.

59. The phalanges are controlled by muscles originating at the tarsal bones and at the metatarsal bones *(Table 7-12)*.

7-12 The size and power of muscle tissue decrease with advancing age *p. 261*

60. Aging reduces the size, elasticity, and power of all muscle tissues. Both exercise tolerance and the ability to recover from muscular injuries decrease with age.

7-13 Exercise produces responses in multiple body systems *p. 262*

61. Exercise integrates the muscular system with the cardiovascular, respiratory, integumentary, nervous, and endocrine systems.

Review Questions

See the blue Answers tab at the back of the book.

Level 1 Reviewing Facts and Terms

Match each item in column A with the most closely related item in column B. Place letters for answers in the spaces provided.

COLUMN A

_____ **1.** Epimysium
_____ **2.** Fascicle
_____ **3.** Endomysium
_____ **4.** Motor end plate
_____ **5.** Transverse tubule
_____ **6.** Actin
_____ **7.** Myosin
_____ **8.** Extensors of the knee
_____ **9.** Sarcomeres
_____ **10.** Tropomyosin
_____ **11.** Recruitment
_____ **12.** Muscle tone
_____ **13.** White muscles
_____ **14.** Flexors of the leg
_____ **15.** Red muscles
_____ **16.** Hypertrophy

COLUMN B

a.   Resting muscle tension
b.   Contractile units
c.   Thin filaments
d.   Surrounds muscle fiber
e.   Muscle enlargement
f.   Surrounds muscle
g.   Slow fibers
h.   Thick filaments
i.   Bundle of muscle fibers
j.   Hamstring muscles
k.   Covers active sites on actin
l.   Transmits action potentials
m.   Fast fibers
n.   Quadriceps muscles
o.   Multiple motor units
p.   Contains ACh receptors

17. Identify the structures in the following figure.

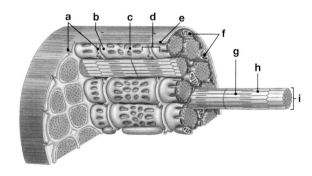

(a) _____   (b) _____
(c) _____   (d) _____
(e) _____   (f) _____
(g) _____   (h) _____
(i) _____

18. A skeletal muscle contains
    (a) connective tissues.   (b) blood vessels and nerves.
    (c) skeletal muscle tissue.   (d) a, b, and c are correct.

19. Label the three visible muscles of the rotator cuff in the following posterior view of the deep muscles that move the arm.

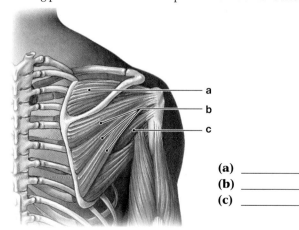

(a) _____
(b) _____
(c) _____

20. What six interlocking steps are involved in the contraction process?

21. What forms of energy reserves are found in resting skeletal muscle cells?

22. What two processes are used to generate ATP from glucose in muscle cells?

Level 2 Reviewing Concepts

23. Areas of the body where no slow fibers would be found include the
- **(a)** back and calf muscles.
- **(b)** eye and hand.
- **(c)** chest and abdomen.
- **(d)** a, b, and c are correct.

24. Describe the basic sequence of events that occurs at a neuromuscular junction.

25. Why is the multinucleate condition important in skeletal muscle fibers?

26. The muscles of the spine include many dorsal extensors but few ventral flexors. Why?

27. What specific structural characteristic makes voluntary control of urination and defecation possible?

28. What types of movements are affected when the hamstrings are injured?

Level 3 Critical Thinking and Clinical Applications

29. Many potent insecticides contain toxins called *organophosphates*, which interfere with the action of the enzyme acetylcholinesterase. Terry is using an insecticide containing organophosphates and is very careless. He does not use gloves or a mask, so he absorbs some of the chemical through his skin and inhales a large amount as well. What signs would you expect to observe in Terry as a result of organophosphate poisoning?

30. The time of a murder victim's death is commonly estimated by the flexibility or stiffness of the body. Explain why this is possible.

31. Makani is interested in building up his thigh muscles, specifically the quadriceps group. What exercises would you recommend to help him accomplish his goal?

8

The Nervous System

Learning Objectives

These objectives tell you what you should be able to do after completing the chapter. They correspond by number to this chapter's sections.

8-1 Describe the anatomical and functional divisions of the nervous system.

8-2 Distinguish between neurons and neuroglia on the basis of structure and function.

8-3 Describe the events involved in the generation and propagation of an action potential.

8-4 Describe the structure of a synapse, and explain the process of nerve impulse transmission at a synapse.

8-5 Describe the three meningeal layers that surround the central nervous system.

8-6 Discuss the roles of gray matter and white matter in the spinal cord.

8-7 Name the major regions of the brain, and describe the locations and functions of each.

8-8 Name the cranial nerves, relate each pair of cranial nerves to its principal functions, and relate the distribution pattern of spinal nerves to the regions they innervate.

8-9 Describe the steps in a reflex arc.

8-10 Identify the principal sensory and motor pathways, and explain how it is possible to distinguish among sensations that originate in different areas of the body.

8-11 Describe the structures and functions of the sympathetic and parasympathetic divisions of the autonomic nervous system.

8-12 Summarize the effects of aging on the nervous system.

8-13 Give examples of interactions between the nervous system and other body systems.

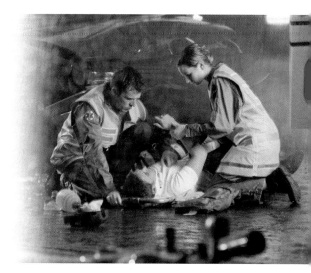

An Introduction to the Nervous System

Two organ systems coordinate organ system activities to maintain homeostasis in response to changing environmental conditions. They are the *nervous system* and the *endocrine system.* The nervous system responds relatively swiftly but briefly to stimuli. In contrast, responses by the endocrine system develop more slowly but last much longer. For example, the nervous system adjusts your body position and moves your eyes across this page. At the same time, the endocrine system is adjusting your body's daily rate of energy use and directing such long-term processes as growth and maturation. (We will consider the endocrine system in Chapter 10.)

The nervous system is your most complex organ system. For example, right now you are consciously reading these words and thinking about them. At the subconscious level (outside your awareness), it is doing much more. Your nervous system is also monitoring the external environment and your internal systems and issuing commands as needed to maintain homeostasis. Yet in a few hours—at mealtime or while you are sleeping—your pattern of nervous system activity will be very different. The change from one pattern of activity to another can take place in almost an instant because neural function relies on electrical events that proceed at great speed.

In this chapter, we examine the structure and function of the nervous system. We will consider its cells through their organization into two major divisions: the *central nervous system* (CNS) and the *peripheral nervous system* (PNS).

8

Build Your Knowledge

Recall that the nervous system directs immediate responses to stimuli (as you saw in **Chapter 1: An Introduction to Anatomy and Physiology**). It usually does so by coordinating the activities of other organ systems. It also provides and interprets sensory information about internal and external conditions. ⤴ **p. 7**

8-1 The nervous system has anatomical and functional divisions

Learning Objective Describe the anatomical and functional divisions of the nervous system.

The **nervous system** carries out three main functions. It (1) monitors the body's internal and external environments, (2) integrates sensory information, and (3) coordinates voluntary and involuntary responses of many other organ systems.

The nervous system has two major anatomical divisions. The **CNS** consists of the *brain* and the *spinal cord.* It integrates and coordinates the processing of sensory data and the transmission of motor commands. The CNS is also the seat of higher functions, such as intelligence, memory, and emotion. All communication between the CNS and the rest of the body takes place through the **PNS**, which includes all the neural tissue *outside* the CNS.

Figure 8-1 presents an overview of the functional relationships of the CNS and PNS. Notice that the PNS itself consists of two divisions. The **afferent division** (*afferens,* to bring to) of the PNS brings sensory information *to* the CNS from *receptors* in body tissues and organs. **Receptors** are sensory structures that either detect changes in the environment (internal or external) or respond to specific stimuli. The **efferent division** (*effero,* to bring out) of the PNS carries motor commands *from* the CNS to muscles and glands. These target organs and tissues respond by *doing* something and are called **effectors**.

The efferent division of the PNS has two parts. The **somatic nervous system (SNS)** controls skeletal muscle contractions. *Voluntary* contractions are under conscious control, such as when you lift a glass of water to your lips. *Involuntary* contractions are simple or complex movements controlled at the subconscious level. For example, if you accidentally place your hand on a hot stove, you will pull it back immediately, even before you notice any pain. This type of automatic response is called a *reflex.*

The **autonomic nervous system (ANS),** or *visceral motor system,* automatically regulates smooth muscle, cardiac muscle, and glandular secretions at the subconscious level. The ANS includes a *sympathetic division* and a *parasympathetic division,* which commonly have opposite effects. For example, activity of the sympathetic division speeds up your heart rate, but the parasympathetic division slows your heart rate.

Figure 8-1 A Functional Overview of the Nervous System.

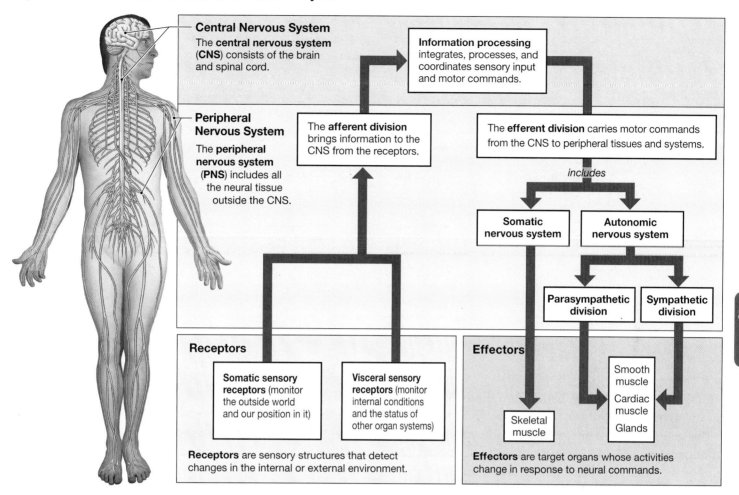

Central Nervous System
The **central nervous system** (**CNS**) consists of the brain and spinal cord.

Information processing integrates, processes, and coordinates sensory input and motor commands.

Peripheral Nervous System
The **peripheral nervous system** (**PNS**) includes all the neural tissue outside the CNS.

The **afferent division** brings information to the CNS from the receptors.

The **efferent division** carries motor commands from the CNS to peripheral tissues and systems.

includes

Somatic nervous system

Autonomic nervous system

Parasympathetic division

Sympathetic division

Receptors

Somatic sensory receptors (monitor the outside world and our position in it)

Visceral sensory receptors (monitor internal conditions and the status of other organ systems)

Receptors are sensory structures that detect changes in the internal or external environment.

Effectors

Skeletal muscle

Smooth muscle
Cardiac muscle
Glands

Effectors are target organs whose activities change in response to neural commands.

CHECKPOINT

1. Identify the two anatomical divisions of the nervous system.
2. Identify the two functional divisions of the peripheral nervous system, and describe their primary functions.
3. What would be the effect of damage to the afferent division of the PNS?

See the blue Answers tab at the back of the book.

8-2 Neurons are specialized for intercellular communication and are supported by cells called neuroglia

Learning Objective Distinguish between neurons and neuroglia on the basis of structure and function.

The nervous system includes all the neural tissue in the body. Neural tissue (introduced in Chapter 4) consists of two kinds of cells, *neurons* and *neuroglia*. ⟳ p. 113 **Neurons** (*neuro-*, nerve) are the basic functional units of the nervous system. All neural functions involve the communication of neurons with one another and with other cells. The **neuroglia** (noo-ROG-lē-uh; *glia*, glue) regulate the environment around neurons, provide a supporting framework for neural tissue, and act as phagocytes. Although they are much smaller cells, neuroglia (also called *glial cells*) far outnumber neurons. Unlike most neurons, most glial cells retain the ability to divide.

Neurons

The General Structure of Neurons

Neurons can have a variety of shapes. **Figure 8-2** shows a *multipolar neuron*, the most common type of neuron in the CNS. A multipolar neuron has (1) a cell body; (2) several branching, sensitive **dendrites**, which receive incoming signals;

Figure 8-2 The Anatomy of a Representative Neuron. The relationships of the four parts of a neuron (cell body, dendrites, axon, and axon terminals) are shown in the multipolar neuron depicted here.

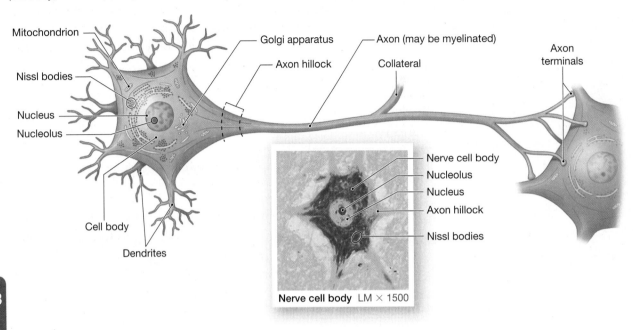

Nerve cell body LM × 1500

and (3) a single long axon, which carries outgoing signals toward (4) one or more **axon terminals**.

The **cell body** contains a large, round nucleus with a prominent nucleolus. The cytoplasm of the cell body contains organelles that provide energy and synthesize organic compounds. The numerous mitochondria, free and fixed ribosomes, and membranes of the rough endoplasmic reticulum (RER) give the cytoplasm a coarse, grainy appearance. Clusters of RER and free ribosomes are known as **Nissl bodies**. They give a gray color to areas containing neuron cell bodies and account for the color of *gray matter* seen in brain and spinal cord dissections.

Projecting from the cell body are a variable number of dendrites and a single large axon. The plasma membrane of the dendrites and cell body is sensitive to chemical, mechanical, or electrical stimulation. In a process described later, such stimulation often leads to the generation of an electrical impulse, or *action potential*, that travels along the axon. Action potentials begin at a thickened region of the cell body called the **axon hillock**. The axon may branch along its length, producing branches called *collaterals*. Axon terminals (also called synaptic terminals and synaptic knobs) are found at the tips of each branch. An axon terminal is part of a **synapse**, a site where a neuron communicates with another cell.

Most neurons lack centrioles, organelles involved in the movement of chromosomes during mitosis. ⮌ p. 70 As a result, typical CNS neurons cannot divide, so they cannot be

replaced if lost to injury or disease. Neural stem cells are present in the adult nervous system, but they are typically inactive. Exceptions occur in the nose, where the regeneration of olfactory (smell) receptors maintains our sense of smell, and in the *hippocampus*, a portion of the brain involved in storing memories. Researchers are studying the processes that trigger neural stem cell activity, with the goal of preventing or reversing neuron loss due to trauma, disease, or aging.

Structural Classification of Neurons

The billions of neurons in the nervous system are variable in form. Based on the relationship of the dendrites to the cell body and axon, neurons are classified into three types (**Figure 8-3**):

1. A **multipolar neuron** has two or more dendrites and a single axon (**Figure 8-3a**). These are the most common neurons in the CNS. All the motor neurons that control skeletal muscles are multipolar. Their axons may be a meter or more in length.

2. In a **unipolar neuron**, the dendrites and axon are continuous, and the cell body lies off to one side (**Figure 8-3b**). In a unipolar neuron, the action potential begins at the base of the dendrites, and the rest of the process is considered an axon. Most sensory neurons of the PNS are unipolar. Their axons can be as long as those of multipolar neurons.

Figure 8-3 A Structural Classification of Neurons. The neurons are not drawn to scale; bipolar neurons are many times smaller than typical unipolar and multipolar neurons. The arrows show the normal direction of an action potential.

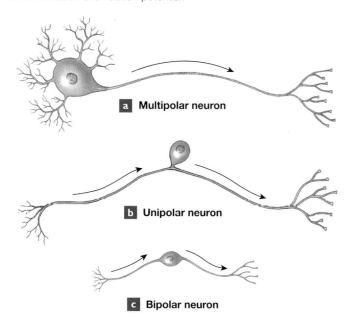

a Multipolar neuron

b Unipolar neuron

c Bipolar neuron

3. **Bipolar neurons** have only one dendrite and one axon, with the cell body between them (**Figure 8-3c**). Bipolar neurons are small and rare. They occur in special sense organs, where they relay information about sight, smell, or hearing from receptor cells to other neurons.

Functional Classification of Neurons

In terms of function, neurons are sorted into three groups: (1) *sensory neurons*, (2) *motor neurons*, and (3) *interneurons*.

SENSORY NEURONS. The approximately 10 million **sensory neurons**, or *afferent neurons*, in the human body form the afferent division of the PNS. Sensory neurons receive information from *sensory receptors* monitoring the external and internal environments and then relay the information to other neurons in the CNS (spinal cord or brain). The receptor may be a dendrite of a sensory neuron or specialized cells of other tissues that communicate with the sensory neuron.

Receptors may be categorized according to the information they detect. Two types of **somatic sensory receptors** detect information about the outside world or our physical position within it.

1. **External receptors** provide information about the external environment in the form of sensations of touch, pressure, pain, and temperature and the more complex senses of taste, smell, sight, equilibrium, and hearing.

2. **Proprioceptors** (prō-prē-ō-SEP-torz; *proprius*, one's own + *capio*, to take) monitor the position and movement of skeletal muscles and joints. **Visceral receptors**, or **internal receptors**, monitor the activities of the digestive, respiratory, cardiovascular, urinary, and reproductive systems. They provide sensations of distension, deep pressure, and pain.

MOTOR NEURONS. The half million **motor neurons**, or *efferent neurons*, of the efferent division carry instructions from the CNS to other tissues, organs, or organ systems. These peripheral targets are called *effectors*. For example, a skeletal muscle is an effector that contracts when it receives neural stimulation. Neurons in the two efferent divisions of the PNS target separate classes of effectors. The **somatic motor neurons** of the SNS innervate skeletal muscles, and the **visceral motor neurons** of the ANS innervate all other effectors, including cardiac muscle, smooth muscle, and glands.

INTERNEURONS. The 20 billion **interneurons**, or *association neurons*, are located entirely within the brain and the spinal cord. Interneurons, as the name implies (*inter-*, between), interconnect other neurons. They are responsible for distributing sensory information and coordinating motor activity. The more complex the response to a given stimulus, the greater the number of interneurons involved. Interneurons also play a role in all higher functions, such as memory, planning, and learning.

Neuroglia

Neuroglia are abundant and diverse. They make up about half of the volume of the nervous system. They are found in both the CNS and PNS, but the CNS has a greater variety of glial cells. The CNS contains four types of neuroglial cells (**Figure 8-4**):

1. **Astrocytes** (AS-trō-sīts; *astro-*, star + *cyte*, cell) are the largest and most numerous neuroglia. These star-shaped cells have varied functions. Astrocytes maintain the *blood-brain barrier* that isolates the CNS from the body's general circulation. Cytoplasmic extensions of the astrocytes end in expanded "feet" that wrap around capillaries. The astrocytes secrete chemicals that cause the capillaries of the CNS to become impermeable to many compounds, such as hormones and amino acids that could interfere with neuron function. Astrocytes also create a structural framework for CNS neurons and perform repairs in damaged neural tissues.

Figure 8-4 Neuroglia in the CNS. This diagrammatic view of neural tissue in the CNS depicts the relationships between neuroglia and neurons.

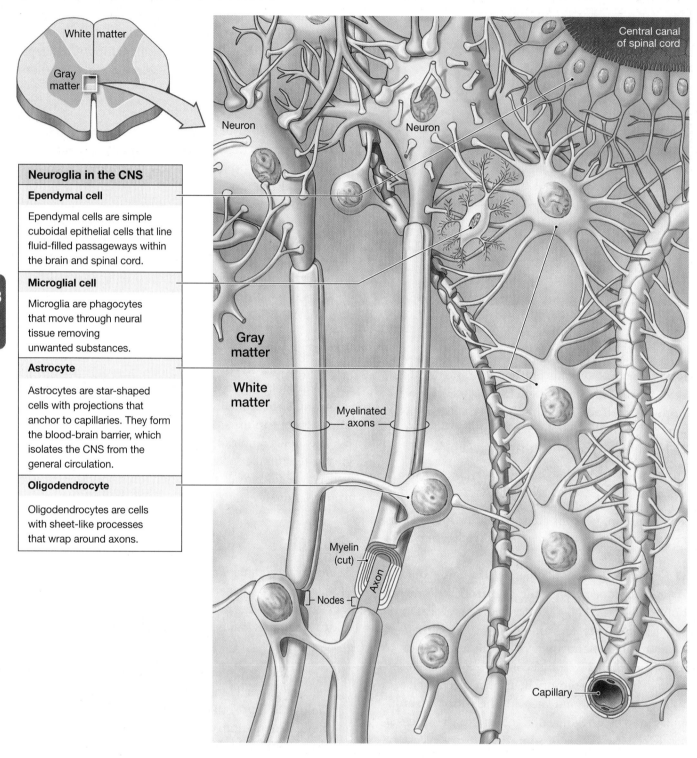

White matter

Gray matter

Central canal of spinal cord

Neuron

Neuron

Gray matter

White matter

Myelinated axons

Myelin (cut)

Axon

Nodes

Capillary

Neuroglia in the CNS	
Ependymal cell	
Ependymal cells are simple cuboidal epithelial cells that line fluid-filled passageways within the brain and spinal cord.	
Microglial cell	
Microglia are phagocytes that move through neural tissue removing unwanted substances.	
Astrocyte	
Astrocytes are star-shaped cells with projections that anchor to capillaries. They form the blood-brain barrier, which isolates the CNS from the general circulation.	
Oligodendrocyte	
Oligodendrocytes are cells with sheet-like processes that wrap around axons.	

2. Oligodendrocytes (ol-i-gō-DEN-drō-sīts; *oligo-*, few) have smaller cell bodies and fewer processes (cytoplasmic extensions) than astrocytes. The plasma membrane at the tip of each process forms a thin, expanded sheet that wraps around an axon. This membranous wrapping is called **myelin** (MĪ-e-lin). It serves as electrical insulation that increases the speed at which an action potential travels along the axon.

Each oligodendrocyte myelinates short segments of several axons, so many oligodendrocytes are needed to coat an entire axon with myelin. Such an axon is said to be **myelinated**. The areas covered in myelin are called **internodes**. The small gaps between adjacent cell processes are called **nodes**, or the *nodes of Ranvier* (rahn-vē-Ā).

Myelin is lipid-rich, and on dissection, areas of the CNS containing myelinated axons appear glossy white. Areas dominated by myelinated axons are known as the **white matter** of the CNS. Not every axon in the CNS is myelinated. Axons without a myelin coating are said to be **unmyelinated**. Areas containing neuron cell bodies, dendrites, and unmyelinated axons make up the **gray matter** of the CNS.

3. **Microglia** (mī-KRŌG-lē-uh) are the smallest and least numerous of the neuroglia in the CNS. Microglia are phagocytic cells derived from white blood cells that migrated into the CNS as the nervous system formed. They perform protective functions such as engulfing cellular waste and pathogens.

4. **Ependymal** (ep-EN-di-mul) **cells** are simple cuboidal epithelial cells that line cavities in the CNS filled with cerebrospinal fluid (CSF). These cavities include the *central canal* of the spinal cord and the chambers, or *ventricles*, of the brain. The lining of epithelial cells is called the **ependyma** (ep-EN-di-muh). Unlike other epithelia, it lacks a basement membrane. In some regions of the brain, the ependyma produces CSF. In other locations, the cilia on ependymal cells help circulate this fluid within and around the CNS.

The PNS contains two types of neuroglia. **Satellite cells** surround and support neuron cell bodies in the PNS, much as astrocytes do in the CNS. The other glial cells in the PNS are **Schwann cells** (**Figure 8-5a**).

Schwann cells cover every axon outside the CNS. Wherever a Schwann cell covers an axon, the outer surface of the Schwann cell is called the *neurilemma* (nū-ri-LEM-uh). Unlike an oligodendrocyte in the CNS, which may myelinate portions of several axons, a Schwann cell can myelinate only one segment of a single axon

(**Figure 8-5a**). However, a Schwann cell can enclose portions of several different unmyelinated axons (**Figure 8-5b**).

Organization of Neurons in the Nervous System

Neuron cell bodies and their axons are not randomly scattered in the CNS and PNS. Instead, they are organized into masses or bundles that have distinct anatomical boundaries and are identified by specific terms (**Figure 8-6**). We will

Figure 8-5 Schwann Cells and Peripheral Axons.

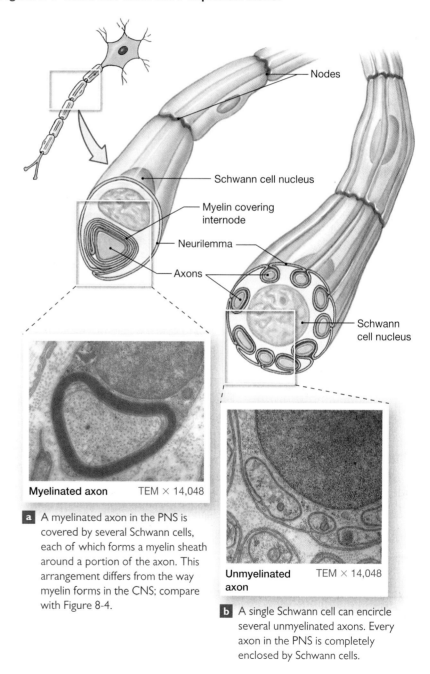

Nodes

Schwann cell nucleus

Myelin covering internode

Neurilemma

Axons

Schwann cell nucleus

Myelinated axon   TEM × 14,048

a A myelinated axon in the PNS is covered by several Schwann cells, each of which forms a myelin sheath around a portion of the axon. This arrangement differs from the way myelin forms in the CNS; compare with Figure 8-4.

Unmyelinated axon   TEM × 14,048

b A single Schwann cell can encircle several unmyelinated axons. Every axon in the PNS is completely enclosed by Schwann cells.

Figure 8-6 Anatomical Organization of the Nervous System.

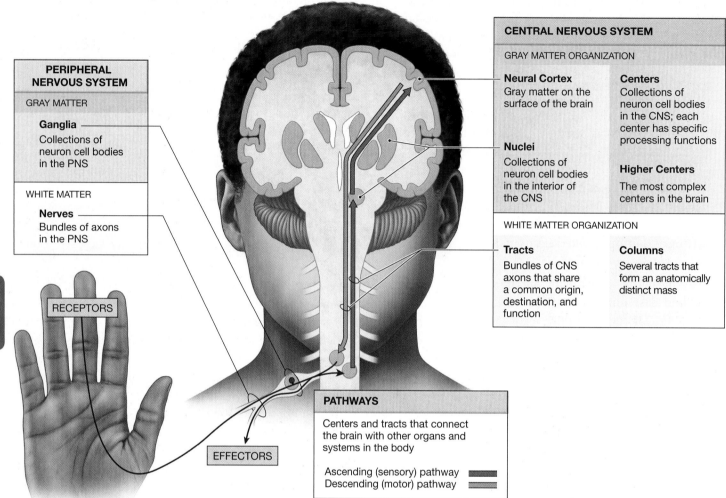

use these terms again, so you may find a brief overview here helpful.

In the PNS:

- Neuron cell bodies (gray matter) are located in **ganglia** (singular, *ganglion*). The neuron cell bodies are surrounded by satellite cells.

- The white matter of the PNS contains axons bundled together in **nerves**. *Spinal nerves* are connected to the spinal cord, and *cranial nerves* are connected to the brain. Both sensory and motor axons may be present in the same nerve.

In the CNS:

- A collection of neuron cell bodies (gray matter) with a common function is called a **center**. A center with a discrete boundary is called a **nucleus**. Portions of the brain

surface are covered by a thick layer of gray matter called **neural cortex** (*cortex*, rind). The term *higher centers* refers to the most complex integration centers, nuclei, and areas of cortex in the brain.

- The white matter of the CNS contains bundles of axons that share common origins, destinations, and functions. These bundles are called **tracts**. Tracts in the spinal cord form larger groups called **columns**.

- **Pathways** include both gray matter and white matter. They link the centers of the brain with the rest of the body. For example, **sensory** (ascending) **pathways** distribute information from sensory receptors to processing centers in the brain. **Motor** (descending) **pathways** begin at CNS centers for motor activity and end at the skeletal muscles they control.

CLINICAL NOTE

Demyelination Disorders

Demyelination is the progressive destruction of myelin sheaths, both in the CNS and PNS. The result is a gradual loss of sensation and motor control that leaves affected body regions numb and paralyzed. One demyelination disorder is **multiple sclerosis** (skler–sis; sklero*sis*, hardness), or **MS**. It affects axons in the optic nerve, brain, and/or spinal cord. Common signs and symptoms of MS include partial loss of vision and problems with speech, balance, and general motor coordination. Other important demyelination disorders include *heavy metal poisoning, Charcot-Marie-Tooth disease*, and *Guillain-Barré syndrome*.

CHECKPOINT

4. Name the structural components of a typical neuron.

5. Examination of a tissue sample reveals unipolar neurons. Are these more likely to be sensory neurons or motor neurons?

6. Identify the neuroglia of the central nervous system.

7. Which type of glial cell would increase in number in the brain tissue of a person with a CNS infection?

8. In the PNS, neuron cell bodies are located in _____ and surrounded by neuroglial cells called _____ cells.

See the blue Answers tab at the back of the book.

8-3 In neurons, a change in the plasma membrane's electrical potential may result in an action potential (nerve impulse)

Learning Objective Describe the events involved in the generation and propagation of an action potential.

The sensory, integrative, and motor functions of the nervous system are dynamic and ever changing. All communications between neurons and other cells take place through their membrane surfaces. These membrane changes are electrical events that proceed at great speed.

The Membrane Potential

A characteristic feature of all living cells is a *polarized* plasma membrane. An undisturbed, or unstimulated, cell has a plasma membrane that is polarized because the membrane separates an excess of positive charges outside the cell from an excess of negative charges inside the cell. When positive and negative charges are held apart, a *potential difference* is said to exist between them. This potential difference is called a **membrane potential**, or *transmembrane potential*, because the charges are separated by a plasma membrane.

The unit of measurement of potential difference is the *volt* (V). Most cars, for example, have 12 V batteries. The membrane potential of cells is much smaller and is usually reported in *millivolts* (mV, thousandths of a volt). The membrane potential of an unstimulated, resting cell is known as its **resting membrane potential**. The resting membrane potential of a neuron is −70 mV. The minus sign indicates that the cytoplasmic surface of the plasma membrane contains an excess of negative charges compared to the extracellular surface.

Factors Responsible for the Membrane Potential

Many factors influence membrane potential. In addition to an imbalance of electrical charges, the intracellular and extracellular fluids differ markedly in chemical and ionic composition. For example, the extracellular fluid contains relatively high concentrations of sodium ions (Na^+) and chloride ions (Cl^-). The intracellular fluid contains high concentrations of potassium ions (K^+) and negatively charged proteins (Pr^-).

The selective permeability of the plasma membrane maintains these differences between the intracellular and extracellular fluids. The proteins within the cytoplasm are too large to cross the membrane. The ions can enter or leave the cell only with the aid of membrane channels and/or carrier proteins. ↪ p. 61 There are many different types of membrane channels:

- Some, called *leak channels*, are always open.

- Others, called *gated channels*, open or close under specific circumstances. For example, gated channels may open or close due to the presence of a specific chemical or a change in membrane potential, or voltage.

Both passive and active processes act across the plasma membrane to determine the membrane potential at any moment. The passive forces are chemical and electrical. Chemical concentration gradients move potassium ions out of the cell and sodium ions into the cell. (These ions move through separate leak channels.) However, it is easier for potassium ions to diffuse through a potassium channel than for sodium ions to diffuse through sodium channels. As a result, potassium ions diffuse out of the cell faster than sodium ions enter the cell.

Electrical forces across the membrane also affect the passive movement of sodium and potassium ions. The overall positive charge on the outer surface of the plasma membrane repels positively charged potassium ions. At the same time, the negatively charged inner membrane surface attracts the positively charged sodium ions. Potassium ions continue to leave the cell, however, because its chemical concentration gradient is stronger than the repelling electrical force.

To maintain a potential difference across the plasma membrane, active processes work both to overcome the combined chemical and electrical forces driving sodium ions into the cell and to maintain the potassium concentration gradient. The resting potential remains stable over time because of the actions of a carrier protein, the sodium–potassium exchange pump. ⤷ p. 66 This ion pump exchanges three intracellular sodium ions for two extracellular potassium ions. At the normal resting membrane potential of −70 mV, sodium ions are ejected as fast as they enter the cell. The cell, therefore, undergoes a net loss of positive charges. As a result, the interior surface of the plasma membrane maintains an excess of negative charges, primarily from negatively charged proteins. **Figure 8-7** shows the plasma membrane at the resting membrane potential.

Changes in the Membrane Potential

Any stimulus that (1) alters membrane permeability to sodium or potassium ions or (2) alters the activity of the exchange pump will disturb the resting membrane potential of a cell. Some stimuli that can affect membrane potential include exposure to specific chemicals, mechanical pressure, changes in temperature, or shifts in the extracellular ion concentrations. Any change in the resting potential can have an immediate effect on the cell. For example, permeability changes in the sarcolemma of a skeletal muscle fiber trigger a contraction. ⤷ p. 199

In most cases, a stimulus opens gated ion channels that are closed when the plasma membrane is at its resting membrane potential. The opening of these channels speeds up ion movement across the plasma membrane and changes the membrane potential. For example, the opening of gated sodium channels speeds up the entry of sodium ions (Na^+) into the cell. As the number of positively charged ions on the inner surface of the plasma membrane increases, the membrane potential shifts toward 0 mV. A shift in this direction is called a **depolarization** of the membrane.

On the other hand, a stimulus that opens gated potassium ion channels shifts the membrane potential away from 0 mV, because additional potassium ions (K^+) will leave the cell. Such a change may take the membrane potential from −70 to −80 mV. This kind of shift is called a **hyperpolarization**.

Figure 8-7 The Resting Membrane Potential.

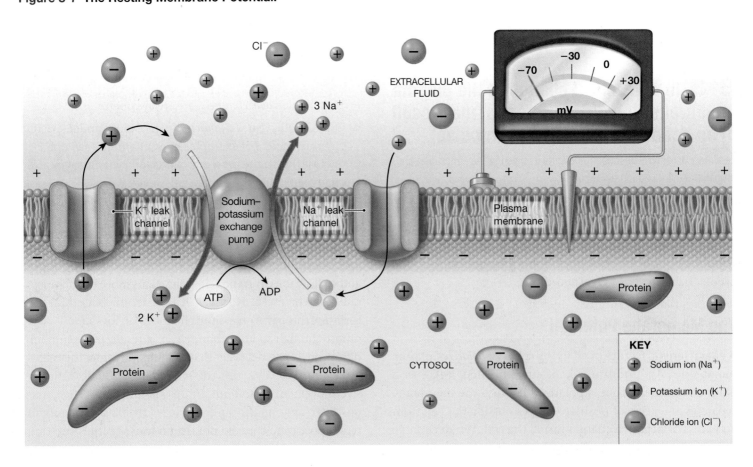

Information transfer between neurons and other cells involves two types of change in membrane potential: graded potentials and action potentials. **Graded potentials**, or *local potentials*, are changes in the membrane potential that cannot spread far from the site of stimulation. For example, if a chemical stimulus to the plasma membrane of a neuron opens gated sodium ion channels at a single site, the sodium ions entering the cell will depolarize the membrane at that location. Attracted to surrounding negative ions, the sodium ions move along the inner surface of the membrane in all directions. The degree of depolarization decreases with distance from the stimulation site. Why? This happens because the cytosol resists ion movement and because some sodium ions are lost as they move back out across the membrane through leak channels.

Graded potentials occur in the plasma membranes of all cells in response to environmental stimuli. They often trigger specific cell functions. For example, a graded potential in the membrane of a gland cell may trigger secretion. However, graded potentials affect too small an area to have an effect on the activities of such large cells as skeletal muscle fibers or neurons. In these cells, graded potentials can influence activities in distant portions of the cell only if they lead to the production of an *action potential*, an electrical signal that affects the surface of the entire membrane.

An **action potential** is a propagated change in the membrane potential of excitable cells. *Excitable cells* are the only cells that have an electrically *excitable membrane* that can be stimulated to propagate action potentials. Excitable membranes contain *voltage-gated channels* that open or close in response to changes in the membrane potential. Skeletal muscle fibers, cardiac muscle cells, and the axons of neurons have excitable membranes.

In a skeletal muscle fiber, the action potential begins at the neuromuscular junction and travels along the entire membrane surface, including the T tubules. ⟳ p. 204 The resulting ion movements trigger a contraction.

In an axon, an action potential usually begins near the axon hillock and travels along the length of the axon toward the axon terminals, where its arrival activates the synapses. An action potential in a neuron is also known as a **nerve impulse**. (We discuss action potentials in cardiac muscle cells in Chapter 12.)

Action potentials are generated by the opening and closing of voltage-gated sodium channels and voltage-gated potassium channels in response to a graded potential. This local depolarization acts like pressure on the trigger of a gun. A gun fires only after a certain minimum pressure has been applied to the trigger. It does not matter whether the pressure builds gradually or is exerted suddenly—when the pressure reaches a critical point, the gun will fire. Whenever the gun fires, the forces that were applied to the trigger have no

Build Your Knowledge

Recall that a single axon of a motor neuron may branch to control more than one skeletal muscle fiber (as you saw in **Chapter 7: The Muscular System**). Each branch ends in an axon terminal that is part of a neuromuscular junction. Each skeletal muscle fiber has only one neuromuscular junction. A motor unit is a single motor neuron and all the muscle fibers it innervates. ⟳ **p. 205**

effect on the speed of the bullet leaving the gun. In an axon, the graded potential is the pressure on the trigger, and the action potential is like the firing of the gun. An action potential will not appear unless the membrane depolarizes to a level known as the **threshold**.

Every stimulus (whether minor or extreme) that brings the membrane to threshold will generate an identical action potential. This concept is called the **all-or-none principle** because a given stimulus either triggers a typical action potential or none at all. The all-or-none principle applies to all excitable membranes.

The Generation of an Action Potential

How is an action potential generated? An action potential begins when the first portion of the excitable axon membrane, called the *initial segment*, depolarizes to threshold. The steps involved in generating an action potential begin with a graded depolarization to threshold (from −70 to −60 mV) and end with a return to the resting potential (−70 mV). The steps are illustrated in **Spotlight Figure 8-8**.

The membrane cannot respond normally to further stimulation during most of these steps. This period is known as the **refractory period** of the membrane. It lasts from the moment the voltage-gated sodium channels open at threshold until the return to the resting potential, or *repolarization*, is complete. The

CLINICAL NOTE

Neurotoxins in Seafood

Potentially deadly forms of poisoning result from eating seafood that contains *neurotoxins*, which are poisons that primarily affect neurons. Several neurotoxins, such as *tetrodotoxin (TTX)* from puffer fish, *saxitoxin (SSX)* from bivalve shellfish, and *ciguatoxin (CTX)* from carnivorous, tropical coral reef fish prevent sodium channels from opening. Motor neurons cannot function under these conditions, and death may result from paralysis of the respiratory muscles.

A neuron receives information on its dendrites and cell body, and communicates that information to another cell at its axon terminal. Because the two ends of the neuron may be a meter apart, such long-range communication relies on action potentials.

Action potentials are propagated changes in the membrane potential that, once started, affect the entire excitable membrane of the axon. Action potentials depend on the presence of voltage-gated channels.

Axon hillock

Initial segment (first portion of excitable axon membrane to reach threshold)

Steps in the generation of an action potential in an axon.
The first step is a graded depolarization caused by the opening of chemically gated sodium ion channels, usually at the axon hillock. The axon membrane colors in steps 1–4 match the colors of the line graph showing changes in the membrane potential.

Resting Potential

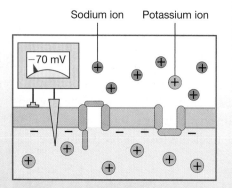

The axon membrane contains both voltage-gated sodium channels and voltage-gated potassium channels that are closed when the membrane is at the resting potential.

1 Depolarization to Threshold

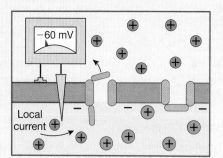

The stimulus that begins an action potential is a graded depolarization large enough to open voltage-gated sodium channels. The opening of the channels occurs at a membrane potential known as the threshold.

2 Activation of Sodium Channels and Rapid Depolarization

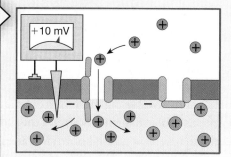

When the voltage-gated sodium channels open, sodium ions rush into the cytosol, and rapid depolarization occurs. The inner membrane surface now contains more positive ions than negative ones, and the membrane potential has changed from −60 mV to a positive value.

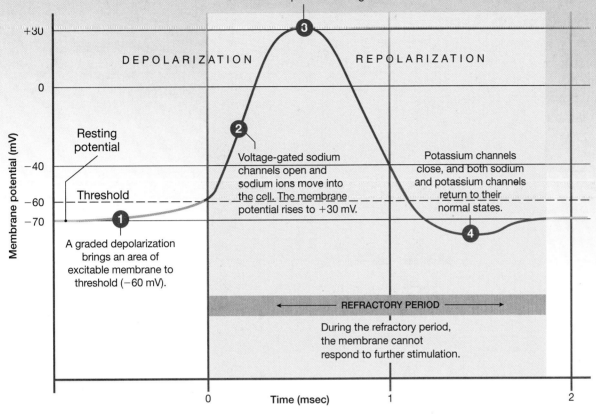

Sodium channels close, voltage-gated potassium channels open, and potassium ions move out of the cell. Repolarization begins.

3

DEPOLARIZATION   REPOLARIZATION

+30

0

−40

−60
−70

Membrane potential (mV)

Resting potential

Threshold

1

A graded depolarization brings an area of excitable membrane to threshold (−60 mV).

2 Voltage-gated sodium channels open and sodium ions move into the cell. The membrane potential rises to +30 mV.

Potassium channels close, and both sodium and potassium channels return to their normal states.

4

REFRACTORY PERIOD

During the refractory period, the membrane cannot respond to further stimulation.

0   Time (msec)   1   2

Changes in the membrane potential at one location during the generation of an action potential. The circled numbers in the graph correspond to the steps illustrated below.

---

3 Inactivation of Sodium Channels and Activation of Potassium Channels

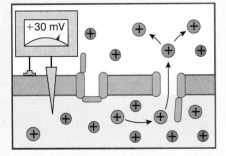

+30 mV

As the membrane potential approaches +30 mV, voltage-gated sodium channels close. This step coincides with the opening of voltage-gated potassium channels. Positively charged potassium ions move out of the cytosol, shifting the membrane potential back toward resting levels. Repolarization now begins.

4 Closing of Potassium Channels

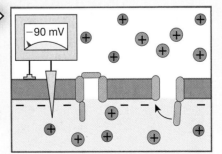

−90 mV

The voltage-gated sodium channels remain inactivated until the membrane has repolarized to near threshold levels. The voltage-gated potassium channels begin closing as the membrane reaches the normal resting potential (about 270 mV). Until all have closed, potassium ions continue to leave the cell. This produces a brief hyperpolarization.

Return to Resting Potential

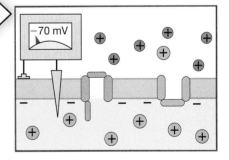

−70 mV

As the voltage-gated potassium channels close, the membrane potential returns to normal resting levels. The action potential is now over, and the membrane is once again at the resting potential.

Continuous Propagation along an Unmyelinated Axon

In an unmyelinated axon, an action potential moves along by continuous propagation. The action potential spreads by depolarizing the adjacent region of the axon membrane. This process continues to spread as a chain reaction down the axon.

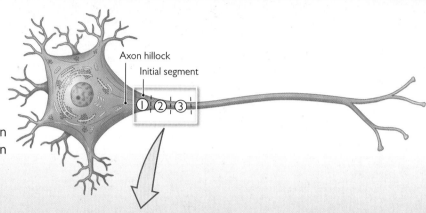

1 As an action potential develops at the initial segment ①, the membrane potential at this site depolarizes to +30 mV.

KEY

- Resting potential
- Graded depolarization
- Rapid depolarization
- Repolarization

2 As the sodium ions entering at ① spread away from the open voltage-gated channels, a graded depolarization quickly brings the membrane in segment ② to threshold.

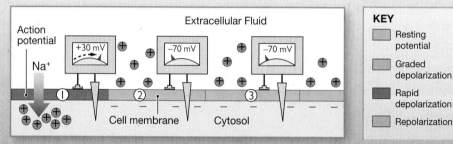

3 An action potential now occurs in segment ② while segment ① begins repolarization.

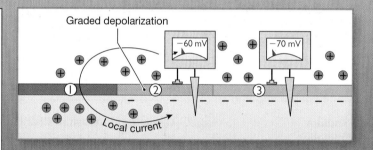

4 As the sodium ions entering at segment ② spread laterally, a graded depolarization quickly brings the membrane in segment ③ to threshold, and the cycle is repeated.

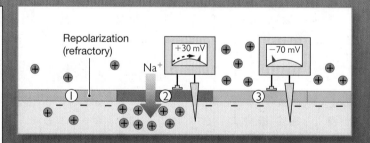

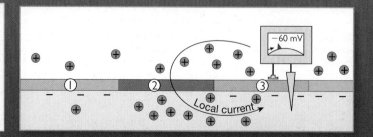

Saltatory Propagation along a Myelinated Axon

Because myelin limits the movement of ions across the axon membrane, the action potential must "jump" from node to node during propagation. This results in much faster propagation along the axon.

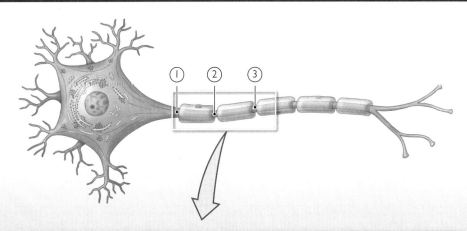

1 An action potential develops at the initial segment ①.

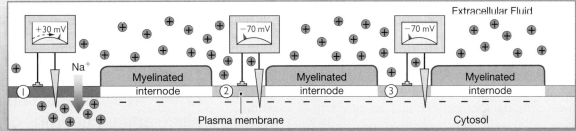

2 A local current produces a graded depolarization that brings the axon membrane at the next node to threshold.

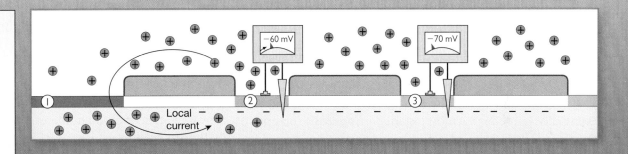

3 An action potential develops at node ②.

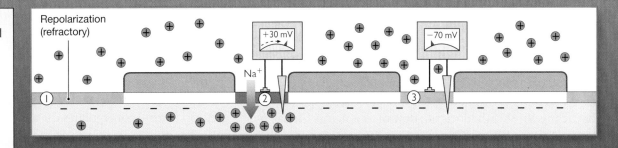

4 A local current produces a graded depolarization that brings the axon membrane at node ③ to threshold.

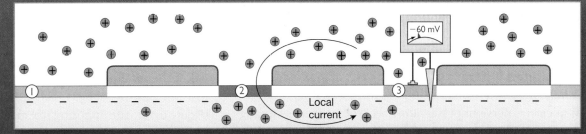

refractory period limits the rate at which action potentials can be generated in an excitable membrane. (The maximum rate of action potential generation is 500–1000 per second.)

Propagation of an Action Potential

An action potential initially involves a relatively small portion of the total membrane surface of the axon. But unlike graded potentials, which diminish rapidly with distance, action potentials affect the entire membrane surface. The basic processes of action potential propagation along unmyelinated and myelinated axons are shown in **Spotlight Figure 8-9** (p. 282). For simplicity, think of the plasma membrane as a series of adjacent segments.

The action potential begins at the axon's initial segment. For a brief moment at the peak of the action potential, the membrane potential becomes positive rather than negative (**1**). A *local current* then develops as the sodium ions begin moving in the cytosol and the extracellular fluid (**2**). The local current of moving sodium ions spreads in all directions, depolarizing adjacent portions of the membrane. (The axon hillock cannot respond with an action potential because it does not have voltage-gated sodium channels.) The process then continues in a chain reaction (**3** and **4**).

Each time a local current develops, the action potential moves forward along the axon. It does not move backward, because the previous segment of the axon is still in the refractory period. As a result, an action potential always proceeds away from its generation site and cannot reverse direction. Eventually, it reaches the most distant portions of the plasma membrane. This form of action potential transmission is known as **continuous propagation**. You might compare continuous propagation to a person walking toward some destination by taking small "baby steps." Progress is made, but slowly. Continuous propagation takes place along unmyelinated axons at a speed of about 1 meter per second (2 mph).

In a myelinated fiber, the axon is wrapped in myelin. This wrapping is complete except at the nodes, where adjacent glial cells contact one another. Between the nodes, the lipids of the myelin sheath block the flow of ions across the membrane. As a result, continuous propagation cannot take place. Instead, when an action potential is initiated by the axon hillock, the local current skips the internode and depolarizes the closest node to threshold (**Spotlight Figure 8-9**). In this way, the action potential jumps from node to node rather than proceeding in a series of small steps. This jumping process is called **saltatory propagation**. Its name comes from *saltare*, the Latin word meaning "to leap." Saltatory propagation carries nerve impulses along an axon at speeds ranging from 18 to 140 meters per second (from 40 to 300 mph). This faster process might be compared to a person jumping over puddles on the way to a destination.

CHECKPOINT

9. What effect would a chemical that blocks the voltage-gated sodium channels in the excitable axon membrane of a neuron have on its ability to depolarize?

10. What effect would decreasing the concentration of extracellular potassium have on the membrane potential of a neuron?

11. List the steps involved in the generation and propagation of an action potential.

12. Two axons are tested for propagation velocities (speeds). One carries action potentials at 50 meters per second, the other at 1 meter per second. Which axon is myelinated?

See the blue Answers tab at the back of the book.

8-4 At synapses, communication takes place among neurons or between neurons and other cells

Learning Objective Describe the structure of a synapse, and explain the process of nerve impulse transmission at a synapse.

Recall that a synapse is a site where a neuron communicates with another cell. In the nervous system, information moves from one location to another in the form of action potentials (nerve impulses) along axons. At the end of an axon, the arrival of an action potential results in the transfer of information to another neuron or to an effector cell. The information transfer takes place through the release of chemicals called **neurotransmitters** from the axon terminal.

The synapse where one neuron communicates with another may be on a dendrite, on the cell body, or along the length of the axon. Synapses between a neuron and another cell type are called **neuroeffector junctions**. As you have learned, a neuron communicates with a muscle cell at a *neuromuscular junction*. ⟲ p. 197 At a *neuroglandular junction*, a neuron controls or regulates the activity of a secretory cell.

Structure of a Synapse

Communication between neurons and other cells takes place in only one direction across a synapse. At a synapse between two neurons, the nerve impulse passes from the axon terminal of the sending neuron, called the **presynaptic neuron**, to the receiving neuron, called the **postsynaptic neuron** (**Figure 8-10**). The opposing plasma membranes are separated by a narrow space called the **synaptic cleft**.

Figure 8-10 The Structure of a Typical Synapse. A diagrammatic view of a typical synapse between two neurons.

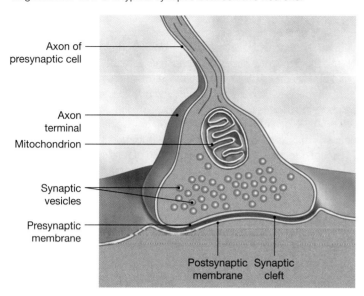

Figure 8-11 The Events at a Cholinergic Synapse.

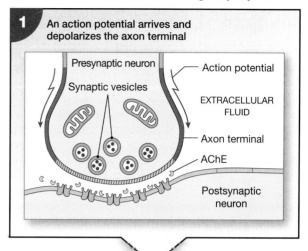

1 An action potential arrives and depolarizes the axon terminal

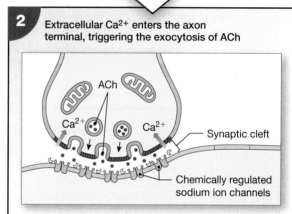

2 Extracellular Ca²⁺ enters the axon terminal, triggering the exocytosis of ACh

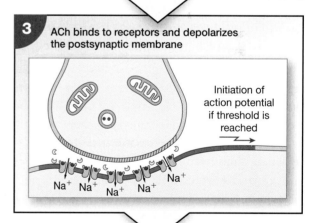

3 ACh binds to receptors and depolarizes the postsynaptic membrane

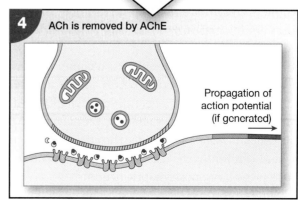

4 ACh is removed by AChE

Each axon terminal contains synaptic vesicles. Each vesicle contains several thousand molecules of a specific neurotransmitter. Upon stimulation, many of these vesicles release their contents into the synaptic cleft. The neurotransmitter then diffuses across the synaptic cleft and binds to receptors on the postsynaptic membrane.

Synaptic Function and Neurotransmitters

There are many different neurotransmitters. The neurotransmitter **acetylcholine**, or **ACh**, is released at **cholinergic synapses**. These synapses are widespread inside and outside of the CNS. The neuromuscular junction (described in Chapter 7) is one example. **Figure 8-11** shows the major events that take place at a cholinergic synapse after an action potential arrives at the presynaptic neuron:

1. ***An action potential arrives and depolarizes the axon terminal.***

2. ***The axon terminal releases the neurotransmitter ACh.*** Depolarization of the presynaptic membrane causes calcium channels to open briefly, allowing extracellular calcium ions to enter the axon terminal. Their entry triggers the exocytosis of the synaptic vesicles and the release of ACh. ACh release stops very quickly, because active transport processes rapidly remove the calcium ions from the cytosol.

3. ***ACh binds to receptors and depolarizes the postsynaptic membrane.*** The binding of ACh to sodium channels causes them to open and allow sodium ions to enter. If the resulting depolarization of the

CLINICAL NOTE

Organophosphate Poisoning

Organophosphates are a class of insecticides used widely in agriculture. Examples of organophosphates include diazinon, orthene, malathion, parathion, and others. In addition, organophosphates have been used as chemical warfare agents since World War II. Most recently, the organophosphate sarin was used in the terrorist attack on a Japanese subway in 1995. The potency of organophosphate compounds varies significantly.

The principle action of the organophosphates is deactivation of the enzyme acetylcholinesterase (cholinesterase) in the nervous system. This leads to the accumulation of acetylcholine at nerve synapses and at the neuromuscular junctions, which results in overstimulation of the acetylcholine receptors. This is followed by paralysis of cholinergic synaptic transmission.

Organophosphates bind irreversibly to cholinesterase, thus inactivating the enzyme. Organophosphates can enter the body through the skin or through the respiratory tract. Acute systemic organophosphate poisoning results in a variety of CNS, muscarinic, nicotinic, and somatic motor manifestations.

CNS symptoms include anxiety, restlessness, tremor, headache, dizziness, mental confusion, and seizures. Muscarinic receptor stimulation causes increased salivation, lacrimation, sweating, urinary incontinence, diarrhea, gastrointestinal system distress, vomiting, and bradycardia. Nicotinic receptor stimulation causes pallor, dilated pupils (mydriasis), and hypertension. Nicotinic stimulation at the neuromuscular junction also causes muscle fasciculations, cramps, and muscle weakness. This can progress to paralysis and a loss of reflexes.

The diagnosis of organophosphate poisoning is made by recognition of the signs and symptoms. Treatment is directed at support of essential functions such as maintenance of the airway and support of respirations. Initially, the drug atropine sulfate is administered. Atropine competes with acetylcholine for the acetylcholine receptors. In severe poisonings, exceedingly large doses of atropine may be required. This helps to reverse muscarinic and CNS symptoms. The antidote for organophosphate poisoning is *pralidoxime (2-PAM)*, which restores cholinesterase activity by regenerating cholinesterase. Pralidoxime also appears to prevent toxicity by detoxifying the remaining organophosphate molecules.

---

postsynaptic membrane reaches threshold, an action potential is generated.

4. ***ACh is removed by AChE.*** The effects on the postsynaptic membrane are temporary. The reason is because the synaptic cleft and postsynaptic membrane contain the enzyme acetylcholinesterase (AChE). ↻ p. 197 AChE removes ACh by breaking it into acetate and choline.

Another common neurotransmitter is **norepinephrine** (nor-ep-i-NEF-rin), or NE. It is important in the brain and in portions of the ANS. NE is also called *noradrenaline*, and synapses releasing NE are described as **adrenergic**.

The neurotransmitters **dopamine** (DŌ-puh-mēn), **gamma aminobutyric** (GAM-ma a-MĒ-nō-bū-TĒR-ik) **acid** (also known as **GABA**), and **serotonin** (ser-o-TŌ-nin) function in the CNS. There are at least 50 other neurotransmitters whose functions are not well understood. In addition, two gases are important neurotransmitters: *nitric oxide* and *carbon monoxide.*

The neurotransmitters released at a synapse may have excitatory or inhibitory effects. Both ACh and NE usually have an excitatory, depolarizing effect on postsynaptic neurons. Like ACh, NE has a temporary effect. It is broken down by an enzyme called *monoamine oxidase.* The effects of dopamine, GABA, and serotonin are usually inhibitory because they tend to hyperpolarize postsynaptic neurons.

Many drugs affect the nervous system by stimulating receptors that otherwise respond only to neurotransmitters. These drugs can have complex effects on perception, motor control, and emotional states.

Whether or not an action potential appears in the postsynaptic neuron depends on the balance between the depolarizing and hyperpolarizing stimuli arriving at any moment. For example, suppose that a neuron will generate an action potential if it receives 10 depolarizing stimuli. That could mean

CLINICAL NOTE

Neurotransmitters

No actual physical connection exists between two nerve cells or between a nerve cell and the organ it innervates. Instead, there is a space, or *synapse*, between nerve cells. Specialized chemicals called *neurotransmitters* conduct the nervous impulse between nerve cells or between a nerve cell and its target organ.

The two neurotransmitters of the autonomic nervous system are *acetylcholine* and *norepinephrine*. Acetylcholine is utilized in the preganglionic nerves of the sympathetic nervous system and in both the preganglionic and postganglionic nerves of the parasympathetic nervous system. Norepinephrine is the postganglionic neurotransmitter of the sympathetic nervous system. Synapses that use acetylcholine as the neurotransmitter are *cholinergic synapses*. Synapses that use norepinephrine as the neurotransmitter are *adrenergic synapses*.

10 active synapses if all release excitatory neurotransmitters. But if, at the same moment, 10 other synapses release inhibitory neurotransmitters, the excitatory and inhibitory effects will cancel one another out. As a result, no action potential would develop.

The activity of a neuron thus depends on the balance between excitation and inhibition. The interactions are extremely complex. Synapses at the cell body and dendrites may involve tens of thousands of other neurons. Some release excitatory neurotransmitters and others release inhibitory neurotransmitters.

Neuronal Pools

As noted earlier, the human body has about 10 million sensory neurons, 20 billion interneurons, and one-half million motor neurons. These individual neurons represent the simplest level of organization within the CNS. However, the integration of sensory and motor information to produce complex responses requires groups of interneurons acting together.

A **neuronal pool** is a group of interconnected interneurons with specific functions. Each neuronal pool has a limited number of input sources and output destinations. Also, each pool may contain excitatory and inhibitory neurons. The output of one pool may stimulate or depress the activity of other pools, or it may exert direct control over motor neurons or peripheral effectors.

Neurons and neuronal pools communicate with one another in several "wiring diagrams," or *neural circuits*. The two simplest circuit patterns are *divergence* and *convergence*. In **divergence**, information spreads from one neuron to several neurons, or from one neuronal pool to multiple neuronal pools (**Figure 8-12a**). Considerable divergence occurs when sensory neurons bring information into the CNS. The sensory information is distributed to different neuronal pools throughout the spinal cord and brain. For example, visual information from the eyes reaches your conscious awareness at the same time it is carried to areas of the brain that control posture and balance at the subconscious level.

Divergence is also involved when you step on a sharp object. That action stimulates sensory neurons that distribute information to a number of neuronal pools. As a result, you might withdraw your foot, shift your weight, move your arms, feel the pain, and shout "Ouch!"—all at the same time.

In **convergence** (**Figure 8-12b**), several neurons synapse on a single postsynaptic neuron. Convergence makes possible both voluntary and involuntary control of some body

Figure 8-12 Two Common Types of Neuronal Pools.

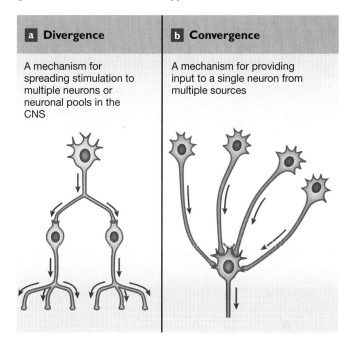

a Divergence	**b** Convergence
A mechanism for spreading stimulation to multiple neurons or neuronal pools in the CNS	A mechanism for providing input to a single neuron from multiple sources

processes. For example, as you read this, the movements of your diaphragm and ribs are being involuntarily, or subconsciously, controlled by respiratory centers in your brain. These centers activate or inhibit motor neurons in your spinal cord that control your respiratory muscles. But those same movements can be controlled voluntarily, or consciously, as when you take a deep breath and hold it. Two neuronal pools are involved, and both synapse on the same motor neurons.

CHECKPOINT

13. Describe the general structure of a synapse.

14. What effect would blocking calcium channels at a cholinergic synapse have on synapse function?

15. What type of neural circuit permits both conscious and subconscious control of the same motor neurons?

See the blue Answers tab at the back of the book.

8-5 The brain and spinal cord are surrounded by three layers of membranes called the meninges

Learning Objective Describe the three meningeal layers that surround the central nervous system.

The CNS consists of the spinal cord and brain. The neural tissue of the CNS is delicate. It also has a very high metabolic rate and requires abundant nutrients and a constant supply of oxygen. At the same time, CNS tissue must be isolated from a variety of compounds in the blood that could interfere with its complex operations. It also needs to be protected against damaging contact with the surrounding bones.

The **meninges** (me-NIN-jēz) are three layers of specialized membranes surrounding the brain and spinal cord (**Figure 8-13**). They provide the CNS tissue with physical stability and shock absorption. Blood vessels branching within these layers deliver needed oxygen and nutrients. At the foramen magnum of the skull, the *cranial meninges* covering the brain are continuous with the *spinal meninges* that surround the spinal cord. The meninges cover cranial nerves as they extend through foramina of the skull and spinal nerves that pass through the intervertebral foramina. The meninges then become continuous with the connective tissues surrounding the peripheral nerves.

The three meningeal layers are the *dura mater*, the *arachnoid*, and the *pia mater*.

The Dura Mater

The tough, fibrous **dura mater** (DOO-ruh MĀ-ter; *dura*, + hard *mater*, mother) forms the outermost covering of

the CNS. The dura mater surrounding the brain consists of two fibrous layers. The outer layer is fused to the periosteum of the skull. In some places, the inner layer is joined with the outer layer. Typically, the two layers are separated by a slender gap that contains tissue fluids and blood vessels (**Figure 8-13a**).

At several locations, the inner layer of the dura mater extends deep into the cranial cavity, forming folded membranous sheets called *dural folds*. The dural folds act like seat belts to hold the brain in position. Large collecting veins known as *dural sinuses* lie between the two layers of a dural fold.

In the spinal cord, the outer layer of the dura mater is not fused to bone. An **epidural space** lies between the dura mater of the spinal cord and the walls of the vertebral canal. This space contains areolar tissue, blood vessels, and adipose tissue (**Figure 8-13b**). Injecting an anesthetic into the epidural space produces a temporary sensory and motor paralysis known as an *epidural block*. This technique has the advantage of affecting only the spinal nerves in the immediate area of the injection. Epidural blocks in the lower lumbar or sacral regions may be used to control pain during childbirth.

Figure 8-13 The Meninges of the Brain and Spinal Cord.

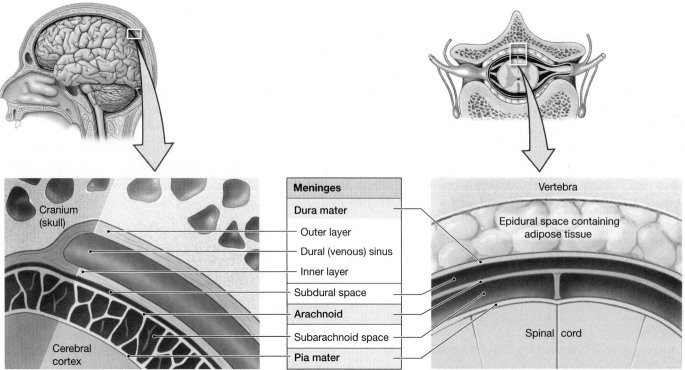

Meninges
Dura mater
Outer layer
Dural (venous) sinus
Inner layer
Subdural space
Arachnoid
Subarachnoid space
Pia mater

Cranium (skull)

Cerebral cortex

Vertebra

Epidural space containing adipose tissue

Spinal cord

a Location and structure of the cranial meninges

b Location and structure of the spinal meninges

CLINICAL NOTE

Burr Holes

Bleeding in the epidural space, called an *epidural hematoma*, usually results from laceration of an artery during blunt head trauma. This causes rapid swelling and compression of the brain. Life-saving emergency treatment may require drilling *burr holes* through the skull over the hematoma to relieve the pressure. Although burr holes are usually performed by neurosurgeons, the emergency physician may have to place them if a neurosurgeon is unavailable.

The Arachnoid

A narrow **subdural space** separates the inner surface of the dura mater from the second meningeal layer, the **arachnoid** (a-RAK-noyd; *arachne*, spider). This intervening space contains a small quantity of lymphatic fluid, which reduces friction between the opposing surfaces. The arachnoid is a layer of squamous epithelial cells. Deep to this layer lies the **subarachnoid space**, which contains a delicate web of collagen and elastic fibers. The subarachnoid space is filled with *CSF*. This fluid acts as a shock absorber and transports dissolved gases, nutrients, chemical messengers, and waste products.

The Pia Mater

The subarachnoid space separates the arachnoid from the innermost meningeal layer, the **pia mater** (*pia*, delicate + *mater*, mother). The pia mater is bound firmly to the underlying neural tissue. The blood vessels servicing the brain and spinal cord run along the surface of this layer, within the subarachnoid space. The pia mater of the brain is highly vascular, and large blood vessels branch over the surface of the brain, supplying the superficial areas of neural cortex. This extensive blood supply is extremely important, for the brain has a very high rate of metabolism. At rest, the 1.4 kg (3.1 lb) brain uses as much oxygen as 28 kg (61.6 lb) of skeletal muscle.

Comparison of epidural and subdural hematomas

CHECKPOINT

16. Identify the three meninges surrounding the CNS.

See the blue Answers tab at the back of the book.

8-6 The spinal cord contains gray matter surrounded by white matter and connects to 31 pairs of spinal nerves

Learning Objective Discuss the roles of gray matter and white matter in the spinal cord.

The spinal cord serves as the major highway for sensory impulses passing to the brain and motor impulses coming from the brain. In addition, the spinal cord integrates information on its own. It controls *spinal reflexes*, automatic motor responses ranging from withdrawal from pain to complex reflex patterns involved in sitting, standing, walking, and running.

CLINICAL NOTE

Epidural and Subdural Hemorrhages

A severe head injury may damage cerebral blood vessels and cause bleeding into the cranial cavity. If blood is forced between the dura mater and the skull, the condition is known as an *epidural hemorrhage*. A *subdural hemorrhage* is bleeding between the dura mater and the arachnoid mater (**Figure 8-14**). These conditions are serious because the blood entering the epidural or subdural spaces compresses and distorts the relatively soft tissues of the brain. The signs and symptoms vary depending on whether an artery or a vein is damaged. Because arterial blood pressure is higher, bleeding from an artery can cause more rapid and severe distortion of neural tissue. There is good reason for adults and children to give their heads added protection by wearing helmets while biking, motorcycling, skiing, skateboarding, and playing various sports.

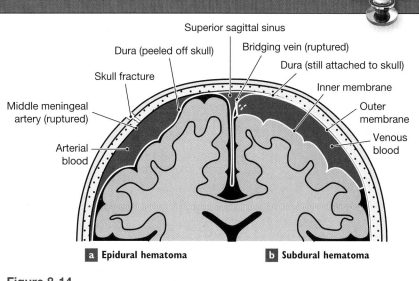

a Epidural hematoma   **b** Subdural hematoma

Figure 8-14

CLINICAL NOTE

Nervous System Infections

Infections of the nervous system can be life threatening. The most common nervous system infection is meningitis. Its causes include viruses, bacteria, fungi, parasites, and prions. Less common CNS infections include encephalitis and brain abscess. CNS infections are classified as acute, subacute, or chronic depending upon the duration of the disease.

Meningitis

Meningitis is an infection of the meninges. Bacterial meningitis is a medical emergency that begins when the causative organisms enter the subarachnoid space. The three principle organisms are *Streptococcal pneumoniae, Haemophilus influenza (type b)*, and *Neisseria meningitidis.* They enter the subarachnoid space, usually through the upper airway, and trigger infection and inflammation. The signs and symptoms of meningitis are fever, headache, altered mental status, photophobia, and stiffness of the neck (meningismus). With meningismus, passive flexion of the neck causes flexion of the hips and knees. This finding, referred to as *Brudzinski's sign*, is due to inflammation of the meninges. *Kernig's sign*, an inability to extend the legs when the knees are flexed, is also due to meningeal inflammation. Brudzinski's sign and Kernig's sign are seen in approximately 50 percent of patients with bacterial meningitis. The diagnosis of meningitis is based on the history, physical examination, and lumbar puncture (spinal tap).

A *lumbar puncture* is an important diagnostic procedure that obtains *cerebrospinal fluid (CSF)* for laboratory analysis. The puncture is usually made between the third and fourth lumbar vertebrae, well below the terminal end of the spinal cord (**Figure 8-15**). The patient is placed in a seated or a lateral

Figure 8-15 Cross Section of the Distal Spine and Spinal Cord That Shows Proper Positioning of a Spinal Needle During Lumbar Puncture. Note that the puncture site is several segments below the terminal end of the spinal cord.

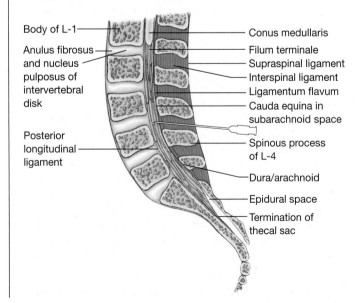

Body of L-1
Anulus fibrosus and nucleus pulposus of intervertebral disk
Posterior longitudinal ligament

Conus medullaris
Filum terminale
Supraspinal ligament
Interspinal ligament
Ligamentum flavum
Cauda equina in subarachnoid space
Spinous process of L-4
Dura/arachnoid
Epidural space
Termination of thecal sac

recumbent position. The skin is cleansed and a sterile spinal needle is slowly inserted through the skin of the lower back into the subarachnoid space. Often, a "pop" can be felt as the needle penetrates the tough dura mater. Once the needle is properly placed, the CSF pressure is measured. Then, approximately 3–4 milliliters of CSF are removed. Spinal fluid is normally clear and does not contain cells. In meningitis, the spinal fluid becomes cloudy due to the presence of white blood cells (*pleocytosis*) and bacteria.

Bacterial meningitis can be rapidly fatal. As soon as the diagnosis is suspected, empiric antibiotics are administered. In adults, *N. meningitidis* and *S. pneumoniae* are the most common organisms. The incidence of *H. influenzae* has steadily declined with the introduction of a vaccine. Infection with *N. meningitidis*, which is referred to as meningiococcemia, is particularly severe. Emergency personnel who have been in close contact with a patient who has meningiococcemia may require prophylactic antibiotics.

Viral Meningitis

The signs and symptoms of viral meningitis are typically less severe than those of bacterial forms. The CSF fluid will typically contain white blood cells, but an infectious organism cannot be seen or cultured. Because of this, viral meningitis is often called aseptic meningitis. Viral meningitis often occurs in winter, and outbreaks are not uncommon. Treatment is supportive.

Unusual Forms of Meningitis

Although viral and bacterial meningitis are by far the most common, some other types of meningitis can be life threatening. The incidence of some infections is increasing due to increasing numbers of patients with incompetent immune systems. These include AIDS patients, patients who have received an organ transplant, and patients who are undergoing chemotherapy treatment for cancer. Often, the causative agent is not infectious and may actually be a part of the body's normal flora, but in patients with immunosuppression from drugs or disease, it can cause infection. Because of this, these types of meningitis are referred to as *opportunistic infections*.

Fungal meningitis is uncommon and, when present, tends to be chronic. Treatment is difficult and often requires long periods of therapy with antifungal drugs. It is most commonly seen in AIDS patients or in others who are immunocompromised.

Tubercular meningitis is being seen with increasing frequency, primarily in AIDS patients. The symptoms include headache, low-grade fever, nausea, vomiting, irritability, difficulty sleeping, and fatigue. As the disease progresses, confusion, stiff neck, behavioral changes, and seizures can occur. Despite the severity, the recovery rate approaches 90 percent if therapy is initiated in time.

Occasionally, meningitis can result from infection with free-living amoebas, particularly Naegleria. These organisms are found in both fresh and brackish water including that from lakes, swimming pools, hot springs, and heating and air conditioning units. Infection occurs when persons swimming in, or exposed to, the water inhale the organism. It invades the olfactory nervous tissue from the nasal cavity. After an incubation period of 2–15 days, the patient develops high fever, severe headache, nausea, vomiting, and meningismus. Rapid progression to seizures and coma occurs, and most patients die within a week. Only four survivors have been reported.

Parasitic Brain Infections

Cestodes are flatworms commonly referred to as tapeworms. The most commonly encountered member of this group is the pork tapeworm (*Taenia solium*). It is a significant problem in developing countries and is occasionally encountered in the United States, especially in immigrants and visitors from Central America and the Middle East.

The larval stage of *T. solium* can cause clinical disease referred to as *cysticercosis*, which can be serious and often fatal. *Taenia* cysts can enter the subcutaneous tissue, the eye, the brain, and the heart and cause seizures and hydrocephalus. Cysticercosis should be considered a possible cause of new-onset seizures in recent immigrants from Central America. It can be identified through computed tomographic scanning of the brain and by isolation of cysts in the stool. Treatment with antiparasitic medications is usually effective if administered in time.

Brain Abscess

Brain abscesses are localized collections of pus within the parenchyma of the brain or spinal cord (**Figure 8–16**). They tend to occur most frequently in men between the ages of 30 and 40 years. They can be caused by open trauma or neurosurgical procedures, by infection that has spread from the middle ear or nose, or by spreading from abscesses elsewhere in the body. AIDS patients are particularly susceptible to brain abscesses caused by the protozoan *Toxoplasma gondii* (*toxoplasmosis*). Treatment of brain abscess generally requires surgical drainage.

Encephalitis

Encephalitis is an acute infection, usually of viral origin, with CNS involvement. Most cases of encephalitis are due to viruses carried by mosquitoes. Outbreaks of encephalitis usually occur in summer. Causative viruses include *Eastern equine encephalitis,*

Figure 8-16 Large Brain Abscess Secondary to Intravenous Injection of Narcotics. Bacteria are introduced to the brain, which results in abscess formation.

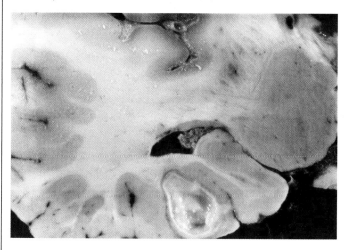

Western equine encephalitis, St. Louis encephalitis, and *California encephalitis*. Encephalitis can also occur as a complication of viral diseases that usually affect other body systems, such as rabies or mononucleosis. Encephalitis is also seen in AIDS patients. Common causative viruses in this population include *herpes virus* and *cytomegalovirus*. The most common signs and symptoms of encephalitis are headache and fever. Delirium, confusion, seizures, and unconsciousness can occur in severe cases. Treatment for epidemic encephalitis is usually supportive. Opportunistic viral infections in AIDS patients are often treated with antiviral drugs.

Prion Diseases

Until recently, scientists thought the smallest particle capable of transmitting disease was a virus. However, researchers have demonstrated that a protein alone is capable of transmitting disease. Protein particles, referred to as prions, have been identified as the causative agent of a group of diseases called *spongiform encephalopathies*. These diseases cause the brain to develop large vacuoles in the cortex and cerebellum, which adversely affect CNS function. It appears that traditional sterilization methods do not inactivate prions and they can remain communicable for long periods of time.

Previously, prion diseases have been rare. However, with the outbreak of mad cow disease in Europe, considerable attention has been focused on them. Mad cow disease, also known as *bovine spongiform encephalopathy (BSE)*, initially appeared in the United Kingdom and has spread to parts of Europe. BSE apparently is transmitted through cattle feed. In the cattle industry, it is not uncommon for cattle feed to contain the byproducts of other cattle. Apparently, parts of infected cattle were unknowingly ground up and mixed in cattle feed and fed to cattle in commercial feedlots. Some cattle that ate the tainted feed developed BSE.

Several human diseases are known to be caused by prions, the most common being *Creutzfeldt-Jakob disease (CJD)*. Prior to the outbreak of BSE, the incidence of CJD was only one person per million per year. However, the incidence has increased since the outbreak of BSE. Now, there appears to be a direct link between BSE and a form of CJD.

Early symptoms of CJD include failing memory, changes in behavior, lack of coordination, and visual disturbances. These are followed by a rapid, progressive dementia, involuntary jerking movements, and progressive motor dysfunction. The duration of CJD from the onset of symptoms to death is usually less than a year. Death is typically caused by secondary pneumonia. There is no treatment or cure for CJD.

Two interesting prion diseases are *fatal familial insomnia (FFI)* and *kuru*. FFI presents with untreatable insomnia, autonomic nervous system dysfunction, and eventually death. It is associated with severe, selective atrophy of the thalamus. Kuru occurs only in isolated tribes in the Fore highlands of New Guinea. In these tribes, the brains of dead relatives were removed and eaten as part of a religious ritual that honors the dead relative. Tribal members ground the brain up into a pale, gray soup, heated it, and ate it. The disease clinically resembles CJD, and some scientists have speculated that the brain tissue was highly infectious, with the causative prion being transmitted through ingestion. An effort by the New Guinea government to curtail cannibalism has caused the incidence of kuru to rapidly decline, and the disease is now almost unknown.

Gross Anatomy

The adult spinal cord (**Figure 8-17a**) is approximately 45 cm (18 in.) long and has a maximum width of roughly 14 mm (0.55 in.). With two exceptions, the diameter of the cord decreases as it extends toward the sacral region. The two exceptions are regions concerned with the sensory and motor control of the limbs. The *cervical enlargement* supplies nerves to the shoulder girdles and upper limbs. The *lumbar enlargement* provides innervation to the pelvis and lower limbs. Inferior to the lumbar enlargement, the spinal cord becomes tapered and conical. A slender strand of fibrous tissue extends from the inferior tip of the spinal cord to the coccyx, serving as an anchor that prevents upward movement.

The spinal cord has a **central canal**, a narrow internal passageway filled with CSF (**Figure 8-17b**). The posterior surface of the spinal cord has a shallow groove, the *posterior median sulcus*. The anterior surface has a deeper groove, the *anterior median fissure.*

The entire spinal cord consists of 31 segments. Each gives rise to a pair of *spinal nerves*. There are 8 cervical, 12 thoracic, 5 lumbar, 5 sacral, and 1 coccygeal spinal segments (**Figure 8-17c**). Each pair of spinal nerves is identified by a letter and number (**Figure 8-17a,c**).

Every spinal segment is associated with a pair of **dorsal root ganglia** (singular: ganglion), which contain the cell bodies of sensory neurons (**Figure 8-17b**). The **dorsal roots** contain the axons of these neurons and bring sensory information to the spinal cord. A pair of **ventral roots** contains the axons of CNS motor neurons that control muscles and glands. On either side, the dorsal and ventral roots from each segment leave the vertebral column between adjacent vertebrae at the *intervertebral foramen.*

Distal to each dorsal root ganglion, the sensory (dorsal) and motor (ventral) roots are bound together into a single **spinal nerve**. All spinal nerves are classified as *mixed nerves* because they contain both sensory and motor fibers. The spinal nerves on either side form outside the vertebral canal, where the ventral and dorsal roots unite. ⟳ p. 162

The spinal cord continues to grow until a person is approximately 4 years old. After age 4, the vertebral column continues to elongate, but the spinal cord does not. As a result, the dorsal and ventral roots gradually grow longer and the correspondence between a spinal cord segment and its adjacent vertebra is lost. This explains why spinal cord segments S_1–S_5 are level with vertebrae T_{12}–L_1 (**Figure 8-17c**).

The adult spinal cord extends only to the level of the first or second lumbar vertebrae. When seen in gross dissection, the long ventral and dorsal roots of spinal nerves inferior to the tip of the spinal cord, plus the cord's threadlike extensions, reminded early anatomists of a horse's tail. With that in mind, they called this complex the *cauda equina* (KAW-duh ek-WĪ-nuh; *cauda*, tail + *equus*, horse).

Sectional Anatomy

The anterior median fissure and the posterior median sulcus mark the division between left and right sides of the spinal cord (**Figure 8-18**). The *gray matter* is dominated by the cell bodies of neurons and glial cells. It forms a rough H, or a butterfly shape, around the narrow central canal. Projections of gray matter, called **horns**, extend outward into the *white matter*, which contains large numbers of myelinated and unmyelinated axons.

Figure 8-18a shows the relationship between the function of a particular nucleus (a collection of sensory or motor cell bodies) and its relative position in the gray matter of the spinal cord. The *posterior gray horns* contain sensory nuclei. The *anterior gray horns* are involved in the motor control of skeletal muscles. Nuclei in the *lateral gray horns* contain the visceral motor neurons that control smooth muscle, cardiac muscle, and glands.

The *gray commissures* anterior and posterior to the central canal interconnect the horns on either side of the spinal cord. The gray and white commissures contain axons that cross from one side of the spinal cord to the other.

The white matter on each side can be divided into three regions, or **columns** (**Figure 8-18a**). The *posterior white columns* extend between the posterior gray horns and the posterior median sulcus. The *anterior white columns* lie between the anterior gray horns and the anterior median fissure. The anterior white columns are interconnected by the *anterior white commissure*. The white matter between the anterior and posterior columns makes up the *lateral white columns*.

Each column contains tracts whose axons carry either sensory information or motor commands. Small tracts carry sensory or motor signals between segments of the spinal cord, and larger tracts connect the spinal cord with the brain. **Ascending tracts** carry sensory information toward the brain. **Descending tracts** convey motor commands into the spinal cord.

CHECKPOINT

17. Damage to which root of a spinal nerve would interfere with motor function?

18. A person with polio has lost the use of his leg muscles. In which area of his spinal cord could you locate the poliovirus-infected motor neurons?

19. Why are spinal nerves also called mixed nerves?

See the blue Answers tab at the back of the book.

Figure 8-17 Gross Anatomy of the Spinal Cord.

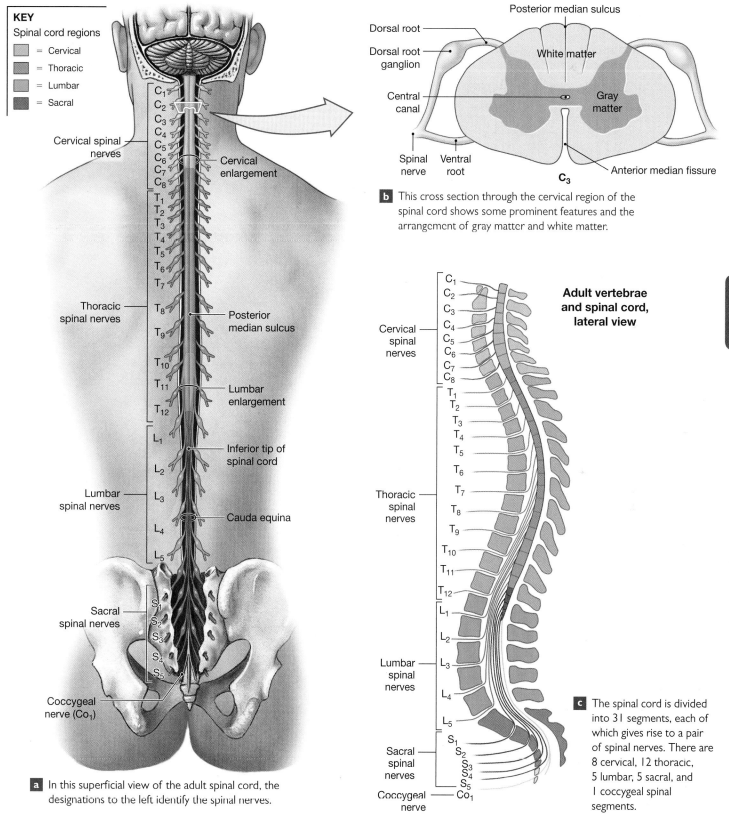

KEY
Spinal cord regions
- ☐ = Cervical
- ☐ = Thoracic
- ☐ = Lumbar
- ☐ = Sacral

a In this superficial view of the adult spinal cord, the designations to the left identify the spinal nerves.

b This cross section through the cervical region of the spinal cord shows some prominent features and the arrangement of gray matter and white matter.

Adult vertebrae and spinal cord, lateral view

c The spinal cord is divided into 31 segments, each of which gives rise to a pair of spinal nerves. There are 8 cervical, 12 thoracic, 5 lumbar, 5 sacral, and 1 coccygeal spinal segments.

Figure 8-18 Sectional Anatomy of the Spinal Cord.

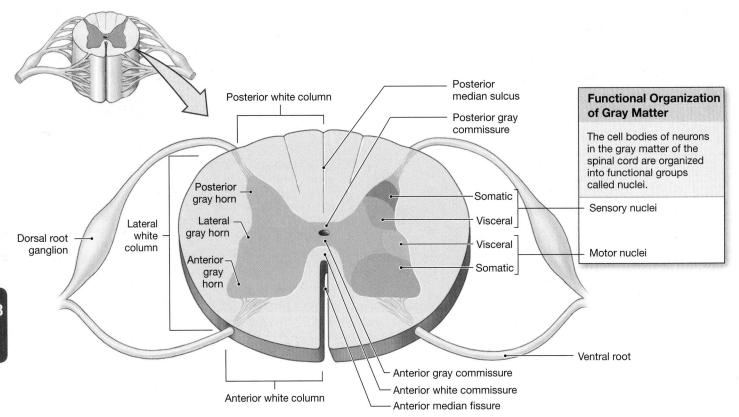

Functional Organization of Gray Matter

The cell bodies of neurons in the gray matter of the spinal cord are organized into functional groups called nuclei.

Sensory nuclei

Motor nuclei

a The left half of this sectional view shows important anatomical landmarks, including the three columns of white matter. The right half indicates the functional organization of the nuclei in the anterior, lateral, and posterior gray horns.

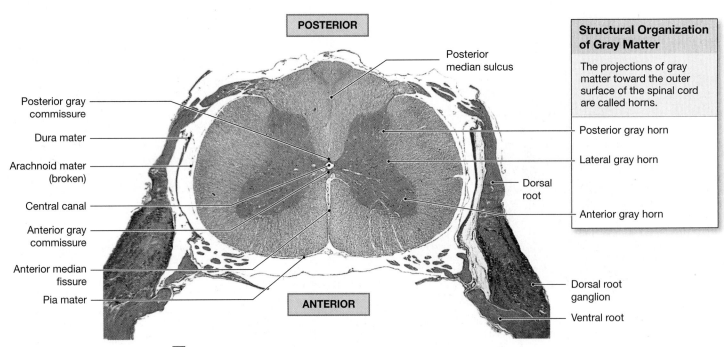

Structural Organization of Gray Matter

The projections of gray matter toward the outer surface of the spinal cord are called horns.

b A micrograph of a section through the spinal cord, showing major landmarks in and surrounding the cord.

CLINICAL NOTE

Spinal Cord Injuries

The spinal cord is well-protected by the vertebral bodies (**Figure 8-19**). Spinal-cord injuries usually are due to vertebral injuries that usually result from the extremes of normal motion such as flexion, extension, rotation, and lateral bending. Damaging mechanisms also include forces transmitted along the axis of the spine: *axial loading* and *distraction*. Finally, spinal injury can result either directly from blunt or penetrating trauma or indirectly when an expanding mass (edema or hematoma) compresses the cord or a disruption of blood supply damages it (**Figure 8-20**). It is possible to have spinal-cord injury without any spinal-column injury.

The bones, ligaments, and joints of the vertebral column may be damaged by hyperflexion or hyperextension. This most frequently occurs in the cervical and lumbar regions. These motions can cause the vertebral column to fracture or dislocate. With fractures, bone fragments can damage the spinal cord. With dislocations, abnormal movement of the vertebrae can compress or even shear the spinal cord.

Spinal-cord injury varies in severity; its classifications include the following:

- *Cord concussion.* A temporary interruption in cordmediated functions.

- *Cord contusion.* Bruising of the neural tissue that results in swelling and temporary loss of cord-mediated functions.

- *Cord compression.* Results from pressure on the cord which causes ischemia. Surgery to decompress the cord is often required to prevent permanent damage.

- *Cord lacerations.* Tearing of the neural tissues from bone fragments or shearing forces. Slight damage may be reversible, but permanent damage can occur if spinal tracts are disrupted.

- *Complete transection.* Severing of the spinal cord that causes permanent loss of function.

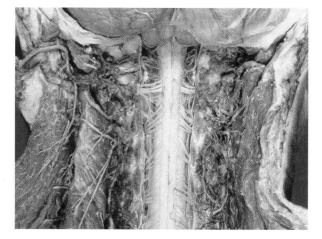

Figure 8-19 Detailed Dissection of the Proximal Spinal Cord that Illustrates Essential Structures and Spinal Nerve Roots.

- *Incomplete transection.* Part of the spinal cord is severed, but some tracts are spared.

- *Cord hemorrhage.* Bleeding into the neural tissues secondary to blood vessel damage following injury.

Several syndromes can develop with spinal-cord injury. These result from partial cord injuries where some spinal tracts are destroyed while others are spared. These syndromes include

- *Anterior-cord syndrome.* Results from compression of the anterior part of the spinal cord, often from hyperflexion of the cervical spine. It causes complete paralysis below the lesion with loss of pain and temperature sensation. Vibratory and light touch ability are spared in this injury.

Figure 8-20 Mechanisms Associated with Cervical Spine, Vertebral, and Spinal-Cord Injury.

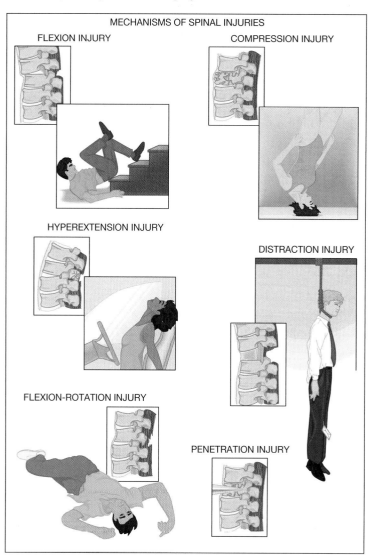

MECHANISMS OF SPINAL INJURIES

FLEXION INJURY

COMPRESSION INJURY

HYPEREXTENSION INJURY

DISTRACTION INJURY

FLEXION-ROTATION INJURY

PENETRATION INJURY

(*Continued*)

- *Central-cord syndrome.* Results from disruption of blood supply to the spinal cord, often due to hyperextension injuries. It causes quadriparesis that is greater in the upper extremities than in the lower extremities. There may be some loss of pain and temperature sensation.

- *Brown-Séquard syndrome.* Results from transection of half of the spinal cord or from unilateral cord compression. It causes spastic paresis and loss of position and vibratory sensation on the affected side and loss of temperature and pain sensation on the opposite side.

- *Cauda equina syndrome.* Results from injury to the cauda equina from lumbar vertebral fractures of herniated discs. It can cause weakness and sensory loss in the lower extremities, sciatica, and possible bowel or bladder dysfunction.

- *Spinal shock.* Results from partial or complete spinal-cord injury at T_6 or above. It causes loss of reflexes, sensation, and flaccid paralysis below the level of the lesion. In addition, there is a flaccid bladder, loss of rectal sphincter tone, bradycardia, and hypotension.

As central nervous system tissues cannot regenerate, spinal-cord injuries are usually permanent. Occasionally, if treated in time, the injury can be minimized by the administration of extremely high doses of corticosteroids. This appears to limit the inflammation associated with the injury and prevent secondary injury from swelling.

Significant research is directed at the biochemical control of nerve growth and regeneration. In addition, electronic devices and computers are being used to stimulate specific muscles and muscle groups. This has allowed persons with spinal cord injuries to walk short distances.

8-7 The brain has several principal structures, each with specific functions

Learning Objective Name the major regions of the brain, and describe the locations and functions of each.

The brain is far more complex than the spinal cord. Its responses to stimuli are also more versatile. The brain contains roughly 20 billion neurons organized into hundreds of neuronal pools. Everything we do and everything we are is the result of brain activity.

The adult human brain contains almost 97 percent of the neural tissue in the body. A "typical" adult brain weighs 1.4 kg (3 lb) and has a volume of 1200 cc (71 in.^{3}). Brain size varies considerably among individuals. The brains of males are, on average, about 10 percent larger than those of females, because of differences in average body size. There is no correlation between brain size and intelligence. Individuals with the smallest brains (750 cc) or largest brains (2100 cc) are functionally normal.

The Major Regions of the Brain

The adult brain has six major regions: (1) the *cerebrum*, (2) the *diencephalon*, (3) the *midbrain*, (4) the *pons*, (5) the *medulla oblongata*, and (6) the *cerebellum*. Major landmarks are indicated in **Figure 8-21**.

The adult brain is dominated in size by the **cerebrum** (se-RĒ-brum or SER-e-brum). The cerebrum is made up of large, paired left and right **cerebral hemispheres** (**Figure 8-21a**). Conscious thoughts, sensations, intellectual functions, memory storage and processing, and complex movements originate in the cerebrum.

The hollow **diencephalon** (dī-en-SEF-a-lon; *dia-*, through + *encephalos*, brain) is connected to the cerebrum (**Figure 8-21c**). Its largest portion is the **thalamus** (THAL-a-mus). The thalamus contains relay and processing centers for sensory information. The **hypothalamus** (*hypo-*, below) is the floor of the diencephalon. It contains centers involved with emotions, autonomic function, and hormone production. A narrow stalk connects the hypothalamus to the *pituitary gland*. The pituitary gland is the primary link between the nervous and endocrine systems. (We will discuss it in Chapter 10.) The **epithalamus** contains another endocrine structure, the *pineal gland*.

The **brain stem** contains three major regions of the brain: the midbrain, pons, and medulla oblongata (**Figure 8-21c**). The brain stem contains important processing centers and relay stations for information headed to or from the cerebrum or cerebellum.

Nuclei in the **midbrain**, or *mesencephalon* (mez-en-SEF-a-lon; *meso-*, middle), process visual and auditory information and generate involuntary motor responses. This region also contains centers that help maintain consciousness.

The **pons** connects the cerebellum to the brain stem (*pons* refers to a bridge). In addition to tracts and relay centers, the pons also contains nuclei involved in somatic and visceral motor control.

The pons is also connected to the **medulla oblongata**, the segment of the brain that is attached to the spinal cord. The medulla oblongata relays sensory information to the thalamus and other brain stem centers. It also contains major centers that regulate autonomic function, such as heart rate, blood pressure, respiration, and digestive activities.

The large cerebral hemispheres and the smaller hemispheres of the **cerebellum** (ser-e-BEL-um) almost completely cover the

Figure 8-21 The Brain.

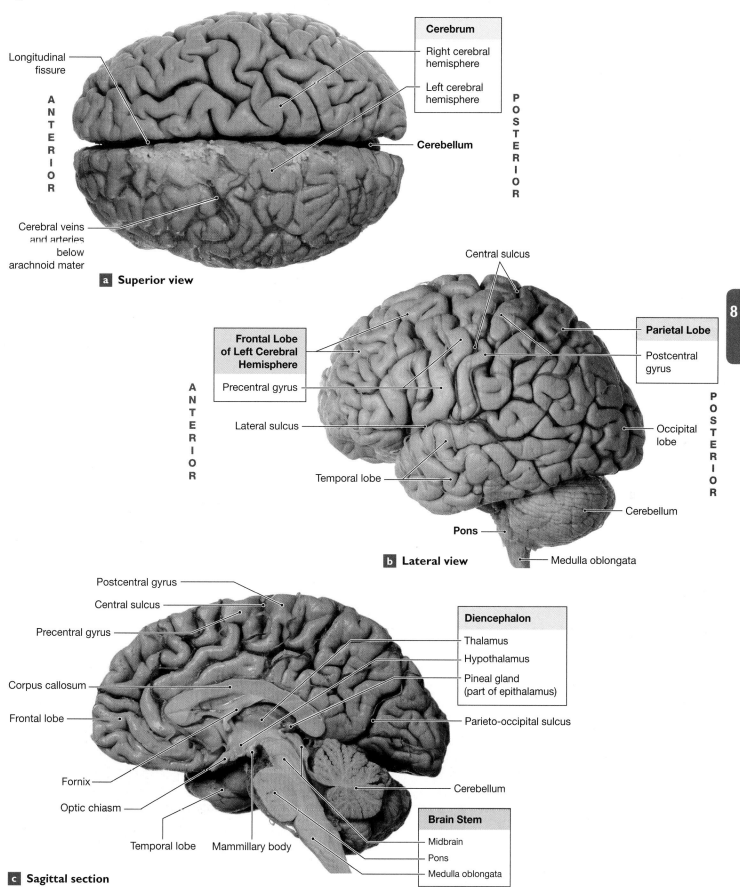

Longitudinal fissure

Cerebrum

Right cerebral hemisphere

Left cerebral hemisphere

Cerebellum

ANTERIOR

POSTERIOR

Cerebral veins and arteries below arachnoid mater

a **Superior view**

Central sulcus

Frontal Lobe of Left Cerebral Hemisphere

Precentral gyrus

Parietal Lobe

Postcentral gyrus

ANTERIOR

POSTERIOR

Lateral sulcus

Occipital lobe

Temporal lobe

Cerebellum

Pons

Medulla oblongata

b **Lateral view**

8

Postcentral gyrus

Central sulcus

Precentral gyrus

Diencephalon

Thalamus

Hypothalamus

Pineal gland (part of epithalamus)

Corpus callosum

Frontal lobe

Parieto-occipital sulcus

Fornix

Cerebellum

Optic chiasm

Brain Stem

Temporal lobe   Mammillary body

Midbrain

Pons

Medulla oblongata

c **Sagittal section**

brain stem (**Figure 8-21b**). The cerebellum adjusts voluntary and involuntary motor activities on the basis of sensory information and stored memories of previous movements.

The Ventricles of the Brain

Recall that the brain and spinal cord contain internal cavities filled with CSF and lined by ependymal cells. ↺ p. 249 The brain has a central passageway that expands to form four chambers called **ventricles** (VEN-tri-kls) (**Figure 8-22**). Each cerebral hemisphere contains a large **lateral ventricle**. These two lateral ventricles are not directly connected. Instead, each communicates with the **third ventricle** of the diencephalon through an opening, the *interventricular foramen*. Rather than a ventricle, the midbrain has a slender canal known as the *cerebral aqueduct*. This passageway connects the third ventricle with the **fourth ventricle**, which extends into the pons and upper portion of the medulla oblongata. Within the medulla oblongata, the fourth ventricle narrows and becomes continuous with the central canal of the spinal cord.

Cerebrospinal Fluid

Cerebrospinal fluid, or **CSF**, fills the ventricles and completely surrounds and bathes the exposed surfaces of the CNS. The CSF has several important functions, including

- *Cushioning the brain and spinal cord against physical trauma.*

- *Supporting the brain.* The brain essentially floats in the CSF. A human brain weighs about 1400 g (3.1 lb) in air but only about 50 g (1.8 oz) when supported by CSF.

- *Transporting nutrients, chemical messengers, and waste products.* Except at the *choroid plexus*, where CSF is produced, the ependymal lining is freely permeable. The CSF is in constant chemical communication with the interstitial fluid that surrounds the neurons and neuroglia of the CNS.

Because free exchange takes place between the interstitial fluid and CSF, changes in CNS function may produce changes in the composition of CSF. Samples of CSF can be obtained through a *lumbar puncture*, or *spinal tap*. Such samples provide useful clinical information about CNS injury, infection, or disease.

A **choroid plexus** (*choroid*, a vascular coat + *plexus*, a network) is a network of permeable capillaries within each ventricle that produces CSF (**Figure 8-23a**). The capillaries of the choroid plexuses are covered by large ependymal cells that secrete CSF at a rate of about 500 mL/day. The total volume of CSF at any given moment is approximately 150 mL. This means that the entire volume of CSF is replaced roughly every 8 hours. Despite this rapid turnover, the composition of CSF is closely regulated. The rate of removal normally keeps pace with the rate of production. If it does not, a variety of clinical problems may appear.

The areas where CSF is formed, its circulatory pathway around the CNS, and its absorption into the venous circulation are shown in **Figure 8-23a**. CSF formed at the

Figure 8-22 The Ventricles of the Brain. The orientation and extent of the ventricles as they would appear if the brain were transparent.

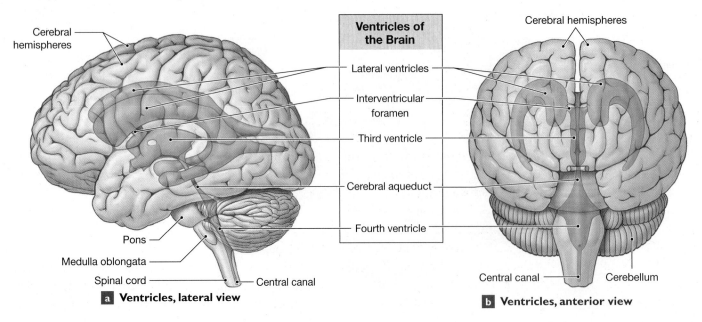

a **Ventricles, lateral view**

b **Ventricles, anterior view**

Figure 8-23 The Formation and Circulation of Cerebrospinal Fluid.

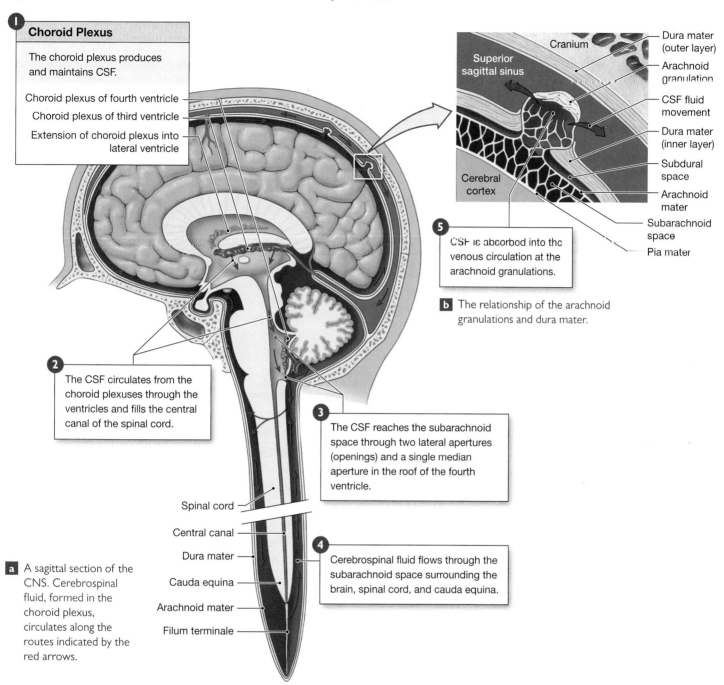

Choroid Plexus

The choroid plexus produces and maintains CSF.

Choroid plexus of fourth ventricle
Choroid plexus of third ventricle
Extension of choroid plexus into lateral ventricle

Dura mater (outer layer)
Cranium
Superior sagittal sinus
Arachnoid granulation
CSF fluid movement
Dura mater (inner layer)
Subdural space
Cerebral cortex
Arachnoid mater
Subarachnoid space
Pia mater

5 CSF is absorbed into the venous circulation at the arachnoid granulations.

b The relationship of the arachnoid granulations and dura mater.

8

2 The CSF circulates from the choroid plexuses through the ventricles and fills the central canal of the spinal cord.

3 The CSF reaches the subarachnoid space through two lateral apertures (openings) and a single median aperture in the roof of the fourth ventricle.

Spinal cord
Central canal
Dura mater
Cauda equina
Arachnoid mater
Filum terminale

4 Cerebrospinal fluid flows through the subarachnoid space surrounding the brain, spinal cord, and cauda equina.

a A sagittal section of the CNS. Cerebrospinal fluid, formed in the choroid plexus, circulates along the routes indicated by the red arrows.

choroid plexuses circulates through the different ventricles and fills the central canal of the spinal cord (**1**) and (**2**). CSF enters the subarachnoid space through openings (*apertures*) in the roof of the fourth ventricle (**3**). CSF then flows through the subarachnoid space surrounding the brain, spinal cord, and cauda equina (**4**). Between the cerebral hemispheres, slender extensions of the arachnoid mater penetrate the inner layer of the dura mater. Clusters of these extensions form **arachnoid granulations**, which project into

the *superior sagittal sinus*, a large cerebral vein (**Figure 8-23b**). Diffusion across the arachnoid granulations returns excess CSF to the venous circulation (**5**).

The Cerebrum

The cerebrum is the largest region of the brain. It is the site where conscious thought and intellectual functions originate. Much of the cerebrum is involved in receiving somatic

CLINICAL NOTE

Hydrocephalus

Hydrocephalus is an abnormal accumulation of cerebrospinal fluid (CSF) within the ventricles of the brain. It results from an imbalance between the amount of CSF that is produced and the rate at which it is absorbed. As the CSF builds up, it causes the ventricles to enlarge and results in increased intracranial pressure (**Figure 8-24**).

Hydrocephalus may be congenital or acquired. The causes of congenital hydrocephalus are complex and believed to be an interaction between environmental and genetic factors. Acquired hydrocephalus may result from intraventricular hemorrhage, meningitis, head trauma, tumors, and cysts. Hydrocephalus is believed to occur in about two out of 1000 births. The incidences of adult-onset hydrocephalus and acquired hydrocephalus are not known.

The symptoms of hydrocephalus vary with age, disease progression, and individual differences in tolerance to CSF. In infancy, the most obvious indication of hydrocephalus is often a rapid increase in head circumference. In older children and adults, symptoms may include headache accompanied by vomiting, nausea, *papilledema* (swelling of the optic disk, which is part of the optic nerve), downward deviation of the eyes (called *sunsetting*), problems with balance, poor coordination, gait disturbance, urinary incontinence, slowing or loss of development (in children), lethargy, drowsiness, irritability, or other changes in personality or cognition, including memory loss.

Hydrocephalus is diagnosed through clinical neurological evaluation and by using cranial imaging techniques such as ultrasonography, computer tomography, magnetic resonance imaging, or pressure-monitoring techniques.

There is no known way to prevent or cure hydrocephalus. The most effective treatment is surgical insertion of a shunt that drains the fluid from the brain, which thus decreases intracranial pressures.

Figure 8-24 Typical Appearance of Infant with Hydrocephalus.

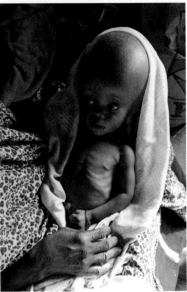

---

sensory information and then exerting voluntary or involuntary control over somatic motor neurons. In general, we are aware of these events. However, most sensory processing and all visceral motor (autonomic) control occur elsewhere in the brain, usually outside our conscious awareness.

The cerebrum includes gray matter and white matter. Gray matter is found in a superficial layer of neural cortex, known as the **cerebral cortex**, and in deeper *basal nuclei*. The white matter lies beneath the neural cortex and surrounds the basal nuclei.

Structure of the Cerebral Hemispheres

A blanket of cerebral cortex ranging from 1 to 4.5 mm (0.04 to 0.18 in.) thickness covers the paired cerebral hemispheres (**Figure 8-25**). This outer surface forms a series of folds, or **gyri** (JĪ-rī; singular, *gyrus*). The gyri are separated by shallow depressions, called **sulci** (SUL-sī), or by deeper grooves, called **fissures**. Gyri increase the surface area of the cerebrum, and thus the number of neurons in the cortex. The total surface area of the cerebral hemispheres is roughly equivalent to 2200 cm^2 (2.5 ft^2) of flat surface.

The two cerebral hemispheres are separated by a deep **longitudinal fissure** (**Figure 8-21a**). Each hemisphere can be divided into well-defined regions, or **lobes**, named after the overlying bones of the skull (**Figures 8-21b** and **8-25**). On each hemisphere, the **central sulcus**, a deep groove, divides the anterior **frontal lobe** from the more posterior **parietal lobe**. The horizontal **lateral sulcus** separates the frontal lobe from the **temporal lobe**. The temporal lobe overlaps the **insula** (IN-sū-luh), an "island" of cortex that is otherwise hidden (**Figure 8-25**). The more posterior **parieto-occipital sulcus** separates the parietal lobe from the **occipital lobe** (**Figure 8-21c**).

In each lobe, some regions are concerned with sensory information and others with motor commands. Additionally, each hemisphere receives sensory information from, and sends motor commands to, the opposite side of the body. As a result, the left cerebral hemisphere controls the right side of the body, and the right cerebral hemisphere controls the left side. This crossing over has no known functional significance.

Motor and Sensory Areas of the Cortex

The major motor and sensory regions of the cerebral cortex are shown in **Figure 8-25**. The central sulcus separates the motor and sensory portions of the cortex. The **precentral gyrus** of the frontal lobe forms the anterior margin of the central sulcus. The surface of this gyrus is the **primary motor cortex**. Neurons of the primary motor cortex direct voluntary movements by controlling somatic motor neurons in the brain stem and spinal cord.

Figure 8-25 Motor and Sensory Regions of the Cerebral Hemispheres. Major anatomical landmarks on the surface of the left cerebral hemisphere are shown. The colored areas represent various motor, sensory, and association areas of the cerebral cortex. (Retractors along the lateral sulcus reveal the insula.)

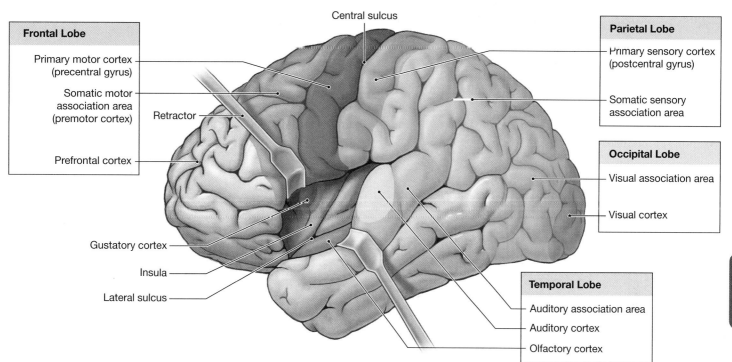

Central sulcus

Frontal Lobe
- Primary motor cortex (precentral gyrus)
- Somatic motor association area (premotor cortex)
- Retractor
- Prefrontal cortex

Gustatory cortex

Insula

Lateral sulcus

Parietal Lobe
- Primary sensory cortex (postcentral gyrus)
- Somatic sensory association area

Occipital Lobe
- Visual association area
- Visual cortex

Temporal Lobe
- Auditory association area
- Auditory cortex
- Olfactory cortex

The **postcentral gyrus** of the parietal lobe forms the posterior margin of the central sulcus. Its surface contains the **primary sensory cortex**. Neurons in this region receive somatic sensory information from touch, pressure, pain, and temperature receptors. We are aware of these sensations only when nuclei in the thalamus relay the information to the primary sensory cortex.

Sensations of sight, taste, sound, and smell arrive at other portions of the cerebral cortex. The **visual cortex** of the occipital lobe receives visual information. The **gustatory cortex** of the frontal lobe receives taste sensations. In the temporal lobe, the **auditory cortex** and **olfactory cortex** receive information about hearing and smell, respectively.

Association Areas

The sensory and motor regions of the cortex are connected to nearby **association areas**. These regions interpret incoming data or coordinate a motor response.

The **somatic sensory association area** monitors activity in the primary sensory cortex. This area allows you to recognize a touch as light as a mosquito landing on your arm. The special senses of smell, sight, and hearing involve separate areas of sensory cortex. Each has its own association area.

The **somatic motor association area**, or **premotor cortex**, is responsible for coordinating learned movements. When you perform a voluntary movement, such as picking up a glass or scanning these lines of type, instructions are relayed to the primary motor cortex by the premotor cortex.

The functional distinctions between the motor and sensory association areas are most evident after localized brain damage has taken place. For example, someone with damage to the premotor cortex might understand written letters and words but be unable to read due to an inability to track along the lines on a printed page. In contrast, someone with a damaged **visual association area** can scan the lines of a printed page but cannot figure out what the letters mean.

Cortical Connections

The various regions of the cerebral cortex are interconnected by the white matter that lies beneath the cerebral cortex. Myelinated axons of different lengths interconnect gyri within a single cerebral hemisphere. Such axons also link the two hemispheres across the **corpus callosum (Figure 8-21c)**. Other bundles of axons link the cerebral cortex with the diencephalon, brain stem, cerebellum, and spinal cord.

Cerebral Processing Centers

"Higher-order" integrative centers receive information from many different association areas. These integrative centers direct extremely complex motor activities and perform complicated analytical functions. Even though integrative centers may be found in both cerebral hemispheres, many are *lateralized*—largely restricted to either the left or the right hemisphere (**Figure 8-26**). Examples of lateralized integrative centers are those concerned with complex processes such as speech, writing, mathematical computation, and understanding spatial relationships.

THE GENERAL INTERPRETIVE AREA. The **general interpretive area**, or *Wernicke's area*, receives information from all the sensory association areas. It plays an essential role in your personality by integrating sensory information and coordinating access to complex visual and auditory memories. This center is present in only one hemisphere, usually the left. Damage to this area affects the ability to interpret what is read or heard, even though the words are understood as individual entities. For example, if your general interpretive area was damaged, you might still understand the meaning of the spoken words *sit* and *here*, because word recognition

Figure 8-26 Hemisphere Lateralization. Some functional differences between the left and right cerebral hemispheres are depicted.

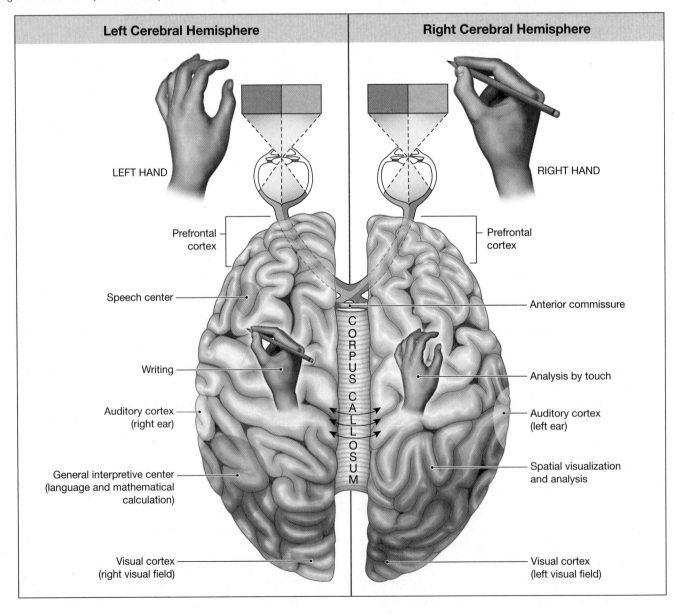

takes place in the auditory association areas. But you would be totally bewildered by the request *sit here.*

THE SPEECH CENTER. Some of the neurons in the general interpretive area connect to the **speech center** *(Broca's area).* This center lies along the edge of the premotor cortex in the same hemisphere as the general interpretive area. The speech center regulates the patterns of breathing and vocalization required for normal speech. A person with a damaged speech center can make sounds but not words.

The motor commands issued by the speech center are adjusted by feedback from the auditory association area. Damage there can cause a variety of speech-related problems. Some affected individuals have difficulty speaking, even though they know exactly which words to use. Others talk constantly but use all the wrong words.

THE PREFRONTAL CORTEX. The **prefrontal cortex** of the frontal lobe (**Figure 8-26**) coordinates information from the association areas of the entire cortex. In doing so, it performs such abstract intellectual functions as predicting the consequences of events or actions. Damage to this area leads to problems in estimating time relationships between events. Questions such as "How long ago did this happen?" or "What happened first?" become difficult to answer.

The prefrontal cortex also has connections with other cortical areas and with other portions of the brain. Feelings of frustration, tension, and anxiety are generated at the prefrontal cortex as it interprets ongoing events and makes predictions about future situations or consequences. If the connections between the prefrontal cortex and other brain regions are severed, the tensions, frustrations, and anxieties are removed. Early in the 1900s this rather drastic procedure, called a *prefrontal lobotomy,* was used to "cure" a variety of mental illnesses, especially those associated with violent or antisocial behavior.

Hemispheric Lateralization

As shown in **Figure 8-26**, each of the two cerebral hemispheres is responsible for specific functions that are not ordinarily performed by the opposite hemisphere. This specialization is called *hemispheric lateralization.* In most people, the left hemisphere contains the general interpretive and speech centers and is responsible for language-based skills (reading, writing, and speaking). In addition, the premotor cortex involved in the control of hand movements is larger on

the left side in right-handed individuals than in left-handed ones. The left hemisphere is also important in performing analytical tasks, such as mathematical calculations and logical decision making. For these reasons, the left hemisphere has been called the dominant hemisphere, or the categorical hemisphere.

The right hemisphere, or *representational hemisphere,* is concerned with spatial relationships and analyses. It analyzes sensory information and relates the body to the sensory environment. Interpretive centers in this hemisphere enable you to identify familiar objects by touch, smell, sight, or taste. The right hemisphere plays a dominant role in recognizing faces and in understanding three-dimensional relationships. It is also important in analyzing the emotional context of a conversation—for instance, distinguishing between the threat "Get lost!" and the question "Get lost?"

Interestingly, there may be a link between handedness and sensory/spatial abilities. An unusually high percentage of musicians and artists are left-handed. The complex motor activities that they perform are directed by the primary motor cortex and association areas of the right cerebral hemisphere. These areas are near the association areas involved with spatial visualization and emotions.

Hemispheric lateralization does not mean that the two hemispheres function independently of each other. Recall that the white fibers of the corpus callosum link the two hemispheres, including their sensory information and motor commands. The corpus callosum alone contains over 200 million axons, carrying an estimated 4 billion impulses per second!

The Electroencephalogram

Various methods have been used to map brain activity and function. The primary sensory cortex and the primary motor cortex have been mapped by direct stimulation in patients undergoing brain surgery. The behavioral changes that follow localized brain injuries or strokes can reveal the functions of other regions of the cerebrum. The activities of specific regions can be examined by noninvasive techniques such as a poistron emission tomographic scan or sequential magnetic resonance imaging scans. ⊃ p. 20

The electrical activity of the brain is commonly monitored to assess brain activity. Neural function depends on electrical events of the plasma membrane of neurons. The brain contains billions of nerve cells, and their activity generates an electrical field that can be measured by placing electrodes on the brain or on the outer surface of the skull. The electrical

Figure 8-27 Brain Waves.

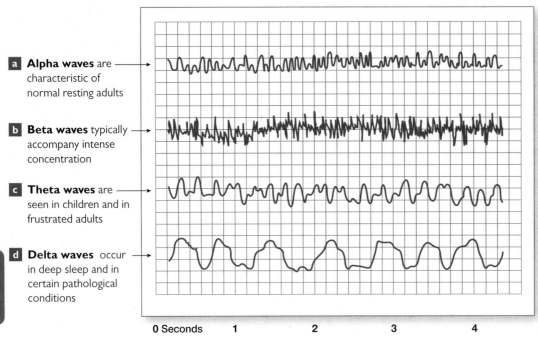

a **Alpha waves** are characteristic of normal resting adults

b **Beta waves** typically accompany intense concentration

c **Theta waves** are seen in children and in frustrated adults

d **Delta waves** occur in deep sleep and in certain pathological conditions

0 Seconds   1   2   3   4

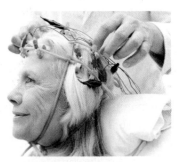

Patient being wired for EEG monitoring

activity changes constantly as nuclei and cortical areas are stimulated or quiet down.

An **electroencephalogram (EEG)** is a printed record of this electrical activity over time. The electrical patterns are called **brain waves**, which can be correlated with the individual's level of consciousness. EEGs can also provide useful diagnostic information regarding brain disorders. Four types of brain wave patterns are shown in **Figure 8-27**.

Memory

What was the topic of the last sentence you read? What is your social security number? How do you open a screw-top jar? To answer these questions, you access *memories*, stored bits of information gathered through experience. **Fact memories** are specific bits of information, such as the color of a stop sign. **Skill memories** are learned motor behaviors. You can probably remember how to light a match

CLINICAL NOTE

Aphasia and Dyslexia

Aphasia (*a–*, without + *phasia*, speech) is a disorder affecting the ability to speak or read. *Global aphasia* results from extensive damage to the general interpretive area or to the associated sensory tracts. Affected individuals cannot speak, read, understand, or interpret the speech of others. Global aphasia often accompanies a severe stroke or tumor that affects a large area of cortex, including the speech and language areas. Recovery is possible when the condition results from *edema* (an abnormal accumulation of fluid) or hemorrhage, but the process often takes months or even years. Lesser degrees of aphasia often follow minor strokes with no initial period of global aphasia. Such individuals can understand spoken and written words and may recover completely.

Dyslexia (*lexis*, diction) is a disorder affecting the comprehension and use of words. Developmental dyslexia affects children. Estimates are that up to 15 percent of children in the United States suffer from some degree of dyslexia. These children have difficulty reading and writing, although their other intellectual functions may be normal or above normal. Their writing looks uneven and unorganized. They typically write letters in the wrong order (*dig* becomes *gid*) or reverse them (*E* becomes Ǝ). Recent evidence suggests that at least some forms of dyslexia result from problems in processing, sorting, and integrating visual or auditory information.

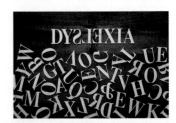

or throw a Frisbee, for example. With repetition, skill memories become incorporated at the unconscious level. Examples include the complex motor patterns involved in skiing or playing the violin. Skill memories related to programmed behaviors, such as eating, are stored in appropriate portions of the brain stem. Complex skill memories involve an integration of motor patterns in the cerebellum and the cerebral cortex.

Memories are often classified according to how long they last. **Short-term memories** do not last long, but while they persist the information can be recalled immediately. Short-term memories contain small bits of information, such as a person's name or a telephone number. Repeating a phone number or other bit of information reinforces the original short-term memory and helps ensure its conversion to a long-term memory. **Long-term memories** remain for much longer periods, in some cases for an entire lifetime. The conversion from short-term to long-term memory is called *memory consolidation*. Some long-term memories fade with time and may require considerable effort to recall. Other long-term memories seem to be part of consciousness, such as your name or the contours of your own body.

Most long-term memories are stored in the cerebral cortex. Conscious motor and sensory memories are referred to the appropriate association areas. For example, visual memories are stored in the visual association area, and memories of voluntary motor activity are kept in the premotor cortex. Special portions of the occipital and temporal lobes retain the memories of faces, voices, and words.

Amnesia refers to the loss of memory as a result of disease or trauma. The type of memory loss depends on the specific regions of the brain affected. For example, damage to the auditory association areas may make it difficult to remember sounds. Damage to thalamic and limbic structures, especially the *hippocampus*, affects memory storage and consolidation.

The Basal Nuclei

While your cerebral cortex is consciously active, other centers of your cerebrum, diencephalon, and brain stem are processing sensory information and issuing motor commands outside your conscious awareness. Many of these activities, which take place at the subconscious level, are directed by the basal nuclei, or *cerebral nuclei*. The **basal nuclei** are masses of gray matter that lie beneath the lateral ventricles, surrounded by the white matter of each cerebral hemisphere (**Figure 8-28**).

The **caudate nucleus** has a massive head and slender, curving tail that follows the curve of the lateral ventricle.

Figure 8-28 The Basal Nuclei.

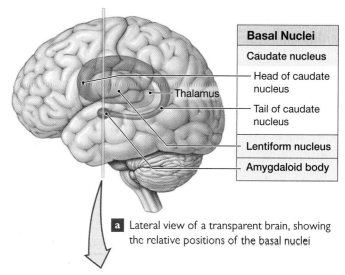

Basal Nuclei
Caudate nucleus
Head of caudate nucleus
Tail of caudate nucleus
Lentiform nucleus
Amygdaloid body

a Lateral view of a transparent brain, showing the relative positions of the basal nuclei

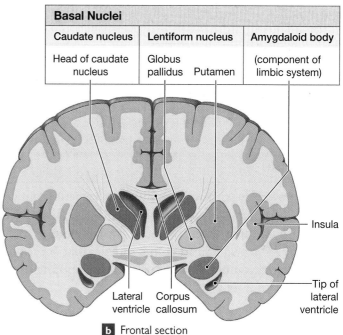

Basal Nuclei		
Caudate nucleus	Lentiform nucleus	Amygdaloid body
Head of caudate nucleus	Globus pallidus Putamen	(component of limbic system)

b Frontal section

The head of the caudate nucleus lies anterior to the **lentiform** (*lens-shaped*) **nucleus**. The lentiform nucleus consists of a medial **globus pallidus** (GL-bus PAL-i-dus; pale globe) and a lateral **putamen** (pū-TĀ-men). Together, the caudate and lentiform nuclei are also called the *corpus striatum* (striated body). Inferior to the caudate and lentiform nuclei is another nucleus, the **amygdaloid** (ah-MIG-da-loyd; *amygdale*, almond) **body**, or amygdala. It is a component of the *limbic system* and is discussed in the next section.

The basal nuclei function in the subconscious control of skeletal muscle tone and the coordination of learned movement patterns. These nuclei do not start a movement—that

CLINICAL NOTE

Seizures

A *seizure* is an episode of abnormal neurological function caused by an abnormal electrical discharge of brain neurons. The seizure is the clinical event experienced by the patient following the abnormal electrical discharge. *Epilepsy* is a clinical syndrome in which an individual is subject to recurrent seizures. The occurrence of one or more seizures indicates an abnormal function of cerebral neurons. Where a cause for attacks in patients who are otherwise normal cannot be determined, seizures are referred to as *primary*, or *idiopathic*. Seizures that result from some identifiable condition, such as brain tumor or brain trauma, are referred to as *secondary seizures*.

Seizures are common and are a frequent reason that EMS is summoned. Most are self-limited and last less than a minute. Seizures can be categorized as generalized or partial depending upon the part of the brain involved. Generalized seizures involve the entire cerebral cortex, and usually begin with a loss of consciousness. This may be the only symptom, or it may be followed by motor activity. *Generalized tonic-clonic seizures* are the most familiar and dramatic seizure type. Often referred to as *grand mal seizures*, generalized tonic-clonic seizures cause the patient to become stiff and fall to the ground. This is followed by alternating contraction and relaxation of the skeletal muscles. Urinary and fecal incontinence is common. A seizure usually lasts 6–90 seconds, and as it ends, the patient is left flaccid

and unconscious. The patient may be confused for up to an hour following the attack (*postictal confusion*). Fatigue is common and may last for hours after the event.

Absence seizures, also called *petit mal seizures*, are very brief, and often last only a few seconds. Absence seizures are generalized seizures in which the patient suddenly loses consciousness without any loss of postural tone. These attacks end abruptly and the patients resume their activities. Often the patient and bystanders are unaware that anything has happened.

Focal seizures are due to electrical discharges that are limited to a portion of the cerebral cortex and are often secondary seizures that result from a lesion in the brain. The effects of focal seizure depend upon the part of the brain involved. If the seizure's focus is in the motor cortex, tonic or clonic muscle contractions that involve a single extremity may result. Sensory hallucinations suggest a focus in the sensory cortex. Visual symptoms, such as flashing lights, suggest a focus in the occipital lobe. Focal seizures isolated in the temporal lobe can cause altered thinking or behavior. Commonly referred to as psychomotor seizures, they can be mistakenly diagnosed as psychiatric disease.

Most seizure disorders can be controlled with medication. Modern anticonvulsant medications have minimal side effects and are highly effective. In fact, most seizures seen in the emergency setting occur because patients fail to take their medication or take it improperly.

---

decision is a voluntary one—but once a movement is under way, the basal nuclei provide the general pattern and rhythm. For example, when you walk, the basal nuclei control the cycles of arm and thigh movements that occur between the time you decide to "start" walking and the time you give the "stop" order.

The Limbic System

The **limbic system** (LIM-bik; *limbus*, border) includes the olfactory cortex, several basal nuclei, gyri, and tracts along the border between the cerebrum and diencephalon (**Figure 8-29**). This system is a functional grouping rather than an anatomical one. The functions of the limbic system include (1) establishing emotional states; (2) linking the conscious, intellectual functions of the cerebral cortex with the unconscious and autonomic functions of the brain stem; and (3) aiding long-term memory storage and retrieval. In short, the sensory cortex, motor cortex, and association areas of the cerebral cortex enable you to perform complex tasks, but it is largely the limbic system that makes you *want* to do them.

The amygdaloid bodies link the limbic system, the cerebrum, and various sensory systems. These nuclei play a role

in regulating heart rate, responding to fear and anxiety, controlling the "fight or flight" response, and linking emotions with specific memories.

Another nucleus, the **hippocampus**, is important in learning and in storing long-term memories. Damage to the hippocampus in Alzheimer's disease interferes with memory storage and retrieval. The **fornix** (FOR-niks, *arch*) is a tract of white matter that connects the hippocampus with the hypothalamus (**Figures 8-21c** and **8-29**).

The limbic system also includes hypothalamic centers that control (1) emotional states, such as rage, fear, and sexual arousal, and (2) reflex movements that can be consciously activated. For example, the limbic system includes the *mammillary bodies* (MAM-i-lar-ē; *mamilla*, a little breast) of the hypothalamus, where many fibers of the fornix end. These nuclei process olfactory sensations and control reflex movements associated with eating, such as chewing, licking, and swallowing.

The Diencephalon

The diencephalon (**Figures 8-21c** and **8-30**) contains switching and relay centers that integrate conscious and unconscious sensory information and motor commands. It

Figure 8-29 The Limbic System. This three-dimensional reconstruction of the limbic system shows the relationships among the system's major components.

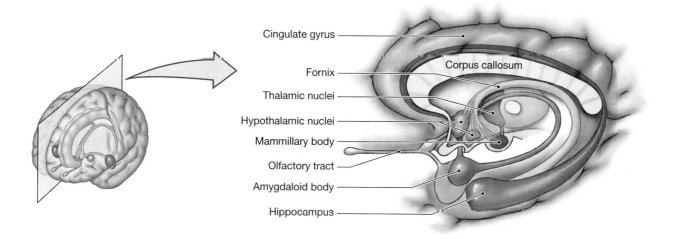

Cingulate gyrus

Corpus callosum

Fornix

Thalamic nuclei

Hypothalamic nuclei

Mammillary body

Olfactory tract

Amygdaloid body

Hippocampus

surrounds the third ventricle and consists of the *epithalamus, thalamus,* and *hypothalamus.*

The Epithalamus

The epithalamus lies superior to the third ventricle, where it forms the roof of the diencephalon. The anterior portion contains an extensive area of choroid plexus. The posterior portion contains the **pineal gland** (**Figure 8-28b**), an endocrine structure that secretes the hormone *melatonin.* Among other functions, melatonin is important in regulating day–night cycles.

The Thalamus

The left thalamus and right thalamus are separated by the third ventricle. Each contains a rounded mass of thalamic nuclei. The thalamus (**Figures 8-21c** and **8-30**) is the final relay point for all ascending sensory information, other than olfactory, that will reach our conscious awareness. It acts as a filter, passing on to the primary sensory cortex only a small portion of the arriving sensory information. The rest is relayed to the basal nuclei and centers in the brain stem. The thalamus also plays a role in coordinating voluntary and involuntary motor commands.

The Hypothalamus

The hypothalamus lies inferior to the third ventricle (**Figure 8-21c**). The hypothalamus contains important control and integrative centers in addition to those associated with the limbic system. Its diverse functions include

1. subconscious control of skeletal muscle contractions associated with rage, pleasure, pain, and sexual arousal;

2. adjusting the activities of autonomic centers in the pons and medulla oblongata (such as heart rate, blood pressure, respiration, and digestive functions);

3. coordinating activities of the nervous and endocrine systems;

4. secreting a variety of hormones, including *antidiuretic hormone* and *oxytocin;*

5. producing the behavioral "drives" involved in hunger and thirst;

6. coordinating voluntary and autonomic functions;

7. regulating normal body temperature; and

8. coordinating the daily cycles of activity.

The Midbrain

The midbrain (**Figure 8-30**) contains various nuclei and bundles of ascending and descending nerve fibers. It includes two pairs of sensory nuclei, or *colliculi* (ko-LIK-ū-lī; singular: *colliculus,* a small hill), involved in processing visual and auditory sensations. The *superior colliculi* control the reflex movements of the eyes, head, and neck in response to visual stimuli, such as a bright light. The *inferior colliculi* control reflex movements of the head, neck, and trunk in response to auditory stimuli, such as a loud noise.

The midbrain also contains motor nuclei for two of the cranial nerves (N III, N IV) involved in the control of eye movements. Descending bundles of nerve fibers on the

Figure 8-30 The Diencephalon and Brain Stem.

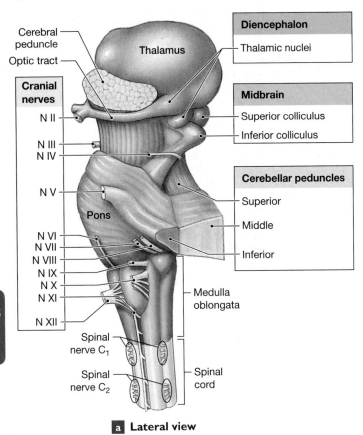

a Lateral view

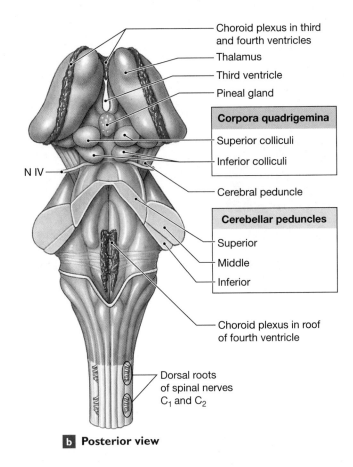

b Posterior view

ventrolateral surface of the midbrain make up the **cerebral peduncles** (*peduncles*, little feet). Some of the descending fibers go to the cerebellum by way of the pons. Others carry voluntary motor commands from the primary motor cortex of each cerebral hemisphere.

The midbrain is also headquarters to one of the most important brain stem components, the **reticular formation**, which regulates many involuntary functions. The reticular formation is a network of interconnected nuclei that extends the length of the brain stem. The reticular formation of the midbrain contains the *reticular activating system (RAS)*. The output of this system directly affects the activity of the cerebral cortex. When the RAS is inactive, so are we. When the RAS is stimulated, so is our state of attention or wakefulness.

Midbrain nuclei that integrate information from the cerebrum and cerebellum control the maintenance of muscle tone and posture. Other midbrain nuclei play an important role in regulating the motor output of the basal nuclei. For example, the *substantia nigra* (NĪ-gruh; black) inhibit the activity of the basal nuclei by releasing the neurotransmitter dopamine. ↰ p. 260 If the substantia nigra are damaged or the neurons secrete less dopamine, the basal nuclei become

more active. The result is a gradual increase in muscle tone and the appearance of symptoms characteristic of *Parkinson's disease*. Persons with Parkinson's disease have difficulty starting voluntary movements because opposing muscle groups do not relax. Instead, they must be overpowered. Once a movement is under way, every aspect must be voluntarily controlled through intense effort and concentration.

The Pons

The pons (**Figure 8-28a**) links the cerebellum with the midbrain, diencephalon, cerebrum, and spinal cord. One group of nuclei within the pons includes the sensory and motor nuclei for four of the cranial nerves (N V–N VIII). Other nuclei are concerned with the involuntary control of the pace and depth of respiration. Tracts passing through the pons link the cerebellum with the brain stem, cerebrum, and spinal cord.

The Cerebellum

The cerebellum (**Figure 8-21b,c**) is an automatic processing center. Like the cerebrum, the cerebellum is composed of white matter covered by a layer of neural cortex (gray matter) called the *cerebellar cortex*. The cerebellum has two important functions:

1. *Adjusting the postural muscles of the body.* The cerebellum coordinates rapid, automatic adjustments to maintain balance and equilibrium.

2. *Programming and fine-tuning movements controlled at the conscious and subconscious levels.* The cerebellum refines learned movement patterns, such as riding a bicycle or playing the piano.

These functions are performed indirectly by regulating activity along motor pathways at the cerebral cortex, basal nuclei, and brain stem. The cerebellum compares the motor commands with proprioceptive information (position sense) and makes adjustments needed to make the movement smooth. The tracts that link the cerebellum with these different regions are the **cerebellar peduncles** (**Figure 8-30**).

The cerebellum can be permanently damaged by trauma or stroke or temporarily affected by drugs such as alcohol. These alterations can produce *ataxia* (a-TAK-sē-uh; *ataxia*, a lack of order), a disturbance in balance.

The Medulla Oblongata

The medulla oblongata (**Figure 8-28**) connects the brain with the spinal cord. It is a very busy place—all communication between the brain and spinal cord involves tracts that ascend or descend through the medulla oblongata. These tracts often synapse in the medulla oblongata at sensory or motor nuclei that act as relay stations and processing centers. In addition to these nuclei, the medulla oblongata contains sensory and motor nuclei associated with five of the cranial nerves (N VIII–N XII).

The portion of the reticular system within the medulla oblongata contains nuclei and centers that regulate vital autonomic functions. These *reflex centers* receive inputs from cranial nerves, the cerebral cortex, and the brain stem. Their output controls or adjusts the activities of the cardiovascular and respiratory systems:

- The **cardiovascular center** adjusts heart rate, the strength of cardiac contractions, and the flow of blood through peripheral tissues. In terms of function, the cardiovascular center is subdivided into a *cardiac center* regulating the heart rate and a *vasomotor center* controlling peripheral blood flow.

- The **respiratory rhythmicity centers** set the basic pace for respiratory movements, and their activity is adjusted by the *respiratory centers* of the pons.

CHECKPOINT

20. Describe one major function of each of the six regions of the brain.

21. The pituitary gland links the nervous and endocrine systems. To which portion of the diencephalon is it attached?

22. How would decreased diffusion across the arachnoid granulations affect the volume of cerebrospinal fluid in the ventricles?

23. Mary suffers a head injury that damages her primary motor cortex. Where is this area located?

24. Which senses would be affected by damage to the temporal lobes of the cerebrum?

25. The thalamus acts as a relay point for all but what type of sensory information?

26. Changes in body temperature stimulate which area of the diencephalon?

27. The medulla oblongata is one of the smallest sections of the brain. Why can damage to it cause death, when similar damage in the cerebrum might go unnoticed?

See the blue Answers tab at the back of the book.

8-8 The PNS connects the CNS with the body's external and internal environments

Learning Objective Name the cranial nerves, relate each pair of cranial nerves to its principal functions, and relate the distribution pattern of spinal nerves to the regions they innervate.

The PNS links the neurons of the CNS to the rest of the body. All sensory information and motor commands are carried by axons of the PNS (**Figure 8-1**, p. 271). These axons are bundled together and wrapped in connective tissue, forming **peripheral nerves**, or simply nerves. Cranial nerves originate from the brain, and spinal nerves connect to the spinal cord. The PNS also includes both the cell bodies and the axons of sensory neurons and motor neurons of the ANS. The cell bodies are clustered together in masses called **ganglia** (singular: *ganglion*) (**Figure 8-6**, p. 276).

The Cranial Nerves

Twelve pairs of **cranial nerves** connect to the brain (**Figure 8-31**). Each cranial nerve has a name related to its appearance or function. Each also has a designation consisting of the letter N (for "nerve") and a Roman numeral (for its position along the longitudinal axis of the brain). For example, N I refers to the first pair of cranial nerves, the olfactory nerves.

Distribution and Function of Cranial Nerves

Functionally, each nerve can be classified as primarily sensory, primarily motor, or mixed (sensory and motor). Many cranial nerves, however, have secondary functions. For example, several cranial nerves (N III, N VII, N IX, and N X) also carry autonomic fibers to PNS ganglia, just as spinal nerves deliver them to ganglia along the spinal cord. Next we consider the distribution and functions of the cranial nerves.

Few people are able to remember the names, numbers, and functions of the cranial nerves without some effort. Many people use mnemonic phrases, such as "Oh, Once One Takes The Anatomy Final, Very Good Vacations Are Heavenly." The first letter of each word represents the name of a cranial nerve.

THE OLFACTORY NERVES (N I). The first pair of cranial nerves, the **olfactory nerves**, are the only cranial nerves attached to the cerebrum. (The rest start or end within nuclei of the diencephalon or brain stem.) These nerves carry special sensory information responsible for the sense of smell. The olfactory nerves originate in the epithelium of the upper nasal cavity and penetrate the cribriform plate of the ethmoid bone to synapse in the *olfactory bulbs* of the brain. ⮌ p. 157 From the olfactory bulbs, the axons of postsynaptic neurons travel within the *olfactory tracts* to the olfactory centers of the brain.

THE OPTIC NERVES (N II). The **optic nerves** carry visual information from the eyes. After passing through the **optic foramina** of the orbits, these nerves intersect at the **optic chiasm** ("a crossing") (**Figure 8-31a,b**) before they continue as the *optic tracts* to nuclei of the left and right thalamus.

THE OCULOMOTOR NERVES (N III). The midbrain contains the motor nuclei controlling the third and fourth cranial nerves. Each **oculomotor nerve** innervates four of the six extrinsic muscles that move an eyeball (the superior, medial, and inferior rectus muscles and the inferior oblique muscle). (Superficial muscles that position or stabilize an organ are called *extrinsic muscles*.) These nerves also carry autonomic fibers to intrinsic eye muscles that control the amount of light entering the eye and the shape of the lens. (Muscles located entirely within an organ are called *intrinsic muscles*.)

THE TROCHLEAR NERVES (N IV). The **trochlear** (TRK-l-ar; *trochlea*, a pulley) **nerves**, the smallest of the cranial nerves, innervate the superior oblique muscles of the eyes. The motor nuclei that control these nerves lie in the midbrain. The name *trochlear* refers to the pulley-shaped, ligamentous sling through which the tendon of the superior oblique muscle passes to reach its attachment on the eyeball (Figure 9-9a, p. 354).

THE TRIGEMINAL NERVES (N V). The pons contains the nuclei associated with cranial nerve V. The **trigeminal** (trī-JEM-i-nal) **nerves** are the largest of the cranial nerves. These nerves provide sensory information from the head and face and motor control over the chewing muscles, such as the temporalis and masseter.

The trigeminal has three major branches. The *ophthalmic branch* provides sensory information from the orbit of the eye, the nasal cavity and sinuses, and the skin of the forehead, eyebrows, eyelids, and nose. The *maxillary branch* provides sensory information from the lower eyelid, upper lip, cheek, nose, upper gums and teeth, palate, and portions of the pharynx. The *mandibular branch* is the largest of the three. It provides sensory information from the skin of the temples, the lower gums and teeth, the salivary glands, and the anterior portions of the tongue. It also provides motor control over the chewing muscles (the temporalis, masseter, and pterygoid muscles). ⮌ p. 219

THE ABDUCENS NERVES (N VI). The **abducens** (ab-DŪ-senz) **nerves** innervate only the lateral rectus, the sixth of the extrinsic eye muscles. The nuclei of the abducens nerves are in the pons. The nerves emerge at the border between the pons and the medulla oblongata and reach the orbit of the eye along with the oculomotor and trochlear nerves. The name *abducens* is based on the action of this nerve's innervated muscle, which abducts the eyeball, causing it to rotate laterally, away from the midline of the body.

THE FACIAL NERVES (N VII). The **facial nerves** are mixed nerves of the face. Their sensory and motor roots emerge from the side of the pons. The sensory fibers monitor proprioceptors in the facial muscles, provide deep pressure sensations over the face, and provide taste information from receptors along the anterior two-thirds of the tongue. The motor fibers produce facial expressions by controlling the superficial muscles of the scalp and face and muscles near

Figure 8-31 The Cranial Nerves.

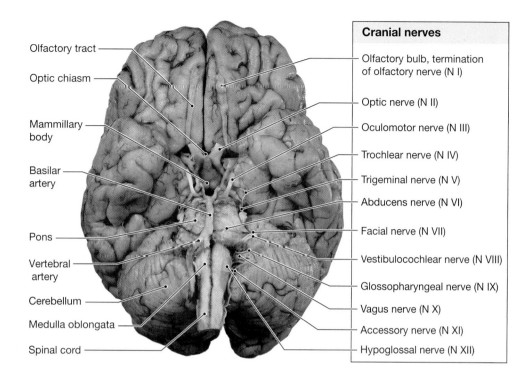

Olfactory tract
Optic chiasm
Mammillary body
Basilar artery
Pons
Vertebral artery
Cerebellum
Medulla oblongata
Spinal cord

Cranial nerves

Olfactory bulb, termination of olfactory nerve (N I)
Optic nerve (N II)
Oculomotor nerve (N III)
Trochlear nerve (N IV)
Trigeminal nerve (N V)
Abducens nerve (N VI)
Facial nerve (N VII)
Vestibulocochlear nerve (N VIII)
Glossopharyngeal nerve (N IX)
Vagus nerve (N X)
Accessory nerve (N XI)
Hypoglossal nerve (N XII)

a Inferior view of the brain

Olfactory tract
Optic chiasm
Infundibulum

b Diagrammatic view showing the attachment of the 12 pairs of cranial nerves

Cranial nerve	Function	Innervation
Olfactory bulb, (end of N I)	Special sensory	Olfactory epithelium
Optic (N II)	Special sensory	Retina of the eye
Oculomotor (N III)	Motor	Inferior, medial, superior rectus, inferior oblique, and intrinsic muscles of the eye
Trochlear (N IV)	Motor	Superior oblique muscle of the eye
Trigeminal (N V)	Mixed	*Sensory:* orbital structures, nasal cavity, skin of forehead, eyelids, eyebrows, nose, lips, gums and teeth; cheek, palate, pharynx, and tongue *Motor:* chewing muscles (temporalis, masseter, pterygoids)
Abducens (N VI)	Motor	Lateral rectus muscle of the eye
Facial (N VII)	Mixed	*Sensory:* taste receptors on anterior 2/3rd of tongue *Motor:* muscles of facial expression, lacrimal (tear) gland, and submandibular and sublingual salivary glands
Vestibulocochlear (N VIII)	Special sensory	Cochlea (receptors for hearing) Vestibule (receptors for motion and balance)
Glossopharyngeal (N IX)	Mixed	*Sensory:* posterior 1/3rd of tongue; pharynx and palate (part); receptors for blood pressure, pH, oxygen, and carbon dioxide *Motor:* pharyngeal muscles, parotid salivary glands
Vagus (N X)	Mixed	*Sensory:* pharynx, auricle and external acoustic meatus (portion of external ear), diaphragm, visceral organs in thoracic and abdominopelvic cavities *Motor:* palatal and pharyngeal muscles and visceral organs in thoracic and abdominopelvic cavities
Accessory (N XI)	Motor	Voluntary muscles of palate, pharynx, and larynx (with vagus nerve); sternocleidomastoid and trapezius muscles
Hypoglossal (N XII)	Motor	Tongue muscles

8

the ear. These nerves also carry autonomic fibers that result in control of the tear glands and salivary glands.

THE VESTIBULOCOCHLEAR NERVES (N VIII). The **vestibulocochlear nerves** monitor the sensory receptors of the internal ear. The pons and medulla oblongata contain nuclei associated with these nerves. Each vestibulocochlear nerve has two parts: (1) a **vestibular nerve** (*vestibulum*, a cavity), which originates at the *vestibule* (the portion of the internal ear concerned with balance sensations) and conveys information on position, movement, and balance; and (2) the **cochlear** (KOK-lē-ar; *cochlea*, snail shell) **nerve**, which monitors the receptors of the cochlea (the portion of the internal ear responsible for the sense of hearing).

THE GLOSSOPHARYNGEAL NERVES (N IX). The **glossopharyngeal** (glos-ō-fah-RIN-jē-al; *glossus*, tongue) **nerves** are mixed nerves innervating the tongue and pharynx. The associated sensory and motor nuclei are in the medulla oblongata. The sensory portion of this nerve provides taste sensations from the posterior third of the tongue. It also monitors blood pressure and dissolved gas concentrations in major blood vessels. The motor portion controls the pharyngeal muscles involved in swallowing. These nerves also carry autonomic fibers that control the parotid salivary glands.

THE VAGUS NERVES (N X). The **vagus** (VĀ-gus; *vagus*, wandering) **nerves** provide sensory information from each auricle and external acoustic meatus (auditory canal), the diaphragm, and taste receptors in the pharynx, and from visceral receptors along the esophagus, respiratory tract, and abdominal organs as far away as the last portions of the large intestine. The associated sensory and motor nuclei of the vagus are located in the medulla oblongata. The sensory information that is provided is vital to the autonomic control of visceral function. We are not consciously aware of these sensations because they are seldom relayed to the cerebral cortex. The motor components of the vagus nerves control skeletal muscles of the soft palate, pharynx, and esophagus and affect cardiac muscle, smooth muscle, and glands of the esophagus, stomach, intestines, and gallbladder.

THE ACCESSORY NERVES (N XI). The **accessory nerves**, sometimes called the *spinal accessory nerves*, are motor nerves that innervate structures in the neck and back. These nerves differ from other cranial nerves in that some of their motor fibers originate in the lateral gray horns of the first five cervical segments of the spinal cord, as well as in the medulla oblongata. All these motor fibers join together in the cranium and exit

as N XI, which then divides into two branches. The internal branch joins the vagus nerve and innervates the voluntary swallowing muscles of the soft palate and pharynx, as well as the laryngeal muscles that control the vocal cords and produce speech. The external branch controls the sternocleidomastoid and trapezius muscles associated with the pectoral girdles. ⊃ pp. 220, 225

THE HYPOGLOSSAL NERVES (N XII). The **hypoglossal** (hī-pō-GLOS-al) **nerves** provide voluntary control over movements of the tongue. The nuclei for these motor nerves are located in the medulla oblongata.

The distribution (innervated structures) and functions of the cranial nerves are summarized in **Figure 8-31b**.

The Spinal Nerves

The 31 pairs of **spinal nerves** are grouped according to the region of the vertebral column from which they originate (**Figure 8-32**). They include 8 pairs of cervical nerves (C_1–C_8), 12 pairs of thoracic nerves (T_1–T_{12}), 5 pairs of lumbar nerves (L_1–L_5), 5 pairs of sacral nerves (S_1–S_5), and 1 pair of coccygeal nerves (Co_1).

Each pair of spinal nerves monitors a specific region of the body surface known as a **dermatome** (**Figure 8-33**). Dermatomes are clinically important because damage or infection of a spinal nerve or of dorsal root ganglia produces a characteristic loss of sensation in the corresponding region of the skin. For example, in *shingles*, a virus that infects dorsal root ganglia causes a painful rash whose distribution corresponds to that of the affected sensory nerves.

Nerve Plexuses

During development, skeletal muscles commonly fuse, forming larger muscles innervated by nerve trunks containing axons derived from several spinal nerves. These compound nerve trunks originate at networks called **nerve plexuses**. The four spinal nerve plexuses and the distribution of some of the major peripheral nerves are shown in **Figure 8-32**.

The **cervical plexus** innervates the muscles of the neck and extends into the thoracic cavity to control the diaphragm, a key respiratory muscle. The **brachial plexus** innervates the pectoral girdles and upper limbs. The **lumbar plexus** and the **sacral plexus** supply the pelvic girdle and lower limbs. These plexuses are sometimes designated the *lumbosacral plexus*.

The nerves arising at the nerve plexuses contain sensory as well as motor fibers. *Peripheral nerve palsies*, also known as *peripheral neuropathies*, are characterized by regional losses of

Figure 8-32 Peripheral Nerves and Nerve Plexuses.

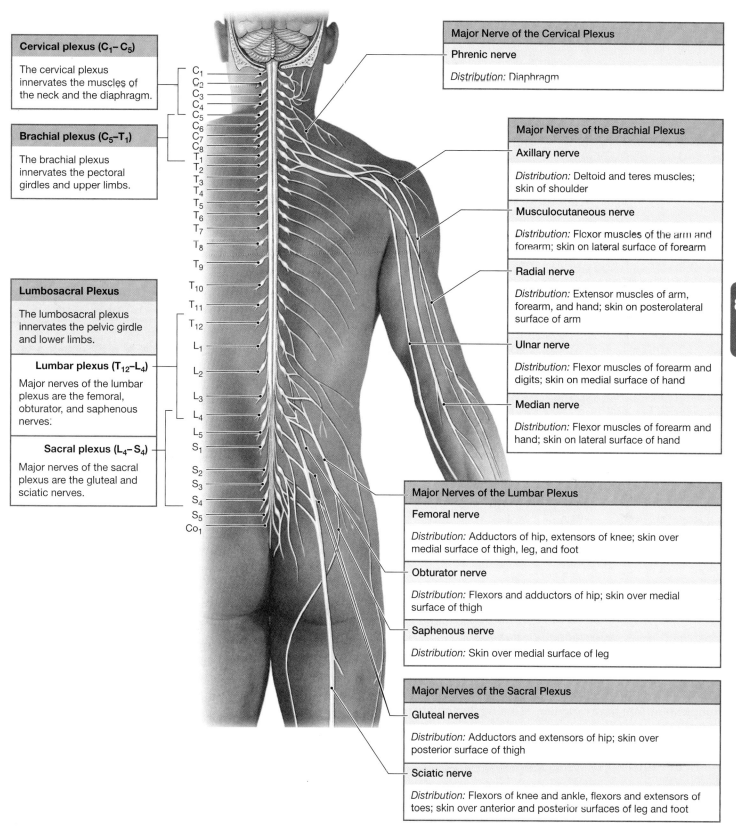

Cervical plexus (C₁– C₅)

The cervical plexus innervates the muscles of the neck and the diaphragm.

Brachial plexus (C₅–T₁)

The brachial plexus innervates the pectoral girdles and upper limbs.

Lumbosacral Plexus

The lumbosacral plexus innervates the pelvic girdle and lower limbs.

Lumbar plexus (T₁₂–L₄)

Major nerves of the lumbar plexus are the femoral, obturator, and saphenous nerves.

Sacral plexus (L₄–S₄)

Major nerves of the sacral plexus are the gluteal and sciatic nerves.

Major Nerve of the Cervical Plexus

Phrenic nerve

Distribution: Diaphragm

Major Nerves of the Brachial Plexus

Axillary nerve

Distribution: Deltoid and teres muscles; skin of shoulder

Musculocutaneous nerve

Distribution: Flexor muscles of the arm and forearm; skin on lateral surface of forearm

Radial nerve

Distribution: Extensor muscles of arm, forearm, and hand; skin on posterolateral surface of arm

Ulnar nerve

Distribution: Flexor muscles of forearm and digits; skin on medial surface of hand

Median nerve

Distribution: Flexor muscles of forearm and hand; skin on lateral surface of hand

Major Nerves of the Lumbar Plexus

Femoral nerve

Distribution: Adductors of hip, extensors of knee; skin over medial surface of thigh, leg, and foot

Obturator nerve

Distribution: Flexors and adductors of hip; skin over medial surface of thigh

Saphenous nerve

Distribution: Skin over medial surface of leg

Major Nerves of the Sacral Plexus

Gluteal nerves

Distribution: Adductors and extensors of hip; skin over posterior surface of thigh

Sciatic nerve

Distribution: Flexors of knee and ankle, flexors and extensors of toes; skin over anterior and posterior surfaces of leg and foot

8

Figure 8-33 Dermatomes. Distributions of dermatomes on the surface of the skin, as seen in the anterior and posterior view. The face is served by cranial nerves, not spinal nerves.

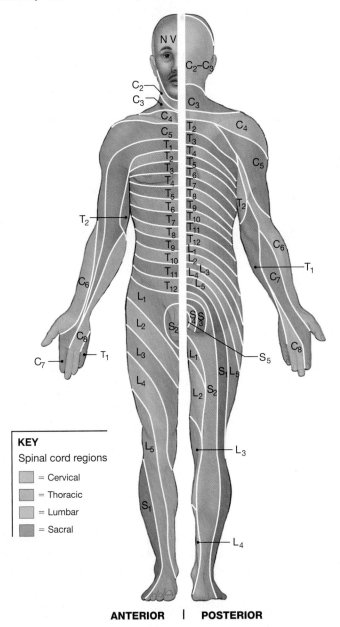

KEY
Spinal cord regions
☐ = Cervical
☐ = Thoracic
☐ = Lumbar
☐ = Sacral

ANTERIOR | POSTERIOR

sensory and motor function as the result of nerve trauma or compression. You have experienced a mild, temporary palsy if your arm or leg has ever "fallen asleep."

CHECKPOINT

28. What signs would you associate with damage to the abducens nerve (N VI)?

29. John is having trouble moving his tongue. His physician tells him it is due to pressure on a cranial nerve. Which cranial nerve is involved?

30. Injury to which nerve plexus would interfere with the ability to breathe?

See the blue Answers tab at the back of the book.

8-9 Reflexes are rapid, automatic responses to stimuli

Learning Objective Describe the steps in a reflex arc.

We can study the CNS and PNS separately, but they work together. To consider the ways the CNS and PNS interact, we begin with simple reflex responses to stimulation. A **reflex** is a rapid, automatic response to a specific stimulus. Reflexes help preserve homeostasis by making rapid adjustments in the function of organs or organ systems. The response shows little variability. Whenever a particular reflex is activated, it usually produces the same motor response.

Simple Reflexes

A reflex involves sensory fibers delivering information from peripheral receptors to the CNS, and motor fibers carrying motor commands to peripheral effectors. The "wiring" of a single reflex is called a **reflex arc**. It begins at a receptor and ends at an effector such as a muscle fiber or gland cell. **Figure 8-34** diagrams the five steps involved in the action of a reflex arc: (1) the arrival of a stimulus and activation of a receptor, (2) the activation of a sensory neuron, (3) information processing by an interneuron, (4) the activation of a motor neuron, and (5) the response by a peripheral effector.

A reflex usually removes or opposes the original stimulus. In **Figure 8-34**, the contracting muscle pulls the hand away from the painful stimulus. This reflex arc is, therefore, an example of *negative feedback*. ↻ p. 10 By opposing potentially harmful changes in the internal or external environment, reflexes play an important role in maintaining homeostasis.

In the simplest reflex arc, a sensory neuron synapses directly on a motor neuron, which performs the information-processing function. Such a reflex is called a **monosynaptic reflex**. Because there is only one synapse, monosynaptic reflexes control the most rapid, stereotyped motor responses of the nervous system. The best-known example is the stretch reflex.

The **stretch reflex** provides automatic regulation of skeletal muscle length. The sensory receptors in the stretch reflex are called **muscle spindles**. They are bundles of small,

Figure 8-34 Events in a Reflex Arc.

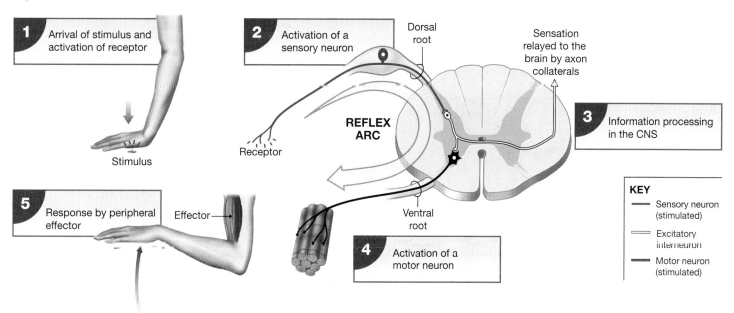

1. Arrival of stimulus and activation of receptor

Stimulus

2. Activation of a sensory neuron

Dorsal root

Sensation relayed to the brain by axon collaterals

REFLEX ARC

Receptor

3. Information processing in the CNS

Ventral root

4. Activation of a motor neuron

5. Response by peripheral effector

Effector

KEY
— Sensory neuron (stimulated)
▭ Excitatory interneuron
— Motor neuron (stimulated)

specialized skeletal muscle fibers scattered throughout skeletal muscles. The stimulus (increasing muscle length) activates a sensory neuron that triggers an immediate motor response (contraction of the stretched muscle) that counteracts the stimulus.

Stretch reflexes are important in maintaining normal posture and balance and in making automatic adjustments in muscle tone. Physicians can use the sensitivity of the stretch reflex to test the general condition of the spinal cord, peripheral nerves, and muscles. For example, in the **patellar reflex**, or *knee-jerk reflex*, a sharp rap on the patellar tendon stretches muscle spindles in the quadriceps muscles (**Figure 8-35**). With so brief a stimulus, the reflexive contraction occurs unopposed and produces a noticeable kick. If this contraction shortens the muscle spindles to less than their original resting lengths, the sensory nerve endings are compressed, the sensory neuron is inhibited, and the leg drops back.

Complex Reflexes

Many spinal reflexes have at least one interneuron between the sensory (afferent) neuron and the motor (efferent) neuron (**Figure 8-34**). Because there are more synapses, such **polysynaptic reflexes** include a longer delay between stimulus and response. But they can produce far more responses because the interneurons can control several muscle groups simultaneously.

Withdrawal reflexes move stimulated parts of the body away from a source of stimulation. Painful stimuli trigger

the strongest withdrawal reflexes, but these reflexes are also initiated by the stimulation of touch or pressure receptors. A **flexor reflex** is a withdrawal reflex affecting the muscles of a limb. If you grab an unexpectedly hot pan on the stove, a dramatic flexor reflex occurs (**Figure 8-36**). When the pain receptors in your hand are stimulated, the sensory neurons activate interneurons in the spinal cord that stimulate motor neurons in the anterior gray horns. As a result, flexor muscles contract and yank your forearm and hand away from the stove. At the same time this response is taking place, pain sensations are ascending to the brain.

When a specific muscle contracts, opposing (antagonistic) muscles are stretched. For example, the flexor muscles that bend the elbow are opposed by extensor muscles, which straighten it out. A potential conflict exists here: Contraction of a flexor muscle should trigger a stretch reflex in the extensors that would cause them to contract, opposing the movement that is under way. Interneurons in the spinal cord prevent such competition through **reciprocal inhibition**. When one set of motor neurons is stimulated, those controlling antagonistic muscles are inhibited.

Integration and Control of Spinal Reflexes

Reflexes are automatic, but higher centers in the brain influence these responses. They do so by facilitating (assisting) or inhibiting the interneurons and motor neurons involved. The sensitivity of a reflex can thus be modified. The facilitation of motor neurons involved in reflexes is

Figure 8-35 A Stretch Reflex. The patellar reflex is a stretch reflex controlled by stretch receptors (muscle spindles) in the muscles that straighten the knee. When a reflex hammer strikes the patellar tendon, the muscle spindles are stretched. This stretching results in a sudden increase in the activity of the sensory neurons, which synapse on motor neurons in the spinal cord. The activation of spinal motor neurons produces an immediate muscle contraction and a reflexive kick.

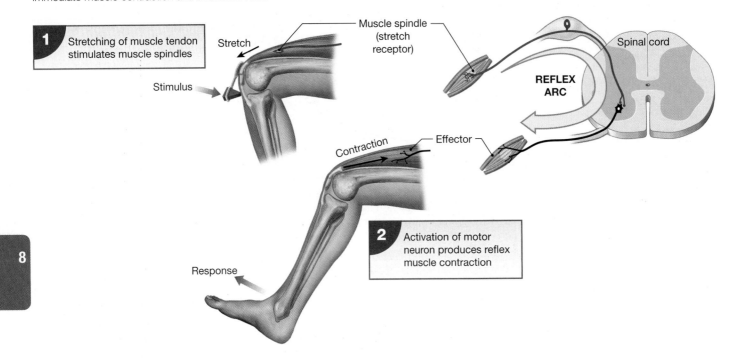

called *reinforcement*. For example, the Jendrassik maneuver is a method used to overemphasize the patellar reflex. To do this, the person hooks the hands together by interlocking the fingers and then tries to pull the hands apart while a light tap is applied to the patellar tendon. This reinforcement produces a big kick rather than a twitch. This distractive technique still produces a larger reflex response even if the individual realizes it is just a distraction.

Other descending fibers have an inhibitory effect on spinal reflexes. Stroking an infant's foot on the side of the sole

Figure 8-36 The Flexor Reflex, a Type of Withdrawal Reflex.

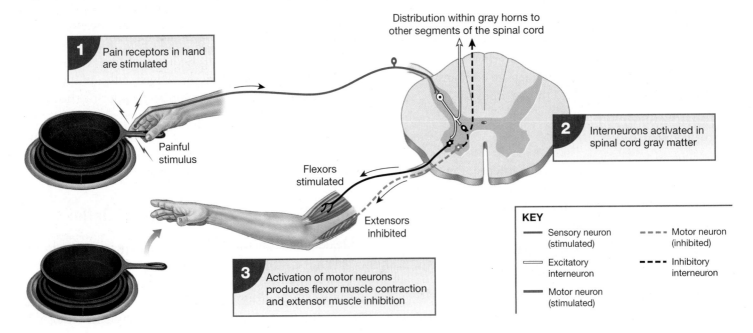

CLINICAL NOTE

Reflexes

Reflex testing can be a useful physical examination tool. A *reflex* is an automatic motor response triggered by a particular stimulus. A *reflex arc* includes a receptor, a sensory neuron, a motor neuron, and an effector. In simple reflex arcs, a sensory neuron interacts directly with a motor neuron. These simple monosynaptic reflexes are quite rapid. They protect parts of the body from injury by withdrawing the affected part when it is exposed to a noxious stimulus, such as heat. The best example of this is the stretch reflex, which provides automatic regulation of skeletal muscle length.

Stretch reflexes can be evaluated by tapping on a part of the muscle with a reflex hammer. The brief stimulus of a hammer tap results in a noticeable contraction in the affected muscle. This response is considered the reflex and is generally graded on a scale of 0–4. **Table 8-1** illustrates the reflex grading scale. Reflexes on one side of the body are usually compared to their corresponding reflexes on the other side of the body. Asymmetry of the reflexes may indicate an abnormality. Testing reflexes provides information about the corresponding spinal segment. The four most commonly examined reflexes are the ankle jerk, biceps reflex, patellar reflex, and abdominal reflex. The ankle jerk reflex evaluates sacral spinal segments S_1 and S_2. The biceps reflex evaluates spinal nerves C_5 and C_6. The patellar reflex examines spinal nerves L_2, L_3, and L_4. The abdominal reflex is a contraction of the abdominal muscles that moves the umbilicus (navel) toward the stimulus. The portion of the abdomen above the umbilicus corresponds to thoracic spinal segments T_8, T_9, and T_{10}, while the portion of the abdomen below the umbilicus corresponds to the thoracic spinal segments T_{10}, T_{11}, and T_{12} (**Figure 8-37**).

A decreased reflex (hyporeflexia), or an absent reflex (areflexia), may be due to temporary or permanent damage to skeletal muscles, dorsal or ventral nerve roots, spinal nerves, the spinal cord, or the brain. An increased reflex (hyperreflexia) usually results from diseases that affect higher centers or descending tracts. In certain patients, a tap on a tendon with a reflex hammer can cause a sustained contraction or several successive contractions, referred to as clonus.

In a pronounced type of hyperreflexia that occurs following severe spinal injury, the motor neurons of the spinal cord lose contact with higher centers in the brain. Initially following the injury is a period of areflexia known as spinal shock. When the reflexes return, they respond in an exaggerated fashion, even to mild stimuli.

Stroking the bottom of the feet along the lateral aspect of the sole should cause plantar flexion of the toes (**Figure 8-38**). If the big toe dorsiflexes and the other toes fan out, this indicates a central nervous system lesion. Known as a *Babinski response*, this reflex should be assessed in all critically ill or critically injured patients.

Figure 8-37 Abdominal Reflex. Gently stroking the skin of the abdomen should cause contraction of the underlying muscles, and move the umbilicus toward the location of the stimulus.

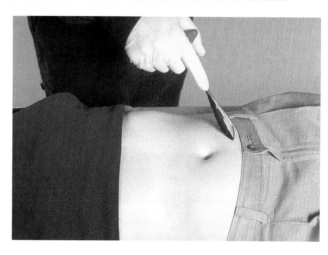

Figure 8-38 Plantar Reflex. Stroking the lateral aspect of the plantar surface of the foot should cause plantar flexion of the toes. Dorsiflexion of the great toe and fanning of the other toes following stimulation is a positive Babinski reflex, which suggests problems with higher centers in the brain.

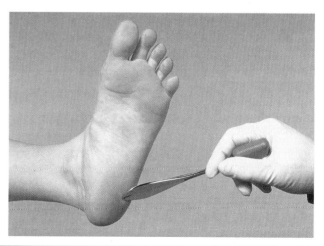

Table 8-1	Reflex Scale
Grade	**Descriptions**
0	No response
+	Diminished, below normal
++	Average, normal
+++	Brisker than normal
++++	Hyperactive, associated with clonus

8

produces a fanning of the toes known as the **Babinski sign**, or *positive Babinski reflex*. This response disappears as descending inhibitory synapses develop, so in adults the same stimulus produces a curling of the toes, called a **plantar reflex**, or *negative Babinski reflex*, after about a one-second delay. If either the higher centers or the descending tracts are damaged, the Babinski sign will reappear. As a result, clinicians often test this reflex if CNS injury is suspected.

Spinal reflexes produce consistent, stereotyped motor patterns that are triggered by specific external stimuli. However, the same motor patterns can also be activated as needed by higher centers in the brain. The use of preexisting motor patterns allows a relatively small number of descending fibers to control complex motor functions. For example, the motor patterns for walking, running, and jumping are directed primarily by neuronal pools in the spinal cord. The descending pathways from the brain facilitate, inhibit, or fine-tune the established patterns.

CHECKPOINT

31. Define reflex.

32. Which common reflex do physicians use to test the general condition of the spinal cord, peripheral nerves, and muscles?

33. Why can polysynaptic reflexes produce more complex responses than can monosynaptic reflexes?

34. After injuring his back lifting a sofa, Tom exhibits a positive Babinski reflex. What does this imply about Tom's injury?

See the blue Answers tab at the back of the book.

Build Your Knowledge

Recall that sensory receptors are present in the dermis and deeper layers of the epidermis (as you saw in **Chapter 5: The Integumentary System**). Dermal nerve fibers monitor these sensory receptors, which provide sensations of touch, pain, pressure, and temperature.⤴ **p. 129**

8-10 Separate pathways carry sensory information and motor commands

Learning Objective Identify the principal sensory and motor pathways, and explain how it is possible to distinguish among sensations that originate in different areas of the body.

The communication among the CNS, the PNS, and organs and organ systems takes place over pathways, nerve tracts, and nuclei that relay sensory and motor information.⤴ p. 250 The names of the major sensory (ascending) and motor (descending) tracts of the spinal cord are based on the destinations of the axons. If the name of a tract begins with *spino-*, the tract starts in the spinal cord and ends in the brain, and it therefore carries sensory information. If the name of a tract ends in *-spinal*, its axons start in the higher centers and end in the spinal cord, bearing motor commands. The rest of the tract's name indicates the associated nucleus or cortical area of the brain.

Table 8-2 lists some examples of sensory and motor pathways, and their functions.

Table 8-2	Sensory and Motor Pathways
Pathway	**Function**
SENSORY	
Posterior column pathway	Delivers highly localized sensations of fine touch, pressure, vibration, and proprioception to the primary sensory cortex
Spinothalamic pathway	Delivers poorly localized sensations of touch, pressure, pain, and temperature to the primary sensory cortex
Spinocerebellar pathway	Delivers proprioceptive information concerning the positions of muscles, bones, and joints to the cerebellar cortex
MOTOR	
Corticospinal pathway	Provides conscious control of skeletal muscles throughout the body
Medial and lateral pathways	Provides subconscious regulation of skeletal muscle tone, controls reflexive skeletal muscle responses to equilibrium sensations and to sudden or strong visual and auditory stimuli

Sensory Pathways

Sensory receptors monitor conditions in the body or the external environment. The information gathered by a sensory receptor arrives in the CNS in the form of action potentials in an afferent (sensory) fiber. The arriving information is called a **sensation**. Most processing of arriving sensations takes place in centers along the sensory pathways in the spinal cord or brain stem. Only about 1 percent of the arriving information reaches the cerebral cortex and our conscious awareness. For example, we usually do not perceive, or feel, the clothes we wear or hear the hum of our car's engine.

The Posterior Column Pathway

One example of an ascending sensory pathway is the **posterior column pathway** (**Figure 8-39**). It sends highly localized ("fine") touch, pressure, vibration, and proprioception (position) sensations to the cerebral cortex. In the process, the information is relayed from one neuron to another.

Sensations travel along the axon of a sensory neuron, reaching the CNS through the dorsal roots of spinal nerves (❶ in **Figure 8-39**). Within the spinal cord, the axons ascend within the posterior column pathway. They synapse in a sensory nucleus of the medulla oblongata. The axons of the neurons in this nucleus (the second neuron in this pathway) cross over to the opposite side of the brain stem before continuing to the thalamus (❷). The location of the synapse in the thalamus depends on the region of the body involved. The thalamic (in this case, third) neuron then relays the information to an appropriate region of the primary sensory cortex (❸).

The sensations arrive at particular locations in the primary sensory cortex. For example, sensory information from the toes reaches one end of the primary sensory cortex, and information from the head reaches the other. As a result, the sensory cortex contains a miniature map of the body surface called a *sensory homunculus* ("little human"). That map is distorted because the area of sensory cortex devoted to a particular region is proportional not to its size, but to the number of sensory receptors the region contains. In other words, it takes many more cortical neurons to process sensory information from the tongue, which has tens of thousands of taste and touch receptors, than it does to analyze sensations from the back, where touch receptors are few and far between.

Figure 8-39 The Posterior Column Pathway. The posterior column pathway carries fine-touch, pressure, vibration, and proprioception sensations to the primary sensory cortex of the cerebral hemisphere on the opposite side of the body. (For clarity, this figure shows only the pathway for sensations originating on the right side of the body.)

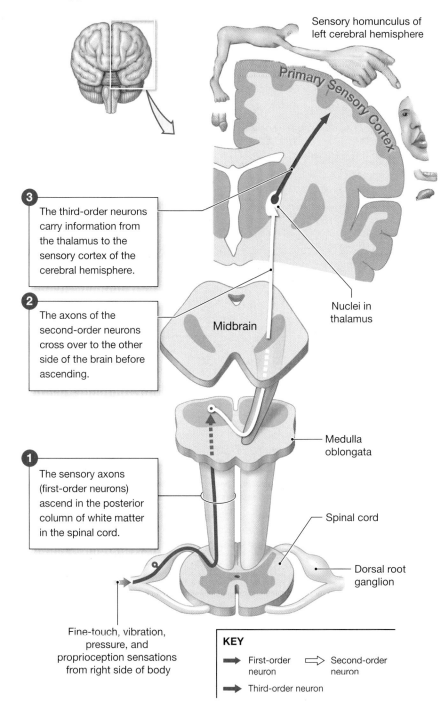

Sensory homunculus of left cerebral hemisphere

Primary Sensory Cortex

❸ The third-order neurons carry information from the thalamus to the sensory cortex of the cerebral hemisphere.

❷ The axons of the second-order neurons cross over to the other side of the brain before ascending.

❶ The sensory axons (first-order neurons) ascend in the posterior column of white matter in the spinal cord.

Nuclei in thalamus

Midbrain

Medulla oblongata

Spinal cord

Dorsal root ganglion

Fine-touch, vibration, pressure, and proprioception sensations from right side of body

KEY

➡ First-order neuron

⇨ Second-order neuron

➡ Third-order neuron

Motor Pathways

In response to information from sensory systems, the CNS issues motor commands that are distributed by the *SNS* and the *ANS* of the efferent division of the PNS (**Figure 8-1**, p. 271). The SNS, under voluntary control, issues somatic motor commands that direct the contractions of skeletal muscles. The motor commands of the ANS occur outside our conscious awareness. They control the smooth muscles, cardiac muscle, and glands.

Three motor pathways provide control over skeletal muscles: the corticospinal pathway, the medial pathway, and the lateral pathway. The corticospinal pathway provides conscious, voluntary control over skeletal muscles. The medial and lateral pathways exert more indirect, subconscious control. **Table 8-2** lists some examples and functions of these motor pathways. We begin our examination of motor pathways with the corticospinal pathway.

The Corticospinal Pathway

The **corticospinal pathway**, sometimes called the *pyramidal system*, provides conscious, voluntary control of skeletal muscles. **Figure 8-40** shows the motor pathway providing voluntary control over the right side of the body. As in the case of the sensory homunculus, in the primary motor cortex the area devoted to a body part does not reflect the size of that part. Instead, the area reflects the number of motor units present in that part of the body. For example, the *motor homunculus* has grossly oversized hands. Their size is an indication of the large number of motor units involved in writing, grasping, and manipulating objects in our environment.

The corticospinal pathway begins at triangular-shaped *pyramidal cells* of the cerebral cortex. The axons of these upper motor neurons extend into the brain stem and spinal cord, where they synapse on lower motor neurons (❶ in **Figure 8-40**). All axons of the corticospinal tracts eventually cross over to reach motor neurons on the opposite side of the body (❷). As a result, the right cerebral hemisphere controls the left side of the body, and the left cerebral hemisphere controls the right side.

The Medial and Lateral Pathways

The **medial and lateral pathways** provide subconscious, involuntary control of muscle tone and movements of the neck, trunk, and limbs. They also coordinate learned movement patterns and other voluntary motor activities (**Table 8-2**). Together, these pathways were known as the

Figure 8-40 The Corticospinal Pathway. The corticospinal pathway originates at the primary motor cortex. Axons of the pyramidal cells of the primary motor cortex descend to reach motor nuclei in the brain stem and spinal cord. Most of the fibers cross over in the medulla oblongata before descending into the spinal cord as the corticospinal tracts.

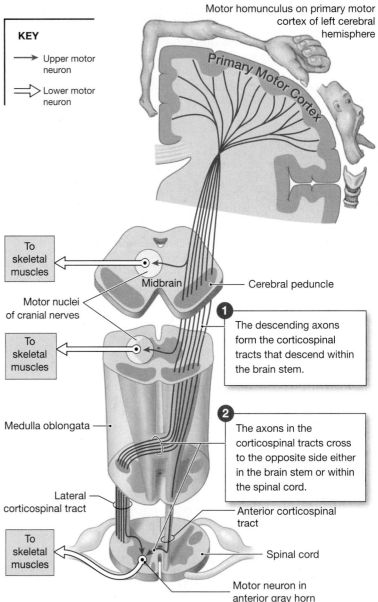

KEY

→ Upper motor neuron

⇒ Lower motor neuron

Motor homunculus on primary motor cortex of left cerebral hemisphere

Primary Motor Cortex

To skeletal muscles

Midbrain

Motor nuclei of cranial nerves

To skeletal muscles

Cerebral peduncle

❶ The descending axons form the corticospinal tracts that descend within the brain stem.

Medulla oblongata

❷ The axons in the corticospinal tracts cross to the opposite side either in the brain stem or within the spinal cord.

Lateral corticospinal tract

To skeletal muscles

Anterior corticospinal tract

Spinal cord

Motor neuron in anterior gray horn

extrapyramidal system because it was thought that they operated independently of and parallel to the *pyramidal system* (the corticospinal pathway). We now know that the control of the body's motor functions is integrated among all three motor pathways.

The components of the medial and lateral pathways are spread throughout the brain. These components include nuclei in the brain stem (midbrain, pons, and medulla oblongata), relay stations in the thalamus, the basal nuclei of the cerebrum, and the cerebellum. Output from the basal

CLINICAL NOTE

Extrapyramidal Motor Syndromes

Several of the drugs used in emergency medicine can cause side effects that involve the *extrapyramidal system (EPS)*. The drugs most frequently implicated are those used in the treatment of nausea and vomiting and in the treatment of acute psychotic disorders. Most belong to a class of medications called *phenothiazines*. These drugs block the neurotransmitter *dopamine* in the brain thus causing EPS.

EPS side effects are similar to the effects of Parkinson's disease but are reversible. They are usually seen in the first few days of treatment and can be misdiagnosed as anxiety. EPS signs and symptoms include muscle spasms of the neck, face, tongue, and back (*dystonia*); a sensation of restlessness (*akathisia*); a shuffling gait; rigidity of the extremities; and drooling. These symptoms can be quite disconcerting for patients and their families.

Treatment usually results in prompt, and often dramatic, reversal of symptoms. Drugs used in the treatment of Parkinson's disease (benztropine) or antihistamines (diphenhydramine) are highly effective.

CLINICAL NOTE

Cerebral Palsy

The term cerebral palsy refers to a number of disorders affecting voluntary motor performance (including speech, movement, balance, and posture) that appear during infancy or childhood and persist throughout life. The cause may be trauma associated with premature or unusually stressful birth; maternal exposure to drugs, including alcohol; or a genetic defect that causes the motor pathways to develop improperly. Problems with labor and delivery result from the compression or interruption of placental circulation or oxygen supplies. If the oxygen concentration of fetal blood declines significantly for as little as 5–10 minutes, CNS function can be permanently impaired.

The cerebral cortex, cerebellum, basal nuclei, hippocampus, and thalamus are likely to be affected. Abnormalities in motor skills, posture and balance, memory, speech, and learning abilities may result.

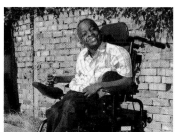

CLINICAL NOTE

Headache

Headache is a common complaint and usually a benign symptom. However, it can be associated with serious disease processes such as meningitis, brain tumor, and uncontrolled hypertension. The several *benign primary headache syndromes* include migraine headache, cluster headaches, and tension headaches.

Migraine Headache

Migraine headache is a common benign primary headache syndrome. It usually begins in the early teenage years and is more common in women than men. Migraine headaches appear to be caused by a particular trigger that sets a chain of events into motion. This complex chain of events includes neurological, vascular, hormonal, and neurotransmitter components. The phases of migraine headache are: (1) initial trigger phase initiated by external factors; (2) an aura with inhibition of neuronal activity in the cortex and a reduction in blood flow; (3) release of chemical substances that affect the blood vessels including serotonin and histamine; and (4) activation of fibers in the fifth cranial nerve (trigeminal nerve), which causes dilation of the dural arteries. These vascular changes cause the typical migraine headache.

Migraine headaches are usually classified as classic migraine or common migraine. In classic migraine, the headache is often preceded by an aura that is due to a slowly expanding area of reduced blood flow. These auras vary from patient to patient but commonly include blurred vision and flashing lights (scotoma). Some patients may report a strange taste or smell. The aura always occurs before the headache begins. In common migraine, the headache develops without a preceding aura.

Migraine headache generally develops slowly and lasts from 4 to 72 hours. It is typically located on one side of the head and pulsates. Physical activity usually worsens migraine headache, and causes the patient to lie motionless. Nausea and vomiting are very common. Sensitivity to light (photophobia) and sound (phonophobia) commonly accompany migraine headache. In rare cases (complex migraine), migraines can cause total blindness, weakness or paralysis of one side of the body, and speech difficulties.

Migraine headaches are a common reason people seek emergency care. Due to a better understanding of the mechanism of migraine, several medications have been developed that will actually abort the headache if administered in time. These medications are most effective if administered as soon as possible following the onset of the aura or the headache. Once the headache has developed, medications for nausea and vomiting and for pain are often required.

(Continued)

Cluster Headache

Cluster headache is characterized by very severe, unilateral pain in the orbit, forehead, or temple. These headaches usually occur in men, with onset typically after age 20. The pain of cluster headache is usually so severe that patients cannot lie still. Generally, they pace and are very restless. Often there will be tearing of the eye or redness of the conjunctiva on the affected side. The headaches usually last from 15 to 180 minutes and generally occur in "clusters" that occur daily on the same side of the face for several weeks. Oxygen is an effective treatment in up to 70 percent of patients, and some of the medications developed for migraine headaches also have proven effective in cluster headaches.

Tension Headache

Tension headache is a common type of headache that occurs in 40–60 percent of the population. The average age of onset is from 25 to 30 years. Tension headache is usually located on both sides of the head and is nonpulsating. Unlike migraine headaches, tension headaches are not associated with nausea and vomiting and are not worsened by physical exertion. Treatment is aimed at alleviating the symptoms.

---

nuclei and cerebellum exerts the highest level of control. For example, their output can stimulate or inhibit (1) other nuclei of these pathways or (2) the activities of pyramidal cells in the primary motor cortex. Also, axons from the upper motor neurons in the medial and lateral pathways synapse on the same motor neurons innervated by the corticospinal pathway.

CHECKPOINT

35. As a result of pressure on her spinal cord, Jill cannot feel touch or pressure on her legs. What sensory pathway is being compressed?

36. The primary motor cortex of the right cerebral hemisphere controls motor function on which side of the body?

37. An injury to the superior portion of the motor cortex would affect the ability to control muscles of which parts of the body?

See the blue Answers tab at the back of the book.

8-11 The autonomic nervous system, composed of the sympathetic and parasympathetic divisions, is involved in the unconscious regulation of body functions

Learning Objective Describe the structures and functions of the sympathetic and parasympathetic divisions of the autonomic nervous system.

Your conscious sensations, plans, and responses are only a tiny fraction of the activities of the nervous system. In practical terms, conscious activities have little to do with our immediate or long-term survival. The **ANS** makes adjustments that are much more important. Without the ANS, a simple night's sleep would be a life-threatening event.

Recall that both the ANS and the SNS are parts of the efferent division of the PNS. As such, they carry motor commands to peripheral effectors. ⊃ p. 245 However, clear anatomical differences exist between them (**Figure 8-41**). In the SNS, lower motor neurons exert direct control over skeletal muscles (**Figure 8-41a**). In the ANS, a second motor neuron always separates the CNS and the peripheral effector (**Figure 8-41b**). We now turn to the ANS.

The ANS motor neurons in the CNS are known as **preganglionic neurons**. They send their axons, called *preganglionic fibers*, to autonomic ganglia outside the CNS. In these ganglia, the axons of preganglionic neurons synapse on **ganglionic neurons**. The axons of the ganglionic neurons are **postganglionic fibers**. These fibers leave the ganglia and innervate cardiac muscle, smooth muscles, glands, and, in some cases, fat cells (adipocytes).

The ANS has two divisions: the sympathetic division and the parasympathetic division. In the **sympathetic division**, preganglionic fibers leave the thoracic and lumbar segments of the spinal cord and synapse in ganglia near the spinal cord (**Figure 8-42**). In this division, the preganglionic fibers are short, and the postganglionic fibers are long. The sympathetic division is often called the "fight or flight" system because it usually stimulates tissue metabolism, increases alertness, and prepares the body to deal with emergencies.

In the **parasympathetic division** of the ANS, preganglionic fibers originate in the brain stem and the sacral segments of the spinal cord (**Figure 8-42**). They synapse on neurons in *terminal ganglia* very close to the target organs, or in *intramural ganglia* (*murus*, wall) embedded within the target organs. In this division, the preganglionic fibers are long, and the postganglionic fibers are short. The parasympathetic division is often regarded as the "rest and repose" or "rest

Figure 8-41 The Organization of the Somatic and Autonomic Nervous Systems.

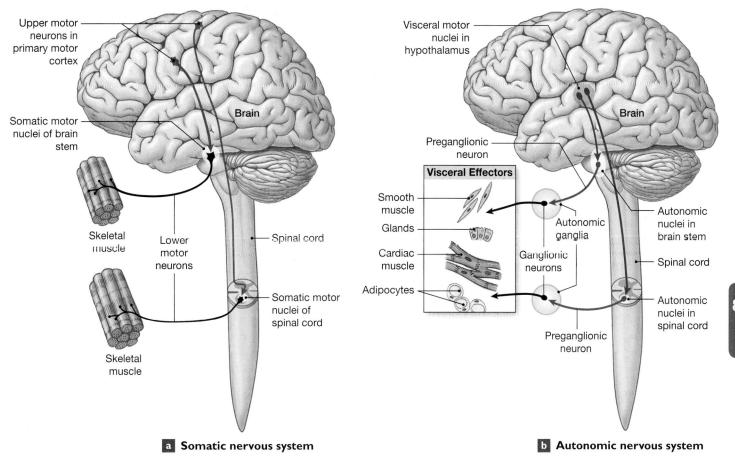

a Somatic nervous system

b Autonomic nervous system

and digest" system because it conserves energy and promotes sedentary activities, such as digestion.

Both divisions of the ANS affect target organs by releasing specific neurotransmitters from their postganglionic fibers. The result may be either stimulation or inhibition of activity, depending on the membrane receptor's response to the neurotransmitter. Some general patterns are worth noting:

- All preganglionic autonomic fibers are cholinergic: They release ACh at their axon terminals. ↺ p. 258 The effects are always excitatory.

- Postganglionic parasympathetic fibers are also cholinergic. However, the effects are excitatory or inhibitory, depending on the nature of the target cell receptor.

- Most postganglionic sympathetic fibers release NE. Neurons that release NE are called *adrenergic*. ↺ p. 260 The effects of NE are usually excitatory.

The Sympathetic Division

The sympathetic division of the ANS (**Figure 8-42**) consists of the following components:

- ***Preganglionic neurons located between segments*** T_1 ***and*** L_2 ***of the spinal cord.*** The cell bodies of these neurons are found in the lateral gray horns. Their short axons enter the ventral roots of these spinal segments.

- ***Ganglionic neurons located in ganglia near the vertebral column.*** Two types of sympathetic ganglia exist. Paired *sympathetic chain ganglia* lie on either side of the vertebral column. They contain neurons that control effectors in the body wall and inside the thoracic cavity. Unpaired *collateral ganglia* lie anterior to the vertebral column. They contain ganglionic neurons that innervate tissues and organs in the abdominopelvic cavity.

- ***The adrenal medullae.*** The center of each adrenal (*ad-*, near *renal*, kidney) gland is known as the **adrenal medulla**, or *suprarenal medulla*. It is a modified sympathetic ganglion. Its neurons have very short axons.

Organization of the Sympathetic Division

Figure 8-42 diagrams the distribution of sympathetic innervation. Note that this distribution is the same on both sides of the body.

THE SYMPATHETIC CHAIN. From spinal segments T_1 to L_2, sympathetic preganglionic fibers join the ventral root of each spinal nerve. All these fibers then exit the spinal nerve to enter the sympathetic chain ganglia (**Figure 8-42**). The fibers diverge extensively, with one preganglionic

Figure 8-42 The Sympathetic Division. The distribution of sympathetic fibers is the same on both sides of the body. For clarity, the innervation of somatic structures is shown to the left, and the innervation of visceral structures to the right.

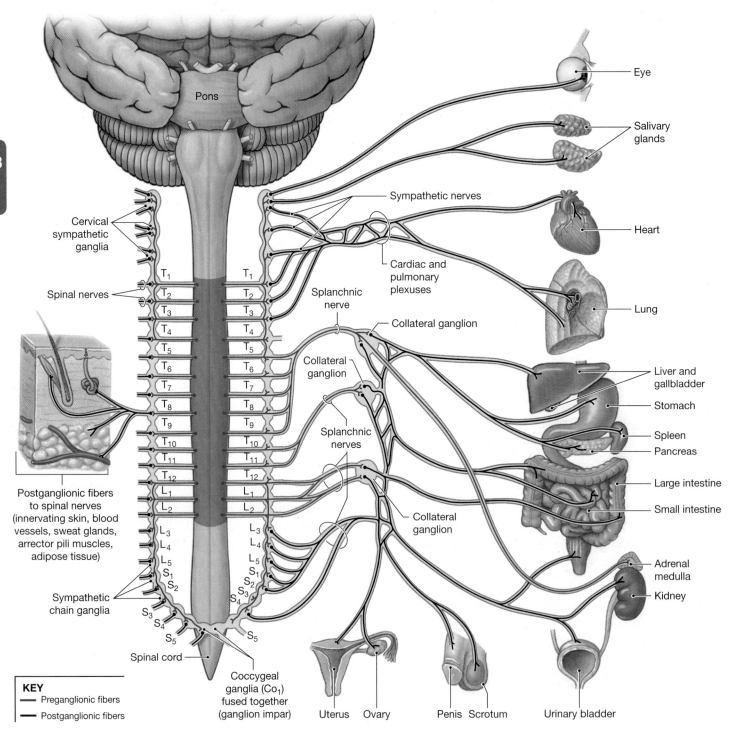

KEY
— Preganglionic fibers
— Postganglionic fibers

fiber synapsing on two dozen or more ganglionic neurons. For motor commands to the body wall, a synapse occurs at the chain ganglia, and then the postganglionic fibers return to the spinal nerve for distribution. For the thoracic cavity, a synapse also occurs at the chain ganglia, but the postganglionic fibers then form nerves that go directly to their targets.

THE COLLATERAL GANGLIA. The abdominopelvic tissues and organs receive sympathetic innervation over preganglionic fibers from lower thoracic and upper lumbar segments that pass through the sympathetic chain without synapsing. Instead, these fibers synapse within three unpaired **collateral ganglia** (**Figure 8-42**). The nerves traveling to the

collateral ganglia are known as *splanchnic nerves.* The postganglionic fibers leave the collateral ganglia and innervate organs throughout the abdominopelvic cavity.

THE ADRENAL MEDULLAE. Preganglionic fibers enter each adrenal gland and proceed to its center, the adrenal medulla. The fibers then synapse on modified neurons with an endocrine function. When stimulated, these cells release the neurotransmitters NE and epinephrine (E) into the bloodstream. The bloodstream carries NE and E throughout the body, where they cause metabolic changes in many different cells. In general, the effects of these neurotransmitters resemble those produced by the stimulation of sympathetic postganglionic fibers.

CLINICAL NOTE

Sympathetic Nervous System

Sympathetic stimulation ultimately results in the release of norepinephrine from postganglionic sympathetic nerves. The norepinephrine crosses the synaptic cleft and interacts with adrenergic receptors on the postsynaptic nerves or target organ. Shortly thereafter, the norepinephrine is either taken up whole by the presynaptic neuron for reuse or broken down by enzyme systems within the synapse. The two most common of these enzyme systems are *monoamine oxidase (MAO)* and *catechol-O-methyltransferase (COMT)* (**Figure 8-43**).

Sympathetic stimulation also results in the release of epinephrine and norepinephrine from the adrenal medulla. These hormones interact with other adrenergic receptors on the membranes

of target organs. This action effectively amplifies the magnitude of the sympathetic response.

The two known types of sympathetic receptors are the adrenergic receptors and the dopaminergic receptors. The adrenergic receptors are generally divided into four types. These four receptors are designated alpha 1 (α_1), alpha 2 (α_2), beta 1 (β_1), and beta 2 (β_2). The α_1 receptors cause peripheral vasoconstriction, mild bronchoconstriction, and stimulation of metabolism. The α_2 receptors are found on the presynaptic surfaces of sympathetic neuroeffector junctions. Stimulation of α_2 receptors is inhibitory. These receptors serve to prevent overrelease of norepinephrine in the synapse. When the level of norepinephrine in the synapse gets high enough, the α_2

Figure 8-43 Norepinephrine Neurotransmission. Norepinephrine is the neurotransmitter of the postganglionic sympathetic nervous system. It is taken up into the presynaptic membrane and broken down by the enzyme monoamine oxidase or catechol-O-methyltransferase.

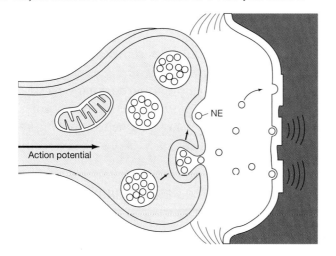

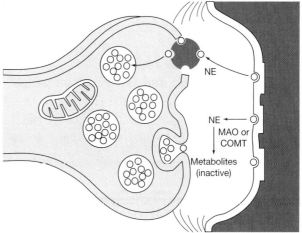

(Continued)

Table 8-3	Primary Actions and Locations of Adrenergic and Dopaminergic Receptors	
Receptor	**Response to Stimulation**	**Location**
Alpha 1 (α_1)	Constriction	Arterioles
	Constriction	Veins
	Mydriasis	Eye
	Ejaculation	Penis
Alpha 2 (α_2)	Inhibition of presynaptic terminals*	
Beta 1 (β_1)	Increased heart rate	Heart
	Increased conductivity	Kidney
	Increased automaticity	
	Increased contractility	
	Renin release	
Beta 2 (β_2)	Bronchodilation	Lungs
	Dilation	Arterioles
	Inhibition of contractions	Uterus
	Tremors	Skeletal muscle
Dopaminergic	Vasodilation (increased blood flow)	Kidney, heart, brain

*Stimulation of α_2 adrenergic receptors inhibits the continued release of norepinephrine from the presynaptic terminal. It is a feedback mechanism that limits the adrenergic response at the synapse. These receptors have no other identified peripheral effects.

receptors are stimulated and norepinephrine release is inhibited. Stimulation of the β_1 receptors causes an increase in heart rate, cardiac contractile force, and cardiac automaticity and conduction. Stimulation of β_2 receptors causes vasodilation and bronchodilation.

Dopaminergic receptors—although not fully understood—evidently cause dilation of the renal, coronary, and cerebral arteries. This helps maintain circulation to critical organs during periods of intense stress. **Table 8-3** describes the chief locations and primary actions of each receptor.

General Functions of the Sympathetic Division

The sympathetic division stimulates tissue metabolism, increases alertness, and prepares the individual for sudden, intense physical activity. Sympathetic innervation by the spinal nerves stimulates sweat gland activity and arrector pili muscles (producing "goose bumps"), reduces circulation to the skin and body wall, speeds up blood flow to skeletal muscles, releases stored lipids from adipose tissue, and dilates the pupils. The activation of the sympathetic nerves to the thoracic cavity accelerates the heart rate, increases the force of cardiac contractions, and dilates the respiratory passageways.

The postganglionic fibers from the collateral ganglia reduce the blood flow to visceral organs that are not important to short-term survival (such as the digestive tract). These fibers also reduce energy use by these organs. In addition, the fibers stimulate the release of stored energy reserves.

The release of NE and E by the adrenal medullae broadens the effects of sympathetic activation to cells not innervated by sympathetic postganglionic fibers. The effects also last much longer than those produced by direct sympathetic innervation.

The Parasympathetic Division

The parasympathetic division of the ANS (**Figure 8-42**) includes the following structures:

- ***Preganglionic neurons in the brain stem and in sacral segments of the spinal cord.*** The midbrain, pons, and medulla oblongata contain autonomic nuclei associated with cranial nerves III, VII, IX, and X. Other autonomic nuclei lie in the lateral gray horns of spinal cord segments S_2 to S_4.
- ***Ganglionic neurons in peripheral ganglia within or adjacent to the target organs.*** Preganglionic fibers of the parasympathetic division do not diverge as extensively as those of the sympathetic division. For this reason, the effects of parasympathetic stimulation are more localized and specific than those of the sympathetic division.

Organization of the Parasympathetic Division

Figure 8-44 diagrams the pattern of parasympathetic innervation. Preganglionic fibers leaving the brain travel within cranial nerves III (oculomotor), VII (facial), IX (glossopharyngeal), and X (vagus). These fibers synapse in terminal

Figure 8-44 The Parasympathetic Division. The distribution of parasympathetic fibers is the same on both sides of the body.

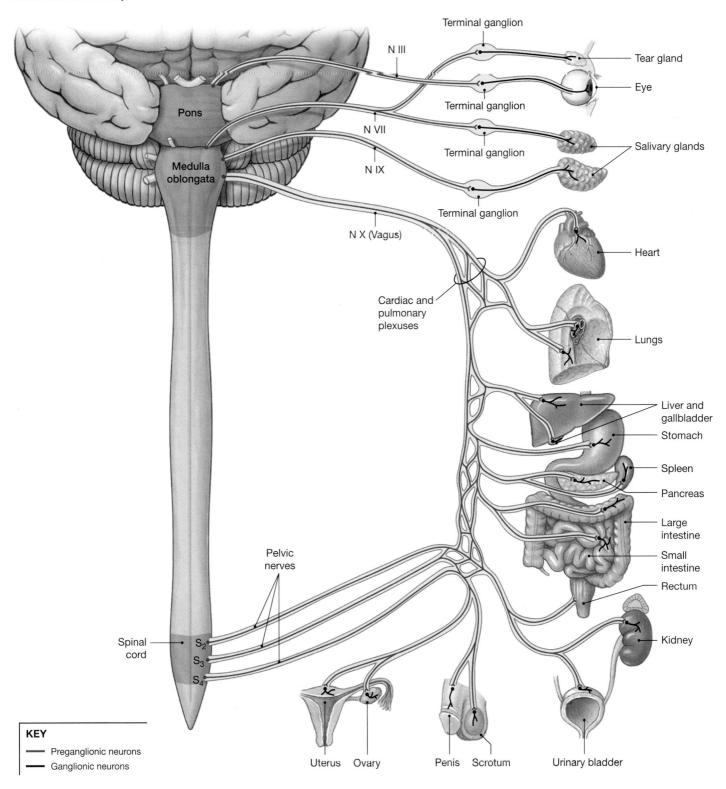

ganglia located in peripheral tissues. Short postganglionic fibers then continue to their targets. The vagus nerves provide preganglionic parasympathetic innervation to ganglia in organs of the thoracic and abdominopelvic cavities. Some of these ganglia are as distant as the last segments of the large intestine. The vagus nerves provide roughly 75 percent of all parasympathetic outflow and innervate most of those organs.

CLINICAL NOTE

Parasympathetic Nervous System

Acetylcholine, which is present in the neuromuscular junction, is the neurotransmitter for the somatic nervous system as well as for the parasympathetic nervous system. Acetylcholine is very short-lived. Within a fraction of a second after its release, it is deactivated by another chemical called *acetylcholinesterase*. Acetylcholinesterase, commonly called *cholinesterase*, breaks acetylcholine into *acetic acid* and *choline*. These two substances are taken back up by the presynaptic neuron and recycled for future use (**Figure 8-45**).

The parasympathetic nervous system has two types of acetylcholine receptors, *nicotinic* and *muscarinic*. Understanding these receptors will significantly aid in understanding the function of many emergency medications. *Nicotinic*$_N$ (neuron) receptors are found in all autonomic ganglia, both parasympathetic and sympathetic, where acetylcholine serves as the neurotransmitter. *Nicotinic*$_M$ (muscle) receptors are found on the neuromuscular junction and initiate muscle contraction as part of somatic nervous system function. *Muscarinic receptors* are found in many organs throughout the body and are primarily responsible for promoting the parasympathetic response. **Table 8-4** summarizes the locations and actions of muscarinic receptors. Because both nicotinic and muscarinic receptors are specific for acetylcholine, they are collectively referred to as cholinergic receptors.

Table 8-4	Location and Effect of Muscarinic Receptors	
Organ	**Functions**	**Location**
Heart	Decreased heart rate	Sinoatrial node
	Decreased conduction rate	Atrioventricular node
Arterioles	Dilation	Coronary
	Dilation	Skin and mucosa
	Dilation	Cerebral
GI tract	Relaxed	Sphincters
	Increased	Motility
	Increased salivation	Salivary glands
	Increased secretion	Exocrine glands
Lungs	Bronchoconstriction	Bronchiole smooth muscle
	Increased mucus production	Bronchial glands
Gallbladder	Contraction	
Urinary bladder	Relaxation	Urinary sphincter
	Contraction	Detrusor muscle
Liver	Glycogen synthesis	
Lacrimal glands	Secretion (increased tearing)	Eye
Eye	Contraction for near vision	Ciliary muscle
	Constriction	Pupil
Penis	Erection	

Figure 8-45 Acetylcholine Neurotransmission. Acetylcholine is the neurotransmitter of the parasympathetic nervous system, the ganglia of the sympathetic nervous system, and the somatic nervous system. It is promptly degraded into acetic acid and choline by the enzyme acetylcholinesterase and those components are taken up by the presynaptic membrane.

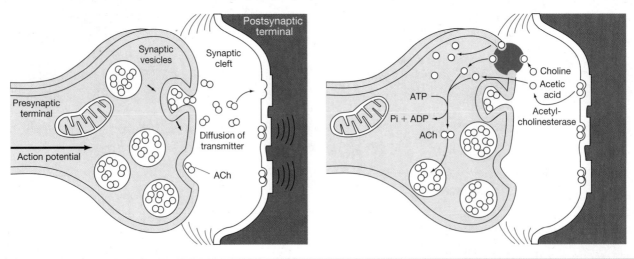

Preganglionic fibers in the sacral segments of the spinal cord carry the sacral parasympathetic output. They do not join the spinal nerves but instead form **pelvic nerves**. These nerves innervate intramural ganglia in the kidney and urinary bladder, the last segments of the large intestine, and the sex organs.

General Functions of the Parasympathetic Division

The functions of the parasympathetic division center on relaxation, food processing, and energy absorption. For example, the parasympathetic division constricts the pupils, increases secretions by the digestive glands, increases smooth muscle activity of the digestive tract, stimulates defecation and urination, constricts respiratory passageways, and reduces heart rate and the force of cardiac contractions. This division has been called the *anabolic system* (*anabole*, a raising up), because its stimulation leads to a general increase in the nutrient content of the blood. In response, cells throughout the body absorb nutrients and use them in growth, cell division, and the storage of energy reserves. The effects of parasympathetic stimulation are usually brief and are restricted to specific organs and sites.

Relationships between the Sympathetic and Parasympathetic Divisions

The sympathetic division has widespread effects, reaching visceral and somatic structures throughout the body. In contrast, the parasympathetic division innervates areas serviced by the cranial nerves and organs in the thoracic and abdominopelvic cavities. Some organs are innervated by one division or the other, but most vital organs receive **dual innervation**. That is, they get instructions from both autonomic divisions. In these cases, the two divisions often have opposing effects. **Table 8-5** provides examples of the effects of either single or dual innervation on selected organs.

CHECKPOINT

38. While out for a brisk walk, Megan is suddenly confronted by an angry dog. Which division of the ANS is responsible for the physiological changes that occur as she turns and runs from the animal?

39. Why is the parasympathetic division of the ANS sometimes referred to as the anabolic system?

40. What effect would loss of sympathetic stimulation have on the flow of air into the lungs?

41. What physiological changes would you expect in a patient who is about to undergo a root canal procedure and is quite anxious about it?

See the blue Answers tab at the back of the book.

8-12 Aging produces various structural and functional changes in the nervous system

Learning Objective Summarize the effects of aging on the nervous system.

Age-related anatomical and physiological changes in the nervous system probably begin by age 30 years and accumulate over time. An estimated 85 percent of individuals above age 65 years lead relatively normal lives, but they exhibit noticeable changes in mental performance and in CNS function. Common age-related anatomical changes include:

- *A reduction in brain size and weight.* This change results primarily from a decrease in the volume of the cerebral cortex. The brains of elderly individuals have narrower gyri and wider sulci than those of young people.

- *A reduction in the number of neurons.* Brain shrinkage has been linked to a loss of cortical neurons. Evidence indicates that the loss of neurons does not occur (at least to the same degree) in brain stem nuclei.

- *A decrease in blood flow to the brain.* With age, the gradual accumulation of fatty deposits in the walls of blood vessels reduces the rate of blood flow through arteries. (This process, called *arteriosclerosis*, affects arteries throughout the body. We discuss it further in Chapter 13.) The reduction in blood flow may not cause a cerebral crisis, but it does increase the chances that the individual will suffer a stroke.

- *Changes in the synaptic organization of the brain.* The number of dendritic branchings and interconnections appears to decrease. Synaptic connections are lost, and neurotransmitter production declines.

- *Intracellular and extracellular changes in CNS neurons.* Many neurons in the brain accumulate abnormal intracellular deposits (pigments or abnormal proteins) that have no apparent function. Extracellular accumulations of proteins (plaques) may also occur. These changes appear to take place in all aging brains. When present in excess, they seem to be associated with clinical abnormalities.

These anatomical changes are linked to impaired neural function. Memory consolidation—the conversion of short-term memory to long-term memory—often becomes more difficult. Other memories, especially those of the recent past, also become more difficult to recall. The sensory systems of the elderly (notably hearing, balance, vision, smell, and taste) become less acute. Light must be brighter, sounds louder, and smells stronger before they are perceived.

Table 8-5	The Effects of the Sympathetic and Parasympathetic Divisions of the ANS on Various Body Structures	
Structure	**Sympathetic Effects**	**Parasympathetic Effects**
EYE		
	Dilation of pupil	Constriction of pupil
	Focusing for near vision	Focusing for distance vision
Tear glands	None (not innervated)	Secretion
SKIN		
Sweat glands	Increases secretion	None (not innervated)
Arrector pili muscles	Contraction, erection of hairs	None (not innervated)
CARDIOVASCULAR SYSTEM		
Blood vessels	Vasoconstriction and vasodilation	None (not innervated)
Heart	Increases heart rate, force of contraction, and blood pressure	Decreases heart rate, force of contraction, and blood pressure
ADRENAL GLANDS		
	Secretion of epinephrine and norepinephrine by adrenal medullae	None (not innervated)
RESPIRATORY SYSTEM		
Airways	Increases diameter	Decreases diameter
Respiratory rate	Increases rate	Decreases rate
DIGESTIVE SYSTEM		
General level of activity	Decreases activity	Increases activity
Liver	Glycogen breakdown, glucose synthesis and release	Glycogen synthesis
SKELETAL MUSCLES		
	Increases force of contraction, glycogen breakdown	None (not innervated)
ADIPOSE TISSUE		
	Lipid breakdown, fatty acid release	None (not innervated)
URINARY SYSTEM		
Kidneys	Decreases urine production	Increases urine production
Urinary bladder	Constricts internal sphincter, relaxes urinary bladder	Tenses urinary bladder, relaxes internal sphincter to eliminate urine
REPRODUCTIVE SYSTEM		
	Increased glandular secretions; ejaculation in males	Erection of penis (males) or clitoris (females)

Reaction times are slowed, and reflexes—even some withdrawal reflexes—weaken or disappear. The precision of motor control decreases, so it takes longer to perform a given motor pattern than it did 20 years earlier.

For roughly 85 percent of the elderly population, these changes do not interfere with their abilities to function. But for as yet unknown reasons, some individuals become incapacitated by progressive CNS changes. These changes, which can include memory loss, an inability to recall new information, and emotional disturbances, are often lumped together as *dementia*.

Dementia is a decline in mental ability characterized by deficits in memory, spatial orientation, language, or personality.

The most common cause of dementia is *Alzheimer's disease* (see the Clinical Note on the next page).

CHECKPOINT

42. What is the major cause of age-related reduction, or shrinkage, of the brain?

See the blue Answers tab at the back of the book.

CLINICAL NOTE

Alzheimer's Disease

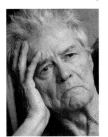

Alzheimer's disease is a progressive disorder characterized by the loss of higher cerebral functions. It is the most common cause of *dementia* in older people. Signs and symptoms may appear at 50–60 years of age or later, but the disease occasionally affects younger people. An estimated 5.2 million people in the United States have some form of the condition, including about 11 percent of those over age 65 years, and 38 percent over age 85 years. The disease causes approximately 100,000 deaths each year. It can also have devastating emotional effects on the patient's immediate family.

In its characteristic form, Alzheimer's disease produces a gradual deterioration of mental organization. The afflicted individual loses memories, verbal and reading skills, and emotional control. As memory losses continue to accumulate, problems become more severe. The affected person may forget relatives, a home address, or how to use the telephone. The loss of memory affects both intellectual and motor abilities. A patient with severe Alzheimer's disease has difficulty performing even the simplest motor tasks. There is no cure for Alzheimer's disease. A few medications and supplements slow its progress in many patients.

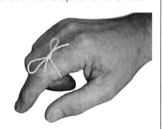

CLINICAL NOTE

Stroke

Stroke, formerly called a *cerebrovascular accident*, is a general term that describes injury or death of brain tissue. Stroke usually results from an interruption of blood supply to the affected area of the brain. The term *brain attack* is used because it compares the physiology of a stroke with that of a heart attack. Strokes are the third most common cause of death and the leading cause of disability.

A stroke results from any disease process that interrupts the blood flow to parts of the brain. The two general categories of stroke are ischemic and hemorrhagic. Ischemic strokes are due to blockage of a blood vessel that supplies a part of the brain. Hemorrhagic strokes occur due to rupture of a blood vessel that supplies a part of the brain (**Figure 8-46**). Approximately 80–85

percent of strokes are ischemic, whereas 15–20 percent are hemorrhagic.

Ischemic strokes can be divided into two general categories: thrombotic and embolic. In *thrombotic strokes* a clot forms at the site of the blockage. Often, the artery is narrowed or irregular due to atherosclerosis, which promotes clot formation. In embolic strokes, the blood clot forms elsewhere in the body, usually in the heart or great vessels, travels through the circulatory system, and ultimately lodges in a cerebral artery, which causes occlusion. Unlike thrombotic strokes, embolic strokes tend to occur in blood vessels that are relatively free of disease or narrowing.

Hemorrhagic strokes tend to occur in younger patients than do ischemic strokes. Most hemorrhagic strokes occur within the substance of the brain (intracerebral hemorrhage) (**Figure 8-47**). Some hemorrhagic strokes, however, will cause bleeding into the subarachnoid space (subarachnoid hemorrhage). In *subarachnoid hemorrhage*, the sudden release of blood under high pressure and the subsequent rise in intracranial pressure (ICP) causes direct cellular injury. Most subarachnoid hemorrhages are due to rupture of *berry aneurysms*. Berry aneurysms are sac-like dilations of blood vessels that supply a part of the brain. They are usually congenital and produce weakened areas of the blood vessel. The highest incidence of berry-aneurysm rupture or bleeding occurs in patients from 20 to 50 years of age.

The signs and symptoms of a stroke depend upon the part or parts of the brain affected. Blockage of one of the smaller cerebral vessels may cause minimal, if any, symptoms. Blockage of a larger cerebral vessel can cause catastrophic symptoms and even death. Blood supply to the brain is derived from two sources: the anterior and posterior circulation. The *anterior circulation* is supplied by the carotid arteries and provides blood to 80 percent of the brain. The *posterior circulation* receives blood from the vertebral arteries. Although the posterior circulation provides only 20 percent of the brain's blood, it supplies critical structures such as

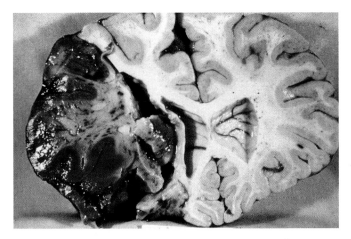

Figure 8-46 Postmortem Specimen That Illustrates Massive Hemorrhagic Stroke That Affects the Vast Majority of One Hemisphere of the Brain.

(Continued)

Figure 8-47 Hemorrhagic Stroke That Involves the Tissues that Adjoin the Lateral Ventricle (Periventricular Hemorrhage).

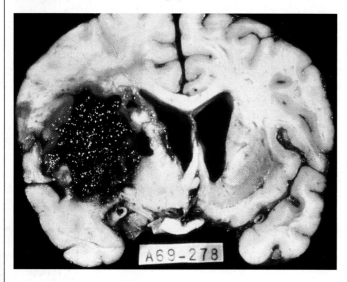

A69-278

8

the brain stem, which is essential for movement, sensation, and normal consciousness.

Because each hemisphere of the brain controls the opposite side of the body, weakness and sensory loss will be noted on the side of the body opposite the stroke. If the dominant hemisphere of the brain is affected, there may be a loss of the ability to speak

(*aphasia*). In right-handed patients and in up to 80 percent of left-handed patients, the left hemisphere is the dominant hemisphere.

Diagnosis of stroke is based on the history, physical examination, and computed tomography (CT). With CT, hemorrhagic strokes are readily identified. Ischemic strokes are more difficult to see in the acute phase. As time progresses, scar tissue replaces the parts of the brain affected, and ischemic lesions become more visible.

Treatment of strokes has changed significantly over the last decade. If treated promptly (usually within three hours), patients with ischemic strokes may be candidates for thrombolytic therapy. A thrombolytic agent, such as *tissue plasminogen activator*, can be administered and may dissolve the clot causing the ischemia. If blood flow can be restored to the affected parts of the brain in time, then the patient may not suffer any permanent injury. Because of this, the concept of "brain attack" has been promoted so that the public will recognize the signs and symptoms of stroke early and get the patient to an appropriate treatment facility.

Transient Ischemic Attacks

Some patients will develop stroke-like symptoms that spontaneously resolve. This is referred to as a *transient ischemic attack (TIA)* and is often a precursor to a full-blown stroke. In most cases of TIA, the symptoms resolve in a few hours, although some may last for 24 hours or more. The occurrence of TIAs prompts a detailed investigation to determine the cause.

CLINICAL NOTE

Neurologic Trauma

Although well protected by bony structures, the brain and spinal cord are susceptible to injury. Injuries are the leading cause of death in persons less than 45 years of age, with approximately half being due to head trauma. *Traumatic brain injury* can be devastating, and cause permanent disability. Young male adults are at greatest risk of neurological trauma, although children and the elderly are at increased risk due to underlying anatomical and physiological factors.

Neurological trauma is usually classified as penetrating or blunt. *Blunt trauma* is more common and results from motor vehicle collisions (MVCs), assaults, and sporting injuries. *Penetrating trauma* is most often due to gunshot or stab wounds. Neurological trauma can also be described as primary or secondary. In *primary injury*, neuronal damage occurs immediately at impact. In *secondary injury*, neuronal damage occurs from minutes to days after the event and results from indirect causes such as brain swelling, lack of oxygen, or inadequate perfusion.

Blunt Trauma

Blunt trauma can cause focal injuries or diffuse injuries, depending upon the location of the force. *Focal injuries* occur at a specific location in the brain, whereas *diffuse injuries* are generalized. Head trauma can cause injury immediately under the point of impact (*coup injury*) or on the opposite side of the brain (*contrecoup*

injury). Contrecoup injury results from the forceful movement of the brain away from the impact, which causes it to impact the interior of the skull opposite the injury. Contrecoup injuries can occur with trauma to the front or back of the head, as well as on either side (**Figure 8-48**).

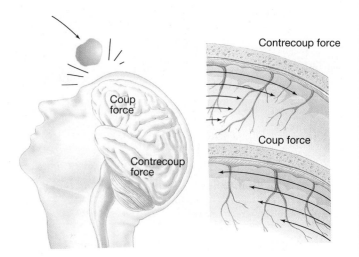

Figure 8-48 Coup and Contrecoup Injuries after Blunt Trauma to the Head.

Diffuse Injuries

During head impact, a shearing, tearing, or stretching force is applied to the nerve fibers and causes damage to the axons. Referred to as *diffuse axonal injury (DAI)*, the damage can range from mild to severe. A concussion is a mild to moderate form of DAI and the most common result of blunt head trauma. In a concussion, there is neuronal dysfunction without underlying anatomical damage. This is characterized by a transient episode of confusion, disorientation, or event amnesia, followed by a rapid return to normal. A brief loss of consciousness can occur. Usually there is no permanent neurological impairment.

Bruising of brain tissue following injury causes moderate DAI. If the cerebral cortex or the reticular activating system is affected, the patient may be rendered unconscious. This injury is more severe than a mild concussion and can cause both short- and long-term signs and symptoms. These include immediate unconsciousness, followed by persistent confusion, inability to concentrate, disorientation, and amnesia.

Severe DAI is caused by mechanical disruption of many axons in both cerebral hemispheres with extension into the brain stem. This injury usually results in coma and causes an increase in intracranial pressure (ICP). Many patients do not survive severe DAI, and those who do survive usually have some degree of permanent neurological impairment.

Focal Injuries

Focal injuries occur at a specific location in the brain and include contusions and intracranial hemorrhages. A *cerebral contusion* is due to capillary bleeding into the substance of the brain at the location of the impact. It can cause confusion and other types of neurological deficits depending upon the location involved. For example, injury to the frontal lobe can cause personality changes.

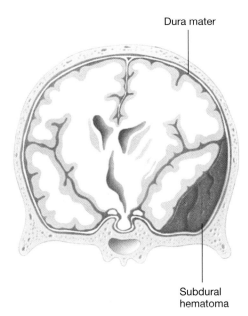

Dura mater

Subdural hematoma

Figure 8-49 Epidural Hematoma. The bleeding usually results from arterial bleeding and can develop rapidly.

Figure 8-50 Subdural Hematoma. The bleeding is usually venous and develops much slower than in epidural hematomas.

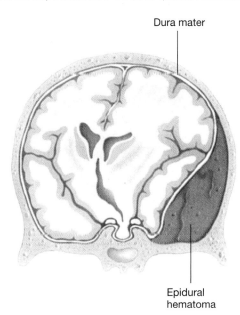

Dura mater

Epidural hematoma

Figure 8-50 Subdural Hematoma. The bleeding is usually venous and develops much slower than in epidural hematomas.

Blunt trauma can cause bleeding at several locations within the brain. Bleeding between the dura mater and the interior surface of the skull is an *epidural hematoma* (**Figure 8-49**). This usually is caused by damage to the middle meningeal arteries from a skull fracture. Because the bleeding is arterial, epidural hematomas develop quickly and can cause herniation of the brain stem if not treated expeditiously. The classic history of an epidural hematoma is for the patient to experience an immediate loss of consciousness after blunt head trauma. The patient then awakens and has a *lucent period* before again falling unconscious as the hematoma expands. However, the classic syndrome occurs in only about 20 percent of patients with epidural hematoma. Treatment is neurosurgical evacuation of the hematoma as soon as possible. Rarely, when neurosurgical care is unavailable, emergency physicians may be required to place burr holes in the skull above the hematoma to prevent brain stem herniation.

Bleeding beneath the dura mater and within the subarachnoid space is a *subdural hematoma*. This type of bleeding occurs very slowly and is usually due to rupture of venous vessels, such as the bridging veins of the dural sinus. Subdural hematoma usually causes few initial signs and symptoms unless the hematoma is large (**Figure 8-50**). Treatment of subdural hematoma is based on its severity. Small hematomas may be monitored with the blood being resorbed over a few days. Large hematomas may require surgical decompression. Associated brain injury is common.

Intracerebral hemorrhage (ICH) results from a ruptured blood vessel within the substance of the brain. Blood loss is usually minimal but particularly damaging. It causes inflammation and swelling of the brain. The signs and symptoms of ICH, which are similar to those of a stroke, depend upon the portion of the brain involved. Treatment is directed at controlling ICP in order to minimize secondary injury.

(Continued)

8

Penetrating Trauma

Penetrating trauma to the brain or spinal cord is potentially devastating. Penetrating injuries are usually due to gunshots or stab wounds or to sharp objects encountered in an MVC. Often, as the penetrating object enters the head, it fractures the skull and carries bone fragments into the substance of the brain. Penetrating injuries can also cause bleeding if a blood vessel is struck during entry. As the brain is exposed to the environment, the possibility of infection exists.

The velocity and energy associated with the penetrating object are major factors in the type of injury encountered. Stab wounds are generally low-velocity and low-energy. Their damage is limited primarily to the point of entry. Small-caliber bullets may not have enough energy to both enter and exit the skull. Instead, after the bullet enters the skull, it strikes the interior surface of the skull on the opposite side and ricochets throughout the brain, which often causes significant tissue damage. High-energy, large-caliber bullets usually have enough energy to penetrate and exit the skull. Because of the tremendous energy associated with these missiles, damage to the brain is significant, and the exit wound destroys a significant part of the skull (**Figure 8-51**). Increased ICP is usually not a concern in penetrating trauma due to the open wound. Penetrating injuries are often fatal. Those who survive often have serious permanent neurological damage.

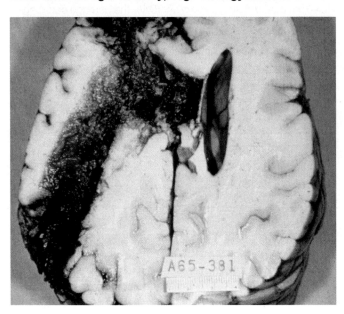

Figure 8-51 Postmortem Specimen that Shows Massive Missile Tract Through the Substance of the Brain after a High-Velocity, High-Energy Gunshot.

8-13 The nervous system is closely integrated with other body systems

Learning Objective Give examples of interactions between the nervous system and other body systems.

The nervous system monitors all other systems and issues commands that adjust their activities.

"Build Your Knowledge: How the NERVOUS SYSTEM integrates with the other body systems presented so far" on p. 297 reviews the major functional relationships between it and the integumentary, skeletal, and muscular systems.

CHECKPOINT

43. Identify the relationships between the nervous system and the other body systems studied so far.

See the blue Answers tab at the back of the book.

RELATED CLINICAL TERMS

amyotrophic lateral sclerosis (ALS): A progressive, degenerative disorder affecting motor neurons of the spinal cord, brain stem, and cerebral hemispheres; commonly known as Lou Gehrig's disease.

cerebrovascular accident (CVA), or *stroke:* A condition in which the blood supply to a portion of the brain is blocked off.

diphtheria (dif-THĒ-rē-uh): A disease that results from a bacterial infection of the respiratory tract. Among other effects, the bacterial toxins damage Schwann cells and cause PNS demyelination.

Hansen's disease (*leprosy***):** A bacterial infection that begins in sensory nerves of the skin and gradually progresses to a motor paralysis of the same regions.

Huntington's disease: An inherited disease marked by a progressive deterioration of mental abilities and by motor disturbances.

meningitis: Inflammation of the meninges involving the spinal cord (*spinal meningitis*) and/or brain (*cerebral meningitis*). It is generally caused by bacterial or viral pathogens.

myelography: A diagnostic procedure in which a radiopaque dye is introduced into the cerebrospinal fluid to obtain an X-ray image of the spinal cord and cauda equina.

neurology: The branch of medicine that deals with the study of the nervous system and its disorders.

neurotoxin: A compound that disrupts normal nervous system function by interfering with the generation or propagation of action potentials. Examples include *tetrodotoxin (TTX), saxitoxin (STX), paralytic shellfish poisoning (PSP),* and *ciguatoxin (CTX).*

paresthesia: An abnormal tingling sensation, usually described as "pins and needles," that accompanies the return of sensation after a temporary palsy.

sciatica (sī-AT-i-kuh): The painful result of compression of the roots of the sciatic nerve.

shingles: A condition caused by the infection of neurons in dorsal root ganglia by the varicella-zoster virus. The primary symptom is a painful rash along the sensory distribution of the affected spinal nerves.

spinal shock: A period of depressed sensory and motor function following any severe injury to the spinal cord.

Build Your Knowledge

How the NERVOUS SYSTEM integrates with the other body systems presented so far

Integumentary System

- The Integumentary System provides sensations of touch, pressure, pain, vibration, and temperature; hair provides some protection and insulation for skull and brain; protects peripheral nerves

- The nervous system controls the contraction of arrector pili muscles and the secretion of sweat glands

Nervous System

The Nervous System is your most complex organ system. It
- monitors the body's internal and external environments
- integrates sensory information
- directs immediate responses to stimuli by coordinating voluntary and involuntary responses of many other organ systems

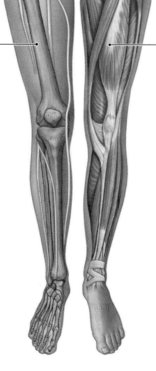

Skeletal System

- The skeletal system provides calcium for neural function and protects the brain and spinal cord

- The nervous system affects bone thickening and maintenance by controlling muscle contractions

Muscular System

- The muscular system expresses emotional states with facial muscles; intrinsic laryngeal muscles permit communication; muscle spindles provide proprioceptive sensations

- The nervous system controls voluntary and involuntary skeletal muscle contractions

8

8 Chapter Review

Summary Outline

An Introduction to the Nervous System *p. 270*

1. Two organ systems—the nervous and endocrine systems—coordinate organ system activity. The nervous system provides swift but brief responses to stimuli. The endocrine system adjusts metabolic operations and directs long-term changes.

8-1 The nervous system has anatomical and functional divisions *p. 270*

2. The **nervous system** includes all the neural tissue in the body. Its major anatomical divisions include the **central nervous system (CNS)** (the brain and spinal cord) and the **peripheral nervous system (PNS)** (all the neural tissue outside the CNS).

3. Functionally, the PNS can be divided into an **afferent division**, which brings sensory information to the CNS, and an **efferent division**, which carries motor commands to muscles and glands. The efferent division includes the **somatic nervous system (SNS)** (voluntary control over skeletal muscle contractions) and the **autonomic nervous system (ANS)** (automatic, involuntary regulation of smooth muscle, cardiac muscle, and glandular activity) *(Figure 8-1)*.

8-2 Neurons are specialized for intercellular communication and are supported by cells called neuroglia *p. 271*

4. There are two types of cells in neural tissue: **neurons**, which are responsible for information transfer and processing, and **neuroglia**, or *glial cells*, which regulate the environment around neurons, provide a supporting framework, and act as phagocytes.

5. **Sensory neurons** form the afferent division of the PNS and deliver information to the CNS. **Motor neurons** stimulate or modify the activity of a peripheral tissue, organ, or organ system. **Interneurons (association neurons)** may be located between sensory and motor neurons; they analyze sensory inputs and coordinate motor outputs.

6. A typical neuron has a cell body, an **axon**, several branching **dendrites**, and axon terminals *(Figure 8-2)*.

7. Neurons may be described as **unipolar, bipolar,** or **multipolar** *(Figure 8-3)*.

8. The four types of neuroglia in the CNS are (1) **astrocytes**, which are the largest and most numerous and maintain the blood–brain barrier; (2) **oligodendrocytes**, which are responsible for the **myelination** of CNS axons; (3) **microglia**, phagocytic cells derived from white blood cells; and (4) **ependymal cells**, with functions related to the *cerebrospinal fluid* (CSF) *(Figure 8-4)*.

9. Nerve cell bodies in the PNS are clustered into **ganglia** (singular: *ganglion*). Their axons are covered by myelin wrappings of **Schwann cells** *(Figure 8-5)*.

10. In the CNS, a collection of neuron cell bodies that share a particular function is called a **center**. A center with a discrete anatomical boundary is called a **nucleus**. Areas of the brain surface are covered by a thick layer of gray matter called the **neural cortex**. The white matter of the CNS contains bundles of axons, or **tracts**, that share common origins, destinations, and functions. Tracts in the spinal cord form larger groups, called *columns (Figure 8-6)*.

11. **Sensory** *(ascending)* **pathways** carry information from peripheral sensory receptors to processing centers in the brain. **Motor** *(descending)* **pathways** extend from CNS centers concerned with motor control to the associated skeletal muscles *(Figure 8-6)*.

8-3 In neurons, a change in the plasma membrane's electrical potential may result in an action potential (nerve impulse) *p. 277*

12. The **resting membrane potential** (or **resting potential**) of an undisturbed nerve cell results from a balance between the rates of sodium ion gain and potassium ion loss achieved by the sodium–potassium exchange pump. Any stimulus that affects this balance will alter the resting potential of the cell *(Figure 8-7)*.

13. An **action potential** appears when the membrane depolarizes to a level known as the **threshold**. The steps involved include depolarization to threshold, the opening of voltage-gated sodium channels and membrane depolarization, the closing of voltage-gated sodium channels and opening of voltage-gated potassium channels, and the return to normal permeability *(Spotlight Figure 8-8)*.

14. In **continuous propagation**, an action potential spreads along the entire excitable membrane surface in a series of small steps. During **saltatory propagation**, the action potential appears to leap from node to node, skipping the intervening myelinated membrane surface *(Spotlight Figure 8-9)*.

8-4 At synapses, communication takes place among neurons or between neurons and other cells *p. 284*

15. A **synapse** is a site where a neuron communicates with another cell through the release of chemicals called **neurotransmitters**. A synapse where neurons communicate with other cell types is a **neuroeffector junction**.

16. Neural communication moves from the **presynaptic neuron** to the **postsynaptic neuron** across the **synaptic cleft** *(Figure 8-10)*.

17. **Cholinergic synapses** release the neurotransmitter **acetylcholine (ACh)**. ACh is broken down in the synaptic cleft by the enzyme **acetylcholinesterase (AChE)** *(Figure 8-11)*.

18. The roughly 20 billion interneurons are organized into **neuronal pools** (groups of interconnected neurons with specific functions). **Divergence** is the spread of information from one neuron to several neurons or from one neuronal pool to several pools. In **convergence**, several neurons synapse on the same postsynaptic neuron *(Figure 8-12)*.

8-5 The brain and spinal cord are surrounded by three layers of membranes called the meninges *p. 287*

19. The CNS is made up of the *spinal cord* and *brain*.

20. Special covering membranes, the **meninges**, protect and support the spinal cord and the delicate brain. The *cranial meninges* (dura mater, arachnoid, and pia mater) are continuous with those of the spinal cord, the *spinal meninges* *(Figure 8-13)*.

21. The **dura mater** covers the brain and spinal cord. The **epidural space** separates the spinal dura mater from the walls of the vertebral canal. The subarachnoid space of the arachnoid layer contains **cerebrospinal fluid** (the CSF), which acts as a shock absorber and a diffusion medium for dissolved gases, nutrients, chemical messengers, and waste products. The **pia mater** is bound to the underlying neural tissue.

8-6 The spinal cord contains gray matter surrounded by white matter and connects to 31 pairs of spinal nerves *p. 289*

22. In addition to relaying information to and from the brain, the spinal cord integrates and processes information on its own.

23. The spinal cord has 31 segments, each associated with a pair of **dorsal root ganglia** and their **dorsal roots**, and a pair of **ventral roots** *(Figures 8-15; 8-17b)*.

24. The white matter contains myelinated and unmyelinated axons; the gray matter contains cell bodies of neurons and glial cells. The projections of gray matter toward the outer surface of the spinal cord are called **horns** *(Figure 8-17a)*.

8-7 The brain has several principal structures, each with specific functions *p. 296*

25. There are six regions in the adult brain: cerebrum, diencephalon, midbrain, pons, medulla oblongata, and cerebellum *(Figure 8-21)*.

26. The central passageway of the brain expands to form four chambers called **ventricles**. Cerebrospinal fluid (CSF) continuously circulates from the ventricles and central canal of the spinal cord into the subarachnoid space of the meninges that surround the CNS *(Figures 8-22; 8-23)*.

27. Conscious thought, intellectual functions, memory, and complex involuntary motor patterns originate in the **cerebrum** *(Figure 8-21)*.

28. The cortical surface of the cerebrum contains **gyri** (elevated ridges) separated by **sulci** (shallow depressions) or deeper grooves (**fissures**). The **longitudinal fissure** separates the two **cerebral hemispheres**. The **central sulcus** marks the boundary between the **frontal lobe** and the **parietal lobe**. Other sulci form the boundaries of the **temporal lobe** and the **occipital lobe** *(Figures 8-21; 8-25)*.

29. Each cerebral hemisphere receives sensory information and generates motor commands that concern the opposite side of the body. The **primary motor cortex** of the **precentral gyrus** directs voluntary movements. The **primary sensory cortex** of the **postcentral gyrus** receives somatic sensory information from touch, pressure, pain, and temperature receptors. **Association areas**, such as the **visual association area** and **premotor cortex** (motor association area), control our ability to understand sensory information and coordinate a motor response *(Figure 8-25)*.

30. The left hemisphere is usually the *categorical hemisphere*, which contains the general interpretive and speech centers and is responsible for language-based skills. The right hemisphere, or *representational hemisphere*, is concerned with spatial relationships and analyses *(Figure 8-26)*.

31. An **electroencephalogram (EEG)** is a printed record of **brain waves** *(Figure 8-27)*.

32. The **basal nuclei** lie within the central white matter and aid in the coordination of learned movement patterns and other somatic motor activities *(Figure 8-28)*.

33. The **limbic system** is a functional grouping rather than an anatomical one. Among other structures, it includes the *hippocampus*, which is involved in memory and learning, and the *mammillary bodies*, which control reflex movements associated with eating. The functions of the limbic system involve establishing emotional states, linking the conscious, intellectual functions of the cerebral cortex with the unconscious and autonomic functions of the brain stem, and aiding long-term memory storage and retrieval *(Figure 8-29)*.

34. The **diencephalon** provides the switching and relay centers needed to integrate the conscious and unconscious sensory and motor pathways. It is made up of the **epithalamus**, which contains the *pineal gland* and *choroid plexus* (a vascular network that produces cerebrospinal fluid), the **thalamus**, and the **hypothalamus** *(Figures 8-21c; 8-30).*

35. The thalamus is the final relay point for ascending sensory information. Only a small portion of the arriving sensory information is passed to the cerebral cortex; the rest is relayed to the basal nuclei and centers in the brain stem *(Figures 8-21c; 8-30).*

36. The hypothalamus contains important control and integrative centers. It can produce emotions and behavioral drives, coordinate activities of the nervous and endocrine systems, secrete hormones, coordinate voluntary and autonomic functions, and regulate body temperature.

37. Three regions make up the **brain stem**. (1) The **midbrain** processes visual and auditory information and generates involuntary somatic motor responses, and contains the *reticular activating system (RAS)*, which directly affects the activity of the cerebral cortex. (2) The **pons** connects the cerebellum to the brain stem and is involved with somatic and visceral motor control. (3) The spinal cord connects to the brain at the **medulla oblongata**, which relays sensory information and regulates autonomic functions *(Figures 8-21c; 8-30).*

38. The **cerebellum** oversees the body's postural muscles and programs and fine-tunes voluntary and involuntary movements. The **cerebellar peduncles** are tracts linking the cerebellum with the brain stem, cerebrum, and spinal cord *(Figures 8-21; 8-30).*

39. The medulla oblongata connects the brain to the spinal cord. Its nuclei relay information from the spinal cord and brain stem to the cerebral cortex. Its reflex centers, including the **cardiovascular center** and the **respiratory rhythmicity centers**, control or adjust the activities of one or more peripheral systems *(Figure 8-30).*

8-8 The PNS connects the CNS with the body's external and internal environments *p. 309*

40. The **peripheral nervous system (PNS)** links the central nervous system (CNS) with the rest of the body; all sensory information and motor commands are carried by axons of the PNS. The sensory and motor axons are bundled together into **peripheral nerves,** or nerves, and clusters of cell bodies, or *ganglia.*

41. The PNS includes cranial nerves and spinal nerves.

42. There are 12 pairs of **cranial nerves**, which connect to the brain, not to the spinal cord *(Figure 8-31).*

43. The **olfactory nerves (N I)** carry sensory information for the sense of smell.

44. The **optic nerves (N II)** carry visual information from special sensory receptors in the eyes.

45. The **oculomotor nerves (N III)** are the primary sources of innervation for four of the six muscles that move the eyeball.

46. The **trochlear nerves (N IV)**, the smallest cranial nerves, innervate the superior oblique muscles of the eyes.

47. The **trigeminal nerves (N V)**, the largest cranial nerves, are mixed nerves with ophthalmic, maxillary, and mandibular branches.

48. The **abducens nerves (N VI)** innervate the sixth extrinsic eye muscle, the lateral rectus.

49. The **facial nerves (N VII)** are mixed nerves that control muscles of the scalp and face. They provide pressure sensations over the face and receive taste information from the tongue.

50. The **vestibulocochlear nerves (N VIII)** contain the vestibular nerves, which monitor sensations of balance, position, and movement, and the cochlear nerves, which monitor hearing receptors.

51. The **glossopharyngeal nerves (N IX)** are mixed nerves that innervate the tongue and pharynx and control swallowing.

52. The **vagus nerves (N X)** are mixed nerves that are vital to the autonomic control of visceral function and have a variety of motor components.

53. The **accessory nerves (N XI)** have an internal branch, which innervates voluntary swallowing muscles of the soft palate and pharynx, and an external branch, which controls muscles associated with the pectoral girdles.

54. The **hypoglossal nerves (N XII)** provide voluntary control over tongue movements.

55. There are 31 pairs of **spinal nerves**: 8 cervical, 12 thoracic, 5 lumbar, 5 sacral, and 1 coccygeal. Each pair monitors a region of the body surface known as a **dermatome** *(Figures 8-32; 8-33).*

56. A **nerve plexus** is a complex, interwoven network of nerves. The four large plexuses are the **cervical plexus**, the **brachial plexus**, the **lumbar plexus**, and the **sacral plexus**. The latter two can be united into a *lumbosacral plexus (Figure 8-32).*

8-9 Reflexes are rapid, automatic responses to stimuli *p. 314*

57. A **reflex** is an automatic involuntary motor response to a specific stimulus.

58. A **reflex arc** is the "wiring" of a single reflex. Five steps are involved in the action of a reflex arc: (1) arrival of a stimulus and activation of a receptor, (2) activation of a

sensory neuron, (3) information processing, (4) activation of a motor neuron, and (5) response by an effector *(Figure 8-34)*.

59. A **monosynaptic reflex** is the simplest reflex arc, in which a sensory neuron synapses directly on a motor neuron that acts as the processing center. A **stretch reflex** is a monosynaptic reflex that automatically regulates skeletal muscle length and muscle tone. The sensory receptors involved are **muscle spindles** *(Figure 8-35)*.

60. **Polysynaptic reflexes**, which have at least one interneuron between the sensory afferent neuron and the motor efferent neuron, have a longer delay between stimulus and response than does a monosynaptic synapse. Polysynaptic reflexes can also produce more complex responses. A **flexor reflex** is a withdrawal reflex affecting the muscles of a limb *(Figure 8-36)*.

61. The brain can facilitate or inhibit reflex motor patterns based in the spinal cord.

8-10 Separate pathways carry sensory information and motor commands *p. 318*

62. The essential communication between the CNS and PNS occurs over pathways that relay sensory information and motor commands *(Table 8-2)*.

63. A **sensation** arrives in the form of an action potential in an afferent fiber. The **posterior column pathway** carries fine touch, pressure, vibration, and proprioceptive sensations. The axons ascend within this pathway and synapse with neurons in the medulla oblongata. These axons then cross over and travel on to the thalamus. The thalamus sorts the sensations according to the region of the body involved and sends them to specific regions of the primary sensory cortex *(Figure 8-39; Table 8-2)*.

64. The **corticospinal pathway** provides conscious skeletal muscle control. The **medial** and **lateral pathways** generally exert subconscious control over skeletal muscles *(Figure 8-40; Table 8-2)*.

8-11 The autonomic nervous system, composed of the sympathetic and parasympathetic divisions, is involved in the unconscious regulation of body functions *p. 322*

65. The autonomic nervous system (ANS) coordinates cardiovascular, respiratory, digestive, excretory, and reproductive functions.

66. **Preganglionic neurons** in the CNS send axons to synapse on **ganglionic neurons** in **autonomic ganglia** outside the CNS. The axons of the ganglionic neurons (postganglionic fibers) innervate cardiac muscle, smooth muscles, glands, and, in some cases, fat cells *(Figure 8-41b)*.

67. Preganglionic fibers from the thoracic and lumbar segments form the **sympathetic division** ("fight or flight" system) of the ANS. Preganglionic fibers leaving the brain and sacral segments form the **parasympathetic division** ("rest and repose" or "rest and digest" system).

68. The sympathetic division consists of preganglionic neurons between segments T_1 and L_2, ganglionic neurons in ganglia near the vertebral column, and specialized neurons in the adrenal gland. Sympathetic ganglia are paired **sympathetic chain ganglia** or unpaired **collateral ganglia** *(Figure 8-42)*.

69. Preganglionic fibers entering the adrenal glands synapse within the **adrenal medullae**. During sympathetic activation, these endocrine organs secrete epinephrine (E) and norepinephrine (NE) into the bloodstream.

70. In a crisis, the entire sympathetic division responds, producing increased alertness, a feeling of energy, increased cardiovascular and respiratory activity, and elevation in muscle tone.

71. The parasympathetic division includes preganglionic neurons in the brain stem and sacral segments of the spinal cord, and ganglionic neurons in peripheral ganglia located within or next to target organs. Preganglionic fibers leaving the sacral segments form **pelvic nerves** *(Figure 8-44)*.

72. The effects produced by the parasympathetic division center on relaxation, food processing, and energy absorption; they are usually brief and restricted to specific sites.

73. The sympathetic division has widespread effects, reaching visceral and somatic structures throughout the body. The parasympathetic division innervates only visceral structures either serviced by cranial nerves or lying within the abdominopelvic cavity. Organs with **dual innervation** receive instructions from both divisions *(Table 8-5)*.

8-12 Aging produces various structural and functional changes in the nervous system *p. 329*

74. Age-related changes in the nervous system include a reduction of brain size and weight, a reduction in the number of neurons, decreased blood flow to the brain, changes in synaptic organization of the brain, and intracellular and extracellular changes in CNS. For roughly 85 percent of the elderly population, these changes do not interfere with their abilities to function.

8-13 The nervous system is closely integrated with other body systems *p. 334*

75. The nervous system monitors all other body systems and issues commands that adjust their activities.

Review Questions

See the blue Answers tab at the back of the book.

Level 1 Reviewing Facts and Terms

Match each item in column A with the most closely related item in column B. Place letters for answers in the spaces provided.

COLUMN A

_____ **1.** Neuroglia
_____ **2.** Autonomic nervous system
_____ **3.** Sensory neurons
_____ **4.** Dual innervation
_____ **5.** Ganglia
_____ **6.** Oligodendrocytes
_____ **7.** Ascending tracts
_____ **8.** Descending tracts
_____ **9.** Saltatory propagation
_____ **10.** Continuous propagation
_____ **11.** Dura mater
_____ **12.** Monosynaptic reflex
_____ **13.** Sympathetic division
_____ **14.** Cerebellum
_____ **15.** Somatic nervous system
_____ **16.** Hypothalamus
_____ **17.** Medulla oblongata
_____ **18.** Choroid plexus
_____ **19.** Parasympathetic division
_____ **20.** Motor neurons

COLUMN B

a. Cover CNS axons with myelin
b. Carry sensory information to the brain
c. Occurs along unmyelinated axons
d. Outermost covering of brain and spinal cord
e. Production of CSF
f. Supporting cells
g. Controls smooth and cardiac muscle, glands, and fat cells
h. Occurs along myelinated axons
i. Link between nervous and endocrine systems
j. Carry motor commands to spinal cord
k. Efferent division of the PNS
l. Controls contractions of skeletal muscles
m. Masses of neuron cell bodies
n. Connects the brain to the spinal cord
o. Stretch reflex
p. Afferent division of the PNS
q. Maintains muscle tone and posture
r. "Rest and digest" division
s. Opposing effects
t. "Fight or flight" division

21. Label the structures in the following diagram of a neuron.

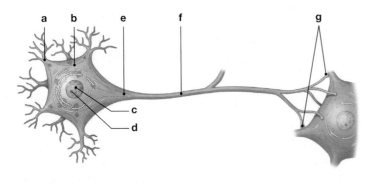

(a) _____
(b) _____
(c) _____
(d) _____
(e) _____
(f) _____
(g) _____

22. Regulation by the nervous system provides
   (a) relatively slow but long-lasting responses to stimuli.
   (b) swift, long-lasting responses to stimuli.
   (c) swift but brief responses to stimuli.
   (d) relatively slow, short-lived responses to stimuli.

23. All the motor neurons that control skeletal muscles are
   (a) multipolar neurons.
   (b) myelinated bipolar neurons.
   (c) unipolar, unmyelinated sensory neurons.
   (d) proprioceptors.

24. Depolarization of a neuron plasma membrane will shift the membrane potential toward
   (a) 0 mV.
   (b) −70 mV.
   (c) −90 mV.
   (d) a, b, and c are correct.

25. Identify the six principal regions of the brain in the following diagram.

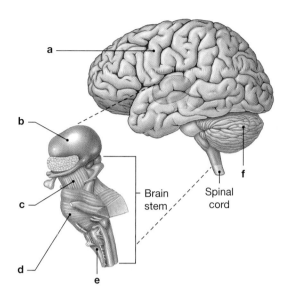

(a) _____   (b) _____

(c) _____   (d) _____

(e) _____   (f) _____

26. The structural and functional link between the cerebral hemispheres and the components of the brain stem is the
   (a) neural cortex.
   (b) medulla oblongata.
   (c) midbrain.
   (d) diencephalon.

27. The ventricles in the brain are filled with
   (a) blood.
   (b) cerebrospinal fluid.
   (c) air.
   (d) neural tissue.

28. Reading, writing, and speaking are dependent on processing in the
   (a) right cerebral hemisphere.
   (b) left cerebral hemisphere.
   (c) prefrontal cortex.
   (d) postcentral gyrus.

29. Establishment of emotional states and related behavioral drives are functions of the
   (a) limbic system.
   (b) pineal gland.
   (c) mammillary bodies.
   (d) thalamus.

30. The final relay point for ascending sensory information that will be projected to the primary sensory cortex is the
   (a) hypothalamus.
   (b) thalamus.
   (c) spinal cord.
   (d) medulla oblongata.

31. Spinal nerves are called mixed nerves because they
   (a) are associated with a pair of dorsal root ganglia.
   (b) exit at intervertebral foramina.
   (c) contain sensory and motor fibers.
   (d) are associated with a pair of dorsal and ventral roots.

32. There is always a synapse between the CNS and the peripheral effector in
   (a) the ANS.
   (b) the SNS.
   (c) a reflex arc.
   (d) a, b, and c are correct.

33. Approximately 75 percent of parasympathetic outflow is provided by the
   (a) pelvic nerves.
   (b) sciatic nerve.
   (c) glossopharyngeal nerves.
   (d) vagus nerve.

34. State the all-or-none principle of action potentials.

35. Using the mnemonic device "Oh, Once One Takes The Anatomy Final, Very Good Vacations Are Heavenly," list the 12 pairs of cranial nerves.

36. How does the emergence of sympathetic preganglionic fibers from the spinal cord differ from the emergence of parasympathetic preganglionic fibers?

Level 2 Reviewing Concepts

37. A graded potential
   (a) decreases with distance from the point of stimulation.
   (b) spreads passively because of local currents.
   (c) may involve either depolarization or hyperpolarization.
   (d) a, b, and c are correct.

38. The loss of positive ions from the interior of a neuron produces
   (a) depolarization.
   (b) threshold.
   (c) hyperpolarization.
   (d) an action potential.

39. Which major part of the brain is associated with respiratory and cardiac activity?

40. Why is response time in a monosynaptic reflex much faster than response time in a polysynaptic reflex?

41. Compare the general effects of the sympathetic and parasympathetic divisions of the ANS on mental alertness, metabolic rate, digestive/urinary function, use of energy reserves, respiratory rate, heart rate/blood pressure, and sweat gland activity.

Level 3 Critical Thinking and Clinical Applications

42. If neurons in the central nervous system lack centrioles and are unable to divide, how can a person develop brain cancer?

43. A police officer has just stopped Bill on suspicion of driving while intoxicated. The officer asks Bill to walk the yellow line on the road and then asks him to place the tip of his index finger on the tip of his nose. Which part of the brain is being tested by these activities? How would these activities indicate Bill's level of sobriety?

44. In some severe cases of stomach ulcers, the branches of the vagus nerve (N X) that lead to the stomach are surgically severed. How might this procedure control the ulcers?

45. Improper use of crutches can produce a condition known as crutch paralysis, which is characterized by a lack of response by the extensor muscles of the arm and a condition known as wrist drop. Which nerve is involved?

46. While playing football, Ramon is tackled hard and suffers an injury to his left leg. As he tries to get up, he finds that he cannot flex his left hip or extend the knee. Which nerve is damaged, and how would this damage affect sensory perception in his left leg?

8

9

The General and Special Senses

Learning Objectives

These objectives tell you what you should be able to do after completing the chapter. They correspond by number to this chapter's sections.

9-1 Explain how the organization of receptors for the general senses and the special senses affects their sensitivity.

9-2 Identify the receptors for the general senses, and describe how they function.

9-3 Describe the sensory organs of smell, and discuss the processes involved in olfaction.

9-4 Describe the sensory organs of taste, and discuss the processes involved in gustation.

9-5 Identify the internal and accessory structures of the eye, and explain their functions.

9-6 Explain how we form visual images and distinguish colors, and discuss how the central nervous system processes visual information.

9-7 Describe the parts of the external, middle, and internal ear, and the receptors they contain, and discuss the processes involved in the senses of equilibrium and hearing.

9-8 Describe the effects of aging on smell, taste, vision, equilibrium, and hearing.

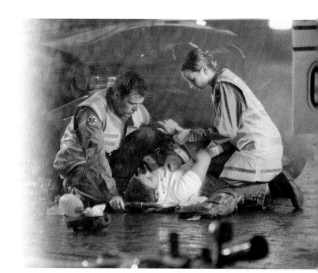

Clinical Notes
Cataracts, p. 361
Visual Acuity, p. 364
Night Blindness, p. 367
Hearing Deficits, p. 378

Spotlight
Refractive Problems, p. 363

An Introduction to General and Special Senses

Our knowledge of the world around us is limited to those characteristics that stimulate our sensory receptors. We may not realize it, but our picture of the environment is incomplete. Colors we cannot see guide insects to flowers. Sounds and smells we cannot detect provide important information to dolphins, dogs, and cats about their surroundings. Moreover, our senses are sometimes deceptive. In cases of phantom limb pain, for example, a person "feels" pain in a missing limb. During an epileptic seizure, a person may experience sights, sounds, or smells that have no physical basis. In this chapter, we discuss the "general senses" that provide information about the body and its environment, and the "special senses" of smell, taste, sight, equilibrium (balance), and hearing.

Build Your Knowledge

What we perceive also varies with the state of our nervous system. Recall that the sympathetic nervous system is often called the "fight or flight" system (as you saw in **Chapter 8: The Nervous System**). During sympathetic activation, you experience an increased state of alertness. In other words, you have a heightened awareness of sensory information. ⊃ **p. 289**

9-1 Sensory receptors connect our internal and external environments with the nervous system

Learning Objective Explain how the organization of receptors for the general senses and the special senses affects their sensitivity.

All sensory information is picked up by *sensory receptors*. **Sensory receptors** are specialized cells or cell processes (extensions) that monitor conditions inside or outside the body.

The simplest receptors are the dendrites (processes) of sensory neurons. The branching tips of these dendrites are called **free nerve endings**. Free nerve endings extend through a tissue the way grass roots extend into the soil. They are sensitive to many types of stimuli. As a result, free nerve endings provide little receptor specificity. For example, a given free nerve ending in the skin may provide the sensation of pain in response to chemicals, pressure, heat, or a cut.

Other receptors are sensitive to one kind of stimulus. For example, a touch receptor is very sensitive to pressure but insensitive to chemical stimuli. A taste receptor is sensitive to dissolved chemicals but insensitive to pressure. The most complex receptors, such as the visual receptors of the eye, are protected by accessory cells and layers of connective tissue. These cells are seldom exposed to any stimulus *except* light and so provide very specific information.

The area monitored by a single receptor cell is its *receptive field* (**Figure 9-1**). Whenever a sufficiently strong stimulus arrives in the receptive field, the CNS receives the information "stimulus arriving at receptor X." The larger the receptive field, the poorer is your ability to localize a stimulus. A touch receptor on the general body surface, for example, may have a receptive field of 7 cm (2.75 in.) in diameter. As a result, you can describe a light touch there affecting only a general area, not an exact spot. On your tongue or fingertips, the receptive fields are less than a millimeter in diameter. In these areas, you can be very precise about the location of a stimulus.

All sensory information arrives at the CNS in the form of action potentials in a sensory (afferent) fiber. In general, the

Figure 9-1 Receptors and Receptive Fields. Each receptor cell monitors a specific area known as the receptive field.

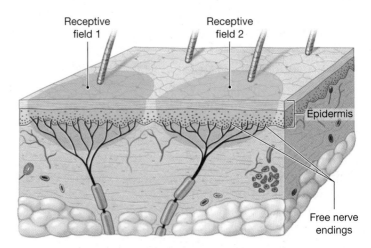

stronger the stimulus, the higher the frequency of action potentials. The arriving information is called a **sensation**.

When sensory information arrives at the CNS, it is routed according to the location and nature of the stimulus. For example, touch, pressure, pain, temperature, and taste sensations arrive at the primary sensory cortex. Information from visual, auditory, and olfactory receptors reaches the visual, auditory, and olfactory regions of the cortex, respectively. A **perception** is the conscious awareness of a sensation.

The CNS interprets the nature of sensory information entirely on the basis of the area of the brain stimulated. The CNS cannot tell the difference between a "true" sensation and a "false" one. For instance, when rubbing your eyes, you may "see" flashes of light. Although the stimulus is physical rather than visual, any activity along the optic nerve is carried to the visual cortex and experienced as a visual perception.

Adaptation is a reduction in sensitivity in the presence of a constant stimulus. Familiar examples are stepping into a hot bath or jumping into a cold lake. Within moments neither temperature seems as extreme as it did at first. Adaptation reduces the amount of information arriving at the cerebral cortex. Most sensory information is routed to centers along the spinal cord or brain stem, potentially triggering such involuntary reflexes as the withdrawal reflexes. ⊃ p. 284 Only about 1 percent of the information provided by afferent fibers reaches the cerebral cortex and our conscious awareness.

Output from higher centers, however, can increase receptor sensitivity or facilitate transmission along a sensory pathway. For example, the *reticular activating system* in the midbrain, which helps focus attention, can heighten or reduce awareness of arriving sensations. ⊃ p. 277 This adjustment of sensitivity can take place under conscious or unconscious direction. When we "listen carefully," our sensitivity to and awareness of auditory stimuli increase. The reverse occurs when we enter a noisy factory or walk along a crowded city street. There we automatically "tune out" the high level of background noise.

The **general senses** include temperature, pain, touch, pressure, vibration, and **proprioception** (body position). The receptors for the general senses occur throughout the body. The **special senses** are smell or **olfaction**, taste or **gustation**, vision, balance or **equilibrium**, and hearing. The receptors for these five special senses are confined to the head and concentrated within specific structures—the sense organs, such as the eye or the ear. In this chapter, we explore both the general senses and the special senses.

CHECKPOINT

1. What is adaptation?
2. Receptor A has a circular receptive field on the skin with a diameter of 2.5 cm. Receptor B has a circular receptive field 7.0 cm in diameter. Which receptor provides more precise sensory information?
3. List the five special senses.

See the blue Answers tab at the back of the book.

9-2 General sensory receptors are classified by the type of stimulus that excites them

Learning Objective Identify the receptors for the general senses, and describe how they function.

Receptors for the general senses are distributed throughout the body. They are relatively simple in structure. We classify them into four types by the nature of the stimulus that excites them: *nociceptors* (pain); *thermoreceptors* (temperature); *mechanoreceptors* (physical distortion); and *chemoreceptors* (chemical concentration).

Pain

Pain receptors, or **nociceptors** (n-s-SEP-trz; *noxa*, harm), are free nerve endings. They are especially common in the superficial portions of the skin, in joint capsules, within the periostea covering bones, and around blood vessel walls. Other deep tissues and most visceral organs contain few nociceptors. Pain receptors have large receptive fields (**Figure 9-1**). As a result, it is often difficult to determine the exact source of a painful sensation.

Nociceptors may be sensitive to (1) extremes of temperature, (2) mechanical damage, or (3) dissolved chemicals, such as those released by injured cells. Very strong stimuli by any of these sources may excite a nociceptor. For that reason, people describing very painful sensations—whether caused by heat, a deep cut, or inflammatory chemicals—use a similar descriptive term, such as "burning."

Once pain receptors in a region are stimulated, two types of axons carry the painful sensations. Myelinated fibers carry very localized sensations of **fast pain** (or *prickling pain*). Examples are pain caused by an injection or a deep cut. These sensations reach the CNS very quickly, where they often trigger somatic reflexes. They are also relayed to the primary sensory cortex and so receive conscious attention. Slower, unmyelinated fibers carry sensations of **slow pain**, or *burning* *and aching pain*. Unlike fast pain sensations, slow pain sensations enable you to identify only the general area involved.

Pain sensations from visceral organs are often perceived as originating at the body surface, generally in those regions innervated by the same spinal nerves. The perception of pain coming from parts of the body that are not actually stimulated is called **referred pain**. The precise process responsible for referred pain is not yet clear, but several clinical examples are shown in **Figure 9-2**. Cardiac pain, for example, is often perceived as originating in the skin of the upper chest and left arm.

Pain receptors continue to respond as long as the painful stimulus remains. However, the perception of the pain can decrease over time. This effect is due to the inhibition of centers in the thalamus, reticular formation, lower brain stem, and spinal cord.

9 Temperature

Temperature receptors, or **thermoreceptors**, are free nerve endings located in the dermis, in skeletal muscles, in the liver, and in the hypothalamus. Cold receptors are three or four times more common than warm receptors. There are no known structural differences between warm and cold thermoreceptors.

Temperature sensations are relayed along the same pathways that carry pain sensations. They are sent to the reticular formation, the thalamus, and (to a lesser extent) the primary sensory cortex. Thermoreceptors are very active when the temperature is changing, but they quickly adapt to a stable temperature. When you enter an air-conditioned classroom on a hot summer day or a warm lecture hall on a brisk fall evening, the temperature may seem extreme at first. Then you quickly become comfortable as adaptation takes place.

Figure 9-2 Referred Pain. Pain sensations from visceral organs are often perceived as arising from areas distant from the actual origin, because the body surface is innervated by the same spinal nerves. Each region of perceived pain is labeled according to the organ at which the pain originates.

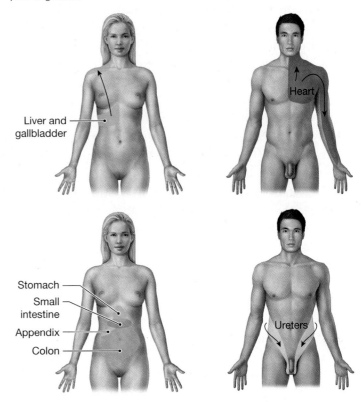

Touch, Pressure, and Position

Mechanoreceptors are sensitive to stimuli such as stretching, compression, or twisting. Distortion of the receptor cell's plasma membrane in response to these stimuli causes mechanically regulated ion channels to open or close. There are three classes of mechanoreceptors: (1) *tactile receptors* (touch), (2) *baroreceptors* (pressure), and (3) *proprioceptors* (position).

CLINICAL NOTE

Pain

Pain is an important symptom in medicine. In fact, over 60 percent of people who present to hospital emergency departments do so because of pain. Despite this, inadequate analgesia continues to be a problem in emergency care, especially in children. Emergency pain management should include pain relief when possible and management of associated anxiety. This must be provided while continuously monitoring the patient's airway, vital signs, and mental status.

The pathophysiology of the pain response is very complex. There are both peripheral and central mediators of pain. The peripheral pain system is activated when nociceptors and free nerve endings register the original noxious stimulus in the peripheral tissues and transmit it to the central nervous system. Several neurotransmitters are involved in the pain response including the excitatory amino acid glutamate and the neuropeptides *neurokinin-A, calcitoningene related peptide*, and *substance P*. Pain signals are integrated in the dorsal horn of the spinal cord. These are relayed to higher centers in the brain including the hypothalamus, thalamus, and the limbic and reticular activating systems. These centers integrate and process pain information, which allows the detection of and perception of pain. Interpretation, identification, and localization of pain also occur at these sites.

Because pain is subjective, it is often difficult to assess. In the emergency setting, it is common to use a pain scale to determine the severity of a patient's pain. The most popular pain scale asks patients to rate their pain on a numeric scale that ranges from 0 to 10; with 0 indicates no pain and 10 indicates the worst possible pain. Pain scale ratings can be monitored to determine the effectiveness of medications and other treatments.

Analgesics are medications that help to alleviate pain. They may work on peripheral pain mediators, central pain mediators, or both. Nonsteroidal anti-inflammatory (NSAID) agents are commonly used for mild to moderate pain. NSAIDs primarily act on peripheral pain mediators and include aspirin, ibuprofen, naproxen, ketoprofen, and many others. These drugs decrease levels of inflammatory mediators, such as prostaglandins, generated at the site of tissue injury. Because they act peripherally, they do not cause sedation or respiratory depression and they do not interfere with bowel or bladder function. Acetaminophen (Tylenol) is also a peripherally acting analgesic. However, unlike the NSAIDs, it does not have anti-inflammatory properties and does not affect platelet aggregation (as does aspirin). Most peripherally acting analgesics must be administered orally or by topical application. The exception is ketorolac (Toradol), which is available for intramuscular or intravenous injection.

Moderate to severe pain usually requires opioid analgesics. Opioid analgesics include morphine, codeine, hydromorphone, meperidine, fentanyl, and others. They are most effective when they are administered parenterally (outside of the digestive system). Common routes of opioid injection are subcutaneous, intramuscular, and intravenous. Several opioids referred to as endorphins and enkephalins occur naturally in the body. These substances serve as natural painkillers. The opiate medications act on the same receptors as the endorphins and enkephalins. Opiate receptors' different shapes influence the fit of the corresponding opiate/opioid molecules. The principle opioid receptors, referred to as mu (μ) receptors, produce analgesia, euphoria, and respiratory depression. The mu receptors can be further classified as mu-1 and mu-2. Mu-1 (μ1) receptors cause analgesia, while mu-2 (μ2) receptors produce constipation, euphoria, physical dependence, and respiratory depression. Several other receptors involved in the central pain response include the delta, sigma, kappa, and epsilon receptors. The delta (δ) receptors also produce analgesia. The sigma (ζ) receptors stimulate respiratory and vasomotor activity as well as hallucinations and dysphoria. The kappa (κ) receptors influence spinal analgesia, sedation, and pupillary constriction. Finally, the epsilon (ε) receptors produce analgesia. Morphine and the other opiate derivatives have an affinity for the mu and kappa receptors.

Peripherally acting and centrally acting analgesics are often mixed to provide highly effective pain control. Usually, these are a combination of an opioid and acetaminophen or an opioid and ibuprofen. In addition, long-term pain control can be provided with delayed-release medications or skin patches that deliver a standard amount of opioid analgesia over 72 hours. Patient comfort and pain control are important aspects of emergency care. Emergency personnel should assess the severity of a patient's pain and expeditiously provide adequate analgesia when possible.

Tactile Receptors

Tactile receptors provide sensations of touch, pressure, and vibration. The distinctions between these sensations are hazy. A touch also represents a pressure, and a vibration is an oscillating touch/pressure stimulus. **Fine touch and pressure receptors** provide detailed information about a source of stimulation, including its exact location, shape, size, texture, and movement. **Crude touch and pressure receptors** provide poor localization. They provide little additional information about the stimulus because they have large receptive fields.

Tactile receptors range in complexity from free nerve endings to specialized sensory complexes with accessory cells and supporting structures. **Figure 9-3** shows six types of tactile receptors in the skin:

1. Free nerve endings sensitive to touch and pressure are located between epidermal cells. There appear to be no structural differences between these receptors and the free nerve endings that provide temperature or pain sensations.

2. Wherever hairs are located, the nerve endings of the **root hair plexus** monitor distortions and movements across the body surface.

3. **Tactile discs**, or *Merkel* (MER-kel) *discs*, are fine touch and pressure receptors. Hairless skin contains large epithelial cells *(Merkel cells)* in its deepest epidermal layer, the stratum basale. The dendrites of a single sensory neuron make close contact with a group of these cells. When compressed, Merkel cells release chemicals that stimulate the neuron.

4. **Tactile corpuscles**, or *Meissner's* (MĪS-nerz) *corpuscles*, give us sensations of fine touch and pressure and low-frequency vibration. They are abundant in the eyelids, lips, fingertips, nipples, and external genitalia. A fibrous capsule surrounds and anchors the corpuscle within the dermis.

5. **Lamellated** (LAM-e-lāt-ed) **corpuscles**, or *pacinian* (pa-SIN-ē-an) *corpuscles*, are large receptors sensitive to deep pressure and to pulsing or high-frequency vibrations. A single dendrite lies within concentric layers of collagen fibers and specialized fibroblasts. These receptors are common in the skin of the fingers, breasts, and external genitalia. They are also present in joint capsules, mesenteries, the pancreas, and the walls of the urethra and urinary bladder.

6. **Ruffini** (roo-FĒ-nē) **corpuscles** are also sensitive to pressure and distortion of the skin, but they are located in the reticular (deep) layer of the dermis. They contain collagen fibers continuous with those in the surrounding dermis.

Figure 9-3 Tactile Receptors in the Skin.

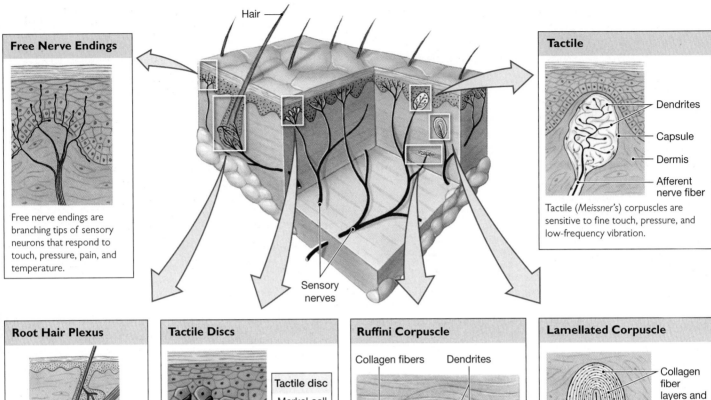

Free Nerve Endings

Free nerve endings are branching tips of sensory neurons that respond to touch, pressure, pain, and temperature.

Hair

Sensory nerves

Tactile

Dendrites

Capsule

Dermis

Afferent nerve fiber

Tactile (*Meissner's*) corpuscles are sensitive to fine touch, pressure, and low-frequency vibration.

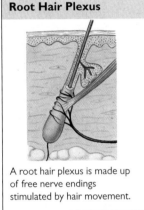

Root Hair Plexus

A root hair plexus is made up of free nerve endings stimulated by hair movement.

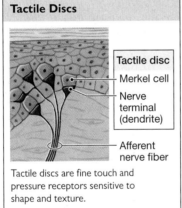

Tactile Discs

Tactile disc

Merkel cell

Nerve terminal (dendrite)

Afferent nerve fiber

Tactile discs are fine touch and pressure receptors sensitive to shape and texture.

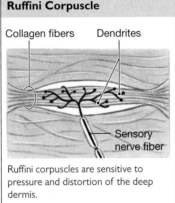

Ruffini Corpuscle

Collagen fibers   Dendrites

Sensory nerve fiber

Ruffini corpuscles are sensitive to pressure and distortion of the deep dermis.

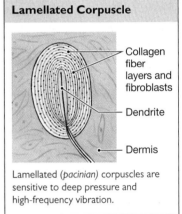

Lamellated Corpuscle

Collagen fiber layers and fibroblasts

Dendrite

Dermis

Lamellated (*pacinian*) corpuscles are sensitive to deep pressure and high-frequency vibration.

Tactile sensations travel through the posterior column and spinothalamic pathways. ↪ p. 286 Infection, disease, and damage to sensory neurons or pathways can alter sensitivity to tactile sensations. The locations of tactile responses may have diagnostic significance. For example, sensory loss along the boundary of a dermatome can help identify the affected spinal nerve or nerves. ↪ p. 281

Baroreceptors

Baroreceptors (bar-ō-rē-SEP-tōrz; *baro-*, pressure) monitor changes in pressure in an organ. They provide information essential to the regulation of autonomic activities. A baroreceptor consists of free nerve endings that branch within the elastic tissues in the wall of an organ that can expand, such as a blood vessel or a portion of the respiratory, digestive, or urinary tract. When the pressure changes, the elastic walls expand or recoil. This movement distorts the dendritic branches and alters the rate of action potential generation. Baroreceptors respond immediately to a change in pressure, but they adapt rapidly, and the output along the afferent fibers gradually returns to normal.

Figure 9-4 shows the locations of some baroreceptors and summarizes their functions in autonomic activities. Baroreceptors monitor blood pressure in the walls of major blood vessels, including the carotid artery (at the *carotid sinus*) and the aorta (at the *aortic sinus*). The information plays a major role in regulating cardiac function and adjusting blood flow to vital tissues. Baroreceptors

Figure 9-4 Baroreceptors and the Regulation of Autonomic Functions.
Baroreceptors at several sites provide information essential to the regulation of various autonomic activities, including blood pressure monitoring, respiration, digestion, urination, and defecation.

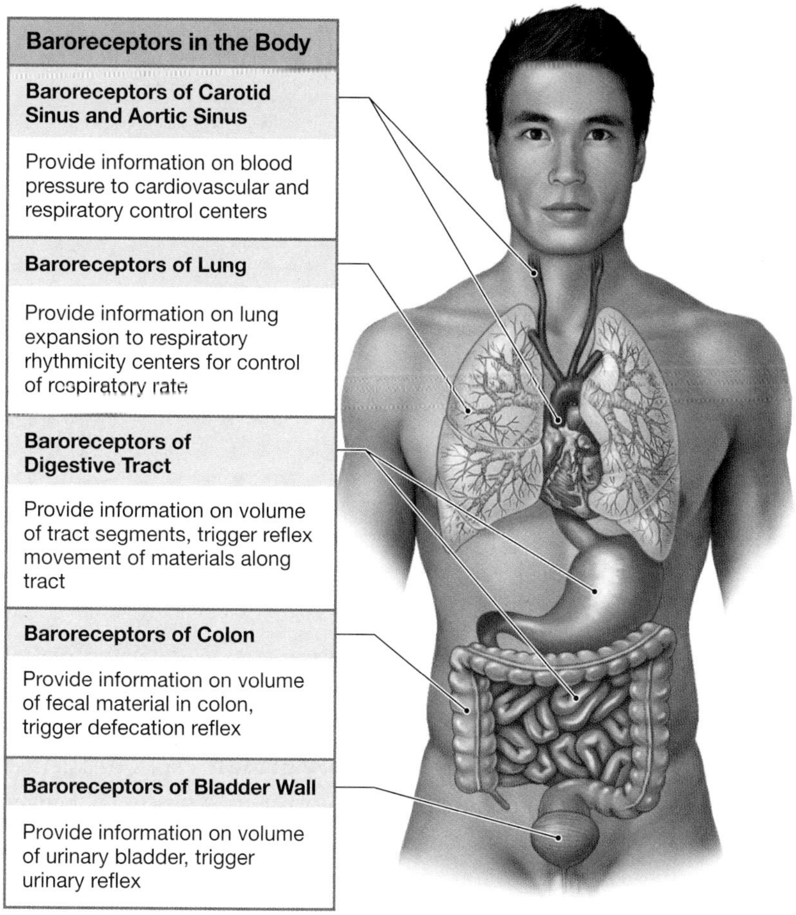

Baroreceptors in the Body

Baroreceptors of Carotid Sinus and Aortic Sinus

Provide information on blood pressure to cardiovascular and respiratory control centers

Baroreceptors of Lung

Provide information on lung expansion to respiratory rhythmicity centers for control of respiratory rate

Baroreceptors of Digestive Tract

Provide information on volume of tract segments, trigger reflex movement of materials along tract

Baroreceptors of Colon

Provide information on volume of fecal material in colon, trigger defecation reflex

Baroreceptors of Bladder Wall

Provide information on volume of urinary bladder, trigger urinary reflex

in the lungs monitor the degree of lung expansion. This information is relayed to the respiratory rhythmicity centers in the brain, which set the pace of respiration. � p. 278 Baroreceptors in the digestive and urinary tracts trigger various visceral reflexes, including actions that move materials along the digestive tract, defecation, and urination.

Proprioceptors

Proprioceptors monitor the position of joints, the tension in tendons and ligaments, and the state of muscular contraction. *Free nerve endings* in joint capsules detect pressure, tension, and movement at the joint. *Golgi tendon organs* lie between a skeletal muscle and its tendon and monitor the strain on a tendon during muscle contraction. *Muscle spindles* monitor the length of a skeletal muscle and trigger stretch reflexes. � p. 284

Proprioceptors do not adapt to constant stimulation. Each receptor continuously sends information to the CNS. Most of this information is processed subconsciously. Only a small proportion of it reaches your conscious awareness. Your sense of body position results from the integration of information from these three types of proprioceptors and from the receptors of the internal ear.

Chemical Detection

Specialized nerve cells called **chemoreceptors** can detect small changes in the concentration of specific chemicals or compounds. They respond only to water-soluble and lipid-soluble substances that are dissolved in body fluids (interstitial fluid, blood plasma, and CSF). Adaptation usually takes place over a few seconds following stimulation. Except for the special senses of taste and smell, there are no well-defined chemosensory pathways in the brain or spinal cord. The chemoreceptors of the general senses send their information to brain stem centers that deal with the autonomic control of respiratory and cardiovascular functions.

The locations of important chemoreceptors are shown in **Figure 9-5**. Neurons within the respiratory centers of the brain respond to the concentrations of hydrogen ions (pH) and carbon dioxide molecules in the cerebrospinal fluid. Chemoreceptors are also found in the **carotid bodies**, near the origin of the internal carotid arteries on each side of the neck, and in the **aortic bodies**, between the major branches of the aortic arch. These receptors monitor the pH, carbon dioxide, and oxygen levels in arterial blood. The afferent fibers leaving the carotid and aortic bodies reach the respiratory centers by traveling within cranial nerves IX (glossopharyngeal) and X (vagus).

CHECKPOINT

4. List the four types of general sensory receptors, and identify the nature of the stimulus that excites each type.

5. Identify the three classes of mechanoreceptors.

6. What would happen if information from proprioceptors in your legs was blocked from reaching the CNS?

See the blue Answers tab at the back of the book.

Figure 9-5 Locations and Functions of Chemoreceptors. Chemoreceptors are located in the CNS (on the ventrolateral surfaces of the medulla oblongata) and in the aortic and carotid bodies. These receptors are involved in the autonomic regulation of respiratory and cardiovascular function.

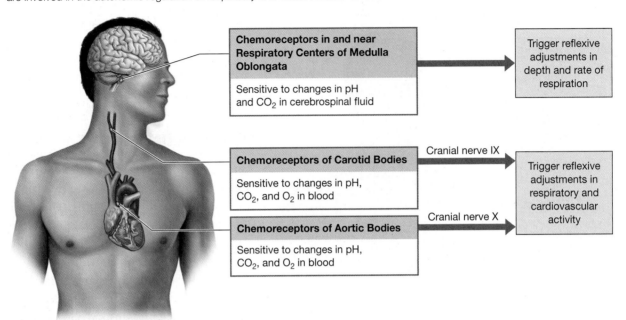

Build Your Knowledge

Recall that there are separate pathways in the spinal cord that carry sensory information (as you saw in **Chapter 8: The Nervous System**). Examples of sensory pathways and the sensations they deliver to the brain include:

- the posterior column pathway (highly localized fine touch, pressure, vibration, and proprioception);
- the spinothalamic pathway (poorly localized touch, pressure, pain, and temperature);
- and the spinocerebellar pathway (proprioceptive information concerning the positions of muscles, bones, and joints). ⊃ **p. 286**

9-3 Olfaction, the sense of smell, involves olfactory receptors responding to chemical stimuli

Learning Objective Describe the sensory organs of smell, and discuss the processes involved in olfaction.

The sense of smell, or *olfaction*, is provided by paired **olfactory organs**. These organs are located in the nasal cavity on either side of the nasal septum (**Figure 9-6a**). Each olfactory organ consists of an **olfactory epithelium** containing **olfactory receptor cells**, supporting cells, and regenerative *basal cells* (stem cells) (**Figure 9-6b**). The underlying *lamina propria* consists of areolar tissue with large **olfactory glands**. ⊃ p. 110 Their secretions absorb water and form a pigmented mucus that covers the epithelium. The mucus is produced in a continuous stream that passes across the surface of the olfactory organs. It prevents the buildup of potentially dangerous or overpowering stimuli. It also keeps the area moist and free from dust or other debris.

When you inhale through your nose, the air swirls within the nasal cavity. A normal, relaxed inhalation carries a small sample (about 2 percent) of the inhaled air to the olfactory organs. If you sniff repeatedly, you increase the flow of air across the olfactory epithelium, intensifying the stimulation of the receptors. However, only the molecules of compounds that can diffuse into the overlying mucus can stimulate the olfactory receptors. Such compounds are "volatile" to some degree; that is, they evaporate easily in air. We don't respond to all airborne chemicals. For example, gases such as oxygen and carbon dioxide, and the poisonous gas, carbon monoxide, are odorless.

The olfactory receptor cells are highly modified neurons. The exposed knob of each receptor cell provides a base for up to 20 cilia-shaped dendrites that extend into the surrounding mucus. Olfactory reception takes place as dissolved chemicals interact with receptors, called *odorant-binding proteins*, on the surfaces of the dendrites.

Odorants are chemicals that stimulate olfactory receptors. The binding of an odorant changes the permeability of the

Figure 9-6 The Olfactory Organs.

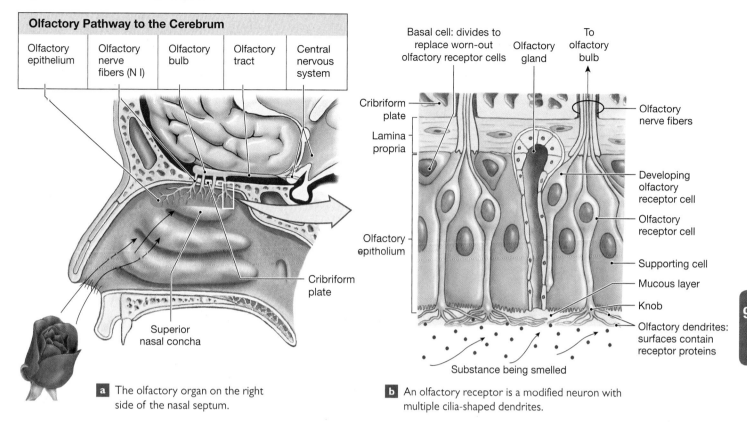

Olfactory Pathway to the Cerebrum				
Olfactory epithelium	Olfactory nerve fibers (N I)	Olfactory bulb	Olfactory tract	Central nervous system

Cribriform plate

Superior nasal concha

a The olfactory organ on the right side of the nasal septum.

Basal cell: divides to replace worn-out olfactory receptor cells

Olfactory gland

To olfactory bulb

Cribriform plate

Lamina propria

Olfactory epithelium

Olfactory nerve fibers

Developing olfactory receptor cell

Olfactory receptor cell

Supporting cell

Mucous layer

Knob

Olfactory dendrites: surfaces contain receptor proteins

Substance being smelled

b An olfactory receptor is a modified neuron with multiple cilia-shaped dendrites.

receptor plasma membrane, producing action potentials. This information is relayed to the central nervous system. The CNS interprets the smell on the basis of the particular pattern of receptor activity.

Approximately 10–20 million olfactory receptor cells are packed into an area of roughly 5 cm^2 (0.8 in.^{2}). If we take into account the surface area of the exposed dendrites, the actual sensory area approaches that of the entire body surface. Yet our olfactory sensitivities cannot compare with those of dogs, cats, or fishes. A German shepherd sniffing for smuggled drugs or explosives has an olfactory receptor surface 72 times greater than that of the nearby customs inspector!

The Olfactory Pathways

The axons leaving the olfactory epithelium collect into 20 or more bundles that penetrate the cribriform plate of the ethmoid bone to reach the **olfactory bulbs** of the cerebrum. There, the first synapse occurs. These bundles are components of the olfactory cranial nerves (I). Axons leaving each olfactory bulb travel along the olfactory tract to reach the olfactory cortex of the cerebrum, the hypothalamus, and portions of the limbic system.

Olfactory stimuli are the only type of sensory information that reaches the cerebral cortex directly. All other sensations

first synapse in processing centers in the thalamus before being relayed. Certain smells can trigger profound emotional and behavioral responses, as well as memories, because of the parallel distribution of olfactory information to the limbic system and hypothalamus. The perfume industry understands the practical implications of these connections and works to develop odors that trigger sexual responses.

CHECKPOINT

7. Define olfaction.

8. How does repeated sniffing help to identify faint odors?

See the blue Answers tab at the back of the book.

9-4 Gustation, the sense of taste, involves taste receptors responding to chemical stimuli

Learning Objective Describe the sensory organs of taste, and discuss the processes involved in gustation.

Gustation, or taste, provides information about the foods and liquids we eat and drink. **Taste receptors**, or *gustatory* (GUS-ta-tor-ē) *receptors*, are distributed over the surface of

Figure 9-7 Gustatory Receptors.

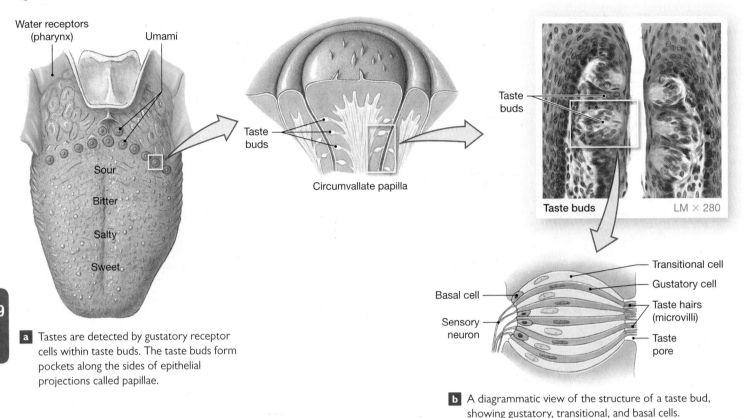

a Tastes are detected by gustatory receptor cells within taste buds. The taste buds form pockets along the sides of epithelial projections called papillae.

b A diagrammatic view of the structure of a taste bud, showing gustatory, transitional, and basal cells.

the tongue and adjacent portions of the pharynx and larynx (**Figure 9-7**). The most important taste receptors are on the tongue. By the time we reach adulthood, those on the pharynx and larynx have become less important.

Taste receptors and specialized epithelial cells form sensory structures called **taste buds**. The taste buds are well protected from the mechanical stress due to chewing. They lie along the sides of epithelial projections called **papillae** (pa-PIL-lē; *papilla*, a nipple-shaped mound). The greatest numbers of taste buds are associated with the large *circumvallate papillae*, which form a V that points toward the base of the tongue.

Each taste bud contains slender sensory receptor cells and basal cells (stem cells). The basal cells continually divide, producing daughter cells that mature in stages—basal, transitional, and mature. The mature cells are called **gustatory receptor cells**, or gustatory cells.

Each gustatory cell extends slender microvilli, sometimes called *taste hairs*, into the surrounding fluids through a narrow opening, the **taste pore**. The process behind gustatory reception seems to parallel that of olfaction. Dissolved chemicals contacting the taste hairs stimulate a change in the membrane potential of the gustatory cell, which leads to action potentials in the sensory neuron.

You are probably already familiar with the four **primary taste sensations**: sweet, salty, sour, and bitter. There is some evidence for differences in sensitivity to tastes along the long axis of the tongue, with greatest sensitivity to salty–sweet anteriorly and to sour–bitter posteriorly (**Figure 9-7a**). However, there are no differences in the structure of the taste buds. Also, taste buds in all portions of the tongue provide all four primary taste sensations.

Two additional tastes, *umami* and *water*, have been discovered in humans. **Umami** (oo-MAH-m) is a pleasant taste corresponding to the flavor of beef broth, chicken broth, and Parmesan cheese. Most people say water has no flavor, yet **water receptors** are present, especially in the pharynx. Their sensory output is processed in the hypothalamus and affects several systems involved in water balance and the regulation of blood volume.

The threshold for receptor stimulation varies for each of the primary taste sensations. Also, the taste receptors respond most readily to unpleasant rather than pleasant stimuli. For example, we are much more sensitive to acids, which taste sour, than to either sweet or salty chemicals. We are even more sensitive to bitter compounds than to acids. This sensitivity has survival value, because acids can damage the mucous membranes of the mouth and pharynx, and many biological toxins have an extremely bitter taste.

The Taste Pathways

Taste buds are monitored by cranial nerves VII (facial), IX (glossopharyngeal), and X (vagus). The sensory afferent fibers of these cranial nerves synapse within a nucleus in the medulla oblongata. There the neurons join axons that carry sensory information on touch, pressure, and proprioception. After another synapse in the thalamus, the information is then carried to the gustatory cortex. ⟲ p. 271

A conscious perception of taste is produced as the information received from the taste buds is combined with other sensory data. Information about the texture of food, along with taste-related sensations such as "peppery" or "spicy hot," is provided by sensory afferents in cranial nerve V (trigeminal). Olfactory information also plays an overwhelming role in taste perception.

The combination of taste and smell is what provides the *flavor*, or distinctive quality of a particular food and drink. You are several thousand times more sensitive to "tastes" when your olfactory organs are fully functional. By contrast, if you have a cold and a stuffy nose, airborne molecules cannot reach your olfactory receptors. Meals taste dull and unappealing, even though your taste buds are responding normally.

CHECKPOINT

9. Define gustation.

10. If you completely dry the surface of your tongue and then place salt or sugar crystals on it, you cannot taste them. Why not?

See the blue Answers tab at the back of the book.

9-5 Internal eye structures contribute to vision, while accessory eye structures provide protection

Learning Objective Identify the internal and accessory structures of the eye, and explain their functions.

We rely more on vision than on any other special sense. Our eyes contain our visual receptors. Eyes are elaborate structures that enable us to detect not only light but also detailed images. We begin our discussion of these complex organs by considering the *accessory structures* that provide protection, lubrication, and support for our eyes.

The Accessory Structures of the Eye

The **accessory structures** of the eye include

1. the eyelids and associated exocrine glands;

2. the superficial epithelium of the eye (**Figure 9-8a**);

3. structures associated with the production, secretion, and removal of tears (**Figure 9-8b**); and

4. the extrinsic eye muscles (**Figure 9-9**).

Figure 9-8 The Accessory Structures of the Eye.

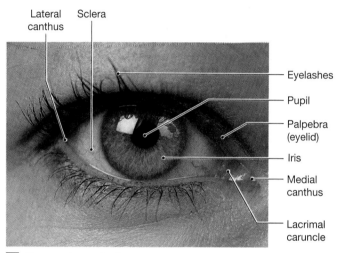

Lateral canthus · Sclera · Eyelashes · Pupil · Palpebra (eyelid) · Iris · Medial canthus · Lacrimal caruncle

a Gross and superficial anatomy of the accessory structures.

Lacrimal gland · Lacrimal gland ducts · Lacrimal pores · Superior lacrimal canal · Lacrimal sac · Inferior lacrimal canal · Nasolacrimal duct · Opening of duct into nasal cavity

b The organization of the lacrimal apparatus.

Figure 9-9 The Extrinsic Eye Muscles.

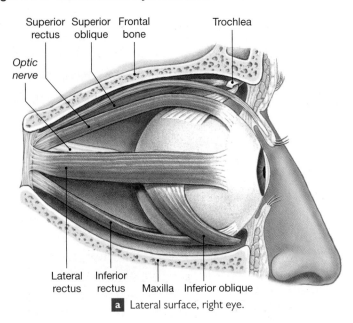

Superior rectus · Superior oblique · Frontal bone · Trochlea

Optic nerve

Lateral rectus · Inferior rectus · Maxilla · Inferior oblique

a Lateral surface, right eye.

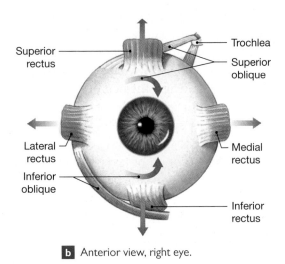

Superior rectus · Trochlea · Superior oblique

Lateral rectus · Medial rectus

Inferior oblique · Inferior rectus

b Anterior view, right eye.

The **eyelids**, or **palpebrae** (pal-PĒ-brē), are a continuation of the skin. Their continual blinking lubricates the surface of the eye. Similar to windshield wipers, they also remove dust and debris. The eyelids can also close firmly to protect the delicate surface of the eye. The upper and lower eyelids are connected at the **medial canthus** (KAN-thus) and the **lateral canthus** (**Figure 9-8a**). The eyelashes are very strong hairs that help prevent foreign matter (including insects) from reaching the surface of the eye.

Several types of exocrine glands protect the eye and its accessory structures. Large sebaceous glands are associated with the eyelashes, as they are with other hairs and hair follicles.⊃ p. 132 Along the inner margins of the eyelids, modified sebaceous glands *(tarsal glands)* secrete a lipid-rich substance that keeps the eyelids from sticking together. At the medial canthus is a soft mass of tissue called the **lacrimal caruncle** (KAR-ung-kul). It contains glands that produce thick secretions that contribute to the gritty deposits occasionally found after a night's sleep. These various glands sometimes become infected by bacteria. An infection in a sebaceous gland of one of the eyelashes, in a tarsal gland, or in one of the sweat glands between the eyelash follicles produces a painful localized swelling known as a **sty**.

The inner surfaces of the eyelids and the outer, white surface of the eye are covered by a thin, transparent mucous membrane called the **conjunctiva** (kon-junk-TĪ-vuh) (**Figure 9-10**). The conjunctiva extends to the edges of the **cornea** (KŌR-nē-uh), a transparent part of the outer fibrous layer of the eye. The cornea is covered by a delicate *corneal epithelium*, which is continuous with the conjunctiva. The conjunctiva contains many free nerve endings and is very sensitive. The painful condition of **conjunctivitis**, or pinkeye, results from damage to and irritation of the conjunctival surface. Its most obvious sign, redness, is due to the dilation of the blood vessels beneath the conjunctival epithelium.

A constant flow of tears keeps the surface of the eyeball moist and clean. Tears reduce friction, remove debris, prevent bacterial infection, and provide nutrients and oxygen to the conjunctival epithelium. The **lacrimal apparatus** produces, distributes, and removes tears (**Figure 9-8b**). Superior and lateral to the eyeball is the **lacrimal gland**, or *tear gland*. It has a dozen or more ducts that empty into the pocket between the eyelid and the eye. About the size of an almond, this gland nestles within a depression in the frontal bone, just inside the orbit. The lacrimal gland normally provides the key ingredients and most of the volume of the tears. Its watery, slightly alkaline secretions also contain *lysozyme*, an enzyme that attacks bacteria. The mixture of secretions from the lacrimal glands, accessory glands, and tarsal glands forms a superficial "oil slick" that assists in lubrication and slows evaporation.

Blinking sweeps tears across the surface of the eye to the medial canthus. Two small pores direct the tears into the **lacrimal canals**, passageways that end at the lacrimal sac (**Figure 9-8b**). From this sac, the **nasolacrimal duct** carries the tears to the nasal cavity.

Six **extrinsic eye muscles**, or *oculomotor* (ok-ū-lō-MŌ-ter) *muscles*, originate on the surface of the orbit and control the position of the eye (**Figure 9-9** and **Table 9-1**). These muscles are the **inferior rectus**, **medial rectus**, **superior rectus**, **lateral rectus**, **inferior oblique**, and **superior oblique**.

Table 9-1	The Extrinsic Eye Muscles (see Figure 9-9)			
Muscle	Origin	Insertion	Action	Innervation
Inferior rectus	Sphenoid bone around optic canal	Inferior, medial surface of eyeball	Eye looks down	Oculomotor nerve (N III)
Medial rectus	Sphenoid bone around optic canal	Medial surface of eyeball	Eye looks medially	Oculomotor nerve (N III)
Superior rectus	Sphenoid bone around optic canal	Superior surface of eyeball	Eye looks up	Oculomotor nerve (N III)
Lateral rectus	Sphenoid bone around optic canal	Lateral surface of eyeball	Eye looks laterally	Abducens nerve (N VI)
Inferior oblique	Maxillary bone at anterior portion of orbit	Inferior, lateral surface of eyeball	Eye rolls, looks up and laterally	Oculomotor nerve (N III)
Superior oblique	Sphenoid bone around optic canal	Superior, lateral surface of eyeball	Eye rolls, looks down and laterally	Trochlear nerve (N IV)

Build Your Knowledge

Recall that a skeletal muscle begins at an origin, ends at an insertion, and contracts to produce a specific action (as you saw in **Chapter 7: The Muscular System**). Generally, a muscle's origin remains stationary and the insertion moves. ⤴**p. 216**

The Eye

The eyes are sophisticated visual instruments. They are more versatile and adaptable than the most expensive cameras, yet compact and durable. Each eye is roughly spherical, has a diameter of nearly 2.5 cm (1 in.), and weighs around 8 g (0.28 oz). The eyeball shares space within the orbit with the extrinsic eye muscles, the lacrimal gland, and the various cranial nerves and blood vessels that service the eye and adjacent areas of the orbit and face. A mass of *orbital fat* cushions and insulates the eye (**Figure 9-10c**).

The eyeball is hollow and filled with fluid. Its interior can be divided into two cavities, anterior and posterior (**Figure 9-10b**). The smaller **anterior cavity** is subdivided into the *anterior chamber* and the *posterior chamber* (**Figure 9-10c**). A clear, watery fluid called the *aqueous humor* fills the anterior cavity. The large **posterior cavity**, or *vitreous chamber*, contains a gelatinous substance called the *vitreous body*. The fluid part of this body is *vitreous humor*. The vitreous body and the aqueous humor help to stabilize the shape of the eye.

The wall of the eye contains three distinct layers, formerly called *tunics*. There is an outer *fibrous layer*, an intermediate *vascular layer*, and a deep *inner layer (retina)* (**Figure 9-10b**).

The Fibrous Layer

The **fibrous layer**, the outermost layer of the eye, consists of the *sclera* (SKLER-uh) and the *cornea*. The fibrous layer (1) provides mechanical support and some degree of physical protection; (2) serves as an attachment site for the extrinsic eye muscles; and (3) assists in the focusing process. The **sclera**, or "white of the eye," is a layer of dense fibrous connective tissue containing both collagen and elastic fibers (**Figure 9-10c**). It is thickest over the posterior surface of the eye and thinnest over the anterior surface. The six extrinsic eye muscles insert on the sclera.

The surface of the sclera contains small blood vessels and nerves that penetrate the sclera to reach internal structures. On the anterior surface of the eye, however, these blood vessels lie under the conjunctiva. The white color of the collagen fibers is visible because this network of capillaries does not carry enough blood to lend an obvious color to the sclera.

The transparent cornea is continuous with the sclera. Unlike the sclera, the collagen fibers of the cornea are organized into a series of layers that does not interfere with the passage of light. The cornea has no blood vessels. Its epithelial cells obtain their oxygen and nutrients from the tears that flow across their surfaces. The cornea has a very restricted ability to repair itself, so corneal injuries must be treated immediately to prevent serious vision losses. Restoring vision after corneal scarring usually requires replacing the cornea through a *corneal transplant*. Such transplants can be performed between unrelated individuals because there are no blood vessels to carry white blood cells, which attack foreign tissues, into the area.

The Vascular Layer

The **vascular layer** contains numerous blood vessels, lymphatic vessels, and the *intrinsic eye muscles*. This middle layer (1) provides a route for blood vessels and lymphatic vessels that supply tissues of the eye; (2) regulates the amount of light entering the eye; (3) secretes and reabsorbs the *aqueous humor* that circulates within the chambers of the eye; and (4) controls the shape of the lens, an essential part of the focusing process.

Figure 9-10 The Sectional Anatomy of the Eye.

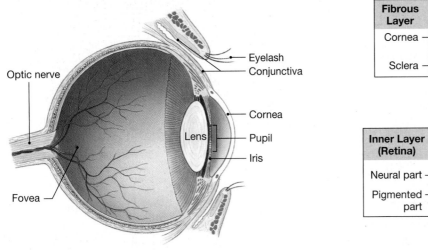

a Sagittal section of left eye.

b Horizontal section of right eye.

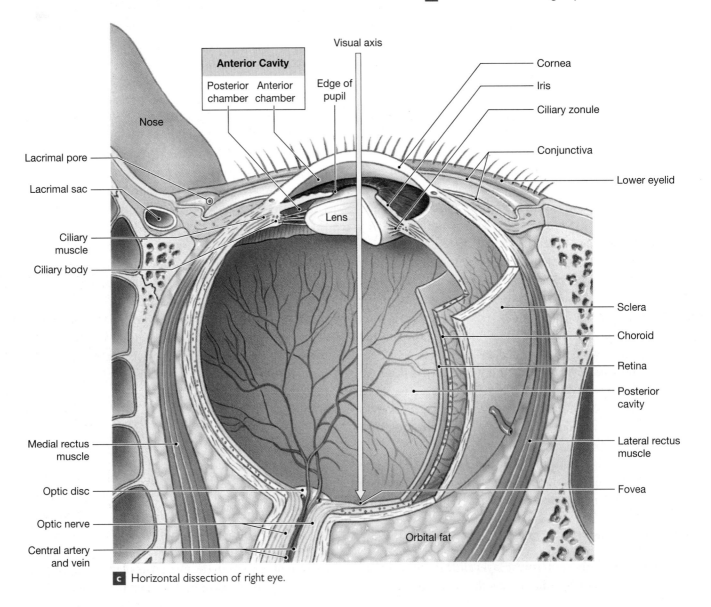

c Horizontal dissection of right eye.

9

CLINICAL NOTE

Anisocoria

Anisocoria, or unequal pupils, is always a concern in the emergency patient. Pupillary constriction is controlled by the *oculomotor nerve (CN III)*. An expanding lesion in the brain can compress the nerve and cause pupillary dilation on the affected side. In a trauma patient, this may indicate an intracranial injury. In a medical patient, anisocoria may indicate intracranial bleeding or tumor. Because of this, the presence of anisocoria requires further investigation.

Anisocoria can be a normal finding. In fact, 20 percent of the general population has some degree of anisocoria. The difference is typically 1 mm or less and is not accompanied by other findings (such as drooping eyelids or extraocular muscle paralysis). Anisocoria may vary from day to day in the same person. Also, many medications, such as decongestants, can cause anisocoria. If necessary, old photographs, such as those on a driver's license, can help determine whether anisocoria is old or new.

The vascular layer includes the *iris*, the *ciliary body*, and the *choroid* (**Figure 9-10b**). The **iris** is visible through the transparent cornea. The iris contains blood vessels, pigment cells, loose connective tissue, and two layers of intrinsic smooth muscle fibers. When these *pupillary muscles* contract, they change the diameter of the central opening, or **pupil**, of the iris. There are two types of pupillary muscles: radial-oriented *dilators* and concentric-oriented *constrictors*. The autonomic nervous system controls both muscle groups. For example, sympathetic activation in response to dim light causes the pupils to dilate, or enlarge. Parasympathetic activation in response to bright light causes the pupils to constrict. ⊃ p. 295

How is eye color determined? Our genes influence the number of melanocytes on the anterior surface and interior of the iris, as well as the presence of melanin granules in the pigmented epithelium on the posterior surface of the iris. (This pigmented epithelium is part of the inner layer, or retina.) When the iris contains few melanocytes, light passes through the iris and bounces off the pigmented epithelium. The eye then appears blue. The irises of green, brown, and very dark brown eyes have increasing numbers of melanocytes. The eyes of people with albinism appear very pale gray or blue gray.

Along its outer edge, the iris attaches to the anterior portion of the **ciliary body**. The ciliary body begins deep to the junction between the cornea and sclera. It extends to the scalloped border that also marks the anterior edge of the thick, neural part of the inner layer (**Figure 9-10c**). Most of the ciliary body consists of the *ciliary muscle*, a ring of smooth muscle that projects into the interior of the eye. Posterior to the iris, the surface of the ciliary body is thrown into folds called *ciliary processes*. The **ciliary zonule** (*suspensory ligament*) is the ring of fibers that attaches the lens to the ciliary processes. The connective tissue fibers hold the lens in place posterior to the iris and centered on the pupil. As a result, light passing through the pupil passes through the center of the lens along the *visual axis*.

The choroid is a vascular layer that separates the fibrous and inner layers posterior to the ciliary body (**Figure 9-10c**). The choroid contains a capillary network that delivers oxygen and nutrients to the inner layer.

The Inner Layer

The **inner layer**, or **retina**, is the innermost layer of the eye. It consists of a thin, outer layer called the *pigmented part* and a thick, inner layer called the *neural part* (**Figure 9-10b**). The pigmented part absorbs light that passes through the neural part, preventing light from bouncing back and producing visual "echoes." The neural part contains

1. the photoreceptors that respond to light,
2. supporting cells and neurons that perform preliminary processing and integration of visual information, and
3. blood vessels supplying tissues that line the posterior cavity.

The two layers of the retina are normally very close together but not tightly interconnected. The pigmented part continues over the ciliary body and iris. The neural part extends anteriorly only up to the ciliary body, forming a cup that establishes the posterior and lateral boundaries of the posterior cavity.

ORGANIZATION OF THE RETINA. The neural part of the retina contains several layers of cells (**Figure 9-11a**). The outermost layer, closest to the wall of the pigmented part of the retina, contains the **photoreceptors**, the cells that detect light. The eye has two main types of photoreceptors: rods and cones.

Rods do not discriminate among colors of light. These very light-sensitive receptors enable us to see in dimly lit rooms, at twilight, or in pale moonlight.

Cones give us color vision. We have three types of cones. Each type contains a different visual pigment: red, green, and blue. The stimulation of various combinations of these cone types provides the perception of different colors. Cones give us sharper, clearer images than rods do, but they require brighter light. When you watch a sunset, you can notice your vision shifting from cone-based vision (a clear image in full color) to rod-based vision (a less distinct image in black and white).

A third type of photoreceptor is the *intrinsically photosensitive retinal ganglion cell*. These non-image-forming cells respond to different levels of brightness. They influence the body's 24-hour circadian rhythm (biological clock).

Figure 9-11 Retinal Organization.

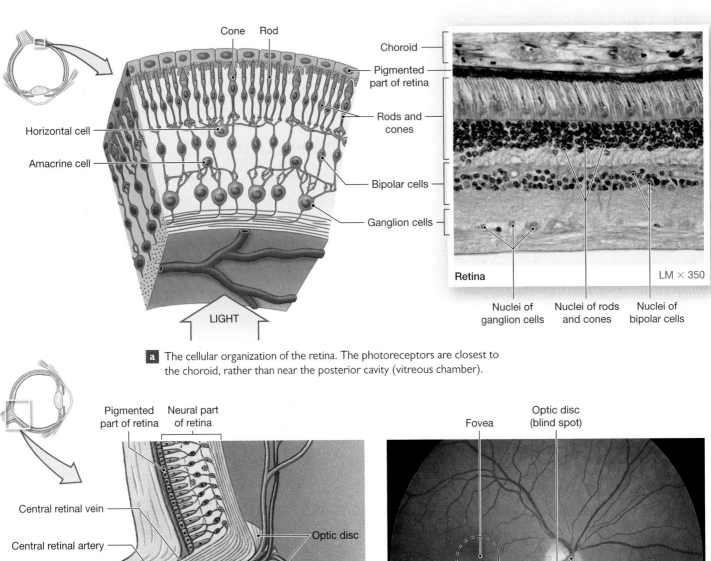

a The cellular organization of the retina. The photoreceptors are closest to the choroid, rather than near the posterior cavity (vitreous chamber).

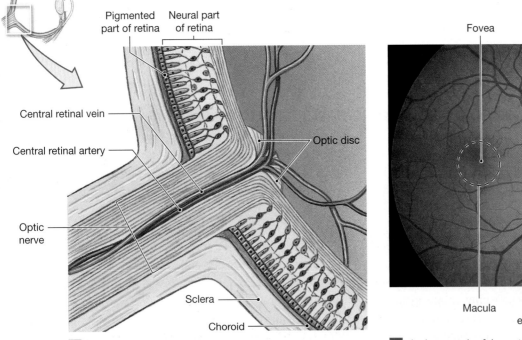

b The optic disc in diagrammatic sagittal section.

c A photograph of the retina as seen through the pupil.

Rods and cones are not evenly distributed across the retina. If you think of the retina as a cup, approximately 125 million rods are found on the sides, and roughly 6 million cones dominate the bottom. Most of these cones are concentrated in the area where the visual image arrives after passing through the cornea and lens. This area, known as the **macula** (MAK-ū-luh; spot), has no rods (**Figure 9-11c**). The very highest concentration of cones is found in the center of the macula in an area called the **fovea** (FŌ-vē-uh; shallow depression), or *fovea centralis*. The fovea is the center of color vision and the site of sharpest vision. When you look directly at an object, its image falls on this portion of the retina. An imaginary line drawn from the center of that object through the center of the lens to the fovea establishes the **visual axis** of the eye (**Figure 9-10c**).

You probably already know something about the way this distribution of cones affects our vision. During the day, when there is enough light to stimulate the cones, you see a very good image. But in very dim light cones cannot function. That is why you can't see a dim star if you stare directly at it. But if you look a little to one side rather than directly at the star, you can see it quite clearly. Shifting your gaze moves the image of the star from the fovea, where it does not provide enough light to stimulate the cones, to the sides of the retina, where it stimulates the more sensitive rods.

Rods and cones synapse with roughly 6 million **bipolar cells** (**Figure 9-11a**). Bipolar cells in turn synapse within the layer of **ganglion cells** adjacent to the posterior cavity. The axons of the ganglion cells deliver the sensory information to the brain.

Horizontal cells and *amacrine* (AM-a-krin) *cells* can regulate communication between photoreceptors and ganglion cells, adjusting the sensitivity of the retina. The effect is comparable to adjusting the contrast on a television. These cells play an important role in the eye's adjustment to dim or brightly lit environments.

THE OPTIC DISC. Axons from an estimated 1 million ganglion cells converge on the **optic disc**, a circular region just medial to the fovea. The optic disc is the origin of the optic nerve (N II) (**Figure 9-11b**). From this point, the axons turn, penetrate the wall of the eye, and proceed toward the diencephalon. Blood vessels that supply the retina pass through the center of the optic nerve and emerge on the surface of the optic disc (**Figure 9-11b,c**). The optic disc has no photoreceptors or other retinal structures. This area is commonly called the **blind spot** because light striking it goes unnoticed.

Why don't you see a blank spot in your field of vision? The reason is because involuntary eye movements keep the visual image moving and allow your brain to fill in the missing information. Try the simple activity in **Figure 9-12** to prove that a blind spot really exists in your field of vision.

The Chambers of the Eye

The ciliary body and lens divide the interior of the eye into the small anterior cavity and the larger posterior cavity, or vitreous chamber (**Figure 9-13**). Recall that the anterior cavity is further subdivided into the **anterior chamber**, which extends from the cornea to the iris, and the **posterior chamber**, between the iris and the ciliary body and lens.

Figure 9-12 A Demonstration of the Presence of a Blind Spot. Close your left eye and stare at the plus sign with your right eye, keeping the plus sign in the center of your field of vision. Begin with the page a few inches away from your eye, and gradually increase the distance. The dot will disappear when its image falls on the blind spot, at your optic disc. To check the blind spot in your left eye, close your right eye, and repeat the sequence while you stare at the dot.

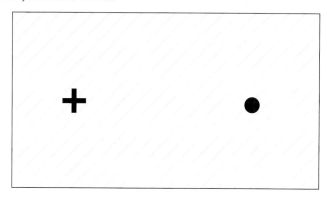

Aqueous humor fills both chambers. This fluid circulates within the anterior cavity, passing from the posterior to the anterior chamber through the pupil. Aqueous humor also circulates within the posterior cavity, but most of this cavity is filled with a clear gelatinous substance known as the **vitreous body**. The vitreous body helps maintain the shape of the eye. It also holds the retina against the choroid.

AQUEOUS HUMOR. Aqueous humor is secreted into the posterior chamber by epithelial cells of the ciliary processes (**Figure 9-13**). Pressure exerted by this fluid helps maintain the shape of the eye. Circulation of aqueous humor transports nutrients and wastes. In the anterior chamber near the edge of the iris, the aqueous humor enters the **scleral venous sinus** (*canal of Schlemm*). This passageway empties into veins in the sclera and returns the aqueous humor to the venous system.

Interference with the normal circulation and reabsorption of aqueous humor leads to greater pressure inside the eye. If this condition, called **glaucoma**, is left untreated, it can eventually produce blindness by distorting the retina and the optic disc.

The Lens

The **lens** lies posterior to the cornea and is held in place by the ciliary zonule that originates on the ciliary body of the choroid. The primary function of the lens is to focus the visual image on the photoreceptors. The lens does so by changing its shape.

THE STRUCTURE OF THE LENS. The transparent lens consists of concentric layers of cells wrapped in a dense fibrous capsule. The cells making up the interior of the lens lack

Figure 9-13 The Circulation of Aqueous Humor. Aqueous humor, which is secreted at the ciliary body, circulates through the posterior and anterior chambers before it is reabsorbed through the scleral venous sinus.

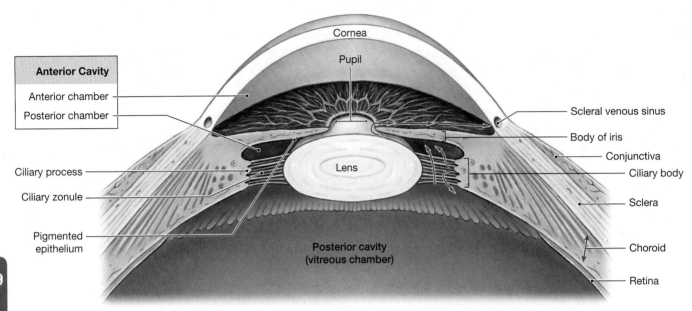

organelles and are filled with transparent proteins. The capsule contains many elastic fibers that, in the absence of any outside force, contract and make the lens spherical. However, tension in the fibers of the ciliary zonule can overpower their contraction and pull the lens into a flattened oval.

LIGHT REFRACTION AND ACCOMMODATION. The eye is often compared to a camera. To provide useful information, the lens of the eye, like a camera lens, must focus the arriving image. To say that an image is "in focus" means that the rays of light arriving from an object strike the sensitive surface of the retina (or the semiconductor device that records light electronically in a digital camera) so as to form a sharp miniature image of the original. If the rays are not perfectly focused, the image will be blurry. Focusing normally occurs in two steps, as light passes first through the cornea and then the lens.

CLINICAL NOTE

Hyphema

Blunt trauma to the eye can rupture one of the blood vessels within the iris, and cause blood to enter the anterior chamber of the eye. Blood in the anterior chamber, called a *hyphema*, is a serious emergency (**Figure 9-14**). The amount of blood in the chamber can range from microscopic to the so-called eight-ball hyphema, where blood fills the entire anterior chamber. Up to one-third of patients will suffer a rebleed within 3–5 days, and these rebleeds are often worse than the original bleed. Complications of hyphema include reduced vision, secondary glaucoma, and staining of the cornea.

Treatment of hyphema includes use of medications that reduce pressure within the anterior chamber and anti-inflammatory medicines. Some patients require hospitalization and complete bed rest for up to 5 days to prevent clot dislodgement and rebleeding. Patients who suffer a hyphema have the best outcome when the injury is promptly recognized and ophthalmologic care is given.

Figure 9-14 Hyphema. Hyphema is the presence of blood in the anterior chamber. Notice the blood level in chamber. Hyphemas can be sight-threatening emergencies

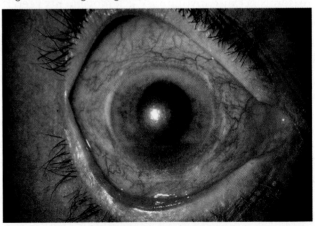

CLINICAL NOTE

Cataracts

The transparency of the lens depends on the transparent proteins maintaining a precise combination of structural and biochemical characteristics. When that balance is disturbed, the lens loses its transparency, a condition known as a cataract. Cataracts can result from drug reactions, injuries, or ultraviolet radiation from sunlight or other sources. Senile cataracts, however, are a natural consequence of aging and the most common form. Over time, the lens becomes less elastic, takes on a yellowish hue, and eventually begins to lose its transparency. As the lens becomes opaque, or "cloudy," the individual needs brighter and brighter reading light, and visual clarity fades. If the lens becomes completely opaque, the person will be functionally blind, even though the photoreceptors are normal. Surgical treatment involves removing the lens and replacing it with an artificial substitute.

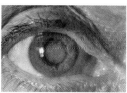

Light is **refracted**, or bent, when it passes from one medium to a medium with a different density. In the human eye, the greatest amount of refraction (bending) occurs when light passes from the air into the cornea, which has a density close to that of water. Then as the light enters the relatively dense lens, the lens provides the extra refraction needed to focus the light rays from an object toward a specific **focal point**—the point at which the light rays converge (**Figure 9-15a**). The distance between the center of the lens and its focal point is the **focal distance** of the lens. Two factors determine the focal distance:

1. *The distance of the object from the lens.* The closer an object is to the lens, the greater the focal distance (**Figure 9-15a,b**).

2. *The shape of the lens.* The rounder the lens, the more refraction occurs. A round lens has a shorter focal distance than a flatter one (**Figure 9-15b,c**).

In the eye, the lens changes shape to keep the focal distance constant so the image remains focused on the retina. **Accommodation** is this process of focusing an image on the retina by changing the shape of the lens (**Figure 9-15d,e**). During accommodation, the lens becomes rounder to focus the image of a nearby object on the retina. The lens becomes flatter to focus the image of a distant object on the retina.

Figure 9-15 Focal Point, Focal Distance, and Visual Accommodation. A lens refracts light toward a specific focal point. The distance from the center of the lens to that point is the focal distance of the lens.

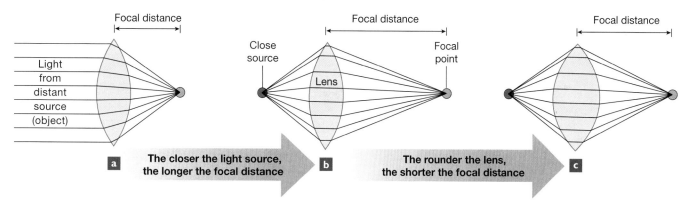

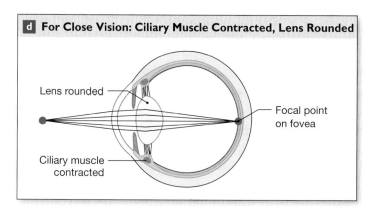

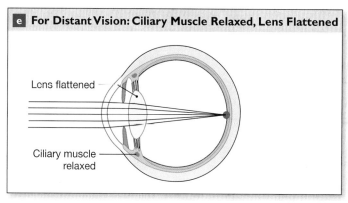

How does the lens change shape? The lens is held in place by the ciliary zonule that originates at the ciliary body. Smooth muscle fibers in the ciliary body encircle the lens and act like sphincter muscles. As you view a nearby object, the ciliary muscle contracts, and the ciliary body moves toward the lens (**Figure 9-15d**). This movement reduces the tension in the ciliary zonule, allowing the elastic capsule to pull the lens into a more rounded shape with greater refractive (bending) power. When you view a distant object, the ciliary muscle relaxes, the ciliary zonule pulls at the circumference of the lens, and the lens becomes flatter (**Figure 9-15e**).

IMAGE FORMATION. The image of an object reaching the retina is a miniature image of the original, but it is upside down and backward. The brain compensates for both aspects of image reversal without our conscious awareness. The reversal takes place because an object we see is really a complex light source having a large number of individual points of light. Light from each point is focused on the retina.

Figure 9-16 Image Formation. (Note that these illustrations are not drawn to scale. In reality, the fovea occupies a small area of the retina, and the projected images are very tiny. Here the crossover of light rays is shown in the lens, but it actually occurs very close to the fovea.)

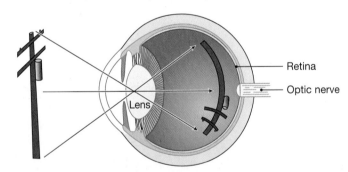

a Light rays projected from a vertical object show why the image arrives upside down. (Note that the image is also reversed.)

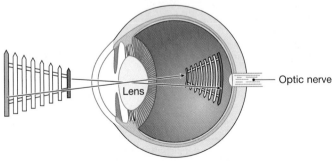

b Light rays projected from a horizontal object show why the image arrives with a left and right reversal. The image also arrives upside down. (As noted in the text, these representations are not drawn to scale.)

Figure 9-16a is a sagittal section through an eye that is looking at a telephone pole. It shows why an image formed on the retina is upside down. Light from the top of the pole is focused on the lower surface of the retina, and light from the bottom of the pole is focused on the upper surface of the retina.

Figure 9-16b is a horizontal section through an eye that is looking at a picket fence. It shows why an image formed on the retina is backward. Light from the left side of the fence falls on the right side of the retina, and light from the right side of the fence falls on the left side of the retina.

If the light passing through the cornea and lens is not refracted properly, the visual image will be distorted. In the condition called **astigmatism**, the degree of curvature in the cornea or lens varies. Minor astigmatism is very common. The image distortion may be so minimal that people are unaware of the condition. Several other visual abnormalities are described in **Spotlight Figure 9-17**.

CHECKPOINT

11. What superficial accessory structure of the eye would be the first to be affected by inadequate tear production?

12. When the lens is more rounded, are you looking at an object that is close to you or far from you?

13. As Malia enters a dimly lit room, most of the available light becomes focused on the fovea of her eye. Will she be able to see very clearly?

See the blue Answers tab at the back of the book.

9-6 Photoreceptors respond to light and change it into electrical signals essential to visual physiology

Learning Objective Explain how we form visual images and distinguish colors, and discuss how the central nervous system processes visual information.

The rods and cones of the retina are called *photoreceptors* because they detect *photons*, basic units of visible light. Light is a form of radiant energy that travels in waves with a characteristic wavelength (distance between wave peaks). Our eyes are sensitive to wavelengths that make up the spectrum of **visible light** (700–400 nm). Remember this spectrum, as seen in a rainbow, by the acronym ROY G. BIV (*Red, Orange, Yellow, Green, Blue, Indigo, Violet*). Color depends on the wavelength of the light. Photons of red light have the longest wavelength and carry the least energy. Photons from the

A camera focuses an image by moving the lens toward or away from the film or semiconductor device. This method cannot work in our eyes, because the distance from the lens to the macula cannot change. We focus images on the retina by changing the shape of the lens to keep the focal distance constant.

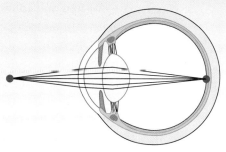

The eye has a fixed focal distance and focuses by varying the shape of the lens.

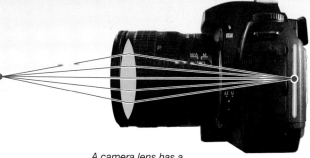

A camera lens has a fixed size and shape and focuses by varying the distance to the film or semiconductor device.

Emmetropia
(normal vision)

In the healthy eye, when the ciliary muscle is relaxed and the lens is flattened, a distant image will be focused on the retina's surface. This condition is called **emmetropia** (*emmetro-*, proper + *opia*, vision).

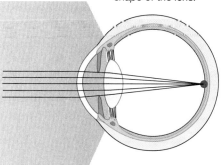

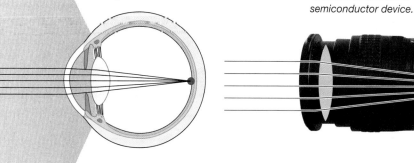

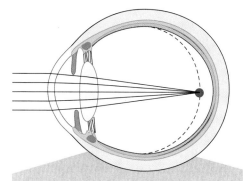

Myopia (nearsightedness)

If the eyeball is too deep or the resting curvature of the lens is too great, the image of a distant object is projected in front of the retina. The person will see distant objects as blurry and out of focus. Vision at close range will be normal because the lens is able to round as needed to focus the image on the retina.

Myopia corrected with a diverging, concave lens

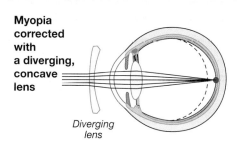

Diverging lens

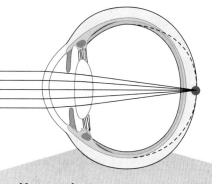

Hyperopia (farsightedness)

If the eyeball is too shallow or the lens is too flat, hyperopia results. The ciliary muscle must contract to focus even a distant object on the retina. And at close range, the lens cannot provide enough refraction to focus an image on the retina. Older people become farsighted as their lenses lose elasticity, a form of hyperopia called **presbyopia** (*presbys*, old man).

Hyperopia corrected with a converging, convex lens

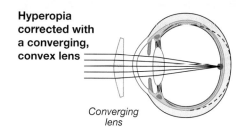

Converging lens

Surgical Correction

Variable success at correcting myopia and hyperopia has been achieved by surgery that reshapes the cornea. In **photorefractive keratectomy** (PRK) a computer-guided laser shapes the cornea to exact specifications. The entire procedure can be done in less than a minute. A variation on PRK is called *LASIK* (*laser-assisted in-situ keratomileusis*). In this procedure, the interior layers of the cornea are reshaped and then re-covered by the flap of original outer corneal epithelium. Roughly 70 percent of LASIK patients achieve normal vision, and LASIK has become the most common form of refractive surgery.

Even after surgery, many patients still need reading glasses, and both immediate and long-term visual problems can occur.

violet portion of the spectrum have the shortest wavelength and carry the most energy.

Rods and Cones

Rods provide the CNS with information about the presence or absence of photons, without regard to wavelength. For this reason, they do not discriminate among colors of light. They are very sensitive, however, and enable us to see in dim conditions.

Cones provide information about the wavelength of photons. Because cones are less sensitive than rods, they function only in relatively bright light. We have three types of cones: *blue cones, green cones*, and *red cones*. Each type contains pigments sensitive to blue, green, or red wavelengths of light. Their stimulation in various combinations accounts for our perception of colors.

Persons unable to distinguish certain colors have a form of **color blindness**. The standard tests for color vision involve picking numbers or letters out of a complex image, such as the one in **Figure 9-18**. Color blindness occurs when one or more classes of cones are absent or nonfunctional. Red-green color blindness is the most common kind. In this condition, the red cones are missing and the individual cannot distinguish red light from green light. Ten percent of all males have some color blindness, but the incidence among females is only around 0.67 percent. Total color blindness is extremely rare. Only one person in 300,000 has no cone pigments of any kind.

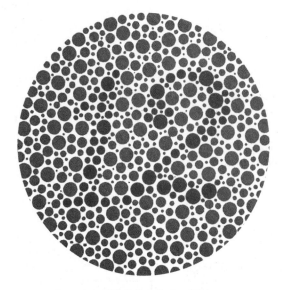

Figure 9-18 A Standard Test for Color Vision. Individuals who lack one or more populations of cones are unable to distinguish the patterned image (the number 12).

Photoreceptor Structure

The structure of rods and cones is compared in **Figure 9-19a**. The *outer segment* of a photoreceptor contains hundreds to thousands of flattened membranous discs. The names *rod* and *cone* refer to the outer segment's shape. The *inner segment* of a photoreceptor contains typical cellular organelles and forms synapses with other cells. In the dark, each photoreceptor continually releases neurotransmitters. The arrival of a photon starts a chain of events that alters the membrane potential of the photoreceptor and changes the rate of neurotransmitter release.

The discs of the outer segment in both rods and cones contain special organic compounds called **visual pigments**. The visual pigments are derived from the compound **rhodopsin** (rō-DOP-sin). Rhodopsin consists of a protein, **opsin**, bound to the pigment **retinal** (RET-i-nal) (**Figure 9-19b**). Retinal is synthesized from **vitamin A**. Retinal is identical in both rods and cones, but a different form of opsin is found in the rods and in each of the three types of cones (red, blue, and green).

Photoreception

The process of *photoreception* is the detection of light. The absorption of photons by visual pigments is the first key step. Photoreception begins when a photon strikes a rhodopsin molecule in the outer segment of a photoreceptor. When the photon is absorbed, a change in the shape of the retinal component activates opsin. Opsin activation starts a chain of enzyme-driven events that alters the rate of neurotransmitter release. This change is the signal that light has struck a photoreceptor at that particular location on the retina.

Shortly after the retinal changes shape, the rhodopsin molecule begins to break down into retinal and opsin, a process

CLINICAL NOTE

Visual Acuity

How well you see, or visual acuity, is rated on the basis of the sight of a "normal" person. A person whose vision is rated 20/20 can see details at a distance of 20 feet as clearly as a "normal" individual would. Vision rated 20/15 is better than average, for at 20 feet the person is able to see details that would be clear to a "normal" eye only at a distance of 15 feet. Conversely, a person with 20/30 vision must be 20 feet from an object to discern details that a person with "normal" vision could make out at a distance of 30 feet.

Figure 9-19 The Structure of Rods and Cones.

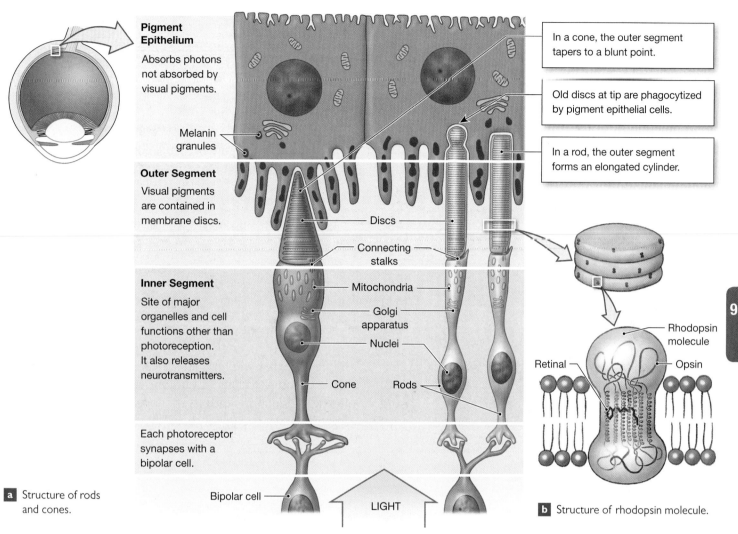

Pigment Epithelium

Absorbs photons not absorbed by visual pigments.

In a cone, the outer segment tapers to a blunt point.

Old discs at tip are phagocytized by pigment epithelial cells.

Melanin granules

In a rod, the outer segment forms an elongated cylinder.

Outer Segment

Visual pigments are contained in membrane discs.

Discs

Connecting stalks

Inner Segment

Site of major organelles and cell functions other than photoreception. It also releases neurotransmitters.

Mitochondria

Golgi apparatus

Nuclei

Cone   Rods

Rhodopsin molecule

Retinal   Opsin

Each photoreceptor synapses with a bipolar cell.

Bipolar cell

LIGHT

a Structure of rods and cones.

b Structure of rhodopsin molecule.

CLINICAL NOTE

Accommodation Problems

In the normal eye, when the ciliary muscles are relaxed and the lens is flattened, a distant image will be focused on the retinal surface (**Figure 9-20a**), which is a condition called *emmetropia* (*emmetro-*, proper measure). However, irregularities in the shape of the lens or cornea can affect refraction and the clarity of the resulting visual image. This condition, called *astigmatism*, can usually be corrected by glasses or special contact lenses.

Figure 9-20 also diagrams two common accommodation problems. If the eyeball is too deep, the image of a distant object will form in front of the retina, and the image will be blurry and out of focus (**Figure 9-20b**). Vision at close range will be normal, because the lens will be able to round up enough to focus the image on the retina. As a result, such individuals are said to be "near-sighted." Their condition is more formally termed *myopia* (*myein*, to shut + *ops*, eye). Myopia can be corrected by placing a diverging lens in front of the eye (**Figure 9-20c**).

If the eyeball is too shallow, *hyperopia* results (**Figure 9-20d**). The ciliary muscles must contract to focus even a distant object on the

retina, and at close range the lens cannot provide enough refraction. These individuals are said to be "farsighted" because they can see distant objects most clearly. Older individuals become far-sighted as their lenses lose elasticity; this form of hyperopia is called *presbyopia* (*presbys*, old man). Hyperopia can be treated by placing a converging lens in front of the eye (**Figure 9-20e**).

Variable success at correcting myopia and hyperopia has been achieved by surgically reshaping the cornea to alter its refractive powers. In *radial keratotomy*, several corneal incisions flatten the surface. Some scarring and localized corneal weakness may occur, and only two-thirds of patients are satisfied with the results. In a newer procedure called *photorefractive keratectomy* (PRK), a computer-guided laser shapes the cornea to exact specifications. Tissue is removed only to a depth of 10–20 μm more than about 10 percent of the cornea's thickness. The entire procedure can be done in less than a minute. Each year, an estimated 100,000 people undergo the PRK procedure in the U.S. Corneal scarring is rare; however, many still need reading glasses, and both immediate and long-term visual problems can occur.

(Continued)

9

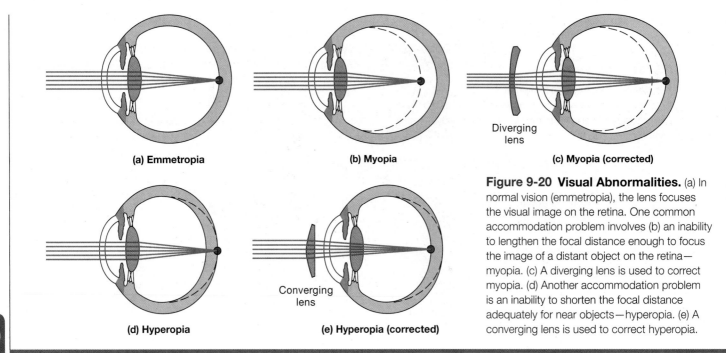

(a) Emmetropia

(b) Myopia

Diverging lens

(c) Myopia (corrected)

Converging lens

(d) Hyperopia

(e) Hyperopia (corrected)

Figure 9-20 Visual Abnormalities. (a) In normal vision (emmetropia), the lens focuses the visual image on the retina. One common accommodation problem involves (b) an inability to lengthen the focal distance enough to focus the image of a distant object on the retina—myopia. (c) A diverging lens is used to correct myopia. (d) Another accommodation problem is an inability to shorten the focal distance adequately for near objects—hyperopia. (e) A converging lens is used to correct hyperopia.

known as **bleaching** (**Figure 9-21**). The retinal must be converted back to its former shape before it can recombine with opsin. This conversion uses energy in the form of ATP, and it takes time. Bleaching contributes to the lingering visual impression that you have after a camera's flash. After an intense exposure to light, a photoreceptor cannot respond to further stimulation until its rhodopsin molecules have been regenerated. As a result, a "ghost" image remains on the retina.

Figure 9-21 Bleaching and Regeneration of Visual Pigments.

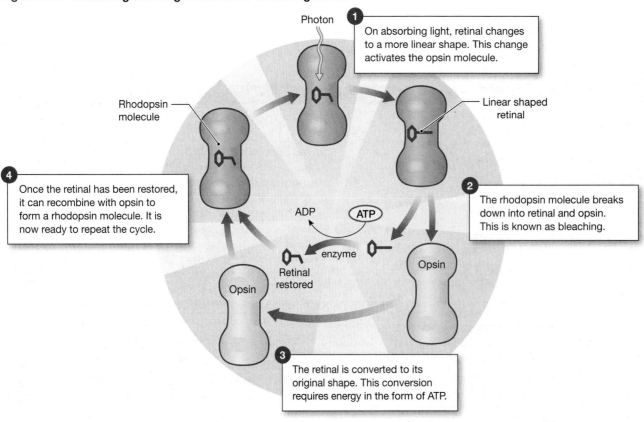

Photon

1 On absorbing light, retinal changes to a more linear shape. This change activates the opsin molecule.

Rhodopsin molecule

Linear shaped retinal

4 Once the retinal has been restored, it can recombine with opsin to form a rhodopsin molecule. It is now ready to repeat the cycle.

ADP   ATP

2 The rhodopsin molecule breaks down into retinal and opsin. This is known as bleaching.

enzyme

Opsin

Opsin

Retinal restored

Opsin

3 The retinal is converted to its original shape. This conversion requires energy in the form of ATP.

CLINICAL NOTE

Night Blindness

The visual pigments of the photoreceptors are synthesized from vitamin A. The body contains vitamin A reserves for several months, and a significant amount is stored in the cells of the pigmented part of the retina. If dietary sources are inadequate, these reserves are gradually exhausted, and the amount of visual pigment in the photoreceptors begins to decline. Daylight vision is affected. However, in daytime, the light is usually bright enough to stimulate any remaining visual pigments in the cones. As a result, the problem first becomes apparent at night, when the dim light cannot activate the rods. This condition, known as night blindness, can be treated by administering vitamin A. The body can convert the carotene pigments in many vegetables to vitamin A. Carrots are a particularly good source of carotene, which explains the old saying that carrots are good for your eyesight.

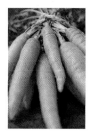

The Visual Pathways

The visual pathways begin at the photoreceptors and end at the visual cortex of the cerebral hemispheres. In other sensory pathways we have examined, at most one synapse lies between a receptor and a sensory neuron that delivers information to the CNS. In the visual pathways, the message must cross two synapses (photoreceptor to bipolar cell, and bipolar cell to ganglion cell). Only then does it move toward the brain. Axons from all the ganglion cells converge on the optic disc, penetrate the wall of the eye, and proceed toward the diencephalon as the optic nerve (N II).

The two optic nerves, one from each eye, meet at the optic chiasm (**Figure 9-22**). From that point, approximately half of the fibers of each optic nerve proceed within the optic tracts toward the thalamic nucleus on the same side of the brain. The other half cross over to reach the thalamic nucleus on the opposite side. These thalamic nuclei act as switching and processing centers. They relay visual information to reflex centers in the brain stem as well as to the cerebral cortex. The visual information received by the *superior colliculi* (midbrain nuclei in the brain stem) controls constriction or dilation of the pupils and reflexes that control eye movement. ⊃ p. 277

The sensation of vision arises from the integration of information arriving at the visual cortex of the cerebrum. The visual cortex of each occipital lobe contains a sensory map of the entire field of vision. As with the primary sensory cortex, the map does not faithfully duplicate the relative areas within the sensory field. For example, the area assigned to the fovea covers about 35 times the surface it would cover if the map were proportionally accurate.

Figure 9-22 The Visual Pathways. At the optic chiasm, a partial crossover of nerve fibers occurs. As a result, each hemisphere receives visual information from the lateral half of the retina on that side and from the medial half of the retina on the opposite side. Visual association areas in the cerebrum integrate this information to develop a composite picture of the entire visual field.

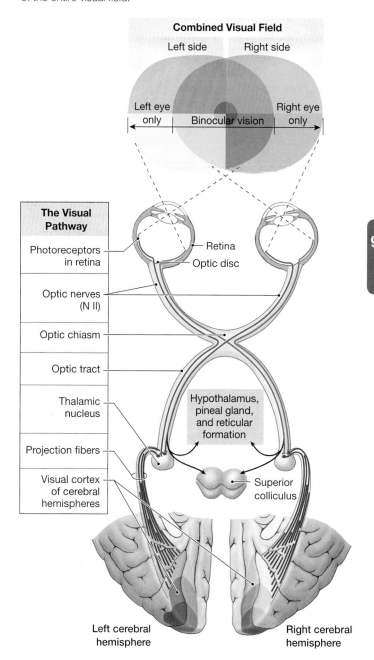

Many centers in the brain stem receive visual information from the thalamic nuclei or over collaterals from the optic tracts. For example, some collaterals bypass the thalamic nuclei and synapse in the hypothalamus. Visual inputs there and at the pineal gland establish a daily pattern of visceral activity that is tied to the day–night cycle. This *circadian* (*circa*, about + *dies*, day) *rhythm* affects your metabolic rate, endocrine function, blood pressure, digestive activities, sleep-wake cycle, and other processes.

CLINICAL NOTE

Eye Emergencies

Vision is one of our most important senses. The eyes are the principle sensory organs of vision, and emergencies that involve the eye can threaten sight. Because of this, detailed evaluation and treatment of emergent eye illnesses and emergencies are essential. Two types of doctors specialize in treating eye disorders: ophthalmologists and optometrists. *Ophthalmologists* are physicians (M.D. or D.O.) who have graduated from medical school and completed a residency in ophthalmology. They specialize in the medical and surgical management of eye disorders. Optometrists are doctors of optometry (O.D.) who have completed four years of optometry school. They primarily perform refractive examinations and prescribe glasses and contact lenses. Optometrists do not perform surgery and, in many states, do not prescribe medication.

Conjunctival Injuries

Acute eye pain or a red eye are the most common initial complaints of patients with an ocular emergency. Injuries to the eye are common. One of the most striking eye injuries is a subconjunctival hemorrhage. Trauma can cause the fragile blood vessels within the conjunctiva to rupture. The bleeding is evident as it occurs over the white of the eye. In addition to trauma, sneezing, coughing, vomiting, and straining can cause a subconjunctival hemorrhage. High blood pressure also can cause a conjunctival hemorrhage. In many cases, a specific cause cannot be identified. Subconjunctival hemorrhages are painless, do not affect vision, generally do not require treatment, and resolve completely within a week or two. Abrasions of the conjunctival membranes, which are also common, heal completely within two to three days (**Figure 9-23**).

Figure 9-23 Conjunctival Abrasion. A conjunctival foreign body and abrasion overlie a large subconjunctival hemorrhage.

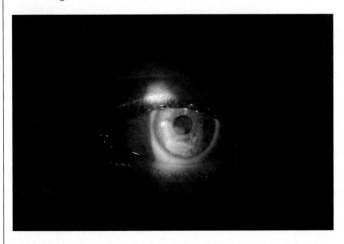

Corneal Injuries

Trauma to the cornea can cause an abrasion. In addition to trauma, corneal abrasions can develop from contact lens wear. Pain, redness, tearing, and light sensitivity usually accompany a corneal abrasion. Assessment of corneal abrasions is often difficult because of the patient's discomfort. Often, these patients feel as though a foreign body is embedded in the eye, and they often worsen the abrasion by trying to remove the perceived foreign body. Usually, a drop or two of topical ophthalmic anesthetic will provide rapid pain relief so that an adequate examination can be carried out. Under magnification, a defect in the cornea can usually be seen. Corneal abrasions can be visualized by staining the eye with fluorescein. The injured cornea takes up the fluorescein, and examination under an ultraviolet light will clearly demonstrate the injury. Corneal abrasions usually heal within a matter of days. Treatment includes analgesics and placement of antibiotic drops or ointment.

Small particles, such as dust or metal fragments, can become embedded in the cornea. These corneal foreign bodies cause an underlying abrasion. Most foreign bodies are superficial and can be removed in the emergency department. A ring of rust may develop around metallic foreign bodies that are embedded more than 24 hours. The rust must be removed or it will permanently scar the cornea. Following removal of a corneal foreign body, it is important to evert the eyelid to make sure a second foreign body is not present.

Blunt Eye Trauma

Blunt trauma to the eye can cause swelling of the lids and the periorbital tissues. A direct blow to the eye can result in a *hyphema*, which is bleeding into the anterior chamber. A hyphema is a serious injury that can result in permanent blindness and should always be evaluated by an ophthalmologist. Hyphemas can cause increased pressures within the eye and permanent injury. The patient's head should be elevated to help decrease intraocular pressure. Spontaneous rebleeding is not uncommon with hyphemas.

Blunt trauma to the eye can sometimes result in a blowout fracture, which is a fracture of the wall or walls of the orbit. Most frequently, the inferior wall of the orbit is fractured into the maxillary sinus. Occasionally, the inferior rectus muscle may be entrapped in the fracture, preventing the eye from moving superiorly (looking up). The patient may report double vision on upward gaze. Blowout fractures require surgical treatment (**Figure 9-24**).

Penetrating Eye Injury

Any injury that penetrates the globe or ruptures the globe is extremely serious. Common causes include BB pellets, lawn mower projectiles, particles from hammering, grinding injuries, knife wounds, and gunshot wounds. Any penetrating injury has the potential for entering the eye. If a ruptured globe is

Figure 9-24 Trauma to the Right Eye. Significant trauma, such as this upper lid laceration, necessitates a detailed examination for other injuries such as a blowout fracture.

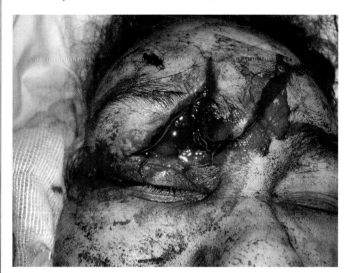

Figure 9-25 Blunt Facial Trauma that Results in Enucleation of the Right Eye. The globe should be carefully protected and the patient transported to a facility with ophthalmological surgery capabilities.

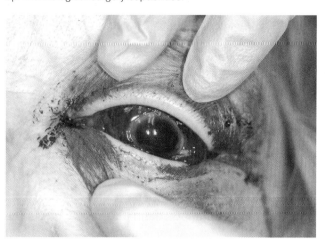

suspected, a protective shield should be immediately placed over the affected eye, and the patient should be kept calm to prevent exacerbating the injury (**Figure 9-25**).

Chemical Injuries

Chemical injuries to the eye are common. The severity of a chemical injury is directly related to the chemical agent involved. To help remove the offending agent immediately following a chemical injury, the eye should be irrigated with copious amounts of water for 10 minutes (if the chemical was an alkali, irrigation is carried out longer until pH of tears returns to normal). Following this, a detailed examination of the affected eye, including possible fluorescein staining, should be carried out to determine the severity of tissue injury.

Ultraviolet Keratitis

Ultraviolet keratitis is severe pain, tearing, light sensitivity, and foreign-body sensation that occurs from 6 to 12 hours after

ocular exposure to a welding arc, tanning lights, or bright snow. Often, the patient is awakened with severe eye pain and tearing. This injury can be extremely painful but responds readily to topical anesthetics. It usually resolves in 24–48 hours.

Acute Glaucoma

Failure of the aqueous humor to enter the canal of Schlemm leads to glaucoma. Although drainage is impaired, the production of aqueous humor continues, and the intraocular pressure begins to rise. As this progresses, the soft tissues within the eye become distorted. *Acute angle-closure glaucoma* is a serious medical emergency. The patient often complains of cloudy vision, eye ache, headache, and frequently nausea and vomiting. Usually, there is no history of glaucoma. Acute angle-closure glaucoma requires hospitalization and treatment with medications that decrease intraocular pressure.

The term *blindness* implies a total absence of vision due to damage to the eyes or to the optic pathways. Common causes of blindness include diabetes mellitus, cataracts, glaucoma, corneal scarring, retinal detachment, accidental injuries, and hereditary factors that are as yet poorly understood.

CHECKPOINT

14. If you had been born without cone cells in your eyes, would you still be able to see? Explain.

15. How could a diet deficient in vitamin A affect vision?

See the blue Answers tab at the back of the book.

9-7 Equilibrium sensations originate within the internal ear, while hearing involves the detection and interpretation of sound waves

Learning Objective Describe the parts of the external, middle, and internal ear, and the receptors they contain, and discuss the processes involved in the senses of equilibrium and hearing.

The *internal ear,* a receptor complex located in the temporal bone of the skull, provides us with the special senses of equilibrium and hearing. ⊃ p. 157 *Equilibrium* informs us of the position of the body in space by monitoring gravity, linear acceleration, and rotation. *Hearing* enables us to detect and interpret sound waves.

The basic receptor process for these senses is the same. The receptors—*hair cells*—are mechanoreceptors. The complex structure of the internal ear and the different arrangements of accessory structures permit hair cells to respond to different stimuli and to provide the input for both senses.

Anatomy of the Ear

The ear is divided into three anatomical regions: the external ear, the middle ear, and the internal ear (**Figure 9-26**). The *external ear* is the visible portion of the ear. It collects and directs sound waves toward the *middle ear*, a chamber located in a thickened portion of the temporal bone. Structures of the middle ear collect and amplify sound waves and transmit them to an appropriate portion of the internal ear. The *internal ear* contains the sensory organs for both hearing and equilibrium.

The External Ear

The **external ear** includes the fleshy and cartilaginous **auricle**, or *pinna*, which surrounds a passageway called the **external acoustic meatus**, or *auditory canal*. The auricle protects the opening of the canal and provides directional sensitivity. Sounds coming from behind the head are blocked by the auricle, but sounds coming from the side or front are collected and channeled into the external auditory meatus. (When you "cup" your ear with your hand to hear a faint sound more clearly, you are exaggerating this effect.)

Ceruminous (se-ROO-mi-nus) **glands** along the external acoustic meatus secrete a waxy material called *cerumen*. It helps prevent the entry of foreign objects and insects. The canal is also lined with many small, outwardly projecting hairs. They trap debris and provide tactile sensations through their root hair plexuses. ↪ p. 309 The waxy

Figure 9-26 The Anatomy of the Ear. The boundaries separating the three regions of the ear (external, middle, and internal) are roughly marked by the dashed lines.

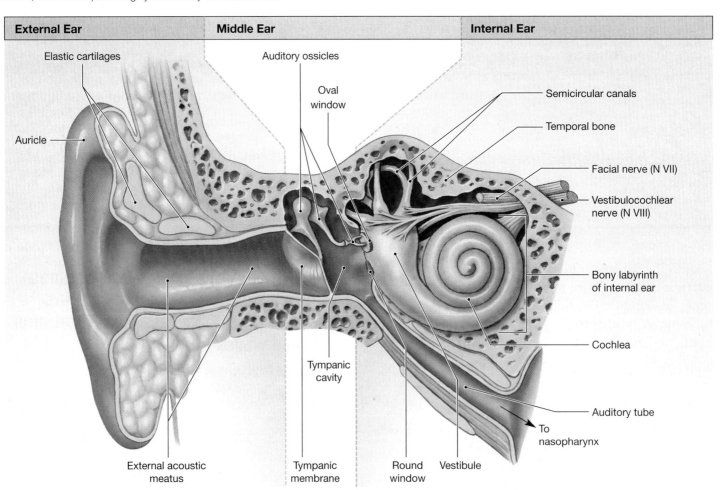

External Ear	Middle Ear	Internal Ear

cerumen also slows the growth of microorganisms and reduces the likelihood of infection.

The external acoustic meatus ends at the **tympanic membrane** (*tympanon*, drum) or *eardrum*. This thin, semitransparent sheet separates the external ear from the middle ear (**Figure 9-26**)

The Middle Ear

The **middle ear**, or *tympanic cavity*, is an air-filled chamber separated from the external acoustic meatus by the tympanic membrane. The middle ear communicates with the superior portion of the pharynx, a region known as the *nasopharynx*, and with *air cells* in the mastoid process of the temporal bone.

The connection with the nasopharynx is the **auditory tube**, also called the *pharyngotympanic tube* or the *Eustachian tube* (**Figure 9-27**). The auditory tube enables the equalization of pressure on either side of the eardrum. Unfortunately, it can also allow microorganisms to travel from the nasopharynx into the middle ear, leading to an unpleasant middle ear infection known as *otitis media*.

THE AUDITORY OSSICLES. The middle ear contains three tiny ear bones, collectively called **auditory ossicles**. These ear bones connect the tympanic membrane with the receptor

complex of the internal ear (**Figure 9-27**). The three auditory ossicles are the malleus, the incus, and the stapes. The **malleus** (*malleus*, hammer) attaches at three points to the interior surface of the tympanic membrane. The middle bone—the **incus** (*incus*, anvil)—attaches the malleus to the inner bone, the **stapes** (*stapes*, stirrup). The base of the stapes almost completely fills the oval window. The *oval window* is a small, membrane-covered opening in the temporal bone that surrounds the internal ear.

Vibration of the tympanic membrane converts arriving sound energy into mechanical movements of the auditory ossicles. The ossicles act as levers that collect the force applied to the tympanic membrane and focus it on the oval window. Because the tympanic membrane is larger and heavier than the delicate membrane of the oval window, the amount of movement is markedly increased.

This amplification in movement enables us to hear very faint sounds. It can also be a problem, however, when we are exposed to very loud noises. In the middle ear, two small muscles protect the eardrum and ossicles from violent movements under noisy conditions. The *tensor tympani* (TEN-sor tim-PAN-ē) *muscle* pulls on the malleus. This action increases the stiffness of the tympanic membrane and reduces the amount of possible movement. The *stapedius* (sta-PĒ-dē-us) *muscle* pulls on the stapes, reducing its movement at the oval window.

The Internal Ear

Receptors within the **internal ear** (**Figures 9-26** and **9-28**) give us our senses of equilibrium and hearing. These receptors are protected by the **bony labyrinth**, whose outer walls are fused with the surrounding temporal bone. The bony labyrinth surrounds and protects the **membranous labyrinth** (*labyrinthos*, network of canals), a collection of tubes and chambers that follow the contours of the bony labyrinth. These tubes and chambers are filled with a fluid called **endolymph** (EN-dō-limf). The receptors lie within the membranous labyrinth. Between the bony and membranous labyrinths flows another fluid, the **perilymph** (PER-i-limf) (**Figure 9-28a**).

The bony labyrinth has three major parts (**Figure 9-28b**):

1. *Vestibule.* The **vestibule** (VES-ti-būl) includes a pair of membranous sacs, the **saccule** (SAK-ūl) and the **utricle** (Ū-tri-kul). Receptors in these sacs provide sensations of gravity and linear acceleration.

2. *Semicircular canals.* The **semicircular canals** enclose slender **semicircular ducts**. Receptors in the

Figure 9-27 The Middle Ear.

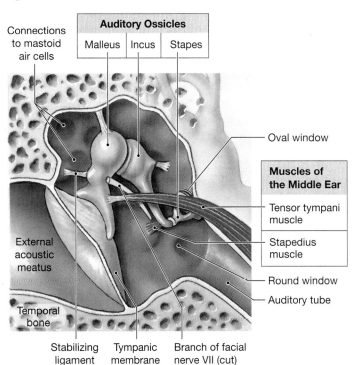

Auditory Ossicles: Malleus | Incus | Stapes

Connections to mastoid air cells

Oval window

Muscles of the Middle Ear
- Tensor tympani muscle
- Stapedius muscle

External acoustic meatus

Round window

Auditory tube

Temporal bone

Stabilizing ligament | Tympanic membrane | Branch of facial nerve VII (cut)

Figure 9-28 The Internal Ear.

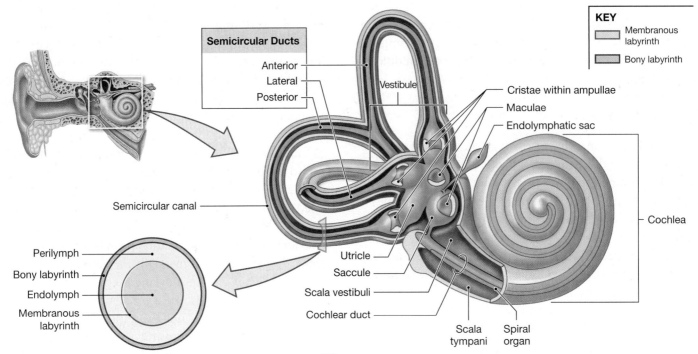

KEY
☐ Membranous labyrinth
☐ Bony labyrinth

Semicircular Ducts
Anterior
Lateral
Posterior

Vestibule

Cristae within ampullae
Maculae
Endolymphatic sac

Cochlea

Semicircular canal

Perilymph
Bony labyrinth
Endolymph
Membranous labyrinth

Utricle
Saccule
Scala vestibuli
Cochlear duct

Scala tympani
Spiral organ

a A section through one of the semicircular canals, showing the relationship between the bony and membranous labyrinths, and the locations of perilymph and endolymph.

b The bony and membranous labyrinths. Areas of the membranous labyrinth containing sensory receptors (cristae, maculae, and spiral organ) are shown in purple.

semicircular ducts are stimulated by rotation of the head. The combination of vestibule and semicircular canals is called the **vestibular complex** because the fluid-filled chambers within the vestibule are continuous with those of the semicircular canals.

3. *Cochlea.* The bony, spiral-shaped **cochlea** (KOK-lē-uh; *cochlea*, snail shell) contains the **cochlear duct** of the membranous labyrinth. Receptors in the cochlear duct provide the sense of hearing. The duct is sandwiched between a pair of perilymph-filled chambers. The entire complex spirals around a central bony hub, much like a snail shell.

The walls of the bony labyrinth are dense bone everywhere except at two small areas near the base of the cochlea. The **round window** is an opening in the bone of the cochlea. A thin membrane spans the opening and separates perilymph in the cochlea from the air-filled middle ear. The membrane spanning the **oval window** is firmly attached to the base of the stapes. Recall that when a sound vibrates the tympanic membrane, the movements are conducted over the malleus and incus to the stapes and oval window. Movement of the stapes ultimately leads to events that stimulate receptors in the cochlear duct, and we hear the sound.

RECEPTOR FUNCTION IN THE INTERNAL EAR. The receptors of the internal ear are called **hair cells**. A representative hair cell

is shown in **Figure 9-29c**. Regardless of location, hair cells are always surrounded by supporting cells and monitored by the dendrites of sensory neurons. Each hair cell communicates with a sensory neuron by continually releasing small quantities of neurotransmitter. The free surface of a hair cell supports 80–100 long microvilli called *stereocilia*. Hair cells do not actively move these stereocilia. Instead, when some external force causes the stereocilia to bend, their movement distorts the cell surface and alters its rate of neurotransmitter release. Displacement of the stereocilia in one direction stimulates the hair cells and increases neurotransmitter release. Displacement in the opposite direction inhibits the hair cells and decreases neurotransmitter release.

Equilibrium

There are two aspects of equilibrium:

1. **dynamic equilibrium**, which aids us in maintaining our balance when the head and body are moved suddenly, and

2. **static equilibrium**, which maintains our posture and stability when the body is motionless.

Hair cells of the vestibular complex provide all equilibrium sensations. The semicircular ducts monitor dynamic equilibrium. They provide information about rotational movements of the head. For example, when you turn your head to the left, receptors in the semicircular ducts tell you how rapid the movement is and in which direction.

The saccule and the utricle monitor static equilibrium. They provide information about the position of your head with respect to gravity. If you stand with your head tilted to one side, receptors in the saccule and utricle will report the angle involved and whether your head is tilting forward or backward. These receptors are also stimulated by sudden changes in velocity. For example, when your car accelerates, these receptors give you the sensation of increasing speed.

The Semicircular Ducts: Rotational Motion

Sensory receptors in the semicircular ducts respond to rotational movements of the head. These hair cells are active during a movement but are quiet when the body is motionless. The **anterior**, **posterior**, and **lateral semicircular ducts** are continuous with the utricle (**Figure 9-29a**). Each semicircular duct contains an **ampulla**, a swollen region that contains the sensory receptors (**Figure 9-29a**). Hair cells attached to the wall of the ampulla form a raised structure known as a

Figure 9-29 The Semicircular Ducts.

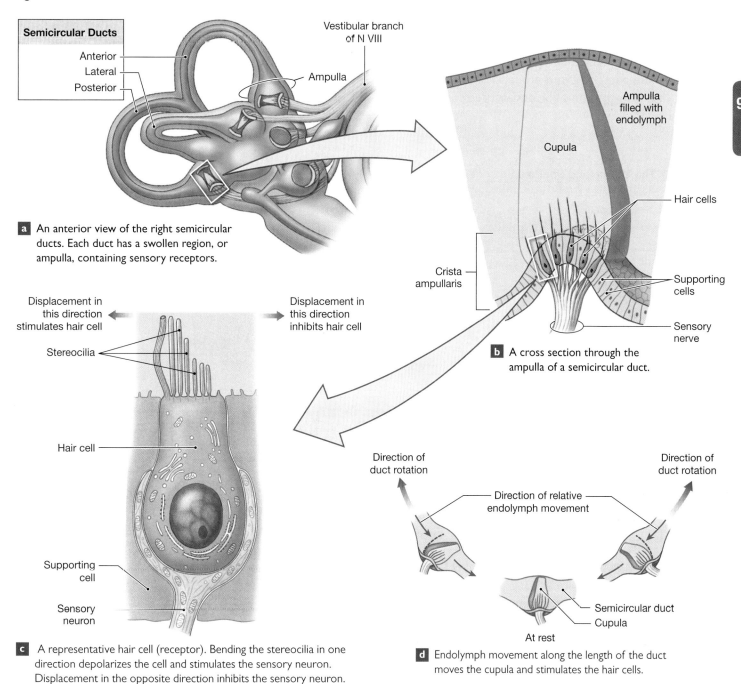

a An anterior view of the right semicircular ducts. Each duct has a swollen region, or ampulla, containing sensory receptors.

b A cross section through the ampulla of a semicircular duct.

c A representative hair cell (receptor). Bending the stereocilia in one direction depolarizes the cell and stimulates the sensory neuron. Displacement in the opposite direction inhibits the sensory neuron.

d Endolymph movement along the length of the duct moves the cupula and stimulates the hair cells.

crista ampullaris, or *crista* (**Figure 9-29b**). The stereocilia of the hair cells are embedded in a gelatinous structure called the **cupula** (KŪ-pū-luh), which nearly fills the ampulla. When the head rotates in the plane of the semicircular duct, movement of the endolymph pushes against this structure and stimulates the hair cells (**Figure 9-29d**).

Each semicircular duct responds to one of three possible rotational movements. To distort the cupula and stimulate the receptors, endolymph must flow along the axis of the duct. Such flow takes place only when there is rotation in that plane. A horizontal rotation, as in shaking the head "no," stimulates the hair cells of the lateral semicircular duct. Nodding "yes" excites receptors of the anterior duct, and tilting the head from side to side activates receptors in the posterior duct. The three planes monitored by the semicircular ducts correspond to the three dimensions in the world around us. The ducts provide accurate information about even the most complex movements.

The Vestibule: Gravity and Linear Acceleration

Receptors in the utricle and saccule respond to gravity and linear acceleration. By responding to gravity, they provide information concerning up and down. Utricle receptors are sensitive to horizontal acceleration. Saccule receptors are sensitive to vertical acceleration. The hair cells of the utricle and saccule are clustered in oval **maculae** (MAK–l; singular *macula*, spot) (**Figure 9-30a**). The hair cell processes in the maculae are embedded in a gelatinous otolithic membrane whose surface contains a thin layer of densely packed calcium carbonate crystals. These calcium carbonate crystals are called **otoliths** (*oto-*, ear + *lithos*, a stone) (**Figure 9-30b**). When the head is in the normal, upright position, the macula in a utricle is oriented horizontally and, in a saccule, vertically. When the head tilts, the pull of gravity on the otoliths shifts their weight to the side, distorting the sensory hairs. The change in receptor activity tells the CNS that the head is no longer level (**Figure 9-30c**).

Figure 9-30 The Utricle and Saccule.

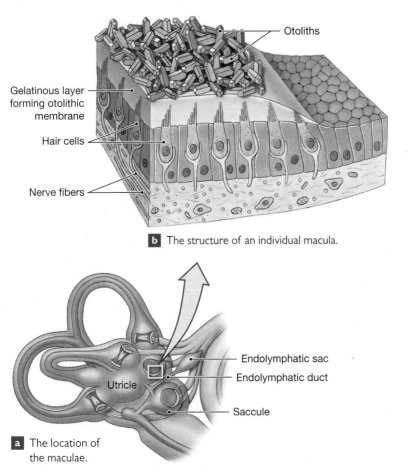

b The structure of an individual macula.

a The location of the maculae.

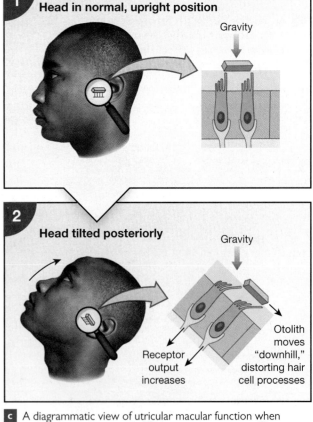

c A diagrammatic view of utricular macular function when the head is held normally ❶ and then tilted back ❷

Otoliths are relatively dense and heavy, and they are connected to the rest of the body only by the sensory processes of the macular hair cells. So whenever the rest of the body makes a sudden movement, the otolith crystals lag behind. For example, you know immediately when an elevator starts downward, because the otoliths within the saccules are displaced upward and bend the stereocilia of the receptor cells. Once they catch up and the elevator has reached a constant speed, you are no longer aware of any movement until the elevator brakes to a halt. As your body slows down, the otoliths of the saccules bend the sensory hairs downward and we "feel" the force of gravity increase.

A similar process accounts for our perception of linear acceleration in a car that speeds up suddenly. The utricle otoliths lag behind, bending the sensory hairs and changing the activity in the sensory neurons. A comparable movement of the otoliths takes place when you raise your chin and gravity pulls the otoliths backward. On the basis of visual information, the brain decides whether the arriving sensations indicate acceleration or a change in head position.

Pathways for Equilibrium Sensations

Sensory neurons monitor hair cells of the vestibule and of the semicircular ducts (**Figure 9-29c**). The fibers of these neurons form the **vestibular branch** of the vestibulocochlear cranial nerve (VIII). These fibers synapse on neurons in the *vestibular nuclei* located at the boundary between the pons and the medulla oblongata. The two vestibular nuclei (1) integrate sensory information arriving from each side of the head; (2) relay information to the cerebellum; (3) relay information to the cerebral cortex, providing a conscious sense of position and movement; and (4) send commands to motor nuclei in the brain stem and in the spinal cord. These reflexive motor commands are distributed to the motor nuclei for cranial nerves involved with eye, head, and neck movements (III, IV, VI, and XI). Descending instructions along the *vestibulospinal tracts* of the spinal cord adjust peripheral muscle tone to complement the reflexive movements of the head or neck.

Hearing

The receptors of the cochlear duct provide us with a sense of hearing. They enable us to detect the quietest whisper, yet they remain functional in a noisy room. The receptors responsible for auditory sensations are hair cells similar to those of the vestibular complex. However, their placement

within the cochlear duct and the organization of the surrounding accessory structures shield them from stimuli other than sound.

In conveying vibrations from the tympanic membrane to the oval window, the auditory ossicles convert sound energy (pressure waves) in air to pressure pulses in the perilymph of the cochlea. These pressure pulses stimulate hair cells along the cochlear spiral. The *frequency* (pitch) of the perceived sound is determined by *which part* of the cochlear duct is stimulated. The *intensity* (volume) of the perceived sound is determined by *how many* hair cells at that location are stimulated.

The Cochlear Duct

In sectional view, the cochlear duct, or **scala media**, lies between a pair of perilymph-filled chambers or *scalae*: the **scala vestibuli** (SKĀ-luh ves-TIB-yū-lē), or *vestibular duct*, and the **scala tympani** (SKĀ-luh TIM-pa-nē), or *tympanic duct* (**Figure 9-31a**). The bony labyrinth encases the outer surfaces of these ducts everywhere except at the oval window (the base of the scala vestibuli) and the round window (the base of the scala tympani). Because these two scalae, or ducts, are interconnected at the tip of the cochlear spiral, they really form one long and continuous perilymph-filled chamber.

THE SPIRAL ORGAN. The hair cells of the cochlear duct are located in the **spiral organ** (*organ of Corti*) (**Figure 9-31b**). This sensory structure sits on the **basilar membrane**, a membrane that separates the cochlear duct from the underlying scala tympani. The hair cells are arranged in a series of longitudinal rows, with their stereocilia in contact with the overlying **tectorial membrane** (tek-TOR-ē-al; *tectum*, roof). This membrane is firmly attached to the inner wall of the cochlear duct. When a portion of the basilar membrane bounces up and down (in response to pressure waves in the perilymph), the stereocilia of the hair cells are pressed up against the tectorial membrane and distorted.

The Hearing Process

Hearing is the perception of sound, but what is sound? It consists of waves of pressure conducted through a medium such as air or water. In air, each pressure wave consists of a region where air molecules are crowded together and adjacent regions where they are farther apart. Physicists use the

Figure 9-31 The Cochlea and Spiral Organ.

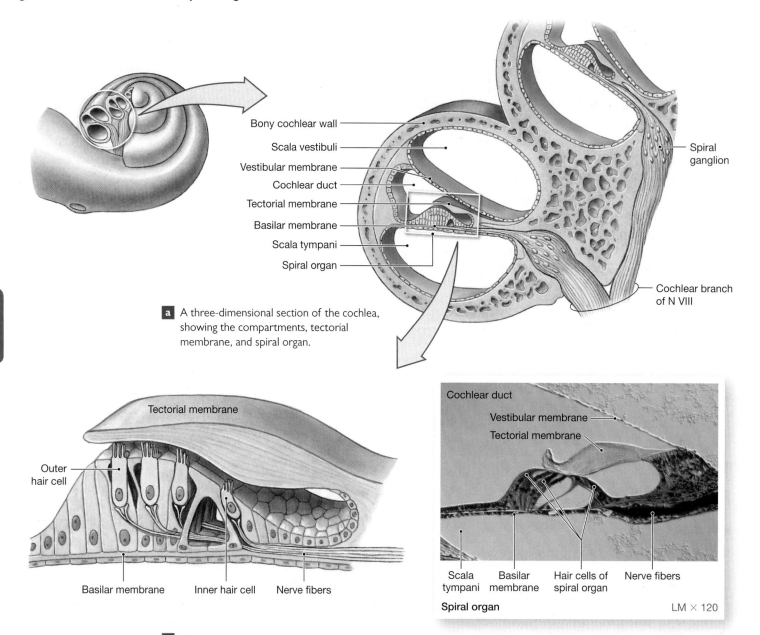

Bony cochlear wall
Scala vestibuli
Vestibular membrane
Cochlear duct
Tectorial membrane
Basilar membrane
Scala tympani
Spiral organ

Spiral ganglion

Cochlear branch of N VIII

a A three-dimensional section of the cochlea, showing the compartments, tectorial membrane, and spiral organ.

Tectorial membrane

Outer hair cell

Basilar membrane   Inner hair cell   Nerve fibers

Cochlear duct
Vestibular membrane
Tectorial membrane

Scala tympani   Basilar membrane   Hair cells of spiral organ   Nerve fibers

Spiral organ   LM × 120

b Diagrammatic and sectional views of the receptor hair cell complex of the spiral organ.

term **cycles** rather than waves, and the number of cycles per second (cps)—or **hertz (Hz)**—represents the **frequency** of the sound.

What we perceive as the **pitch** of a sound (how high or low it is) is our sensory response to its frequency. A sound of high frequency (high pitch) might have a frequency of 15,000 Hz or more. A sound of low frequency (low pitch) could have a frequency of 100 Hz or less.

The amount of energy, or power, of a sound determines its *intensity*, or volume (loudness). Intensity is reported in **decibels** (DES-i-belz). Some examples of different sounds and their intensities include a soft whisper (30 decibels), a

refrigerator (50 decibels), a gas lawnmower (90 decibels), a chain saw (100 decibels), and a jet plane (140 decibels).

Hearing can be divided into six basic steps, diagrammed in **Figure 9-32**.

❶ *Sound waves arrive at the tympanic membrane.* They enter the external acoustic meatus and travel toward the tympanic membrane. Sound waves approaching the side of the head have direct access to the tympanic membrane on that side. Sounds arriving from another direction must bend around corners or pass through the auricle or other body tissues.

Figure 9-32 Sound and Hearing. Steps in the reception of sound and the process of hearing.

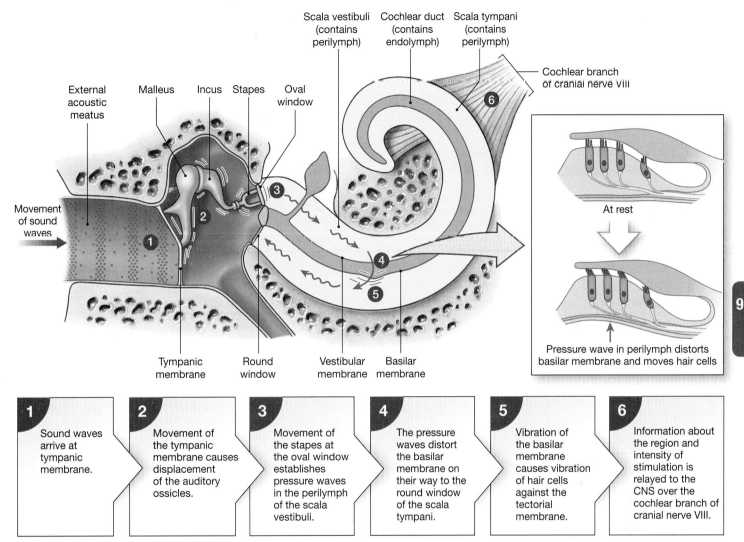

Scala vestibuli (contains perilymph)

Cochlear duct (contains endolymph)

Scala tympani (contains perilymph)

Cochlear branch of cranial nerve VIII

External acoustic meatus

Malleus

Incus

Stapes

Oval window

Movement of sound waves

Tympanic membrane

Round window

Vestibular membrane

Basilar membrane

At rest

Pressure wave in perilymph distorts basilar membrane and moves hair cells

1 Sound waves arrive at tympanic membrane.

2 Movement of the tympanic membrane causes displacement of the auditory ossicles.

3 Movement of the stapes at the oval window establishes pressure waves in the perilymph of the scala vestibuli.

4 The pressure waves distort the basilar membrane on their way to the round window of the scala tympani.

5 Vibration of the basilar membrane causes vibration of hair cells against the tectorial membrane.

6 Information about the region and intensity of stimulation is relayed to the CNS over the cochlear branch of cranial nerve VIII.

2 *Movement of the tympanic membrane causes displacement of the auditory ossicles.* The tympanic membrane provides the surface for sound collection. It vibrates to sound waves with frequencies between approximately 20 and 20,000 Hz. When the tympanic membrane vibrates, so do the malleus, incus, and stapes.

3 *The movement of the stapes at the oval window establishes pressure waves in the perilymph of the scala vestibuli.* When the stapes moves, it applies pressure to the perilymph of the scala vestibuli. Because the rest of the cochlea is sheathed in bone, pressure applied at the oval window can be relieved only at the round window. When the stapes moves inward, the membrane spanning the round window bulges outward. As the stapes moves in and out, vibrating at the frequency of the sound at the tympanic membrane, it creates pressure waves within the perilymph.

4 *The pressure waves distort the basilar membrane on their way to the round window of the scala tympani.* These pressure waves cause movement in the basilar membrane. The basilar membrane does not have the same structure throughout its length. Near the oval window, it is narrow and stiff. At its terminal end, it is wider and more flexible. As a result, the location of maximum stimulation varies with the frequency of the sound. High-frequency sounds vibrate the basilar membrane near the oval window. The lower the frequency of the sound, the farther from the oval window is the area of maximum distortion. The actual *range* of movement at a given location depends on the amount of force applied by the stapes. The louder the sound, the more the basilar membrane moves.

5 *Vibration of the basilar membrane causes hair cells to vibrate against the tectorial membrane.* The vibration of the affected region of the basilar membrane

9

pushes hair cells against the tectorial membrane. The displacement of the hair cells results in the release of neurotransmitters and the stimulation of sensory neurons. The hair cells are arranged in several rows. A very soft sound may stimulate only a few hair cells in a portion of one row. As the volume of a sound increases, not only do these hair cells become more active, but additional hair cells—at first in the same row and then in adjacent rows—are stimulated as well. In this way, the number of hair cells responding in a given region of the spiral organ provides information on the intensity of the sound.

6 *Information about the region and intensity of stimulation is relayed to the CNS over the cochlear branch of cranial nerve VIII.* The cell bodies of the sensory neurons that monitor the cochlear hair cells are located at the center of the bony cochlea (**Figure 9-31a**) in the *spiral ganglion*. Their afferent fibers (axons) form the**cochlear branch** of the vestibulocochlear nerve (N VIII). It carries information to the cochlear nuclei of the medulla oblongata for distribution to other centers in the brain.

Auditory Pathways

At the medulla oblongata, fibers from the sensory neurons synapse at the cochlear nucleus on that side (**Figure 9-33**). From there, information ascends to both *inferior colliculi* of the midbrain. This midbrain processing center coordinates a number of responses to acoustic stimuli, including auditory reflexes involving skeletal muscles of the head, face, and trunk. For example, these reflexes automatically turn your head and your eyes toward the source of a sudden loud noise.

Before reaching the cerebral cortex and your conscious awareness, ascending auditory sensations synapse in the thalamus. Thalamic fibers then deliver the information to the auditory cortex of the temporal lobe. In effect, the auditory cortex contains a map of the spiral organ. High-frequency sounds activate one portion of the cortex, and low-frequency sounds affect another.

Most of the auditory information from one cochlea is projected to the auditory complex of the cerebral hemisphere on the opposite side of the brain. However, each auditory cortex also receives information from the cochlea on that side. These interconnections enable you to localize left/right sounds.

An individual whose auditory cortex is damaged will respond to sounds and have normal acoustic reflexes, but will find it difficult or impossible to interpret the sounds and

CLINICAL NOTE

Hearing Deficits

Probably more than 6 million people in the United States alone have at least a partial hearing deficit. Conductive deafness results from conditions in the external or middle ear that block the normal transfer of vibrations from the tympanic membrane to the

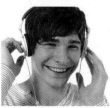

oval window. An external acoustic meatus plugged by built-up wax or trapped water may cause a temporary hearing loss. Scarring or perforation of the tympanic membrane and immobilization of one or more of the auditory ossicles are more serious causes of conductive deafness.

In nerve deafness, the problem lies within the cochlea or somewhere along the auditory pathway. The vibrations are reaching the oval window and entering the perilymph, but the receptors either cannot respond or their response cannot reach its CNS destinations. Very loud (high-intensity) sounds, for example, can produce nerve deafness by breaking stereocilia off the surfaces of the hair cells. (The reflex contraction of the tensor tympani and stapedius muscles in response to a dangerously loud noise occurs in less than 0.1 second, but this may not be fast enough.) Drugs such as the aminoglycoside antibiotics (*neomycin* or *gentamicin*) may diffuse into the endolymph and kill hair cells. Hair cells and sensory nerves can also be damaged by bacterial infection. For this reason, potential side effects of drug treatment must be balanced against the severity of infection.

Many treatment options are available for conductive deafness. Treatment options for nerve deafness are relatively limited. Early diagnosis improves the chances for successful treatment because many of these problems become progressively worse.

recognize a pattern in them. Damage to the adjacent association area does not affect the ability to detect tones and patterns but produces an inability to comprehend their meaning.

Auditory Sensitivity

Our hearing abilities are remarkable, but it is difficult to assess the absolute sensitivity of the system. The range from the softest audible sound to the loudest tolerable blast represents a trillionfold increase in power. The receptor process is so sensitive that if we were to remove the stapes, we could, in theory, hear air molecules bouncing off the oval window. We never utilize our full auditory potential, because body movements and our internal organs produce squeaks, groans, thumps, and other sounds that are tuned out by adaptation. When other environmental noises fade away, the level of adaptation drops and the system becomes increasingly

Figure 9-33 Pathways for Auditory Sensations.

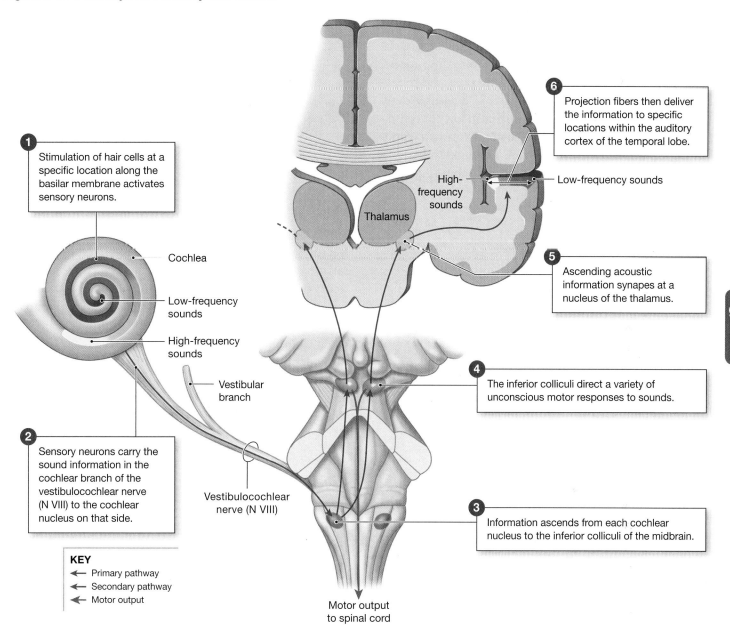

1 Stimulation of hair cells at a specific location along the basilar membrane activates sensory neurons.

Cochlea

Low-frequency sounds

High-frequency sounds

Vestibular branch

2 Sensory neurons carry the sound information in the cochlear branch of the vestibulocochlear nerve (N VIII) to the cochlear nucleus on that side.

Vestibulocochlear nerve (N VIII)

KEY
← Primary pathway
← Secondary pathway
← Motor output

High-frequency sounds

Thalamus

Low-frequency sounds

6 Projection fibers then deliver the information to specific locations within the auditory cortex of the temporal lobe.

5 Ascending acoustic information synapses at a nucleus of the thalamus.

4 The inferior colliculi direct a variety of unconscious motor responses to sounds.

3 Information ascends from each cochlear nucleus to the inferior colliculi of the midbrain.

Motor output to spinal cord

9

sensitive. If we relax in a quiet room, our heartbeat seems to get louder and louder as the auditory system adjusts to the lower level of background noise.

CHECKPOINT

16. If the round window were not able to bulge out with increased pressure in the perilymph, how would sound perception be affected?

17. How would the loss of stereocilia from the hair cells of the spiral organ affect hearing?

See the blue Answers tab at the back of the book.

9-8 Aging is accompanied by a noticeable decline in the special senses

Learning Objective Describe the effects of aging on smell, taste, vision, equilibrium, and hearing.

The general lack of replacement of neurons leads to an inevitable decline in sensory function with age. Increases in stimulus strength can compensate for part of this functional decline, but the loss of axons that conduct sensory action potentials cannot be compensated for so easily. Next we consider the toll aging takes on various special senses.

9

Smell and Aging

Unlike populations of other neurons, the population of olfactory receptor cells is regularly replaced by the division of stem cells in the olfactory epithelium. Despite this process, the total number of receptors declines with age, and the remaining receptors become less sensitive. As a result, elderly individuals have difficulty detecting odors in low concentrations. This drop in the number of receptors explains a grandmother's tendency to use too much perfume and why a grandfather's aftershave lotion seems so overpowering. They must use more to be able to smell it.

Taste and Aging

Tasting ability declines with age due to the thinning of mucous membranes and a reduction in the number and sensitivity of taste buds. We begin life with more than 10,000 taste buds, but that number begins declining dramatically by the age of 50 years. In addition, aging individuals also experience a decline in the number of olfactory receptor cells. As a result, many elderly people find their food bland and unappetizing. Children, however, find the same food too spicy.

Vision and Aging

Various disorders of vision are associated with normal aging. The most common ones involve the lens and the neural part of the retina. With age, the lens loses its elasticity and stiffens. As a result, seeing close-up objects becomes more difficult, and older individuals become farsighted—a condition called *presbyopia*. ↻ p. 324 For example, the inner limit of clear vision, known as the *near point of vision*, changes from 7–9 cm (2.8–3.5 in.) in children to 15–20 cm (5.9–7.9 in.) in young adults, and typically reaches 83 cm (32.7 in.) by age 60. As noted earlier, advancing age is the most common cause of the loss of transparency in the lens known as *senile cataracts*. ↻ p. 321 In addition, a gradual loss of rods takes place with age. This loss explains why individuals over age 60 years need almost twice as much light for reading than individuals at age 40 years.

The leading cause of blindness in persons over 50 is *macular degeneration*. This condition involves the growth and proliferation of blood vessels in the retina. Blood leaking from these abnormal vessels causes retinal scarring and a loss of photoreceptors. The vascular proliferation begins in the macula, the area of the retina correlated with the clearest vision. As the cones there deteriorate, color vision and the center of the visual field are affected.

Equilibrium and Aging

Problems with equilibrium, or balance, increase with age. An important health concern for people over the age of 60 years is falling. Falls cause more than 95 percent of hip fractures. Complications following a hip fracture can be disastrous. It is estimated that 20 percent of hip fracture patients die within a year of their injury. Good balance relies on sensory input from the vestibular complex (vestibule and semicircular canals) and visual and proprioceptive receptors. From about age 55 years, there is a decrease in the number of nerve cells in the vestibular complex. Damage to the vestibular complex by any cause may lead to dizziness and balance problems. However, problems in balance due to the gradual, age-related loss of vestibular nerve cells are not accompanied by dizziness.

Hearing and Aging

Hearing is generally affected less by aging than are the other senses. However, it becomes more difficult to hear high-pitched sounds because the tympanic membrane loses some of its elasticity. The progressive loss of hearing that occurs with aging is called *presbycusis* (prez-bē-KŪ-sis; *presbys*, old man + *akousis*, hearing).

CHECKPOINT

18. How can a given food be both too spicy for a child and too bland for an elderly individual?

19. Explain why we have an increasingly difficult time seeing close-up objects as we age.

See the blue Answers tab at the back of the book.

RELATED CLINICAL TERMS

analgesic: A drug that relieves pain without eliminating sensitivity to other stimuli, such as touch or pressure.

anesthesia: A total or partial loss of sensation.

Ménière's disease: A condition in which high fluid pressures rupture the walls of the membranous labyrinth, resulting in acute vertigo (an inappropriate sense of motion) and inappropriate auditory sensations.

nystagmus: Abnormal eye movements that may appear after the brain stem or internal ear is damaged.

ophthalmology (of-thal-MOL-o-jē)**:** The study of the eye and its diseases.

retinitis pigmentosa: A group of inherited retinopathies (see the next term) characterized by the progressive deterioration of photoreceptors, eventually resulting in blindness.

retinopathy (ret-i-NOP-ah-thē)**:** A disease or disorder of the retina.

scotomas (skō-TŌ-muhz)**:** Abnormal blind spots in the field of vision (that is, those not caused by the optic disc).

Snellen chart: A printed chart of block letters in graduated type sizes used to measure visual acuity.

strabismus: Deviations in the alignment of the eyes to each other. One or both eyes are turned inward or outward.

synesthesia: Abnormal condition in which sensory nerve messages connect to the wrong centers of the brain. For example, touching an object may produce the perception of a sound, while hearing a tone may produce the visualization of a color.

9 Chapter Review

Summary Outline

9-1 Sensory receptors connect our internal and external environments with the nervous system *p. 344*

1. The **general senses** are temperature, pain, touch, pressure, vibration, and proprioception. The receptors for these sensations are distributed throughout the body. Receptors for the **special senses** (smell, taste, vision, balance, and hearing) are located in specialized areas or in sense organs.

2. A *sensory receptor* is a specialized cell that, when stimulated, sends a sensation to the CNS. The simplest receptors are **free nerve endings**. The most complex have specialized accessory structures that isolate the receptors from all but a specific type of stimulus.

3. Each receptor cell monitors a specific *receptive field (Figure 9-1)*.

4. Sensory information is relayed in the form of action potentials in a sensory (afferent) fiber. In general, the larger the stimulus, the greater is the frequency of action potentials. The CNS interprets the nature of the arriving sensory information on the basis of the area of the brain stimulated.

5. **Adaptation**—a reduction in sensitivity in the presence of a constant stimulus—involves changes in receptor sensitivity or inhibition along sensory pathways.

9-2 General sensory receptors are classified by the type of stimulus that excites them *p. 345*

6. **Nociceptors** respond to a variety of stimuli usually associated with tissue damage. The two types of painful sensations are **fast pain**, or *prickling pain*, and **slow pain**, or *burning and aching pain*.

7. The perception of pain in parts of the body that are not actually stimulated is called **referred pain** *(Figure 9-2)*.

8. **Thermoreceptors** respond to changes in temperature.

9. **Mechanoreceptors** respond to physical distortion of, contact with, or pressure on their plasma membranes. **Tactile receptors** respond to touch, pressure, and vibration. **Baroreceptors** respond to pressure changes in the walls of blood vessels, the digestive and urinary tracts, and the lungs. **Proprioceptors** respond to positions of joints and muscles.

10. **Fine touch and pressure receptors** provide detailed information about a source of stimulation; **crude touch and pressure receptors** are poorly localized. Important tactile receptors include the *root hair plexus, tactile discs, tactile (Meissner's) corpuscles, lamellated (pacinian) corpuscles*, and *Ruffini corpuscles (Figure 9-3)*.

11. Baroreceptors in the walls of major arteries and veins respond to changes in blood pressure, and those along the digestive tract help coordinate reflex activities of digestion *(Figure 9-4)*.

12. Proprioceptors monitor the position of joints, tension in tendons and ligaments, and the state of muscular contraction. Proprioceptors include Golgi tendon organs and muscle spindles.

13. In general, **chemoreceptors** respond to water-soluble and lipid-soluble substances dissolved in the surrounding fluid. They monitor the chemical composition of body fluids *(Figure 9-5)*.

9

9-3 Olfaction, the sense of smell, involves olfactory receptors responding to chemical stimuli *p. 350*

14. The **olfactory organs** consist of an **olfactory epithelium** containing **olfactory receptor cells** (neurons sensitive to chemicals dissolved in the overlying mucus), supporting cells, and *basal cells* (stem cells). Their surfaces are coated with the secretions of the **olfactory glands** (*Figure 9-6*).

15. The olfactory receptors are modified neurons.

16. The olfactory system has extensive limbic and hypothalamic connections.

9-4 Gustation, the sense of taste, involves taste receptors responding to chemical stimuli *p. 351*

17. **Taste (gustatory) receptors** are clustered in **taste buds**. Each taste bud contains **gustatory receptor cells**, which extend *taste hairs* through a narrow **taste pore** (*Figure 9-7*).

18. Taste buds are associated with **papillae**, epithelial projections on the superior surface of the tongue (*Figure 9-7*).

19. The **primary taste sensations** are sweet, salty, sour, and bitter. Receptors for umami and water are also present (*Figure 9-7*).

20. The taste buds are monitored by cranial nerves that synapse within a nucleus of the medulla oblongata.

9-5 Internal eye structures contribute to vision, while accessory eye structures provide protection *p. 353*

21. The **accessory structures** of the eye include the eyelids and associated exocrine glands, the superficial epithelium of the eye, structures associated with the production and removal of tears, and the extrinsic eye muscles.

22. An epithelium called the **conjunctiva** covers most of the exposed surface of the eye except the transparent **cornea**.

23. The secretions of the **lacrimal gland** bathe the conjunctiva and contain *lysozyme* (an enzyme that attacks bacteria). Tears reach the nasal cavity after passing through the **lacrimal canals**, the **lacrimal sac**, and the **nasolacrimal duct** (*Figure 9-8*).

24. Six **extrinsic eye muscles** control external eye movements: the **inferior** and **superior rectus**, the **lateral** and **medial rectus**, and the **superior** and **inferior obliques** (*Figure 9-9; Table 9-1*).

25. The eye has three layers: an outer fibrous layer, a vascular layer, and a deeper inner layer. Most of the ocular surface is covered by the **sclera** (a dense fibrous connective tissue), which is continuous with the cornea, both of which are part of the **fibrous layer** (*Figure 9-10*).

26. The **vascular layer** includes the **iris**, the **ciliary body**, and the **choroid**. The iris forms the boundary between the eye's anterior and posterior chambers. The iris regulates the amount of light entering the eye. The ciliary body contains the *ciliary muscle* and the *ciliary processes*, which attach to the **ciliary zonule** (*suspensory ligament*) of the **lens** (*Figure 9-10*).

27. The **inner layer**, or **retina**, consists of an outer *pigmented part* and an inner *neural part*. The neural part contains the two types of image-forming **photoreceptors**, the **rods** and **cones**, and associated neurons (*Figures 9-10, 9-11*).

28. Cones are densely clustered in the **fovea** (the site of sharpest vision), at the center of the **macula** (*Figure 9-11*).

29. From the photoreceptors, the information is relayed to **bipolar cells**, then to **ganglion cells**, and to the brain by the optic nerve. Horizontal cells and amacrine cells modify the signals passed between other retinal components (*Figure 9-11*).

30. The ciliary body and lens divide the interior of the eye into a large **posterior cavity** and a smaller **anterior cavity**. The anterior cavity is subdivided into the **anterior chamber**, which extends from the cornea to the iris, and a **posterior chamber** between the iris and the ciliary body and lens. The posterior cavity contains the gelatinous *vitreous body*, which helps stabilize the shape of the eye and supports the retina (*Figure 9-13*).

31. **Aqueous humor** circulates within the eye and re-enters the circulation after diffusing through the walls of the anterior chamber and into veins of the sclera through the **scleral venous sinus** (canal of Schlemm) (*Figure 9-13*).

32. The lens, held in place by the ciliary zonule, focuses a visual image on the retinal receptors. Light is refracted (bent) when it passes through the cornea and lens. During **accommodation**, the shape of the lens changes to focus an image on the retina (*Figures 9-14, 9-15, Spotlight Figure 9-16*).

9-6 Photoreceptors respond to light and change it into electrical signals essential to visual physiology *p. 362*

33. Light is radiated in waves with a characteristic wavelength. A *photon* is a single energy packet of visible light. Rods respond to almost any photon, regardless of its energy content (wavelength). Cones have characteristic ranges of wavelength sensitivity and provide color vision. **Color blindness** is the inability to detect certain colors (*Figures 9-17, 9-18*).

34. Each photoreceptor contains an outer segment with membranous **discs** containing **visual pigments**. Light is absorbed by the visual pigments, which are derivatives of **rhodopsin** (**opsin** plus the pigment **retinal**, which is synthesized from **vitamin A**). A photoreceptor responds to light by changing its rate of neurotransmitter release and thereby altering the activity of a bipolar cell (*Figures 9-18, 9-19*).

35. Visual information is relayed from photoreceptors to bipolar cells to ganglion cells within the retina. The axons of ganglion cells converge at the optic disc and leave the eye as the optic nerve. A partial crossover occurs at the optic chiasm before the information reaches a nucleus in the thalamus on each side of the brain. From these nuclei, visual information is relayed to the visual cortex of the occipital lobe, which contains a sensory map of the field of vision (*Figure 9-20*).

9-7 Equilibrium sensations originate within the internal ear, while hearing involves the detection and interpretation of sound waves *p. 369*

36. The senses of equilibrium (**dynamic equilibrium** and **static equilibrium**) and hearing are provided by the receptors of the **internal ear**. Its chambers and canals contain the fluid **endolymph**. The **bony labyrinth** surrounds and protects the **membranous labyrinth**, and the space between them contains the fluid **perilymph**. The bony labyrinth consists of the **vestibule**, the **semicircular canals** (receptors in the vestibule and semicircular canals provide the sense of equilibrium), and the **cochlea** (where receptors provide the sense of hearing). The structures and air spaces of the **external ear** and **middle ear** help capture and transmit sound to the cochlea (*Figures 9-26–28*).

37. The external ear includes the **auricle** (*pinna*), which surrounds the entrance to the **external acoustic meatus**, which ends at the **tympanic membrane** (*eardrum*) (*Figures 9-26, 9-27*).

38. The middle ear is connected to the nasopharynx by the **auditory tube** (*pharyngotympanic tube* or *Eustachian tube*). The middle ear encloses and protects the **auditory ossicles** (*Figures 9-26, 9-27*).

39. The vestibule includes a pair of membranous sacs, the **saccule** and **utricle**, whose receptors provide sensations of gravity and linear acceleration (static equilibrium). The semicircular canals contain the **semicircular ducts**, whose receptors provide sensations of rotation (dynamic equilibrium). The cochlea contains the **cochlear duct**, an elongated portion of the membranous labyrinth, whose receptors provide the sense of hearing (*Figure 9-28*).

40. The basic receptors of the internal ear are **hair cells**, whose surfaces support *stereocilia*. Hair cells provide information about the direction and strength of mechanical stimuli (*Figure 9-29c*).

41. The **anterior, posterior**, and **lateral semicircular ducts** are attached to the utricle. Each semicircular duct contains a sensory organ, the **crista ampullaris**. The stereocilia of its hair cells contact the **cupula**, a gelatinous mass that is distorted when endolymph flows along the axis of the duct (*Figures 9-29a,b,d*).

42. In the saccule and utricle, hair cells cluster within **maculae**, where their stereocilia contact a gelatinous otolithic membrane covered by **otoliths** (calcium carbonate crystals). When the head tilts, the otoliths shift, and the resulting distortion in the sensory hairs signals the CNS (*Figure 9-30*).

43. The vestibular receptors activate sensory neurons whose axons form the **vestibular branch** of the vestibulocochlear nerve (VIII).

44. The **cochlear duct** lies between the **scala vestibuli** (*vestibular duct*) and the **scala tympani** (*tympanic duct*). The hair cells lie within the **spiral organ** (*organ of Corti*) (*Figure 9-31*).

45. Sound waves travel toward the tympanic membrane, which vibrates; the auditory ossicles amplify and conduct the vibrations to the internal ear. Movement at the oval window applies pressure to the perilymph of the scala vestibuli (*Figures 9-31, 9-32*).

46. Pressure waves distort the **basilar membrane** and push the hair cells of the spiral organ (organ of Corti) against the **tectorial membrane** (*Figure 9-31*).

47. The sensory neurons are located in the **spiral ganglion** of the cochlea. Afferent fibers of sensory neurons form the **cochlear branch** of the vestibulocochlear nerve (VIII), synapsing at their respective left or right cochlear nucleus (*Figure 9-33*).

9-8 Aging is accompanied by a noticeable decline in the special senses *p. 379*

48. As part of aging, there are (1) gradual reductions in smell and taste sensitivity, (2) a tendency toward *presbyopia* and cataract formation in the eyes, (3) problems with equilibrium, or balance, that may lead to falling and hip fractures, and (4) a progressive loss of hearing (*presbycusis*).

Review Questions

See the blue Answers tab at the back of the book.

Level 1 Reviewing Facts and Terms

Match each item in column A with the most closely related item in column B. Place letters for answers in the spaces provided.

COLUMN A

_____ **1.** Myopia

_____ **2.** Fibrous layer

_____ **3.** Nociceptors

_____ **4.** Proprioceptors

_____ **5.** Cones

_____ **6.** Accommodation

_____ **7.** Tympanic membrane

_____ **8.** Thermoreceptors

COLUMN B

a. Pain receptors

b. Temperature receptors

c. Sclera and cornea

d. Rotational movements

e. Provide information on joint position

f. Color vision

g. Site of sharpest vision

h. Active in dim light

COLUMN A

_____ **9.** Rods

_____ **10.** Olfaction

_____ **11.** Fovea

_____ **12.** Hyperopia

_____ **13.** Maculae

_____ **14.** Semicircular ducts

COLUMN B

i. Eardrum

j. Change in lens shape to focus retinal image

k. Nearsighted

l. Farsighted

m. Sense of smell

n. Gravity and acceleration receptors

15. Identify the structures in the following horizontal section of the right eye.

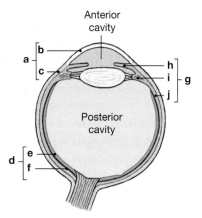

(a) _____   (b) _____

(c) _____   (d) _____

(e) _____   (f) _____

(g) _____   (h) _____

(i) _____   (j) _____

16. Regardless of the nature of a stimulus, sensory information must be sent to the central nervous system in the form of
   (a) dendritic processes.
   (b) action potentials.
   (c) neurotransmitter molecules.
   (d) generator potentials.

17. A reduction in sensitivity in the presence of constant stimulus is called
   (a) transduction.   **(b)** sensory coding.
   (c) line labeling.   **(d)** adaptation.

18. Mechanoreceptors that detect pressure changes in the walls of blood vessels and in portions of the digestive, reproductive, and urinary tracts are
   (a) tactile receptors.
   (b) baroreceptors.
   (c) proprioceptors.
   (d) free nerve endings.

19. Examples of proprioceptors that monitor the position of joints and the state of muscular contraction are
   (a) lamellated and tactile corpuscles.
   (b) carotid and aortic sinuses.
   (c) tactile discs and Ruffini corpuscles.
   (d) Golgi tendon organs and muscle spindles.

20. Molecules of volatile compounds in the nasal cavity stimulate
   (a) gustatory cells.
   (b) olfactory receptors.
   (c) rod cells.
   (d) tactile receptors.

21. Taste receptors are also known as
   (a) tactile discs.
   (b) gustatory receptors.
   (c) hair cells.
   (d) olfactory receptors.

22. The function of tears produced by the lacrimal apparatus is to
   (a) keep conjunctival surfaces moist and clean.
   (b) reduce friction and remove debris from the eye.
   (c) provide nutrients and oxygen to the conjunctival epithelium.
   (d) a, b, and c are correct.

23. The thickened gel-like substance that helps support the structure of the eyeball is the
   (a) vitreous body.   **(b)** aqueous humor.
   (c) cupula.   **(d)** perilymph.

24. The sclera is considered to be a part of the
   (a) vascular layer.
   (b) fibrous layer.
   (c) inner layer.
   (d) a, b, and c are correct.

25. At sunset your visual system adapts to
   (a) fovea vision.
   (b) rod-based vision.
   (c) macular vision.
   (d) cone-based vision.

26. The malleus, incus, and stapes are the tiny ear bones located in the
   (a) external ear.
   (b) middle ear.
   (c) internal ear.
   (d) membranous labyrinth.

27. Receptors in the saccule and utricle provide sensations of
   (a) balance and equilibrium.
   (b) hearing.
   (c) vibration.
   (d) gravity and linear acceleration.

28. Identify the structures of the external, middle, and internal ear in the following figure.

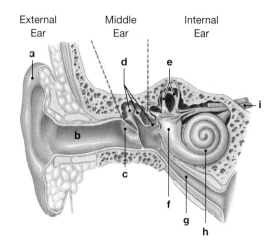

External Ear   Middle Ear   Internal Ear

(a) _____   (b) _____
(c) _____   (d) _____
(e) _____   (f) _____
(g) _____   (h) _____
(i) _____

29. The spiral organ is located within the of the internal ear.
  (a) Utricle   (b) Bony labyrinth
  (c) Vestibule   (d) Cochlea

30. What three types of mechanoreceptors respond to stretching, compression, twisting, or other distortions of the cell membrane?

31. Identify six types of tactile receptors found in the skin and their sensitivities.

32. (a) What structures make up the fibrous layer of the eye?
  (b) What are the functions of the fibrous layer?

33. What structures are parts of the vascular layer of the eye?

34. What six basic steps are involved in the process of hearing?

Level 2 Reviewing Concepts

35. The CNS interprets sensory information entirely on the basis of the
  (a) strength of the action potential.
  (b) number of action potentials.
  (c) area of brain stimulated.
  (d) a, b, and c are correct.

36. If the auditory cortex is damaged, the individual will respond to sounds and have normal acoustic reflexes, but
  (a) the sounds may produce nerve deafness.
  (b) the auditory ossicle may be immobilized.
  (c) sound interpretation and pattern recognition may be impossible.
  (d) normal transfer of vibration to the oval window is inhibited.

37. Distinguish between the general senses and the special senses in the human body.

38. In what form does the CNS receive a stimulus detected by a sensory receptor?

39. What is the usual result if a sebaceous gland of an eyelash or a tarsal gland becomes infected?

40. Jane makes an appointment with the optometrist for a vision test. Her test results for visual acuity are reported as 20/15. What does this test result mean? Is a rating of 20/20 better or worse?

Level 3 Critical Thinking and Clinical Applications

41. You are at a park watching some deer 35 feet away from you. Your friend taps you on the shoulder to ask a question. As you turn to look at your friend, who is standing 2 feet away, what changes would your eyes undergo?

42. After attending a Fourth of July fireworks extravaganza, Millie finds it difficult to hear normal conversation, and her ears keep "ringing." What is causing her hearing problems?

43. After riding the express elevator from the twentieth floor to the ground floor, for a few seconds you still feel as if you are descending, even though you have obviously come to a stop. Why?

The Endocrine System

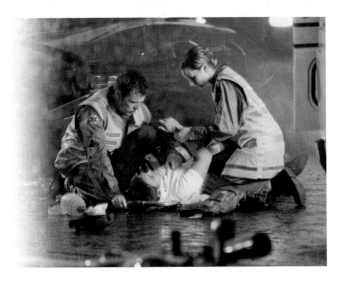

Learning Objectives

These objectives tell you what you should be able to do after completing the chapter. They correspond by number to this chapter's sections.

10-1 Explain the role of intercellular communication in homeostasis, and describe the complementary roles of the endocrine and nervous systems.

10-2 Contrast the major structural classes of hormones, and explain the general processes and effects of hormone action on target organs.

10-3 Describe the location, hormones, and functions of the pituitary gland.

10-4 Describe the location, hormones, and functions of the thyroid gland.

10-5 Describe the location, hormones, and functions of the parathyroid glands.

10-6 Describe the location, hormones, and functions of the adrenal glands.

10-7 Describe the location of the pineal gland, and discuss the functions of the hormone it produces.

10-8 Describe the location, hormones, and functions of the pancreas.

10-9 Discuss the functions of the hormones produced by the kidneys, heart, thymus, testes, ovaries, and adipose tissue.

10-10 Explain how hormones interact to produce coordinated physiological responses, and describe how the endocrine system responds to stress and is affected by aging.

10-11 Give examples of interactions between the endocrine system and other body systems.

An Introduction to the Endocrine System

The human body contains about 30 chemical messengers known as hormones. They regulate activities such as sleep, body temperature, hunger, and stress management. These hormones are products of the endocrine system, which, along with the nervous system, controls and coordinates our body processes.

In this chapter, we introduce the components and functions of the endocrine system. We also explore the interactions between the nervous and endocrine systems.

Build Your Knowledge

Recall that the endocrine system directs long-term changes in the activities of other organ systems (as you saw in **Chapter 1: An Introduction to Anatomy and Physiology**). Both the endocrine and nervous systems act to maintain homeostasis as environmental conditions change. The nervous system responds relatively quickly to stimuli. On the other hand, endocrine system responses develop more slowly but last much longer. ↺ **p. 8**

10-1 Homeostasis is preserved through intercellular communication

Learning Objective Explain the role of intercellular communication in homeostasis, and describe the complementary roles of the endocrine and nervous systems.

To maintain homeostasis, every cell in the body must communicate with its neighbors and with cells and tissues in distant portions of the body. Most of this communication involves chemical messages. Each cell continually "talks" to its neighbors by releasing chemicals into the extracellular fluid. These chemicals tell cells what their neighbors are doing at any given moment. As a result, tissue function is coordinated at the local level.

Cellular communication also takes place over greater distances. It is coordinated by both the nervous and endocrine systems. The nervous system functions somewhat like a telecommunications company, with a cable network carrying high-speed "messages" from one location to another inside the body. The source and the destination are quite specific, and the effects are short lived. This form of communication is ideal for crisis management. If you are in danger of being hit by a speeding bus, the nervous system can coordinate and direct your leap to safety.

Many life processes, however, require long-term cellular communication. The endocrine system provides this type of regulation, which uses chemical messengers called *hormones* to relay information and instructions between cells. In such

communication, hormones are like messages, and the cardiovascular system is e-mail. A hormone released into the bloodstream is distributed throughout the body. Each hormone has **target cells**, specific cells that have the receptors that bind and "read" the hormonal message when it arrives. But hormones are really like e-mail spam—cells throughout the body are exposed to them whether or not they have the necessary receptors. At any moment, each individual cell can respond to only a few of the hormones present. The other hormones are ignored, because the cell lacks the receptors needed to read the messages they contain.

A single hormone can alter the metabolic activities of multiple tissues and organs at the same time because target cells can be anywhere in the body. The effects may be slow to appear, but they often persist for days. This persistence makes hormones effective in coordinating cell, tissue, and organ activities on a sustained, long-term basis. For example, circulating hormones keep body water content and levels of electrolytes and organic nutrients within normal limits 24 hours a day throughout our entire lives.

Cells can respond to several different hormones at the same time, as long as they have the proper receptors. The result is a further alteration in cellular operations. Gradual changes in the quantities and identities of circulating hormones can produce complex changes in physical structure and physiological capabilities. Examples are the processes of embryonic and fetal development, growth, and puberty.

Viewed broadly, the differences between the nervous and endocrine systems seem relatively clear. In fact, these broad organizational and functional distinctions are the basis for treating them as two separate systems. Yet when we consider them in detail, we see that the two systems function in parallel ways:

- Both systems rely on the release of chemicals that bind to specific receptors on target cells.

- Both systems share various chemical messengers. For example, norepinephrine and epinephrine are called *hormones* when released into the bloodstream, and *neurotransmitters* when released across synapses.

- Both systems are regulated mainly by negative feedback processes.

- Both systems share a common goal: to maintain homeostasis by coordinating and regulating the activities of other cells, tissues, organs, and systems.

CHECKPOINT

1. List four similarities between the nervous and endocrine systems.

See the blue Answers tab at the back of the book.

10-2 The endocrine system regulates physiological processes through the binding of hormones to receptors

Learning Objective Contrast the major structural classes of hormones, and explain the general processes and effects of hormone action on target organs.

The **endocrine system** includes all the endocrine cells and tissues of the body. **Endocrine cells** are glandular secretory cells that release their secretions into the extracellular fluid (as noted in Chapter 4). This feature distinguishes them from exocrine cells, which secrete onto epithelial surfaces. ⊃ p. 93 The chemicals released by endocrine cells may affect adjacent cells only—as is the case of *local hormones* such as *prostaglandins*—or they may affect cells throughout the body. We define **hormones** as chemical messengers that are released in one tissue and transported by the bloodstream to target cells in other tissues.

The tissues and organs of the endocrine system, and some of the major hormones they produce, are introduced in **Figure 10-1**. Some of these organs, such as the pituitary gland, have endocrine secretion as a primary function. Others, such as the pancreas, have many other functions besides endocrine secretion. We consider such endocrine organs in more detail in chapters on other systems.

The Structure of Hormones

We can divide hormones into three groups based on their chemical structure:

1. ***Amino acid derivatives.*** Some hormones are relatively small molecules that are structurally similar to amino acids. (Amino acids, the building blocks of proteins, were introduced in Chapter 2.) ⊃ p. 43 This group includes *epinephrine, norepinephrine*, the *thyroid hormones*, and *melatonin*.

2. ***Peptide hormones.*** **Peptide hormones** consist of chains of amino acids. These molecules range from short chain polypeptides, such as *antidiuretic hormone (ADH)* and *oxytocin*, to small proteins such as *growth hormone (GH)* and *prolactin*. This is the largest class of hormones. It includes all the hormones secreted by the hypothalamus, pituitary gland, heart, kidneys, thymus, digestive tract, and pancreas.

3. ***Lipid derivatives.*** There are two classes of lipid-based hormones: steroid hormones and eicosanoids (-kō-sa-noydz). **Steroid hormones** are lipids that are structurally similar to cholesterol (a lipid introduced in Chapter 2). ⊃ p. 42 Steroid hormones are released by the reproductive organs and the adrenal glands. Insoluble in water, steroid hormones are bound to specific transport proteins in blood. **Eicosanoids** are fatty acid–based compounds derived from the 20-carbon fatty acid *arachidonic* (a-rak-i-DON-ik) *acid*. Eicosanoids coordinate local cellular activities and affect enzymatic processes (such as blood clotting) in extracellular fluids. They include the **prostaglandins**.

Build Your Knowledge

Recall that the major types of lipids are fatty acids, fats, steroids, and phospholipids (as you saw in **Chapter 2: The Chemical Level of Organization**). Fatty acids are long chains of carbon atoms with attached hydrogen atoms and end in a carboxyl group (—COOH). When a fatty acid is in solution, only the carboxyl end dissolves in water. Steroids are large molecules composed of four connected rings of carbon atoms. They differ in the carbon chains that are attached to this basic structure. ⊃ **p. 40**

Hormone Action

Proteins determine all cellular structures and functions. Structural proteins give a cell its general shape and internal structure, and enzymes direct the cell's metabolism. Hormones alter cellular operations by changing the *types, activities, locations,* or *quantities* of important enzymes and structural proteins in various target cells.

What determines a target cell's sensitivity to a given hormone? The presence or absence of a specific target cell receptor for that hormone is the key to the target cell's sensitivity

(**Figure 10-2**). The way that a hormone alters cellular activities depends on whether its receptors are located on the target cell's plasma membrane or inside the cell (**Figure 10-3**).

Hormones and Plasma Membrane Receptors

The receptors for epinephrine, norepinephrine, peptide hormones, and eicosanoids are in the plasma membranes of their target cells (**Figure 10-3a**). However, hormones that bind to plasma membrane receptors (also called membrane receptors) cannot directly affect the activities inside the

Figure 10-1 Organs and Tissues of the Endocrine System.

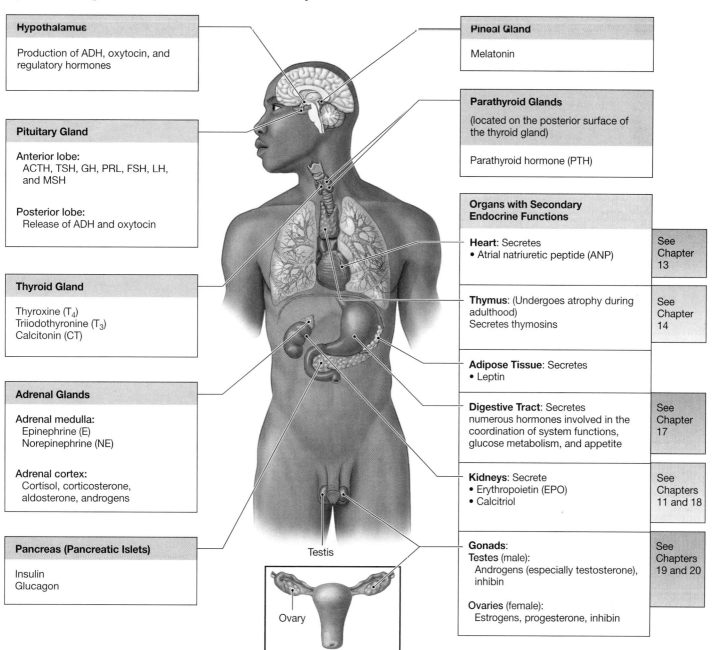

Hypothalamus

Production of ADH, oxytocin, and regulatory hormones

Pituitary Gland

Anterior lobe:
ACTH, TSH, GH, PRL, FSH, LH, and MSH

Posterior lobe:
Release of ADH and oxytocin

Thyroid Gland

Thyroxine (T_4)
Triiodothyronine (T_3)
Calcitonin (CT)

Adrenal Glands

Adrenal medulla:
Epinephrine (E)
Norepinephrine (NE)

Adrenal cortex:
Cortisol, corticosterone, aldosterone, androgens

Pancreas (Pancreatic Islets)

Insulin
Glucagon

Testis

Ovary

Pineal Gland

Melatonin

Parathyroid Glands

(located on the posterior surface of the thyroid gland)

Parathyroid hormone (PTH)

Organs with Secondary Endocrine Functions

Heart: Secretes
• Atrial natriuretic peptide (ANP)

See Chapter 13

Thymus: (Undergoes atrophy during adulthood)
Secretes thymosins

See Chapter 14

Adipose Tissue: Secretes
• Leptin

Digestive Tract: Secretes numerous hormones involved in the coordination of system functions, glucose metabolism, and appetite

See Chapter 17

Kidneys: Secrete
• Erythropoietin (EPO)
• Calcitriol

See Chapters 11 and 18

Gonads:
Testes (male):
Androgens (especially testosterone), inhibin

Ovaries (female):
Estrogens, progesterone, inhibin

See Chapters 19 and 20

10

Figure 10-2 The Role of Target Cell Receptors in Hormone Action. For a hormone to affect a target cell, that cell must have receptors that can bind the hormone and initiate a change in cellular activity. The hormone shown here affects skeletal muscle tissue but not neural tissue, because only the muscle tissue has the appropriate receptors.

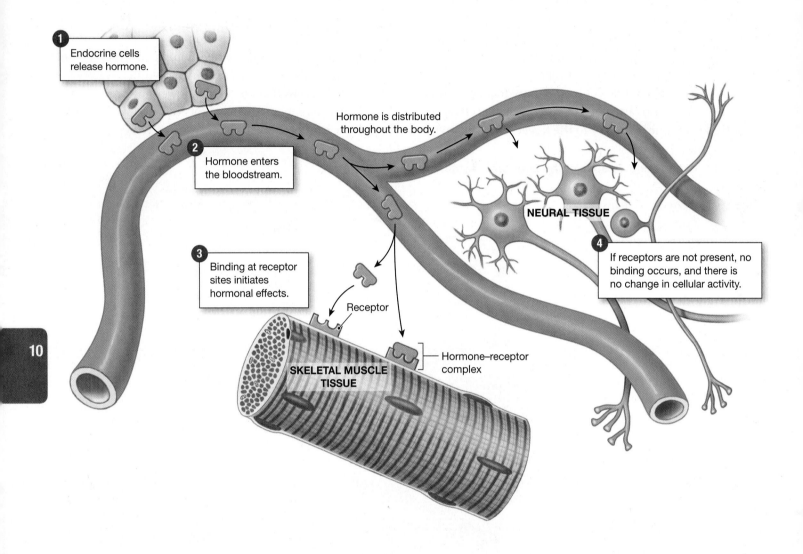

1 Endocrine cells release hormone.

Hormone is distributed throughout the body.

2 Hormone enters the bloodstream.

NEURAL TISSUE

3 Binding at receptor sites initiates hormonal effects.

4 If receptors are not present, no binding occurs, and there is no change in cellular activity.

Receptor

Hormone–receptor complex

SKELETAL MUSCLE TISSUE

target cell. Instead, communication between the hormone and the cell uses both first and second messengers. A **first messenger** is the hormone that binds to a receptor on the plasma membrane surface. A **second messenger** is an intermediary molecule that forms due to a hormone-receptor interaction.

The link between the first messenger and the second messenger usually involves a **G protein**, an enzyme complex coupled to a receptor on the plasma membrane. The G protein is activated when a hormone binds to the receptor at the membrane surface. Its activation gives rise to second messengers in the cell. The second messenger in turn may activate or inhibit enzymes inside the cell, but the net result is a change in the cell's metabolic activities. (Roughly

80 percent of prescription drugs target receptors coupled to G proteins.)

When a small number of hormone molecules bind to membrane receptors, thousands of second messengers may be formed in a cell. This process, called *amplification*, magnifies the effect of a hormone on the target cell.

One of the most important second messengers is **cyclic-AMP (cAMP)** (**Figure 10-3a**). Its formation depends on an activated G protein, which activates an enzyme called **adenylate cyclase**. Adenylate cyclase converts ATP to a ring-shaped molecule of cAMP. Cyclic-AMP then functions as a second messenger, typically by activating a kinase (KĪ-nās). Kinases are enzymes that attach a high-energy phosphate group (PO_4^{3-}) to another molecule in a process called *phosphorylation*.

Figure 10-3 Processes of Hormone Action.

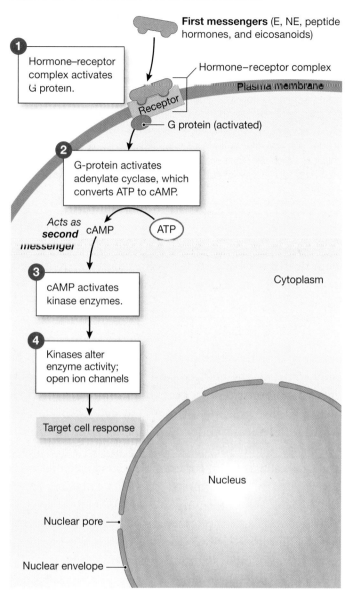

First messengers (E, NE, peptide hormones, and eicosanoids)

1 Hormone–receptor complex activates G protein.

Hormone–receptor complex

Receptor

Plasma membrane

G protein (activated)

2 G-protein activates adenylate cyclase, which converts ATP to cAMP.

*Acts as **second** messenger* cAMP ATP

3 cAMP activates kinase enzymes.

Cytoplasm

4 Kinases alter enzyme activity; open ion channels

Target cell response

Nucleus

Nuclear pore

Nuclear envelope

a Nonsteroidal hormones, such as epinephrine (E), norepinephrine (NE), peptide hormones, and eicosanoids, bind to membrane receptors and activate G proteins. They exert their effects on target cells through a second messenger, such as cAMP, which alters the activity of enzymes present in the cell.

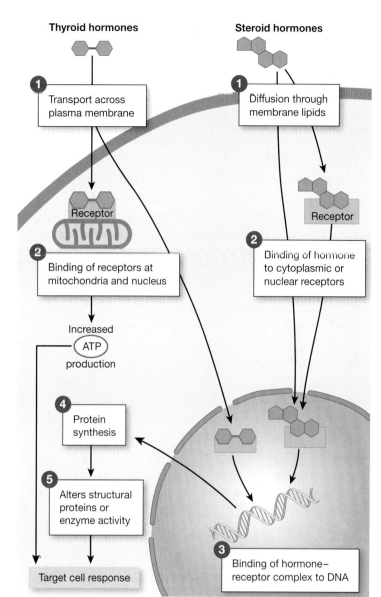

Thyroid hormones   **Steroid hormones**

1 Transport across plasma membrane

1 Diffusion through membrane lipids

Receptor   Receptor

2 Binding of receptors at mitochondria and nucleus

2 Binding of hormone to cytoplasmic or nuclear receptors

Increased ATP production

4 Protein synthesis

5 Alters structural proteins or enzyme activity

3 Binding of hormone–receptor complex to DNA

Target cell response

b Thyroid hormones are transported across the target cell's plasma membrane and either bind to receptors in the nucleus or to receptors on mitochondria. Steroid hormones enter a target cell by diffusion and bind to receptors in the cytoplasm or nucleus. In the nucleus, both steroid and thyroid hormone–receptor complexes directly affect gene activity and protein synthesis. Thyroid hormones also increase the rate of ATP production in the cell.

Generally, cAMP activates kinases that phosphorylate proteins. The effect on the target cell depends on the nature of the proteins affected. For example, the phosphorylation of certain membrane proteins can open ion channels. In the cytoplasm, many enzymes can be activated only by phosphorylation. As a result, a single hormone can have one effect in one target tissue and quite different effects in other target tissues.

The effects of cAMP are usually very short-lived, because another enzyme in the cell, *phosphodiesterase (PDE)*, inactivates cAMP by converting it to adenosine monophosphate (AMP). In a few instances, the activation of a G protein can *lower* the concentration of cAMP within the cell by stimulating PDE activity. The decline in cAMP has an inhibitory effect on the cell because without phosphorylation, key enzymes remain inactive.

Cyclic-AMP is one of the most common second messengers, but there are many others. Important examples are *calcium ions* and *cyclic-GMP*, a derivative of the high-energy compound *guanosine triphosphate.*

Hormones and Intracellular Receptors

Thyroid hormones and steroid hormones cross the plasma membrane before binding to receptors inside the cell (intracellular receptors) (**Figure 10-3b**). Thyroid hormones cross the plasma membrane primarily by a carrier-mediated transport process. Once within the cell, thyroid hormones bind to receptors within the nucleus or on mitochondria. The resulting *hormone–receptor complexes* in the nucleus activate specific genes or change the rate of mRNA transcription. As a result, metabolic activity increases due to changes in the nature or number of enzymes in the cytoplasm. Thyroid hormones bound to mitochondria increase the mitochondrial rates of ATP production.

Steroid hormones diffuse rapidly through the lipid portion of the plasma membrane and bind to intracellular receptors in the cytoplasm or nucleus. The resulting *hormone–receptor complex* then activates or inactivates specific genes. By this process, steroid hormones can alter the rate of DNA transcription in the nucleus. In this way, they change the pattern of protein synthesis and the structure or function of the cell. For example, the sex hormone testosterone stimulates the production of enzymes and proteins in skeletal muscle fibers, increasing muscle size and strength.

The Secretion and Distribution of Hormones

Hormones are released where capillaries are abundant. The hormones quickly enter the bloodstream for distribution throughout the body. Within the blood, hormones may circulate freely or travel bound to special transport proteins. A freely circulating hormone remains functional for less than one hour, and sometimes for as little as two minutes. It is inactivated when (1) it diffuses out of the bloodstream and binds to receptors on target cells, (2) it is absorbed and broken down by certain liver or kidney cells, or (3) it is broken down by enzymes in the plasma or interstitial fluids.

Steroid hormones and thyroid hormones remain in circulation much longer because almost all become attached to special transport proteins. For each hormone, an equilibrium

CLINICAL NOTE

Endocrine Emergencies

The symptoms of endocrine emergencies (**Figure 10-4**) can usually be assigned to one of two basic categories: symptoms of underproduction (inadequate hormonal effects) or symptoms of overproduction (excessive hormonal effects). The observed symptoms may reflect either abnormal hormone production (hyposecretion or hypersecretion) or abnormal cellular sensitivity. These conditions are interesting because they highlight the significance of normally "silent" hormonal contributions.

occurs between the bound hormones and the small number remaining in a free state. As the free hormones are removed, they are replaced by the release of bound hormones.

The Control of Endocrine Activity

Endocrine activity—specifically, hormone secretion—is mainly controlled by negative feedback. That is, a stimulus triggers the production of a hormone whose direct or indirect effects reduce the intensity of the stimulus. ⟳ p. 10

In the simplest case, endocrine activity may be controlled by *humoral* ("liquid") *stimuli*—changes in the composition of the extracellular fluid. For example, blood calcium levels are controlled by two hormones, *parathyroid hormone (PTH)* and *calcitonin.* When calcium levels in the blood decrease, PTH is released, and the responses of target cells increase blood calcium levels. When calcium levels in the blood increase, calcitonin is released, and the responses of target cells decrease blood calcium levels.

Endocrine activity may also be controlled by *hormonal stimuli*—changes in the levels of circulating hormones. Such control may involve one or more intermediary steps and two or more hormones.

Finally, endocrine control can be triggered by *neural stimuli* that result when a neurotransmitter arrives at a neuroglandular junction. An important example of endocrine activity linked to neural stimuli involves the activity of the hypothalamus.

The hypothalamus provides the highest level of endocrine control. It acts as an important link between the nervous and endocrine systems. Coordinating centers in the hypothalamus regulate the activities of the nervous and endocrine systems in three ways (**Figure 10-4**):

Figure 10-4 Hypothalamic Control over Endocrine Function.

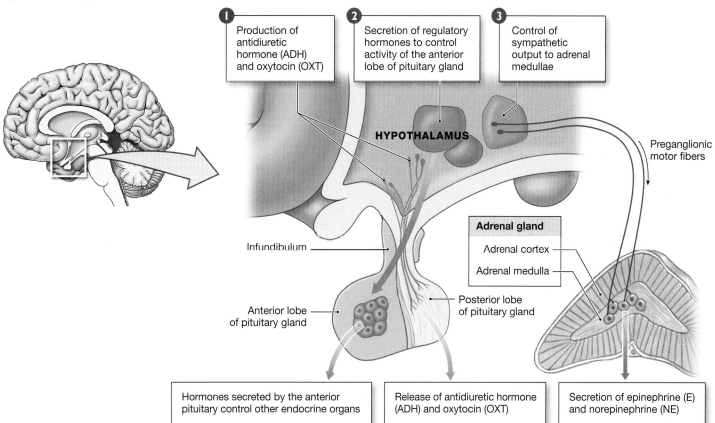

1. ***The hypothalamus secretes two hormones directly into the general circulation.*** Neurons in the hypothalamus synthesize two hormones—ADH and oxytocin—which are transported along axons to the posterior lobe of the pituitary gland. From there, they are released into the bloodstream for distribution throughout the body. ⤴ p. 276

2. ***The hypothalamus secretes two classes of regulatory hormones.*** **Regulatory hormones** are special hormones that control endocrine cells in the anterior lobe of the pituitary gland. **Releasing hormones (RH)** stimulate the synthesis and secretion of one or more hormones in the anterior lobe. **Inhibiting hormones (IH)** prevent the synthesis and secretion of pituitary hormones. The hormones released by the anterior lobe of the pituitary gland control other endocrine glands.

3. ***The hypothalamus controls sympathetic output to the adrenal medullae.*** The hypothalamus contains autonomic nervous system centers that control the endocrine cells of the adrenal medullae (the interior of the adrenal glands) through sympathetic innervation. ⤴ p. 292 When the sympathetic division is activated, the adrenal medullae release hormones into the bloodstream.

CHECKPOINT

2. Define hormone.

3. What primary factor determines each cell's sensitivities to hormones?

4. How would the presence of a molecule that blocks adenylate cyclase affect the activity of a hormone that produces cellular effects through cAMP?

5. Why is cAMP described as a second messenger?

6. What are the three types of stimuli that control hormone secretion?

See the blue Answers tab at the back of the book.

10-3 The bilobed pituitary gland is an endocrine organ that releases nine peptide hormones

Learning Objective Describe the location, hormones, and functions of the pituitary gland.

The **pituitary gland**, or **hypophysis** (hī-POF-i-sis), is a small, oval gland nestled within the *sella turcica*, a depression in the sphenoid bone of the skull (**Figure 10-5**). It hangs beneath the hypothalamus, connected by a slender stalk, the **infundibulum** (in-fun-DIB-ū-lum; funnel). The pituitary gland has a complex structure, with distinct anterior and posterior lobes. It secretes nine important peptide hormones. Seven come from the anterior lobe and two from the posterior lobe. All nine bind to membrane receptors. All also use cAMP as a second messenger.

The Anterior Lobe of the Pituitary Gland

The **anterior lobe** of the pituitary gland contains endocrine cells surrounded by an extensive capillary network. The hormones secreted by the endocrine cells of the anterior lobe enter the bloodstream through the capillaries. This capillary network is part of the *hypophyseal portal system*.

The Hypophyseal Portal System

The hypothalamus controls the production of hormones in the anterior lobe of the pituitary gland by secreting regulatory hormones. These hormones are released by hypothalamic neurons near the attachment of the infundibulum. There the hormones enter a network of highly permeable capillaries. Before leaving the hypothalamus, this capillary network unites to form a series of slightly larger vessels that descend to the anterior lobe and then form a second capillary network (**Figure 10-6**).

The circulatory arrangement illustrated in **Figure 10-6**, in which blood flows from one capillary bed to another, is very unusual. Typically, blood flows from the heart through increasingly smaller arteries to a capillary network and then returns to the heart through increasingly larger veins. Blood vessels that link two capillary networks—including the vessels between the hypothalamus and the anterior lobe—are called *portal vessels*. Here, the portal vessels have the structure of veins, so they are also called *portal veins*. The entire complex is termed a **portal system**.

Portal systems ensure that all the blood entering the portal vessels reaches certain target cells before returning to the general circulation. Portal systems are named after their destinations, so this particular network is called the **hypophyseal** (hī-pō-FIZ-ē-al) **portal system**.

Figure 10-5 The Location and Anatomy of the Pituitary Gland.

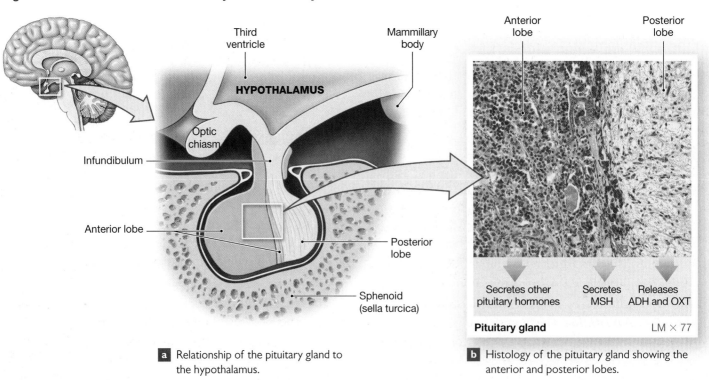

a Relationship of the pituitary gland to the hypothalamus.

b Histology of the pituitary gland showing the anterior and posterior lobes.

Figure 10-6 The Hypophyseal Portal System and the Blood Supply to the Pituitary Gland.

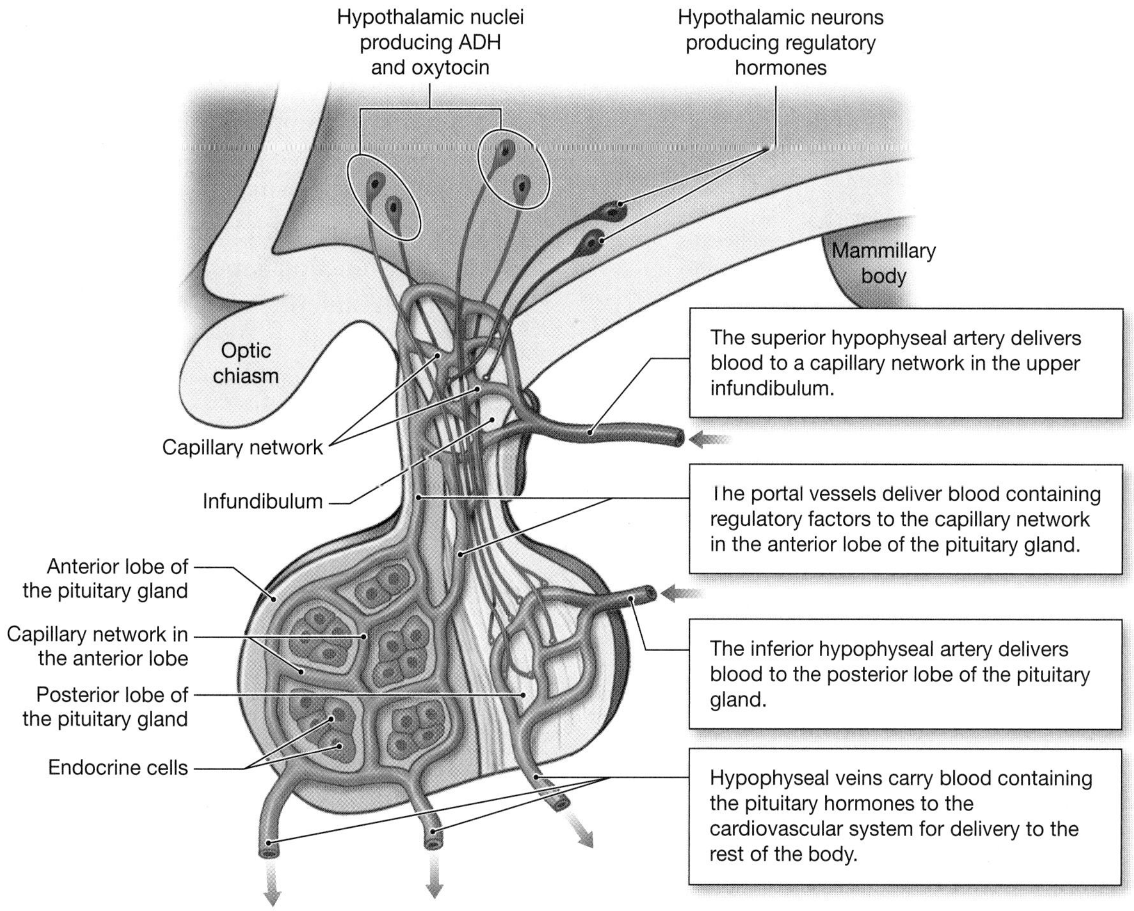

Hypothalamic Control of the Anterior Lobe

The regulatory hormones released at the hypothalamus travel directly to the anterior lobe by the hypophyseal portal system. An endocrine cell in the anterior lobe of the pituitary may be controlled by RH, IH, or some combination of the two.

Negative feedback regulates the rate of regulatory hormone secretion by the hypothalamus. The basic regulatory patterns are diagrammed in **Figure 10-7**. We will refer to these patterns in the following description of pituitary hormones. Many of these regulatory hormones are called *tropic hormones* (*tropos*, a turning) because they "turn on" other endocrine glands or support the functions of other organs.

Hormones of the Anterior Lobe

The anterior lobe of the pituitary gland produces seven hormones. The first four described in the following list regulate the production of hormones by other endocrine glands.

1. **Thyroid-stimulating hormone (TSH)**, or *thyrotropin*, targets the thyroid gland and triggers the release of thyroid hormones. TSH is released in response to *thyrotropin-releasing hormone (TRH)* from the hypothalamus. As circulating concentrations of thyroid hormones rise, the rates of TRH and TSH production decline (**Figure 10-7a**).

2. **Adrenocorticotropic hormone (ACTH)**, or *corticotropin*, stimulates the release of steroid hormones by the *adrenal cortex*, the outer portion of the adrenal glands. ACTH specifically targets cells producing hormones called *glucocorticoids* (gloo-kō-KOR-ti-koydz), which affect glucose metabolism. ACTH release occurs under the stimulation of *corticotropin-releasing hormone (CRH)* from the hypothalamus. A rise in glucocorticoid levels causes a decline in the production of ACTH and CRH. This type of negative feedback control is similar to that for TSH (**Figure 10-7a**).

The hormones called **gonadotropins** (gō-nad-ō-TRŌ-pinz) regulate the activities of the male and female *gonads*. (These organs—the testes in males and the ovaries

Figure 10-7 Negative Feedback Control of Endocrine Secretion.

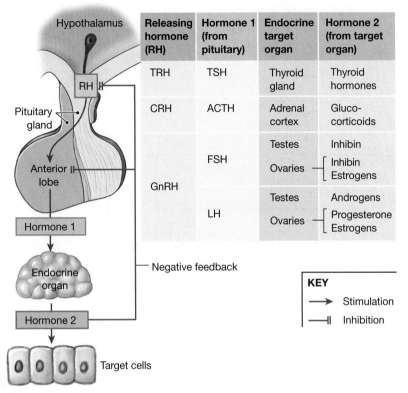

Releasing hormone (RH)	Hormone 1 (from pituitary)	Endocrine target organ	Hormone 2 (from target organ)
TRH	TSH	Thyroid gland	Thyroid hormones
CRH	ACTH	Adrenal cortex	Gluco-corticoids
GnRH	FSH	Testes	Inhibin
		Ovaries	Inhibin / Estrogens
	LH	Testes	Androgens
		Ovaries	Progesterone / Estrogens

KEY

→ Stimulation

⊣ Inhibition

a A typical pattern of regulation when multiple endocrine organs are involved. The hypothalamus produces a releasing hormone (RH) to stimulate hormone production by other glands; control occurs by negative feedback.

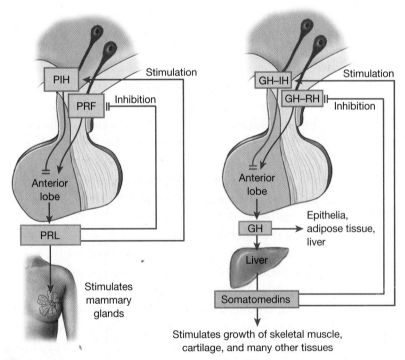

b Variations on the theme outlined in part (a). Left: The regulation of prolactin (PRL) production by the anterior lobe. In this case, the hypothalamus produces both a releasing factor (PRF) and an inhibiting hormone (PIH); when one is stimulated, the other is inhibited. Right: the regulation of growth hormone (GH) production by the anterior lobe; when GH–RH release is inhibited, GH–IH release is stimulated.

in females—produce reproductive cells as well as hormones.) The production of gonadotropins is stimulated by *gonadotropin-releasing hormone (GnRH)* from the hypothalamus. An abnormally low production of gonadotropins produces *hypogonadism*. Children with this condition will not undergo sexual maturation. Adults with hypogonadism cannot produce functional sperm (males) or ova (females). The anterior lobe produces two gonadotropins: follicle-stimulating hormone (FSH) and luteinizing (LŪ-tē-i-nīz-ing) hormone (LH).

3. **FSH** promotes follicle development in females, and, with luteinizing hormone, stimulates the secretion of estrogens by ovarian cells. In males, FSH supports sperm production in the testes. A peptide hormone called *inhibin*, released by the cells of the testes and ovaries, inhibits the release of FSH and GnRH through negative feedback comparable to that for TSH (**Figure 10-7a**).

4. **LH** induces *ovulation*, the production of reproductive cells in females. It also promotes the secretion by the ovaries of estrogens and *progesterone*, which prepare the body for possible pregnancy. In males, LH is sometimes called *interstitial cell-stimulating hormone* because it stimulates the interstitial cells of the testes to produce sex hormones. These male sex hormones are called **androgens** (AN-drō-jenz; *andros*, man). The most important one is *testosterone*. LH production, like FSH production, is stimulated by GnRH from the hypothalamus. Estrogens, progesterone, and androgens inhibit GnRH production (**Figure 10-7a**).

5. **Prolactin** (prō-LAK-tin; *pro-*, before + *lac*, milk), or **PRL**, works with other hormones to stimulate mammary gland development. In pregnancy and during the period of nursing following delivery, PRL also stimulates milk production by the mammary glands. Prolactin's effects in human males are poorly understood, but it may help regulate androgen production. The production of PRL is stimulated by prolactin-releasing factor (PRF) from the hypothalamus. Circulating

PRL then stimulates prolactin-inhibiting hormone from the hypothalamus and also inhibits the secretion of PRF. This regulatory pattern is diagrammed in **Figure 10-7b**.

6. **GH**, also called *human growth hormone (hGH)* or *somatotropin* (*soma*, body), stimulates cell growth and replication by speeding up the rate of protein synthesis. Skeletal muscle cells and chondrocytes (cartilage cells) are particularly sensitive to GH. Virtually every tissue responds to some degree, however.

GH stimulates growth through two processes—indirect and direct. The primary process is indirect, and best understood. Liver cells respond to GH by synthesizing and releasing **somatomedins**, or *insulin-like growth factors*. These peptide hormones bind to receptor sites on a variety of plasma membranes. Somatomedins increase the rates at which amino acids are taken up and combined into new proteins. These effects develop almost immediately after GH is released. They are particularly important after a meal, when blood glucose and amino acid concentrations are high.

The direct actions of GH are more selective. They play a role in mobilizing energy reserves. They usually do not occur until after blood glucose and amino acid concentrations have returned to normal levels:

- In epithelia and connective tissues, GH stimulates stem cell divisions and the differentiation of daughter cells. (Somatomedins then stimulate the growth of these daughter cells.)
- In adipose tissue, GH stimulates the breakdown of stored fats and the release of fatty acids into the blood. In turn, many tissues stop breaking down glucose and start breaking down fatty acids to generate ATP. This process is termed a glucose-sparing effect.
- In the liver, GH stimulates the breakdown of glycogen reserves and the release of glucose into the bloodstream. Blood glucose concentrations rise higher than normal because most tissues are now metabolizing fatty acids.

The production of GH is regulated by *growth hormone-releasing hormone (GH–RH)* and *growth hormone–inhibiting hormone (GH–IH)* from the hypothalamus. Somatomedins stimulate GH–IH and inhibit GH–RH. This regulatory process is summarized in **Figure 10-7b**.

7. **Melanocyte-stimulating hormone (MSH)** stimulates the melanocytes in the skin to increase their production of melanin. ⟲ p. 126 MSH is important in the control of skin and hair pigmentation in fishes, amphibians, reptiles, and many mammals other than primates. In humans, MSH is produced locally, within sun-exposed skin. The MSH-producing cells of the pituitary gland in adult humans are virtually nonfunctional, and the circulating blood usually does not contain MSH. However, the human pituitary secretes MSH (1) during fetal development, (2) in very young children, (3) in pregnant women, and (4) in certain diseases. The functions of MSH under these circumstances are not known. The administration of a synthetic form of MSH causes darkening of the skin, so MSH has been suggested as a means of obtaining a "sunless tan."

The Posterior Lobe of the Pituitary Gland

The **posterior lobe** of the pituitary gland contains axons from two different groups of hypothalamic neurons. One group synthesizes ADH. The other synthesizes oxytocin. These hormones are transported within axons along the infundibulum to the posterior lobe, as indicated in **Figure 10-6**.

ADH, also known as *vasopressin*, is released when the body is low on water. Stimuli for its release include a rise in the concentration of solutes in the blood (an increased osmotic concentration) or a fall in blood volume or pressure. Specialized neurons in the hypothalamus, called *osmoreceptors*, detect a rise in osmotic concentration. The osmoreceptors then stimulate the hypothalamic neurons that release ADH.

Diuresis (dī-ū-RĒ-sis) typically indicates the production of a large volume of urine. The primary function of ADH is to decrease the amount of water lost in the urine. With losses minimized, any water absorbed from the digestive tract will be retained, reducing the concentration of solutes. ADH also causes *vasoconstriction*, a constriction of peripheral blood vessels that helps increase blood pressure. Alcohol inhibits ADH release, which explains the increased fluid excretion that follows when someone drinks alcoholic beverages.

In women, **oxytocin** (*okytokos*, swift birth), or **OXT**, stimulates smooth muscle contractions in the wall of the uterus, promoting labor and delivery. Until the final stages of pregnancy, the uterine muscles are insensitive to oxytocin, but they become more sensitive as the time of delivery approaches. The stimulation of uterine muscles by oxytocin helps maintain and complete normal labor and childbirth (discussed in Chapter 20).

Oxytocin also promotes the ejection of milk by the mammary glands. After delivery, oxytocin stimulates the contraction of special contractile cells surrounding the secretory cells and ducts of the mammary glands. In the "milk letdown" reflex, oxytocin is secreted in response to suckling and triggers the release of milk from the breasts.

Oxytocin's functions in sexual activity remain uncertain, but circulating oxytocin levels are known to rise during sexual arousal and peak at orgasm in both sexes. In men, oxytocin stimulates smooth muscle contraction in the walls of the sperm duct and prostate gland. These actions may be important in *emission*, the ejection of prostate secretions, sperm, and the secretions of other glands into the male reproductive tract before ejaculation. In women, oxytocin released during intercourse may stimulate smooth muscle contractions in the uterus and vagina that promote the transport of sperm toward the uterine tubes.

Figure 10-8 and **Table 10-1** summarize important information about the hormones of the pituitary gland.

CLINICAL NOTE

Vasopressin

Antidiuretic hormone (ADH), also called *vasopressin*, is one of two hormones secreted by the posterior pituitary. It decreases the amount of water lost through the kidney and causes constriction of peripheral blood vessels (vasoconstriction). Both mechanisms serve to increase the blood pressure.

When vasopressin is given in unnaturally high doses, much higher than those needed for its ADH effects, its vasoconstrictive properties are enhanced. Because of this, vasopressin can be used to treat certain types of medical conditions. The side effects include nausea, intestinal cramps, the urge to defecate, bronchial constriction, and pallor of the skin. In women, it can also cause uterine contractions.

CLINICAL NOTE

Diabetes Insipidus

Diabetes (*diabetes*, to pass through) occurs in several forms. All are characterized by excessive urine production (polyuria). Most forms result from endocrine abnormalities, but diabetes can be caused by physical damage to the kidneys. The two most important forms are diabetes mellitus and diabetes insipidus. (Diabetes mellitus is described on p. 366.)

Diabetes insipidus (*insipidus*, tasteless) develops when the posterior lobe of the pituitary gland no longer releases adequate amounts of ADH or the kidneys fail to respond to ADH. Water conservation at the kidneys is impaired, and excessive amounts of water are lost in the urine. As a result, the individual is constantly thirsty—a condition known as polydipsia (*dipsa*, thirst)—but the body does not retain the fluids consumed. Mild cases may not require treatment, as long as fluid and electrolyte intake keep pace with urinary losses. In severe cases, fluid losses can reach 10 liters per day, and a fatal dehydration will occur unless treatment is provided.

CHECKPOINT

7. If a person were dehydrated, how would the amount of ADH released by the posterior lobe of the pituitary gland change?

8. A blood sample contains elevated levels of somatomedins. Which pituitary hormone would you also expect to be elevated?

9. What effect would elevated circulating levels of cortisol, a hormone from the adrenal cortex, have on the pituitary secretion of ACTH?

See the blue Answers tab at the back of the book.

10-4 The thyroid gland lies inferior to the larynx and requires iodine for hormone synthesis

Learning Objective Describe the location, hormones, and functions of the thyroid gland.

The **thyroid gland** lies anterior to the trachea and just inferior to the *thyroid* ("shield-shaped") *cartilage*, which forms most of the anterior surface of the larynx (**Figure 10-9a**). The two lobes of the thyroid gland are united by a slender connection, the *isthmus* (IS-mus). An extensive blood supply gives the thyroid gland a deep red color.

Thyroid Follicles and Thyroid Hormones

The thyroid gland contains numerous **thyroid follicles**, spheres lined by a simple cuboidal epithelium (**Figure 10-9b,c**). The cavity within each follicle contains a viscous *colloid*, a fluid containing large amounts of suspended proteins and thyroid hormones. A network of capillaries surrounds each follicle. They deliver nutrients and regulatory hormones to the glandular cells and pick up their secretory products and metabolic wastes.

Thyroid hormones are manufactured by the follicular epithelial cells and stored within the follicle cavities. Under TSH stimulation from the anterior lobe of the

Figure 10-8 Pituitary Hormones and Their Targets.

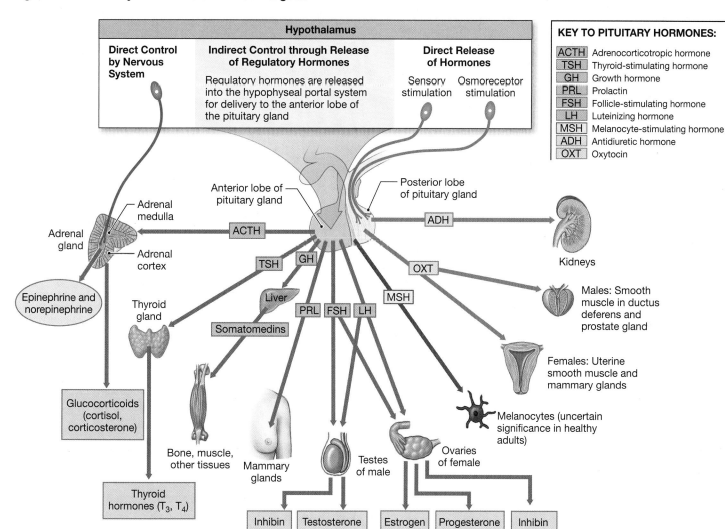

pituitary gland, the epithelial cells remove hormones from the follicle cavities and release them into the bloodstream. However, almost all the released thyroid hormones are unavailable because they become attached to plasma proteins in the blood. Only the remaining unbound thyroid hormones, a small percentage of the total released, are free to be transported into target cells in body tissues. As the concentration of unbound hormone molecules decreases, the plasma proteins release additional bound hormone. The bound thyroid hormones are a substantial reserve. In fact, the bloodstream normally contains more than a week's supply of thyroid hormones.

The thyroid hormones are derived from molecules of the amino acid tyrosine to which iodine atoms have been attached. The hormone **thyroxine** (thī-ROKS-ēn) contains

four atoms of iodine. It is also known as *tetraiodothyronine* (tet-ra-ī-ō-dō-THĪ-rō-nēn), or **T4**. Thyroxine accounts for roughly 90 percent of all thyroid secretions. **Triiodothyronine**, or **T3**, is a related, more potent molecule containing three iodine atoms.

Thyroid hormones affect almost every cell in the body. Inside a cell, they bind to receptor sites on mitochondria and in the nucleus (**Figure 10-3b**). The binding of thyroid hormones to mitochondria increases the rate of ATP production. Thyroid hormone–receptor complexes in the nucleus activate genes coding for the synthesis of enzymes involved in glycolysis and energy production. As a result, rates of metabolism and oxygen consumption increase in the cell. The effect is called the **calorigenic effect** (*calor*, heat) of thyroid hormones because the cell consumes more

Table 10-1	The Pituitary Hormones	
Pituitary Lobe/Hormone	**Target**	**Hormonal Effects**
ANTERIOR LOBE		
Thyroid-stimulating hormone (TSH)	Thyroid gland	Secretion of thyroid hormones
Adrenocorticotropic hormone (ACTH)	Adrenal cortex	Secretion of glucocorticoids (cortisol, corticosterone)
Gonadotropins:		
Follicle-stimulating hormone (FSH)	Follicle cells of ovaries	Secretion of estrogen, follicle development
	Nurse cells of testes	Sperm maturation
Luteinizing hormone (LH)	Follicle cells of ovaries	Ovulation, formation of corpus luteum, secretion of progesterone
	Interstitial cells of testes	Secretion of testosterone
Prolactin (PRL)	Mammary glands	Production of milk
Growth hormone (GH)	**All cells**	**Growth, protein synthesis, lipid mobilization and catabolism**
Melanocyte-stimulating hormone (MSH)	Melanocytes of skin	Increased melanin synthesis in epidermis
POSTERIOR LOBE		
Antidiuretic hormone (ADH)	Kidneys	Reabsorption of water, elevation of blood volume and pressure
Oxytocin (OXT)	Uterus, mammary glands (females)	Labor contractions, milk ejection
	Sperm duct and prostate gland (males)	Contractions of sperm duct and prostate gland

energy (and energy use is measured in *calories*). When the metabolic rate increases, more heat is generated and body temperature rises. In growing children, thyroid hormones are essential to normal development of the skeletal, muscular, and nervous systems.

Normal production of thyroid hormones establishes the background rates of cellular metabolism. These hormones exert their primary effects on active tissues and organs, including skeletal muscles, the liver, the heart, and the kidneys. Overproduction or underproduction of thyroid hormones can, therefore, cause very serious metabolic problems. In many parts of the world, inadequate dietary iodine intake leads to an inability to synthesize thyroid hormones. Under these conditions, TSH stimulation continues, and the thyroid follicles become distended with nonfunctional secretions. The result is an enlarged thyroid gland, or *goiter*. Goiters vary in size, and a large goiter can interfere with breathing and swallowing. This is seldom a problem in the United States where the typical American diet provides roughly three times the minimum daily requirement of iodine. Much of the excess is due to the addition of iodine to table salt (iodized salt), which is consumed in large quantities in processed foods.

The C Cells of the Thyroid Gland and Calcitonin

C cells, or *parafollicular cells*, are endocrine cells sandwiched between the follicle cells and their basement membrane (see **Figure 10-9b,c**). C cells produce the hormone **calcitonin**. Calcitonin helps regulate calcium ion concentrations in body fluids.

The control of calcitonin secretion is independent of the hypothalamus or pituitary gland. As **Figure 10-10** shows, C cells release calcitonin when the calcium ion (Ca^{2+}) concentration of the blood rises above normal. The target organs are the bones and the kidneys. Calcitonin inhibits osteoclasts (which slows the release of calcium from bone) and stimulates calcium excretion by the kidneys. The resulting reduction in blood calcium levels eliminates the stimulus and "turns off" the C cells.

Calcitonin is most important during childhood, when it stimulates active bone growth and calcium deposition in the skeleton. It also acts to reduce the loss of bone mass during prolonged starvation and during late pregnancy, when the maternal skeleton competes with the developing fetus for absorbed calcium ions. The role of calcitonin in healthy nonpregnant adults is unclear.

Figure 10-9 The Thyroid Gland.

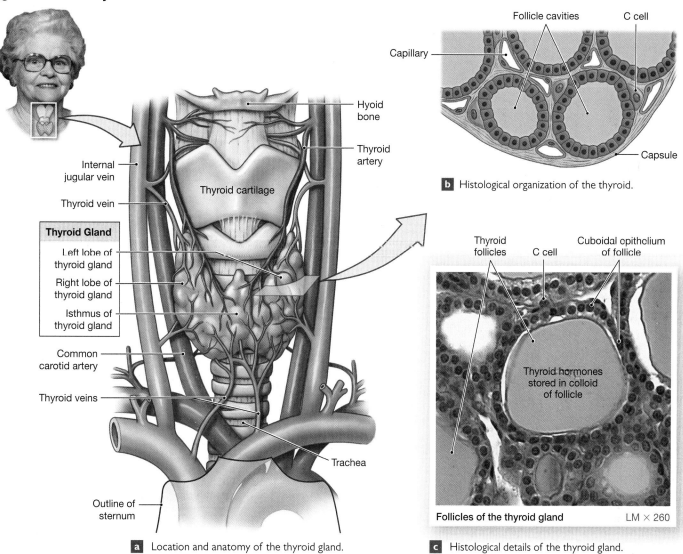

b Histological organization of the thyroid.

a Location and anatomy of the thyroid gland.

Follicles of the thyroid gland — LM × 260

c Histological details of the thyroid gland.

We have seen the importance of calcium ions in controlling muscle cell and nerve cell activities.⤴ pp. 202, 259 Calcium ion concentrations also affect the sodium permeabilities of excitable membranes. At high calcium levels, sodium permeability decreases, and membranes become less responsive. Such problems are relatively rare, because under normal conditions, calcium levels seldom rise enough to trigger calcitonin secretion.

Most homeostatic adjustments prevent lower-than-normal calcium ion concentrations. Low calcium concentrations are dangerous because sodium permeabilities then increase, and muscle cells and neurons become extremely excitable. If calcium levels fall too far, convulsions or muscular spasms can result. Such disastrous events are prevented by the actions of the parathyroid glands.

CHECKPOINT

10. Identify the hormones of the thyroid gland.

11. What signs and symptoms would you expect to see in an individual whose diet lacks iodine?

12. When a person's thyroid gland is removed, signs of decreased thyroid hormone concentration do not appear until about one week later. Why?

See the blue Answers tab at the back of the book.

Figure 10-10 The Homeostatic Regulation of Calcium Ion Concentrations.

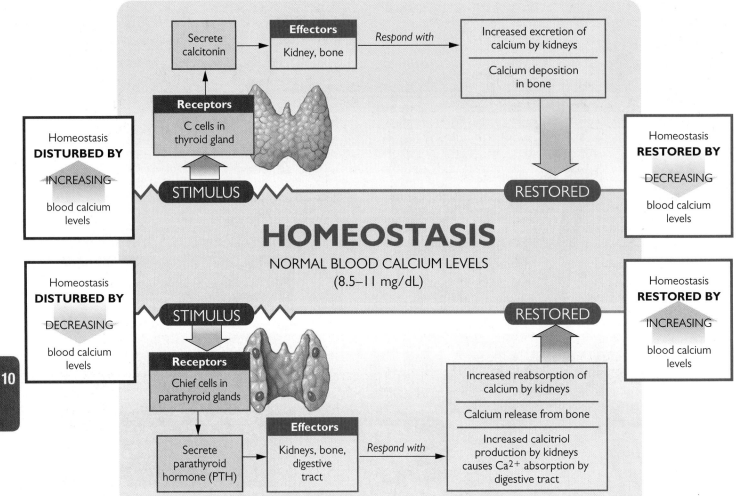

CLINICAL NOTE

Disorders of the Thyroid Gland

Disorders of the thyroid gland are typically chronic conditions. However, you may see patients with acute complications of thyroid disorders. The most common of these are:

- *Hyperthyroidism.* The presence of excess thyroid hormones in the blood.
- *Thyrotoxic crisis.* A condition that reflects prolonged exposure of body organs to excess thyroid hormones, with resultant changes in structure and function. Thyrotoxicosis is generally caused by Graves' disease.
- *Hypothyroidism.* The presence of inadequate thyroid hormones in the blood.
- *Myxedema.* A condition that reflects long-term exposure to inadequate levels of thyroid hormones, with resultant changes in structure and function.

The risk factors for developing thyroid dysfunction include:

- Female sex
- Older age
- Personal history:
  - Goiter
  - Previous surgery or radiotherapy that affects the thyroid gland
  - Other autoimmune diseases, including diabetes mellitus, vitiligo, pernicious anemia, and leukotrichia
  - Use of lithium or compounds that contain iodine
- Family history:
  - Thyroid disease
  - Pernicious anemia
  - Diabetes mellitus
  - Primary adrenal insufficiency

Figure 10-11 The Thyroid Loop. The hypothalamus controls the anterior pituitary, which in turn controls the thyroid gland. Negative feedback loops prevent the oversecretion of hormones.

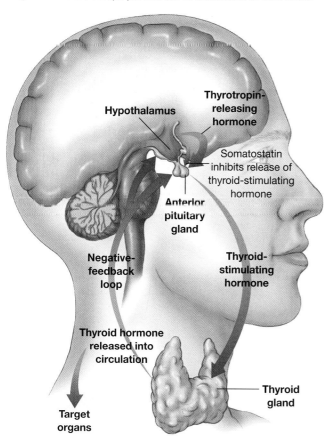

Table 10-2	Common Signs and Symptoms of Thyroid Disease	
Hypothyroidism	**Hyperthyroidism**	
Fatigue	Fatigue	
Weight gain	Weight loss	
Cold intolerance	Heat intolerance	
Skin dry	Skin moist (hyperhidrous)	
Hair dryness and/or loss	Hair fine and silky	
Depression	Nervousness	
Dementia	Insomnia	
	Tremor	
Muscle cramps and myalgia	Muscle weakness	
	Dyspnea	
Bradycardia	Tachycardia	
	Palpations	
Constipation	Hyperdefecation	
Infertility		
Edema		
Menstrual irregularity (hypermenorrhea common)	Menstrual irregularity (hypermenorrhea common)	

Source: "American Thyroid Association Guidelines for Detection of Thyroid Dysfunction." *Archives of Internal Medicine* 160 (2000): 1573–75.

The thyroid gland is controlled by the anterior pituitary gland through the release of thyroid-stimulating hormone (TSH). The anterior pituitary, in turn, is controlled by the hypothalamus through the release of thyrotropin-releasing hormone. An increased level of TSH results in increased thyroid function, while a decreased level results in a decline. A negative feedback loop exists between the thyroid gland and the anterior pituitary gland and hypothalamus (**Figure 10-11**). **Table 10-2** compares common signs and symptoms of hypothyroidism and hyperthyroidism.

Graves' Disease

Excess circulating thyroid hormones result from Graves' disease. Roughly 15 percent of Graves' patients have a close relative with the disease, which suggests a strong hereditary role in predisposition to the disorder. In addition, Graves' disease is about six times more common in women than in men, with onset typically in young adulthood (20s and 30s).

Graves' disease has an autoimmune origin. Autoantibodies are generated that stimulate thyroid tissue to produce excessive amounts of thyroid hormones (**Figure 10-12**). The resultant changes in organ function are responses to either excess thyroid hormones or to the autoantibodies themselves.

The signs and symptoms of Graves' disease include agitation, emotional lability, insomnia, poor heat tolerance, weight loss despite increased appetite, weakness, dyspnea, and tachycardia

or new-onset atrial fibrillation in the absence of a cardiac history. Nervous system symptoms tend to be more common in younger adults, whereas serious cardiovascular symptoms tend to predominate in older individuals. Prolonged exposure of orbital tissues to the pathological thyroid-stimulating autoantibodies can cause exophthalmos (protrusion of the eyeballs), whereas interaction of autoantibodies with thyroid tissue often produces diffuse goiter (a generally enlarged thyroid gland).

Cardiac dysfunction is probably the most likely context in which an emergency call may arise from thyrotoxicosis, usually caused by Graves' disease. Use of β-adrenergic blockers such as propranolol may temporarily reduce cardiac stress, but make sure the patient does not have heart failure or asthma before considering use. Glucocorticoid therapy (namely, dexamethasone) is sometimes helpful in quickly reducing the level of circulating T_4.

Thyrotoxic Crisis (Thyroid Storm)

Thyrotoxic crisis, or thyroid storm, is a life-threatening emergency that can be fatal within as few as 48 hours if untreated. It is usually associated with severe physiological stress (e.g., trauma, infection), less often with psychological stress. You may also encounter thyroid storm secondary to overdose of thyroid hormone medication in a hypothyroid individual.

The mechanisms that underlie thyrotoxic crisis are poorly understood. An acute increase in the levels of thyroid hormones does not appear to be the cause. More likely, thyroid storm is

(Continued)

Figure 10-12 Graves' Disease. Hyperthyroidism results in an increase in the levels of circulating thyroid hormone.

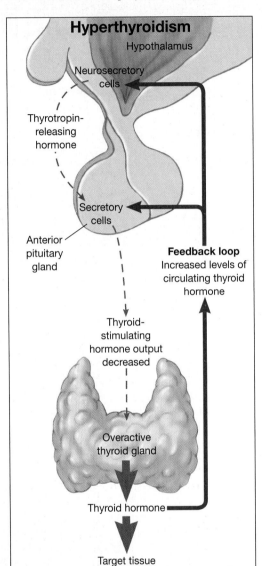

Figure 10-13 Hypothyroidism. Hypothyroidism results from a decrease in the levels of circulating thyroid hormones.

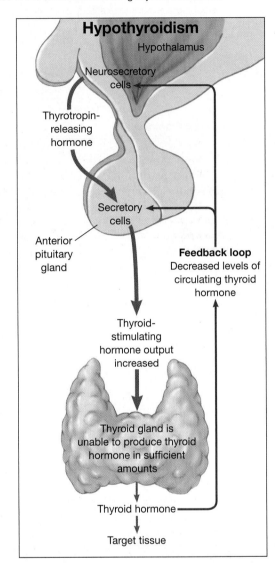

caused by a shift of thyroid hormone in the blood from the protein-bound (biologically inactive) to the free (biologically active) state. This significantly increases the amount of active hormone in the circulation, and thus stimulates the thyroid gland.

The signs and symptoms associated with thyrotoxic crisis reflect the patient's extreme hypermetabolic state and increased activity of the sympathetic nervous system. The syndrome is characterized by high fever (106°F/41°C or higher), irritability, delirium or coma, tachycardia, hypotension, vomiting, and diarrhea. A less severe presentation may also occur, with slight fever and marked lethargy.

In the presence of the signs and symptoms of thyrotoxic crisis, field management is largely focused on supportive care: oxygenation, ventilatory assistance, fluid resuscitation, and cardiac monitoring. Glucocorticoids and β-adrenergic blockers may be

helpful, especially if transport times are long. Transport should be expedited for definitive therapy that blocks the high blood levels of thyroid hormones.

Hypothyroidism and Myxedema

Hypothyroidism can be congenital or acquired and can affect both sexes. The recent increase in incidence of hypothyroidism in middle-aged women may reflect better diagnostics, a true rise in incidence, or both. Advanced myxedema in middle-aged and elderly individuals is the condition you are most likely to see in the emergency setting.

Hypothyroidism creates a low metabolic state, and early signs reflect poor organ function and poor response to challenges such as exercise or infection (**Figure 10-13**). Over time, untreated severe hypothyroidism causes the additional sign of myxedema, which is a thickening of connective tissue in the skin and other tissues, including the heart. Patients with myxedema may progress into a hypothermic, stuporous state called *myxedema coma*, which can be fatal if respiratory depression occurs. Triggers for progression to myxedema coma include infection, trauma, a cold environment, or exposure to central nervous system depressants such as alcohol or certain drugs.

Early signs of hypothyroidism may be subtle. Symptoms may be as slight as fatigue and slowed mental function attributed falsely to aging. Typically, patients with hypothyroidism or myxedema show lethargy, cold intolerance, constipation, decreased mental function, or decreased appetite with increased weight. In addition, the relaxation stage of deep tendon reflexes is slowed. The classic appearance of myxedema is an unemotional, puffy-faced, and pale individual with thinned hair, enlarged tongue, and cool skin that looks and feels like dough. Myxedema coma may be difficult to identify. Note if the history is consistent with

hypothyroidism and look for the physical appearance of myxedema. Other signs include profound hypothermia (temperatures as low as 75°F/24°C are not uncommon), low amplitude bradycardia, and carbon dioxide retention.

These signs and symptoms may alert you to the possible presence of myxedema. Keep in mind that heart failure due to the combination of age, atherosclerosis, and myxedematous enlargement is not uncommon, so focus on maintaining the ABCs and closely monitoring cardiac and pulmonary status. Most patients with myxedema coma require intubation and ventilatory assistance. Active rewarming is contraindicated due to the risk of cardiac dysrhythmias and cardiovascular collapse secondary to vasodilatation. Although IV access is important, limit fluids because fluid and electrolyte imbalance is common and cardiac function is compromised. IV therapy should be guided by appropriate laboratory studies. Expedite transport to an appropriate facility for definitive treatment.

10-5 The four parathyroid glands, embedded in the posterior surfaces of the thyroid gland, secrete parathyroid hormone to elevate blood calcium levels

Learning Objective Describe the location, hormones, and functions of the parathyroid glands.

Two tiny pairs of **parathyroid glands** are embedded in the posterior surfaces of the thyroid gland (**Figure 10-14**). A capsule of connective tissue fibers separates each parathyroid gland

Figure 10-14 The Parathyroid Glands.

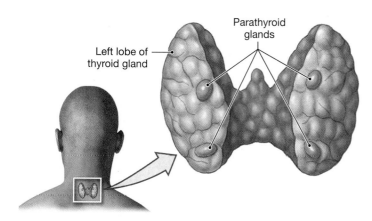

from the cells of the thyroid gland. The parathyroid glands have at least two cell populations. The **parathyroid (chief) cells** produce PTH. The functions of the other cell type are unknown.

Like the C cells of the thyroid, the chief cells monitor the concentration of circulating calcium ions. When the Ca^{2+} concentration falls below normal, the chief cells secrete **PTH**, or *parathormone* (see **Figure 10-10**). PTH acts on the same target organs as calcitonin, but it produces the opposite effects. PTH stimulates osteoclasts, inhibits the bone-building functions of osteoblasts, and reduces urinary excretion of calcium ions. PTH also stimulates the kidneys to form and secrete the hormone *calcitriol*. This hormone promotes the absorption of Ca^{2+} and PO_4^{3-} by the digestive tract.

Information concerning the hormones of the thyroid and parathyroid glands is summarized in **Table 10-3**.

CHECKPOINT

13. Identify the hormone secreted by the parathyroid glands.

14. Removal of the parathyroid glands would result in decreased blood concentrations of what important mineral?

See the blue Answers tab at the back of the book.

Table 10-3	Hormones of the Thyroid Gland and Parathyroid Glands		
Gland/Cells	**Hormone(s)**	**Targets**	**Hormonal Effects**
THYROID			
Follicular epithelium	Thyroxine (T_4), triiodothyronine (T_3)	Most cells	Increased energy use, oxygen consumption, growth, and development
C cells	Calcitonin (CT)	Bone, kidneys	Decreased calcium ion concentrations in body fluids (see Figure 10-10)
PARATHYROIDS			
Chief cells	Parathyroid hormone (PTH)	Bone, kidneys	Increased calcium ion concentrations in body fluids (see Figure 10-10)

10-6 The adrenal glands, consisting of a cortex and a medulla, cap each kidney and secrete several hormones

Learning Objective Describe the location, hormones, and functions of the adrenal glands.

A yellow, pyramid-shaped **adrenal** (ad-RĒ-nal; *ad-*, near + *renes*, kidneys) **gland**, or *suprarenal gland*, sits on the superior border of each kidney (**Figure 10-15a**). Each adrenal gland has two parts with separate functions: an outer *adrenal cortex* and an inner *adrenal medulla* (**Figure 10-15b**).

The Adrenal Cortex

The yellowish color of the **adrenal cortex** is due to stored lipids, especially cholesterol and various fatty acids. The adrenal cortex produces more than two dozen steroid hormones. They are collectively called **corticosteroids**. In the bloodstream, these hormones are bound to transport proteins. Corticosteroids are vital. If the adrenal glands are destroyed or removed, the individual will die unless corticosteroids are administered. These hormones affect metabolism in many different tissues, so overproduction or underproduction of any of the corticosteroids will have severe consequences.

Each of the three distinct regions or zones of the adrenal cortex synthesizes specific corticosteroids (**Figure 10-15c**). The outer *zona glomerulosa* (glō-mer-ū-LŌ-suh) produces *mineralocorticoids*. The middle *zona fasciculata* (fa-sik-ū-LA-tuh) produces glucocorticoids. The inner *zona reticularis* (re-tik-ū-LAR-is) produces *androgens*.

Mineralocorticoids (MCs)

The **MCs** affect the electrolyte composition of body fluids. **Aldosterone** (al-DOS-ter-ōn) is the principal MC of the adrenal cortex. It stimulates the conservation of sodium ions and the elimination of potassium ions by targeting cells that regulate the ionic composition of excreted fluids.

Specifically, aldosterone causes the retention of sodium by preventing the loss of sodium ions in urine, sweat, saliva, and digestive secretions. The retention of sodium ions is accompanied by a loss of potassium ions. Secondarily, the reabsorption of sodium ions results in the osmotic reabsorption of water at the kidneys, sweat glands, salivary glands, and pancreas. Aldosterone also increases the sensitivity of salt receptors in the tongue, resulting in greater interest in consuming salty foods.

Aldosterone secretion occurs in response to a drop in blood sodium content, blood volume, or blood pressure, or to a rise in blood potassium levels. Aldosterone release also occurs in response to *angiotensin II* (*angeion*, vessel + *teinein*, to stretch). We will discuss this hormone later in the chapter.

Glucocorticoids

The steroid hormones, collectively known as **glucocorticoids**, affect glucose metabolism. The three most important glucocorticoids are **cortisol** (KOR-ti-sol; also called *hydrocortisone*), **corticosterone** (kor-ti-KOS-te-rōn), and **cortisone**.

Glucocorticoid secretion takes place under ACTH stimulation and is regulated by negative feedback (**Figure 10-7a**). Glucocorticoids speed up the rates of glucose synthesis and glycogen formation, especially in the liver. Skeletal muscle and adipose tissues respond by releasing amino acids and fatty acids into the blood, respectively. The liver synthesizes glucose with the amino acids, and other tissues begin to break down fatty acids instead of glucose. This process is another example of a *glucose-sparing effect* that results in an increase in blood glucose levels (p. 355).

Figure 10-15 The Adrenal Gland and Adrenal Hormones.

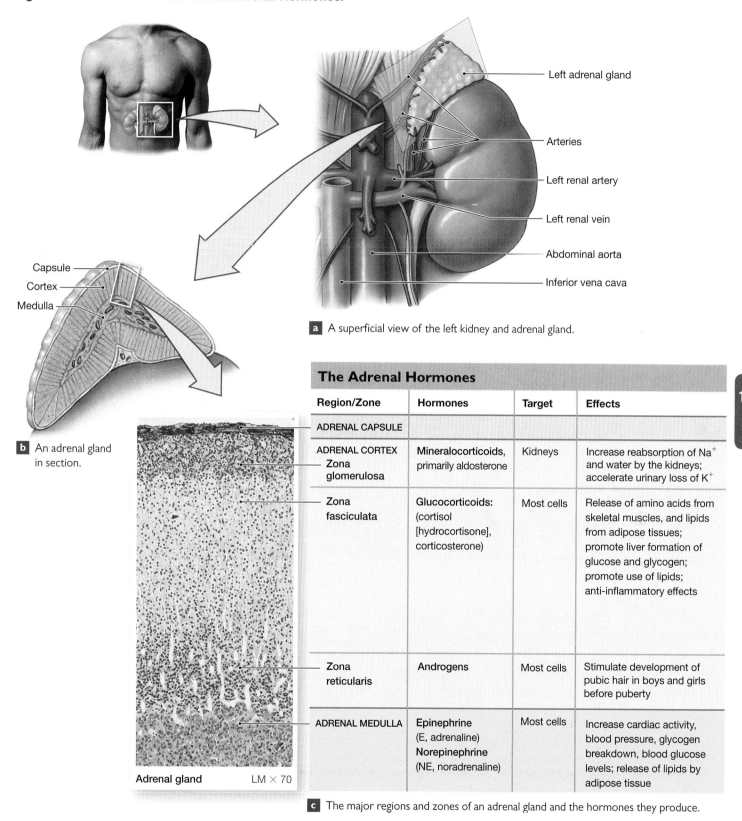

a A superficial view of the left kidney and adrenal gland.

b An adrenal gland in section.

Adrenal gland LM × 70

The Adrenal Hormones

Region/Zone	Hormones	Target	Effects
ADRENAL CAPSULE			
ADRENAL CORTEX Zona glomerulosa	**Mineralocorticoids,** primarily aldosterone	Kidneys	Increase reabsorption of Na^+ and water by the kidneys; accelerate urinary loss of K^+
Zona fasciculata	**Glucocorticoids:** (cortisol [hydrocortisone], corticosterone)	Most cells	Release of amino acids from skeletal muscles, and lipids from adipose tissues; promote liver formation of glucose and glycogen; promote use of lipids; anti-inflammatory effects
Zona reticularis	Androgens	Most cells	Stimulate development of pubic hair in boys and girls before puberty
ADRENAL MEDULLA	**Epinephrine** (E, adrenaline) **Norepinephrine** (NE, noradrenaline)	Most cells	Increase cardiac activity, blood pressure, glycogen breakdown, blood glucose levels; release of lipids by adipose tissue

c The major regions and zones of an adrenal gland and the hormones they produce.

Glucocorticoids also show *anti-inflammatory* effects. That is, they inhibit the activities of white blood cells and other components of the immune system. "Steroid creams" are often used to control irritating allergic rashes, such as those produced by poison ivy. Injections of glucocorticoids may be used to control more severe allergic reactions. On the negative side, GCs slow wound healing and suppress immune defenses against infectious organisms. For this reason, the topical steroids used to treat superficial rashes should never be applied to open wounds.

Androgens

The adrenal cortex in both sexes produces small quantities of **androgens**, the sex hormones produced in large quantities by the testes in males. Once in the bloodstream, some of the androgens are converted to estrogens, the dominant sex hormones in females. Adrenal androgens stimulate the development of pubic hair in boys and girls before puberty. Adrenal androgens are not important in adult men. In adult women they produce more muscle mass and blood cell formation, and support the sex drive.

The Adrenal Medulla

The **adrenal medulla** is pale gray or pink, due in part to the many blood vessels in the area. It contains large, rounded cells similar to those found in other sympathetic ganglia.

These cells are innervated by preganglionic sympathetic fibers. The secretory activities of the adrenal medullae are controlled by the sympathetic division of the ANS. ⟳ p. 292

The adrenal medulla contains two populations of secretory cells. One produces **epinephrine** (or *adrenaline*). The other produces **norepinephrine** (or *noradrenaline*) (**Figure 10-15c**). These hormones are continuously released at a low rate, but sympathetic stimulation speeds up the rate of discharge dramatically.

Epinephrine makes up 75–80 percent of the secretions from the medulla. The rest is norepinephrine. Receptors for epinephrine and norepinephrine are found on skeletal muscle fibers, adipocytes, liver cells, and cardiac muscle fibers. In skeletal muscles, these hormones trigger a mobilization of glycogen reserves and speed up the breakdown of glucose to provide ATP. This combination results in increased muscular power and endurance. In adipose tissue, stored fats are broken down to fatty acids. In the liver, glycogen molecules are converted to glucose. The fatty acids and glucose are then released into the bloodstream for use by peripheral tissues. The heart responds to adrenal medulla hormones by increasing the rate and force of cardiac contractions.

The metabolic changes that follow epinephrine and norepinephrine release peak 30 seconds after adrenal stimulation and linger for several minutes. As a result, the effects produced by stimulation of the adrenal medullae outlast the other signs of sympathetic activation.

CLINICAL NOTE

Disorders of the Adrenal Glands

Two disorders of the adrenal cortex, Cushing's syndrome and Addison's disease, can play a part in medical emergencies or complicate responses to trauma. Cushing's syndrome is caused by excessive adrenocortical activity, while Addison's disease is caused by deficient adrenocortical activity.

Hyperadrenalism (Cushing's Syndrome)

Cushing's syndrome is a relatively common disorder of the adrenal glands. It usually affects middle-aged persons and is more common in women than in men. It results from excess glucocorticoids, primarily cortisol, which can be due to abnormalities in the anterior pituitary gland or in the adrenal cortex. It also can be due to treatment with glucocorticoids, such as prednisone. Check the history to note any recent steroid treatment for nonendocrine conditions such as cancer or rheumatologic disorders.

Long-term exposure to excess glucocorticoids produces numerous changes. Metabolically, cortisol is an antagonist to insulin. Gluconeogenesis is prominent, with profound protein catabolism. The body's handling of fats is altered; because of this, atherosclerosis and hypercholesterolemia are common. Over time,

diabetes mellitus also may develop. Cortisol's mineralocorticoid activity causes sodium retention and increased blood volume. Increased vascular sensitivity to catecholamines occurs, and this may also contribute to hypertension. Potassium loss through the kidneys may cause hypokalemia. Cortisol's anti-inflammatory and immunosuppressive properties predispose the patient to infection.

Regardless of its cause, the presenting signs and symptoms of hyperadrenalism are the same. The earliest sign is weight gain, particularly through the trunk of the body, face, and neck. A "moon-faced" appearance often develops (**Figure 10-16**). The accumulation of fat on the upper back is occasionally referred to as a buffalo hump. Skin changes are also very common and may be an early clue to potential problems. These include the skin's thinning to an almost transparent appearance, a tendency to bruise easily, delayed healing from even minor wounds, and development of facial hair among women (hirsutism). Mood swings and impaired memory or concentration are also common.

Although you probably will not see patients with acute hyperadrenal crisis, you are likely to encounter patients with signs and symptoms of Cushing's syndrome. Remember that these patients

Figure 10-16 Facial Features of Cushing's Syndrome.

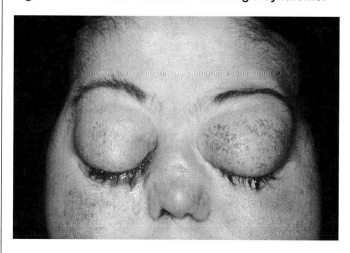

have a higher incidence of cardiovascular disease, including hypertension and stroke. Pay particular attention to skin preparation when starting IV lines because of the patient's fragile skin and susceptibility to infection. Note any observations indicative of Cushing's syndrome in your report and relay them to hospital staff.

Adrenal Insufficiency (Addison's Disease)

Addison's disease is due to cortical destruction. Addison's has become less common as its former leading causes, such as tuberculosis, have come under control. Currently, over 90 percent of Addison's disease cases are due to autoimmune disease. As with Graves' disease, which is another autoimmune disorder, heredity plays a prominent role in an individual's predisposition for Addison's disease. In fact, patients with Addison's are more likely than average to have other autoimmune disorders, including Graves' disease.

Destruction of the adrenal cortex results in minimal production of all three classes of hormones: glucocorticoids, mineralocorticoids, and androgens. Low mineralocorticoid activity is key to the changes of Addison's, which causes major disturbances in water and electrolyte balance. Increased sodium excretion in urine results in low blood volume, and potassium retention can cause hyperkalemia and ECG changes. Many cases of adrenal insufficiency are due to therapy with steroids such as prednisone, which can completely suppress normal adrenal function. Sudden cessation of the drug may trigger symptoms of Addison's disease or even an Addisonian crisis, with cardiovascular collapse.

Addison's disease is characterized by changes related to low corticosteroid activity: progressive weakness, fatigue, decreased appetite, and weight loss. Hyperpigmentation of the skin and mucous membranes, particularly in sun-exposed areas, is also characteristic.

Acute stresses, such as infection or trauma, may tip Addison's patients into a metabolic failure called Addisonian crisis, which is characterized by profound hypotension and electrolyte imbalances. Many patients will have gastrointestinal problems such as vomiting or diarrhea, which will exacerbate electrolyte imbalances, low blood volume, and hypotension and increase the potential for cardiac dysrhythmias. Be alert for this potentially life-threatening emergency, and include it in your list of possible causes of unexplained cardiovascular collapse, particularly if the history suggests primary Addison's disease or Addison's disease secondary to drug therapy.

The patient may reveal the presence of Addison's disease during the history, or the disease's signs and symptoms may lead you to suspect its presence. Focus emergency management on maintaining the ABCs and on closely monitoring cardiac and oxygenation status as well as blood-glucose level. Hypoglycemia poses its own threat. Assess blood-glucose levels and administer 25–50 grams of 50 percent dextrose to patients with blood glucose levels less than 50 mg/dL or those with altered mental status. Obtain a baseline 12-lead ECG to check for dysrhythmias related to electrolyte imbalance. Be aggressive in fluid resuscitation. Follow your local protocol or contact medical direction for specific orders based on your patient's presentation. Expedite transport to an appropriate facility for definitive treatment.

10

CHECKPOINT

15. Identify the two regions of the adrenal gland, and list the hormones secreted by each.

16. What effect would elevated cortisol levels have on blood glucose levels?

See the blue Answers tab at the back of the book.

10-7 The pineal gland, attached to the third ventricle, secretes melatonin

Learning Objective Describe the location of the pineal gland, and discuss the functions of the hormone it produces.

The **pineal gland** lies in the posterior portion of the roof of the third ventricle. ↺ p. 276 It contains neurons, glial cells, and secretory cells that synthesize the hormone **melatonin** (mel-a-TŌ-nin). Branches of the axons making up the visual pathways enter the pineal gland and affect the rate of melatonin production. The rate is lowest during daylight hours and highest at night.

Several functions have been suggested for melatonin in humans. It may:

- **Inhibit reproductive function.** In some mammals, melatonin slows the maturation of sperm, ova, and reproductive organs. The significance of this effect in humans remains unclear. Circumstantial evidence suggests that melatonin may play a role in the timing of human sexual maturation. For example, melatonin levels in the blood decline at puberty. Also, pineal tumors that eliminate melatonin production cause premature puberty in young children.

- **Protect against damage by free radicals.** Melatonin is a very effective antioxidant. It may protect CNS neurons from *free radicals*, such as nitric oxide (NO) or hydrogen peroxide (H_2O_2), that may form in active neural tissue. (Free radicals are highly reactive atoms or molecules that contain unpaired electrons in their outer electron shell.) ⊃ p. 73

- **Establish day–night cycles of activity.** Because its activity is cyclical, the pineal gland may also be involved in maintaining basic *circadian rhythms*—daily changes in physiological processes that follow a regular day–night pattern. Increased melatonin secretion in darkness has been suggested as a primary cause of *seasonal affective disorder*. This condition can develop during the winter in people who live at high latitudes, where sunshine is scarce or lacking. It is characterized by changes in mood, eating habits, and sleeping patterns.

CHECKPOINT

17. Increased amounts of light would inhibit the production of which hormone?

18. List three possible functions of melatonin.

See the blue Answers tab at the back of the book.

10-8 The endocrine pancreas produces insulin and glucagon, hormones that regulate blood glucose levels

Learning Objective Describe the location, hormones, and functions of the pancreas.

The **pancreas** lies in the J-shaped loop between the stomach and proximal portion of the small intestine (**Figure 10-17**). It is a slender, pale organ with a nodular (lumpy) consistency (**Figure 10-17a**). It contains both exocrine and endocrine cells. The pancreas is primarily a digestive organ whose exocrine cells make digestive enzymes. (We discuss the **exocrine pancreas** in Chapter 16.)

Cells of the **endocrine pancreas** form clusters known as **pancreatic islets**, or the *islets of Langerhans* (LAN-ger-hanz). The islets are scattered among the exocrine cells (**Figure 10-17b**) and account for only about 1 percent of all pancreatic cells. Each islet contains several cell types. The two most important are alpha and beta cells. **Alpha cells** produce the hormone **glucagon** (GLOO-ka-gon), which raises blood glucose levels. **Beta cells** produce **insulin** (IN-suh-lin), which lowers blood glucose levels. Glucagon and insulin regulate blood glucose levels in much the same way PTH and calcitonin control blood calcium levels.

Figure 10-18 diagrams the hormonal regulation of blood glucose levels. Glucose is the preferred energy source for most cells in the body. Under normal conditions, it is the only energy source for neurons. When blood glucose levels rise above normal homeostatic levels, beta cells release insulin. Insulin stimulates the transport of glucose across plasma membranes into target cells. The plasma membranes of almost all cells in the body contain insulin receptors. The only exceptions are (1) neurons and red blood cells, which cannot metabolize nutrients other than glucose; (2) epithelial cells of the kidney tubules, where glucose is reabsorbed; and (3) epithelial cells of the intestinal lining, where glucose is obtained from the diet.

When glucose is abundant, all cells use it as an energy source rather than amino acids and lipids. The breakdown of glucose molecules generates ATP, which is used to build proteins and to increase energy reserves. Insulin also stimulates

Figure 10-17 The Endocrine Pancreas.

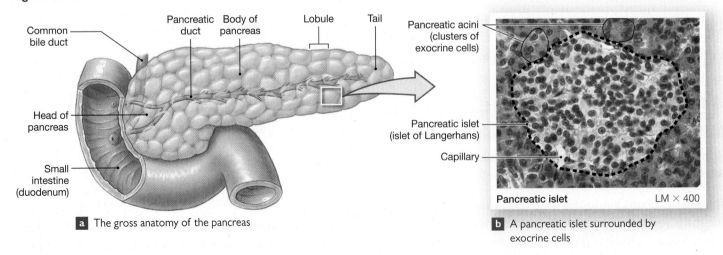

a The gross anatomy of the pancreas

b A pancreatic islet surrounded by exocrine cells

Pancreatic acini (clusters of exocrine cells)

Pancreatic islet (islet of Langerhans)

Capillary

Pancreatic islet   LM × 400

Common bile duct

Pancreatic duct

Body of pancreas

Lobule

Tail

Head of pancreas

Small intestine (duodenum)

Figure 10-18 The Regulation of Blood Glucose Concentrations.

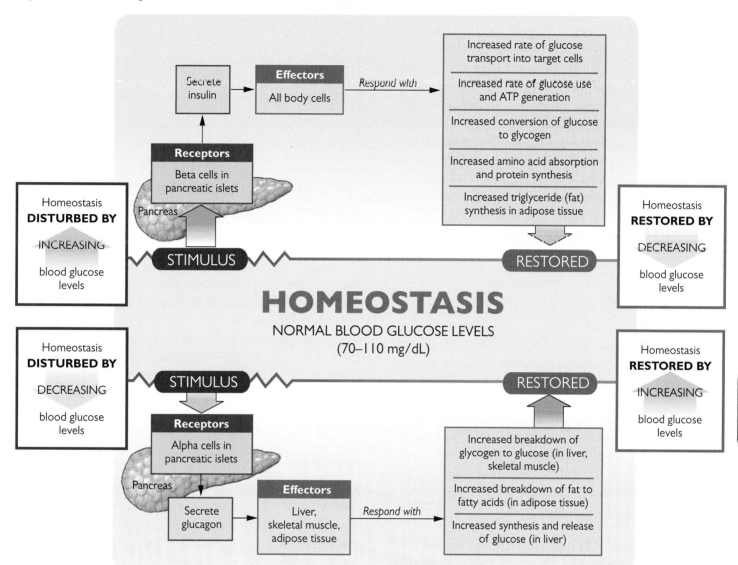

amino acid absorption and protein synthesis. This effect helps to maintain glucose levels by preventing the conversion of amino acids to glucose. Insulin also stimulates adipocytes (fat cells) to increase their rates of triglyceride (fat) synthesis and storage. In the liver and in skeletal muscle fibers, insulin also speeds up the formation of glycogen.

In summary, the pancreas secretes insulin when glucose is abundant. Insulin stimulates glucose use to support growth and to establish carbohydrate (glycogen) and lipid (triglyceride) reserves. The increased use of glucose reduces blood glucose levels to within normal limits (**Figure 10-18**).

When glucose concentrations fall below normal homeostatic levels, alpha cells release glucagon to mobilize energy reserves. Skeletal muscles and liver cells break down glycogen into glucose. The glucose molecules are either used for energy (in skeletal muscle fibers) or released into the bloodstream (by liver cells). Adipose tissue breaks down triglycerides (fat) into fatty acids that are released into the bloodstream for use by other tissues. Liver cells take in amino acids from the bloodstream, convert them to glucose, and release the glucose into the bloodstream. As a result, blood glucose concentrations rise toward normal levels

(Figure 10-18). The interplay between insulin and glucagon both stabilizes blood glucose levels and prevents competition between neural tissue and other tissues for limited glucose supplies.

Pancreatic alpha and beta cells are sensitive to blood glucose concentrations. For this reason, glucagon and insulin can be secreted without endocrine or nervous system instructions. Yet because the islet cells are very sensitive to variations in blood glucose levels, any hormone that affects blood glucose concentrations will indirectly affect the production of insulin and glucagon. Insulin and glucagon production are also influenced by autonomic activity. Parasympathetic stimulation enhances insulin release. Sympathetic stimulation inhibits insulin release and promotes glucagon release.

Diabetes Mellitus

Whether glucose is absorbed across the digestive tract or manufactured and released by the liver, very little glucose leaves the body intact once it has entered the circulation. Glucose does get filtered out of the blood at the kidneys, but virtually all of it is reabsorbed, so urinary glucose losses are negligible. However, in *diabetes mellitus*, glucose builds up in the blood and urine as a result of faulty glucose metabolism. The two types of diabetes are *Type 1 diabetes* (previously known as *juvenile diabetes*) and *Type 2 diabetes*. This disorder is discussed in the Clinical Note: Diabetes Mellitus on p. 366.

Build Your Knowledge

Recall that glucose ($C_6H_{12}O_6$) is the most important "fuel" in the body (as you saw in **Chapter 2: The Chemical Level of Organization**). Carbohydrates are most important as sources of energy, and our tissues can break down most of them. You learned that the major types of carbohydrates are monosaccharides, disaccharides, and polysaccharides. Glucose and other monosaccharides, and disaccharides (such as sucrose), dissolve readily in water. Polysaccharides are the largest carbohydrate molecules. Glycogen is a polysaccharide composed of interconnected glucose molecules. Like most large polysaccharides, glycogen will not dissolve in water or body fluids. Both liver and muscle cells make and store glycogen. ⟳ **pp. 38, 39**

CHECKPOINT

19. Identify two important types of cells in the pancreatic islets and the hormones produced by each.

20. Which pancreatic hormone causes skeletal muscle and liver cells to convert glucose to glycogen?

21. What effect would increased levels of glucagon have on the amount of glycogen stored in the liver?

See the blue Answers tab at the back of the book.

10-9 Many organs have secondary endocrine functions

Learning Objective Discuss the functions of the hormones produced by the kidneys, heart, thymus, testes, ovaries, and adipose tissue.

Many organs that are part of other body systems have secondary endocrine functions. Examples are the intestines (digestive system), the kidneys (urinary system), the heart (cardiovascular system), the thymus (lymphatic system), and the gonads—the testes in males and ovaries in females (reproductive system). We include the endocrine functions of adipose tissue in this section, although all the details have yet to be worked out.

The Intestines

The intestines process and absorb nutrients. They also release a variety of hormones that coordinate the activities of the digestive system. Local hormones control most digestive processes, but the autonomic nervous system can influence the pace of digestive activities. (We describe these hormones in Chapter 16.)

The Kidneys

The kidneys release the steroid hormone *calcitriol*, the peptide hormone *erythropoietin*, and the enzyme *renin*. Calcitriol is important to calcium ion homeostasis. Erythropoietin and renin are involved in the regulation of blood pressure and blood volume.

The kidneys secrete **calcitriol** in response to PTH. Calcitriol synthesis depends on the availability of vitamin D_3, which may be synthesized in the skin or absorbed from the diet. The liver absorbs vitamin D_3 and converts it to an intermediary product that is released into the circulation and absorbed by the kidneys. Calcitriol stimulates the absorption of calcium and phosphate ions across the intestinal lining of the digestive tract.

CLINICAL NOTE

Diabetes Mellitus

The disease diabetes mellitus is marked by inadequate insulin activity in the body. Insulin is critical to maintaining normal blood glucose levels. Glucose is important for all cells, but it is especially critical for brain cells. In fact, glucose is the only substance that brain cells can readily and efficiently use as an energy source. In addition, insulin enables the body to store energy as glycogen, protein, and fat.

Diabetes mellitus, or sugar diabetes, is a common and ancient serious disease. Over 8 million Americans have been diagnosed with diabetes, and U.S. health experts believe nearly the same number of the populace may be living with undiagnosed diabetes. The disease was named in ancient times by Greek physicians who noted that affected persons produced large volumes of urine that attracted bees and other insects, hence *diabetes* (meaning "to siphon," or "to pass through") for excessive urine production and *mellitus* (meaning "honey sweet") for the presence of sugar in the urine.

Diabetes mellitus is typically categorized as Type I diabetes or Type II diabetes. In addition, diabetes can also be classified as primary or secondary. Secondary diabetes is due to another cause and is uncommon; it affects only about 1 percent of diabetics. Causes include drugs, infections, genetic disorders, other endocrine disorders, and immune-mediated diseases. Gestational diabetes, which occurs only during pregnancy, affects about 4 percent of pregnancies. Careful control of blood glucose levels in gestational diabetes is essential in preventing fetal cardiac and nervous system abnormalities. Untreated gestational diabetes is a major cause of large birth weight infants (macrosomia). Gestational diabetes must be treated with insulin, as oral hypoglycemic medications cross the placental barrier and adversely affect the developing fetus.

Type I Diabetes Mellitus

Type I diabetes mellitus is characterized by the destruction of the beta (β) cells of the pancreas, which usually leads to absolute insulin deficiency. Type I diabetes is commonly called juvenile-onset diabetes because of the average age at diagnosis. The term *insulin-dependent diabetes mellitus* also is used because patients require regular insulin injections to maintain glucose homeostasis. This type of diabetes is less common than Type II diabetes, but it is more serious. Diabetes is regularly among the 10 leading causes of death in the United States and Type I diabetes accounts for most diabetes-related deaths.

Heredity is important in determining who will be predisposed to develop Type I diabetes. Although the cause of Type I diabetes is often unclear, viral infection, production of autoantibodies directed against beta cells, and genetically determined early deterioration of beta cells are all possible causes. Regardless, the immediate cause of the disease is destruction of beta cells in the islets of Langerhans in the pancreas.

In untreated Type I diabetes, blood-glucose levels rise because, without adequate insulin, cells cannot take up the circulating glucose. Hyperglycemia in the range of 300–500 milligrams per deciliter is not uncommon. As glucose spills into the urine, large amounts of water are lost through osmotic diuresis. Catabolism of fat becomes significant as the body switches to fatty acids as the primary energy source. Overall, this pathophysiology accounts for the constant thirst (polydipsia), excessive urination (polyuria), ravenous appetite (polyphagia), weakness, and weight loss associated with untreated Type I diabetes. Ketosis can occur as the result of fat catabolism, and it may proceed to frank diabetic ketoacidosis (DKA), a medical emergency that you will encounter in the field.

Treatment of Type I diabetes requires the administration of insulin. Tight control of blood glucose levels minimizes many of the long-term complications of diabetes mellitus. To achieve this, insulin dosing must be individualized based upon the patient's activities of daily living. Frequent dosing of short- and medium-acting insulin provides tighter control of blood-glucose levels than a single daily dose of long-term or mixed insulin. Selected patients can benefit from an insulin pump that slowly administers insulin over a 24-hour period as programmed based on the patient's daily activities.

Type II Diabetes Mellitus

Type II diabetes mellitus, also called adult-onset diabetes or non-insulin-dependent diabetes, is associated with a moderate decline in insulin production accompanied by a markedly deficient response to the insulin present in the body. Some Type II patients will predominantly have insulin resistance with relative insulin deficiency, while others will have a predominantly secretory defect with insulin resistance.

Heredity may also play a role in predisposition to Type II diabetes. In addition, obese persons are more likely to develop Type II diabetes, and obesity probably plays a role in development of the disease. Increased weight (and increased size of fat cells) causes a relative deficiency in the number of insulin receptors per cell, which makes fat cells less responsive to insulin. This type of diabetes is far more common than Type I diabetes, and accounts for about 90 percent of cases of diabetes mellitus. It is also less serious. The major risk factors for Type II diabetes mellitus are:

- Family history of diabetes (i.e., parents or siblings with diabetes)
- Obesity (≥ 20 percent over desired body weight or body mass index ≥ 27 kg/m^2)
- Race or ethnicity with high risk of diabetes (e.g., African American, Hispanic American, Native American, Asian American, Pacific Islander)
- Age ≥ 45 years
- Previously identified impaired fasting glucose or impaired glucose tolerance
- Hypertension (≥ 140/90 mmHg)
- Hyperlipidemia (HDL cholesterol level ≤ 35 mg/dL [0.90 mmol/L] or triglyceride level ≥ 250 mg/dL [2.82 mmol/L] or both)
- History of gestational diabetes or delivery of baby over 9 lb (4.1 kg)

Untreated Type II diabetes typically presents with a lower level of hyperglycemia and fewer major signs of metabolic disruption

(Continued)

than Type I diabetes. For instance, limited glucose use is usually sufficient to keep the body from switching to fats as the primary energy source. Thus, diabetic ketoacidosis (DKA) is uncommon in these patients. However, a complication called *nonketotic hyperosmolar coma* can occur, and you may see it as a medical emergency.

Medical treatment of Type II diabetes is less intensive than for Type I diabetes. Initial therapy often consists of dietary change and increased exercise in an attempt to improve body weight. If nonpharmacological therapy is insufficient to bring blood glucose levels down to the normal range, oral hypoglycemic agents may be prescribed. These drugs stimulate insulin secretion by beta cells and promote an increase in the number of insulin receptors per cell. In some cases, however, control may eventually require use of insulin.

Emergency Complications of Diabetes

Some of the complications of diabetes mellitus are medical emergencies and require prompt intervention. These include diabetic hypoglycemia (insulin shock), ketoacidosis (diabetic coma), and nonketotic hyperosmolar coma.

Hypoglycemia (Insulin Shock)

Hypoglycemia, or low blood glucose, is a medical emergency. It can occur when a patient takes too much insulin, eats too little to match an insulin dose, or physically overexerts and uses almost all of the available blood glucose. As the duration of hypoglycemia lengthens, the risk increases that brain cells will be permanently damaged or killed due to lack of glucose. Although brain cells can adapt to use fats as an energy source, this adaptation requires hours to develop, and the switch to fat-based metabolism cannot correct any damage already incurred. This is why every second counts in treating hypoglycemia.

Hypoglycemia, or insulin shock, reflects high insulin and low blood-glucose levels. Regardless of the reason for low blood sugar, insulin causes almost all remaining blood glucose to be taken up by cells. Because of the high level of insulin, glucagon may be ineffective in raising blood-glucose levels. In prolonged fasts, almost half the glucose normally produced through gluconeogenesis is of renal origin. This activity is stimulated by epinephrine. Diabetic patients with kidney failure may be predisposed to hypoglycemia because of a lack of renal gluconeogenesis.

The signs and symptoms of hypoglycemia are many and varied. Altered mental status is the most important. As blood-glucose levels fall, the patient may display inappropriate anger (even rage) or display a bizarre behavior. Sometimes the patient may be placed in police custody for such behavior or be involved in an automobile collision. Physical signs may include diaphoresis and tachycardia. If the blood glucose falls to a critically low level, the patient may have a hypoglycemic seizure or become comatose. In contrast to DKA, hypoglycemia can develop quickly. A clear change in mental status can occur without warning. Always consider hypoglycemia when encountering a patient with bizarre behavior. Additionally, hypoglycemia can cause symptoms that resemble a CVA (hypoglycemic hemiparesis), which is why blood sugar evaluation is mandatory prior to treating for stroke.

Figure 10-19 Intravenous Glucose Administration. Patients with confirmed or suspected hypoglycemia must receive glucose before brain cells are injured.

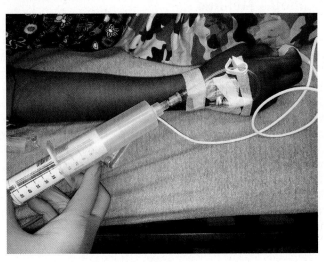

In suspected cases of hypoglycemia, perform the initial assessment quickly. Look for a medical identification device, such as a MedicAlert bracelet. If possible, determine blood-glucose level. Because of the urgency of this emergency, most paramedic units must be able to perform this task or to rush a blood sample along with the patient. If the blood-glucose level is less that 60 mg/dL, a dextrose solution should be administered intravenously (**Figure 10-19**). If the patient is conscious and able to swallow, glucose administration may be provided orally with orange juice, sugared soft drinks, or commercially available glucose pastes.

When an IV cannot be started, hypoglycemic patients may improve following the administration of glucagon, which can be administered intramuscularly. This is a much slower process and will work only if adequate stores of glycogen are available. Glucagon must be reconstituted immediately prior to administration.

Diabetic Ketoacidosis (Diabetic Coma)

DKA is a serious, potentially life-threatening complication associated with Type I diabetes. It occurs when profound insulin deficiency is coupled with increased glucagon and stress hormone activity. It may occur as the initial presentation of severe diabetes, as a result of patient noncompliance with insulin injections, or as the result of physiologic stress, such as surgery, a myocardial infarction, or serious infection.

DKA reflects amplification of the same physiological mechanisms as ketosis. In the initial phase of DKA, profound hyperglycemia develops because of lack of insulin. Body cells cannot take in glucose for normal metabolic processes. Gluconeogenesis, which is the compensatory mechanism for low glucose levels within cells, only contributes more blood glucose. The consequent loss of glucose in the urine, accompanied by loss of water through osmotic diuresis, produces significant dehydration.

As the body switches to fat-based metabolism, the blood levels of ketones rise. The ketone load accounts for the observed acidosis. By the time the characteristic decrease in pH from about 7.4 to about 6.9 has occurred, the patient is within hours of death if left untreated. The onset of clinically obvious DKA is slow, and lasts from 12 to 24 hours. In the initial phase, signs of osmotic diuresis appear, including increased urine production and dry, warm skin and mucous membranes. The individual often has excessive hunger and thirst coupled with a progressive sense of general malaise. Volume depletion induces tachycardia and feelings of physical weakness.

As ketoacidosis develops, a rapid deep breathing pattern termed Kussmaul's respirations appears. This major compensatory mechanism for acidosis helps expel carbon dioxide (CO_2) from the body. The breath itself may have a fruity or acetone-like smell as some blood acetone is expelled through the lungs. The blood profile includes not only hyperglycemia and acidic pH but also multiple electrolyte abnormalities. Low bicarbonate levels (HCO_3^-) reflect loss of acid-base buffer via Kussmaul's respirations. Low potassium levels may be found secondary to diuresis, with marked hypokalemia that increases the risk for cardiac dysrhythmias or death. Over time, mental function declines and frank coma may occur. A fever is not characteristic of ketoacidosis. If present, it is a sign of infection.

The treatment for a patient suffering from DKA is essentially the same as for any other patient who has mental impairment or is unconscious. The sweet, fruity odor of ketones occasionally can be detected in the breath. If possible, the blood glucose level should be determined. It is not uncommon for patients with ketoacidosis to have blood-glucose levels well in excess of 300 mg/dL. Prehospital treatment of DKA includes airway maintenance and fluid resuscitation to counteract dehydration. Often, the DKA patient will require several liters of an isotonic fluid. Definitive treatment includes insulin administration and correction of electrolyte deficiencies.

Nonketotic Hyperosmolar Coma

Nonketotic hyperosmolar coma (NKHC) is a serious complication associated with Type II diabetes. Typically, both insulin and glucagon activity are present. NKHC develops when two conditions occur: sustained hyperglycemia causes osmotic diuresis sufficient to produce marked dehydration, and water intake is inadequate to replace lost fluids. Renal or peritoneal dialysis, high-osmolarity feeding supplements, infection, and certain drugs also can be associated with development of NKHC.

As sustained hyperglycemia develops, glucose spills into the urine, which causes osmotic diuresis and resultant dehydration. The level of hyperglycemia is often much higher than is seen in DKA (up to 1000 mg/dL). However, insulin activity in patients with NKHC is usually sufficient to prevent significant production of ketone bodies. Inadequate fluid replacement results in characteristic signs and symptoms.

The mortality rate for NKHC coma is higher than for ketoacidosis: it ranges from 40 to 70 percent. The higher mortality rate may be due to the lack of early signs and symptoms that would bring patients with ketoacidosis to the attention of family or healthcare professionals.

The onset of NKHC is even slower than that of ketoacidosis; development often occurs over several days. Early signs include increased urination and increased thirst. Subsequent volume depletion can result in orthostatic hypotension when the patient gets out of bed, along with other signs such as dry skin and mucous membranes, as well as tachycardia. The patient may become lethargic, confused, or enter frank coma. Kussmaul's respirations are rarely seen because of the lack of ketoacidosis.

Prehospital treatment of the patient suffering from NKHC is essentially the same as of any other patient who has mental impairment or is unconscious. Distinguishing DKA from NKHC is often difficult in the field. Therefore, the prehospital treatment of both emergencies is identical, and transportation should be expedited.

Erythropoietin (e-rith-rō-POY-e-tin); *erythros*, red + *poiesis*, making), or **EPO**, is released by the kidneys in response to low oxygen levels in kidney tissues. EPO stimulates the red bone marrow to produce red blood cells. The increase in the number of red blood cells elevates blood volume. Because these cells transport oxygen, this increase improves oxygen delivery to peripheral tissues. (We will consider EPO again in Chapter 11.)

Renin (RĒ-nin) is released by specialized kidney cells in response to a decline in blood volume, blood pressure, or both. Once in the bloodstream, renin starts an enzymatic chain reaction, known as the *renin-angiotensin-aldosterone system (RAAS)*. RAAS leads to the formation of the hormone **angiotensin II**. Angiotensin II stimulates the secretion of aldosterone (by the adrenal cortex) and ADH (by the posterior lobe of the pituitary gland). This combination restricts salt and water loss by the kidneys. Angiotensin II also stimulates thirst and elevates blood pressure. Because renin plays a leading role in the formation of angiotensin II, many physiological and endocrinological references consider renin to be a hormone. (We will discuss the *renin–angiotensin–aldosterone system* in Chapters 13 and 18.)

The Heart

The endocrine cells in the heart are cardiac muscle cells in the walls of the *right atrium*; this chamber receives blood from the largest veins. If blood volume becomes too great, these cardiac muscle cells are stretched, stimulating them to release the hormone **atrial natriuretic peptide (ANP)** (nā-trē-ū-RET-ik; *natrium*, sodium + *ouresis*, making water).

In general, the effects of ANP oppose those of angiotensin II. ANP promotes the loss of sodium ions and water by the kidneys. It also inhibits renin release and ADH and aldosterone secretion. As a result of ANP secretion, both blood volume and pressure decline. (We discuss ANP further when we consider the control of blood pressure and volume in Chapter 13.)

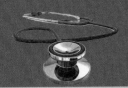

CLINICAL NOTE
DIABETES MELLITUS

Untreated diabetes mellitus disrupts metabolic activities throughout the body. Clinical problems arise because the tissues involved are experiencing an energy crisis—in essence, most of the tissues are responding as they would during chronic starvation, breaking down lipids and even proteins because they are unable to absorb glucose from their surroundings. Problems involving abnormal changes in blood vessel structure are particularly dangerous. An estimated 25.8 million people in the United States have some form of diabetes.

Retinal Damage

The proliferation of capillaries and hemorrhaging at the retina may cause partial or complete blindness. This condition is called **diabetic retinopathy**.

Early Heart Attacks

Degenerative blockages in cardiac circulation can lead to early heart attacks. For a given age group, heart attacks are three to five times more likely in people with diabetes than in nondiabetic people.

Peripheral Nerve Problems

Abnormal blood flow to neural tissues is probably responsible for a variety of neural problems with peripheral nerves, including abnormal autonomic function. These disorders are collectively termed **diabetic neuropathies**.

Kidney Degeneration

Degenerative changes in the kidneys, a condition called **diabetic nephropathy**, can lead to kidney failure.

Diabetes Mellitus

Diabetes mellitus (mel-Ī-tus; *mellitum*, honey), is characterized by glucose concentrations that are high enough to overwhelm the reabsorption capabilities of the kidneys. (The presence of abnormally high glucose levels in the blood in general is called **hyperglycemia** [hī-per-glī-SĒ-mē-ah].) Glucose appears in the urine (**glycosuria**; glī-kō-SYŪ-rē-a), and urine volume generally becomes excessive (**polyuria**).

subdivided into

Type 1 Diabetes

Type 1 is characterized by inadequate insulin production by the pancreatic beta cells. Persons with Type 1 diabetes require insulin to live and usually require multiple injections daily, or continuous infusion through an insulin pump or other device. This form of diabetes accounts for approximately 5 percent of cases. It usually develops in children and young adults.

Type 2 Diabetes

Type 2 is the most common form of diabetes mellitus. Most people with this form of diabetes produce normal amounts of insulin, at least initially, but their tissues do not respond properly, a condition known as insulin resistance. Type 2 diabetes is associated with obesity. Weight loss through diet and exercise can be an effective treatment, especially when coupled with oral medicines.

Peripheral Tissue Damage

Blood flow to the distal portions of the limbs is reduced, and peripheral tissues may suffer as a result. For example, a reduction in blood flow to the feet can lead to tissue death, ulceration, infection, and loss of toes or a major portion of one or both feet.

CLINICAL NOTE

Natriuretic Peptides

Natriuretic peptides are a group of naturally occurring substances that counteract the effects of the renin-angiotensin system. They cause vasodilation, stimulate the kidneys to increase sodium excretion (natriuresis), and water loss. They appear to be effective in the management of congestive heart failure because they decrease preload and promote sodium and water loss.

Three types of natriuretic peptides have been identified:

- *Atrial natriuretic peptide (ANP)*. ANP is produced in the atria. The identification of ANP was the first indication that the heart also has some endocrine function.
- *Brain natriuretic peptide (BNP)*. BNP is synthesized in the ventricles but named BNP as it was first identified in the porcine brain.
- *C-type natriuretic peptide (CNP)*. CNP is produced in the brain.

Both ANP and BNP are released in response to atrial and ventricular stretch, respectively. They cause vasodilation, inhibition of aldosterone secretion from the adrenal cortex, and inhibition of renin in the kidney. Both ANP and BNP will cause natriuresis and a reduction in intravascular volume. These effects are amplified by antagonism of antidiuretic hormone. The physiologic effects of CNP are different from those of ANP and BNP. CNP has a hypotensive effect, but no direct diuretic or natriuretic actions.

In the emergency setting, BNP can be measured in the blood. An elevated BNP is suggestive of congestive heart failure. The higher the level of BNP the more severe is the heart failure.

The Thymus

The **thymus** is located in the *mediastinum*, generally just deep to the sternum. In a newborn infant, the thymus is relatively enormous, often extending from the base of the neck to the superior border of the heart. As the child grows, the thymus continues to enlarge slowly, reaching a maximum weight of about 40 g (1.4 oz) just before puberty. After puberty, it gradually diminishes in size. By the age of 50 years, the thymus may weigh less than 12 g (0.4 oz).

The thymus produces several hormones that are important in developing and maintaining immune defenses. They are collectively known as **thymosins** (THĪ-mō-sinz). It has been suggested that the gradual decrease in the size and secretory abilities of the thymus may make elderly people more susceptible to disease. (We consider the structure of the thymus and the functions of the thymosins in Chapter 14.)

The Gonads

Information about the reproductive hormones of the testes and ovaries is presented in **Table 10-4**.

The Testes

In males, the **interstitial cells** of the testes produce the steroid hormones known as androgens. Recall that **testosterone** (tes-TOS-ter-ōn) is the most important androgen. It promotes the production of functional sex cells (sperm), maintains the secretory glands of the male reproductive tract, and determines secondary sex characteristics such as the distribution of facial hair and body fat. Testosterone also affects metabolic activities throughout the body. It stimulates protein synthesis and muscle growth, and it produces aggressive behavioral responses. During embryonic development, the production of testosterone affects the development of male reproductive ducts, external genitalia, and CNS structures, including hypothalamic nuclei that will later affect sexual behaviors.

Nurse cells in the testes support the formation of functional sperm. Under FSH stimulation, nurse cells secrete the hormone **inhibin**. Recall that this hormone inhibits the secretion of FSH by the anterior lobe of the pituitary gland.

Table 10-4	Hormones of the Reproductive System		
Structure/Cells	**Hormone**	**Primary Target**	**Effects**
TESTES			
Interstitial cells	Androgens	Most cells	Support functional maturation of sperm, protein synthesis in skeletal muscles, male secondary sex characteristics, and associated behaviors
Nurse cells	Inhibin	Anterior lobe of pituitary gland	Inhibits secretion of FSH
OVARIES			
Follicular cells	Estrogens	Most cells	Support follicle maturation, female secondary sex characteristics, and associated behaviors
	Inhibin	Anterior lobe of pituitary gland	Inhibits secretion of FSH
Corpus luteum	Progesterone	Uterus, mammary glands	Prepares uterus for implantation of embryo; prepares mammary glands for secretory functions

Throughout adult life, inhibin and FSH interact to maintain sperm production at normal levels.

The Ovaries

In the ovaries, female sex cells (*oocytes*) develop in specialized structures called **follicles**, under stimulation by FSH. (An oocyte is an immature ovum, or egg cell. Upon fertilization, the oocyte matures to become an *ovum*.) Follicle cells surrounding the oocyte produce **estrogens** (ES-trō-jenz), steroid hormones that support the maturation of the egg cell and stimulate the growth of the lining of the uterus. Under FSH stimulation, follicle cells secrete inhibin, which suppresses FSH release through a negative feedback process similar to that in males.

At ovulation, a mature follicle in an ovary releases an oocyte. The remaining follicle cells then form a **corpus luteum** that releases a mixture of estrogens and **progesterone** (prō-JES-ter-ōn). Progesterone speeds up the movement of fertilized eggs along the uterine tubes and prepares the uterus for the arrival of a developing embryo. In combination with other hormones, it also causes the mammary glands to enlarge.

The production of androgens, estrogens, and progesterone is controlled by regulatory hormones released by the anterior lobe of the pituitary gland. During pregnancy, the placenta functions as an endocrine organ, working with the ovaries and the pituitary gland to promote normal fetal development and delivery.

Adipose Tissue

Recall that adipose tissue is a type of loose connective tissue (introduced in Chapter 4). ⟳ p. 104 Adipose tissue produces a peptide hormone called **leptin**, which has several functions. Its best known function is the negative feedback control of appetite. When you eat, adipose tissue absorbs glucose and lipids and synthesizes triglycerides (fats) for storage. At the same time, it releases leptin into the bloodstream. Leptin binds to neurons in the hypothalamus involved with emotion and appetite control. The result is a sense of fullness (satiation) and the suppression of appetite.

Leptin must be present for normal levels of GnRH and gonadotropin synthesis to take place. This explains why (1) thin girls commonly enter puberty relatively late, (2) an increase in body fat content can improve fertility, and (3) women stop menstruating when their body fat content becomes very low.

CHECKPOINT

22. Identify the two hormones secreted by the kidneys, and describe their functions.

23. Describe the action of renin.

24. Identify a hormone released by adipose tissue.

See the blue Answers tab at the back of the book.

10-10 Hormones interact to produce coordinated physiological responses

Learning Objective Explain how hormones interact to produce coordinated physiological responses, and describe how the endocrine system responds to stress and is affected by aging.

We usually study hormones individually, but the extracellular fluids contain a mixture of hormones. Their concentrations change daily and even hourly. When a cell receives instructions from two different hormones at the same time, four outcomes are possible:

- *Antagonistic effects.* The two hormones may have **antagonistic (opposing) effects**, as is the case for PTH and calcitonin, or insulin and glucagon.

- *Synergistic effects.* The two hormones may have additive effects, in which case the net result is greater than the effect that each would produce acting alone. In some cases, the net result is greater than the *sum* of their individual effects. An example of such a **synergistic** (sin-er-JIS-tik; *syn*, together + *ergon*, work) **effect** is the glucose-sparing action of GH and glucocorticoids. ⟳ pp. 355, 362

- *Permissive effects.* Hormones can have a **permissive effect** on other hormones. In such cases, one hormone must be present if a second hormone is to produce its effects. For example, epinephrine has no apparent effect on energy consumption unless thyroid hormones are also present in normal concentrations.

- *Integrative effects.* Hormones may also produce different but complementary results in a given tissue or organ. These **integrative effects** are important in coordinating the activities of diverse physiological systems. The differing effects of calcitriol and PTH on tissues involved in calcium metabolism are an example.

The next few sections focus on how hormones interact to control normal growth, reactions to stress, alterations of behavior, and the effects of aging. More detailed discussions can be found in chapters on cardiovascular function, metabolism, excretion, and reproduction.

Hormones and Growth

Normal growth requires the cooperation of several endocrine organs. Six hormones—GH, thyroid hormones, insulin, PTH, calcitriol, and reproductive hormones—are especially important. Many others also have secondary effects on growth rates and patterns.

- **GH.** The effects of GH on protein synthesis and cellular growth are most apparent in children. GH supports their muscular and skeletal development. In adults, GH helps to maintain normal blood glucose levels and to mobilize lipid reserves in adipose tissues. GH is not the primary hormone involved, however. An adult with a GH deficiency but normal levels of thyroxine, insulin, and glucocorticoids will have no physiological problems.

- **Thyroid hormones.** Normal growth also requires appropriate levels of thyroid hormones. If these hormones are absent during fetal development or for the first year of life, the nervous system fails to develop normally. Developmental delay results. If thyroxine concentrations decline later in life but before puberty, normal skeletal development does not continue.

- **Insulin.** Growing cells need adequate supplies of energy and nutrients. Without insulin, the passage of glucose and amino acids across plasma membranes stops or is drastically reduced.

- **Parathyroid hormone and calcitriol.** PTH and calcitriol promote the absorption of calcium for building bone. Without adequate levels of both hormones, bones can enlarge but will be poorly mineralized, weak, and flexible. For example, rickets is a condition typically resulting from inadequate production of calcitriol due to vitamin D_3 deficiency in growing children. As a result, the lower limb bones are so weak that they bend under the body's weight. ↺ p. 148

- **Reproductive hormones.** The presence or absence of sex hormones (androgens in males, estrogens in females) affects the activities of osteoblasts in key locations and the growth of specific cell populations. Androgens and estrogens stimulate cell growth and differentiation in their target tissues, but the targets differ. The differential growth induced by each accounts for gender-related differences in skeletal proportions and secondary sex characteristics.

10

CLINICAL NOTE

Hormones and Athletic Performance

The use of hormones to improve athletic performance is banned by the International Olympic Committee, the U.S. Olympic Committee, the National Collegiate Athletic Association, Major League Baseball, and the National Football League. The American Medical Association and the American College of Sports Medicine condemn the practice. A significant number of amateur and professional athletes, however, persist in this dangerous practice. Synthetic forms of testosterone are used most often, but athletes may use any combination of testosterone, growth hormone, erythropoietin (EPO), and a variety of synthetic hormones.

The use of *anabolic steroids* or androgens has become popular with many amateur and professional athletes. The goal of steroid use is to increase muscle mass, endurance, and "competitive spirit." A steroid, such as *androstenedione*, is converted to testosterone in the body. One justification for this steroid use is the unfounded opinion that compounds made in the body are not only safe, but good for you. In reality, the use of natural or synthetic androgens in abnormal amounts carries unacceptable health risks. Androgens produce several complications. These include (1) premature closure of epiphyseal cartilages;

(2) liver dysfunctions (such as jaundice and liver tumors); (3) in males, prostate gland enlargement, urinary tract obstructions, testicular atrophy, and infertility; and (4) in females, irregular menstrual periods and changes in body hair distribution. Links to heart attacks, impaired heart function, and strokes have also been suggested. Finally, androgen abuse can cause a generalized depression of the immune system.

EPO is sometimes used by endurance athletes, such as cyclists and marathon runners, to boost the number of oxygen-carrying red blood cells in the bloodstream. This effect increases the oxygen content of the blood, but it also makes the blood more viscous. For this reason, the heart must work harder to push the "thick" blood through the blood vessels. This effort can result in death due to heart failure or stroke in young and otherwise healthy individuals.

The effects of androgens and EPO are reasonably well understood. Drug testing is now widespread in amateur and professional sports, but athletes seeking "an edge" are experimenting with drugs not easily detected by standard tests. The effects of these drugs are difficult to predict.

Hormones and Stress

Any condition—physical or emotional—that threatens homeostasis is a form of **stress**. Stresses may be (1) physical, such as illness or injury; (2) emotional, such as depression or anxiety; (3) environmental, such as extreme heat or cold; or (4) metabolic, such as starvation. Many stresses are opposed by specific homeostatic adjustments. For example, a decline in body temperature leads to shivering or changes in the pattern of blood flow, which can restore normal body temperature.

In addition, the body has a *general* response to stress that can take place while other, more specific, responses are under way. A wide variety of stress-causing factors produce the same basic pattern of hormonal and physiological adjustments. These responses are part of the **general adaptation syndrome (GAS)**, also known as the **stress response**. The GAS has three phases: the *alarm phase*, the *resistance phase*, and the *exhaustion phase*. These phases are described in **Spotlight Figure 10-20**.

Hormones and Behavior

As we have seen, the hypothalamus regulates many endocrine functions. Its neurons also monitor the levels of many circulating hormones. Other portions of the brain that affect how we act, or behave, are also quite sensitive to hormonal stimulation.

The clearest demonstrations of the behavioral effects of specific hormones involve individuals whose endocrine glands are oversecreting or undersecreting. But even normal changes in circulating hormone levels can cause behavioral changes. In *precocious* (premature) *puberty*, sex hormones are produced at an inappropriate time, perhaps as early as age five or six. Not only does an affected child begin to develop adult secondary sex characteristics, but the child's behavior also changes. The "nice little kid" disappears, and the child becomes aggressive and assertive due to the effects of sex hormones on CNS function. In normal teenagers, these behaviors are usually attributed to environmental stimuli, such as peer pressure, but here we can see that they have a physiological basis as well. In adults, changes in the mixture of hormones reaching the CNS can affect intellectual capabilities, memory, learning, and emotional states.

Hormones and Aging

The endocrine system undergoes relatively few functional changes with age. The most dramatic exception is the decline in the concentration of reproductive hormones. (We noted

CLINICAL NOTE

The Physiologic Response to Stress

EMS is an inherently stressful profession. *Stress* can be defined as any condition within the body that threatens *homeostasis*. The word *stress* also refers to a "hardship or strain," or a "physical or emotional response to a stimulus." A person's reactions to stress are individual and varied. They are affected by previous exposure to the *stressor* (a stimulus that causes stress), the perception of the event, general life events, and personal coping skills.

Adapting to stress is a dynamic and evolving process. The body has a general physiological response to stress. In fact, all stressors produce the same basic pattern of hormonal and physiological adjustments. The stress response is called the *general adaptation syndrome* and consists of three basic phases: *alarm, resistance,* and *exhaustion* (see Spotlight **Figure 10-20**). At the end comes a period of rest and recovery.

- *Stage I: Alarm.* The alarm phase is the "fight-or-flight" response. It occurs when the body physically and rapidly prepares to defend itself against a threat, whether real or imagined. Hormones begin to flood the body via the sympathetic nervous system under the control of the hypothalamus. *Epinephrine* and *norepinephrine* from the adrenal medulla increase the heart rate and blood pressure, dilate the pupils, increase the blood sugar level, slow digestion, and dilate the bronchial tree.

In addition, the pituitary gland begins releasing *adrenocorticotropic hormones* that stimulate the adrenal cortex.

- *Stage II: Resistance.* If the stress lasts longer than a few hours, the individual will enter the resistance phase. The glucocorticoid hormones dominate this stage, although other hormones are involved. Energy demands remain higher because of increased production of the glucocorticoids, epinephrine, growth hormone, and thyroid hormone. These serve to maintain an elevated level of blood glucose, which facilitates the mobilization of lipid and protein, the conservation of glucose for the brain and neural tissues, and the synthesis and release of glucose by the liver. In this stage, the individual beings to cope with the stress. Over time, the individual may become desensitized or adapted to stressors. Late in this stage, physiological parameters, such as blood pressure and pulse rate, may return to normal.

- *Stage III: Exhaustion.* When the resistance phase ends, the homeostatic regulatory mechanisms break down and the exhaustion phase begins. Prolonged exposure to the same stressors leads to exhaustion of an individual's ability to resist and adapt. Resistance to all stressors declines, and susceptibility to physical and psychological ailments increases. A period of rest and recovery is necessary for a healthy outcome. Unless corrective actions are taken, organ system failure will begin.

ALARM

Alarm Phase ("Fight or Flight")

The **alarm phase** is an immediate response to stress, or crisis. The dominant hormone is epinephrine, and its secretion is part of a generalized sympathetic activation.

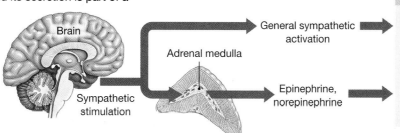

Brain

Adrenal medulla

Sympathetic stimulation

General sympathetic activation

Epinephrine, norepinephrine

Immediate Short-Term Responses to Crises

- Increases mental alertness
- Increases energy use by all cells
- Mobilizes glycogen and lipid reserves
- Changes circulation
- Reduces digestive activity and urine production
- Increases sweat gland secretion
- Increases heart rate and respiratory rate

RESISTANCE

Resistance Phase

The **resistance phase** begins if a stress lasts longer than a few hours. Glucocorticoids (GCs) are the dominant hormones of the resistance phase. GCs and other hormones act to shift tissue metabolism away from glucose, thus increasing its availability to neural tissue.

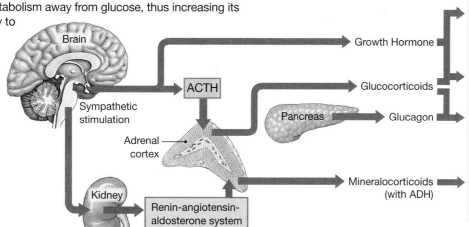

Brain

Sympathetic stimulation

ACTH

Adrenal cortex

Kidney

Renin-angiotensin-aldosterone system

Growth Hormone

Glucocorticoids

Pancreas

Glucagon

Mineralocorticoids (with ADH)

Long-Term Metabolic Adjustments

- Mobilizes remaining energy reserves: Lipids are released by adipose tissue; amino acids are released by skeletal muscle
- Conserves glucose: Peripheral tissues (except neural) break down lipids to obtain energy
- Elevates blood glucose concentrations: Liver synthesizes glucose from other carbohydrates, amino acids, and lipids
- Maintains blood volume: Conservation of salts and water, loss of K^+ and H^+

EXHAUSTION

Exhaustion Phase

The body's lipid reserves are sufficient to maintain the resistance phase for weeks or even months. But when the resistance phase ends, homeostatic regulation breaks down and the **exhaustion phase** begins. Without immediate corrective actions, the ensuing failure of one or more organ systems will prove fatal.

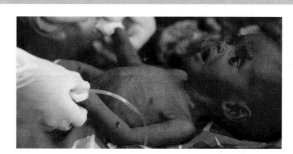

Collapse of Vital Systems

- Exhaustion of lipid reserves
- Cumulative structural or functional damage to vital organs
- Inability to produce glucocorticoids
- Failure of electrolyte balance

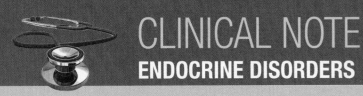
Endocrine disorders fall into two basic categories: inadequate hormonal effects and excessive hormonal effects. The observed signs and symptoms may reflect either abnormal hormone production (hyposecretion or hypersecretion) or abnormal target cell sensitivity. Characteristic features of some important endocrine disorders are described in the table below.

An Overview of Some Important Endocrine Disorders

Hormone	Results of Underproduction or Tissue Insensitivity	Principal Signs and Symptoms	Results of Overproduction or Tissue Hypersensitivity	Principal Signs and Symptoms
Growth hormone (GH)	Pituitary growth failure	Delayed growth, abnormal fat distribution, low blood glucose hours after a meal	Gigantism, acromegaly	Excessive growth
Thyroxine (T$_4$), Triiodothyroxine (T$_3$)	Congenital hypothyroidism, hypothyroidism, myxedema	Low metabolic rate, low body temperature, impaired physical and mental development	Hyperthyroidism, Graves disease	High metabolic rate and body temperature
Insulin	Diabetes mellitus (Type 1)	High blood glucose, impaired glucose use, glycosuria	Excess insulin production	Low blood glucose levels, possibly causing coma
Glucocorticoids Example: cortisol	Addison disease	Inability to tolerate stress, mobilize energy reserves, or maintain normal blood glucose levels	Cushing disease	Excessive breakdown of tissue proteins and lipid reserves, impaired glucose metabolism
Estrogens (females)	Hypogonadism	Sterility, lack of secondary sex characteristics	Precocious puberty	Premature sexual maturation and related behavioral changes
Androgens (males)	Hypogonadism	Sterility, lack of secondary sex characteristics	Precocious puberty	Premature sexual maturation and related behavioral changes

Congenital hypothyroidism results from thyroid hormone insufficiency during pregnancy.

A **goiter**, or enlarged thyroid gland, can be associated with thyroid hyposecretion due to iodine insufficiency in adults.

Acromegaly results from the overproduction of growth hormone after puberty, when most of the epiphyseal cartilages have fused. Bone shapes change and cartilaginous areas of the skeleton enlarge. Note the broad facial features and enlarged lower jaw.

Addison disease I is caused by hyposecretion of corticosteroids, especially glucocorticoids. Pigment changes result from stimulation of melanocytes by ACTH, which is structurally similar to MSH

Cushing disease is caused by hypersecretion of glucocorticoids. Lipid reserves are mobilized, and adipose tissue accumulates in the cheeks and at the base of the neck.

the effects of these hormonal changes on the skeletal system in Chapter 6. ⟲ p. 152 We will continue the discussion in Chapter 20.)

Blood and tissue concentrations of many other hormones, including TSH, thyroid hormones, ADH, PTH, prolactin, and glucocorticoids, do not change with increasing age. Circulating hormone levels may remain within normal limits, but some endocrine tissues become less responsive to stimulation. For example, in elderly individuals, less GH and insulin are secreted after a carbohydrate-rich meal. The reduction in levels of GH and other tropic hormones affects tissues throughout the body. These hormonal effects are associated with the reductions in bone density and muscle mass noted in earlier chapters.

Finally, age-related changes in peripheral tissues may make them less responsive to some hormones. This loss of sensitivity has been documented for glucocorticoids and ADH.

CHECKPOINT

25. Insulin decreases blood glucose levels and glucagon increases blood glucose levels. This is an example of which type of hormonal interaction?

26. The lack of which hormones would inhibit skeletal formation?

27. What are the dominant hormones of the resistance phase of the general adaptation syndrome, and in what ways do they act?

See the blue Answers tab at the back of the book.

10-11 Extensive integration occurs between the endocrine system and other body systems

Learning Objective Give examples of interactions between the endocrine system and other body systems.

The endocrine system provides long-term regulation and adjustments of homeostatic processes that affect many body functions. For all systems, the endocrine system adjusts metabolic rates and use of substrates, such as glucose, triglycerides, and amino acids. It also regulates growth and development.

Build Your Knowledge: How the ENDOCRINE SYSTEM integrates with the other body systems presented so far on p. 374 reviews the major functional relationships between it and the integumentary, skeletal, muscular, and nervous systems.

CHECKPOINT

28. Discuss the general role of the endocrine system in the functioning of other body systems.

29. Discuss the functional relationship between the endocrine system and the muscular system.

See the blue Answers tab at the back of the book.

Related Clinical Terms

adrenalectomy: Surgical removal of an adrenal gland.

endocrinology (EN-dō-kri-NOL-ō-jē)**:** The study of hormones, hormone-secreting tissues and glands, and their roles in physiological and disease processes in the body.

Hashimoto's disease: Disorder that affects the thyroid gland, also known as chronic lymphocytic thyroiditis, causing the immune system to attack the thyroid gland. It is the most common cause of hypothyroidism in the United States.

hypocalcemic tetany: Muscle spasms affecting the face and upper extremities; caused by low calcium ion (Ca^{2+}) concentrations in body fluids.

hypophysectomy: Surgical removal of the pituitary gland.

myxedema: In adults, the effects of hyposecretion of thyroid hormones, including subcutaneous swelling, hair loss, dry skin, low body temperature, muscle weakness, and slowed reflexes.

posttraumatic stress disorder (PTSD): A common anxiety disorder that develops after being exposed to a life-threatening situation or terrifying event.

thyroidectomy: Surgical removal of all or part of the thyroid gland.

thyrotoxicosis: A condition caused by the oversecretion of thyroid hormones (*hyperthyroidism*). Signs and symptoms include increases in metabolic rate, blood pressure, and heart rate; excitability and emotional instability; and lowered energy reserves.

Build Your Knowledge
How the ENDOCRINE SYSTEM integrates with the other body systems presented so far

Integumentary System

• The integumentary system protects superficial endocrine organs; epidermis synthesizes vitamin D_3

• The endocrine system secretes sex hormones that stimulate sebaceous gland activity, influence hair growth, fat distribution, and apocrine sweat gland activity; PRL that stimulates development of mammary glands; adrenal hormones that alter dermal blood flow; MSH that stimulates melanocyte activity

Skeletal System

• The skeletal system protects endocrine organs, especially in brain, chest, and pelvic cavity

• The endocrine system regulates skeletal growth with several hormones; calcium homeostasis regulated by parathyroid hormone and calcitonin; sex hormones speed growth and closure of epiphyseal cartilages at puberty and help maintain bone mass in adults

Muscular System

• The muscular system provides protection for some endocrine organs

• The endocrine system secretes hormones that adjust muscle metabolism, energy production, and growth; regulate calcium and phosphate levels in body fluids; speed skeletal muscle growth

Nervous System

• The nervous system produces hypothalamic hormones that directly control pituitary secretions and indirectly control secretions of other endocrine organs; controls adrenal medullae; secretes ADH and oxytocin

• The endocrine system secretes several hormones that affect neural metabolism and brain development; hormones that help regulate fluid and electrolyte balance; reproductive hormones that influence CNS development and behaviors

Endocrine System

The endocrine system provides long-term regulation and adjustments of homeostatic processes that affect many body functions. It:
• regulates fluid and electrolyte balance
• regulates cell and tissue metabolism
• regulates growth and development
• regulates reproductive functions
• responds to stressful stimuli through the general adaptation syndrome (GAS)

10

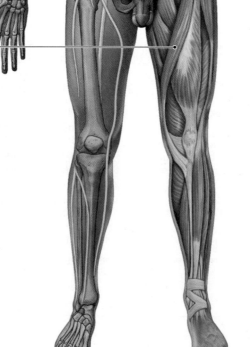

10 Chapter Review

Summary Outline

10-1 Homeostasis is preserved through intercellular communication p. 387

1. In general, the nervous system performs short-term "crisis management," whereas the endocrine system regulates longer-term, ongoing metabolic processes. Endocrine cells release **hormones**, chemicals that alter the metabolic activities of many different tissues and organs *(Figure 10-1)*.

10-2 The endocrine system regulates physiological processes through the binding of hormones to receptors p. 388

2. Hormones can be divided into three groups based on chemical structure: amino acid derivatives, peptide hormones, and lipid derivatives.

3. *Amino acid derivatives* are structurally similar to amino acids; they include *epinephrine, norepinephrine, thyroid hormones*, and *melatonin*.

4. **Peptide hormones** are chains of amino acids.

5. There are two classes of *lipid derivatives*: **steroid hormones**, lipids that are structurally similar to cholesterol, and **eicosanoids**, fatty acid–based hormones that include **prostaglandins**.

6. Hormones exert their effects by modifying the activities of **target cells** (peripheral cells that are sensitive to that particular hormone) *(Figure 10-2)*.

7. Receptors for amino acid–derived hormones, peptide hormones, and fatty acid–derived hormones are in the plasma membranes of target cells. In this case, the hormone acts as a **first messenger** that causes the formation of a **second messenger** in the cytoplasm. Thyroid and steroid hormones cross the plasma membrane and bind to intracellular receptors in the cytoplasm or nucleus. Thyroid hormones also bind to mitochondria, where they increase the rate of ATP production *(Figure 10-3)*.

8. Hormones may circulate freely or be carried by transport proteins. Free hormones are rapidly removed from the bloodstream.

9. The most direct patterns of endocrine control involve negative feedback to the endocrine cells resulting from changes in the extracellular fluid.

10. The hypothalamus regulates the activities of the nervous and endocrine systems in three ways: (1) It synthesizes and secretes two hormones into the bloodstream at the posterior lobe of the pituitary gland; (2) it secretes **regulatory** hormones that control the activities of endocrine cells in the anterior lobe of the pituitary gland; and (3) it exerts direct neural control over the endocrine cells of the adrenal medullae *(Figure 10-4)*.

10-3 The bilobed pituitary gland is an endocrine organ that releases nine peptide hormones p. 394

11. The **pituitary gland** (*hypophysis*) releases nine important peptide hormones; all bind to membrane receptors, and most use cyclic-AMP as a second messenger *(Figure 10-5)*.

12. Hypothalamic neurons release regulatory factors into the surrounding interstitial fluids, which then enter highly permeable capillaries.

13. The **hypophyseal portal system** ensures that all the blood entering the *portal vessels* will reach target cells in the anterior lobe of the pituitary gland before returning to the general circulation *(Figure 10-6)*.

14. The rate of regulatory hormone secretion by the hypothalamus is regulated through negative feedback *(Figure 10-7)*.

15. The seven hormones of the **anterior lobe** of the pituitary gland are (1) **thyroid-stimulating hormone (TSH)**, which triggers the release of thyroid hormones; (2) **adrenocorticotropic hormone (ACTH)**, which stimulates the release of glucocorticoids by the adrenal gland; (3) **follicle-stimulating hormone (FSH)**, which stimulates estrogen secretion and egg development in females and sperm production in males; (4) **luteinizing hormone (LH)**, which causes ovulation and progesterone production in females and **androgen** production in males; (5) **prolactin (PRL)**, which stimulates the development of the mammary glands and the production of milk; (6) **growth hormone (GH)**, which stimulates cell growth and replication by triggering the release of somatomedins from liver cells; and (7) **melanocyte-stimulating hormone (MSH)**, which may be secreted during fetal development, early childhood, pregnancy, or certain diseases. MSH stimulates melanocytes to produce melanin.

16. The **posterior lobe** of the pituitary gland contains the axons of hypothalamic neurons that produce **antidiuretic hormone (ADH)** and **oxytocin (OXT)**. ADH decreases the amount of water lost at the kidneys. In females, oxytocin stimulates smooth muscle cells in the uterus and contractile cells in the mammary glands. In males, it stimulates contractions of smooth muscles in the sperm duct and prostate gland *(Figure 10-8; Table 10-1)*.

10-4 **The thyroid gland lies inferior to the larynx and requires iodine for hormone synthesis** *p. 398*

17. The **thyroid gland** lies near the **thyroid cartilage** of the larynx and consists of two lobes *(Figure 10-9)*.

18. The thyroid gland contains numerous **thyroid follicles**. Thyroid follicles release several hormones, including **thyroxine (T4)** and **triiodothyronine (T3)** *(Table 10-3)*.

19. Thyroid hormones exert a **calorigenic effect**, which enables us to adapt to cold temperatures.

20. The **C cells** of the follicles produce **calcitonin (CT)**, which helps lower calcium ion concentrations in body fluids *(Table 10-3)*.

10-5 **The four parathyroid glands, embedded in the posterior surfaces of the thyroid gland, secrete parathyroid hormone to elevate blood calcium levels** *p. 405*

21. Four **parathyroid glands** are embedded in the posterior surfaces of the thyroid gland. The **chief cells** of the parathyroid produce **parathyroid hormone (PTH)** in response to lower than normal concentrations of calcium ions. Chief cells and the C cells of the thyroid gland maintain calcium levels within relatively narrow limits (Figures 10-10, 10-14; *Table 10-3*).

10-6 **The adrenal glands, consisting of a cortex and a medulla, cap each kidney and secrete several hormones** *p. 406*

22. A single **adrenal gland**, or *suprarenal gland*, lies along the superior border of each kidney. Each gland, which is surrounded by a fibrous capsule, can be subdivided into the superficial adrenal cortex and the inner adrenal medulla *(Figure 10-15)*.

23. The **adrenal cortex** manufactures steroid hormones called **corticosteroids**. The cortex produces (1) **glucocorticoids**—notably, **cortisol, corticosterone,** and **cortisone**, which, in response to ACTH, affect glucose metabolism; (2) **mineralocorticoids**—principally **aldosterone**, which, in response to *angiotensin II*, restricts sodium and water losses at the kidneys, sweat glands, digestive tract, and salivary glands; and (3) androgens *(Figure 10-15)*.

24. The **adrenal medulla** produces **epinephrine** and **norepinephrine** *(Figure 10-15)*.

10-7 **The pineal gland, attached to the third ventricle, secretes melatonin** *p. 409*

25. The **pineal gland** synthesizes **melatonin**. Melatonin appears to (1) slow the maturation of sperm, eggs, and reproductive organs; (2) protect neural tissue from free radicals; and (3) establish daily circadian rhythms.

10-8 **The endocrine pancreas produces insulin and glucagon, hormones that regulate blood glucose levels** *p. 410*

26. The **pancreas** contains both exocrine and endocrine cells. The **exocrine pancreas** secretes an enzyme-rich fluid that functions in the digestive tract. Cells of the endocrine pancreas form clusters called **pancreatic islets** *(islets of Langerhans)*, containing alpha cells (which produce the hormone **glucagon**) and **beta cells** (which produce **insulin**) *(Figure 10-17)*.

27. Insulin lowers blood glucose levels by increasing the rate of glucose uptake and its use. Glucagon raises blood glucose levels by increasing the rates of glycogen breakdown and glucose synthesis in the liver *(Figure 10-18)*.

10-9 **Many organs have secondary endocrine functions** *p. 412*

28. The intestines release hormones that coordinate digestive activities.

29. Endocrine cells in the kidneys produce two hormones and an enzyme important in calcium metabolism and in the maintenance of blood volume and blood pressure.

30. **Calcitriol** stimulates calcium and phosphate ion absorption along the digestive tract.

31. **Erythropoietin (EPO)** stimulates red blood cell production by the red bone marrow.

32. **Renin** activity leads to the formation of **angiotensin II**, the hormone that stimulates the production of aldosterone in the adrenal cortex.

33. Specialized muscle cells in the heart produce **atrial natriuretic peptide (ANP)** when blood pressure or blood volume becomes excessive.

34. The **thymus** produces several hormones called **thymosins**, which play a role in developing and maintaining normal immune defenses.

35. The **interstitial cells** of the paired testes in males produce androgens and **inhibin**. The androgen testosterone is the most important sex hormone in males *(Table 10-4)*.

36. In females, oocytes (immature eggs) develop in **follicles**. Follicle cells surrounding the oocytes produce **estrogens** and inhibin. After ovulation, these cells reorganize into a **corpus luteum** that releases a mixture of estrogens and **progesterone**. If pregnancy occurs, the placenta functions as an endocrine organ *(Table 10-4)*.

37. Adipose tissue secretes **leptin**, which functions in the negative feedback control of appetite.

10-10 **Hormones interact to produce coordinated physiological responses** *p. 418*

38. The endocrine system functions as an integrated unit, and hormones often interact. These interactions may have (1) **antagonistic** (opposing) effects, (2) **synergistic** (additive) effects,

(3) **permissive** effects, or (4) **integrative** effects, in which hormones produce different but complementary results.

39. Normal growth requires the cooperation of several endocrine organs. Six hormones are especially important: growth hormone, thyroid hormones, insulin, parathyroid hormone, calcitriol, and reproductive hormones.

40. Any condition that threatens homeostasis is a **stress**. Our bodies respond to a variety of stress-causing factors through the **general adaptation syndrome (GAS)**. The GAS is divided into three phases: (1) the **alarm phase**, under the direction of the sympathetic division of the ANS; (2) the **resistance phase**, dominated by glucocorticoids; and (3) the **exhaustion phase**, the eventual breakdown of homeostatic regulation and failure of one or more organ systems (*Spotlight Figure 10-20*).

41. Many hormones affect the functional state of the nervous system, producing changes in mood, emotional states, and various behaviors.

42. The endocrine system undergoes relatively few functional changes with advancing age. The most dramatic endocrine change is a decline in the concentration of reproductive hormones.

10-11 Extensive integration occurs between the endocrine system and other body systems *p. 423*

43. The endocrine system affects all organ systems by adjusting metabolic rates and substrate use, and regulating growth and development.

Review Questions

See the blue Answers tab at the back of the book.

Level 1 Reviewing Facts and Terms

Match each item in column A with the most closely related item in column B. Place letters for answers in the spaces provided.

COLUMN A

_____ **1.** Thyroid gland
_____ **2.** Pineal gland
_____ **3.** Polyuria
_____ **4.** Parathyroid gland
_____ **5.** Thymus gland
_____ **6.** Adrenal cortex
_____ **7.** Heart
_____ **8.** Endocrine pancreas
_____ **9.** Gonadotropins
_____ **10.** Hypothalamus
_____ **11.** Pituitary gland
_____ **12.** Growth hormone

COLUMN B

a. Islets of Langerhans
b. Atrophies by adulthood
c. Atrial natriuretic peptide
d. Stimulates cell growth and protein synthesis
e. Melatonin
f. Hypophysis
g. Excessive urine production
h. Calcitonin
i. Secretes regulatory hormones
j. FSH and LH
k. Secretes androgens, mineralocorticoids, and glucocorticoids
l. Stimulated by low calcium levels

13. Identify the endocrine glands and tissues in the diagram on the right.

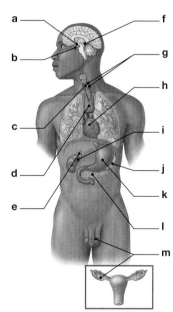

(a) _____ **(b)** _____
(c) _____ **(d)** _____
(e) _____ **(f)** _____
(g) _____ **(h)** _____
(i) _____ **(j)** _____
(k) _____ **(l)** _____
(m) _____

14. Adrenocorticotropic hormone (ACTH) stimulates the release of
    (a) thyroid hormones by the hypothalamus.
    (b) gonadotropins by the adrenal glands.
    (c) somatotropins by the hypothalamus.
    (d) steroid hormones by the adrenal glands.

15. FSH production in males supports
    (a) maturation of sperm by stimulating nurse cells.
    (b) development of muscles and strength.
    (c) production of male sex hormones.
    (d) increased desire for sexual activity.

16. The hormone that induces ovulation in women and promotes the ovarian secretion of progesterone is
    (a) interstitial cell-stimulating hormone.
    (b) estradiol.
    (c) luteinizing hormone.
    (d) prolactin.

17. The two hormones released by the posterior lobe of the pituitary gland are
    (a) somatotropin and gonadotropin.
    (b) estrogen and progesterone.
    (c) growth hormone and prolactin.
    (d) antidiuretic hormone and oxytocin.

18. The primary function of antidiuretic hormone (ADH) is to
    (a) increase the amount of water lost at the kidneys.
    (b) decrease the amount of water lost at the kidneys.
    (c) dilate peripheral blood vessels to decrease blood pressure.
    (d) increase absorption along the digestive tract.

19. The element required for normal thyroid function is
    (a) magnesium.
    (b) calcium.
    (c) potassium.
    (d) iodine.

20. Reduced fluid losses in the urine due to retention of sodium ions and water is a result of the action of
    (a) insulin.
    (b) calcitonin.
    (c) aldosterone.
    (d) cortisone.

21. The adrenal medullae produce the hormones
    (a) cortisol and cortisone.
    (b) epinephrine and norepinephrine.
    (c) corticosterone and testosterone.
    (d) androgens and progesterone.

22. What seven hormones are released by the anterior lobe of the pituitary gland?

23. What are the effects of calcitonin and parathyroid hormone on blood calcium levels?

24. (a) What three phases of the general adaptation syndrome (GAS) constitute the body's response to stress? (b) What endocrine secretions play dominant roles in each of the first two phases?

Level 2 Reviewing Concepts

25. What is the primary difference in the ways the nervous and endocrine systems communicate with their target cells?

26. In what ways can hormones modify the activities of their target cells?

27. What possible results occur when a cell receives instructions from two different hormones at the same time?

28. How would blocking the activity of phosphodiesterase (PDE) affect a cell that responds to hormonal stimulation by the cAMP second messenger system?

Level 3 Critical Thinking and Clinical Applications

29. Roger has been extremely thirsty. He drinks numerous glasses of water every day and urinates a great deal. Name two disorders that could produce these signs and symptoms. What test could a clinician perform to determine which disorder Roger has?

30. Julie is pregnant but is not receiving prenatal care. She has a poor diet consisting mostly of fast food. She drinks no milk, preferring colas instead. How will this situation affect Julie's level of parathyroid hormone?

The Cardiovascular System: Blood

Learning Objectives

These objectives tell you what you should be able to do after completing the chapter. They correspond by number to this chapter's sections.

11-1 Describe the components and major functions of blood, and list the physical characteristics of blood.

11-2 Describe the composition and functions of plasma.

11-3 List the characteristics and functions of red blood cells, describe the structure and function of hemoglobin, describe how red blood cell components are recycled, and explain erythropoiesis.

11-4 Discuss the factors that determine a person's blood type, and explain why blood typing is important.

11-5 Categorize the various white blood cells on the basis of their structures and functions, and discuss the factors that regulate their production.

11-6 Describe the structure, function, and production of platelets.

11-7 Describe the processes that control blood loss after an injury.

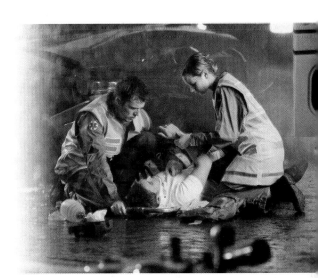

Clinical Notes
Abnormal Hemoglobin, p. 436
Hemolytic Disease of the
   Newborn, p. 443
Abnormal Hemostasis, p. 450

Spotlight
The Composition of Whole Blood,
   pp. 432–433

An Introduction to the Cardiovascular System

Your body is constantly exchanging chemicals with its external environment. The lining of the digestive tract absorbs nutrients, gases move across the thin epithelium of the lungs, and wastes are excreted in the feces and urine. These chemical exchanges rapidly affect every cell, tissue, and organ because of our internal transport network, the **cardiovascular system**.

We can compare the cardiovascular system to the cooling system of a car. Both systems circulate a fluid (blood versus water) with a pump (the heart versus a water pump). Both carry a fluid in flexible tubing (the blood vessels versus radiator hoses). The cardiovascular system is far more complicated, but either system can malfunction due to fluid losses, pump failures, or damaged tubing.

The cardiovascular system is the first organ system to become fully operational. The heart begins beating by the end of the third week of embryonic life. At that time, most other systems have barely begun to develop. Before then, embryos don't need cardiovascular systems because diffusion across their exposed surfaces takes place rapidly enough to meet their demands. When an embryo has reached a few millimeters in length, however, diffusion is too slow for developing tissues. At that stage, the cardiovascular system begins serving as a rapid-transport system for oxygen, nutrients, and waste products. When the heart starts beating, blood begins circulating. The embryo can now make more efficient use of the nutrients from the mother's bloodstream, and the embryo's size doubles in the next week.

We consider the nature of the circulating blood in this chapter. (We discuss the heart in Chapter 12 and the blood vessels in Chapter 13. In Chapter 14, we consider the lymphatic system, a defense system closely connected to the cardiovascular system.)

Build Your Knowledge

Recall that blood is a fluid connective tissue (as you saw in **Chapter 4: The Tissue Level of Organization**). Like all connective tissues, blood has three components: (1) specialized cells, (2) extracellular protein fibers, and (3) a ground substance. The extracellular fibers and ground substance form the matrix that surrounds the cells. In blood, the ground substance is a fluid. The watery matrix is called plasma. The plasma proteins are dissolved and usually do not form insoluble fibers. つ **pp. 102, 106**

11-1 Blood has several important functions and unique physical characteristics

Learning Objective: Describe the components and major functions of blood, and list the physical characteristics of blood.

The circulating fluid of the body is **blood**, a specialized connective tissue that contains cells suspended in a fluid matrix. つ p. 106 Blood has five major functions:

1. **Transporting dissolved gases, nutrients, hormones, and metabolic wastes.** Blood carries oxygen from the lungs to the body's tissues, and carbon dioxide from these tissues to the lungs. Blood distributes nutrients absorbed by the digestive tract or released from storage in adipose tissue or in the liver. It carries hormones from endocrine glands toward their target cells. It also absorbs and carries the wastes produced by active cells to the kidneys for excretion.

2. **Regulating the pH and ion composition of interstitial fluids.** Diffusion between interstitial fluids and blood eliminates local deficiencies or excesses of ions such as calcium or potassium. Blood also absorbs and neutralizes the acids generated by active tissues, such as lactic acid produced by skeletal muscle.

3. **Restricting fluid losses at injury sites.** Blood contains enzymes and factors that respond to breaks in vessel walls by initiating the process of *blood clotting*. A blood clot acts as a temporary patch that prevents further fluid loss.

4. **Defending against toxins and pathogens.** Blood transports white blood cells (WBCs), specialized cells that migrate into body tissues to fight infections or remove debris. Blood also delivers *antibodies*, special proteins that attack invading organisms or foreign compounds.

5. Stabilizing body temperature. Blood absorbs the heat generated by active skeletal muscles and redistributes it to other tissues. If body temperature is high, blood is directed toward the skin surface, where heat is lost to the environment. If body temperature is too low, warm blood is directed to the brain and other temperature sensitive organs.

Composition of Blood

Spotlight Figure 11-1 (pp. 432–433) describes the composition of whole blood, which is made up of *plasma* and *formed elements* (blood cells and cell fragments). The components of whole blood may be separated, or **fractionated**, for analytical or clinical purposes.

Whole blood from any source—veins, capillaries, or arteries—has the same basic physical characteristics:

- **Temperature.** The temperature of blood is roughly 38°C (100.4°F), slightly above normal body temperature.

- **Viscosity.** Blood is five times as viscous ("thick") as water. It is five times stickier, more cohesive, and resistant to flow than water. The high viscosity results from interactions among the dissolved proteins, formed elements, and water molecules in plasma.

- **pH.** Blood is slightly alkaline, with a pH between 7.35 and 7.45 (average: 7.4). ⤺ p. 36

Blood Collection and Analysis

Fresh whole blood is usually collected from a superficial vein, such as the median cubital vein on the anterior surface of the elbow. This procedure is called **venipuncture** (VĒN-i-punk-chur; *vena,* vein + *punctura,* a piercing). It is a common sampling technique because (1) superficial veins are easy to locate; (2) the walls of veins are thinner than those of arteries of comparable size; and (3) blood pressure in the veins is relatively low, so the puncture wound seals quickly. The most common clinical procedures examine venous blood.

Blood from peripheral capillaries can be obtained by puncturing the tip of a finger, an ear lobe, or (in infants) the great toe or heel of the foot. A small drop of capillary blood can be used to prepare a *blood smear,* a thin film of blood on a microscope slide. The blood smear is then stained with special dyes to show different types of formed elements.

An **arterial puncture**, or "arterial stick," may be required for evaluating the efficiency of gas exchange at the lungs. Samples are usually drawn from the radial artery at the wrist or the brachial artery at the elbow.

CHECKPOINT

1. List five major functions of blood.

2. What two components make up whole blood?

3. Why is venipuncture a common technique for obtaining a blood sample?

See the blue Answers tab at the back of the book.

11-2 Plasma, the fluid portion of blood, contains significant quantities of plasma proteins

Learning Objective: Describe the composition and functions of plasma.

Plasma and interstitial fluid account for most of the volume of extracellular fluid in the body. Plasma makes up about 55 percent of the volume of whole blood. As shown in **Spotlight Figure 11-1**, the components of plasma include plasma proteins (7%), other solutes (1%), and water (92%).

Plasma Proteins

The proteins in plasma are in solution (dissolved). The three primary types are *albumins* (al-BŪ-minz), *globulins* (GLOB-ū-linz), and *fibrinogen* (fī-BRIN-ō-jen). They make up more than 99 percent of the plasma proteins.

Albumins make up the majority of the plasma proteins. For this reason, their presence is important in maintaining the osmotic pressure of plasma. Globulins are the second most abundant proteins in plasma. They include antibodies and transport proteins. Antibodies attack foreign proteins and pathogens. Transport proteins bind small ions, hormones, or compounds that might otherwise be lost at the kidneys or that have very low solubility in water. One example is *thyroid-binding globulin,* which binds and transports thyroid hormones.

Both albumins and globulins can bind to lipids, such as triglycerides, fatty acids, or cholesterol. These lipids are not themselves water soluble, but the protein–lipid combination readily dissolves in plasma. In this way, the cardiovascular system transports insoluble lipids to peripheral tissues. Globulins involved in lipid transport are called *lipoproteins* (LĪ-pō-prō-tēnz).

Fibrinogen, the third type of plasma protein, functions in blood clotting. Under certain conditions, fibrinogen molecules interact to form large, insoluble strands of **fibrin** (FĪ-brin). These strands form insoluble fibers that provide the basic framework for a blood clot. If steps are not taken to prevent clotting in a blood sample, the conversion of fibrinogen

A Fluid Connective Tissue

Blood is a fluid connective tissue. It consists of a matrix called **plasma** (PLAZ-muh) and formed elements (cells and cell fragments). The term **whole blood** refers to the combination of both plasma and the formed elements. The cardiovascular system of an adult male contains 5–6 liters (5.3–6.4 quarts) of whole blood; that of an adult female contains 4–5 liters (4.2–5.3 quarts). The sex differences in blood volume primarily reflect differences in average body size.

PLASMA

Plasma, the matrix of blood, makes up about 55 percent of the volume of whole blood. In many respects, the composition of plasma resembles that of interstitial fluid. This similarity exists because water, ions, and small solutes are continuously exchanged between plasma and interstitial fluids across the walls of capillaries. The primary differences between plasma and interstitial fluid involve (1) the levels of oxygen and carbon dioxide (due to the respiratory activities of tissue cells), and (2) the concentrations and types of dissolved proteins (because plasma proteins cannot cross capillary walls).

Plasma		
55% (Range 46–63%)	Plasma Proteins	7%
	Other Solutes	1%
	Water	92%

consists of +

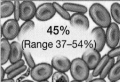

Formed Elements		
45% (Range 37–54%)	Platelets	< .1%
	White Blood Cells	< .1%
	Red Blood Cells	99.9%

The **hematocrit** (he-MAT-ō-krit) is the percentage of whole blood volume contributed by formed elements. The normal hematocrit, or **packed cell volume (PCV)**, in adult males is 46 and in adult females is 42. The sex difference in hematocrit primarily reflects the fact that androgens (male hormones) stimulate red blood cell production, whereas estrogens (female hormones) do not.

Formed elements are blood cells and cell fragments that are suspended in plasma. These elements account for about 45 percent of the volume of whole blood. Three types of formed elements exist: platelets, white blood cells, and red blood cells. Formed elements are produced through the process of **hemopoiesis** (hēm-ō-poy-Ē-sis), also called **hematopoiesis**. Two populations of stem cells—myeloid stem cells and lymphoid stem cells—are responsible for the production of formed elements.

FORMED ELEMENTS

Plasma Proteins

Plasma proteins are in solution (dissolved) rather than forming insoluble fibers like those in other connective tissues, such as loose connective tissue or cartilage. On average, each 100 mL of plasma contains 7.6 g of protein, almost five times the concentration in interstitial fluid. The large size and globular shapes of most blood proteins prevent them from crossing capillary walls, so they remain trapped within the bloodstream. The liver synthesizes and releases more than 90% of the plasma proteins. These include all albumins, fibrinogen, and most globulins.

Albumins (al-BŪ-minz) make up roughly 60% of the plasma proteins. As the most abundant plasma proteins, they are major contributors to the osmotic pressure of plasma.

Globulins (GLOB-ū-linz) account for approximately 35% of the proteins in plasma. Important plasma globulins include antibodies and transport globulins. **Antibodies**, also called **immunoglobulins** (i-mū-nō-GLOB-ū-linz), attack foreign proteins and pathogens. **Transport globulins** bind small ions, hormones, and other compounds.

Fibrinogen (fī-BRIN-ō-jen) functions in clotting, and normally accounts for roughly 4% of plasma proteins. Under certain conditions, fibrinogen molecules interact, forming large, insoluble strands of **fibrin** (FĪ-brin) that form the basic framework for a blood clot.

Plasma also contains enzymes and hormones whose concentrations vary widely.

Other Solutes

Other solutes are generally present in concentrations similar to those in the interstitial fluids. However, because blood is a transport medium there may be differences in nutrient and waste product concentrations between arterial blood and venous blood.

Organic Nutrients: Organic nutrients are used for ATP production, growth, and maintenance of cells. This category includes lipids (fatty acids, cholesterol, glycerides), carbohydrates (primarily glucose), amino acids, and vitamins.

Electrolytes: Normal extracellular ion composition is essential for vital cellular activities. The major plasma electrolytes are Na^+, K^+, Ca^{2+}, Mg^{2+}, Cl^-, HCO_3^-, HPO_4^-, and SO_4^{2-}.

Organic Wastes: Waste products are carried to sites of breakdown or excretion. Examples of organic wastes include urea, uric acid, creatinine, bilirubin, and ammonium ions.

Platelets

Platelets are small, membrane-bound cell fragments that contain enzymes and other substances important to clotting.

White Blood Cells

White blood cells (**WBCs**), or **leukocytes** (LOO-kō-sīts; *leukos*, white + *-cyte*, cell), participate in the body's defense mechanisms. There are five classes of leukocytes, each with slightly different functions that will be explored later in the chapter.

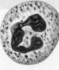 Neutrophils

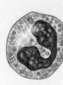 Eosinophils

 Basophils

 Lymphocytes

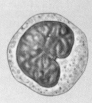 Monocytes

Red Blood Cells

Red blood cells (**RBCs**), or **erythrocytes** (e-RITH-rō-sīts; *erythros*, red + *-cyte*, cell), are the most abundant blood cells. These specialized cells are essential for the transport of oxygen in the blood.

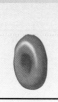

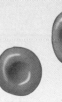

(a soluble protein) to fibrin (an insoluble protein) will take place. This conversion removes the clotting proteins, leaving a fluid known as **serum**.

The liver synthesizes more than 90 percent of the plasma proteins, including all albumins and fibrinogen and most globulins. For this reason, liver disorders can alter the composition and functional properties of the blood. For example, some forms of liver disease can lead to uncontrolled bleeding due to the inadequate synthesis of fibrinogen and other plasma proteins involved in clotting.

CHECKPOINT

4. List the three major types of plasma proteins.

5. What would be the effects of a decrease in the amount of plasma proteins?

See the blue Answers tab at the back of the book.

11-3 Red blood cells, formed by erythropoiesis, contain hemoglobin that can be recycled

Learning Objective: List the characteristics and functions of red blood cells, describe the structure and function of hemoglobin, describe how red blood cell components are recycled, and explain erythropoiesis.

Red blood cells (RBCs), or **erythrocytes**, account for 99.9 percent of the formed elements. RBCs give whole blood its deep red color because they contain the red pigment *hemoglobin*, which binds and transports oxygen and carbon dioxide.

Abundance of Red Blood Cells

Roughly one-third of all cells in the human body are RBCs. A standard blood test reports the number of RBCs per microliter (µL) of whole blood as the *RBC count*. In adult males, 1 (µL) or 1 cubic millimeter (mm^3), of whole blood contains roughly 5.4 million RBCs. In adult females, 1 microliter contains about 4.8 million. A single drop of whole blood contains some 260 million RBCs. The blood of an average adult has 25 trillion RBCs.

The *hematocrit* is the percentage of whole blood volume occupied by formed elements (**Spotlight Figure 11-1**). The hematocrit is measured after a blood sample has been spun in a centrifuge to make all the formed elements come out of suspension. After centrifugation, the WBCs and platelets form a very thin *buffy coat* above a thick layer of RBCs. The hematocrit closely approximates the volume of RBCs because whole blood contains roughly 1000 red

blood cells for each WBC. For this reason, hematocrit values are often reported as the *volume of packed red cells*, or simply the *PCV*.

Many conditions can affect the hematocrit. The hematocrit increases, for example, during dehydration (when plasma volume is reduced) or after *erythropoietin* (*EPO*) stimulation. ⮌ p. 367 The hematocrit decreases as a result of internal bleeding or problems with RBC formation. So, the hematocrit alone does not provide specific diagnostic information. However, a change in hematocrit is an indication that more specific tests are needed.

Structure of RBCs

RBCs are specialized to transport oxygen and carbon dioxide within the bloodstream. As **Figure 11-2** shows, each RBC is a biconcave disc with a thin central region and a thick outer margin. This unusual shape has two important effects on RBC function: (1) It gives each RBC a relatively large surface area to volume ratio, which increases the rate of diffusion between the cytoplasm and the surrounding plasma; and (2) it enables RBCs to bend and flex to squeeze through narrow capillaries.

A RBCs is very different from the "typical cell" we discussed in Chapter 3. During their formation, RBCs lose most of their organelles, including nuclei, ribosomes, and mitochondria. They retain only the cytoskeleton. Without a nucleus or ribosomes, circulating RBCs can neither divide nor synthesize structural proteins or enzymes. As a result, the RBCs cannot make repairs, so their life span is relatively short—only about 120 days.

With few organelles and no way to synthesize proteins, their energy demands are low. Without mitochondria, RBCs obtain the energy they need through anaerobic metabolism, relying on glucose absorbed from the surrounding plasma. This characteristic makes RBCs relatively inefficient in terms of energy use. However, it ensures that absorbed oxygen will be carried to peripheral tissues, not "stolen" by mitochondria in the cytoplasm.

Hemoglobin Structure and Function

A mature RBC consists of a cell membrane enclosing a mass of transport proteins. Molecules of **hemoglobin** (HĒ-mō-glō-bin) **(Hb; Hgb)** account for over 95 percent of an RBC's intracellular proteins. Hemoglobin is responsible for the cell's ability to transport oxygen and carbon dioxide.

Figure 11-2 The Anatomy of Red Blood Cells.

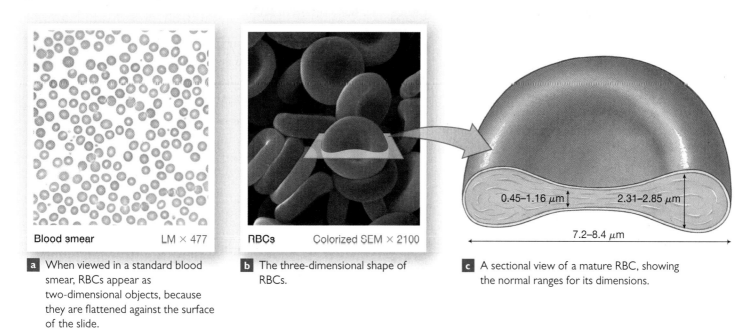

Blood smear   LM × 477

RBCs   Colorized SEM × 2100

0.45–1.16 μm   2.31–2.85 μm

7.2–8.4 μm

a When viewed in a standard blood smear, RBCs appear as two-dimensional objects, because they are flattened against the surface of the slide.

b The three-dimensional shape of RBCs.

c A sectional view of a mature RBC, showing the normal ranges for its dimensions.

Hemoglobin molecules have a complex quaternary structure. A hemoglobin molecule consists of four globular protein subunits, arranged in two pairs. The members of each pair are composed of slightly different polypeptide chains. ⟳ p. 44 Each of the four globular subunits includes a single molecule of an organic pigment called **heme**. A heme molecule holds an iron ion in such a way that it can interact with an oxygen molecule (O_2). The iron–oxygen interaction is very weak, and the two can easily separate. RBCs containing hemoglobin with bound oxygen give blood a bright red color. When oxygen is not bound to hemoglobin, the RBCs give blood a dark red, almost burgundy, color.

The amount of oxygen bound in each RBC depends on the conditions in the surrounding plasma. When oxygen is abundant in the plasma, hemoglobin molecules gain oxygen until all their heme molecules are occupied. As plasma oxygen levels decline, plasma carbon dioxide levels are usually rising. Under these conditions, heme molecules release their oxygen, and the globin portions of each hemoglobin molecule begins to bind carbon dioxide molecules in a process that is just as reversible as the binding of oxygen to heme.

As RBCs circulate, they are exposed to varying concentrations of oxygen and carbon dioxide. At the lungs, diffusion brings oxygen into the plasma and removes carbon dioxide. The hemoglobin molecules in RBCs respond by absorbing oxygen and releasing carbon dioxide. In peripheral tissues, active cells consume oxygen and produce carbon dioxide.

As blood flows through these areas, the situation is reversed. Oxygen diffuses out of the plasma, and carbon dioxide diffuses in. Under these conditions, hemoglobin releases its bound oxygen and binds carbon dioxide.

Normal activity levels can be sustained only when tissue oxygen levels are kept within normal limits. The blood of a person who has a low hematocrit, or whose RBCs have a reduced hemoglobin content, has a reduced oxygen-carrying capacity. This condition is called **anemia**. Symptoms of anemia include premature muscle fatigue, weakness, and a general lack of energy.

RBC Life Span and Circulation

RBCs are exposed to severe physical stresses. A single round-trip from the heart, through the peripheral tissues, and back to the heart takes less than a minute. In that time, an RBC is forced along vessels where it bounces off the walls, collides with other RBCs, and is squeezed through tiny capillaries. With all this wear and tear and no capacity for repair, either its plasma membrane ruptures or some other damage occurs.

Phagocytes of the spleen, liver, or red bone marrow detect the damage and engulf the RBC. The elimination of RBCs usually goes unnoticed because new ones enter the circulation at a comparable rate. About 1 percent of the circulating RBCs are replaced each day, and approximately 3 million new RBCs enter the circulation each second!

Build Your Knowledge

Recall that phagocytosis is a process in which solid, extracellular materials are packaged into a vesicle for transport into a cell (as you saw in **Chapter 3: Cell Structure and Function**). Phagocytosis is also called "cell eating." Large particles are brought into the cell as cytoplasmic extensions (pseudopodia) surround and engulf the particle and move it into the cell. Phagocytes are cells that perform phagocytosis. They engulf substances such as bacteria, viruses, cellular debris, and other foreign material. ⟳ **p. 68**

Hemoglobin Recycling

Most of the components of RBCs are recycled, including their hemoglobin. Macrophages (phagocytic cells) in the liver, spleen, and red bone marrow play a role in recycling these components. These phagocytes engulf RBCs and also detect and remove hemoglobin molecules from RBCs that rupture, or **hemolyze** (HĒ-mō-līz). Hemoglobin remains intact only inside an RBC. If the hemoglobin released by *hemolysis* is not phagocytized, it will not be recycled. Instead, this hemoglobin breaks down in the blood. The individual polypeptide chains are then filtered from the blood by the kidneys and lost in the urine. Fortunately, only about 10 percent of RBCs undergo *hemolysis* in the bloodstream. When large numbers of RBCs do break down in the bloodstream, the urine can turn red or brown, a condition called **hemoglobinuria**.

The recycling of hemoglobin and turnover of RBCs is shown in **Figure 11-3**. Once a macrophage has engulfed and broken down an RBC, each part of a hemoglobin molecule has a different fate:

1. **The four globular proteins of each hemoglobin molecule are broken apart into their component amino acids.** These amino acids are either metabolized by the cell or released into the bloodstream for use by other cells.

2. **Iron is extracted from heme molecules.** It may be stored in the macrophage or released into the bloodstream, where it binds to **transferrin** (tranz-FER-in), a plasma transport protein. RBCs developing in the red bone marrow use amino acids and transferrins from the bloodstream to synthesize new hemoglobin molecules. Excess transferrins are removed in the liver and spleen, where the iron is stored in special protein–iron complexes.

3. **After being stripped of its iron, each heme molecule is converted to biliverdin** (bil-i-VER-din). Biliverdin is an organic compound with a green color. (Bad bruises commonly appear greenish because biliverdin forms in the blood-filled tissues.) Biliverdin is then converted to **bilirubin** (bil-i-ROO-bin), an orange-yellow pigment, and released into the bloodstream. Liver cells absorb the bilirubin and normally release it into the small intestine within the bile. Bilirubin reaching the large intestine is converted to related pigment molecules, called *urobilins* (ūr-ō-BĪ-lins) and *stercobilins* (ster-kō-BĪ-lins). Some are absorbed into the bloodstream and excreted into urine. These bilirubin-derived pigments produce the yellow color of urine and the brown color of feces.

If the bile ducts are blocked (by gallstones, for example) or the liver cannot absorb or excrete bilirubin, its levels rise in the bloodstream. Bilirubin then diffuses into peripheral

CLINICAL NOTE

Abnormal Hemoglobin

Abnormal hemoglobin characterizes several inherited disorders. Two of the best known are *thalassemia* and *sickle cell anemia (SCA)*.

The various forms of thalassemia (thal-ah-SĒ-me-uh) result from an inability to produce adequate amounts of the globular proteins that make up hemoglobin. This slows the rate of RBC production. The reduced oxygen-carrying capacity of the blood leads to problems in growth and development. Individuals with severe thalassemia need frequent *transfusions*—the administration of blood components—to maintain adequate numbers of RBCs.

SCA results from a mutation affecting the amino acid sequence of one of the two types of globular proteins of the hemoglobin molecule. When blood contains an abundance of oxygen, the hemoglobin molecules and the RBCs that carry them appear normal. But when the defective hemoglobin gives up enough of its bound oxygen, nearby hemoglobin molecules interact and the cells become stiff and curved. This "sickling" makes the cells more fragile and easily damaged. RBCs can also become stuck in capillaries as sickling occurs. This blocks blood flow, and nearby tissues become oxygen starved.

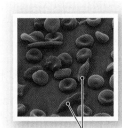

Sickling in Red Blood Cells

Figure 11-3 Recycling of Hemoglobin.

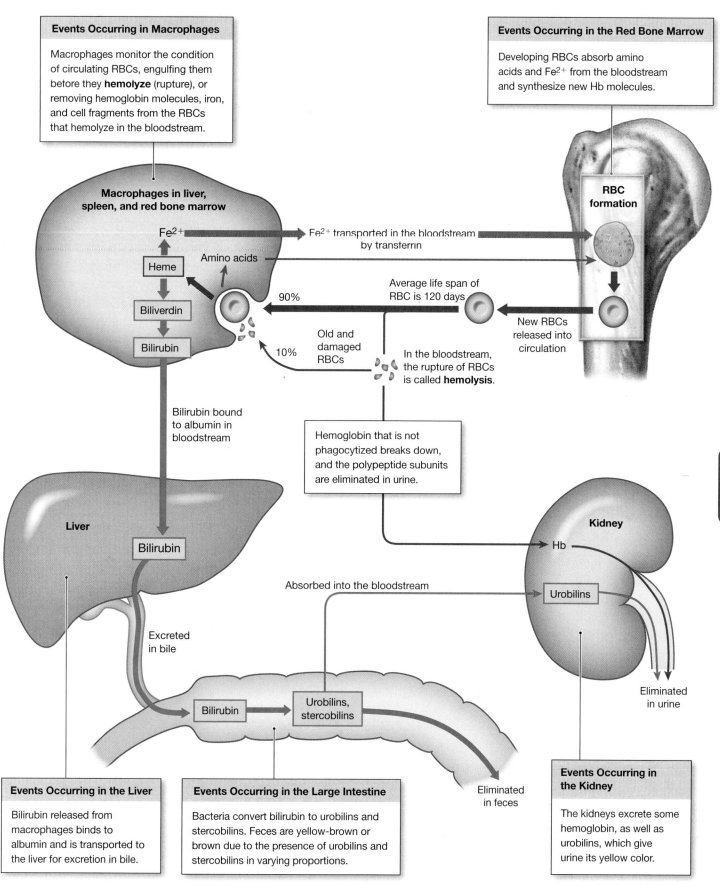

Events Occurring in Macrophages

Macrophages monitor the condition of circulating RBCs, engulfing them before they **hemolyze** (rupture), or removing hemoglobin molecules, iron, and cell fragments from the RBCs that hemolyze in the bloodstream.

Events Occurring in the Red Bone Marrow

Developing RBCs absorb amino acids and Fe²⁺ from the bloodstream and synthesize new Hb molecules.

RBC formation

Macrophages in liver, spleen, and red bone marrow

Fe²⁺

Fe²⁺ transported in the bloodstream by transferrin

Heme

Amino acids

Biliverdin

90%

Average life span of RBC is 120 days

New RBCs released into circulation

Bilirubin

10%

Old and damaged RBCs

In the bloodstream, the rupture of RBCs is called **hemolysis**.

Bilirubin bound to albumin in bloodstream

Hemoglobin that is not phagocytized breaks down, and the polypeptide subunits are eliminated in urine.

Liver

Bilirubin

Excreted in bile

Absorbed into the bloodstream

Eliminated in urine

Kidney

Hb

Urobilins

Bilirubin

Urobilins, stercobilins

Eliminated in feces

Events Occurring in the Liver

Bilirubin released from macrophages binds to albumin and is transported to the liver for excretion in bile.

Events Occurring in the Large Intestine

Bacteria convert bilirubin to urobilins and stercobilins. Feces are yellow-brown or brown due to the presence of urobilins and stercobilins in varying proportions.

Events Occurring in the Kidney

The kidneys excrete some hemoglobin, as well as urobilins, which give urine its yellow color.

11

tissues, producing a combination of signs (yellow skin and eyes) called **jaundice** (JAWN-dis).

The recycling of the components of an individual RBC following hemolysis or phagocytosis is a remarkably efficient process. For example, roughly 26 mg of iron are incorporated into hemoglobin molecules each day, but a dietary iron supply of 1–2 mg can keep pace with the incidental losses in the feces and urine.

Gender and Iron Reserves

Any impairment in iron uptake or metabolism can cause serious clinical problems because RBC formation will be affected. Women are especially dependent on a normal dietary supply of iron because their iron reserves are smaller than those of men. The body of a normal man contains around 3.5 g of iron (in the ionic form Fe^{2+}). Of that amount, 2.5 g is bound to the hemoglobin of circulating RBCs. The rest is stored in the liver and red bone marrow. In women, total body iron content averages 2.4 g, with roughly 1.9 g in RBCs. Thus, a woman's iron reserves are only 0.5 g, half that of a typical man. If dietary supplies of iron are inadequate, hemoglobin production slows, and symptoms of *iron-deficiency anemia* appear.

The buildup of too much iron in the liver and in cardiac muscle tissue can also cause problems. Excessive iron in cardiac muscle cells has been linked to heart disease.

RBC Formation

Embryonic blood cells appear in the bloodstream during the third week of development. These cells divide repeatedly, rapidly increasing in number. The vessels of the embryonic *yolk sac* are the primary sites of blood formation for the first eight weeks of development. As other organ systems appear, some of the embryonic blood cells move out of the bloodstream and into the liver, spleen, thymus, and bone marrow. These embryonic cells differentiate into stem cells that divide to produce blood cells.

From the second to fifth months of development, the liver and spleen are the primary sites of hemopoiesis (blood cell formation and differentiation). As the skeleton enlarges, the bone marrow becomes increasingly important. In adults, red bone marrow is the only site of RBC production, as well as the primary site of WBC formation.

RBC formation, or **erythropoiesis** (e-rith-rō-poy-Ē-sis), takes place only in *red bone marrow*, or **myeloid tissue** (MĪ-e-loyd; *myelos*, marrow). This tissue is located in the vertebrae, sternum, ribs, scapulae, pelvis, and proximal limb bones. Other marrow areas contain a fatty tissue known as *yellow bone marrow.* Under extreme stimulation, such as a severe and sustained blood loss, areas of yellow marrow can convert to red marrow. This change increases the rate of RBC formation.

Stages in RBC Maturation

RBCs mature in a series of stages. Blood specialists, known as **hematologists** (hē-ma-TOL-o-jists), have named key stages. Like all formed elements, RBCs result from the divisions of **hemocytoblasts**, or **hematopoietic stem cells**, in red bone marrow (**Figure 11-4**). In giving rise to the cells that ultimately become RBCs, the hemocytoblasts produce **myeloid stem cells**. Some of these cells develop through a series of stages to become mature erythrocytes (see left side of **Figure 11-4**).

Erythroblasts are very immature RBCs that are actively synthesizing hemoglobin. After roughly four days of differentiation, each erythroblast sheds its nucleus and becomes a **reticulocyte** (re-TIK-ū-lō-sīt). After two or three more days in the red bone marrow synthesizing proteins, reticulocytes enter the bloodstream. At this time, they can still be detected in a blood smear with stains that only combine with RNA. Normally, reticulocytes account for about 0.8 percent of the circulating erythrocytes. After 24 hours in circulation, the reticulocytes complete their maturation and resemble other mature RBCs.

The Regulation of Erythropoiesis

For erythropoiesis to proceed normally, the red bone marrow must have adequate supplies of amino acids, iron, and vitamins (including B_{12}, B_6, and folic acid) for protein synthesis. We obtain **vitamin B_{12}** from dairy products and meat, but its absorption requires *intrinsic factor* produced in the stomach. Without vitamin B_{12} from the diet, normal stem cell divisions cannot take place, and *pernicious anemia* results.

Erythropoiesis is stimulated directly by the hormone EPO and indirectly by several hormones, including thyroxine, androgens, and growth hormone. **EPO**, also called *erythropoiesis-stimulating hormone*, is formed by the kidneys and liver. It appears in the plasma when peripheral tissues, especially the kidneys, are exposed to low oxygen concentrations (**Figure 11-5**). A low oxygen level in tissues is called **hypoxia** (hī-POKS-ē-uh; *hypo-*, below + *oxy-*, presence of oxygen). EPO is released (1) during anemia, (2) when blood flow to the kidneys declines, (3) when the oxygen content

Figure 11-4 The Origins and Differentiation of Red Blood Cells, Platelets, and White Blood Cells.
Hemocytoblast divisions give rise to myeloid stem cells or lymphoid stem cells. Lymphoid stem cells produce the various lymphocytes. Myeloid stem cells produce progenitor cells that divide to produce the other classes of formed elements. The targets of EPO and colony-stimulating factors (CSFs) are also indicated.

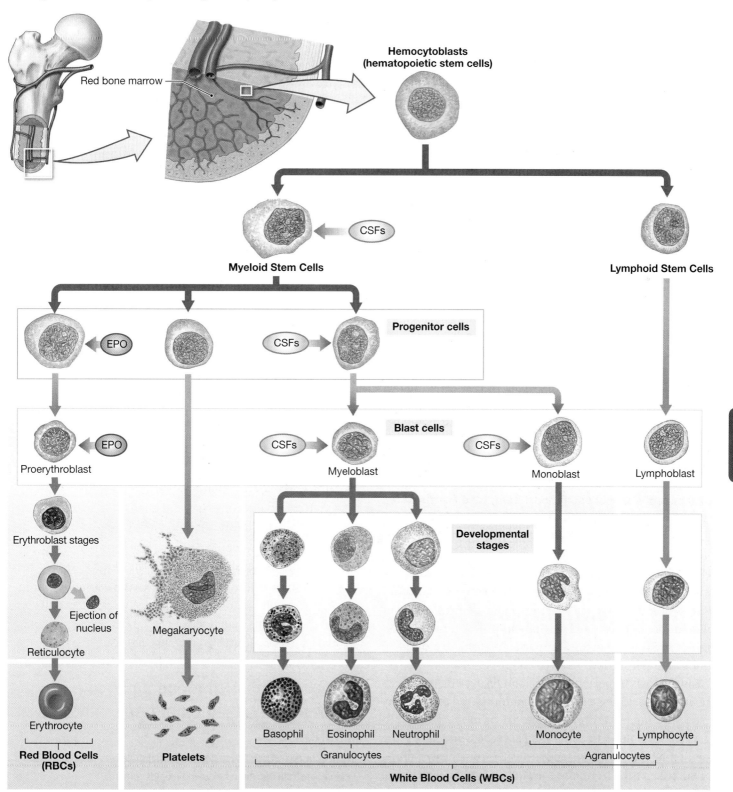

Figure 11-5 The Role of EPO in the Stimulation of Erythropoiesis. Tissues (especially the kidneys) deprived of oxygen release erythropoietin (EPO). EPO accelerates the division of stem cells and the maturation of erythroblasts. More red blood cells then enter the circulation, improving the delivery of oxygen to peripheral tissues.

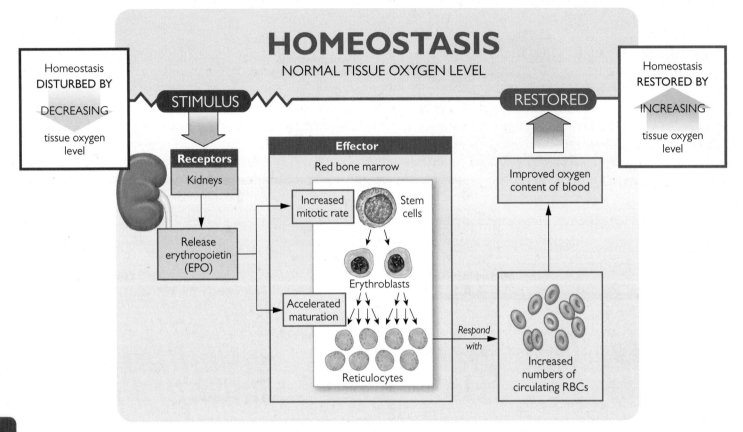

of air in the lungs declines (due to disease or high altitude), and (4) when the respiratory surfaces of the lungs are damaged. Once in the bloodstream, EPO travels to red bone marrow, where it stimulates stem cells and developing RBCs.

EPO has two major effects: (1) It stimulates increased cell division rates in erythroblasts and in the stem cells that produce erythroblasts; and (2) it speeds up the maturation of RBCs, primarily by increasing the rate of hemoglobin synthesis. Under maximum EPO stimulation, red bone marrow can increase the rate of RBC formation tenfold, to around 30 million cells per second.

This ability is important to a person recovering from a severe blood loss. However, if EPO is administered to a healthy person, the hematocrit may rise to 65 or more. The resulting increase in blood viscosity increases the workload on the heart, which can lead to sudden death from heart failure. Similar risks result from *blood doping,* in which athletes reinfuse packed RBCs removed at an earlier date. Their goal is to improve oxygen delivery to muscles, thereby enhancing performance.

CHECKPOINT

6. Describe hemoglobin.

7. How would the hematocrit change after an individual suffered a significant blood loss?

8. In what way would a disease that causes liver damage affect the level of bilirubin in the blood?

9. Keith develops a blockage in his renal arteries that restricts blood flow to his kidneys. What effect will this have on his hematocrit?

See the blue Answers tab at the back of the book.

11-4 The ABO blood types and Rh system are based on antigen–antibody responses

Learning Objective: Discuss the factors that determine a person's blood type, and explain why blood typing is important.

Antigens are substances (most often proteins) that can trigger a protective defense process called an *immune response.* The plasma membranes of all your cells contain surface antigens, substances that your immune defenses recognize as "normal." In other words, your immune system ignores these substances rather than attacking them as "foreign."

The presence or absence of specific surface antigens in RBC membranes determines your **blood type**. Your genetic makeup determines which antigens occur on your RBCs. RBCs have at least 50 kinds of surface antigens, but three are of particular importance: **A, B,** and **Rh** (or **D**).

Based on RBC surface antigens, there are four blood types (**Figure 11-6a**). **Type A** blood has antigen A only, **type B** has antigen B only, **type AB** has both A and B, and **type O** has neither A nor B. Individuals with these blood types are not evenly distributed throughout the world. The average percentages for various populations in the United States are given in **Table 11-1**.

The term **Rh positive** (Rh$^+$) indicates the presence of the Rh antigen on the surface of RBCs. The term **Rh negative** (Rh$^-$) indicates the absence of this antigen. When an individual's complete blood type is recorded, the term *Rh* is usually omitted. The data are reported as O negative (O$^-$), A positive (A$^+$), and so on. In the general U.S. population, blood types are distributed approximately as follows: O$^+$, 38 percent; A$^+$, 34 percent; B$^+$, 9 percent; O$^-$, 7 percent; A$^-$, 6 percent; AB$^+$, 3 percent; B$^-$, 2 percent; and AB$^-$, 1 percent.

Figure 11-6 Blood Types and Cross-Reactions.

Type A	Type B	Type AB	Type O
Type A blood has RBCs with surface antigen A only.	**Type B** blood has RBCs with surface antigen B only.	**Type AB** blood has RBCs with both A and B surface antigens.	**Type O** blood has RBCs lacking both A and B surface antigens.
Surface antigen A	Surface antigen B		
If you have type A blood, your plasma contains anti-B antibodies, which will attack Type B surface antigens.	If you have type B blood, your plasma contains anti-A antibodies, which will attack Type A surface antigens.	If you have type AB blood, your plasma has neither anti-A nor anti-B antibodies.	If you have type O blood, your plasma contains both anti-A and anti-B antibodies.

a Blood type depends on the presence of surface antigens (agglutinogens) on RBC surfaces. The plasma contains antibodies (agglutinins) that will react with foreign surface antigens.

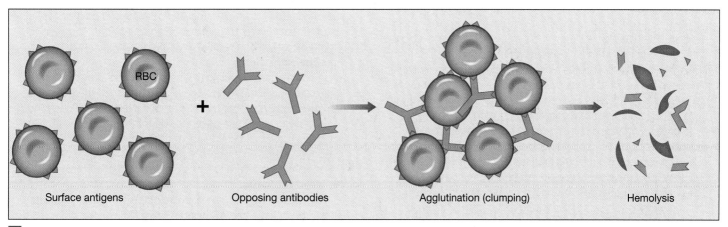

Surface antigens + Opposing antibodies → Agglutination (clumping) → Hemolysis

b In a cross-reaction, antibodies react with their target antigens causing agglutination and hemolysis of the affected RBCs. In this example, anti-B antibodies encounter B surface antigens, which cause the RBCs bearing the B surface antigens to clump together and break up.

Table 11-1	Differences in Blood Group Distribution				
	Percentage with Each Blood Type				
Population	**O**	**A**	**B**	**AB**	**Rh⁺**
U.S. (AVERAGE)	46	40	10	4	85
African American	49	27	20	4	92
Caucasian	45	40	11	4	85
Chinese American	42	27	25	6	100
Filipino American	44	22	29	6	100
Hawaiian	46	46	5	3	100
Hispanic	57	31	10	2	92
Japanese American	31	39	21	10	100
Korean American	32	28	30	10	100
Native North American	79	16	4	<1	100
Native South American	100	0	0	0	100
Australian Aborigine	44	56	0	0	100

As we noted previously, your immune system ignores the surface antigens—also called *agglutinogens* (a-glū-TIN-ō-jenz)—on your own RBCs. However, your plasma contains antibodies, or *agglutinins* (a-GLŪ-ti-ninz), that will attack surface antigens on RBCs of a different blood type (**Figure 11-6a**). That is, the plasma of individuals with type A blood contains circulating anti-B antibodies, which will attack type B surface antigens. The plasma of type B individuals contains anti-A antibodies, which will attack type A surface antigens. Similarly, type AB individuals lack antibodies against either A or B

surface antigens. The plasma of type O individuals has both anti-A and anti-B antibodies.

Based on the presence of these antibodies, the blood types of donor and recipient are identified before blood is transfused. If an individual receives blood of a different blood type, antibodies in the recipient's plasma meet their specific antigen on the donated RBCs, and a **cross-reaction** occurs (**Figure 11-6b**). Initially the binding of antigens and antibodies causes the foreign RBCs to clump together—a process called **agglutination** (a-gloo-ti-NĀ-shun). Then the RBCs may break up, or *hemolyze.* Clumps and fragments of RBCs under attack from antibodies form drifting masses that can plug small vessels in the kidneys, lungs, heart, or brain, damaging or destroying tissues. Such cross-reactions, or *transfusion reactions*, can be avoided by ensuring that the blood types of donor and recipient are **compatible**.

In practice, the surface antigens on the donor's cells are more important in determining compatibility than are the antibodies in the donor's plasma. Unless large volumes of whole blood or plasma are transferred, cross-reactions between the donor's plasma and the recipient's blood cells will fail to produce significant agglutination. Packed RBCs, with a minimal amount of plasma, are commonly transfused. Even when whole blood is transfused, the plasma is diluted through mixing with the recipient's relatively large plasma volume.

CLINICAL NOTE

Emergency Transfusions

Blood is a precious commodity and must be utilized so that it can provide the most benefit for the greatest number of people. A unit of whole blood consists of approximately 450 milliliters of blood with about 65 grams of hemoglobin. In current medical practice, it is uncommon to administer whole blood. Instead, the blood is separated into its various elements, and those elements are administered as needed. Elements derived from whole blood include the red blood cells (RBCs) (*packed RBCs*), *platelets, granulocytes,* and plasma (*fresh frozen plasma*). Patients receive only the blood elements that they need. A patient who has sustained hemorrhage, for instance, will receive packed RBCs and crystalloid fluids, while a patient with a platelet disorder will receive platelet transfusion.

In order to prevent a *hemolytic transfusion reaction*, blood must be tested for compatibility between the donor and the recipient. Blood products are tested for the major antigens (AB and Rh). In addition, they are tested for minor antigen compatibility. The analysis and selection of blood products for transfusion is a time-consuming process called *typing* and *crossmatching.* In a critical emergency, there may not be time to wait for blood typing and crossmatching. In these situations, Type O-negative (O⁻)

blood can be safely administered. Type O⁻ blood does not contain the A, B, or Rh antigen. Thus, it will not induce a hemolytic reaction in a patient with a different blood type. Because of this, persons with Type O⁻ blood are referred to as *universal donors.*

Persons who have type AB blood are referred to as *universal recipients.* They have both the A and B antigens on their RBCs and thus lack circulating antibodies against both A and B. In an emergency, they can receive any type of blood, as they already have the antibodies.

In an emergency setting, if time permits, it is preferred to wait until the blood is fully typed and crossmatched. If there is not adequate time for this, the patient can be given *type-specific blood.* Type-specific blood has been tested for the major (ABO and Rh) antigens. It has not been tested for the minor antigens. Finally, as described above, in critical situations, the patient may be given un-crossmatched Type O⁻ blood until typing and crossmatching have been completed.

Platelets do not contain any minor blood antigens. Platelets should be of the same ABO and Rh type. They are rapidly destroyed by the body and must be frequently administered.

CLINICAL NOTE

Hemolytic Disease of the Newborn

Genes from both parents determine the surface antigens on a person's RBCs. For this reason, a child's blood type can differ from that of either parent. During pregnancy, when fetal and maternal circulatory systems are closely intertwined, the mother's antibodies may cross the placenta, attacking and destroying fetal RBCs. The resulting condition is called hemolytic disease of the newborn (HDN). Some forms are quite dangerous and others so mild as to remain undetected.

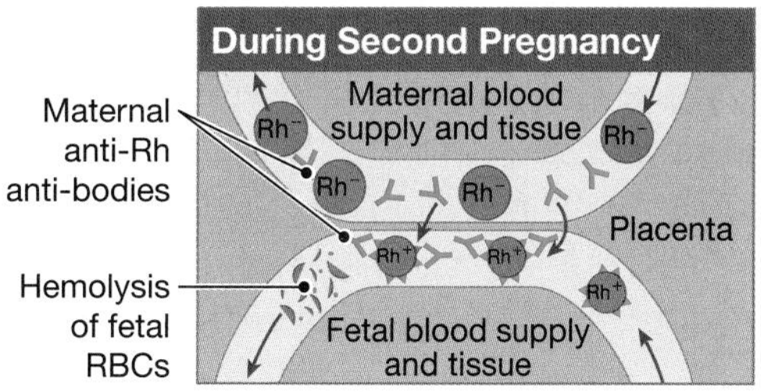

The sensitization that causes HDN usually takes place during delivery. Bleeding at the placenta and uterus exposes an Rh-negative mother to an Rh-positive fetus' Rh antigens. This event can trigger the production of anti-Rh

During Second Pregnancy

Maternal anti-Rh anti-bodies

Maternal blood supply and tissue

Placenta

Hemolysis of fetal RBCs

Fetal blood supply and tissue

antibodies in the mother. The first Rh-positive infant is not affected because these antibodies are not produced in large amounts until after delivery. However, a sensitized Rh-negative mother will produce massive amounts of anti-Rh antibodies in response to a second Rh-positive fetus. These antibodies attack fetal RBCs, producing a dangerous anemia.

Fortunately, it is possible to prevent the mother's anti-Rh antibody production. This is done by administering such antibodies (under the name RhoGAM) to the mother in weeks 26–28 of pregnancy and during and after delivery. These antibodies destroy any fetal RBCs that cross the placenta before they can stimulate a maternal immune response.

Unlike the case for type A and type B individuals, the plasma of an Rh-negative individual does not normally contain anti-Rh antibodies. These antibodies are present only if the individual has been *sensitized* by previous exposure to Rh-positive RBCs. Such exposure can occur accidentally, during a transfusion. It can also occur in a normal pregnancy when an Rh-negative mother carries an Rh-positive fetus.

Testing for Blood Compatibility

Testing for blood compatibility normally involves two steps: (1) a determination of blood type, and (2) a *cross-match test.* The standard test for blood type categorizes a blood sample on the basis of the three RBC surface antigens most likely to produce dangerous cross-reactions (**Figure 11-7**). The test involves mixing drops of blood with solutions containing anti-A, anti-B, and anti-Rh antibodies and noting any cross-reactions.

For example, if the RBCs clump together when exposed to anti-A and anti-B, the individual has type AB blood. If no reactions take place, the person must be type O. The presence or absence of the Rh antigen is also noted, and the individual is classified as Rh-positive or Rh-negative. In the most common type—type O-positive (O^+)—the RBCs lack surface antigens A and B, but they do have the Rh antigen. Standard blood typing of both donor and recipient can be completed in a matter of minutes.

In an emergency (such as a severe gunshot wound), a patient may require 5 liters or more of blood. In such cases, type O blood can be safely administered to a victim of any blood type because type O RBCs lack A and B surface antigens. Type O (especially O^-) individuals are sometimes called *universal*

donors because their blood cells are unlikely to produce severe cross-reactions in a recipient. Type AB individuals were once called *universal recipients* because they lack anti-A or anti-B antibodies, which would attack donated RBCs. This term is no longer used largely because reliable blood supplies and quick compatibility testing typically allow type AB blood to be given to type AB recipients.

Still, cross-reactions can occur, even to type O^- blood, because at least 48 other possible antigens are present. Whenever time and facilities permit, further testing is done

Figure 11-7 Blood Type Testing. Test results for blood samples from four individuals. Drops of blood are mixed with solutions containing antibodies to the surface antigens A, B, and Rh (D). Clumping occurs when the sample contains the corresponding surface antigen(s). The blood types of the individuals are shown on the right.

Anti-A	Anti-B	Anti-Rh	Blood type
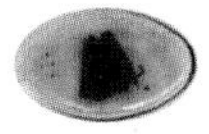	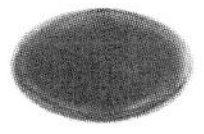	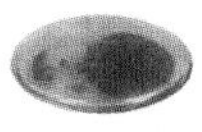	A^+
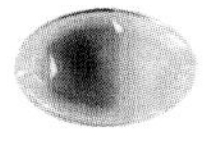	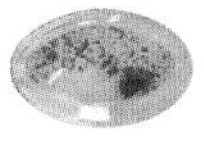	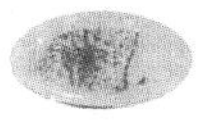	B^+
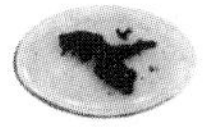	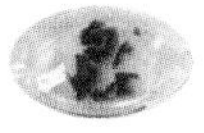	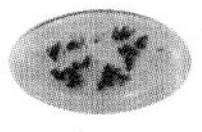	AB^+
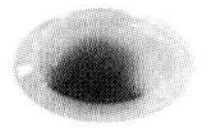	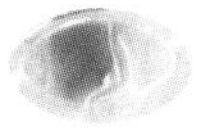	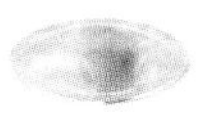	O^-

CLINICAL NOTE

Blood Transfusion Reactions

Human red blood cell membranes contain hundreds of different antigenic structures. Great care is taken to ensure that blood products match the intended recipient before transfusion is undertaken. All blood products are tested to determine the ABO blood type and for the presence of the Rh antigen, as well as for several minor antigens. Blood that has been tested and deemed suitable for transfusion to a patient is said to be crossmatched. This means that the blood product in question has the lowest possible likelihood of causing a transfusion reaction.

Blood transfusion reactions can develop quite rapidly and are sometimes fatal. Transfusion reactions are usually classified as immune or nonimmune. Immune reactions are antibody-mediated reactions directed against a blood component. Nonimmune reactions include such complications as circulatory overload or transmission of an infectious agent.

A common type of blood transfusion reaction is the hemolytic reaction, in which red blood cell antibodies lyse (rupture) red cells within the circulatory system. This allows the contents of the cell to spill into the circulatory system. Hemoglobin can collect in the urine and adversely affect renal function. Patients with hemolytic reactions often complain of flushing, pain at the infusion site, chest or back pain, restlessness, anxiety, nausea, or diarrhea. Fever and chills are common findings. Shock and renal failure also can occur. Treatment of a hemolytic transfusion reaction should begin with termination and removal of the product being transfused, which should be returned to the laboratory to determine the cause of the reaction. Fluids should be administered to maintain adequate renal output. On occasion, it may be necessary to administer a diuretic such as furosemide (Lasix) or an osmotic diuretic such as mannitol (Osmotrol) in order to maintain renal function and prevent fluid overload. Intravenous antihistamines and corticosteroids are sometimes required. Analgesics and anti-inflammatory agents may be required for the treatment of pain as well as fever and chills.

Nonimmune transfusion reactions are managed by treating the underlying problem. Circulatory overload is treated with fluid restriction and diuretics as needed. Infections are treated based on the type of infection present.

to ensure complete compatibility. **Cross-match testing** involves exposing the donor's RBCs to a sample of the recipient's plasma under controlled conditions. Another way to avoid compatibility problems is to replace lost blood with synthetic blood substitutes, which do not contain surface antigens that can trigger a cross-reaction.

Because blood groups are inherited, blood tests are also used as paternity tests and in crime detection. Results from such tests can only prove that a particular person is *not* a certain child's father or is *not* guilty of a specific crime. It is impossible, for example, for an adult with type AB blood to be the parent of an infant with type O blood.

CHECKPOINT

10. Which blood type(s) can be safely transfused into a person with type AB blood?

11. Why can't a person with type A blood safely receive blood from a person with type B blood?

See the blue Answers tab at the back of the book.

11-5 The various types of white blood cells contribute to the body's defenses

Learning Objective: Categorize the various white blood cells on the basis of their structures and functions, and discuss the factors that regulate their production.

WBCs, also known as **leukocytes**, can be distinguished from RBCs by their larger size and the presence of a nucleus and other organelles. WBCs also lack hemoglobin. They help defend the body against invasion by pathogens. WBCs also remove toxins, wastes, and abnormal or damaged cells.

Traditionally, WBCs have been divided into two groups based on their appearance after staining: (1) *granulocytes* (with abundant stained "granules") and (2) *agranulocytes* (with few, if any, stained granules). This scheme is convenient but somewhat misleading. In reality, the granules in granulocytes are secretory vesicles and lysosomes. The agranulocytes also contain vesicles and lysosomes, but they are quite small and difficult to see with a light microscope.

Typical WBCs in the circulating blood are shown in **Figure 11-8**. *Neutrophils, eosinophils,* and *basophils* are granulocytes. *Monocytes* and *lymphocytes* are agranulocytes.

A typical microliter of blood contains 5000–10,000 WBCs, compared with 4.2 to 6.3 million RBCs. Most of the WBCs in the body are located in connective tissue proper or in organs of the lymphatic system. Circulating WBCs are only a small fraction of the total WBC population.

WBC Circulation and Movement

Unlike RBCs, WBCs circulate for only a short portion of their life span. WBCs migrate through the loose and dense connective tissues of the body. They use the bloodstream to travel from one organ to another and for rapid transportation to areas of invasion or injury. WBCs can detect the chemical signs of damage to surrounding tissues. When

Figure 11-8 White Blood Cells.

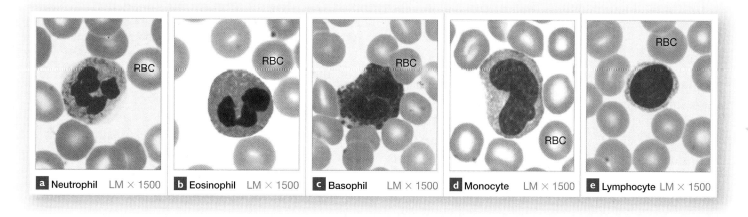

| **a** Neutrophil LM × 1500 | **b** Eosinophil LM × 1500 | **c** Basophil LM × 1500 | **d** Monocyte LM × 1500 | **e** Lymphocyte LM × 1500 |

problems are detected, they leave the bloodstream and enter the damaged area.

Circulating WBCs have four characteristics:

1. *All are capable of amoeboid movement. Amoeboid movement* is a gliding motion due to the flow of cytoplasm into slender cellular processes extended in the direction of movement. This mobility allows WBCs to move along the walls of blood vessels and through surrounding tissues.

2. *All can migrate out of the bloodstream.* WBCs can enter surrounding tissue by squeezing between adjacent epithelial cells in the capillary wall. This process is called **diapedesis** (dī-a-pe-DĒ-sis).

3. *All are attracted to specific chemical stimuli.* This characteristic, called **positive chemotaxis** (kē-mō-TAK-sis), guides WBCs to invading pathogens, damaged tissues, and other active WBCs.

4. *Neutrophils, eosinophils, and monocytes are capable of phagocytosis.* These cells can engulf pathogens, cell debris, or other materials. Neutrophils and eosinophils are sometimes called *microphages* to distinguish them from the larger macrophages in connective tissues. Macrophages are monocytes that have moved out of the bloodstream and become actively phagocytic. ⤴ p. 68

Types of WBCs

Neutrophils, eosinophils, basophils, and monocytes are part of the body's *nonspecific defenses.* A variety of stimuli activate such defenses, which do not discriminate between one type of threat and another.

Lymphocytes, in contrast, are responsible for *specific defenses*, which mount a counterattack against specific types of

Build Your Knowledge

Recall that one function of connective tissue is defense of the body (as you saw in **Chapter 4: The Tissue Level of Organization**). Connective tissue proper contains fixed (resident) and free (migrating) macrophages, or "big eater," phagocytic cells. In addition to the free macrophages, other phagocytic and antibody-producing white blood cells move through connective tissue proper. Their numbers increase if the tissue is damaged, as does the production of antibodies. Antibodies are proteins that destroy invading microorganisms or foreign substances. ⤴ **pp. 102–103**

invading pathogens or foreign proteins. We discuss specific and nonspecific defenses in Chapter 14.

Neutrophils

About 50–70 percent of the circulating WBCs are **neutrophils** (NOO-trō-filz). This name reflects the fact that their granules are chemically neutral and thus are difficult to stain with either acidic or basic dyes. A mature neutrophil has a very dense, contorted nucleus with two to five lobes resembling beads on a string (**Figure 11-8a**).

Neutrophils are usually the first WBCs to arrive at an injury site. They are very active phagocytes, specializing in attacking and digesting bacteria. Most neutrophils have a short life span. They survive in the bloodstream for only about 10 hours. When actively engulfing debris or pathogens, they may last 30 minutes or less. A neutrophil dies after engulfing one to two dozen bacteria, but its breakdown releases chemicals that attract other neutrophils to the site. A mixture of dead neutrophils, cellular debris, and other waste products forms the *pus* of infected wounds.

Eosinophils

Eosinophils (ē-ō-SIN-ō-filz) have granules that stain darkly with eosin, a red dye. They usually represent 2–4 percent of circulating WBCs. They are similar in size to neutrophils. Their deep red granules and a two-lobed nucleus make them easy to identify (**Figure 11-8b**). Eosinophils attack objects that are coated with antibodies. They will engulf antibody-marked bacteria, protozoa, or cellular debris, but their primary mode of attack is the exocytosis of toxic compounds. These compounds include nitric oxide and cytotoxic enzymes. These cells increase dramatically in number during a parasitic infection or an allergic reaction. Eosinophils are also attracted to sites of injury, where they release enzymes that reduce inflammation produced by mast cells and neutrophils. In this way, they help to control the spread of inflammation to nearby tissues.

Basophils

Basophils (BĀ-sō-filz) have numerous granules that stain darkly with basic dyes. In a standard blood smear, the granules are a deep purple or blue (**Figure 11-8c**). These cells are somewhat smaller than neutrophils or eosinophils and are relatively rare. They account for less than 1 percent of the circulating WBC population. Basophils migrate to sites of injury and cross the capillary wall into damaged tissues, where they discharge their granules into the interstitial fluids. The granules contain the chemicals *heparin*, which prevents blood clotting, and *histamine*, which dilates blood vessels. These chemicals enhance the local inflammation initiated by mast cells. ⟳ p. 114 Other chemicals released by stimulated basophils attract eosinophils and other basophils to the area.

Monocytes

Monocytes (MON-ō-sīts) are nearly twice the size of a typical erythrocyte. The nucleus is large and commonly oval or shaped like a kidney bean (**Figure 11-8d**). Monocytes normally account for 2–8 percent of circulating WBCs. They remain in circulation for only about 24 hours before entering peripheral tissues to become tissue macrophages. These migrating monocytes are called *free macrophages* to distinguish them from the immobile *fixed macrophages* in many connective tissues. ⟳ p. 103 They are aggressive phagocytes, often attempting to engulf items as large as or larger than themselves. Active monocytes release chemicals that attract and stimulate neutrophils, additional monocytes, and other phagocytes, and also draw fibroblasts to the region. The fibroblasts then begin to produce scar tissue, which walls off the injured area.

Lymphocytes

Typical **lymphocytes** (LIM-fō-sīts) are slightly larger than RBCs and contain a relatively large nucleus surrounded by a thin halo of cytoplasm (**Figure 11-8e**). Lymphocytes account for 20–40 percent of the WBC population in blood. Lymphocytes migrate continuously from the bloodstream, through peripheral tissues, and back to the bloodstream. Circulating lymphocytes represent a very small fraction of the entire WBC population. At any moment, most lymphocytes are in connective tissues and in organs of the lymphatic system. They protect the body and its tissues, but they do not rely on phagocytosis. Some kinds of lymphocytes directly attack foreign cells and abnormal body cells. Others secrete antibodies into the circulation. The antibodies can attack foreign cells or proteins in distant parts of the body.

The Differential Count and Changes in WBC Abundance

A variety of disorders, including infections, inflammation, and allergic reactions, cause characteristic changes in the circulating populations of WBCs. By examining a stained blood smear, we can obtain a **differential count** of the WBC population. The values reported indicate the number of each type of cell in a sample of 100 WBCs.

The normal range of abundance for each WBC type is shown in **Table 11-2**. The term **leukopenia** (loo-kō-PĒ-nē-uh; *penia,* poverty) indicates reduced numbers of WBCs. **Leukocytosis** (loo-kō-sī-TŌ-sis) refers to excessive numbers of WBCs. A modest leukocytosis is normal during an infection. Extreme leukocytosis (WBC counts of 100,000/μL or more) generally indicates some form of **leukemia** (loo-KĒ-mē-uh), a cancer of blood-forming tissues. Only some of the many types of leukemia are characterized by leukocytosis. Other indications are the presence of abnormal or immature WBCs.

WBC Formation

Stem cells that produce WBCs originate in the red bone marrow, from the division of hemocytoblasts. Hemocytoblasts produce (1) lymphoid stem cells, which give rise to lymphocytes;

Table 11-2	Formed Elements of the Blood			
	Cell	**Abundance (average number per µL)**	**Functions**	**Remarks**
	RED BLOOD CELLS	5.2 million (range: 4.4–6.3 million)	Transport oxygen from lungs to tissues, and carbon dioxide from tissues to lungs	Remain in bloodstream; 120-day life expectancy; amino acids and iron recycled; produced in red bone marrow
	WHITE BLOOD CELLS	7000 (range: 5000–10,000)		
	Neutrophils	4150 (range: 1800–7300) Differential count: 50–70 percent	Phagocytic: Engulf pathogens or debris in tissues, release cytotoxic enzymes and chemicals	Move into tissues after several hours; survive minutes to days, depending on tissue activity; produced in red bone marrow
	Eosinophils	165 (range: 0–700) Differential count: 2–4 percent	Phagocytic: Engulf antibody-labeled materials, release cytotoxic enzymes, reduce inflammation; increase during allergic and parasitic situations	Move into tissues after several hours; survive minutes to days, depending on tissue activity; produced in red bone marrow
	Basophils	44 (range: 0–150) Differential count: <1 percent	Enter damaged tissues and release histamine and other chemicals that promote inflammation	Survival time unknown; assist mast cells of tissues in producing inflammation; produced in red bone marrow
	Monocytes	456 (range: 200–950) Differential count: 2–8 percent	Enter tissues to become macrophages; engulf pathogens or debris	Move into tissues after 1–2 days; survive months or longer; primarily produced in red bone marrow
	Lymphocytes	2185 (range: 1500–4000) Differential count: 20–40 percent	Cells of lymphatic system, providing defense against specific pathogens or toxins	Survive months to decades; circulate from blood to tissues and back; produced in red bone marrow and lymphatic tissues
	PLATELETS	350,000 (range: 150,000–500,000)	Hemostasis: Clump together and stick to vessel wall (platelet phase); activate intrinsic pathway of coagulation phase	Remain in bloodstream or in vascular organs (such as the spleen); remain intact for 7–12 days; produced by megakaryocytes in red bone marrow

and (2) myeloid stem cells, which give rise to all the other types of formed elements (**Figure 11-4**, p. 439). Granulocytes (basophils, eosinophils, and neutrophils) complete their development in myeloid (red bone marrow) tissue. Monocytes begin their differentiation in red bone marrow, enter the bloodstream, and complete development when they become free macrophages in peripheral tissues. Each of these cell types goes through a characteristic series of developmental stages.

The process of lymphocyte production is called **lymphopoiesis**. Many of the lymphoid stem cells responsible for the production of lymphocytes migrate from the red bone marrow to peripheral **lymphatic tissues**, including the thymus, spleen, and lymph nodes. As a result, lymphocytes are produced in these organs as well as in the red bone marrow.

Various hormones are involved in the regulation of WBC populations. Hormones called *colony-stimulating factors (CSFs)* regulate WBCs other than lymphocytes. Four CSFs have been identified. Each targets single stem cell lines or groups of stem

cell lines (**Figure 11-4**, p. 439). Before a person reaches maturity, hormones from the thymus gland (thymosins) promote the differentiation of one type of lymphocyte, the *T cells*. In adults, the production of lymphocytes is regulated by exposure to antigens such as foreign proteins, cells, and toxins. When antigens appear, lymphocyte production escalates. (We describe the control processes in Chapter 14.)

CHECKPOINT

12. Identify the five types of white blood cells.

13. Which type of white blood cell would you find in the greatest numbers in an infected cut?

14. Which type of cell would you find in elevated numbers in a person producing large amounts of circulating antibodies to combat a virus?

15. How do basophils respond to an injury?

See the blue Answers tab at the back of the book.

11

11-6 Platelets, disc-shaped structures formed from megakaryocytes, function in the clotting process

Learning Objective: Describe the structure, function, and production of platelets.

Platelets (PLĀT-lets) are among the formed elements. In nonmammalian vertebrates, platelets are nucleated cells called **thrombocytes** (THROM-bō-sīts; *thrombos*, clot). In humans, these formed elements are cell fragments rather than individual cells. For this reason, the term *platelet* is preferred when referring to our blood.

Red bone marrow contains enormous cells with large nuclei called **megakaryocytes** (meg-a-KAR-ē-ō-sīts; *megas*, big + *karyon*, nucleus + *-cyte*, cell) (**Figure 11-4**). Megakaryocytes continuously shed cytoplasm in small membrane-enclosed packets. These packets are the platelets that enter the bloodstream. Platelets initiate the clotting process and help close injured blood vessels. They play a major part in a vascular *clotting system*, detailed in the next section.

Platelets are continuously replaced. Each platelet circulates for 9–12 days before being removed by phagocytes. Each microliter of circulating blood contains 150,000–500,000 platelets. The average concentration is 350,000/μL. About one-third of the platelets in the body are in the spleen and other blood-rich organs, rather than in the bloodstream. These reserves are mobilized during severe bleeding.

An abnormally low platelet count (80,000/μL or less) is known as *thrombocytopenia* (throm-bō-sī-tō-PĒ-nē-uh). This condition usually results from excessive platelet destruction or inadequate platelet production. Clinical signs include bleeding along the digestive tract, within the skin, and occasionally inside the CNS. In *thrombocytosis* (throm-bō-sī-TŌ-sis), platelet counts can exceed 1,000,000/μL. Thrombocytosis usually results from accelerated platelet formation in response to infection, inflammation, or cancer.

CHECKPOINT

16. Explain the difference between platelets and thrombocytes.

17. List the primary functions of platelets.

See the blue Answers tab at the back of the book.

11-7 Hemostasis involves vascular spasm, platelet plug formation, and blood coagulation

Learning Objective: Describe the processes that control blood loss after an injury.

Hemostasis (*haima*, blood + *stasis*, halt), the stopping of bleeding, halts the loss of blood through the walls of damaged vessels. At the same time, it establishes a framework for tissue repairs.

Phases of Hemostasis

Hemostasis has three overlapping phases: the *vascular phase*, the *platelet phase*, and the *coagulation phase*. In reality, hemostasis is a complex cascade, or chain reaction. Many things happen at once, and all of them interact to some degree.

1. **The Vascular Phase.** The walls of blood vessels contain smooth muscle and an inner lining of simple squamous epithelium known as an **endothelium** (en-dō-THĒ-lē-um). Breaking open the wall of a blood vessel, such as by cutting, triggers a contraction in the smooth muscle fibers in the vessel wall that decreases the vessel's diameter (**Figure 11-9 ❶**). This local contraction, called a *vascular spasm*, can slow or even stop the loss of blood through the wall of a small vessel. The vascular spasm lasts about 30 minutes, a period called the **vascular phase** of hemostasis. The membranes of endothelial cells at the injury site also become "sticky." A tear in a small artery or vein may be partially sealed off by the attachment of endothelial cells on either side of the break. In small capillaries, the cells may stick together and block the opening completely.

2. **The Platelet Phase.** The platelets begin to attach to the sticky endothelial surfaces and exposed collagen fibers within 15 seconds of the injury (**Figure 11-9 ❷**). These attachments mark the start of the **platelet phase** of hemostasis. Platelets also stick to one another and form a mass called a *platelet plug*. The plug may close the break in the vessel wall, if the damage is not severe or occurs in a small blood vessel.

3. **The Coagulation Phase.** The **coagulation phase** does not start until 30 seconds or more after the vessel has been damaged (**Figure 11-9 ❸**). **Coagulation**, or *blood clotting*, involves a complex sequence of steps leading to the conversion of circulating fibrinogen into the insoluble protein fibrin. As the fibrin network grows, blood cells and additional platelets are trapped

Figure 11-9 The Vascular, Platelet, and Coagulation Phases of Hemostasis.

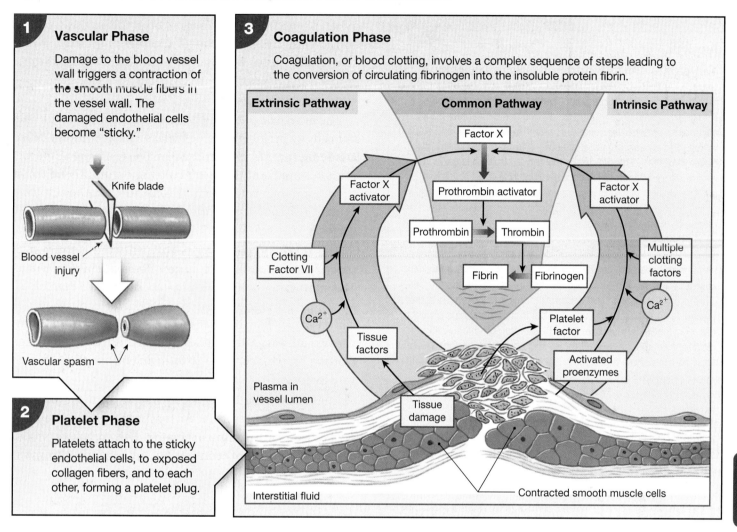

1 Vascular Phase

Damage to the blood vessel wall triggers a contraction of the smooth muscle fibers in the vessel wall. The damaged endothelial cells become "sticky."

Knife blade

Blood vessel injury

Vascular spasm

2 Platelet Phase

Platelets attach to the sticky endothelial cells, to exposed collagen fibers, and to each other, forming a platelet plug.

3 Coagulation Phase

Coagulation, or blood clotting, involves a complex sequence of steps leading to the conversion of circulating fibrinogen into the insoluble protein fibrin.

Extrinsic Pathway | Common Pathway | Intrinsic Pathway

Factor X

Factor X activator

Prothrombin activator

Factor X activator

Clotting Factor VII

Prothrombin — Thrombin

Multiple clotting factors

Ca^{2+}

Fibrin — Fibrinogen

Tissue factors

Platelet factor

Ca^{2+}

Plasma in vessel lumen

Activated proenzymes

Tissue damage

Interstitial fluid

Contracted smooth muscle cells

within the fibrous tangle, forming a **blood clot** that effectively seals off the damaged portion of the vessel (**Figure 11-10**).

Figure 11-10 The Structure of a Blood Clot.

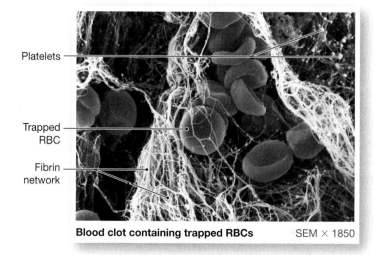

Platelets

Trapped RBC

Fibrin network

Blood clot containing trapped RBCs   SEM × 1850

The Clotting Process

Normal blood clotting cannot occur unless the plasma contains the necessary **clotting factors**, which include calcium ions and 11 different plasma proteins. Many of these proteins are *proenzymes* (inactive enzymes). When converted to active enzymes, they direct essential reactions in the clotting response. The liver synthesizes most of the circulating clotting proteins.

During the coagulation phase, the clotting proteins interact in sequence. One protein is converted into an enzyme that activates a second protein and so on, in a chain reaction, or *cascade*. A blood clot forms as a result of the cascades of the *extrinsic, intrinsic,* and *common pathways* (**Figure 11-9 3**). The extrinsic pathway begins outside the bloodstream, in the vessel wall. The intrinsic pathway begins in the bloodstream. These two pathways join at the common pathway through the activation of Factor X, a clotting protein produced by the liver.

11

CLINICAL NOTE

Aspirin

Acetylsalicylic acid, more commonly called *aspirin*, was introduced in 1899. Now, over a century later, it remains an important drug—not only in medicine, but in emergency medicine. Aspirin has been widely used as an analgesic for minor aches and pains, as an antipyretic, and anti-inflammatory agent. Aspirin inhibits the aggregation of platelets—often a precursor to the development of a blood clot or thrombus. Thus, it is used in long-term low doses to prevent heart attacks.

Low-dose, long-term aspirin irreversibly blocks the formation of thromboxane A_2 in platelets, producing an inhibitory effect on platelet aggregation. This blood-thinning property makes aspirin useful for reducing the incidence of heart attacks and strokes. The American Heart Association recommends aspirin use for patients who have signs and symptoms of a myocardial infarction, unstable angina, ischemic stroke, or transient ischemic attacks, if not contraindicated. This recommendation is based on sound evidence from clinical trials that show that aspirin helps prevent the recurrence of such events as heart attack, hospitalization for recurrent angina, second strokes, and so on (secondary prevention). Studies show that aspirin also helps prevent these events from occurring in people at high risk (primary prevention),

The prehospital administration of aspirin can save lives. However, several studies report that it remains underused in the prehospital setting. Paramedics should remember to consider aspirin for patients with chest pain and those with symptoms of stroke or transient ischemic attack.

The Extrinsic, Intrinsic, and Common Pathways

When a blood vessel is damaged, both the extrinsic and intrinsic pathways are activated. Clotting is initiated by the shorter and faster extrinsic pathway. The slower, intrinsic pathway reinforces the initial clot, making it larger and more effective.

The **extrinsic pathway** begins when damaged endothelial cells or peripheral tissues release a glycoprotein called **tissue factor**. The greater the damage, the more tissue factor is released and the faster clotting occurs. Tissue factor then combines with calcium ions and another clotting protein (Factor VII) to form an enzyme that can activate Factor X.

The **intrinsic pathway** begins with the activation of proenzymes exposed to collagen fibers at the injury site. This pathway proceeds with the assistance of a *platelet factor* released by aggregating platelets. Platelets also release a variety of other factors that speed up the reactions of the intrinsic pathway. After a series of linked reactions, activated clotting proteins combine to form an enzyme that can activate Factor X.

The **common pathway** begins when enzymes from either pathway activate Factor X. Factor X then activates a complex called **prothrombin activator**. This complex converts the proenzyme **prothrombin** to the enzyme **thrombin**

CLINICAL NOTE

Abnormal Hemostasis

Hemostasis involves a complex chain of events, and any disorder that affects any individual clotting factor can disrupt the entire process. As a result, managing many clinical conditions involves controlling or manipulating the clotting process.

Excessive Coagulation

If the clotting process is not well controlled, clots will form in the circulation rather than at an injury site. These blood clots drift downstream until plasmin digests them or they become lodged in a small blood vessel. A drifting blood clot is a type of embolus (EM-bo-lus; *embolos*, plug; *emboli* plural), an abnormal mass within the bloodstream. (Other common emboli are drifting air bubbles and fat globules.) When an embolus lodges in a blood vessel, it blocks circulation to the area downstream, killing the affected tissues. The resulting condition is called embolism.

An embolus in the arterial system can lodge in the capillaries in the brain, causing a tissue-damaging event known as a *stroke*. An embolus in the venous system is likely to lodge in the capillaries in the lung. There it causes a *pulmonary embolism*.

A thrombus is a blood clot attached to the inner surface of a vessel wall. It begins to form when platelets stick to the wall of an intact blood vessel. Often the platelets are attracted to roughened areas called *plaques*, where endothelial and smooth muscle cells contain large quantities of lipids. The blood clot gradually enlarges, projecting into the vessel's channel (or *lumen*) and reducing its diameter. Eventually the vessel may be completely blocked, or a large chunk of the clot may break off, creating an equally dangerous embolus.

Prevention of these conditions generally includes exercises to increase blood flow and reduce pooling of blood, and pharmacologic or natural "blood thinners."

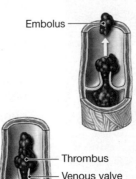

Embolus —

— Thrombus
— Venous valve

Inadequate Coagulation

Hemophilia (hē-mō-FĒL-ē-uh) is an inherited disorder characterized by the inadequate production of clotting factors. About one person in 10,000 has hemophilia. Males account for 80–90 percent of those affected. In hemophilia, production of a single clotting factor (most often Factor VIII in the intrinsic clotting pathway) is inadequate. The severity of the condition depends on the degree of underproduction. In severe cases, extensive bleeding accompanies the slightest mechanical stresses and occurs spontaneously at joints and around muscles.

Transfusions of clotting factors can reduce or control the effects of hemophilia. To obtain adequate amounts of clotting factors, however, plasma samples from many individuals must

be pooled (combined). This procedure makes treatment very expensive. It also increases the risk of blood-borne infections such as hepatitis or AIDS. Gene-splicing techniques have been used to manufacture Factor VIII. As methods are developed to synthesize other clotting factors, treatment of the various forms of hemophilia will become safer and cheaper.

(THROM-bin). Thrombin then completes the clotting process by converting fibrinogen to fibrin.

The thrombin formed in the common pathway also acts to increase the rate of clot formation. Thrombin stimulates the formation of tissue factor and the release of platelet factor by platelets. The presence of these factors further stimulates both the extrinsic and intrinsic pathways. This positive feedback loop accelerates the clotting process, and speed can be very important in reducing blood loss after a severe injury. ↪ p. 12

Calcium ions and a single vitamin, **vitamin K**, affect almost every aspect of the clotting process. All three pathways (intrinsic, extrinsic, and common) require the presence of calcium ions, so any disorder that lowers plasma Ca^{2+} concentrations will also impair blood clotting. Adequate amounts of vitamin K must be present for the liver to synthesize four

of the clotting factors (including prothrombin). For this reason, a vitamin K deficiency leads to the breakdown of the common pathway, and inactivates the clotting system. We obtain roughly half of our daily requirement of vitamin K from the diet. Bacteria in the large intestine manufacture the other half.

Clot Retraction and Removal

Once the fibrin network has appeared, platelets and RBCs stick to the fibrin strands. During **clot retraction**, the platelets then contract, pulling the torn edges of the vessel closer together. This process also reduces the size of the damaged area, making it easier for fibroblasts, smooth muscle cells, and endothelial cells in the area to complete repairs.

CLINICAL NOTE

Blood Banking and Transfusion

Each year in the U.S. approximately 13.9 million units of whole blood are donated and are transfused into approximately 4.5 million patients (**Figure 11-11**). Typically, each donated unit of blood, referred to as *whole blood*, is separated, or *fractionated*, into multiple components, and each component is generally transfused into different individuals according to their specific needs. The components of whole blood include red blood cells (RBCs), plasma, platelets, white blood cells (WBCs), and plasma derivatives.

Red Blood Cells

RBCs are the most recognizable component of whole blood. The RBCs, also called *erythrocytes*, contain hemoglobin, which transports oxygen. With an average life of approximately 120 days, RBCs are continuously being produced and broken down by the body and are ultimately removed by the spleen. RBC transfusions, often called *packed cells*, are used in the treatment of acute blood loss and anemia.

Plasma

The plasma is the liquid portion of the blood in which the red cells, white cells, and platelets are suspended. It is a protein-salt solution that is 90 percent water. Plasma contains *albumin*, which is the principle protein in the blood. In addition, it contains *fibrinogen* and other proteins that are part of the clotting system, and

globulins, which include the antibodies that aid in fighting infection. Plasma is administered to patients with bleeding disorders.

Figure 11-11 Modern Blood Banking. Modern blood banking techniques have made transfusion a safe procedure. Liquid blood can remain in storage for up to 42 days before it must be discarded.

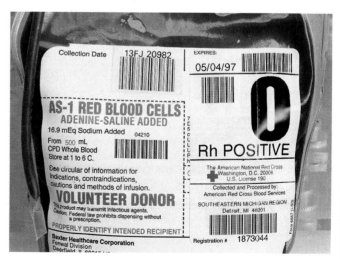

(Continued)

Cryoprecipitated AHF (cryoprecipitate) is the part of the plasma that contains certain clotting factors, including Factor VIII, fibrinogen, von Willebrand factor, and Factor XIII. Cryoprecipitated AHF is removed from plasma by freezing and then slowly thawing the plasma. Used only when specific factor concentrates are unavailable, it helps to control bleeding in individuals with hemophilia and von Willebrand's disease.

Platelets

Platelets, also called *thrombocytes*, are small blood components that aid in the clotting process by adhering to the lining of blood vessels. Platelets are manufactured in the bone marrow and remain viable in the circulation for an average of 9–10 days before being removed by the spleen. Units of platelets for transfusion are prepared by using a centrifuge to separate the platelets from plasma. Platelets can also be obtained through *apheresis*, a procedure in which blood is drawn from a patient, the platelets are removed, and the other blood components are returned to the patient. Platelets are used to treat thrombocytopenia or conditions that involve an abnormality in platelet function.

White Blood Cells

WBCs, also called *leukocytes*, are responsible for protecting the body from invasion by foreign substances such as bacteria, viruses, fungi, and parasites. The majority of WBCs are produced in the bone marrow. There are several types of WBCs, which have been previously detailed in the text. WBCs must be used within 24 hours after collection. They are most frequently used for infections that are unresponsive to antibiotic therapy. However, the effectiveness of WBC transfusions is still not clear.

Plasma Derivatives

Plasma derivatives are concentrates of specific plasma proteins prepared from pools of many donors through a process known as *fractionation.* They are usually heat-treated or washed with a solvent-detergent that kills certain viruses including HIV and hepatitis B and C. Plasma derivatives include:

- Factor VIII concentrate
- Factor IX concentrate
- Anti-inhibitor coagulation complex
- Albumin
- Immune globulins (including Rh immune globulin)
- Antithrombin III concentrate
- Alpha 1-proteinase inhibitor complex

Blood transfusions may be either allogenic or autologous. In *allogenic* blood transfusions, blood is transfused to someone other than the donor. In *autologous* transfusions, the blood donor and transfusion recipient are the same individual. The most common autologous donation is the preoperative donation of blood for transfusion back to the donor during elective surgery. Blood can be stored in its liquid form for up to 42 days. Preoperative autologous donation is not allowed within 72 hours of surgery due to the time necessary to recover from donation.

11

CLINICAL NOTE

Heparin and Fibrinolytic Therapy

The localized formation of a blood clot (thrombosis) is a normal part of the body's repair and healing response. A physiological thrombus serves to limit hemorrhage that results from microscopic or macroscopic vascular injury. Physiological thrombus is counterbalanced by physiological anticoagulation and physiological fibrinolysis. In the normal setting, a physiological thrombus is confined to the immediate area of injury and does not obstruct blood flow to critical areas. Certain pathological conditions can lead to thrombus formation. In addition, under pathological conditions, a thrombus can expand into otherwise normal blood vessels, and obstruct blood flow to critical tissues. An abnormal thrombus can occur anywhere in the body but is particularly problematic when it causes acute coronary syndrome, deep vein thrombosis, pulmonary embolism, acute nonhemorrhagic stroke, or blockage of peripheral arteries.

A thrombus in a coronary artery interrupts blood supply to a portion of the myocardium, which results in acute coronary syndrome. Likewise, the formation of a thrombus within the vessels of the brain can cause a stroke. The time from blockage of the vessel until irreversible tissue injury occurs is short. In the setting of acute myocardial infarction, treatment must be provided in six hours or less in order to be most effective. When fibrinolytics are administered to treat non-hemorrhagic strokes, they generally must be administered within three hours.

Therapy for abnormal thrombosis uses drugs that can be divided into three categories. The first is fibrinolytic agents that break down the offending thrombus (*thrombolysis*). Another is anticoagulants, which are agents that help prevent thrombus formation. Finally, antiplatelet drugs, which inhibit platelet aggregation, are helpful in preventing clot formation. All three categories play essential roles in emergency medicine.

- *Fibrinolytic therapy.* Fibrinolytic agents are able to dissolve preformed arterial and venous thrombi and restore blood flow to the affected tissues. They are derived from bacteria (streptokinase) or from recombinant DNA technology (tissue plasminogen activator, tPA). The effects of fibrinolytic therapy impact the entire body. Because of this, complications, most notably bleeding, can occur. Patients must be carefully screened before receiving fibrinolytic therapy to ensure that the possible benefits exceed the risks.

- *Anticoagulation therapy.* Anticoagulants are drugs that inhibit clot formation. They do not affect a clot that has already formed. These drugs are administered to patients at increased risk of clot formation or following removal of a clot. Heparin and warfarin (Coumadin) are the most frequently used. Heparin must be administered by injection, while warfarin must be administered orally. Recently, newer forms of heparin have been created that are much easier to administer and do not require frequent blood testing. These agents, called *low-molecular-weight heparins (LMWHs)*, include enoxaparin (Fragmin), dalteparin (Lovenox), and ardeparin (Fraxiparine). These drugs can be administered once or twice daily, and allow selected patients to be treated in the outpatient setting.

• *Antiplatelet therapy.* In addition to anticoagulants and fibrinolytics, several other agents are beneficial in preventing thrombosis. Aspirin, which is a mainstay of medical therapy, inhibits platelet function and aggregation; it is inexpensive and highly effective. A new class of antiplatelet agents is the adenosine diphosphate (ADP) inhibitors. These agents are potent inhibitors of platelet aggregation through a mechanism that differs from aspirin. Drugs in this class include: abciximab (Reopro), eptifibatide (Integrilin), and tirofibin (Aggrastat).

These agents are being used with increasing frequency in the treatment of acute coronary syndrome.

Other thrombotic disorders, including deep venous thrombosis, pulmonary embolism, and peripheral arterial occlusion, benefit from these new therapies. With the development of safer and easier-to-administer medications, the use of fibrinolytics and anticoagulants in prehospital care is increasing.

As the repairs proceed, the clot gradually dissolves in a process called **fibrinolysis** (fī-bri-NOL-i-sis). The process begins when two enzymes activate the proenzyme **plasminogen** (plaz-MIN-ō-jen). These enzymes are thrombin, produced by the common pathway, and **tissue plasminogen activator**, or **t-PA**, released by damaged tissues at the site of the injury. The activation of plasminogen produces the enzyme **plasmin** (PLAZ-min), which begins digesting the fibrin strands and breaking down the clot.

CHECKPOINT

18. A sample of red bone marrow has fewer than normal numbers of megakaryocytes. What body process would you expect to be impaired as a result?

19. Two alternate pathways of interacting clotting proteins lead to coagulation, or blood clotting. How is each pathway initiated?

20. What are the effects of a vitamin K deficiency on blood clotting (coagulation)?

See the blue Answers tab at the back of the book.

RELATED CLINICAL TERMS

blood bank: Place where blood is collected, typed, separated into components, stored, and prepared for transfusion to recipients.

dyscrasia: An abnormal condition, especially of the blood.

ecchymosis: Skin discoloration caused by the escape of blood into tissues from ruptured blood vessels.

hematology (HĒM-ah-tol-o-jē)**:** The study of blood and its disorders.

hematuria (hē-ma-TOO-rē-uh)**:** The presence of red blood cells in the urine.

heterologous marrow transplant: The transplantation of bone marrow from one individual to another to replace bone marrow destroyed during cancer therapy.

hypervolemic: Having an excessive blood volume.

hypovolemic: Having a low blood volume.

normovolemic (nor-mō-vō-LĒ-mik)**:** Having a normal blood volume.

phlebotomy (fle-BOT-o-mē)**:** The process of withdrawing blood from a vein.

polycythemia (po-lē-sī-THĒ-mē-uh)**:** An elevated number of red blood cells in the blood; signs include a high hematocrit and a high hemoglobin concentration.

septicemia: A dangerous condition in which bacteria and bacterial toxins are distributed throughout the body in the bloodstream.

11 Chapter Review

Summary Outline

An Introduction to the Cardiovascular System *p. 430*

1. The **cardiovascular system** enables the rapid transport of nutrients, waste products, respiratory gases, and cells within the body.

11-1 Blood has several important functions and unique physical characteristics *p. 430*

2. **Blood** is a specialized fluid connective tissue. Its functions include (1) transporting dissolved gases, nutrients, hormones, and metabolic wastes; (2) regulating the pH and ion composition of the interstitial fluids; (3) restricting fluid losses at injury sites; (4) defending against pathogens and toxins; and (5) regulating body temperature by absorbing and redistributing heat.

3. Blood contains **plasma** and **formed elements—red blood cells (RBCs), white blood cells (WBCs),** and **platelets.** The plasma and formed elements make up whole blood, which can be **fractionated** for analytical or clinical purposes. The formed elements account for about 45 percent of the volume of blood *(Spotlight Figure 11-1).*

4. **Hemopoiesis,** or **hematopoiesis,** is the process by which all formed elements are produced. *Myeloid stem cells* and *lymphoid stem cells* divide to form all three types of formed elements.

11-2 Plasma, the fluid portion of blood, contains significant quantities of plasma proteins *p. 431*

5. Plasma accounts for about 55 percent of the volume of blood. Roughly 92 percent of plasma is water *(Spotlight Figure 11-1).*

6. Compared with interstitial fluid, plasma has a higher dissolved oxygen concentration and more dissolved proteins. The three classes of plasma proteins are *albumins, globulins,* and *fibrinogen.*

7. **Albumins** constitute about 60 percent of plasma proteins. **Globulins** make up roughly 35 percent of plasma proteins. They include **antibodies (immunoglobulins),** which attack foreign proteins and pathogens, and **transport proteins,** which bind ions, hormones, and other compounds. In the clotting reaction, soluble **fibrinogen** molecules are converted to insoluble **fibrin.** The removal of clotting proteins from plasma leaves a fluid called **serum.**

11-3 Red blood cells, formed by erythropoiesis, contain hemoglobin that can be recycled *p. 434*

8. Red blood cells **(RBCs),** or **erythrocytes,** account for slightly less than half of the blood volume and 99.9 percent of the formed elements. The **hematocrit** value is the percentage of formed elements within whole blood *(Spotlight Figure 11-1).*

9. RBCs transport oxygen and carbon dioxide within the bloodstream. They are highly specialized cells with a large surface area to volume ratio. They lack many organelles and usually degenerate after 120 days in the bloodstream *(Figure 11-2).*

10. Molecules of **hemoglobin (Hb)** account for over 95 percent of RBC proteins. Hemoglobin is a globular protein formed from four subunits. Each subunit contains a single molecule of **heme.** Each heme has an iron atom that can reversibly bind an oxygen molecule. Phagocytes recycle hemoglobin from damaged or dead RBCs *(Figure 11-4).*

11. **Erythropoiesis,** the formation of RBCs, occurs mainly in the **red bone marrow (myeloid tissue)** in adults. RBC formation increases under stimulation by **erythropoietin (EPO),** or erythropoiesis-stimulating hormone. EPO release occurs when peripheral tissues, especially the kidneys, are exposed to low oxygen concentrations. Stages in RBC development include **erythroblasts** and **reticulocytes** *(Figures 11-4, 11-5).*

11-4 The ABO blood types and Rh system are based on antigen–antibody responses *p. 440*

12. **Blood type** is determined by the presence or absence of three specific **surface antigens** (*agglutinogens*) in the plasma membranes of RBCs: antigens A, B, and Rh (D). Antibodies (*agglutinins*) in the plasma of individuals of some blood types can react with surface antigens on the RBCs of different blood types. Anti-Rh antibodies are synthesized only after an Rh-negative individual becomes sensitized to the Rh surface antigen *(Figures 11-6, 11-7; Table 11-1).*

11-5 The various types of white blood cells contribute to the body's defenses *p. 444*

13. White blood cells (WBCs), or **leukocytes,** defend the body against pathogens and remove toxins, wastes, and abnormal or damaged cells.

14. White blood cells exhibit amoeboid movement, **diapedesis** (the ability to move through vessel walls), and **positive chemotaxis** (an attraction to specific chemicals). Some WBCs are phagocytic.

15. *Granulocytes* (granular leukocytes) are *neutrophils, eosinophils,* and *basophils*. About 50–70 percent of circulating WBCs are **neutrophils**, which are highly mobile phagocytes. The much less common **eosinophils** are phagocytes attracted to foreign substances that have reacted with circulating antibodies. Their primary mode of attack is the exocytosis of toxic compounds. The relatively rare **basophils** migrate to damaged tissues and release histamine and heparin, aiding the inflammation response *(Figure 11-8; Table 11-2)*.

16. *Agranulocytes* (agranular leukocytes) are *monocytes* and *lymphocytes*. **Monocytes** that migrate into peripheral tissues become free macrophages. Most **lymphocytes** are in the tissues and organs of the **lymphatic system**, where they function in the body's specific defenses. Different classes of lymphocytes attack foreign cells directly, produce antibodies, and destroy abnormal body cells *(Figure 11-8; Table 11-2)*.

17. Granulocytes and monocytes are produced by **myeloid stem cells** in the red bone marrow. **Lymphoid stem cells** responsible for **lymphopoiesis** (production of lymphocytes) also originate in the bone marrow, but many migrate to lymphatic tissues *(Figure 11-4)*.

18. Various hormones are involved in regulating WBC populations. *Colony-stimulating factors* (*CSFs*) are hormones that regulate WBC populations other than lymphocytes *(Figure 11-4)*.

11-6 Platelets, disc-shaped structures formed from megakaryocytes, function in the clotting process *p. 448*

19. **Megakaryocytes** in the red bone marrow release packets of cytoplasm (platelets) into the circulating blood. Platelets are essential to the clotting process *(Figure 11-4; Table 11-2)*.

11-7 Hemostasis involves vascular spasm, platelet plug formation, and blood coagulation *p. 448*

20. **Hemostasis** prevents the loss of blood through the walls of damaged vessels.

21. The initial step of hemostasis, the **vascular phase**, is a period of local contraction of vessel walls resulting from a *vascular spasm* at the injury site. The **platelet phase** follows as platelets stick to damaged surfaces. The third phase of hemostasis is the **coagulation phase** *(Figure 11-9)*.

22. The coagulation phase occurs as factors released by platelets and endothelial cells interact with **clotting factors** (through either the **extrinsic pathway**, the **intrinsic pathway**, or the **common pathway**) to form a **blood clot** *(Figures 11-9, 11-10)*.

23. During **clot retraction,** platelets contract, pulling the torn edges of a damaged blood vessel closer together. During **fibrinolysis**, the clot gradually dissolves through the action of **plasmin**, the activated form of circulating **plasminogen**.

11

Review Questions

See the blue Answers tab at the back of the book.

Level 1 Reviewing Facts and Terms

Match each item in column A with the most closely related item in column B. Place letters for answers in the spaces provided.

COLUMN A

_____ 1. Interstitial fluid
_____ 2. Hemopoiesis
_____ 3. Stem cells
_____ 4. Hypoxia
_____ 5. Surface antigens
_____ 6. Antibodies
_____ 7. Diapedesis
_____ 8. Leucopenia
_____ 9. Agranulocyte
_____ 10. Leukocytosis
_____ 11. Granulocyte
_____ 12. Thrombocytopenia

COLUMN B

a. Hemocytoblasts
b. Abundant WBCs
c. Agglutinogens
d. Neutrophil
e. WBC migration
f. Extracellular fluid
g. Monocyte
h. Few WBCs
i. Low platelet count
j. Agglutinins
k. Process of blood cell formation
l. Low oxygen concentration

13. Blood temperature is approximately _____, and blood pH averages _____.
   (a) 98.6°F, 7.0   (b) 104°F, 7.8
   (c) 100.4°F, 7.4   (d) 96.8°F, 7.0

14. Plasma contributes approximately _____ percent of the volume of whole blood, and water accounts for _____ percent of the plasma volume.
   (a) 55, 92   (b) 25, 55
   (b) 92, 55   (d) 35, 72

15. Identify the five types of white blood cells in the following micrographs.

(a)   (b)   (c)

(d)   (e)

(a) _____
(b) _____
(c) _____
(d) _____
(e) _____

16. The formed elements of the blood include
  (a) plasma, fibrin, and serum.
  (b) albumins, globulins, and fibrinogen.
  (c) WBCs, RBCs, and platelets.
  (d) a, b, and c are correct.

17. When the clotting proteins are removed from plasma, _____ remains.
  (a) fibrinogen   **(b)** fibrin
  (c) serum   **(d)** heme

18. In an adult, the only site of red blood cell production, and the primary site of white blood cell formation, is the
  (a) liver.   **(b)** spleen.
  (c) thymus.   **(d)** red bone marrow.

19. The most numerous WBCs found in a differential count of a "normal" individual are
  (a) neutrophils.   **(b)** basophils.
  (c) lymphocytes.   **(d)** monocytes.

20. Stem cells responsible for the process of lymphopoiesis are located in the
  (a) thymus and spleen. **(b)** lymph nodes.
  (c) red bone marrow.   **(d)** a, b, and c are correct.

21. The first step in the process of hemostasis is
  (a) coagulation.   **(b)** the platelet phase.
  (c) fibrinolysis.   **(d)** vascular spasm.

22. The complex sequence of steps leading to the conversion of fibrinogen to fibrin is called
  (a) fibrinolysis.   **(b)** clotting.
  (c) retraction.   **(d)** the platelet phase.

23. Name the three major types of plasma proteins and identify their functions.

24. What type(s) of antibodies does the plasma contain for each of the following blood types?
  (a) type A   **(b)** type B
  (c) type AB   **(d)** type O

25. What four characteristics of WBCs are important to their response to tissue invasion or injury?

26. What contribution from the intrinsic and/or extrinsic pathways is necessary for the common pathway to begin?

27. Distinguish between an embolus and a thrombus.

Level 2 Reviewing Concepts

28. Dehydration would
  (a) cause an increase in the hematocrit.
  (b) cause a decrease in the hematocrit.
  (c) have no effect on the hematocrit.
  (d) cause an increase in plasma volume.

29. Erythropoietin directly stimulates RBC formation by
  (a) increasing rates of mitotic divisions in erythroblasts.
  (b) speeding up the maturation of red blood cells.
  (c) accelerating the rate of hemoglobin synthesis.
  (d) a, b, and c are correct.

30. A person with type A blood has
  (a) anti-A antibodies in the plasma.
  (b) B antigens in the plasma.
  (c) A antigens on red blood cells.
  (d) anti-B antibodies on red blood cells.

31. Hemolytic disease of the newborn can result if
  (a) the mother is Rh-positive and the father is Rh-negative.
  (b) both the father and the mother are Rh-negative.
  (c) both the father and the mother are Rh-positive.
  (d) an Rh-negative woman carries an Rh-positive fetus.

32. How do red blood cells differ from typical body cells?

Level 3 Critical Thinking and Clinical Applications

33. Which of the formed elements would you expect to increase after you have donated a pint of blood?

34. Why do many individuals with advanced kidney disease become anemic?

35. In the disease mononucleosis ("mono"), the spleen enlarges because of increased numbers of phagocytes and other cells. Common signs and symptoms of this disease include pale complexion, a tired feeling, and a lack of energy sometimes to the point of not being able to get out of bed. What might cause each of these signs and symptoms?

11

The Cardiovascular System: The Heart

Learning Objectives

These objectives tell you what you should be able to do after completing the chapter. They correspond by number to this chapter's sections.

12-1 Describe the anatomy of the heart, including blood supply and pericardium structure, and trace the flow of blood through the heart, identifying the major blood vessels, chambers, and heart valves.

12-2 Explain the events of an action potential in cardiac muscle, describe the conducting system of the heart, and identify the electrical events recorded in a normal electrocardiogram.

12-3 Explain the events of the cardiac cycle, and relate the heart sounds to specific events in this cycle.

12-4 Define cardiac output, describe the factors that influence heart rate and stroke volume, and explain how adjustments in stroke volume and cardiac output are coordinated at different levels of physical activity.

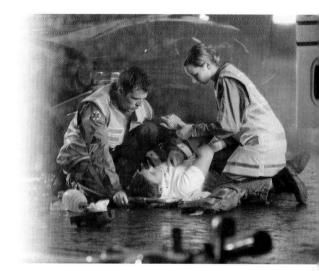

Clinical Notes

Valvular Heart Disease, p. 467
Abnormal Conditions Affecting Cardiac Output, p. 482

Spotlight

The Heart: Internal Anatomy and Blood Flow, p. 464

The Heart's Role in the Cardiovascular System

Our body cells rely on the surrounding interstitial fluid for oxygen, nutrients, and waste disposal. Conditions in the interstitial fluid are kept stable through continuous exchange between the peripheral tissues and circulating blood. If the blood stops moving, its oxygen and nutrient supplies are quickly exhausted. Its capacity to absorb wastes is soon saturated, and neither hormones nor white blood cells can reach their targets. Thus, all cardiovascular functions ultimately depend on the heart. This muscular organ beats approximately 100,000 times each day. It pumps roughly 8000 liters of blood—enough to fill forty 55-gallon drums, or nearly 8500 quart-sized milk cartons. Despite its impressive workload, the heart is a small organ, about the size of a clenched fist.

Blood flows through a network of blood vessels that extend between the heart and peripheral tissues. Those blood vessels make up two circuits. The **pulmonary circuit** carries blood to and from the gas exchange surfaces of the lungs. The **systemic circuit** transports blood to and from the rest of the body (**Figure 12-1**). Each circuit begins and ends at the heart, and blood travels through them in sequence. Thus, blood returning to the heart from the systemic circuit must complete the pulmonary circuit before re-entering the systemic circuit.

Arteries, or *efferent* vessels, carry blood away from the heart. **Veins**, or *afferent* vessels, return blood to the heart. **Capillaries** are small, thin-walled vessels between the smallest arteries and the smallest veins. Their thin walls permit the exchange of nutrients, dissolved gases, and wastes between the blood and surrounding tissues.

The heart contains four muscular chambers. Two are associated with each circuit. The **right atrium** (Ā-trē-um; entry chamber; plural, *atria*) receives blood from the systemic circuit, and passes it to the **right ventricle** (VEN-tri-kl; little belly), which then pumps blood into the pulmonary circuit. The **left atrium** collects blood from the pulmonary circuit, and empties it into the **left ventricle**, which pumps blood into the systemic circuit. When the heart beats, the two atria contract together first, then the ventricles. The two ventricles contract at the same time. They eject equal volumes of blood into the pulmonary and systemic circuits.

We begin this chapter by examining the structural features that enable the heart to perform so reliably. We then consider the physiological processes that regulate the activities of the heart to meet the body's ever-changing needs.

12

Build Your Knowledge

Recall that the cardiovascular system was our example organ system when we examined the relationships among the various levels of organization of the human body (as you saw in **Chapter 1: An Introduction to Anatomy and Physiology**). Contractile proteins and their atoms represent the chemical level. Cardiac cells containing those proteins represent the cellular level. Cardiac tissue made up of cardiac cells represents the tissue level. The heart containing cardiac tissue and other tissues represents the organ level. The heart, blood, and blood vessels represent the organ system level. つ **pp. 5, 8**

12-1 The heart is a four-chambered organ, supplied by coronary circulation, that pumps oxygen-poor blood to the lungs and oxygen-rich blood to the rest of the body

Learning Objective Describe the anatomy of the heart, including blood supply and pericardium structure, and trace the flow of blood through the heart, identifying the major blood vessels, chambers, and heart valves.

The heart is located near the anterior chest wall, directly behind the sternum (**Figure 12-2a**). It sits in the anterior portion of the *mediastinum*, the connective tissue mass between the two pleural cavities (see **Figure 1-10c**, p. 18). The mediastinum also contains the *great vessels* (the largest arteries and veins in the body), thymus, esophagus, and trachea.

The heart is surrounded by the **pericardial** (per-i-KAR-dē-al) **cavity**. The lining of the pericardial cavity is a serous membrane called the **pericardium**. つ p. 111 To visualize the relationship between the heart and the pericardial cavity, imagine pushing your fist toward the center of a large balloon (**Figure 12-2b**). The balloon represents the pericardium, and your fist represents the heart. Your wrist, where the balloon folds back on itself, corresponds to the **base** of the heart

Figure 12-1 An Overview of the Cardiovascular System.

Driven by the pumping of the heart, blood flows through separate pulmonary and systemic circuits. Each circuit begins and ends at the heart and contains arteries, capillaries, and veins.

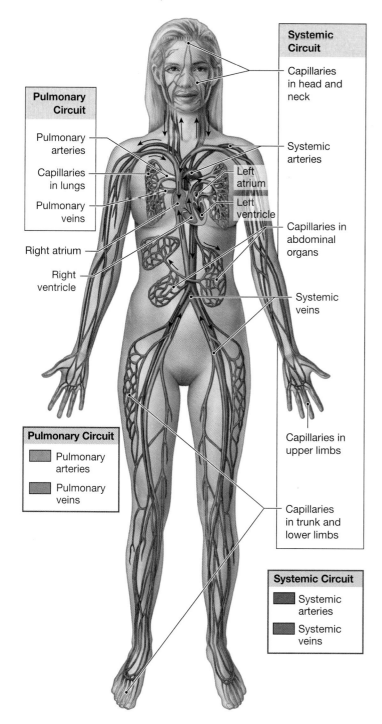

Systemic Circuit

- Capillaries in head and neck
- Systemic arteries
- Left atrium
- Left ventricle
- Capillaries in abdominal organs
- Systemic veins
- Capillaries in upper limbs
- Capillaries in trunk and lower limbs

Pulmonary Circuit

- Pulmonary arteries
- Capillaries in lungs
- Pulmonary veins
- Right atrium
- Right ventricle

Pulmonary Circuit

- Pulmonary arteries
- Pulmonary veins

Systemic Circuit

- Systemic arteries
- Systemic veins

(**Figure 12-2a**). The air space inside the balloon corresponds to the pericardial cavity.

The *pericardial sac* is a dense network of collagen fibers that stabilizes the positions of the pericardium, heart, and associated vessels in the mediastinum. The pericardium can be subdivided into the visceral pericardium and the parietal pericardium. The **visceral pericardium**, or **epicardium**, covers the outer surface of the heart. The **parietal pericardium** lines the inner surface of the pericardial sac (**Figure 12-2b**). The space between the parietal and visceral surfaces is the pericardial cavity. It normally contains a small quantity of *pericardial fluid* secreted by the pericardial (serous) membranes. The fluid acts as a lubricant, reducing friction between the opposing surfaces as the heart beats.

The Surface Anatomy of the Heart

We can use several external features of the heart to identify its four chambers (**Figure 12-3a,b,c**). The two atria have relatively thin muscular walls and are highly expandable. When not filled with blood, the outer portion of each atrium deflates into a lumpy, wrinkled flap. This expandable extension of an atrium is called an **auricle** (AW-ri-kl; *auris,* ear). The **coronary sulcus**, a deep groove, marks the border between the atria and the ventricles. Shallower depressions—the **anterior interventricular sulcus** and **posterior interventricular sulcus**—mark the boundary between the left and right ventricles. Substantial amounts of fat generally lie within these three sulci (SUL-sī). In addition to fat, they also contain the major arteries and veins that carry blood to and from the cardiac muscle.

The great vessels are connected to the superior base of the heart. The inferior, pointed tip of the heart is the **apex** (Ā-peks) (**Figure 12-2a**). A typical heart measures approximately 12.5 cm (5 in.) from the attached base to the apex.

The heart sits at an angle to the longitudinal axis of the body. It is also rotated slightly toward the left, so the anterior surface primarily consists of the right atrium and right ventricle (**Figure 12-3a,b,d**). The wall of the left ventricle forms much of the posterior surface between the base and the apex of the heart (**Figure 12-3b**).

The Heart Wall

The wall of the heart contains three distinct layers: an outer epicardium, a middle myocardium, and an inner endocardium (**Figure 12-4a**). The **epicardium** is the visceral pericardium that covers the outer surface of the heart. This serous membrane consists of an exposed epithelium and an underlying layer of areolar tissue that is attached to the myocardium. The **myocardium**, or muscular wall of the heart, contains cardiac muscle tissue, blood vessels, and nerves. The cardiac muscle tissue of the myocardium forms bands that wrap around the atria in a figure eight pattern and spiral into the walls of the ventricles (**Figure 12-4b**).

12

Figure 12-2 The Location of the Heart in the Thoracic Cavity.

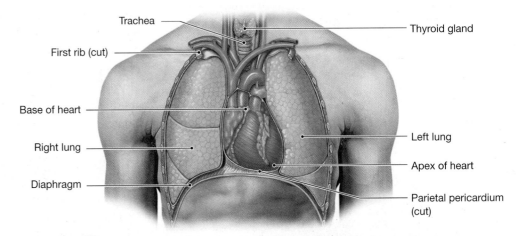

Trachea — Thyroid gland

First rib (cut) —

Base of heart —

Right lung —

Diaphragm —

— Left lung

— Apex of heart

— Parietal pericardium (cut)

a An anterior view of the chest, showing the position of the heart and major blood vessels relative to the lungs and diaphragm.

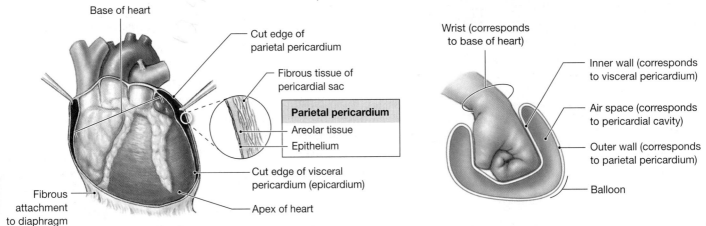

Base of heart

— Cut edge of parietal pericardium

— Fibrous tissue of pericardial sac

| Parietal pericardium |
| Areolar tissue |
| Epithelium |

— Cut edge of visceral pericardium (epicardium)

Fibrous attachment to diaphragm

— Apex of heart

Wrist (corresponds to base of heart)

— Inner wall (corresponds to visceral pericardium)

— Air space (corresponds to pericardial cavity)

— Outer wall (corresponds to parietal pericardium)

— Balloon

b The pericardial cavity surrounding the heart is formed by the visceral pericardium and the parietal pericardium. The relationship between the heart and the pericardial cavity can be likened to a fist pushed into a balloon.

This arrangement results in squeezing and twisting contractions that increase the pumping efficiency of the heart. The heart's inner surfaces, including the heart valves, are covered by the **endocardium** (en-dō-KAR-dē-um), which is made up of a simple squamous epithelium and underlying areolar tissue. The squamous epithelial lining of the cardiovascular system is called an *endothelium*. The endothelium of the heart is continuous with the endothelium of the attached great vessels. ⊃ p. 397

Cardiac Muscle Cells

Typical cardiac muscle cells are shown in **Figure 12-4c,d**. These cells are smaller than skeletal muscle fibers. They contain a single, centrally located nucleus. Like skeletal muscle fibers, each cardiac muscle cell contains myofibrils, and

contraction involves the shortening of individual sarcomeres. Cardiac muscle cells are almost totally dependent on aerobic metabolism for the energy needed to continue contracting. Many mitochondria and abundant reserves of myoglobin (to store oxygen) support their energy needs. Energy reserves are stored as glycogen and lipids.

Each cardiac muscle cell is in contact with several others at specialized sites known as **intercalated** (in-TER-ka-lā-ted) **discs.** ⊃ p. 113 At these sites, the interlocking membranes of adjacent cells are held together by desmosomes and linked by gap junctions. ⊃ p. 93 The desmosomes help convey the force of contraction from cell to cell, increasing their efficiency as they "pull together" during a contraction. The gap junctions provide for the movement of ions and small molecules, enabling action potentials to travel rapidly from cell to cell.

12

Figure 12-3 The Position and Surface Anatomy of the Heart.

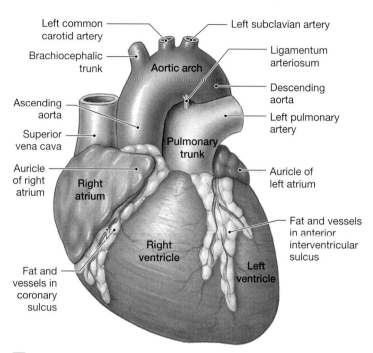

a   Major anatomical features on the anterior surface.

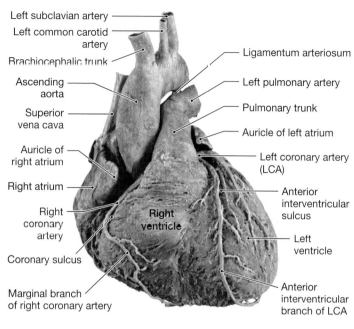

b   Anterior surface of the heart, cadaver dissection.

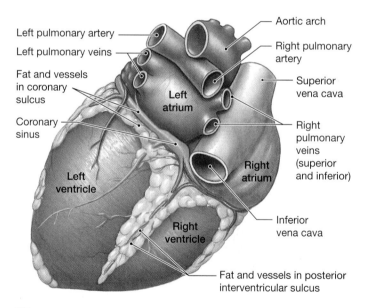

c   Major landmarks on the posterior surface. Coronary arteries (which supply the heart itself) are shown in red; coronary veins are shown in blue.

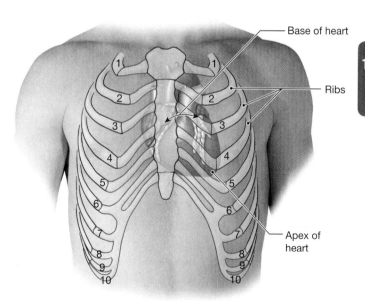

d   Heart position relative to the rib cage.

Connective Tissue in the Heart

The connective tissues of the heart include abundant collagen and elastic fibers that wrap around each cardiac muscle cell and tie together adjacent cells. These fibers (1) provide support for cardiac muscle fibers, blood vessels, and nerves of the myocardium; (2) add strength and prevent overexpansion of the heart; and (3) help the heart return to normal shape after contractions. Connective tissue also forms the *cardiac skeleton* of the heart, discussed in a later section.

Figure 12-4 The Heart Wall and Cardiac Muscle Tissue.

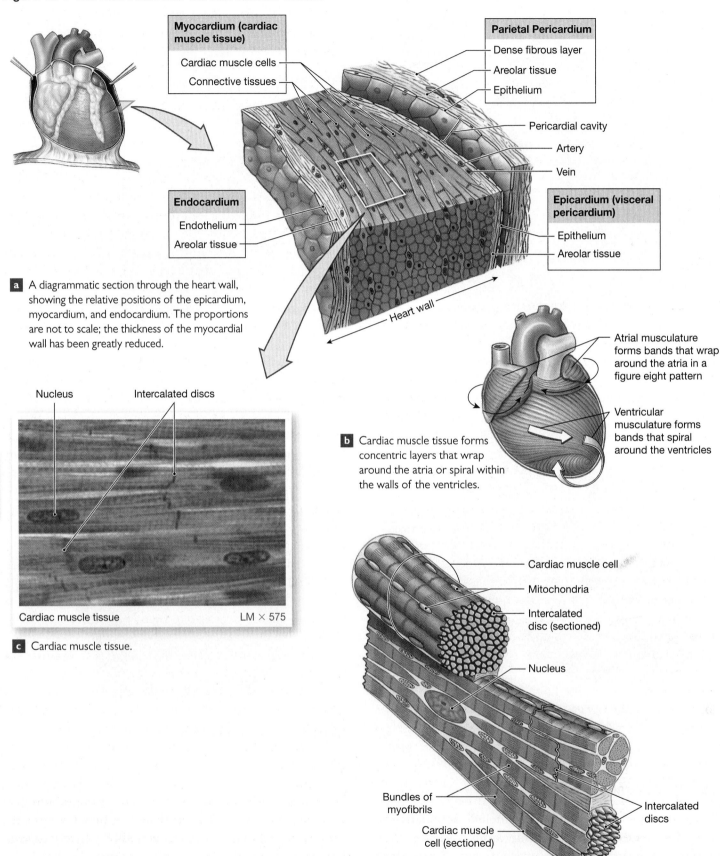

Myocardium (cardiac muscle tissue)
- Cardiac muscle cells
- Connective tissues

Parietal Pericardium
- Dense fibrous layer
- Areolar tissue
- Epithelium

- Pericardial cavity
- Artery
- Vein

Endocardium
- Endothelium
- Areolar tissue

Epicardium (visceral pericardium)
- Epithelium
- Areolar tissue

Heart wall

a A diagrammatic section through the heart wall, showing the relative positions of the epicardium, myocardium, and endocardium. The proportions are not to scale; the thickness of the myocardial wall has been greatly reduced.

Nucleus   Intercalated discs

Cardiac muscle tissue   LM × 575

c Cardiac muscle tissue.

Atrial musculature forms bands that wrap around the atria in a figure eight pattern

Ventricular musculature forms bands that spiral around the ventricles

b Cardiac muscle tissue forms concentric layers that wrap around the atria or spiral within the walls of the ventricles.

- Cardiac muscle cell
- Mitochondria
- Intercalated disc (sectioned)
- Nucleus

Bundles of myofibrils

Cardiac muscle cell (sectioned)

Intercalated discs

d Cardiac muscle cells.

CLINICAL NOTE

Chagas' Disease

In many parts of Central and South America, heart disease is the number one cause of death. But, unlike the United States and Canada, the type of heart disease seen in those areas is called *Chagas' disease* and is due to infection by the parasite *Trypanosoma cruzi*. Thought to infect over 16 million persons, it is spread through the bite of an insect known as the "kissing bug." The initial signs and symptoms are mild. However, 10–20 years later, the patient develops an enlarged heart and dysrhythmias and eventually dies from heart failure.

Internal Anatomy and Organization

The four chambers of the heart are shown in sectional view in **Spotlight Figure 12-5**. The two atria are separated by the **interatrial septum** (*septum,* wall). The two ventricles are separated by the **interventricular septum**. Both septa are muscular partitions. **Atrioventricular (AV) valves** are folds of fibrous tissue that extend into the openings between the atria and the ventricles. They function as one-way valves, permitting blood to flow only in one direction: from the atria to the ventricles.

The right atrium receives blood from the systemic circuit through two large veins, the superior vena cava (VĒ-na KĀ-vuh; plural, *venae cavae*) and the inferior vena cava and a smaller vein, the coronary sinus (**Spotlight Figure 12-5**). The **superior vena cava** delivers blood from the head, neck, upper limbs, and chest. The **inferior vena cava** carries blood from the rest of the trunk, the viscera, and the lower limbs. The *cardiac veins* draining the myocardium of the heart return deoxygenated blood to the **coronary sinus**. This large, thin-walled vein opens into the right atrium slightly below the connection with the inferior vena cava.

The opening of the coronary sinus lies near the posterior edge of the interatrial septum. From the fifth week of embryonic development until birth, an oval opening, the *foramen ovale*, penetrates the interatrial septum. Before birth, the foramen ovale allows blood to flow from the right atrium to the left atrium while the lungs are developing (see **Figure 13–21**, p. 520). At birth, the foramen ovale closes. The opening is permanently sealed off within the first year. A small depression called the *fossa ovalis* remains in the adult heart (**Spotlight Figure 12-5**). Occasionally, the foramen ovale remains open even after birth. Under these conditions, contractions of the left atrium push blood back into the pulmonary circuit. This leads to heart enlargement and eventual heart failure and death if the condition is not surgically corrected.

Blood travels from the right atrium into the right ventricle through a broad opening bounded by three flaps of fibrous tissue. These flaps, or **cusps**, are part of the **right AV valve**, also known as the **tricuspid** (trī-KUS-pid; *tri-,* three + *cuspis,* point) **valve** (**Spotlight Figure 12-5**). Each cusp is braced by connective tissue fibers called **chordae tendineae** (KOR-dē TEN-di-nē-ē; "tendinous cords"). These fibers are connected to **papillary** (PAP-i-ler-ē) **muscles**, cone-shaped projections on the inner surface of the ventricle. The contraction of these muscles tenses the chordae tendineae, limiting the movement of the cusps and preventing the backflow of blood into the right atrium. The internal surface of the right and left ventricles have muscular ridges called the *trabeculae carneae* (tra-BEK-ū-lē KAR-nē-ē; *carneus,* fleshy).

Blood leaving the right ventricle flows into the **pulmonary trunk**, the start of the pulmonary circuit. The **pulmonary valve**, or *pulmonary semilunar* (*semi-,* half + *luna,* moon; a crescent, or half-moon, shape) *valve*, guards the entrance to this efferent trunk. Once in the pulmonary trunk, blood flows into the **left** and **right pulmonary arteries**. These vessels branch repeatedly within the lungs before supplying the capillaries where gas exchange occurs. From these respiratory capillaries, oxygenated blood moves into the **left** and **right pulmonary veins**, which deliver it to the left atrium.

The pulmonary trunk is attached to the **aortic arch** by a fibrous band called the *ligamentum arteriosum* (**Spotlight Figure 12-5**). It is all that remains of an important fetal blood vessel that once linked the pulmonary and systemic circuits.

Like the right atrium, the left atrium has an external auricle and a valve, the **left AV valve**, or **bicuspid** (bī-KUS-pid) **valve**. As the name *bicuspid* implies, the left AV valve contains two cusps, rather than three. Clinicians often call this valve the **mitral** (MĪ-tral; *mitre,* a bishop's hat) **valve**.

The internal organization of the left ventricle resembles that of the right ventricle. A pair of papillary muscles braces the chordae tendineae that insert on the bicuspid valve. Muscular ridges also line the internal surface of the left ventricle. Blood leaves the left ventricle through the **aortic valve**, or *aortic semilunar valve*, and passes into the **ascending aorta**, the start of the systemic circuit.

12

This diagrammatic frontal section through the heart shows its major landmarks and the path of blood flow (marked by arrows) through the atria, ventricles, and associated blood vessels. Red arrows represent oxygenated blood, and blue arrows represent deoxygenated blood.

As you can see, the right atrium communicates with the right ventricle, and the left atrium with the left ventricle. The atria are separated by the **interatrial septum**. The ventricles are separated by the much thicker **interventricular septum**. Each septum is a muscular partition. Atrioventricular (AV) valves, folds of fibrous tissue, extend into the openings between the atria and ventricles. These valves permit blood to flow in only one direction: from the atria to the ventricles.

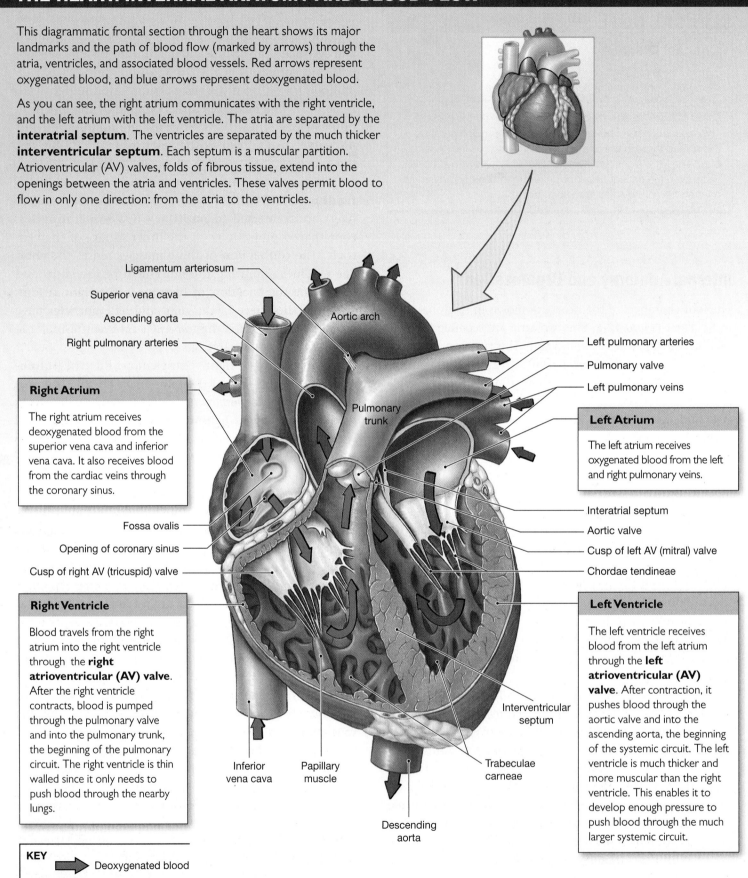

Ligamentum arteriosum

Superior vena cava

Ascending aorta

Right pulmonary arteries

Aortic arch

Left pulmonary arteries

Pulmonary valve

Left pulmonary veins

Pulmonary trunk

Right Atrium

The right atrium receives deoxygenated blood from the superior vena cava and inferior vena cava. It also receives blood from the cardiac veins through the coronary sinus.

Left Atrium

The left atrium receives oxygenated blood from the left and right pulmonary veins.

Fossa ovalis

Opening of coronary sinus

Cusp of right AV (tricuspid) valve

Interatrial septum

Aortic valve

Cusp of left AV (mitral) valve

Chordae tendineae

Right Ventricle

Blood travels from the right atrium into the right ventricle through the **right atrioventricular (AV) valve**. After the right ventricle contracts, blood is pumped through the pulmonary valve and into the pulmonary trunk, the beginning of the pulmonary circuit. The right ventricle is thin walled since it only needs to push blood through the nearby lungs.

Left Ventricle

The left ventricle receives blood from the left atrium through the **left atrioventricular (AV) valve**. After contraction, it pushes blood through the aortic valve and into the ascending aorta, the beginning of the systemic circuit. The left ventricle is much thicker and more muscular than the right ventricle. This enables it to develop enough pressure to push blood through the much larger systemic circuit.

Inferior vena cava

Papillary muscle

Interventricular septum

Trabeculae carneae

Descending aorta

KEY

➡ Deoxygenated blood

➡ Oxygenated blood

Structural Differences between the Left and Right Ventricles

The function of each atrium is to collect blood returning to the heart and deliver that blood to the attached ventricle. With very similar demands, the two atria look almost identical. But the demands on the right and left ventricles are very different, and the two have significant structural differences.

The lungs are close to the heart, and the pulmonary arteries and veins are relatively short and wide. For these reasons, the right ventricle normally does not need to push very hard to propel blood through the pulmonary circuit. The wall of the right ventricle is relatively thin (**Spotlight Figure 12-5**). In sectional view, the right ventricle resembles a pouch attached to the massive wall of the left ventricle. When the right ventricle contracts, it acts like a bellows pump, squeezing the blood against the left ventricle and then out through the pulmonary semilunar valve. This action moves blood very efficiently with minimal effort, but it develops relatively low pressures.

A comparable pumping arrangement would not work well for the left ventricle. Four to six times as much pressure must be exerted to push blood around the systemic circuit as around the pulmonary circuit. The left ventricle has an extremely thick muscular wall and is round in cross section. When this ventricle contracts, it shortens and narrows. That is, (1) the distance between the heart's base and apex decreases, and (2) the diameter of the ventricular chamber decreases. (The effect is similar to simultaneously squeezing and rolling up the end of a toothpaste tube.) More than enough pressure is generated to open the aortic valve and eject blood into the ascending aorta.

As the powerful left ventricle contracts, it also bulges into the right ventricular cavity. This action helps force blood out of the right ventricle. Individuals with severe damage to their right ventricle may survive, because the left ventricle helps push blood through the pulmonary circuit.

The Heart Valves

As we have seen, the heart has two pairs of one-way valves that prevent the backflow of blood as the chambers contract. Let's look at the structure and function of these heart valves.

THE ATRIOVENTRICULAR VALVES. The atrioventricular valves prevent the backflow of blood from the ventricles into the atria. The chordae tendineae and papillary muscles play important roles in the normal function of the AV valves. When the ventricles are relaxed, the chordae tendineae are loose

CLINICAL NOTE

Mitral Valve Prolapse

Minor abnormalities in valve shape are relatively common. For example, an estimated 10 percent of normal individuals ages 14–30 have some degree of *mitral valve prolapse*. In this condition, the cusps of the left AV valve (the mitral valve) do not close properly. The problem may stem from abnormally long (or short) chordae tendineae or malfunctioning papillary muscles. Because the valve does not work perfectly, some regurgitation occurs during the contraction of the left ventricle. Most individuals with mitral valve prolapse are completely asymptomatic; they live normal, healthy lives unaware of any circulatory malfunction.

and the AV valve offers no resistance to the flow of blood from atrium to ventricle (**Figure 12-6a**). When the ventricles contract, blood moving back toward the atrium swings the cusps together, closing the valves (**Figure 12-6b**). During ventricular contraction, tension in the papillary muscles and chordae tendineae keeps the cusps from swinging into the atrium. This action prevents the backflow, or **regurgitation**, of blood into the atrium each time the ventricle contracts. A small amount of regurgitation often occurs, even in normal individuals. The swirling blood creates a soft but distinctive sound called a *heart murmur.*

THE SEMILUNAR VALVES. The pulmonary and aortic semilunar valves prevent the backflow of blood from the pulmonary trunk and ascending aorta into the right and left ventricles, respectively. Unlike the AV valves, the semilunar valves do not require muscular bracing, because the arterial walls do not contract and the relative positions of the cusps are stable. When the semilunar valves close, the three symmetrical cusps in each valve support one another like the legs of a tripod, preventing the movement of blood back into the ventricles (**Figure 12-6a**).

Saclike expansions of the base of the ascending aorta occur next to each cusp of the aortic semilunar valve. These sacs, called **aortic sinuses**, prevent the cusps from sticking to the wall of the aorta when the valve opens (**Figure 12-6b**). The *right* and *left coronary arteries* originate at the aortic sinuses.

The Cardiac Skeleton of the Heart

The **cardiac skeleton**, or *fibrous skeleton*, of the heart consists of dense bands of tough, elastic connective tissue that encircle the bases of the large blood vessels carrying blood

Figure 12-6 The Valves of the Heart. Red (oxygenated) and blue (deoxygenated) arrows indicate blood flow into and out of a ventricle; thin red arrows, blood flow into an atrium; and green arrows, ventricular contraction.

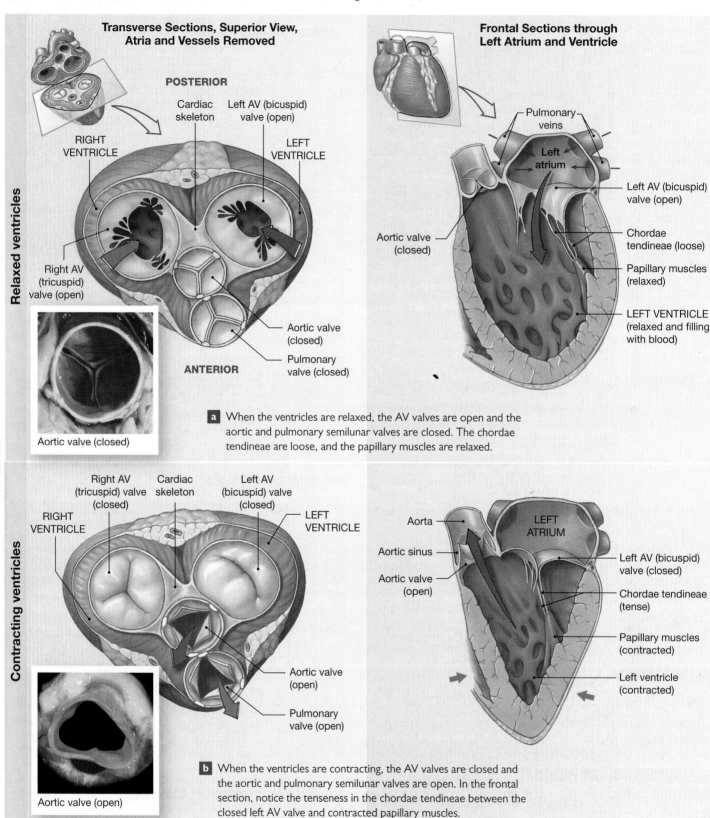

Transverse Sections, Superior View, Atria and Vessels Removed

POSTERIOR

Cardiac skeleton

Left AV (bicuspid) valve (open)

RIGHT VENTRICLE

LEFT VENTRICLE

Right AV (tricuspid) valve (open)

Aortic valve (closed)

Pulmonary valve (closed)

ANTERIOR

Aortic valve (closed)

Frontal Sections through Left Atrium and Ventricle

Pulmonary veins

Left atrium

Aortic valve (closed)

Left AV (bicuspid) valve (open)

Chordae tendineae (loose)

Papillary muscles (relaxed)

LEFT VENTRICLE (relaxed and filling with blood)

a When the ventricles are relaxed, the AV valves are open and the aortic and pulmonary semilunar valves are closed. The chordae tendineae are loose, and the papillary muscles are relaxed.

Right AV (tricuspid) valve (closed)

Cardiac skeleton

Left AV (bicuspid) valve (closed)

RIGHT VENTRICLE

LEFT VENTRICLE

Aortic valve (open)

Pulmonary valve (open)

Aortic valve (open)

Aorta

Aortic sinus

Aortic valve (open)

LEFT ATRIUM

Left AV (bicuspid) valve (closed)

Chordae tendineae (tense)

Papillary muscles (contracted)

Left ventricle (contracted)

b When the ventricles are contracting, the AV valves are closed and the aortic and pulmonary semilunar valves are open. In the frontal section, notice the tenseness in the chordae tendineae between the closed left AV valve and contracted papillary muscles.

Relaxed ventricles

Contracting ventricles

12

CLINICAL NOTE

Valvular Heart Disease

Minor abnormalities in valve shape are relatively common. For example, an estimated 10 percent of normal individuals ages 14–30 have some degree of mitral valve prolapse. In this condition, the cusps of the left AV valve (the mitral valve) do not close properly. The problem may stem from abnormally long (or short) chordae tendineae or malfunctioning papillary muscles. Because the valve does not work perfectly, some regurgitation takes place when the left ventricle contracts. Most individuals with mitral valve prolapse have no symptoms. They live normal healthy lives unaware of any circulatory malfunction.

Serious valve problems are very dangerous because they reduce pumping efficiency. If valve function deteriorates such that the heart cannot maintain adequate circulatory flow, symptoms of valvular heart disease appear. Congenital defects may be responsible, but in many cases the condition develops following *carditis*, an inflammation of the heart. In severe cases, the only option may be to replace the damaged valve with a prosthetic one. One relatively common cause of carditis is rheumatic (roo-MA-tik) fever, an inflammatory autoimmune response to an infection by streptococcal bacteria. It most often occurs in children.

away from the heart (*pulmonary trunk* and *aorta*) and each of the heart valves (**Figure 12-6**). The cardiac skeleton stabilizes the position of the heart valves and also physically isolates the atrial muscle tissue from the ventricular muscle tissue. This isolation is important to normal heart function because it means that the timing of ventricular contraction relative to atrial contraction can be precisely controlled.

The Blood Supply to the Heart

The heart works continuously, so cardiac muscle cells require reliable supplies of oxygen and nutrients. The **coronary circulation** supplies blood to the muscle tissue of the heart (**Figure 12-7**). During maximum exertion, the heart's demand for oxygen rises considerably. The blood flow to the heart may then increase up to nine times that of resting levels.

The left and right **coronary arteries** originate at the base of the aorta at the aortic sinuses (**Figure 12-7a**). Blood pressure here is the highest in the systemic circuit. This high pressure ensures a continuous flow of blood to meet the demands of active cardiac muscle. The right coronary artery supplies blood to the right atrium and to portions of both ventricles. The left coronary artery supplies blood to the left ventricle, left atrium, and interventricular septum.

Each coronary artery gives rise to two branches. The right coronary artery forms the *marginal* and *posterior interventricular* (*descending*) arteries. The left coronary artery forms

12

Figure 12-7 The Coronary Circulation.

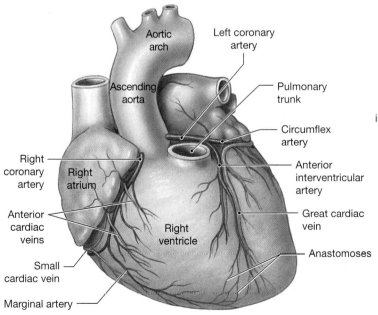

a Coronary vessels supplying and draining the anterior surface of the heart.

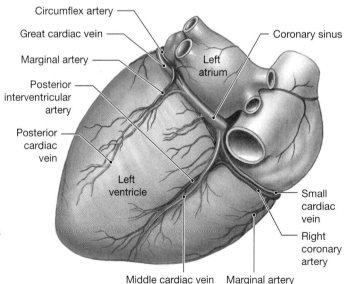

b Coronary vessels supplying and draining the posterior surface of the heart.

the *circumflex* and *anterior interventricular* (*descending*) arteries. The anterior interventricular artery supplies small tributaries continuous with those of the posterior artery. Such interconnections between arteries are called **anastomoses** (a-nas-tō-MŌ-sēz; *anastomosis,* outlet). Because the arteries are interconnected in this way, alternate pathways exist for the blood supply to reach cardiac muscle.

The **great** and **middle cardiac veins** carry blood away from the coronary capillaries. They drain into the **coronary sinus**, a large, thin-walled vein in the posterior portion of the coronary sulcus. The coronary sinus opens into the right atrium near the base of the inferior vena cava (**Spotlight Figure 12-5**).

An area of dead tissue caused by an interruption in blood flow is called an **infarct**. In a **myocardial** (mī-ō-KAR-dē-al) **infarction**, or *heart attack*, the coronary circulation becomes blocked, and cardiac muscle cells die from lack of oxygen. Heart attacks most often result from severe *coronary artery disease,* a condition characterized by the buildup of fatty deposits in the walls of the coronary arteries.

CHECKPOINT

1. Damage to the semilunar valve of the right ventricle would affect blood flow into which vessel?

2. What prevents the AV valves from swinging into the atria?

3. Why is the left ventricle more muscular than the right ventricle?

See the blue Answers tab at the back of the book.

12-2 Contractile cells and the conducting system produce each heartbeat, and an electrocardiogram records the associated electrical events

Learning Objective Explain the events of an action potential in cardiac muscle, describe the conducting system of the heart, and identify the electrical events recorded in a normal electrocardiogram.

In a single **heartbeat**, the entire heart—atria and ventricles—contracts in a coordinated manner so that blood flows in the correct direction at the proper time. Each time the heart beats, the contractions of individual cardiac muscle cells take place first in the atria and then in the ventricles. Two types of cardiac muscle cells are involved in a normal heartbeat: (1) *Contractile cells* produce the powerful contractions that propel blood, and (2) specialized noncontractile muscle cells of the *conducting system* control and coordinate the activities of the contractile cells.

12

CLINICAL NOTE

Coronary Artery Disease

The initial biological process in the progression of coronary artery disease is the development of microscopic *atherosclerosis.* Atherosclerosis is a form of *arteriosclerosis* where soft deposits of intra-arterial fat and fibrin cause thickening and hardening of the arterial wall. The initial occurrence in this process is an endothelial injury, followed by a series of pathological events that lead to the development of a fatty streak on the lining of the vessel. These lesions can be found in the walls of most people's arteries, even young children's. They are reversible with treatment that lowers *low-density lipoprotein* levels. Once formed, however, fatty streaks produce toxic oxygen radicals and cause inflammatory changes that result in progressive damage to the arterial wall.

The next stage of *atherogenesis* is the incorporation of fibrous tissue and damaged smooth muscle cells into the area that forms a *fibrous plaque* or *fibroadenoma.* This causes further endothelial dysfunction, necrosis of underlying vessel tissue, and narrowing of the vessel lumen. As the plaque continues to develop, it can ulcerate or rupture because of the mechanical shear forces and continued necrosis of the vessel wall. Platelets aggregate and adhere to the vessel surface, which simultaneously activates the coagulation cascade. In severe cases, a thrombus (blood clot) can form, completely obstructing the vessel lumen and resulting in tissue ischemia and infarction.

The rate of progression of atherosclerosis can be significantly influenced by specific conditions and behaviors referred to as *risk factors* including age, gender, tobacco use, diabetes, obesity, hypertension, and many others. Atherosclerosis is a disease spectrum with various events that occur along the continuum. Cardiac arrest and myocardial infarction (heart attack) are, in the vast majority of cases, end points in a decades-long evolution of atherosclerotic arterial disease (**Figure 12-8**). The rate of progression of atherosclerosis is the primary determinant of the age at which myocardial infarction or sudden death occurs. Control or elimination of risk factors can usually be achieved by establishing positive health attitudes and behaviors, especially in the young. Significant modifications in risk factors can occur by exercise, smoking cessation, dietary modifications, control

Figure 12-8 Cardiac Arrest. Acute myocardial infarction and cardiac arrest are often the end points of atherosclerotic arterial disease over a number of decades.

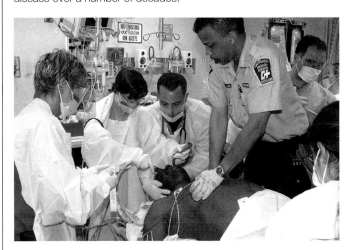

of hypertension, and use of medications to reduce lipid levels, blood pressure, and platelet aggregation. Atherosclerotic heart disease is a disease that must be identified and controlled in order to assure long-term health.

Acute Coronary Syndrome

Our knowledge and treatment of acute myocardial infarction (AMI) has evolved dramatically over the past decade. We now recognize that AMI and unstable angina are part of a spectrum of clinical disease referred to as *acute coronary syndrome*. Most patients with acute coronary syndrome have some level of underlying atherosclerotic coronary artery disease. Often, an atheromatous plaque will rupture and block the artery, or a thrombus (blood clot) will form and block blood flow through the affected vessel. The degree and duration of the occlusion determine the type of infarction. The severity of the infarction can

Figure 12-9 Myocardial Infarction. Blockage of a coronary artery results in injury and death to the myocardial tissue supplied by that artery.

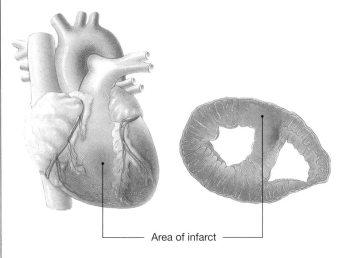

Area of infarct

Figure 12-10 Nuclear Medicine Scan of the Heart That Illustrates Good Ventricular Function. Nuclear medicine technology allows detailed examination of cardiac perfusion and function.

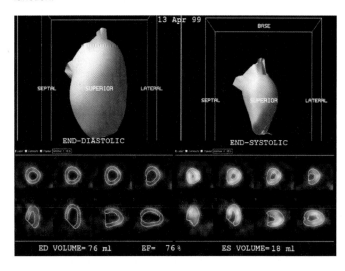

Figure 12-11 Coronary Arteriography.

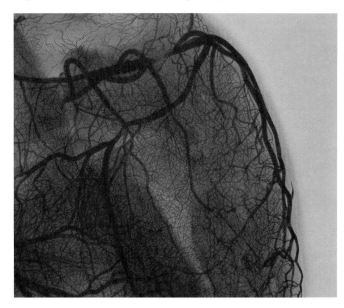

be reduced if collateral blood vessels supply some blood to the tissues distal to the obstruction.

Initially following coronary artery occlusion, the myocardial tissue supplied by the affected artery will become ischemic (**Figures 12-9 to 12-11**). If blood flow is restored in time, myocardial ischemia will resolve without permanent muscle injury; however, if myocardial ischemia continues, then actual tissue injury will begin. Tissue injury may or may not be reversed with the restoration of blood flow. Finally, if blood flow is interrupted long enough, then irreversible tissue damage (myocardial infarction) will occur (**Figure 12-12**).

(Continued)

Figure 12-12 Evolving Myocardial Infarction. The center of the lesion is the zone of infarction where tissue death has actually occurred. Adjacent to that is the zone of injury where some recovery is possible. At the periphery of the lesion is the zone of ischemia where actual tissue injury has not yet occurred.

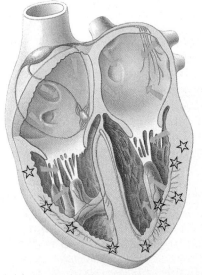

Zone of ischemia

Zone of injury

Zone of infarction

as result of absence

Myocardial ischemia causes ST segment depression with or without T wave inversion as result of altered repolarization

Myocardial injury causes ST segment elevation with or without loss of R wave

Myocardial infarction causes deep Q waves of depolarization current from dead tissue and receding currents from opposite side of heart

The signs and symptoms of acute coronary syndrome are due to coronary artery occlusion and related muscle injury and death. They include chest pain, difficulty breathing, sweating (diaphoresis), nausea, vomiting, and dizziness.

Half of all patients who die of AMI do so early, usually before they reach a hospital. Most of these patients develop *dysrhythmias*, which are irregularities in their heart's electrical activity, some of which can be immediately fatal. Common dysrhythmias associated with myocardial ischemia and sudden death are *ventricular fibrillation* or *ventricular tachycardia*. In ventricular fibrillation, no organized electrical activity occurs, and the myocardial muscle mass simply quivers, or fibrillates (**Figure 12-13**). Thus, no myocardial contraction takes place. Ventricular fibrillation can be effectively treated by defibrillation, which is the rapid application of an electrical countershock (**Figure 12-14**). Defibrillation stops the irregular electrical activity of the heart and allows the normal pacemaker of the heart to resume control. Defibrillator technology has evolved significantly. Now, portable defibrillators are completely automated and readily available. Persons who learn CPR and basic life support are now trained in the use of an automated defibrillator.

Reperfusion

One of the most significant advances in emergency medicine over the last decade has been the development of reperfusion therapy, which is the process of restoring blood flow through an occluded artery. This can be achieved with medications, surgery, or both. Initially limited to acute myocardial infarction, reperfusion therapy is being used now in the treatment of selected stroke patients and patients with large blood clots in the lungs (pulmonary emboli).

The 12-lead electrocardiogram (ECG) is a major tool in diagnosing acute coronary syndrome. It is also used to stratify, or triage, patients into one of three groups for treatment:

1. ST segment elevation or new left bundle branch block (LBBB)
2. ST segment depression (>1 millimeter) or T wave inversion
3. Nondiagnostic or normal ECG

Patients who have signs and symptoms consistent with acute coronary syndrome and have demonstrable high-risk ECG changes (ST segment elevation or new left bundle

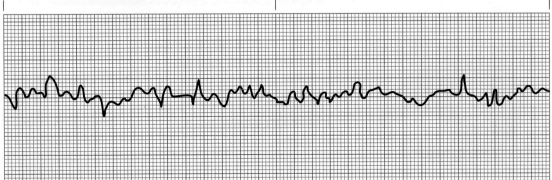

Figure 12-13 Physiology of Ventricular Fibrillation and ECG. Ventricular fibrillation is a lethal dysrhythmia where cells throughout the heart fire in an uncoordinated fashion, resulting in loss of the heart's pumping action.

Figure 12-14 EMS-Provided Defibrillation. Defibrillation can be life saving in the treatment of sudden death and acute coronary syndrome when complicated by ventricular fibrillation or ventricular tachycardia.

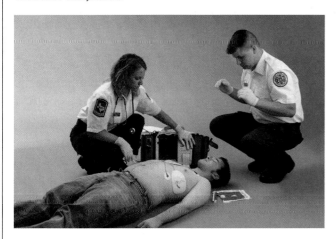

branch block) should be considered candidates for thrombolytic therapy. Patients who meet the screening criteria and whose symptoms have been present for six hours or less should receive thrombolytic therapy. The thrombolytic agent varies depending upon local recommendations. Regardless of the agent, the patient should be monitored for the development of adverse effects such as intracranial hemorrhage. In addition to thrombolytic agents, patients usually will receive aspirin, heparin (blood thinner), beta blockers, and nitroglycerin. The treatment is based upon the assessment of the patient's overall condition.

Patients who have signs and symptoms consistent with acute coronary syndrome and demonstrable moderate-risk ECG changes (ST segment depression or T wave inversion) should be considered as strongly suspicious for myocardial ischemia. These patients should be treated with heparin, aspirin, beta blockers, and nitroglycerin. Some patients in this category might benefit from glycoprotein IIb/IIIa inhibitors. These agents provide benefits beyond those of aspirin and heparin. A commonly used drug from this classification is abciximab (ReoPro). Aggrastat and Integrilin are also commonly used in the non-catheterization setting.

Finally, patients who have signs and symptoms consistent with acute coronary syndrome but do not have demonstrable ECG changes or have a normal ECG should receive aspirin and other therapy as appropriate. The concept of risk-stratification in acute coronary syndrome is designed to ensure that patients receive the best possible therapy as quickly as possible.

Revascularization

Following thrombolytic therapy, or when thrombolytic therapy is not indicated or is ineffective, patients should be referred for coronary angiography and possible interventional therapy. In many cases, emergent cardiac catheterization is superior to thrombolytic therapy. It allows visualization of the coronary artery anatomy including the degree and magnitude of vessel blockage.

While in the cardiac catheterization lab for coronary angiography, patients with atherosclerotic lesions and occlusions suitable for angioplasty can be treated. The process, called *percutaneous transluminal coronary angioplasty*, involves introducing a small catheter into the affected artery. An uninflated balloon catheter is placed at the site of the lesion, or lesions, and then inflated. This compresses the atheromatous plaque and increases the size of the vessel lumen. This procedure may need to be repeated several times until the artery remains open. If the vessel will not remain adequately open following balloon angioplasty, a metal stent can be placed at the site of the lesion. The metal stent is compressed for placement. Once placed, the stent is released and expands to hold back the plaque, which restores patency to the blood vessel. Other technologies, such as intraluminal lasers and rotary files that break down inflammatory and atheromatous plaques, are used occasionally.

Some patients have severe and diffuse atherosclerotic coronary artery disease. Their coronary angiograms reveal multiple regions of obstruction that make angioplasty impossible. These patients are evaluated for *coronary artery bypass grafting (CABG)*. CABG is a major procedure that requires that the sternum be split, the heart stopped (cardioplegia), and the patient placed on a bypass pump for the duration of the surgery. The medial aspect of the leg is opened and a part of the saphenous vein is harvested for the bypass grafts. The grafts are prepared and sewn into the aorta, just above the aortic valve. The distal end is then attached to the diseased coronary artery distal to the blockage. Some patients require multiple grafts. It is not uncommon to perform four or five grafts in one operation. In younger patients, arteries in the chest, such as the internal mammary artery, are used to provide blood to one of the new grafts. New technologies are making the surgical procedure less invasive, which shortens the patient's hospitalization and recovery period. In "keyhole surgery" a small camera and the necessary surgical instruments are introduced through several small incisions in the chest. This operation is referred to as "off pump" surgery because the entire procedure is performed while the heart remains beating. This significantly lessens the patient's pain and decreases the hospital stay because the patient has several small incisions instead of two large ones.

Contractile Cells

Contractile cells form the bulk of the heart's muscle tissue (about 99 percent of all cardiac muscle cells). In both cardiac muscle cells and skeletal muscle fibers, an action potential leads to the appearance of Ca^{2+} among the myofibrils, and Ca^{2+} binding to troponin on the thin filaments begins a contraction. However, skeletal and cardiac muscle cells differ in the duration of action potentials, the source of Ca^{2+}, and the duration of the resulting contraction.

What happens in cardiac muscle cells? The resting potential of a ventricular contractile cell is about -90 mV. An action potential begins when the plasma membrane of the ventricular muscle cell reaches threshold, usually about

−75 mV The typical stimulus is the excitation of an adjacent muscle cell. Once threshold has been reached, the action potential proceeds in three basic steps (**Figure 12-15a**):

❶ Rapid depolarization. At threshold, voltage-gated sodium channels open. The influx of sodium ions rapidly depolarizes the sarcolemma (plasma membrane). The sodium channels close when the membrane potential reaches a value between +20 and +30 mV.

❷ The plateau. A partial repolarization takes place as some K^+ leave the cell before most K^+ channels close. Voltage-gated calcium channels then open and *extracellular* calcium ions enter the cytosol. The calcium channels remain open for a relatively long period—roughly 175 ms. The inflow of positive charges (Ca^{2+}) and reduced outflow of K^+ delay repolarization, causing the membrane potential to remain near 0 mV for an extended period. This portion of the action

potential is called the *plateau*. The extracellular calcium ions initiate contraction, as well as delaying repolarization. Their increased concentration within the cell also triggers the release of Ca^{2+} from reserves in the sarcoplasmic reticulum (SR), which continue the contraction.

❸ Repolarization. As the plateau continues, calcium channels begin closing and potassium channels begin opening. As these channels open, potassium ions (K^+) rush out of the cell. The net result is a rapid repolarization that restores the resting potential.

In contrast, in a skeletal muscle fiber, the 10-msec action potential of a rapid depolarization is immediately followed by a rapid repolarization. This brief action potential ends as the related twitch contraction begins (**Figure 12-15b, top**). The twitch contraction is short and ends as the SR reclaims the Ca^{2+} it released.

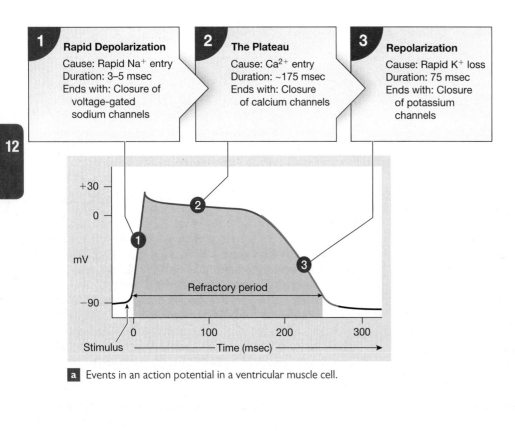

1 Rapid Depolarization	**2** The Plateau	**3** Repolarization
Cause: Rapid Na⁺ entry Duration: 3–5 msec Ends with: Closure of voltage-gated sodium channels	Cause: Ca²⁺ entry Duration: ~175 msec Ends with: Closure of calcium channels	Cause: Rapid K⁺ loss Duration: 75 msec Ends with: Closure of potassium channels

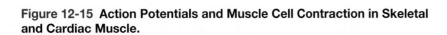

a Events in an action potential in a ventricular muscle cell.

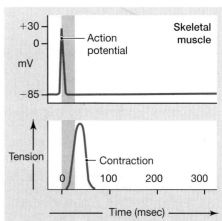

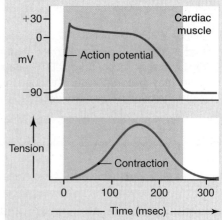

b Action potentials and twitch contractions in a skeletal muscle (above) and cardiac muscle (below). The shaded areas indicate the duration of the refractory periods.

Figure 12-15 Action Potentials and Muscle Cell Contraction in Skeletal and Cardiac Muscle.

In a cardiac muscle cell, the action potential is prolonged because Ca^{2+} continues to enter the cell throughout the plateau (**Figure 12-15b, bottom**). As a result, the period of muscle contraction continues until the plateau ends. As the calcium channels close, the intracellular calcium ions are absorbed by the SR or are pumped out of the cell, and the muscle cell relaxes.

The complete depolarization–repolarization process, or action potential, in a cardiac muscle cell lasts 250–300 msec, some 25–30 times as long as an action potential in a skeletal muscle fiber (**Figure 12-15b**). The membrane cannot respond to further stimulation until it repolarizes, so the refractory period of a cardiac muscle cell membrane is relatively long. For this reason, a normal cardiac muscle cell is limited to a maximum rate of about 200 contractions per minute.

In skeletal muscle fibers, the refractory period ends before the muscle fiber develops peak tension and relaxes. As a result, twitches can build on one another until tension reaches a sustained peak, a state called *tetanus.* ⟳ p. 205 In cardiac muscle cells, the refractory period continues until relaxation is under way. A summation of twitches is therefore not possible. Tetanic contractions cannot take place in a normal cardiac muscle cell, regardless of the frequency and intensity of stimulation. This feature is absolutely vital because a heart in tetany could not pump blood.

The Conducting System

Unlike skeletal muscle, cardiac muscle tissue contracts on its own, without neural or hormonal stimulation. This ability is called *automaticity*, or *autorhythmicity*. It is also characteristic of some types of smooth muscle tissue (discussed in Chapter 7). ⟳ p. 212

In the heart's normal pattern of activity, contractions follow a precise sequence: The atria contract first, followed by the ventricles. The heart's **conducting system** coordinates cardiac contractions. This system is a network of specialized cardiac muscle cells that initiates and distributes electrical impulses (**Figure 12-16a**). The network is made up of two types of cardiac muscle cells that do not contract, *nodal cells* and *conducting cells*. **Nodal cells** establish the rate of cardiac contraction. They are located at the *sinoatrial (SA)* and *atrioventricular (AV)* nodes. **Conducting cells** interconnect the two nodes and distribute the contractile stimulus throughout the myocardium. In the ventricles, the conducting cells include those in the *AV bundle* and the *bundle branches*, as well as the *Purkinje fibers*.

Nodal cells are unusual because their plasma membranes depolarize spontaneously and generate action potentials at regular intervals. Nodal cells are electrically coupled to one another, to conducting cells, and to normal cardiac muscle cells. As a result, when an action potential is initiated in a nodal cell, it sweeps through the conducting system. The signal reaches all of the cardiac muscle tissue and causes a coordinated contraction. In this way, nodal cells determine the heart rate.

Not all nodal cells depolarize at the same rate. The normal rate of contraction is established by **pacemaker cells**, the nodal cells that reach threshold first. These pacemaker cells are located in the **sinoatrial** (sī-nō-Ā-trē-al) **node (SA node)**, or *cardiac pacemaker*. It is a tissue mass embedded in the posterior wall of the right atrium near the entrance of the superior vena cava (**Figure 12-16a**). Pacemaker cells depolarize rapidly and spontaneously, generating 70–80 action potentials per minute. This results in a heart rate of 70–80 beats per minute (bpm).

Once the stimulus for a contraction is generated at the SA node, it must be distributed so that (1) the atria contract together, before the ventricles; and (2) the ventricles contract together, in a wave that begins at the apex and spreads toward the base. When the ventricles contract in this way, blood is pushed toward the base of the heart into the aorta and pulmonary trunk.

The cells of the SA node are electrically connected to those of the larger **atrioventricular** (ā-trē-ō-ven-TRIK-ū-lar) **node** by conducting cells in the atrial walls (**Figure 12-16a**). The AV nodal cells also depolarize spontaneously, but they generate only 40–60 action potentials per minute. Under normal circumstances, before an AV cell depolarizes to threshold spontaneously, it is stimulated by an action potential generated by the SA node. However, if the AV node does not receive this action potential, it will then become the pacemaker of the heart and establish a heart rate of 40–60 beats per minute.

The AV node is located in the floor of the right atrium near the opening of the coronary sinus. From there the action potentials travel to the **AV bundle**, also known as the *bundle of His* (pronounced *hiss*). This bundle of conducting cells extends along the interventricular septum before dividing into **left** and **right bundle branches**. These branches extend to the apex of the heart, turn, and radiate across the inner surfaces of the left and right ventricles. Then specialized **Purkinje** (pur-KIN-jē) **fibers** (*Purkinje cells*) convey the impulses to the contractile cells of the ventricular myocardium.

12

Figure 12-16 The Conducting System of the Heart.

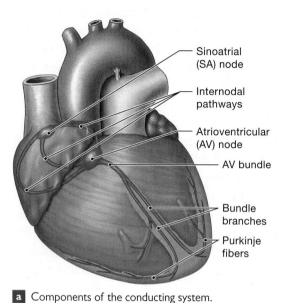

Sinoatrial (SA) node

Internodal pathways

Atrioventricular (AV) node

AV bundle

Bundle branches

Purkinje fibers

a Components of the conducting system.

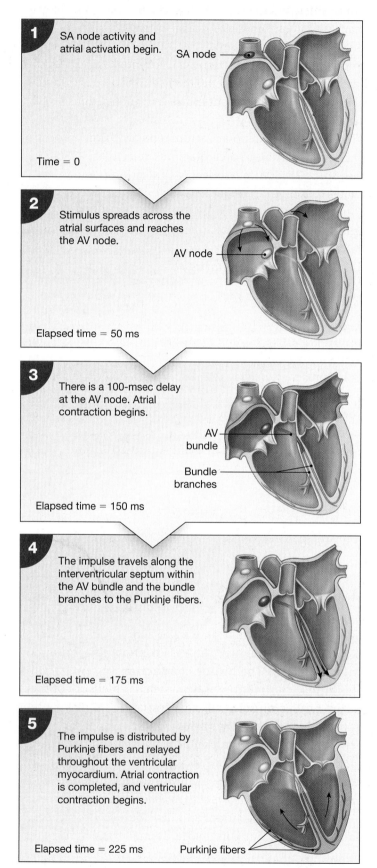

1 SA node activity and atrial activation begin.

SA node

Time = 0

2 Stimulus spreads across the atrial surfaces and reaches the AV node.

AV node

Elapsed time = 50 ms

3 There is a 100-msec delay at the AV node. Atrial contraction begins.

AV bundle

Bundle branches

Elapsed time = 150 ms

4 The impulse travels along the interventricular septum within the AV bundle and the bundle branches to the Purkinje fibers.

Elapsed time = 175 ms

5 The impulse is distributed by Purkinje fibers and relayed throughout the ventricular myocardium. Atrial contraction is completed, and ventricular contraction begins.

Elapsed time = 225 ms   Purkinje fibers

b The stimulus for contraction is conducted through the heart in a predictable sequence of events (steps 1–5).

The path of an impulse from its initiation at the SA node through the heart is shown in **Figure 12-16b**. Atrial activation begins at the SA node (**Figure 12-16b ①**). It takes an action potential roughly 50 msec to travel from the SA node to the AV node over the conducting pathways. Along the way, the conducting cells pass the contractile stimulus to cardiac muscle cells of the right and left atria. The action potential then spreads across the atrial surfaces through cell-to-cell contact (**Figure 12-16b ②**). The stimulus affects only the atria because the cardiac skeleton electrically isolates the atria from the ventricles everywhere except at the AV bundle. ↻ p. 412

At the AV node, the impulse slows down. Another 100 msec pass before it reaches the AV bundle (**Figure 12-16b ③**). This delay is important because the atria must be contracting, and blood must be moving, before the ventricles are stimulated. Once the impulse enters the AV bundle, it flashes down the interventricular septum, along the bundle branches, and into the ventricular myocardium along the Purkinje fibers (**Figure 12-16b ④**). Within 75 msec, the stimulus to begin a contraction reaches all of the ventricular muscle cells (**Figure 12-16b ⑤**).

Abnormal pacemaker function can cause a number of clinical problems. **Bradycardia** (brād-ē-KAR-dē-uh; *bradys,* slow) is a condition in which the heart rate is slower than normal (less than 60 bpm). **Tachycardia** (tak-ē-KAR-dē-uh; *tachys,* swift) is a faster than normal heart rate (100 bpm or more). In some cases, an abnormal conducting cell or ventricular muscle cell may begin generating action potentials so rapidly that they override those of the SA or AV node. The origin of such abnormal signals is called an **ectopic (ek-TOP-ik; out of place) pacemaker**. The action potentials may completely bypass the conducting system and disrupt the timing of ventricular contractions. Such conditions are commonly diagnosed with the aid of an *electrocardiogram,* which we discuss next.

CLINICAL NOTE

Defibrillation

Defibrillation is used to treat life-threatening dysrhythmias such as ventricular fibrillation and nonperfusing ventricular tachycardia. Defibrillation is the delivery of sufficient electrical energy to the heart to depolarize the myocardial muscle mass and at the same time causes minimal electrical injury to the heart. This allows a pacemaker cell within the heart to resume its rhythmic firing, and restores a normal electrical pattern. A shock will not terminate the dysrhythmia if the energy or current is too low. Functional and structural damage to the heart can occur if the energy or current are too high.

When first developed, defibrillators were extremely large units that operated on standard electrical current. These older units used alternating current (AC) and were limited to hospitals. In the 1970s, portable defibrillators that could be used in the prehospital setting were developed. These units utilized direct current (DC) but were extremely heavy and bulky, often weighing 40 pounds or

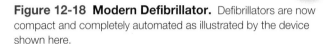

Figure 12-18 Modern Defibrillator. Defibrillators are now compact and completely automated as illustrated by the device shown here.

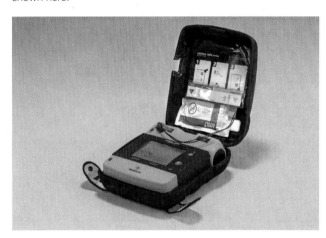

more (**Figure 12-17**). Battery technology was limited and the unit required recharging immediately after use. Now, defibrillators are available that are approximately the size of a notebook. Many are completely automated, which allows use by nonmedical personnel (**Figure 12-18**).

Technology has also allowed the development of a defibrillator unit that can be permanently implanted in patients deemed at risk for life-threatening dysrhythmias. These devices, referred to as *implanted automatic cardioverter-defibrillators (IACDs)*, have become the treatment of choice for sudden cardiac death. They have reduced mortality from 30 to 45 percent per year to less than 2 percent per year. The IACD consists of a pulse generator, a lead system with both sensing and shocking electrodes, integrated circuitry to analyze the cardiac rhythm and trigger defibrillation, and a power supply. The life span of these units is approximately eight years depending upon the frequency of discharge.

Today, there are three general types of external defibrillators: automated external defibrillators (AEDs), semi-automated external defibrillators (SAEDs), and manual defibrillators. Automated units simply require application of the electrodes and turning on the device. Semi-automated units require that the operator press a button to deliver the electrical shock as directed by the device. These extremely automated units are designed for use by first

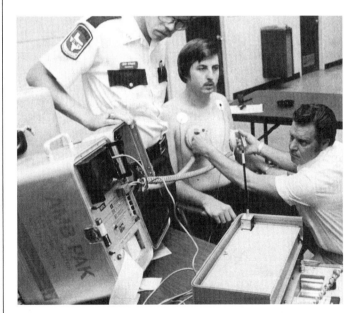

Figure 12-17 Early Portable Defibrillator. Defibrillator and EMS technology has evolved significantly. This 1975 photo shows a portable defibrillator/monitor that weighed nearly 40 pounds. The large device at the bottom of the screen is a Motorola Apcor radio modified to operate as a mobile telephone.

(Continued)

12

responders and nonmedical personnel. Most airlines now carry automated external defibrillators on flights longer than three hours. Soon, all large commercial passenger aircraft will carry these devices. The manual units are designed for use by trained medical personnel. They usually have several other features including continuous cardiac monitoring, synchronized cardioversion, hardcopy recording, and external cardiac pacing. Newer units allow recording and monitoring of a 12-lead ECG. They also contain a diagnostic module that provides a computerized interpretation of the ECG tracing.

The ability to defibrillate a fibrillating heart depends primarily on the electrical current delivered to the myocardium. All modern defibrillators use direct current (DC) and store the energy in a capacitor that discharges when triggered by the operator. Factors that impede the flow of energy to the myocardium include resistance to current flow by the chest wall (transthoracic impedance) and internal loss of energy within the defibrillator. The current delivered to the myocardium is a function of the energy delivered by the defibrillator, the electrical impedance within the device and chest, and the duration of current flow:

$$\text{Energy} = \text{current} \times \text{impedance} \times \text{duration}$$

$$(\text{Joules} = \text{amperes} \times \text{ohms} \times \text{seconds})$$

An increase in either current or duration will increase the energy. An increase in transthoracic impedance (resistance to current flow) will reduce the delivered current.

Modern defibrillators deliver energy, or current, in waveforms. The energy levels vary with the type of device and type of waveform it uses. Modern defibrillators use two types of waveforms: monophasic and biphasic (**Figure 12-19**). For years the standard DC waveform was monophasic, and delivered current in one direction only. Biphasic waveforms, in contrast, deliver current that flows in a positive direction for a specific duration and then flows in a negative direction for the remaining millisecond of the electrical discharge. A biphasic waveform has been demonstrated to be superior in patients who have implantable cardioverter-defibrillators. However, research has not determined whether a biphasic waveform provides any advantage in external defibrillators. The recommended energy settings for defibrillation with a monophasic-type machine start at 200 Joules, then increase to 300 Joules with the second shock,

Figure 12-19 Examples of Defibrillator Waveforms. The top waveform is monophasic, the lower waveform is biphasic. With a biphasic waveform, current travels in a positive direction for the first part of the energy delivery and then in a negative direction for the remainder.

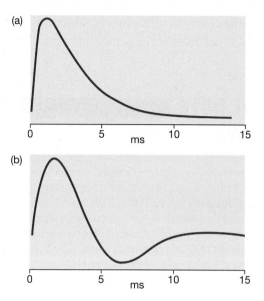

and increase again to 360 Joules with the third and subsequent shocks. The optimum energy for biphasic-type machines has not been clearly identified.

Many of the manual defibrillator/monitors can provide synchronized cardioversion. This technology, monitors the patient's ECG, electronically marks the QRS complex, and triggers the shock at precisely the proper time in the cardiac cycle to depolarize the heart. Because the shock targets the vulnerable period, the amount of energy needed to depolarize the myocardium is markedly less. The electrical events in the heart are powerful enough to be detected by electrodes placed on the body surface. A recording of these events is an **electrocardiogram** (ē-lek-trō-KAR-dē-ō-gram), also called an **ECG** or **EKG**. Each time the heart beats, a wave of depolarization spreads through the atria, pauses at the AV node, then travels down the interventricular septum to the apex, turns, and spreads through the ventricular myocardium toward the base.

An ECG combines information obtained from electrodes placed at different locations on the body surface. Clinicians can use an ECG to assess the performance of specific nodal, conducting, and contractile components. When a portion of the heart has been damaged by a heart attack, for example, the ECG will reveal an abnormal pattern of impulse conduction.

The appearance of the ECG tracing varies with the placement of the monitoring electrodes, or *leads*. The important features of an electrocardiogram as analyzed with the leads in one of the standard configurations are shown in **Figure 12-20**:

- A small **P wave** accompanies the depolarization of the atria. The atria begin contracting about 25 msec after the start of the P wave.

- A **QRS complex** appears as the ventricles depolarize. This electrical signal is relatively strong because the mass of the ventricular muscle is much larger than that of the atria. The ventricles begin contracting shortly after the peak of the R wave.

- A smaller **T wave** indicates ventricular repolarization. Atrial repolarization is not apparent because it takes place while the ventricles are depolarizing, and the QRS complex masks the electrical events.

Analyzing an ECG involves measuring the size of the voltage changes and determining the temporal (time) relationships of the various components. Attention usually focuses on the amount of depolarization occurring during the P wave and the QRS complex. For example, a smaller than normal electrical signal can mean that the mass of the heart muscle has decreased. In contrast, excessively strong depolarizations can mean that the heart muscle has become enlarged.

The times between waves are reported as *segments* and *intervals*. Segments generally extend from the end of one wave to the start of another. Intervals are more variable, but always include at least one entire wave. Commonly used segments and intervals are labeled in **Figure 12-20b**. The names, however, can be somewhat misleading. For example:

● The **P–R interval** extends from the start of atrial depolarization to the start of the QRS complex (ventricular depolarization) rather than to R, because in abnormal ECGs

Figure 12-20 An Electrocardiogram.

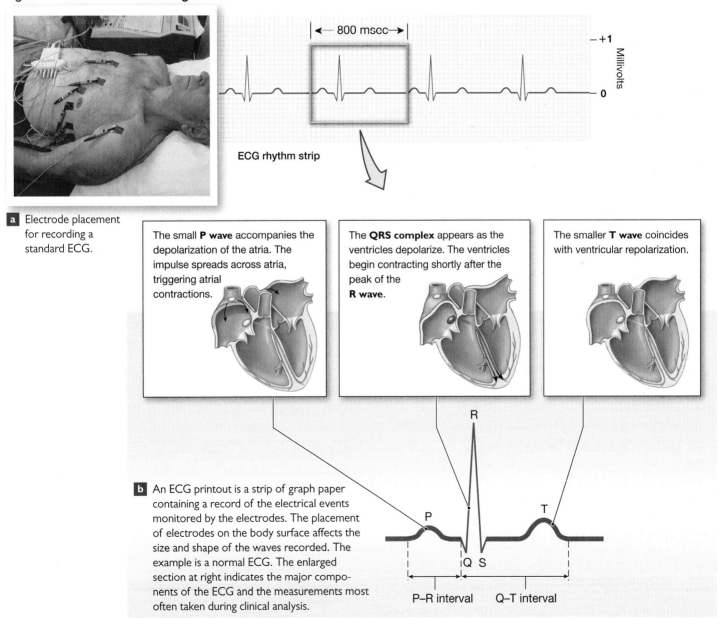

a Electrode placement for recording a standard ECG.

b An ECG printout is a strip of graph paper containing a record of the electrical events monitored by the electrodes. The placement of electrodes on the body surface affects the size and shape of the waves recorded. The example is a normal ECG. The enlarged section at right indicates the major components of the ECG and the measurements most often taken during clinical analysis.

the peak at R can be difficult to determine. Extension of the P–R interval to more than 200 msec can indicate damage to the conducting pathways or AV node.

- The **Q–T interval** indicates the time required for the ventricles to undergo a single cycle of depolarization and repolarization. It is usually measured from the end of the P–R interval rather than from the bottom of the Q wave. The Q–T interval can be lengthened by electrolyte disturbances, some medications, conduction problems, *coronary ischemia* (inadequate blood supply to the heart), or myocardial damage. A congenital heart defect that can cause sudden death without warning may be detectable as a prolonged Q–T interval.

Electrocardiogram analysis is useful in detecting and diagnosing **cardiac arrhythmias** (ā-RITH-mē-az), abnormal patterns of cardiac activity. Momentary arrhythmias are not inherently dangerous, and about 5 percent of the normal population experiences a few abnormal heartbeats each day. Clinical problems appear when the arrhythmias reduce the heart's pumping efficiency. Serious arrhythmias can indicate damage to the myocardium, injuries to the pacemaker or conduction pathways, exposure to drugs, or variations in the electrolyte composition of the extracellular fluids.

CHECKPOINT

4. How does the fact that cardiac muscle does not undergo tetanus (as skeletal muscle does) affect the functioning of the heart?

5. If the cells of the SA node did not function, how would the heart rate be affected?

6. Why is it important for impulses from the atria to be delayed at the AV node before they pass into the ventricles?

7. What might cause an increase in the size of the QRS complex in an electrocardiogram?

See the blue Answers tab at the back of the book.

12-3 Events during a complete heartbeat make up a cardiac cycle

Learning Objective Explain the events of the cardiac cycle, and relate the heart sounds to specific events in this cycle.

A brief resting phase follows each heartbeat. It allows time for the chambers to relax and prepare for the next heartbeat. The period between the start of one heartbeat and the start

of the next is a single **cardiac cycle** (Figure 12-21). It includes alternating periods of contraction and relaxation. For any one chamber of the heart, the cardiac cycle can be divided into two phases. During contraction, or **systole** (SIS-tō-lē), the chamber squeezes blood into an adjacent chamber or into an arterial trunk. Systole is followed by relaxation, or **diastole** (dī-AS-tō-lē). During diastole, the chamber fills with blood and prepares for the start of the next cardiac cycle.

Fluids move from an area of higher pressure to one of lower pressure. During the cardiac cycle, the pressure within each chamber rises during systole and falls during diastole. An increase in pressure in one chamber causes the blood to flow to another chamber (or vessel) where the pressure is lower. The atrioventricular and semilunar valves ensure that blood flows in one direction only during the cardiac cycle.

The correct pressure relationships among the heart chambers depend on the careful timing of contractions. The pacemaking and conduction systems normally provide the required interval of time between atrial systole and ventricular systole. If the atria and ventricles were to contract simultaneously, blood could not leave the atria because the AV valves would be closed. In the normal heart, atrial systole and atrial diastole are slightly out of phase with ventricular systole and diastole.

CLINICAL NOTE

Emergency Cardiac Care

Emergency cardiac care (ECC) is a comprehensive system designed to deal with sudden, often life-threatening events that affect the cardiovascular, cerebrovascular, and respiratory systems. ECC specifically includes:

1. Recognition of the early warning signs of a heart attack and stroke, efforts to prevent complications, reassurance of the victim, activation of the EMS system, and prompt availability of monitoring equipment.
2. Provision of immediate basic life support (BLS) and cardiopulmonary resuscitation (CPR) at the scene when needed.
3. Provision of advanced cardiac life support at the scene as quickly as possible to defibrillate if necessary and to stabilize the victim prior to transport.
4. Transfer of the stabilized victim to a hospital where definitive cardiac care can be provided.

The key link in the ECC system is the layperson who recognizes the medical emergency, summons EMS, and provides initial CPR and other BLS measures.

Advanced prehospital care and paramedic practice were first developed to treat life-threatening cardiac emergencies. Now, in addition to ECC, paramedics treat all types of medical and traumatic emergencies and provide effective on-scene stabilization.

Figure 12-21 The Cardiac Cycle. Thin black arrows indicate blood flow, and green arrows indicate contractions. Times noted in the figure are for a heart rate of 75 bpm.

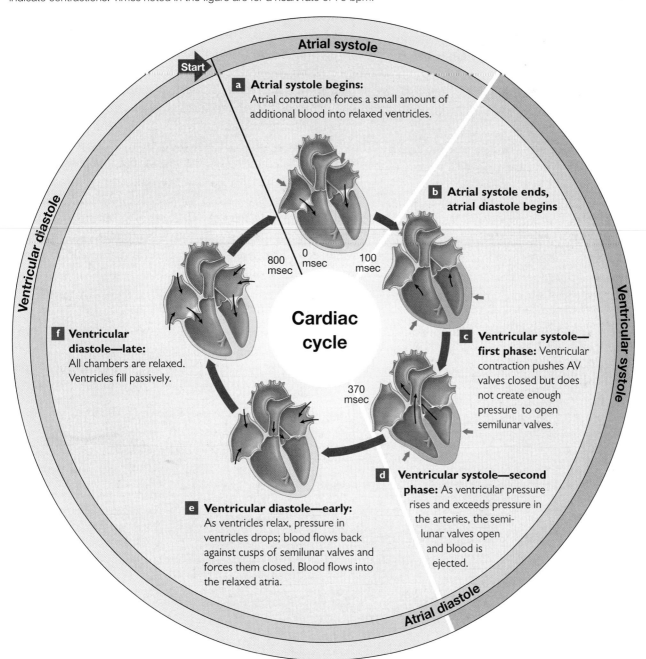

Phases of the Cardiac Cycle

The phases of the cardiac cycle—atrial systole, atrial diastole, ventricular systole, and ventricular diastole—are diagrammed in **Figure 12-21** for a heart rate of 75 bpm. When the cardiac cycle begins, all four chambers are relaxed, the atria are filled with blood, and the ventricles are partially filled with blood.

The cardiac cycle begins with atrial systole. During this phase, the atria contract, completely filling the ventricles with blood (**Figure 12-21a**). Atrial systole lasts 100 msec. As atrial systole ends, atrial diastole and ventricular systole begin (**Figure 12-21b**). As pressures in the ventricles rise above those in the atria, the AV valves swing shut (**Figure 12-21c**). But blood cannot begin moving into the arterial trunks until ventricular pressures exceed the arterial pressures. At this point, the blood pushes open the semilunar valves and flows into the aorta and pulmonary trunk (**Figure 12-21d**). This blood flow continues for the duration of ventricular systole, and lasts approximately 270 msec in a resting adult.

The heart then enters ventricular diastole. This phase lasts 530 msec (the 430 msec remaining in this cardiac cycle, plus the first 100 msec of the next when the atria are contracting (**Figure 12-21e**). When ventricular diastole begins, ventricular pressures decline rapidly. As they fall below the pressures of the arterial trunks, the semilunar valves close. Ventricular pressures continue to drop. As they fall below atrial pressures, the AV valves open and blood flows from the atria into the ventricles. Both atria and ventricles are now relaxed in diastole. Blood now flows from the major veins through the relaxed atria and into the ventricles (**Figure 12-21f**).

By the time atrial systole marks the start of another cardiac cycle, the ventricles are roughly 70 percent filled. Atrial systole actually makes a relatively minor contribution to ventricular volume. This fact explains why individuals can survive quite normally when their atria have been so severely damaged that they can no longer function. In contrast, damage to one or both ventricles can leave the heart unable to maintain adequate blood flow. A condition of *heart failure* then exists. In this condition, the heart weakens and peripheral tissues suffer from oxygen and nutrient deprivation.

Heart Sounds

Clinicians use a **stethoscope** to listen for normal and abnormal heart sounds. There are four **heart sounds**, named S_1 through S_4 (**Figure 12-22**). If you listen to your own heart with a stethoscope, you hear the familiar "lubb-dupp" that accompanies each heartbeat. These two sounds (S_1 and S_2) come from the actions of the heart valves. The *first heart sound* ("lubb") is produced as the AV valves close and the semilunar valves open. It marks the start of ventricular systole and lasts a little longer than the second sound. The *second heart sound*, "dupp," occurs at the beginning of ventricular diastole, when the semilunar valves close. *Third* and *fourth heart sounds* (S_3 and S_4) may be audible as well, but they are usually very faint. They are seldom detectable in healthy adults. These sounds are associated with atrial contraction and blood flowing into the ventricles rather than with valve action.

CHECKPOINT

8. Provide the alternative terms for the contraction and relaxation of heart chambers.

9. Is the heart always pumping blood when pressure in the left ventricle is rising? Explain.

10. What events cause the "lubb-dupp" heart sounds as heard with a stethoscope?

See the blue Answers tab at the back of the book.

12

Figure 12-22 Heart Sounds.

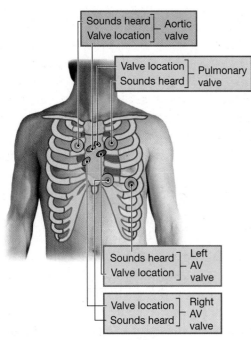

a Placements of a stethoscope for listening to the different sounds produced by individual valves.

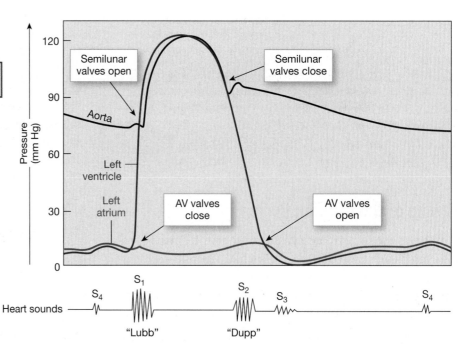

b The relationship between heart sounds and key events in the cardiac cycle.

CLINICAL NOTE

Blunt Myocardial Injury

Blunt trauma to the myocardium can result in injuries that range from contusions to concussion. In a myocardial contusion, blunt trauma to the anterior chest transmits energy to the underlying heart. The most common cause of blunt myocardial injury is high-speed motor-vehicle collisions, often with crushing of the steering wheel. This can result in focal myocardial edema, interstitial hemorrhage, and occasionally subendocardial hemorrhage. The portions of the heart most frequently affected are the anterior right ventricular wall, the anterior interventricular septum, and the anterior/apical aspect of the left ventricle.

A myocardial contusion usually causes chest pain similar to that seen in angina pectoris. There is often tachycardia associated with rhythm and conduction disturbances. Severe injuries can cause a reduction in cardiac output. Myocardial contusions can cause abnormalities in the ECG such as ST segment elevation in the leads over the injured myocardium. In some cases, an elevation of cardiac enzymes is often seen. Most patients who sustain a myocardial contusion have complete recovery within three to six weeks.

Commotio Cordis

A *myocardial concussion*, often called *commotio cordis*, is a blow to the myocardium where no obvious gross or microscopic injury can be found. However, the patient can develop a life-threatening dysrhythmia, such as ventricular fibrillation, and die. Myocardial concussion usually results from a direct force to the chest, often a seemingly minor blow during sporting activities. The sports most frequently associated with *commotio cordis* are karate, hockey, softball, and baseball. Young male athletes aged 5–18 years are particularly at risk for this catastrophe. Death is usually instantaneous. In animal models, *commotio cordis* has been reproduced. The patient develops ventricular fibrillation immediately upon impact. The chest impact must fall within the vulnerable period of the cardiac cycle (during repolarization just before peaking of the T wave) to induce ventricular fibrillation. Successful resuscitation has been documented with prompt defibrillation, cardiopulmonary resuscitation, or application of a precordial thump. *Commotio cordis* is an extremely rare cause of death. The personal, physiological, and cardiovascular benefits of athletics far outweigh the risks. When possible, protective pads and similar devices should be used by those who are at increased risk.

12-4 Heart dynamics examines the factors that affect cardiac output

Learning Objective Define cardiac output, describe the factors that influence heart rate and stroke volume, and explain how adjustments in stroke volume and cardiac output are coordinated at different levels of physical activity.

The term *heart dynamics*, or *cardiodynamics*, refers to the movements and forces generated during cardiac contractions. Each time the heart beats, the two ventricles eject equal amounts of blood. **Stroke volume (SV)** is the amount of blood ejected by a ventricle during a single beat. The stroke volume can vary from beat to beat, so physicians are often more interested in the **cardiac output (CO)**, or the amount of blood pumped by the left ventricle in 1 minute. Cardiac output provides an indication of the blood flow through peripheral tissues. Adequate blood flow is needed to maintain homeostasis.

We can calculate cardiac output by multiplying the heart rate (HR) by the average stroke volume (SV):

$$\underset{\substack{\text{cardiac output} \\ \text{(mL/min)}}}{\text{CO}} = \underset{\substack{\text{heart rate} \\ \text{(beats/min)}}}{\text{HR}} \times \underset{\substack{\text{stroke volume} \\ \text{(mL/beat)}}}{\text{SV}}$$

For example, if the heart rate is 75 beats per minute (bpm) and the average stroke volume is 80 mL per beat, the cardiac output will be:

$$\begin{aligned} \text{CO} &= 75 \text{ beats/min} \times 80 \text{ mL/beat} \\ &= 6000 \text{ mL/min (6 L/min)} \end{aligned}$$

This value represents a cardiac output that equals the total volume of blood of an average adult every minute. Cardiac output is highly variable, however, because a normal heart can increase both its rate of contraction and its stroke volume. When necessary, stroke volume in a normal heart can almost double. The heart rate can increase by 250 percent. When both increase together, the cardiac output can increase by 500–700 percent, or up to 30 liters per minute.

Cardiac output is precisely regulated so that peripheral tissues receive an adequate blood supply under a variety of conditions. The primary factors that regulate cardiac output often affect both heart rate and stroke volume at the same time. These factors include *blood volume reflexes, autonomic innervation*, and *hormones*. Secondary factors include various drugs, the concentration of ions in the extracellular fluid, and body temperature (see the Clinical Note "Abnormal Conditions Affecting Cardiac Output").

Blood Volume Reflexes

Cardiac muscle contraction is an active process, but relaxation is entirely passive. The force needed to return cardiac muscle to its precontracted length comes from the blood

CLINICAL NOTE

Abnormal Conditions Affecting Cardiac Output

The SA node sets the basic rhythm of heart contraction, but various drugs, abnormal variations in extracellular ion concentrations, and changes in body temperature can alter this rhythm. Several drugs, including caffeine and nicotine, have a stimulating effect that causes an increase in heart rate. Caffeine acts directly on the conducting system. It increases the rate of depolarization at the SA node. Nicotine directly stimulates the activity of sympathetic neurons that innervate the heart.

Disorders affecting ion concentrations can affect cardiac output by changing the stroke volume, the heart rate, or both. Changes in extracellular calcium ion concentrations mainly affect the strength and duration of cardiac contractions, and thus stroke volume. If these calcium concentrations are elevated, the condition is called hypercalcemia. Cardiac muscle cells become extremely excitable, and their contractions become powerful and prolonged. In extreme cases, the heart goes into an extended state of contraction that is usually fatal. When

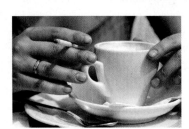

calcium levels are abnormally low, the condition is called hypocalcemia. Contractions become very weak and may stop altogether.

Abnormal extracellular potassium ion concentrations can change heart rate. They do so by altering the resting membrane potential of nodal cells at the SA node. When potassium concentrations are high in hyperkalemia, cardiac contractions become weak and irregular. When the potassium levels are abnormally low in hypokalemia, heart rate is slowed.

Temperature changes also affect metabolic operations throughout the body. For example, a lowered body temperature slows the rate of depolarization at the SA node, lowers heart rate, and reduces the strength of cardiac contractions. (In open-heart surgery, the exposed heart may be deliberately chilled until it stops beating.) An elevated body temperature increases heart rate and contractile force—one reason why your heart seems to race and pound when you have a fever.

pouring into the heart, aided by the elasticity of the cardiac skeleton. As a result, there is a direct relationship between the amount of blood entering the heart and the amount of blood ejected during the next contraction.

Two heart reflexes respond to changes in blood volume. One of these occurs in the right atrium and affects heart rate. The other is a ventricular reflex that affects stroke volume.

The **atrial reflex** (*Bainbridge reflex*) adjusts heart rate in response to an increase in the **venous return**, the flow of venous blood into the heart. Venous return varies in response to alterations in cardiac output, peripheral circulation, and other factors that affect the rate of blood flow through the venae cavae. How does the atrial reflex work? The entry of blood stimulates stretch receptors in the right atrial walls. This triggers a reflexive increase in heart rate through increased sympathetic activity. As a result of sympathetic stimulation, the cells of the SA node depolarize faster and heart rate increases.

The amount of blood pumped out of a ventricle with each heartbeat (the stroke volume) depends not only on venous return but also on the **filling time**—the duration of ventricular diastole, when blood can flow into the ventricles. Filling time depends primarily on the heart rate. The faster the heart rate, the shorter the filling time.

Over the range of normal activities, the greater the volume of blood entering the ventricles, the more powerful the contraction and the greater the stroke volume. In a resting individual, venous return is relatively low and the walls are not stretched much. As a result, the ventricles develop little power, and stroke volume is low. What happens if venous return suddenly increases (that is, more blood flows into the heart)? The myocardium stretches farther, the ventricles produce greater force upon contraction, and stroke volume increases.

This general rule of "more in = more out" is known as the **Frank–Starling principle**. It is named for the physiologists who first demonstrated the relationship. Its major effect is that the output of blood from the left and right ventricles is balanced under a variety of conditions.

Autonomic Innervation

As we have noted, the pacemaker cells of the SA node establish the basic heart rate. However, the autonomic nervous system (ANS) can modify this heart rate. Both the sympathetic and parasympathetic divisions of the ANS innervate the heart (**Figure 12-23**). Postganglionic sympathetic fibers extend from neuron cell bodies located in the cervical and upper thoracic ganglia. The vagus nerves (N X) carry parasympathetic preganglionic fibers to small ganglia near the heart. Both ANS divisions innervate the SA and AV nodes and atrial muscle cells. Both also innervate ventricular muscle cells, but sympathetic fibers far outnumber parasympathetic fibers.

12

Figure 12-23 Autonomic Innervation of the Heart.

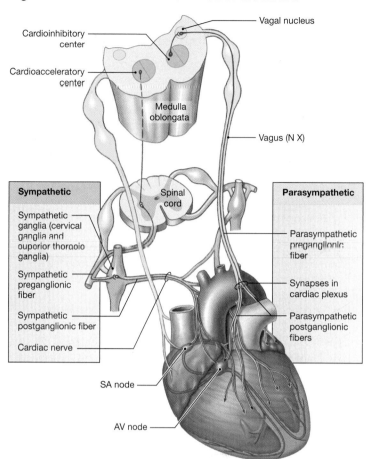

Autonomic Effects on Heart Rate

Autonomic effects on heart rate primarily reflect the responses of the SA node to acetylcholine (ACh) and to norepinephrine (NE). ACh released by parasympathetic motor neurons lowers the heart rate. NE released by sympathetic neurons increases the heart rate. A more sustained rise in heart rate follows the release of epinephrine (E) and NE by the adrenal medullae during sympathetic activation.

Autonomic Effects on Stroke Volume

The ANS also affects stroke volume by altering *contractility*, the amount of force produced during a contraction. The ANS does so through the release of NE, E, and ACh:

- ***NE and E increase contractility.*** The sympathetic release of NE at synapses in the myocardium and the release of NE and E by the adrenal medullae stimulate cardiac muscle cell metabolism. This change increases the force of ventricular contraction. The result is an increase in stroke volume.

![Build Your Knowledge]

Build Your Knowledge

Recall that the autonomic nervous system (ANS) is an efferent division of the peripheral nervous system (PNS). It carries motor commands from the central nervous system (CNS) to cardiac muscle, smooth muscle, and glands (as you saw in **Chapter 8: The Nervous System**). The motor commands of the ANS occur outside our conscious awareness. The ANS motor neurons in the CNS are known as preganglionic neurons. Their axons synapse on ganglionic neurons in PNS ganglia. The axons of the ganglionic neurons are called postganglionic fibers. The ANS includes a sympathetic division and a parasympathetic division, which commonly have opposite effects. ⟲ **p. 289**

CLINICAL NOTE

The Denervated Heart

Cardiac transplantation is now a fairly common procedure; many transplants last 15–20 years with proper care. It is important to remember that the transplanted heart is a denervated heart. That is, when the heart is removed from the donor, the autonomic nerves that control the heart are severed and cannot be reattached upon transplant into the recipient. Thus, there is no nervous control of the transplanted heart although there is evidence that some nervous control develops over time in a small percentage of patients.

In the transplanted heart, the resting heart rate is controlled by the heart's intrinsic pacemaker system and the autonomic nervous system through hormonal influence. This delicate balance keeps the heart functioning at the appropriate rate. Also, the modification of these systems is responsible for the change in heart rate in the appropriate direction. It has been shown that the parasympathetic nervous system is the major controlling factor in the resting state. Early after transplantation, the rate must be supported by administered drugs (chronotropes) or pacing. Later, circulating endogenous catecholamines support the resting heart rate. In the transplanted denervated heart, the resting rate is faster than normal due to the loss of parasympathetic inhibition.

The transplanted heart responds to exercise as expected by increasing its rate. However, the rate of increase is delayed just as the decrease of heart rate. The mechanism implicated in the increase of heart rate is the release of catecholamines from the peripheral nervous system.

12

- ***ACh decreases contractility.*** The primary effect of parasympathetic ACh release is inhibition, causing the force of cardiac contractions to decrease. The greatest reduction in contractile force takes place in the atria, because parasympathetic innervation is relatively limited in the ventricles. The result is a decrease in stroke volume.

Both autonomic divisions are normally active at a steady background level, releasing ACh and NE both at the nodes and into the myocardium. Thus, cutting the vagus nerves increases heart rate, and sympathetic blocking agents slow heart rate. Through dual innervation and adjustments in autonomic tone, the ANS can make very delicate adjustments in cardiovascular function.

The Coordination of Autonomic Activity

The *cardiac center* of the medulla oblongata contains the autonomic headquarters for cardiac control. ⮌ p. 278 It includes sympathetic and parasympathetic centers. The **cardioacceleratory center** controls sympathetic motor neurons that increase heart rate. The adjacent **cardioinhibitory center** controls the parasympathetic motor neurons that slow heart rate (**Figure 12-23**). Information about the status of the cardiovascular system arrives at the cardiac center over visceral sensory fibers accompanying the vagus nerves and the sympathetic nerves of the cardiac plexus.

The cardiac center responds to changes in blood pressure and in the arterial concentrations of dissolved oxygen and carbon dioxide. These changes are monitored by baroreceptors and chemoreceptors innervated by the glossopharyngeal (N IX) and vagus nerves. A decline in blood pressure or oxygen concentrations or an increase in carbon dioxide levels usually means that the oxygen demands of peripheral tissues have increased. The cardiac center then calls for an increase in cardiac output, and the heart works harder.

Build Your Knowledge

Recall that the medulla oblongata is the region of the brain that is attached to the spinal cord (as you saw in **Chapter 8: The Nervous System**). One of its roles is to relay sensory information to the thalamus and other brain stem centers. It also contains major centers that regulate autonomic function, such as heart rate, blood pressure, respiration, and digestive activities. ⮌ p. 268

CLINICAL NOTE

Extracellular Ions, Temperature, and Cardiac Output

Changes in extracellular calcium ion concentrations primarily affect the strength and duration of cardiac contractions and, thus, stroke volume. If such calcium concentrations are elevated *(hypercalcemia)*, cardiac muscle cells become extremely excitable, and their contractions become powerful and prolonged. In extreme cases, the heart goes into an extended state of contraction that is usually fatal. When calcium levels are abnormally low *(hypocalcemia)*, the contractions become very weak and may cease altogether.

Abnormal extracellular potassium ion concentrations alter the resting potential at the SA node and primarily change the heart rate. When potassium concentrations are high *(hyperkalemia)*, cardiac contractions become weak and irregular. When the extracellular concentration of potassium is abnormally low *(hypokalemia)*, heart rate is reduced.

Temperature changes affect metabolic operations throughout the body. For example, a lowered body temperature slows the rate of depolarization at the SA node, lowers the heart rate, and reduces the strength of cardiac contractions. An elevated body temperature accelerates the heart rate and the contractile force—one reason why your heart seems to race and pound when you have a fever.

In addition to making automatic adjustments in response to sensory information, the cardiac center can be influenced by higher centers, especially centers in the hypothalamus. For this reason, changes in emotional state (such as rage, fear, or arousal) have an immediate effect on heart rate.

Hormones

Recall that E and NE secreted by the adrenal medullae act to increase both heart rate and force of contraction. Thyroid hormones and glucagon also act to increase heart rate and force of contraction. Before synthetic drugs were available, glucagon was widely used to stimulate heart function.

Various drugs that affect the contractility of the heart have been developed for use in cardiac emergencies and to treat heart disease. Drugs that act by increasing the Ca^{2+} concentration within cardiac muscle cells, such as *digitalis* and related drugs, result in an increase in the force of contractions. Many drugs used to treat hypertension (high blood pressure) act to decrease contractility.

CHECKPOINT

11. Define cardiac output.

12. If the cardioinhibitory center of the medulla oblongata were damaged, which division of the autonomic nervous system would be affected, and how would the heart be influenced?

13. What effect would stimulating the acetylcholine receptors of the heart have on cardiac output?

14. What effect does increased venous return have on stroke volume?

15. Why is it a potential problem if the heart beats too rapidly?

See the blue Answers tab at the back of the book.

RELATED CLINICAL TERMS

angina pectoris (an-JĪ-nuh PEK-tor-is): Severe chest pain resulting from temporary ischemia (local loss of blood supply) whenever the heart's workload increases (as during exertion or stress).

balloon angioplasty: A technique for reducing the size of a coronary plaque by compressing it against the arterial walls using a catheter with an inflatable collar.

cardiac tamponade: A condition, resulting from pericardial irritation and inflammation, in which fluid collects in the pericardial sac, restricting movement of the heart and cardiac output.

cardiology (kar-dē-OL-o-jē): The study of the heart, its functions, and its diseases.

coronary arteriography: The production of an X-ray image of coronary circulation after the introduction of a radiopaque dye into one of the coronary arteries through a catheter; the resulting image is a *coronary angiogram*.

coronary artery bypass graft (CABG): The routing of blood around an obstructed coronary artery (or one of its branches) by a vessel transplanted from another site in the body.

coronary thrombosis: The presence of a thrombus (clot) in a coronary artery; may cause circulatory blockage resulting in a heart attack.

defibrillator: A device used to eliminate atrial or ventricular fibrillation (uncoordinated contractions) and restore normal cardiac rhythm.

echocardiography: Ultrasound analysis of the heart and of the blood flow through the great vessels.

heart block: An impairment of conduction in the heart in which damage to conduction pathways (due to mechanical distortion, ischemia, infection, or inflammation) disrupts the heart's normal rhythm.

pericarditis: Inflammation of the pericardium.

12 Chapter Review

Summary Outline

The Heart's Role in the Cardiovascular System *p. 458*

1. The blood vessels of the cardiovascular system can be subdivided into the **pulmonary circuit** (which carries blood to and from the lungs) and the **systemic circuit** (which transports blood to and from the rest of the body). **Arteries** carry blood away from the heart; **veins** return blood to the heart. **Capillaries** are tiny vessels between the smallest arteries and smallest veins *(Figure 12-1)*.

2. The heart has four chambers: the **right atrium, right ventricle, left atrium,** and **left ventricle.**

12-1 · The heart is a four-chambered organ, supplied by coronary circulation, that pumps oxygen-poor blood to the lungs and oxygen-rich blood to the rest of the body *p. 458*

3. The heart is surrounded by the **pericardial cavity**, which is lined by the **pericardium.** The **visceral pericardium (epicardium)** covers the heart's outer surface. The **parietal** pericardium lines the inner surface of the *pericardial sac*, which surrounds the heart *(Figure 12-2)*.

4. The **coronary sulcus**, a deep groove, marks the boundary between the atria and ventricles. The **anterior** and **posterior interventricular sulci** mark the boundary between the left and right ventricles *(Figure 12-3)*.

5. The bulk of the heart consists of the muscular **myocardium**. The **endocardium** lines the inner surfaces of the heart, and the **epicardium** covers the outer surface *(Figure 12-4a,b)*.

6. **6. Cardiac muscle cells** are interconnected by **intercalated discs**, which convey the force of contraction from cell to cell and conduct action potentials *(Figure 12-4c,d)*.

7. The atria are separated by the **interatrial septum**, and the ventricles are separated by the **interventricular septum.** The right atrium receives blood from the systemic circuit by two large veins, the **superior vena cava** and **inferior vena cava** *(Spotlight Figure 12-5)*.

8. Blood flows from the right atrium into the right ventricle through the **right atrioventricular (AV) valve (tricuspid valve).** This opening is bounded by three **cusps** of fibrous tissue braced by the tendinous **chordae tendineae,** which are connected to **papillary muscles** (*Spotlight Figure 12-5*).

9. Blood leaving the right ventricle enters the **pulmonary trunk** after passing through the **pulmonary semilunar valve.** The pulmonary trunk divides to form the **left** and **right pulmonary arteries.** The **left** and **right pulmonary veins** return oxygenated blood to the left atrium. Blood leaving the left atrium flows into the left ventricle through the **left atrioventricular (AV) valve (bicuspid valve** or **mitral valve).** Blood leaving the left ventricle passes through the **aortic semilunar valve** and into the systemic circuit through the **aorta** (*Spotlight Figure 12-5*).

10. Anatomical differences between the ventricles reflect the functional demands on them. The wall of the right ventricle is relatively thin. The left ventricle has a massive muscular wall.

11. Valves normally permit blood flow in only one direction, preventing the **regurgitation** (backflow) of blood (*Figure 12-6*).

12. The connective tissues of the heart and **cardiac skeleton** support the heart's contractile cells and valves (*Figure 12-6*).

13. The **coronary circulation** meets the high oxygen and nutrient demands of cardiac muscle cells. The two coronary arteries originate at the base of the aorta. Arterial **anastomoses**—interconnections between arteries—ensure a constant blood supply. The **great** and **middle cardiac veins** carry blood from the coronary capillaries to the **coronary sinus** (*Figure 12-7*).

12-2 Contractile cells and the conducting system produce each heartbeat, and an electrocardiogram records the associated electrical events *p. 415*

14. Two general classes of cardiac cells are involved in the normal heartbeat: *contractile cells* and cells of the conducting system.

15. Cardiac muscle cells have a long refractory period, so rapid stimulation produces isolated contractions (twitches) rather than tetanic contractions (*Figure 12-15*).

16. The conducting system includes **nodal cells** and **conducting cells.** The conducting system initiates and distributes electrical impulses within the heart. Nodal cells establish the rate of cardiac contraction. **Pacemaker cells** are nodal cells that reach threshold first. Conducting cells distribute the contractile stimulus to the general myocardium.

17. Unlike skeletal muscle, cardiac muscle contracts without neural or hormonal stimulation. Pacemaker cells in the **sinoatrial (SA) node** (*cardiac pacemaker*) normally establish the rate of contraction. From the SA node, impulses travel

to the **atrioventricular (AV) node** and then to the **AV bundle,** which divides into **bundle branches.** From there, **Purkinje fibers** convey the impulses to the ventricular myocardium (*Figure 12-16*).

18. A recording of electrical activities in the heart is an **electrocardiogram (ECG or EKG).** Important landmarks of an ECG include the **P wave** (atrial depolarization), **QRS complex** (ventricular depolarization), and **T wave** (ventricular repolarization) (*Figure 12-20*).

12-3 Events during a complete heartbeat make up a cardiac cycle *p. 420*

19. A **cardiac cycle** consists of **systole** (contraction) followed by **diastole** (relaxation). Both ventricles contract at the same time, and they eject equal volumes of blood (*Figure 12-21*).

20. The closing of the heart valves and the rushing of blood through the heart cause characteristic **heart sounds** (*Figure 12-22*).

12-4 Heart dynamics examines the factors that affect cardiac output *p. 422*

21. *Heart dynamics,* or *cardiodynamics,* refers to the movements and forces generated during contractions. The amount of blood ejected by a ventricle during a single beat is the **stroke volume (SV).** The amount of blood pumped by the left ventricle each minute is the **cardiac output (CO).**

22. The major factors that affect cardiac output are blood volume reflexes, autonomic innervation, and hormones.

23. Blood volume reflexes are stimulated by changes in **venous return,** the amount of blood entering the heart. The **atrial reflex** speeds up the heart rate when entering blood stretches the walls of the right atrium. Ventricular contractions become more powerful and increase stroke volume when the ventricular walls are stretched (the **Frank–Starling principle**).

24. The basic heart rate is established by pacemaker cells, but it can be modified by the ANS (*Figure 12-23*).

25. Acetylcholine (ACh) released by parasympathetic motor neurons lowers heart rate and stroke volume. Norepinephrine (NE) released by sympathetic neurons increases heart rate and stroke volume.

26. Epinephrine (E) and norepinephrine, hormones released by the adrenal medullae during sympathetic activation, increase both heart rate and stroke volume. Thyroid hormones and glucagon also act to increase cardiac output.

27. The **cardioacceleratory center** in the medulla oblongata activates sympathetic neurons; the **cardioinhibitory center** governs the activities of the parasympathetic neurons. These sympathetic and parasympathetic cardiac centers receive inputs from higher centers and from receptors monitoring blood pressure and the levels of dissolved gases.

Review Questions

See the blue Answers tab at the back of the book.

Level 1 Reviewing Facts and Terms

Match each item in column A with the most closely related item in column B. Place letters for answers in the spaces provided.

COLUMN A

_____ **1.** Epicardium
_____ **2.** Right AV valve
_____ **3.** Left AV valve
_____ **4.** Anastomoses
_____ **5.** Myocardial infarction
_____ **6.** SA node
_____ **7.** Systole
_____ **8.** Diastole
_____ **9.** Cardiac output
_____ **10.** HR slower than usual
_____ **11.** HR faster than normal
_____ **12.** Atrial reflex

COLUMN B

a. Heart attack
b. Cardiac pacemaker
c. Tachycardia
d. HR × SV
e. Tricuspid valve
f. Bradycardia
g. Mitral valve
h. Interconnections between arteries
i. Visceral pericardium
j. Increased venous return
k. Contractions of heart chambers
l. Relaxation of heart chambers

13. Identify the superficial structures in the following diagram of the heart.

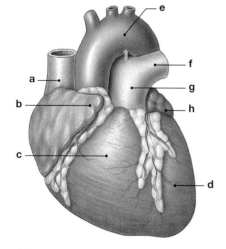

(a) _____ (b) _____
(c) _____ (d) _____
(e) _____ (f) _____
(g) _____ (h) _____

14. The blood supply to the heart is provided by the
   (a) systemic circulation.
   (b) pulmonary circulation.
   (c) coronary circulation.
   (d) coronary portal system.

15. The autonomic centers for cardiac function are located in
   (a) myocardial tissue of the heart.
   (b) cardiac center of the medulla oblongata.
   (c) the cerebral cortex.
   (d) a, b, and c are correct.

16. The simple squamous epithelium covering the valves of the heart is called
   (a) epicardium. **(b)** endocardium.
   (c) myocardium. **(d)** endothelium.

17. The structure that permits blood flow from the right atrium to the left atrium while the lungs are developing is the
   (a) foramen ovale. **(b)** interatrial septum.
   (c) coronary sinus. **(d)** fossa ovalis.

18. Identify the structures in the following diagram of a sectional view of the heart.

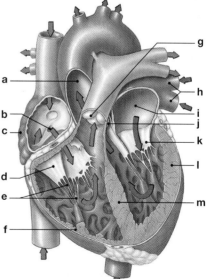

(a) _____
(b) _____
(c) _____
(d) _____
(e) _____
(f) _____
(g) _____
(h) _____
(i) _____
(j) _____
(k) _____
(l) _____
(m) _____

19. Blood leaves the left ventricle by passing through the
   (a) aortic semilunar valve.
   (b) pulmonary semilunar valve.
   (c) mitral valve.
   (d) tricuspid valve.

20. The QRS complex of the ECG is produced when the
   (a) atria depolarize.
   (b) ventricles depolarize.
   (c) ventricles repolarize.
   (d) atria repolarize.

21. During diastole, the chambers of the heart
   (a) undergo a sharp increase in pressure.
   (b) contract and push blood into an adjacent chamber.
   (c) relax and fill with blood.
   (d) reach a pressure of approximately 120 mm Hg.

22. What roles do the chordae tendineae and papillary muscles have in the normal function of the AV valves?

23. What are the principal heart valves, and what is the function of each?

24. Trace the normal path of an electrical impulse (action potential) through the conducting system of the heart.

25. (a) What is the cardiac cycle? (b) What phases and events are necessary to complete the cardiac cycle?

Level 2 Reviewing Concepts

26. Tetanic muscle contractions cannot occur in a normal cardiac muscle cell because
   (a) cardiac muscle tissue contracts on its own.
   (b) there is no neural or hormonal stimulation.
   (c) the refractory period lasts until the muscle cell relaxes.
   (d) the refractory period ends before the muscle cell reaches peak tension.

27. The amount of blood forced out of the heart depends on the
   (a) degree of stretching at the end of ventricular diastole.
   (b) contractility of the ventricle.
   (c) amount of pressure required to eject blood.
   (d) a, b, and c are correct.

28. Cardiac output cannot increase indefinitely because
   (a) available filling time becomes shorter as the heart rate increases.
   (b) the cardiac center adjusts the heart rate.
   (c) the rate of spontaneous depolarization decreases.
   (d) the ion concentrations surrounding pacemaker plasma membranes decrease.

29. Describe the relationships of the four chambers of the heart to the pulmonary and systemic circuits.

30. What are the sources and clinical significance of the heart sounds?

31. (a) What effect does sympathetic stimulation have on the heart? (b) What effect does parasympathetic stimulation have on the heart?

Level 3 Critical Thinking and Clinical Applications

32. A patient's ECG tracing shows a consistent pattern of two P waves followed by a normal QRS complex and T wave. What is the cause of this abnormal wave pattern?

33. The following measurements were made on two individuals (the values recorded remained stable for one hour):
   Person A: heart rate, 75 bpm; stroke volume, 60 mL
   Person B: heart rate, 90 bpm; stroke volume, 95 mL
   Which person has the greater venous return? Which person has the longer ventricular filling time?

34. Karen is taking the medication *verapamil*, a drug that blocks the calcium channels in cardiac muscle cells. What effect should this medication have on Karen's stroke volume?

12

The Cardiovascular System: Blood Vessels and Circulation

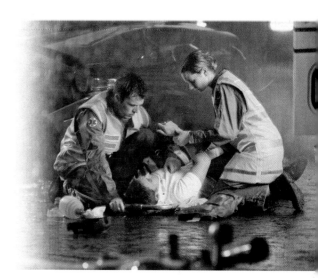

Learning Objectives

These objectives tell you what you should be able to do after completing the chapter. They correspond by number to this chapter's sections.

13-1 Distinguish among the types of blood vessels based on their structure and function.

13-2 Explain the processes that regulate blood flow through blood vessels, and discuss the processes that regulate movement of fluids between capillaries and interstitial spaces.

13-3 Describe the control processes that interact to regulate blood flow and pressure in tissues, and explain how the activities of the cardiac, vasomotor, and respiratory centers are coordinated to control blood flow through tissues.

13-4 Explain the cardiovascular system's homeostatic response to exercise and hemorrhaging.

13-5 Describe the three general functional patterns seen in the pulmonary and systemic circuits.

13-6 Identify the major arteries and veins of the pulmonary circuit.

13-7 Identify the major arteries and veins of the systemic circuit.

13-8 Identify the differences between fetal and adult circulation patterns, and describe the changes in the patterns of blood flow that occur at birth.

13-9 Discuss the effects of aging on the cardiovascular system.

13-10 Give examples of interactions between the cardiovascular system and other body systems.

An Introduction to Blood Vessels and Circulation

We have already examined the composition of blood and the structure and function of the heart, whose pumping action keeps blood in motion (Chapters 11 and 12). Here we consider the vessels that carry blood to peripheral tissues, and the nature of the exchange that takes place between the blood and interstitial fluids.

In this chapter, we first examine the structure of arteries, capillaries, and veins. Then we explore their functions, the basic principles of cardiovascular regulation, and the distribution of the body's major blood vessels.

Build Your Knowledge

Recall that the surface of the skin, the epidermis, lacks blood vessels. Its cells depend on the exchange of nutrients, dissolved gases, and wastes with capillaries in the dermis (as you saw in **Chapter 5: The Integumentary System**). Arteries supplying the skin form two networks in the dermis. One is a deep cutaneous plexus, and the other is a superficial subpapillary plexus. Loops of capillaries extending from the subpapillary plexus provide the sites where materials are exchanged with epidermal cells by diffusion. Blood in the capillaries drains into small veins of the subpapillary plexus. These veins then empty into those of the cutaneous plexus. ⟲ **p. 129**

13-1 Arteries, arterioles, capillaries, venules, and veins differ in size, structure, and function

Learning Objective Distinguish among the types of blood vessels based on their structure and function.

Blood circulates throughout the body, moving from the heart through the tissues and back to the heart in blood vessels. Blood leaves the heart by way of the pulmonary trunk, which begins at the right ventricle, and the aorta, which begins at the left ventricle. Each of these vessels has an internal diameter of around 2.5 cm (1 in.). These vessels branch repeatedly, forming the major **arteries** that carry blood to body organs. Within these organs, further branching creates several hundred million tiny arteries, or **arterioles** (ar-TĒR-ē-ōls). The arterioles send blood into more than 10 billion **capillaries**. These capillaries are barely the diameter of a single red blood cell. The capillaries form extensive, branching networks. If all the capillaries in an average adult's body were placed end to end, their combined length would be more than 25,000 miles, enough to circle the planet.

The vital functions of the cardiovascular system take place at the capillary level. *Chemical and gaseous exchange between the blood and interstitial fluid takes place across capillary walls.* Tissue cells rely on capillary diffusion to obtain nutrients and oxygen and to remove metabolic wastes such as carbon dioxide and urea.

Blood flowing out of a capillary network first enters **venules** (VEN-ūls), the smallest vessels of the venous system. These slender vessels merge to form small **veins**. Blood then passes through medium-sized and large veins before reaching the venae cavae (in the systemic circuit) or the pulmonary veins (in the pulmonary circuit) (see **Figure 12-1**, p. 459).

The Structure of Vessel Walls

The walls of arteries and veins are made up of three layers containing different tissues (**Figure 13-1**):

1. The **tunica intima** (IN-ti-muh), or *tunica interna*, is the innermost layer of a blood vessel. It includes an endothelium with its basement membrane and a surrounding layer of connective tissue with elastic fibers.

2. The **tunica media** is the middle layer. It contains sheets of smooth muscle within loose connective tissue containing collagen and elastic fibers. Collagen fibers bind the tunica media to the tunica intima and tunica externa. When its smooth muscles contract, vessel diameter decreases. When they relax, vessel diameter increases.

3. The outer **tunica externa** (eks-TER-nuh), or *tunica adventitia* (ad-ven-TISH-uh), forms a sheath of connective tissue around the vessel. Its collagen fibers may intertwine with those of adjacent tissues, stabilizing and anchoring the blood vessel.

Figure 13-1 A Comparison of a Typical Artery and a Typical Vein. In general, for a vessel of a given size, an artery has a thicker wall and smaller lumen than a vein.

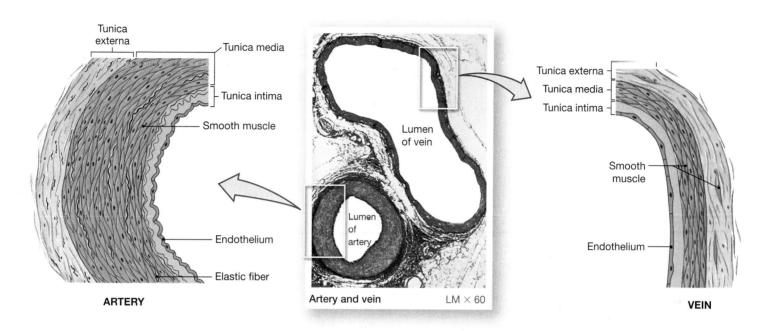

Arteries and veins supplying the same region lie side by side (**Figure 13-1**). Such a sectional view clearly shows the greater wall thickness characteristic of arteries. The thicker tunica media of an artery contains more elastic fibers and smooth muscle cells than does that of a vein. The elastic fibers enable arterial vessels to resist the pressure generated by the heart as it forces blood into the arterial network. The smooth muscle provides a means of actively controlling vessel diameter. Arterial smooth muscle is under the control of the sympathetic division of the autonomic nervous system. When stimulated, these muscles in the vessel wall contract, and the artery constricts in a process called **vasoconstriction**. When these muscles relax, the diameter of the artery and its central opening, or *lumen*, increase in a process called **vasodilation**.

Arteries

On its way from the heart to the capillaries, blood passes through elastic arteries, muscular arteries, and arterioles (**Figure 13-2**).

Elastic arteries are large, extremely resilient vessels with internal diameters up to 2.5 cm (1 in.). The pulmonary trunk and aorta, and their major arterial branches, are elastic arteries. The walls of elastic arteries contain a tunica media dominated by elastic fibers rather than smooth muscle cells. For this reason, elastic arteries are able to absorb the pressure changes of the cardiac cycle. During ventricular systole,

blood pressure rises quickly as additional blood is pushed into the systemic circuit. Over this period, the elastic arteries are stretched, and their diameter increases. During ventricular diastole, arterial blood pressure declines, and the elastic fibers recoil to their original dimensions. The net result is that the expansion of the arteries dampens the rise in pressure during ventricular systole, and the arterial recoil slows the decline in pressure during ventricular diastole. If the arteries were solid pipes rather than elastic tubes, pressures would rise much higher during systole. Pressures would also fall much lower during diastole.

Muscular arteries, also known as *medium-sized arteries* or *distribution arteries,* distribute blood to skeletal muscles and internal organs. A typical muscular artery has an internal diameter of approximately 0.4 cm (0.16 in.). The external carotid arteries of the neck are one example. The thick tunica media in a muscular artery contains more smooth muscle cells and fewer elastic fibers than does an elastic artery (**Figure 13-2**).

Arterioles, with an internal diameter of about 30 μm (0.03 mm), are much smaller than muscular arteries. The tunica media of an arteriole consists of one to two layers of smooth muscle cells. The diameter of the smaller muscular arteries and arterioles changes in response to local conditions, such as low oxygen levels, or to sympathetic or endocrine stimulation. Such changes in diameter alter blood pressure and the rate of flow through dependent tissues.

13

Figure 13-2 The Structure of the Various Types of Blood Vessels. The different types of blood vessels have different diameters, wall thicknesses, and lumen sizes. Note that the wall of a capillary is only one cell thick. This wall consists of an endothelium and a basement membrane.

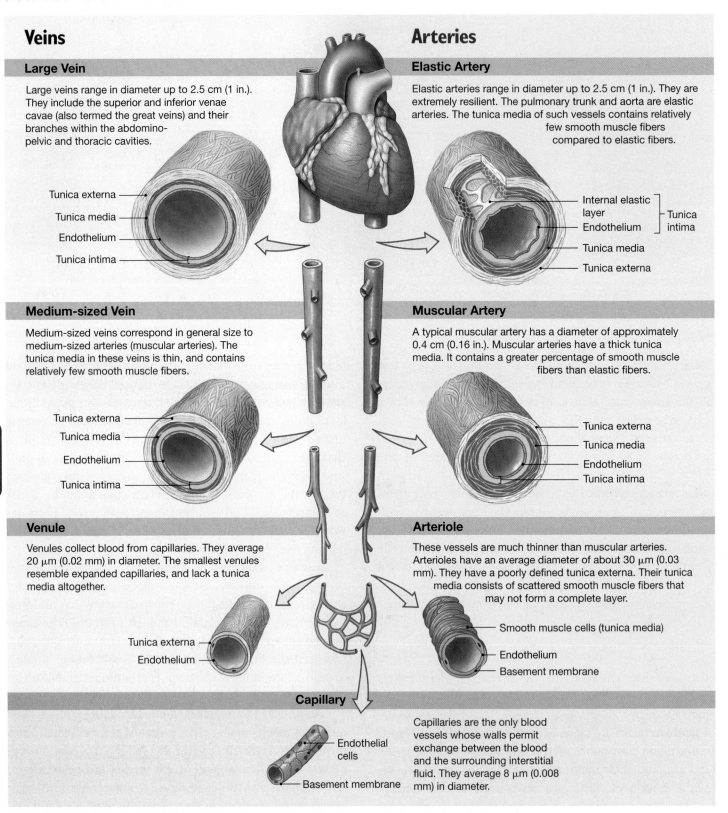

Veins

Large Vein

Large veins range in diameter up to 2.5 cm (1 in.). They include the superior and inferior venae cavae (also termed the great veins) and their branches within the abdomino-pelvic and thoracic cavities.

Tunica externa
Tunica media
Endothelium
Tunica intima

Medium-sized Vein

Medium-sized veins correspond in general size to medium-sized arteries (muscular arteries). The tunica media in these veins is thin, and contains relatively few smooth muscle fibers.

Tunica externa
Tunica media
Endothelium
Tunica intima

Venule

Venules collect blood from capillaries. They average 20 μm (0.02 mm) in diameter. The smallest venules resemble expanded capillaries, and lack a tunica media altogether.

Tunica externa
Endothelium

Arteries

Elastic Artery

Elastic arteries range in diameter up to 2.5 cm (1 in.). They are extremely resilient. The pulmonary trunk and aorta are elastic arteries. The tunica media of such vessels contains relatively few smooth muscle fibers compared to elastic fibers.

Internal elastic layer
Endothelium — Tunica intima
Tunica media
Tunica externa

Muscular Artery

A typical muscular artery has a diameter of approximately 0.4 cm (0.16 in.). Muscular arteries have a thick tunica media. It contains a greater percentage of smooth muscle fibers than elastic fibers.

Tunica externa
Tunica media
Endothelium
Tunica intima

Arteriole

These vessels are much thinner than muscular arteries. Arterioles have an average diameter of about 30 μm (0.03 mm). They have a poorly defined tunica externa. Their tunica media consists of scattered smooth muscle fibers that may not form a complete layer.

Smooth muscle cells (tunica media)
Endothelium
Basement membrane

Capillary

Endothelial cells
Basement membrane

Capillaries are the only blood vessels whose walls permit exchange between the blood and the surrounding interstitial fluid. They average 8 μm (0.008 mm) in diameter.

13

Capillaries

When we think of the cardiovascular system, we usually think first of the heart or the great blood vessels attached to it. But the microscopic capillaries that spread throughout most tissues do the real work of the cardiovascular system. The reason is that capillaries are the *only* blood vessels whose walls permit exchange between the blood and the surrounding interstitial fluid. Capillary walls are relatively thin, so diffusion distances are short, and exchange can take place quickly. In addition, the small diameter of capillaries slows blood flow, allowing time for the diffusion or active transport of materials across capillary walls.

A typical capillary consists of a single layer of endothelial cells inside a basement membrane (**Figure 13-2**). There

CLINICAL NOTE

Arteriosclerosis

Arteriosclerosis (ar-tēr-ē-ō-skler-Ō-sis; *skleros*, hard) is a thickening and toughening of arterial walls. Many people know it as "hardening of the arteries." Complications related to it account for about half of all deaths in the United States. The effects of arteriosclerosis are varied. For example, arteriosclerosis of coronary vessels is responsible for *coronary artery disease.* ⟳ p. 414 Arteriosclerosis of arteries supplying the brain can lead to strokes.

Arteriosclerosis takes two major forms:

1. Focal calcification is the deposition of calcium salts following the gradual degeneration of smooth muscle in the tunica media. Some focal calcification is part of the aging process. It may also develop in association with *atherosclerosis.*

2. Atherosclerosis (ath-er-ō-skler-Ō-sis; *athero-,* a pasty deposit) is the formation of lipid deposits in the tunica media associated with damage to the endothelial lining. It is the most common form of arteriosclerosis.

Many factors may contribute to the development of atherosclerosis. Lipid levels in the blood are one major factor. Atherosclerosis tends to develop in people whose blood contains elevated levels of lipids, specifically cholesterol. Cholesterol is transported to peripheral tissues in protein–lipid complexes called *lipoproteins.* (We will discuss the various types of lipoproteins in Chapter 17.) When cholesterol-rich lipoproteins remain in circulation for an extended period, circulating monocytes begin removing them from the bloodstream. Eventually the monocytes become filled with lipid droplets. Now called foam cells, they attach themselves to the endothelial lining of blood vessels. These cells then release growth factors that stimulate smooth muscle cells near the tunica intima to divide, thickening the vessel wall.

Other monocytes then invade the area, migrating between the endothelial cells. As these changes take place, the monocytes, smooth muscle fibers, and endothelial cells begin phagocytizing lipids as well. The result is an atherosclerotic plaque, a fatty mass of tissue that projects into the lumen of the vessel. At this point, the plaque has a relatively simple structure, and evidence suggests that the process can be reversed with appropriate dietary adjustments.

If the conditions persist, the endothelial cells become swollen with lipids, and gaps appear in the endothelial lining. Platelets now begin sticking to the exposed collagen fibers. This platelet adhesion and aggregation lead to the formation of a localized blood clot that further restricts arterial blood flow. The structure of the plaque is now relatively complex. Plaque growth can be halted, but the structural changes are permanent. A typical plaque is shown in b and c. A normal artery appears in a.

Elderly individuals, especially elderly men, are most likely to develop atherosclerotic plaques. In addition to age, sex, and high blood cholesterol levels, other important risk factors include high blood pressure, cigarette smoking, diabetes mellitus, obesity, and stress.

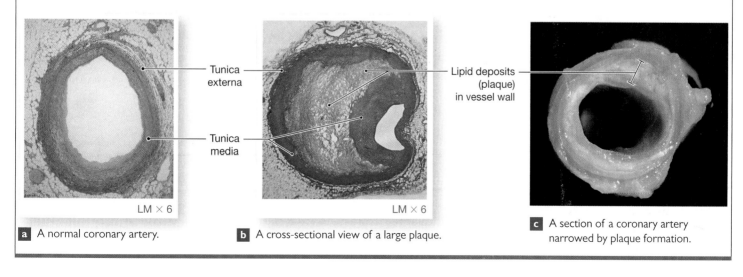

Tunica externa

Tunica media

Lipid deposits (plaque) in vessel wall

LM × 6

LM × 6

a A normal coronary artery.

b A cross-sectional view of a large plaque.

c A section of a coronary artery narrowed by plaque formation.

13

is no tunica externa and no tunica media. The average internal diameter of a capillary is 8 μm (0.008 mm), very close to that of a red blood cell. In most regions of the body, the endothelium forms a complete lining. Most substances enter or leave the capillary by diffusing across endothelial cells or through gaps between them. Water, small solutes, and lipid-soluble materials can easily diffuse into the surrounding interstitial fluid. In a few areas (notably, the choroid plexus of the brain, the hypothalamus, and filtration sites in the kidneys), small pores in the endothelial cells also permit the passage of relatively large molecules, including proteins.

Capillaries do not function as individual units. Instead, they function as part of an interconnected network called a **capillary bed** (**Figure 13-3**). A single arteriole usually gives rise to dozens of capillaries. In turn, capillaries collect into several *venules,* the smallest vessels of the venous system. A **precapillary sphincter**, a band of smooth muscle, guards the entrance to each capillary. Contraction of the smooth muscle fibers narrows the diameter of the capillary's entrance and reduces the flow of blood. The relaxation of the sphincter dilates the opening, allowing blood to enter the capillary more rapidly.

Blood usually flows from arterioles to venules at a constant rate, but the blood flow within any single capillary can be quite variable. Each precapillary sphincter undergoes cycles of activity, alternately contracting and relaxing perhaps a dozen times each minute. As a result of this cyclical change—called **vasomotion** (*vaso-,* vessel)—blood flow within any given capillary is intermittent rather than a steady and constant stream. The net effect is that blood may reach the venules by one route now and by a quite different route later.

This process is controlled at the tissue level, as smooth muscle fibers respond to local changes in the concentrations of chemicals and dissolved gases in the interstitial fluid. For example, when dissolved oxygen levels decline within a tissue, the capillary sphincters relax, and blood flow to the area increases. Such control at the tissue level is called *autoregulation.*

Figure 13-3 The Organization of a Capillary Bed.

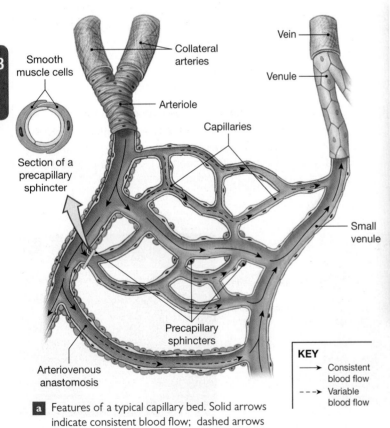

Smooth muscle cells

Collateral arteries

Arteriole

Capillaries

Section of a precapillary sphincter

Small venule

Precapillary sphincters

Arteriovenous anastomosis

KEY
→ Consistent blood flow
- - → Variable blood flow

a Features of a typical capillary bed. Solid arrows indicate consistent blood flow; dashed arrows indicate variable or pulsating blood flow.

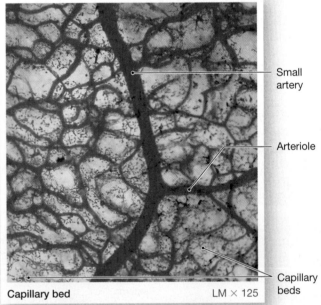

Vein

Venule

Small artery

Arteriole

Capillary beds

Capillary bed   LM × 125

b This micrograph shows a number of capillary beds.

Sometimes alternate routes for blood flow are formed by an **anastomosis** (a-nas-tō-MŌ-sis; "outlet"; plural, *anastomoses*), the joining of blood vessels. Under certain conditions, blood completely bypasses a capillary bed through an **arteriovenous** (ar-tēr-ē-ō-VĒ-nus) **anastomosis**, a vessel that connects an arteriole to a venule (**Figure 13-3a**). In other cases, a single capillary bed is supplied by an **arterial anastomosis**, in which multiple arteries fuse before giving rise to arterioles. An arterial anastomosis serves as an insurance policy for capillary beds. If one artery is compressed or blocked, the others can continue to deliver blood to the capillary bed, and dependent tissues will not be damaged. Arterial anastomoses are found in the brain, in the coronary circulation, and in many other sites as well. ⟳ p. 414

Veins

Veins collect blood from all tissues and organs and return it to the heart. Veins are classified on the basis of their internal diameters. **Venules** are the thinnest. An average venule has an internal diameter of 20 μm (0.02 mm). Those smaller than 50 μm (0.05 mm) lack a tunica media, and resemble expanded capillaries (**Figure 13-2**).

Medium-sized veins are comparable in size to muscular arteries. They range from 2 to 9 mm (0.08 to 0.35 in.) in internal diameter. Their tunica media contains several smooth muscle layers. The relatively thick tunica externa has longitudinal bundles of elastic and collagen fibers.

Large veins include the two venae cavae and their tributaries in the abdominopelvic and thoracic cavities. In these veins, the thin tunica media is surrounded by a thick tunica externa made of a mixture of elastic and collagen fibers.

Veins have relatively thin walls because the blood pressure inside them is low. The blood pressure in venules and medium-sized veins is so low that it cannot overcome the force of gravity. In the limbs, medium-sized veins contain **valves**, folds of tunica intima that project from the vessel wall. They function like the valves in the heart, preventing the backflow of blood (**Figure 13-4**). As long as the valves work normally, any body movement that compresses a vein will push blood toward the heart, improving *venous return.* ⟳ p. 422 If the walls of the veins near the valves weaken or become stretched and distorted, the valves may not work properly. Blood then pools in the veins, and the vessels become distended. The effects range from mild discomfort and a cosmetic problem, as in superficial *varicose veins* in the thighs and legs, to painful distortion of adjacent tissues, as in *hemorrhoids*, swollen veins in the lining of the anal canal.

Figure 13-4 The Function of Valves in the Venous System. Valves in the walls of medium-sized veins prevent the backflow of blood. The compression of veins by the contraction of adjacent skeletal muscles helps maintain venous blood flow.

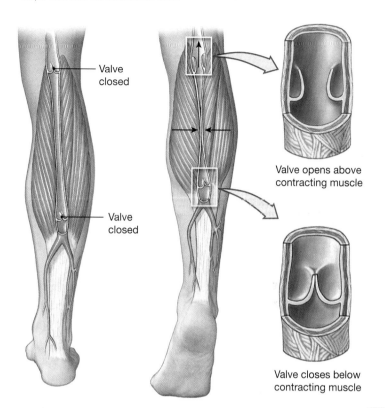

Valve closed

Valve closed

Valve opens above contracting muscle

Valve closes below contracting muscle

CHECKPOINT

1. List the five general classes of blood vessels.
2. A cross section of tissue shows several small, thin-walled vessels with very little smooth muscle tissue in the tunica media. Which type of vessels are these?
3. What effect would relaxation of precapillary sphincters have on blood flow through a tissue?
4. Why are valves found in veins, but not in arteries?

See the blue Answers tab at the back of the book.

13-2 Pressure and resistance determine blood flow and affect rates of capillary exchange

Learning Objective Explain the processes that regulate blood flow through blood vessels, and discuss the processes that regulate movement of fluids between capillaries and interstitial spaces.

The primary function of the parts of the cardiovascular system (the blood, heart, and blood vessels) is to maintain an adequate blood flow through the capillaries in the tissues and organs of the body. Under normal circumstances, blood flow equals cardiac output. When cardiac output goes up, so does blood flow through capillary beds. When cardiac output declines, blood flow is reduced. But the flow of blood through capillaries also depends on two additional factors—*pressure* and *resistance*—as we discuss next.

Factors Affecting Blood Flow

To keep blood moving in the body, the heart must generate enough pressure to overcome the resistance to blood flow in the pulmonary and systemic circuits. Pressure and resistance both affect blood flow to the tissues, but they have opposing effects. In general terms, blood flow and pressure are directly related. That is, when pressure increases, flow increases. Blood flow and resistance are inversely related. So, when resistance increases, flow decreases.

Pressure

Liquids, including blood, cannot be compressed. For this reason, a force exerted against a liquid generates a fluid pressure, or hydrostatic pressure, that is conducted in all directions. If pressures differ from one place to another, a liquid will flow from an area of higher pressure toward an area of lower pressure. The flow rate is directly proportional to the pressure difference. The greater the difference in pressure, the faster the flow.

However, the absolute pressure is less important than the *pressure gradient*—the difference in pressure from one end of the vessel to the other. The largest pressure gradient is found in the systemic circuit between the base of the aorta (where blood leaves the left ventricle) and the entrance to the right atrium (where blood returns to the heart). This pressure difference, called the *circulatory pressure*, averages about 100 mm Hg (millimeters of mercury, a standard unit of pressure). This relatively high circulatory pressure serves primarily to force blood through the arterioles and into the capillaries.

We can divide circulatory pressure into three components: (1) *arterial pressure* (routinely measured on a person's arm and commonly referred to as **blood pressure**); (2) *capillary pressure*; and (3) *venous pressure*. Shortly we will discuss each component of circulatory pressure.

Resistance

Resistance is any force that opposes movement. In the cardiovascular system, resistance opposes the movement of blood. For blood to flow, the circulatory pressure must be great enough to overcome the **total peripheral resistance**, the resistance of the entire cardiovascular system. The steepest decline in pressure within the cardiovascular system—about 65 mm Hg—occurs in the arterial network because of the high resistance of the arterioles. The resistance of the arterial system is termed **peripheral resistance**. Sources of peripheral resistance include *vascular resistance, viscosity,* and *turbulence.*

VASCULAR RESISTANCE. Vascular resistance is the resistance of the blood vessels to blood flow. It is the largest component of peripheral resistance. *The most important factor in vascular resistance is friction between the blood and the vessel walls.* The amount of friction depends on the length and diameter of the vessel. Friction increases with increasing vessel length, because longer vessels have a larger surface area in contact with the blood. Friction also increases with decreasing vessel diameter. For this reason, in small-diameter vessels, nearly all the blood is slowed down by friction with the vessel walls. Vessel length cannot ordinarily be changed, so vascular resistance is controlled by changing the diameter of blood vessels. Such changes take place through the contraction or relaxation of smooth muscle in the vessel walls.

Most of the vascular resistance occurs in arterioles, which are extremely muscular. The walls of an arteriole with a 30-μm internal diameter, for example, can have a 20-μm-thick layer of smooth muscle. Local, neural, and hormonal stimuli that stimulate or inhibit contractions of this smooth muscle tissue can adjust the diameters of these vessels. A small change in diameter can produce a very large change in resistance.

VISCOSITY. Viscosity is the resistance to flow caused by interactions among molecules and suspended materials in a liquid. Liquids of low viscosity, such as water, flow at low pressures. Thick, syrupy liquids such as molasses flow only under higher pressures. Whole blood has a viscosity about five times that of water. ⊃ p. 381 This viscosity is due to its plasma proteins and blood cells.

Under normal conditions, the viscosity of blood remains stable. But disorders that affect the hematocrit or the plasma protein content can change blood viscosity and increase or decrease peripheral resistance. For example, in **anemia**, the hematocrit is reduced due to inadequate production of hemoglobin, RBCs, or both. As a result, both the oxygen-carrying capacity and the viscosity of the blood are reduced. A reduction in blood viscosity can also result from protein deficiency diseases, in which the liver cannot synthesize normal amounts of plasma proteins.

TURBULENCE. Blood usually flows through a vessel smoothly. The slowest flow is near the walls, and the fastest flow is at the center of the vessel. High flow rates, irregular surfaces due to injury or disease processes, or sudden changes in vessel diameter upset this smooth flow, creating eddies and swirls. This result, called **turbulence**, increases resistance and slows blood flow.

Turbulence normally occurs when blood flows between the heart's chambers and from the heart into the aorta and pulmonary trunk. In addition to increasing resistance, this turbulence generates the *third* and *fourth heart sounds* often heard through a stethoscope. Turbulent blood flow across damaged or misaligned heart valves produces the sound of *heart murmurs.* ⟳ p. 412

The Interplay between Pressure and Resistance

Neural and hormonal control processes regulate blood pressure, keeping it relatively stable. Adjustments in the peripheral resistance of vessels supplying specific organs allow the rate of blood flow to be precisely controlled. An example is the increase in blood flow to skeletal muscles during exercise (discussed in Chapter 7). ⟳ p. 237 That increase results from a drop in the peripheral resistance of the arteries supplying active muscles. Of the three sources of resistance, only vascular resistance can be adjusted by the nervous or endocrine systems

to regulate blood flow. Viscosity and turbulence, which also affect peripheral resistance, are normally constant.

Cardiovascular Pressures within the Systemic Circuit

Pressure varies along the path of blood flow within the systemic circuit. Systemic pressures are highest in the aorta, peaking at around 120 mm Hg, and lowest at the venae cavae, averaging about 2 mm Hg (**Figure 13-5**). Next we consider pressures in the arterial network. We then examine how pressure in the capillaries drives the exchange of substances between the bloodstream and body tissues before we consider pressures in the venous system.

Blood Pressure (Arterial Pressure)

The pressure in large and small arteries fluctuates, rising during ventricular systole and falling during ventricular diastole (**Figure 13-5**). **Systolic pressure** is the peak blood pressure measured during ventricular systole. **Diastolic pressure** is the minimum blood pressure at the end of ventricular diastole. In recording blood pressure, we separate systolic and diastolic pressures by a slash mark, as in "120/80" (read as "one twenty over eighty"). A **pulse** is a rhythmic pressure oscillation that accompanies each heartbeat. The difference between the systolic and diastolic pressures is the **pulse pressure** (*pulsus,* stroke).

13

CLINICAL NOTE

Hypertension

A consistent elevation of the blood pressure is called *hypertension*. Approximately 50 million people in the U.S. have hypertension. The diagnosis is made when the average of two or more diastolic blood pressure measurements taken on two different occasions is 90 mm Hg or higher or when the average of two or more systolic blood pressure measurements taken on two different occasions is 130 mm Hg or higher.

The blood pressure is a function of cardiac output and peripheral vascular resistance. An increase in cardiac output, peripheral vascular resistance, or both will increase the blood pressure. A specific cause of hypertension has not been determined. However, both genetic and environmental factors appear responsible for its development.

Chronic hypertension damages the walls of systemic blood vessels. Prolonged vasoconstriction and high pressures within these vessels, particularly the arteries and arterioles, cause the vessels to thicken and strengthen to withstand the stress.

Treatment of hypertension depends on the severity. Exercise, dietary changes, weight control, and medications can keep blood pressure under control and reduce the long-term complications.

Figure 13-5 Pressures within the Systemic Circuit.
Notice the general reduction of circulatory pressure within the systemic circuit and the elimination of the pulse pressure in the arterioles.

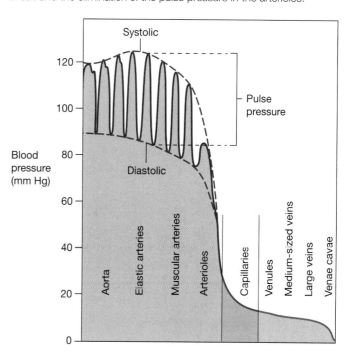

Build Your Knowledge

Recall that diffusion is a passive transport process (as you saw in **Chapter 3: Cell Structure and Function**). Passive transport processes move ions or molecules across the plasma membrane without any energy being expended by the cell. Osmosis is a special term for the diffusion of water across a selectively permeable membrane that separates two solutions of differing solute concentrations. During osmosis, water moves into the solution with the higher solute concentration. ⤸ **pp. 61, 63**

Pulse pressure lessens as the distance from the heart increases. As noted earlier, the average pressure declines due to friction between the blood and the vessel walls. The pulse pressure fades because arteries are elastic tubes rather than solid pipes. Much as a balloon's walls expand when

air enters, the elasticity of the arteries allows them to expand with blood during systole. When diastole begins and blood pressures fall, the arteries recoil to their original dimensions. This arterial recoil adds an extra push to the flow of blood because the aortic semilunar valve prevents blood from returning to the heart. The magnitude of this effect, called *elastic rebound*, is greatest near the heart and drops in succeeding arterial sections.

By the time blood reaches a precapillary sphincter, no pressure oscillations remain. The blood pressure is about 35 mm Hg (**Figure 13-5**). Along the length of a typical capillary, blood pressure gradually falls from about 35 mm Hg to roughly 18 mm Hg, the pressure at the start of the venous system.

Capillary Pressures and Capillary Exchange

The pressure of blood within a capillary bed is called **capillary pressure**. Blood pushes against capillary walls, just as it does in arteries. But unlike other blood vessel walls, capillary walls are quite permeable to small ions, nutrients, organic wastes, dissolved gases, and water. These materials exit, but most are reabsorbed by the capillaries. The remainder, about 3.6 liters (0.95 gallons) of water and solutes, flows through peripheral tissues each day. It then enters the **lymphatic vessels** of the lymphatic system, which empty into the bloodstream (**Figure 13-6**).

This continuous movement and exchange of water and solutes out of the capillaries, through the body tissues, and then back into the bloodstream has four important functions:

1. *Communication.* It maintains constant communication between blood plasma and interstitial fluid. Together, they account for most of the volume of extracellular fluid in the body.

2. *Distribution.* It speeds the distribution of nutrients, hormones, and dissolved gases throughout tissues.

3. *Transport.* It assists in the transport of insoluble lipids and tissue proteins that cannot enter the bloodstream by crossing capillary walls.

4. *Defense.* It flushes bacterial toxins and other chemical stimuli to lymphatic tissues and organs responsible for providing immunity to disease.

Figure 13-6 Forces Acting across Capillary Walls. At the arterial end of the capillary, capillary hydrostatic pressure (CHP) is greater than blood osmotic pressure (BOP), so fluid moves out of the capillary (filtration). Near the venule, CHP is lower than BOP, so fluid moves into the capillary (reabsorption).

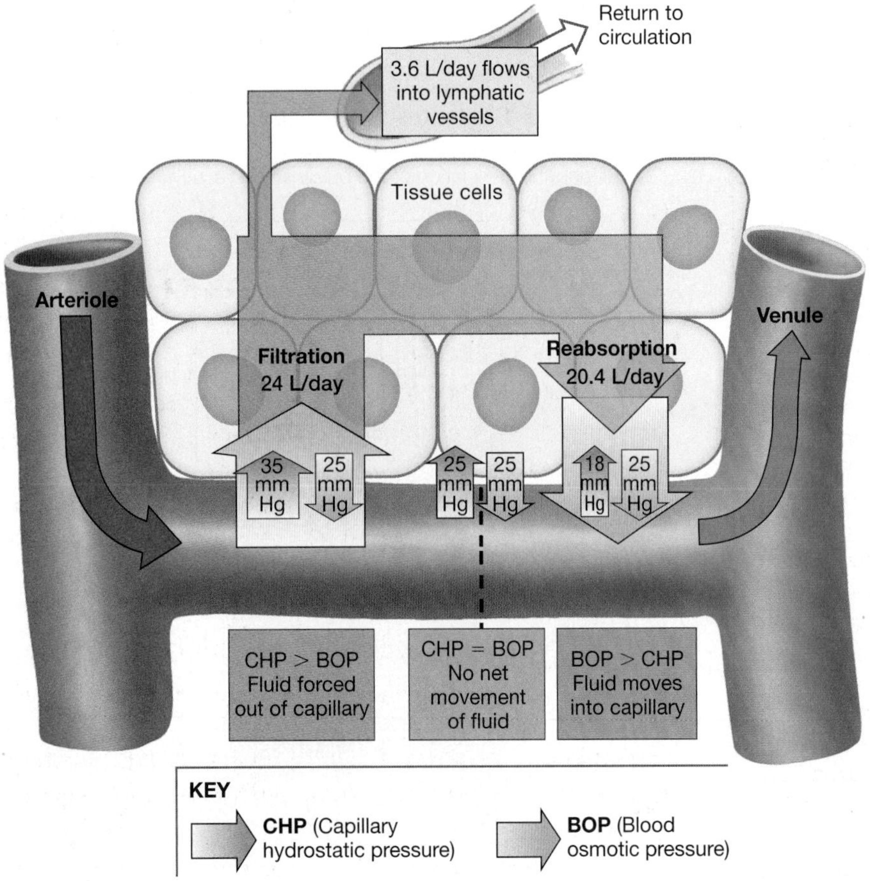

Return to circulation

3.6 L/day flows into lymphatic vessels

Tissue cells

Arteriole

Venule

Filtration 24 L/day

Reabsorption 20.4 L/day

35 mm Hg | 25 mm Hg | 25 mm Hg | 25 mm Hg | 18 mm Hg | 25 mm Hg

CHP > BOP
Fluid forced out of capillary

CHP = BOP
No net movement of fluid

BOP > CHP
Fluid moves into capillary

KEY

CHP (Capillary hydrostatic pressure)

BOP (Blood osmotic pressure)

Capillary exchange between the plasma and interstitial fluid plays a key role in homeostasis. The most important processes that move materials across capillary walls are diffusion, filtration, and reabsorption.

Diffusion is the net movement of ions or molecules from an area where their concentration is higher to an area where their concentration is lower. Solute molecules tend to diffuse across the capillary endothelium, driven by their individual concentration gradients. Water-soluble materials—including ions and small organic molecules such as glucose, amino acids, or urea—diffuse through small spaces between adjacent endothelial cells. (Larger water-soluble molecules, such as plasma proteins, cannot normally leave the bloodstream.) Lipid-soluble materials—including steroids, fatty acids, and dissolved gases—diffuse across the endothelium, passing through the membrane lipids.

Filtration is the removal of solutes as a solution flows across a porous membrane. Solutes too large to pass through the pores are filtered out of the solution. The driving force of filtration is hydrostatic pressure. As we saw earlier, it pushes water from an area of higher pressure to an area of lower pressure. Water molecules move when driven by either hydrostatic (fluid) pressure or osmotic pressure. ⟲ p. 64

In *capillary filtration*, water and small solutes are forced across a capillary wall, leaving larger solutes and suspended proteins in the bloodstream (**Figure 13-6**). At a capillary, the hydrostatic pressure, or *capillary hydrostatic pressure (CHP)*, is greatest at the arterial end (35 mm Hg) and least at the venous end (18 mm Hg). As a result, filtration is greatest at the start of a capillary, where the CHP is highest, and declines along the length of the capillary as CHP falls.

Reabsorption takes place as the result of osmosis. *Osmosis* refers to the diffusion of water across a selectively permeable membrane. When such a membrane separates two solutions of differing solute concentrations, water moves into the solution with the higher solute concentration. The force of this water movement is called *osmotic pressure*. Because blood contains more dissolved proteins than does interstitial fluid, its osmotic pressure is higher, and water tends to move from the interstitial fluid into the blood. ⟲ p. 64 The osmotic pressure of blood (25 mm Hg) is constant along the length of the capillaries. Thus, CHP tends to push water out of the capillary, and blood osmotic pressure tends to reabsorb water, or pull it back in (**Figure 13-6**).

CLINICAL NOTE

Capillary Physiology

What happens at the capillary level to a bleeding accident victim? Or to a dehydrated person lost in the desert? In both cases, the decrease in blood volume causes a drop in blood pressure. In the second case, however, the loss in blood volume is also accompanied by a rise in blood osmotic pressure, because as water is lost, the blood becomes more concentrated. In both cases, a net movement of water from the interstitial fluid to the bloodstream takes place, and blood volume increases. This process is known as a *recall of fluids*.

The opposite situation is edema (e-DĒ-muh), an abnormal accumulation of interstitial fluid in the tissues. Localized edema often occurs around a bruise, for example. Damage to capillaries at the injury site allows plasma proteins to leak into the interstitial fluid, which decreases the osmotic pressure of the blood and elevates that of the tissues. More water then moves into the tissue, resulting in edema. In the U.S. population, serious cases of edema most often result from an increase in pressure in the arterial system, the venous system, or both. This condition often occurs during *congestive heart failure (CHF)*.

Heart failure occurs when cardiac output cannot meet the circulatory demands of the body. In CHF, the left ventricle can no longer keep up with the right ventricle. Blood flow backs up (becomes congested) in the pulmonary circuit. This situation makes the right ventricle work harder, further elevating pulmonary arterial pressures and forcing blood through the lungs and into the weakened left ventricle. The increased blood pressure in the pulmonary vessels leads to *pulmonary edema,* a buildup of fluids in the lungs.

Venous Pressure

Pressure at the start of the venous system (18 mm Hg) is only about one-fifth of the pressure at the start of the arterial system (100 mm Hg) (**Figure 13-5**). Yet the blood must still travel through a vascular network that is just as complex as the arterial system before returning to the heart. However, venous pressures are low, but the veins offer little resistance. For this reason, once blood enters the venous system, pressure declines very slowly.

As blood travels through the venous system toward the heart, the veins become larger, resistance drops further, and the flow rate increases. Pressures at the entrance to the right atrium fluctuate, but average about 2 mm Hg. This means that the driving force pushing blood through the venous system is a mere 16 mm Hg (18 mm Hg in the venules − 2 mm Hg in the venae cavae = 16 mm Hg). In comparison, a pressure of 65 mm Hg acts along the arterial system (100 mm Hg at the aorta − 35 mm Hg at the capillaries = 65 mm Hg)

13

When you are lying down, a pressure gradient of 16 mm Hg is sufficient to maintain venous flow. But when you are standing, venous blood in regions below the heart must overcome gravity as it ascends within the inferior vena cava (IVC). Two factors help overcome gravity and propel venous blood toward the heart:

1. *Muscular compression.* The contractions of skeletal muscles near a vein compress it, helping push blood toward the heart. The valves in medium-sized veins ensure that blood flow occurs in one direction only (**Figure 13-4**, p. 495).

2. *The respiratory pump.* As you inhale, your thoracic cavity expands, reducing pressures within the pleural cavities. This drop in pressure draws air into the lungs. At the same time, it also pulls blood into the IVC and right atrium from smaller veins in the abdominal cavity and lower body, increasing venous return. During exhalation, the increased pressure that forces air out of the lungs compresses the venae cavae, pushing blood into the right atrium.

During exercise, both factors work together to increase venous return and push cardiac output to maximal levels. However, when a person stands at attention, with knees locked and leg muscles immobile, these factors are impaired. The reduction in venous return leads to a fall in cardiac output. The blood supply to the brain is in turn reduced, sometimes enough to cause *fainting,* a temporary loss of consciousness. The person then collapses, but once the body is horizontal, both venous return and cardiac output return to normal.

The mechanisms involved in the regulation of cardiovascular function include the following (**Figure 13-8**):

- *Autoregulation.* Changes in tissue conditions act directly on precapillary sphincters to alter peripheral resistance, producing local changes in the pattern of blood flow within capillary beds. Such autoregulation causes immediate, localized homeostatic adjustments. If autoregulation is unable to normalize tissue conditions, neural and endocrine mechanisms are activated.

- *Neural mechanisms.* Neural mechanisms respond to changes in arterial pressure or blood gas levels at specific sites. When those changes occur, the autonomic nervous system adjusts cardiac output and peripheral resistance to maintain adequate blood flow.

- *Endocrine mechanisms.* The endocrine system releases hormones that enhance short-term adjustments and direct long-term changes in cardiovascular performance.

Short-term responses adjust cardiac output and peripheral resistance to stabilize blood pressure and blood flow to tissues. Long-term adjustments involve alterations in blood volume that affect cardiac output and the transport of oxygen and carbon dioxide to and from active tissues.

CHECKPOINT

5. Identify the factors that contribute to total peripheral resistance.

6. In a healthy person, where is blood pressure greater: at the aorta or at the inferior vena cava? Explain.

7. While standing in the hot sun, Sally begins to feel light-headed and then faints. Explain what happened.

See the blue Answers tab at the back of the book.

13-3 Cardiovascular regulation involves autoregulation, neural processes, and endocrine responses

Learning Objective Describe the control processes that interact to regulate blood flow and pressure in tissues, and explain how the activities of the cardiac, vasomotor, and respiratory centers are coordinated to control blood flow through tissues.

Homeostatic processes regulate cardiovascular activity to ensure that tissue blood flow, also called *tissue perfusion*, meets the demand for oxygen and nutrients. The factors that affect tissue blood flow are (1) cardiac output, (2) peripheral resistance, and (3) blood pressure. We discussed cardiac output in Chapter 12. ⮌ p. 422 We considered peripheral resistance and pressure earlier in this chapter.

Most cells are relatively close to capillaries. When a group of cells becomes active, the circulation to that region must increase to deliver the oxygen and nutrients they need and to carry away the waste products and carbon dioxide they generate. The goal of cardiovascular regulation is to ensure that these blood flow changes take place (1) at an appropriate time, (2) in the right area, and (3) without drastically altering blood pressure and blood flow to vital organs.

The processes involved in regulating cardiovascular function include the following:

- *Autoregulation.* Changes in tissue conditions act directly on precapillary sphincters to alter peripheral resistance, producing local changes in the pattern of blood flow within capillary beds. Autoregulation causes

CLINICAL NOTE

Vital Signs

Vital signs are outward indicators of what is going on inside the body. They include blood pressure (BP), heart rate, respiratory rate, and temperature. These measurements provide a great deal of information about a patient's condition and should be measured frequently.

The *pulse rate* is a measure of the number of times the heart beats per minute. The pulse is best measured where an artery lies close to the body's surface and crosses over a bone. Common locations for pulse determination are illustrated in **Figure 13-7a**. To measure the pulse rate, locate a suitable site and palpate the pulse. Then, count the number of pulse waves that occur in one minute. Alternatively, you can count the number of pulse waves in 30 seconds and multiply by two. In order to ensure accuracy, it is not recommended that intervals less than 30 seconds be measured.

The *respiratory rate* is a measure of the number of times a person breathes in one minute. To measure the respiratory rate, have the patient assume a comfortable position. While the patient is at rest, count the number of respirations that occur in one minute. People will alter their respiratory pattern if they feel it is being watched, so it is best to distract the patient. Skilled personnel will often take a patient's wrist and measure the pulse. Then while still holding the wrist, they will count the respiratory rate while the patient thinks that the pulse is being measured.

The *BP* is a function of the amount of blood being pumped by the heart (cardiac output) and the peripheral vascular resistance. To determine the BP, a *blood pressure cuff (sphygmomanometer)* is placed on the arm 3−4 cm above the elbow (**Figure 13-7b**). A stethoscope is placed over the brachial artery. The blood pressure cuff is inflated to approximately 30 mm Hg above the point where it occludes the brachial artery and stops the flow of blood. Then, the pressure in the cuff is slowly released. When the pressure in the cuff falls below systolic pressure, blood flow resumes in the artery and produces *Korotkoff sounds*. As the pressure falls, the vessel remains open longer and the sounds in the artery change. When the cuff pressure falls below the diastolic pressure, blood flow becomes continuous and the Korotkoff sounds disappear completely.

The *temperature* is not often measured in EMS. However, electronic thermometers have made this a simple procedure. The temperature is measured in the mouth (under the tongue), rectally, or through the ear (tympanic membrane). Normal body temperature is 37°C (98.6°F).

Figure 13-7 Checking the Pulse and Blood Pressure.

(a) Several pressure points can be used to monitor the pulse or control peripheral bleeding. **(b)** A sphygmomanometer and a stethoscope are used to check an individual's blood pressure.

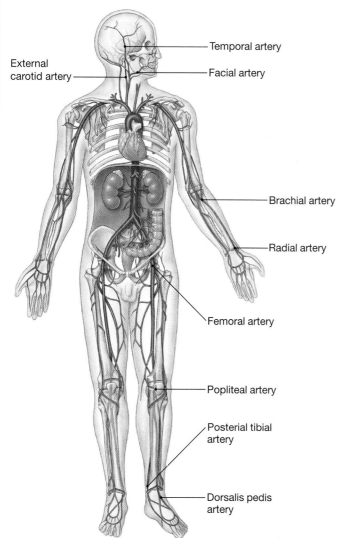

External carotid artery

Temporal artery

Facial artery

Brachial artery

Radial artery

Femoral artery

Popliteal artery

Posterial tibial artery

Dorsalis pedis artery

(a)

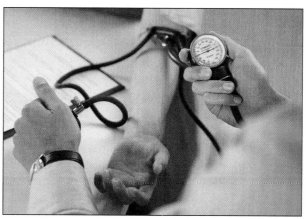

(b)

13

immediate, localized homeostatic adjustments. If autoregulation fails to normalize tissue conditions, then neural and endocrine processes are activated.

- *Neural processes.* The nervous system responds to changes in arterial pressure or blood gas levels sensed at specific sites. When those changes take place, the autonomic nervous system adjusts cardiac output and peripheral resistance to maintain adequate blood flow.

- *Endocrine processes.* The endocrine system releases hormones that enhance short-term adjustments and direct long-term changes in cardiovascular performance.

Short-term responses adjust cardiac output and peripheral resistance to stabilize blood pressure and blood flow to tissues. Long-term adjustments involve alterations in blood volume that affect cardiac output and the transport of oxygen and carbon dioxide to and from active tissues.

The regulatory relationships that compensate for a reduction in blood pressure and blood flow are diagrammed in **Figure 13-8**.

Autoregulation of Blood Flow within Tissues

Under normal resting conditions, cardiac output remains stable. Peripheral resistance within individual tissues is adjusted by precapillary sphincters to control local blood flow.

The smooth muscles of precapillary sphincters respond automatically to certain changes in the local environment. Such changes may take place in oxygen and carbon dioxide levels or the presence of specific chemicals. For example, when oxygen is abundant, the smooth muscle cells in the sphincters contract and slow the flow of blood. As the cells take up and use O_2, tissue oxygen supplies dwindle, carbon dioxide levels rise, and pH falls. These chemical changes signal the smooth muscle cells in the precapillary sphincters to relax, and blood flow increases. Similarly, changes involving other chemicals can trigger the relaxation of precapillary sphincters, increasing blood flow. These triggers include the presence of histamine at an injury site during inflammation, and the release of nitric oxide by capillary endothelial cells stimulated by high shear forces along the capillary walls.

Factors that promote the dilation of precapillary sphincters are called **vasodilators**. Those that stimulate the constriction of precapillary sphincters are called **vasoconstrictors**. Together, such factors control blood flow in a single capillary bed. In high concentrations, these factors also affect arterioles, increasing or decreasing blood flow to all the capillary beds in a given region. Such an event often triggers a neural response, because significant changes in blood flow to one region of the body immediately affect circulation to other regions.

Neural Control of Blood Pressure and Blood Flow

The nervous system adjusts cardiac output and peripheral resistance to maintain adequate blood flow to vital tissues and organs. The *cardiovascular center* of the medulla oblongata is responsible for these regulatory activities. ⟲ p. 278 This center includes the *cardiac center* and the *vasomotor center*. The cardiac center has a *cardioacceleratory center*, which increases cardiac output through sympathetic innervation (as noted in Chapter 12). The cardiac center also has a *cardioinhibitory center*, which reduces cardiac output through parasympathetic innervation. ⟲ p. 424

The vasomotor center of the medulla oblongata primarily controls the diameters of arterioles through sympathetic innervation. Inhibition of the vasomotor center leads to vasodilation (dilation of arterioles), reducing peripheral resistance. Stimulation of the vasomotor center causes vasoconstriction (constriction of peripheral arterioles). Very strong stimulation causes **venoconstriction** (constriction of peripheral veins). Both types of constriction increase peripheral resistance.

The *cardiovascular center* detects changes in tissue demand by monitoring arterial blood, especially blood pressure, pH, and dissolved gas concentrations. *Baroreceptor reflexes* respond to changes in blood pressure. *Chemoreceptor reflexes* respond to changes in chemical composition. Negative feedback regulates these reflexes: The stimulation of a receptor by an abnormal condition leads to a response that counteracts the stimulus and restores normal conditions.

Baroreceptor Reflexes

Baroreceptors monitor the degree of stretch in the walls of expandable organs. ⟲ p. 310 The baroreceptors involved in cardiovascular regulation are found in the walls of (1) the **carotid sinuses**, expanded chambers near the bases of the *internal carotid arteries* of the neck (**Figure 13-9a**, p. 504); (2) the **aortic sinuses**, pockets in the walls of the aorta adjacent to the heart

Figure 13-8 Short-Term and Long-Term Cardiovascular Responses.

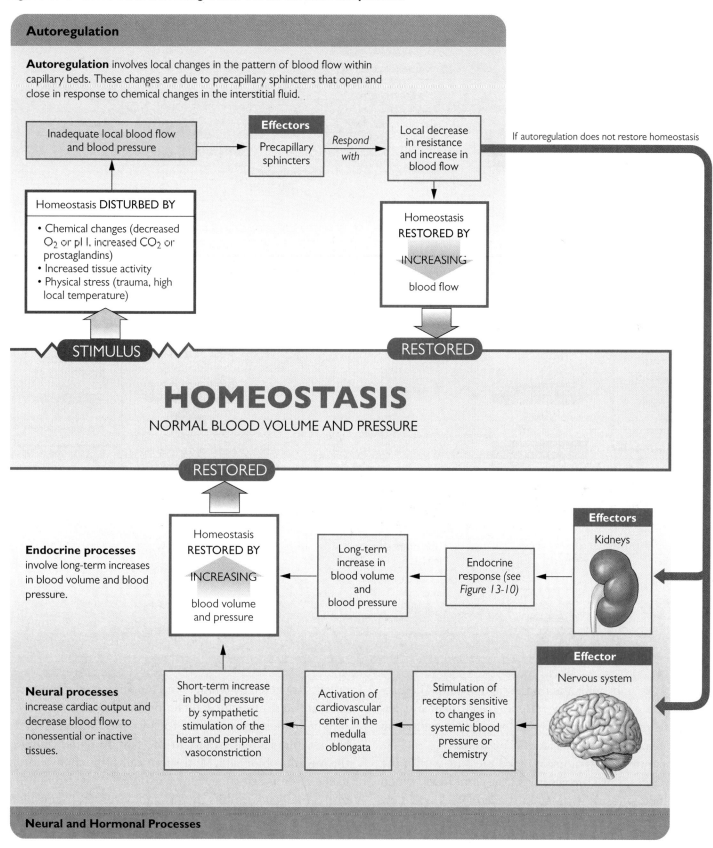

Autoregulation

Autoregulation involves local changes in the pattern of blood flow within capillary beds. These changes are due to precapillary sphincters that open and close in response to chemical changes in the interstitial fluid.

Inadequate local blood flow and blood pressure

Effectors
Precapillary sphincters

Respond with

Local decrease in resistance and increase in blood flow

If autoregulation does not restore homeostasis

Homeostasis DISTURBED BY
• Chemical changes (decreased O₂ or pI I, increased CO₂ or prostaglandins)
• Increased tissue activity
• Physical stress (trauma, high local temperature)

Homeostasis RESTORED BY INCREASING blood flow

STIMULUS

RESTORED

HOMEOSTASIS
NORMAL BLOOD VOLUME AND PRESSURE

RESTORED

Endocrine processes involve long-term increases in blood volume and blood pressure.

Homeostasis RESTORED BY INCREASING blood volume and pressure

Long-term increase in blood volume and blood pressure

Endocrine response *(see Figure 13-10)*

Effectors
Kidneys

Neural processes increase cardiac output and decrease blood flow to nonessential or inactive tissues.

Short-term increase in blood pressure by sympathetic stimulation of the heart and peripheral vasoconstriction

Activation of cardiovascular center in the medulla oblongata

Stimulation of receptors sensitive to changes in systemic blood pressure or chemistry

Effector
Nervous system

Neural and Hormonal Processes

Figure 13-9 The Baroreceptor Reflexes of the Carotid and Aortic Sinuses.

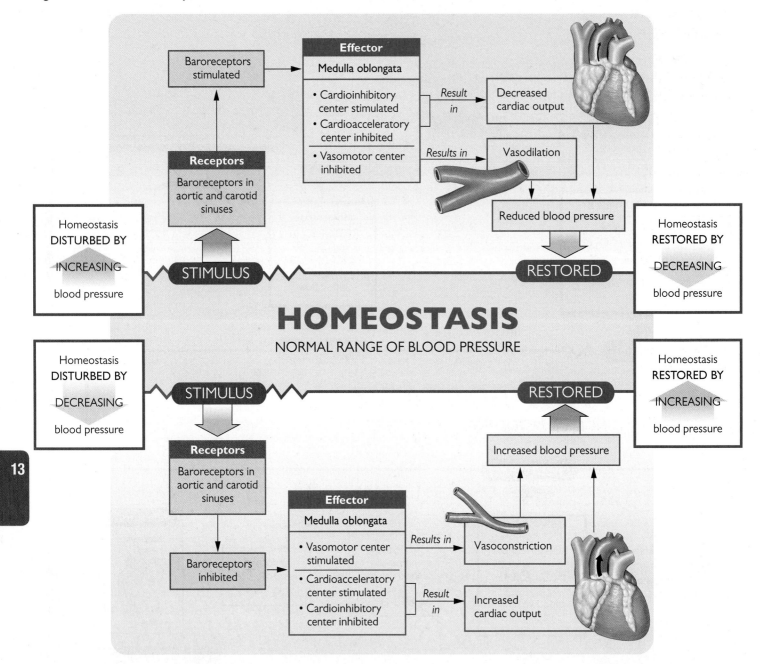

(see **Figure 12-6b**, p. 466); and (3) the right atrium. These receptors initiate **baroreceptor reflexes** (*baro-,* pressure), autonomic reflexes that adjust cardiac output and peripheral resistance to maintain normal arterial pressures.

Aortic baroreceptors monitor blood pressure within the ascending aorta. Any changes trigger the *aortic reflex*, which adjusts blood pressure to maintain adequate blood flow through the systemic circuit. Carotid sinus baroreceptors trigger reflexes that maintain adequate blood flow to the brain. These receptors are extremely sensitive because blood flow to the brain must remain constant. The baroreceptor

reflexes triggered by changes in blood pressure at the aortic and carotid sinuses are diagrammed in **Figure 13-9**.

When blood pressure rises, the increased output from the baroreceptors alters activity in the cardiovascular center of the medulla oblongata. More specifically, this change inhibits the cardioacceleratory center, stimulates the cardioinhibitory center, and inhibits the vasomotor center (**Figure 13-9**). Two effects result:

1. *A decrease in cardiac output.* Under the command of the cardioinhibitory center, the vagus nerves release acetylcholine at the sinoatrial (SA) node. This parasympathetic stimulation reduces the rate and force of cardiac contractions.

2. ***Widespread peripheral vasodilation.*** The inhibition of the vasomotor center leads to dilation of peripheral arterioles throughout the body.

This combination of reduced cardiac output and decreased peripheral resistance then lowers blood pressure.

When blood pressure falls below normal, baroreceptor output is reduced (**Figure 13-9**). This change has two major effects that work together to raise blood pressure:

1. ***An increase in cardiac output.*** Reduced baroreceptor activity stimulates the cardioacceleratory center, inhibits the cardioinhibitory center, and stimulates the vasomotor center. The cardioacceleratory center stimulates sympathetic neurons to the SA node, atrioventricular node, and general myocardium. This sympathetic stimulation increases heart rate and stroke volume. As a result, cardiac output increases immediately.

2. ***A widespread peripheral vasoconstriction.*** Vasomotor activity, also carried by sympathetic motor neurons, produces rapid vasoconstriction. This change increases peripheral resistance.

These adjustments—increased cardiac output and increased peripheral resistance—work together to elevate blood pressure.

Atrial baroreceptors monitor blood pressure at the end of the systemic circuit—at the venae cavae and the right atrium. The *atrial reflex* is a response to the stretching of the wall of the right atrium. ⟲ p. 422 Normally, the heart pumps blood into the aorta at the same rate at which it arrives at the right atrium. A rise in blood pressure at the atrium means that blood is arriving at the heart faster than it is being pumped out. The atrial baroreceptors correct the situation by stimulating the cardioacceleratory center, increasing cardiac output until the backlog of venous blood is removed. Atrial pressure then returns to normal.

Chemoreceptor Reflexes

The **chemoreceptor reflexes** respond to changes in carbon dioxide, oxygen, or pH levels in blood and cerebrospinal fluid (CSF) (**Figure 13-10**). The chemoreceptors involved are

Figure 13-10 The Chemoreceptor Reflexes.

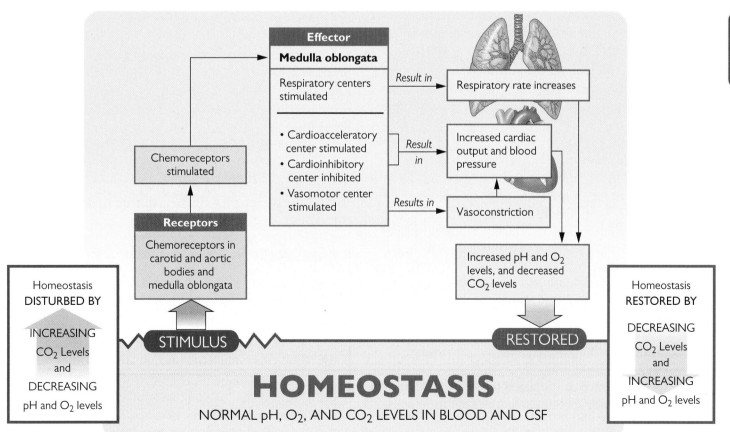

sensory neurons. They are found in the **carotid bodies** (located in the neck near the carotid sinuses) and in the **aortic bodies** (near the arch of the aorta). ⟳ p. 311 These receptors monitor the chemical composition of the arterial blood. Other chemoreceptors on the surface of the medulla oblongata monitor the composition of the CSF.

Chemoreceptors are activated by a decrease in pH or in plasma O_2, or by an increase in CO_2. Any of these changes leads to a stimulation of the cardioacceleratory and vasomotor centers. This elevates arterial pressure and increases blood flow through peripheral tissues. Chemoreceptor output also affects the respiratory centers in the medulla oblongata. As a result, a rise in blood flow and blood pressure is associated with an elevated respiratory rate. The coordination of cardiovascular and respiratory activity is vital, because accelerating tissue blood flow is useful only if the blood contains adequate oxygen. In addition, an increase in the respiratory rate speeds up venous return through the action of the respiratory pump. ⟳ p. 439

Hormones and Cardiovascular Regulation

The endocrine system regulates cardiovascular performance in both the short term and long term. In the short term, epinephrine (E) and norepinephrine (NE) from the adrenal medullae stimulate cardiac output and peripheral vasoconstriction. Long-term cardiovascular regulation involves other hormones. These are antidiuretic hormone (ADH), angiotensin II, erythropoietin (EPO), and atrial natriuretic peptide (ANP) (introduced in Chapter 10). ⟳ pp. 355, 367 Their roles in the regulation of blood pressure and blood volume are diagrammed in **Figure 13-11**.

Antidiuretic Hormone

ADH is released at the posterior lobe of the pituitary gland. This happens in response to a decrease in blood volume, an increase in the osmotic concentration of the plasma, or the presence of angiotensin II (**Figure 13-11**). The immediate result is peripheral vasoconstriction that elevates blood pressure. ADH also has a water-conserving effect on the kidneys, thereby preventing a reduction in blood volume.

Angiotensin II

Angiotensin II is formed in the blood following the release of the enzyme renin by specialized kidney cells in response to a fall in blood pressure (**Figure 13-11**). Renin starts an enzymatic chain reaction that ultimately converts an inactive plasma protein, *angiotensinogen*, to the hormone angiotensin II. Angiotensin II stimulates cardiac output and triggers arteriole constriction, which in turn elevates systemic blood pressure almost immediately. This hormone also stimulates the pituitary gland to secrete ADH, and the adrenal cortex to secrete aldosterone.

ADH and aldosterone have complementary effects. ADH stimulates water conservation at the kidneys. Aldosterone stimulates sodium ion retention and potassium ion loss by the kidneys. In addition, angiotensin II stimulates thirst. The presence of ADH and aldosterone ensures that the additional water consumed will be retained, increasing blood volume.

Erythropoietin

The kidneys release EPO when blood pressure falls or when the oxygen content of the blood becomes abnormally low (**Figure 13-11**). EPO stimulates red blood cell production. The result is increased blood volume and improved oxygen-carrying capacity of the blood.

Atrial Natriuretic Peptide

In contrast to the three hormones just described, ANP release is stimulated by *increased* blood pressure (**Figure 13-11**). The cardiac muscle cells in the wall of the right atrium produce ANP when they are stretched by excessive venous return. ANP reduces blood volume and blood pressure by (1) increasing the loss of sodium ions by the kidneys; (2) promoting water losses by increasing the volume of urine; (3) reducing thirst; (4) blocking the release of ADH, aldosterone, E, and NE; and (5) stimulating peripheral vasodilation. As blood volume and blood pressure decrease, the stresses on the atrial walls are removed. ANP production then ceases.

CHECKPOINT

8. Describe the actions of vasodilators and vasoconstrictors.

9. How would applying slight pressure to the common carotid artery affect your heart rate?

10. What effect would the vasoconstriction of the renal artery have on blood pressure and blood volume?

See the blue Answers tab at the back of the book.

Figure 13-11 The Hormonal Regulation of Blood Pressure and Blood Volume.

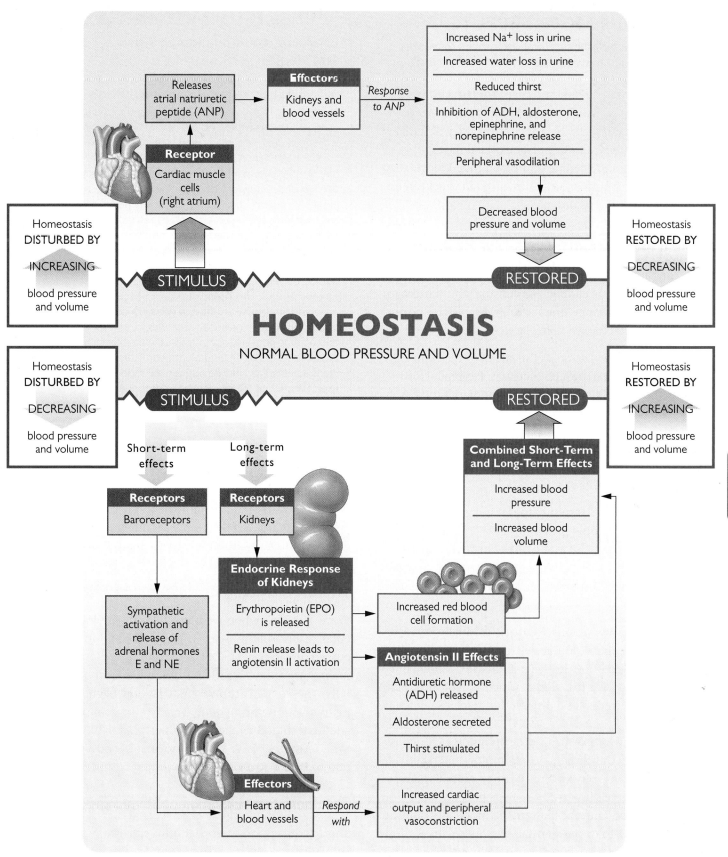

13-4 The cardiovascular system adapts to physiological stress

Learning Objective Explain the cardiovascular system's homeostatic response to exercise and hemorrhaging.

In our day-to-day lives, the components of the cardiovascular system—the blood, heart, and blood vessels—work together in an integrated way. In this section, we will see how this adaptable system maintains homeostasis in response to two common stresses: exercise and blood loss. We will also look at the physiological processes involved in shock, an important cardiovascular disorder.

Exercise and the Cardiovascular System

At rest, cardiac output averages about 5.8 liters per minute. During exercise, both cardiac output and the pattern of blood distribution change dramatically. As exercise begins, several interrelated changes take place:

- *Extensive vasodilation occurs* as the rate of oxygen consumption in skeletal muscles increases. Peripheral resistance drops, blood flow through the capillaries increases, and blood enters the venous system at a faster rate.

- *Venous return increases* as skeletal muscle contractions squeeze blood along the peripheral veins. A faster breathing rate also pulls blood into the venae cavae by the respiratory pump.

- *Cardiac output rises* in response to (1) the rise in venous return (the Frank–Starling principle) and (2) atrial stretching (the atrial reflex). ⊃ pp. 422–423 The increased cardiac output keeps pace with the greater demand. Arterial pressures are maintained despite the drop in peripheral resistance.

This regulation by venous feedback gradually increases cardiac output to about double resting levels. The increase supports faster blood flow to skeletal muscles, cardiac muscle, and the skin. Over this range, which is typical of light exercise, the pattern of blood distribution remains relatively unchanged.

At higher levels of exertion, other physiological adjustments take place as the cardiac and vasomotor centers activate the sympathetic nervous system. Cardiac output increases toward maximal levels (up to 20–25 liters per minute), blood pressure increases, and the pattern of blood distribution shifts. Blood flow to "nonessential" organs (such as those of the digestive system) becomes severely restricted. This shift helps to increase blood flow to active skeletal muscles.

CLINICAL NOTE

Exercise, Cardiovascular Fitness, and Health

Cardiovascular performance improves significantly with training. Trained athletes have larger hearts and stroke volumes than do nonathletes. These functional changes are important. Recall that cardiac output is equal to stroke volume times heart rate. So, for a given cardiac output, a person with a larger stroke volume has a lower heart rate. A professional athlete at rest can maintain normal blood flow to peripheral tissues at a heart rate as low as 32 bpm (beats per minute), compared with about 80 bpm for a nonathlete. And, when necessary, the athlete's cardiac output can increase to levels 50 percent higher than those of nonathletes.

If you are not a trained athlete, regular exercise still has several beneficial effects. Even a modest exercise routine (jogging 5 miles per week, for example) can lower total blood cholesterol levels. High cholesterol is one of the major risk factors for atherosclerosis, which leads to cardiovascular disease and strokes. In addition, a healthy lifestyle— regular exercise, a balanced diet, weight control, and no smoking—reduces stress, lowers blood pressure, and slows plaque formation. Large-scale statistical studies indicate that regular moderate exercise can cut the incidence of heart attacks almost in half.

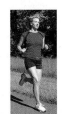

When you exercise at maximal levels, your blood essentially races among your skeletal muscles, lungs, and heart. Blood flow to most tissues is diminished, but that to the skin increases further, because body temperature continues to climb. Only the blood supply to the brain is unaffected.

The Cardiovascular Response to Hemorrhage

What happens when we bleed? Recall the local cardiovascular reaction to a break in the wall of a blood vessel discussed in Chapter 11. ⊃ p. 397 When the clotting response fails to prevent a significant blood loss and blood pressure falls, the entire cardiovascular system begins making adjustments. The immediate, short-term goal is to maintain adequate blood pressure and peripheral blood flow. The long-term goal is to restore normal blood volume (lower half of **Figure 13-11**).

The Short-Term Elevation of Blood Pressure

Short-term responses appear almost as soon as blood pressure starts to decline. For example, the carotid and aortic reflexes increase cardiac output and cause peripheral

CLINICAL NOTE

Shock

Shock (hypoperfusion) is a state of inadequate tissue perfusion and is often the end product of many disease and injury processes. During shock, body tissues are deprived of oxygen and essential nutrients. At the same time, carbon dioxide and other waste products accumulate. Regardless of the cause, shock results from one of three physiological problems. These include an inadequate pump (cardiogenic shock), inadequate fluid (hypovolemic shock), or an inadequate container (neurogenic shock). All of these can result in a fall in blood pressure and, ultimately, inadequate tissue perfusion.

Cardiogenic shock occurs when the heart fails as an effective pump. This is a complication of heart attack or congestive heart failure. *Hypovolemic shock* results from the loss of blood or plasma from the intravascular space. It is seen following severe hemorrhage, burns, crush injuries, and severe nausea and vomiting. *Neurogenic shock* occurs when autonomic control of peripheral

blood vessels is lost, resulting in marked dilation and a marked decrease in peripheral vascular resistance. This can be seen following a spinal-cord injury where nerve fibers are severed. It can also be seen in severe allergic reactions (*anaphylactic shock*) where histamine and other chemical mediators cause marked peripheral vascular dilation and loss of plasma from the capillaries. Thus, anaphylactic shock involves problems with both fluid loss and peripheral vascular dilation. Another form of neurogenic shock, *septic shock,* occurs following a severe bacterial infection, whereby bacteria release potent *endotoxins* that cause marked peripheral vasodilation that results in shock.

The signs and symptoms of shock, which can often be subtle, include altered mental status; pale, cool, clammy skin; nausea and vomiting, increased pulse rate, increased respiratory rate, and a fall in blood pressure. A fall in blood pressure is considered a late sign. Shock is best treated when it is promptly identified and emergency interventions are provided before the blood pressure falls.

---

vasoconstriction. When you donate blood at a blood bank, the amount collected is usually 500 mL, roughly 10 percent of your total blood volume. Such a loss initially causes a drop in cardiac output. However, the vasomotor center quickly improves venous return and restores cardiac output to normal levels by mobilizing a large *venous reservoir* of slowly moving blood from the digestive organs that drains into the liver, through venoconstriction (see **Figure 13-11** on p. 507). This venous compensation can restore normal arterial pressures and peripheral blood flow after losses of 15–20 percent of total blood volume.

With a more substantial blood loss, cardiac output is maintained by increasing the heart rate, often to 180–200 bpm. Sympathetic activation assists by constricting the muscular arteries and arterioles, which elevates blood pressure. Sympathetic activation also causes the adrenal medullae to secrete E and NE. At the same time, the posterior lobe of the pituitary gland releases ADH, and the fall in blood pressure in the kidneys causes the release of renin. This enzyme, in turn, activates angiotensin II. Both E and NE increase cardiac output. In combination with ADH and angiotensin II, they cause a powerful vasoconstriction that raises blood pressure and improves peripheral blood flow.

The Long-Term Restoration of Blood Volume

After serious hemorrhaging, several days may pass before blood volume returns to normal. When short-term responses are unable to maintain normal cardiac output and blood pressure, the decline in capillary blood pressure triggers a

recall of fluids from the interstitial spaces. ⮌ p. 439 Over this period, ADH and aldosterone promote fluid retention and reabsorption at the kidneys, preventing further reductions in blood volume. Thirst increases, and additional water is absorbed across the digestive tract. This intake of fluid increases blood volume and ultimately replaces the interstitial fluids "borrowed" at the capillaries. EPO targets the red bone marrow, stimulating red blood cells to mature. These cells increase blood volume and improve oxygen delivery to peripheral tissues.

13

CHECKPOINT

11. Why does blood pressure increase during exercise?

12. Name the immediate and long-term problems related to the cardiovascular response to hemorrhaging.

13. Explain the role of aldosterone and ADH in long-term restoration of blood volume.

See the blue Answers tab at the back of the book.

13-5 The pulmonary and systemic circuits of the cardiovascular system exhibit three general functional patterns

Learning Objective Describe the three general functional patterns seen in the pulmonary and systemic circuits.

Recall that the cardiovascular system is divided into the **pulmonary circuit** and the **systemic circuit**. ⮌ p. 405 The pulmonary circuit is made up of arteries and veins that transport blood between the heart and the lungs. This circuit begins at the right ventricle and ends at the left atrium. The systemic circuit is made up of arteries that transport oxygenated blood and nutrients to all other organs and tissues, and veins that return deoxygenated blood to the heart. This circuit begins at the left ventricle and ends at the right atrium. **Figure 13-12** summarizes the main distribution routes within the pulmonary and systemic circuits.

Figure 13-12 An Overview of the Pattern of Circulation.

RA stands for right atrium; LA for left atrium.

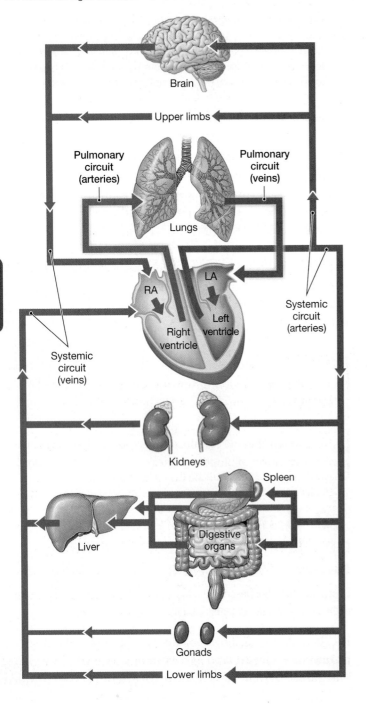

We will examine the vessels of these two circuits in the following pages. Three general functional patterns of blood vessels are worth noting:

1. The distribution of arteries and veins on the left and right sides of the body is usually identical—except near the heart, where large vessels connect to the atria or ventricles. For example, the distribution of the *left* and *right subclavian, axillary, brachial,* and *radial arteries* parallels the *left* and *right subclavian, axillary, brachial,* and *radial veins.*

2. A single vessel may have several name changes as it crosses specific anatomical boundaries. For example, the *external iliac artery* becomes the *femoral artery* as it leaves the trunk and enters the thigh.

3. Tissues and organs are usually serviced by several arteries and veins. Often, anastomoses between adjacent arteries or veins reduce the impact of a temporary or even permanent *occlusion* (blockage) of a single blood vessel.

CHECKPOINT

14. Identify the two circuits of the cardiovascular system.

15. Identify the three general functional patterns of the body's blood vessels.

See the blue Answers tab at the back of the book.

13-6 In the pulmonary circuit, deoxygenated blood enters the lungs in arteries, and oxygenated blood leaves the lungs in veins

Learning Objective Identify the major arteries and veins of the pulmonary circuit.

Blood entering the right atrium has just returned from peripheral capillary beds. There it released oxygen and absorbed carbon dioxide. After traveling through the right atrium and right ventricle, blood enters the **pulmonary trunk** (*pulmo-,* lung), the start of the pulmonary circuit (**Figure 13-13**). (By convention, several large arteries are called *trunks.*) At the lungs, oxygen is replenished, and carbon dioxide is released. The oxygenated blood returns to the heart for distribution by the systemic circuit.

The pulmonary circuit is quite short, compared with the systemic circuit. The base of the pulmonary trunk and the lungs are only about 15 cm (6 in.) apart.

Figure 13-13 The Pulmonary Circuit.

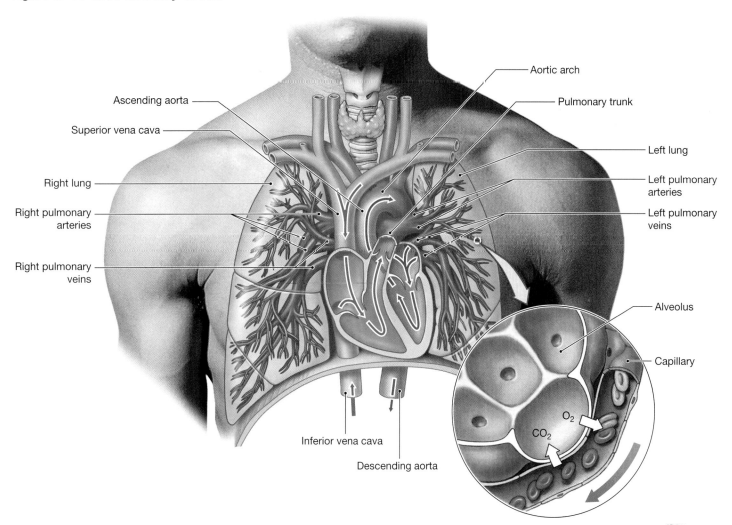

- Ascending aorta
- Superior vena cava
- Right lung
- Right pulmonary arteries
- Right pulmonary veins
- Aortic arch
- Pulmonary trunk
- Left lung
- Left pulmonary arteries
- Left pulmonary veins
- Alveolus
- Capillary
- O_2
- CO_2
- Inferior vena cava
- Descending aorta

13

CLINICAL NOTE

Acute Pulmonary Embolism

Acute pulmonary embolism (PE) occurs when a blood clot or other particle lodges in a pulmonary artery and blocks blood flow through that vessel. Pulmonary emboli may be composed of air, fat, amniotic fluid, or blood clots. Factors that predispose a patient to blood clots include prolonged immobilization, thrombophlebitis (inflammation and clots in a vein), use of certain medications, and atrial fibrillation. Long periods of travel in airplanes and automobiles increase an individual's chances of developing a PE.

When a PE blocks the blood flow through a pulmonary vessel, the right heart must pump against increased resistance, which in turn increases pulmonary capillary pressure (**Figure 13-11**). The area of the lung supplied by the occluded vessel then stops functioning, and gas exchange decreases. The larger the volume of the lung affected, the more significant the problems with gas exchange.

The signs and symptoms of pulmonary embolism depend upon the size of the obstruction. The patient who suffers from an acute PE may report a sudden onset of severe and unexplained dyspnea that may or may not be associated with chest pain. The signs and symptoms of an acute PE can be subtle and easily overlooked. The diagnosis can be made using several imaging techniques. A frequently used test is the ventilation/perfusion scan (V/Q scan), for which the patient inhales radioactive material and also has radioactive material injected into his or her venous system. Two sets of images of the patient's lungs are obtained, one that shows pulmonary ventilation through the respiratory tree and the other that shows pulmonary perfusion in the pulmonary circulatory system. Areas of the lung that are ventilated but not perfused indicate a PE. The gold standard for the diagnosis of PE is a pulmonary arteriogram that will show any blockage in the pulmonary circulation. Pulmonary angiograms are higher risk procedures than V/Q scans and require specialized facilities.

The treatment of a PE varies depending upon its size. With small to moderate emboli, the patient will usually receive a blood thinner and be closely monitored in the hospital. Large emboli, as evidenced by marked hypoxia and low blood pressure, may require thrombolytic therapy. In most severe cases, the affected pulmonary artery is catheterized and a thrombolytic agent is injected directly into the affected vessel.

The arteries of the pulmonary circuit differ from those of the systemic circuit in that they carry deoxygenated blood. (For this reason, color-coded diagrams usually show the pulmonary arteries in blue, the same color as systemic veins.) As the pulmonary trunk curves over the superior border of the heart, it gives rise to the **left** and **right pulmonary arteries**. These large arteries enter the lungs and then branch repeatedly, giving rise to smaller and smaller arteries.

The smallest branches, the *pulmonary arterioles*, provide blood to capillary networks that surround small air pockets, or **alveoli** (al-VĒ-ō-lī; *alveolus*, sac). The walls of alveoli are thin enough for gas exchange to take place between the capillary blood and inhaled air.

As oxygenated blood leaves the *alveolar capillaries*, it enters venules, which in turn unite to form larger vessels leading to the **pulmonary veins**. These four veins (two from each lung) empty into the left atrium, completing the pulmonary circuit.

CHECKPOINT

16. Name the blood vessels that enter and exit the lungs, and note whether they contain primarily oxygenated or deoxygenated blood.

17. Trace the path of a drop of blood through the lungs, beginning at the right ventricle and ending at the left atrium.

See the blue Answers tab at the back of the book.

13-7 The systemic circuit carries oxygenated blood from the left ventricle to tissues other than the lungs' exchange surfaces, and returns deoxygenated blood to the right atrium

Learning Objective Identify the major arteries and veins of the systemic circuit.

The systemic circuit supplies the capillary beds in all parts of the body not serviced by the pulmonary circuit. This circuit begins at the left ventricle and ends at the right atrium. At any moment, the systemic circuit contains about 84 percent of total blood volume. **Spotlight Figure 13-17** provides an overview of the arterial and venous systems of the systemic circuit.

Systemic Arteries

Spotlight Figure 13-17a shows the locations of the major systemic arteries.

The Ascending Aorta

The first systemic vessel and largest artery is the aorta. The **ascending aorta** begins at the aortic semilunar valve of the left ventricle. The *left* and *right coronary arteries* originate near its base (see **Figure 12-7**, p. 467). The **aortic arch** curves across the superior surface of the heart, connecting the ascending aorta with the **descending aorta** (Figure 13-14).

CLINICAL NOTE

Aneurysm

An *aneurysm* is a bulging in the weakened wall of a blood vessel. Aneurysms are at risk for rupture, and rupture of aneurysms in the brain, aorta, or heart can be rapidly fatal. The several types of aneurysms include

- Atherosclerotic
- Dissecting
- Infectious
- Congenital
- Traumatic

Most aneurysms result from atherosclerosis and involve the aorta because the blood pressure there is higher than at any other vessel in the body (**Figures 13-14, 13-15**). An aneurysm usually occurs gradually. Eventually, blood surges into the aortic wall through a tear in the aortic *tunica intima*. Infectious aneurysms are most commonly associated with syphilis and are rare in the U.S. Congenital aneurysms can occur with several disease states, such as Marfan's syndrome, which is a hereditary disease that affects the connective tissue. Aortic aneurysm occurs in people with Marfan's syndrome because it involves the connective tissue within the vessel wall. Those affected may experience sudden death, usually from spontaneous rupture of the aorta, often at a fairly young age. Aortic aneurysms can occur in the chest or in the abdomen. Thoracic aortic aneurysms usually involve the arch of the aorta. They cause symptoms by eroding into nearby structures. Rupture of a thoracic aortic aneurysm is usually a catastrophic event.

Abdominal Aortic Aneurysm

Abdominal aortic aneurysm usually results from atherosclerosis and occurs most frequently in the aorta, below the renal arteries and above the bifurcation of the common iliac arteries (**Figure 13-16**). It is 10 times more common in men than in women and most prevalent between ages 60 and 70. Many abdominal aortic aneurysms are detected by physical exam or by diagnostic imaging (X-rays, ultrasound). Nondissecting aneurysms less than 5 cm in diameter are usually monitored. Larger aneurysms, or those that are rapidly expanding, require surgical repair.

Figure 13-14 Normal Artery. Post-mortem specimen of a large artery, opened to reveal minimal atherosclerotic changes.

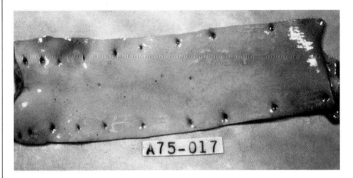

Figure 13-15 Atherosclerotic Changes. Marked atherosclerosis in a medium-sized artery that causes turbulent blood flow and marked blood flow resistance.

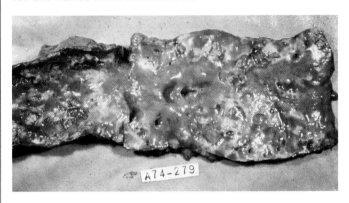

The signs and symptoms of an abdominal aneurysm include

- Abdominal pain
- Back and flank pain
- Hypotension
- Urge to defecate, caused by the retroperitoneal leakage of blood

Rupture or leaking of an aortic aneurysm is a surgical emergency. Patients suspected of having this condition should be promptly taken to surgery for repair and grafting. Massive transfusion of blood in these cases is common.

Figure 13-16 Abdominal Aortic Aneurysm. Most abdominal aortic aneurysms occur below the level of the branches of the renal arteries and extend down to the bifurcation of the iliac arteries. Rupture can cause rapid exsanguination that will be rapidly fatal without emergency surgical repair.

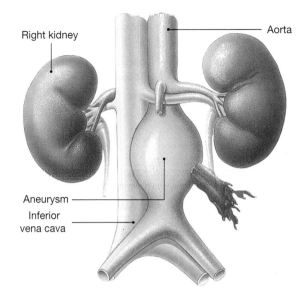

Dissecting Aneurysm

Some aneurysms will begin to dissect within the wall of the blood vessel. Most dissecting aortic aneurysms result from degenerative changes in the smooth muscle and elastic tissue of the aortic tunica media that can result in hematoma and, subsequently, aneurysm. The original tear often is due to *cystic medial necrosis*, which is a degenerative disease of connective tissue commonly associated with hypertension and to a certain extent, aging. Predisposing factors include hypertension, which is present in 75–85 percent of cases. It occurs more frequently in patients older than 40–50, although it can occur in younger individuals, especially pregnant women. A tendency for this disease also runs in families.

Of dissecting aortic aneurysms, 67 percent involve the ascending aorta. Once dissection has started, it can extend to all of the abdominal aorta as well as its branches, including the coronary arteries, aortic valve, subclavian arteries, and carotid arteries. The aneurysm can rupture at any time, usually into the pericardial or pleural cavity, which often causes death.

Arteries of the Aortic Arch

Three elastic arteries—the **brachiocephalic** (br-k–se-FAL-ik) **trunk**, the **left common carotid**, and the **left subclavian** (sub-CLĀ-vē-an)—originate along the aortic arch. They deliver blood to the head, neck, shoulders, and upper limbs (**Figures 13-18** and **13-19**). The brachiocephalic trunk ascends for a short distance before branching to form the **right common carotid artery** and the **right subclavian artery**. Note that we have only one brachiocephalic trunk, and that the left common carotid and left subclavian arteries arise separately from the aortic arch. In terms of their peripheral distribution, however, the vessels on the left side are mirror images of those on the right side. Because most of the major arteries are paired, with one artery of each pair on either side of the body, the descriptions that follow will not use the terms *right* and *left*.

Systemic Arteries

This figure is an overview of the major systemic arteries. Note that all arteries of the systemic circuit originate from the aorta, the large elastic artery extending from the left ventricle of the heart. When naming vessels, several large arteries are called *trunks*. Systemic arterial trunks include the *thyrocervical*, *brachiocephalic*, and *celiac trunks*. (The *pulmonary trunk* of the pulmonary circuit in Figure 13-12 is another example.)

To reduce clutter here, and in the figures that follow, "artery" will not be repeated in every label. Because most of the major arteries are paired, with one artery of each pair on either side of the body, the terms "right" and "left" will appear in figure labels only when the arteries on both sides are labeled.

KEY

■ Arteries
■ Superficial veins
■ Deep veins

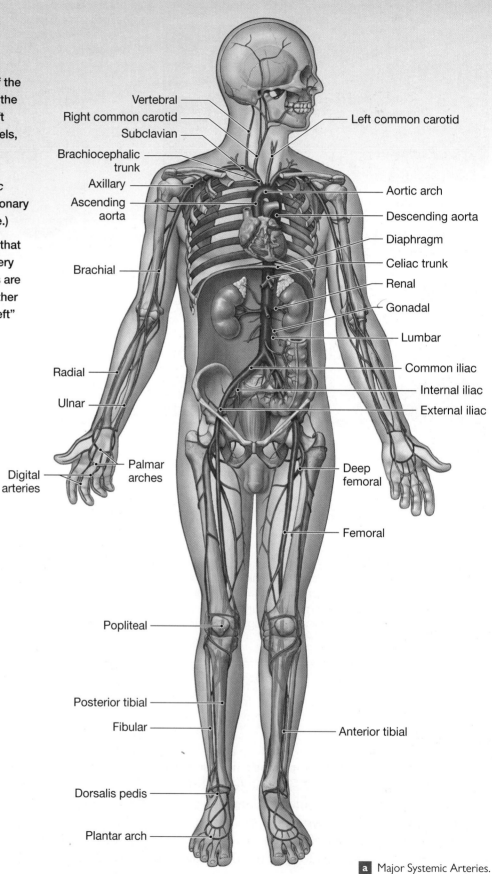

Vertebral
Right common carotid
Subclavian
Brachiocephalic trunk
Axillary
Ascending aorta
Brachial
Radial
Ulnar
Digital arteries
Palmar arches

Left common carotid
Aortic arch
Descending aorta
Diaphragm
Celiac trunk
Renal
Gonadal
Lumbar
Common iliac
Internal iliac
External iliac
Deep femoral
Femoral

Popliteal
Posterior tibial
Fibular
Anterior tibial
Dorsalis pedis
Plantar arch

a Major Systemic Arteries.

Systemic Veins

Vertebral
External jugular
Internal jugular
Subclavian
Brachiocephalic
Axillary
Cephalic
Brachial
Basilic
Radial
Median antebrachial
Ulnar
Palmar venous arches
Digital veins
Great saphenous
Popliteal
Small saphenous
Fibular
Plantar venous arch
Dorsal venous arch

Superior vena cava
Intercostal veins
Diaphragm
Inferior vena cava
Renal
Gonadal
Lumbar veins
Common iliac
Internal iliac
External iliac
Deep femoral
Femoral
Posterior tibial
Anterior tibial

This figure is an overview of the major systemic veins. Note that veins of the systemic circuit merge into two large veins: the superior vena cava, which collects systemic blood from the head, chest, and upper limbs, and the inferior vena cava, which collects systemic blood from all structures inferior to the diaphragm.

To reduce clutter here, and in the figures that follow, "vein" will not be repeated in every label. The same name often applies to both the artery and the vein servicing a particular structure or region. Additionally, "right" and "left" will appear in figure labels only when the veins on both sides are shown.

One significant difference between the systemic arteries and veins is the distribution of major veins in the neck and limbs. Arteries in these areas are located deep beneath the skin, protected by bones and surrounding soft tissues. In contrast, the neck and limbs usually have two sets of peripheral veins, one superficial and the other deep. This dual venous drainage is important for controlling body temperature. In hot weather, venous blood flows through superficial veins, where heat can easily be lost. In cold weather, blood is routed to the deep veins to minimize heat loss.

b Major Systemic Veins.

515

Figure 13-18 Arteries of the Chest and Upper Limb.

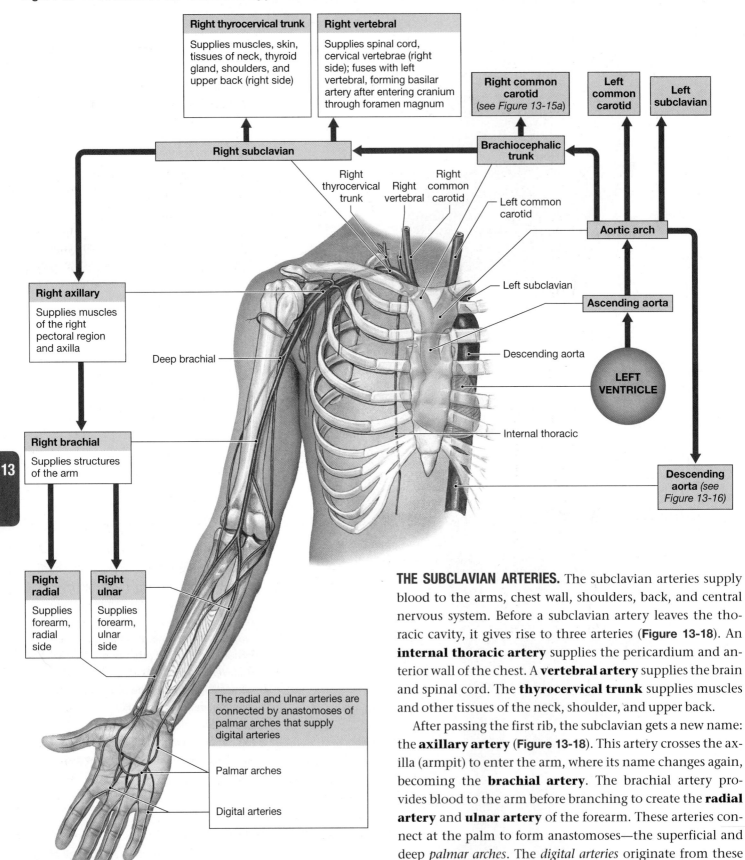

Right thyrocervical trunk	**Right vertebral**
Supplies muscles, skin, tissues of neck, thyroid gland, shoulders, and upper back (right side)	Supplies spinal cord, cervical vertebrae (right side); fuses with left vertebral, forming basilar artery after entering cranium through foramen magnum

Right common carotid (see Figure 13-15a)

Left common carotid

Left subclavian

Right subclavian

Brachiocephalic trunk

Right thyrocervical trunk

Right vertebral

Right common carotid

Left common carotid

Aortic arch

Left subclavian

Right axillary

Supplies muscles of the right pectoral region and axilla

Ascending aorta

Deep brachial

Descending aorta

LEFT VENTRICLE

Right brachial

Supplies structures of the arm

Internal thoracic

Descending aorta (see Figure 13-16)

Right radial	**Right ulnar**
Supplies forearm, radial side	Supplies forearm, ulnar side

The radial and ulnar arteries are connected by anastomoses of palmar arches that supply digital arteries

Palmar arches

Digital arteries

THE SUBCLAVIAN ARTERIES. The subclavian arteries supply blood to the arms, chest wall, shoulders, back, and central nervous system. Before a subclavian artery leaves the thoracic cavity, it gives rise to three arteries (**Figure 13-18**). An **internal thoracic artery** supplies the pericardium and anterior wall of the chest. A **vertebral artery** supplies the brain and spinal cord. The **thyrocervical trunk** supplies muscles and other tissues of the neck, shoulder, and upper back.

After passing the first rib, the subclavian gets a new name: the **axillary artery** (**Figure 13-18**). This artery crosses the axilla (armpit) to enter the arm, where its name changes again, becoming the **brachial artery**. The brachial artery provides blood to the arm before branching to create the **radial artery** and **ulnar artery** of the forearm. These arteries connect at the palm to form anastomoses—the superficial and deep *palmar arches*. The *digital arteries* originate from these anastomoses.

Figure 13-19 Arteries of the Neck, Head, and Brain.

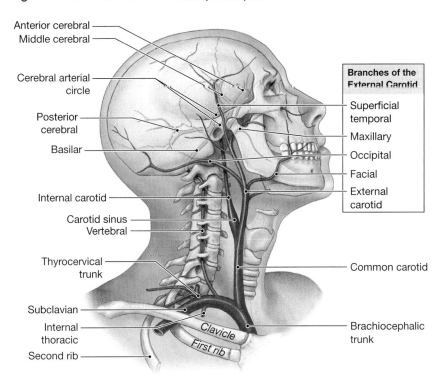

Branches of the External Carotid
Superficial temporal
Maxillary
Occipital
Facial
External carotid

a The general circulation pattern of arteries supplying the neck and superficial structures of the head.

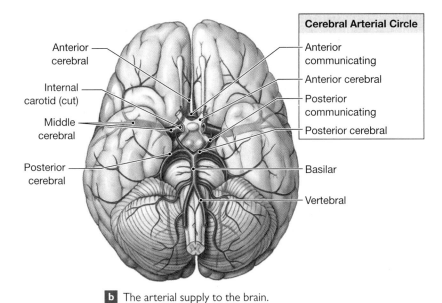

Cerebral Arterial Circle
Anterior communicating
Anterior cerebral
Posterior communicating
Posterior cerebral

b The arterial supply to the brain.

THE CAROTID ARTERY AND THE BLOOD SUPPLY TO THE BRAIN.

The common carotid arteries ascend deep in the tissues of the neck. Each common carotid artery divides into an **external carotid** and an **internal carotid artery** (**Figure 13-19a**). The external carotid artery can usually be located by pressing gently along either side of the windpipe (trachea) until a strong pulse is felt. The external carotid arteries supply blood to the pharynx, esophagus, larynx, and face. The internal carotid arteries enter the skull to deliver blood to the brain and the eyes.

The brain is extremely sensitive to changes in blood supply. An interruption of blood flow for several seconds will produce unconsciousness. After four minutes, permanent neural damage may result. Such circulatory crises are rare, however, because blood reaches the brain by two routes: through the vertebral arteries, and through the internal carotid arteries.

The vertebral arteries ascend within the transverse foramina of the cervical vertebrae and penetrate the skull at the foramen magnum. Inside the cranium, they fuse to form a large **basilar artery**, which continues along the ventral surface of the brain. This artery gives rise to the vessels shown in **Figure 13-19b**.

The internal carotid arteries normally supply the arteries of the anterior half of the cerebrum. The rest of the brain receives blood from the vertebral arteries. But this pattern of blood flow can easily change, because the internal carotids and the basilar artery are interconnected. They form a ring-shaped anastomosis in the **cerebral arterial circle**, or *circle of Willis*, which encircles the infundibulum (stalk) of the pituitary gland. With this arrangement, the brain can receive blood from either the carotid or the vertebral arteries. For this reason, the chances of a serious interruption of blood flow are reduced.

The Descending Aorta

The **descending aorta** is continuous with the aortic arch. The diaphragm divides the descending aorta into a superior **thoracic aorta** and an inferior **abdominal aorta** (**Figure 13-20**). The thoracic aorta travels within the mediastinum, providing blood to the intercostal arteries, which carry blood to the vertebral column area and the body wall. The thoracic aorta also gives rise to arteries that supply tissues of the lungs not involved in gas exchange, the esophagus, pericardium, and other mediastinal structures. Near the diaphragm, the **phrenic** (FREN-ik) **arteries** deliver blood to the muscular diaphragm, which separates the thoracic and abdominopelvic cavities.

13

CLINICAL NOTE

Acute Arterial Occlusion

An acute arterial occlusion is the sudden occlusion of arterial blood flow due to trauma, thrombosis, tumor, embolus, or idiopathic means. Emboli are probably the most common cause of acute arterial occlusion. They can arise from within a chamber of the heart (mural emboli), as from a thrombus in the left ventricle, from an atrial thrombus secondary to atrial fibrillation, or from a thrombus caused by abdominal aortic atherosclerosis. Arterial occlusions most commonly involve vessels in the abdomen or lower extremities.

Acute arterial occlusions are usually treated by an embolectomy, which is the surgical removal of the clot. In this procedure, a balloon catheter or similar device is inserted in the artery distal to the obstruction. The balloon is inflated, the catheter is withdrawn, and the embolus is removed from the vessel lumen.

The abdominal aorta delivers blood to all the abdominopelvic organs and structures (**Figure 13-20**). The **celiac** (SĒ-lē-ak) **trunk**, **superior mesenteric** (mez-en-TER-ik) **artery**, and **inferior mesenteric artery** arise on the anterior surface of the abdominal aorta. These three vessels provide blood to the digestive organs. The celiac trunk divides into three branches that deliver blood to the liver, gallbladder, stomach, and spleen. The liver is supplied by a branch of the common hepatic, called the *hepatic artery proper*. The superior mesenteric artery supplies the pancreas, small intestine, and most of the large intestine. The inferior mesenteric delivers blood to the last portion of the large intestine and rectum.

Paired **gonadal** (gō-NAD-al) **arteries** originate between the superior and inferior mesenteric arteries. In males they are called *testicular arteries*. In females, they are *ovarian arteries*. The **adrenal arteries** and **renal arteries** arise along the lateral surface of the abdominal aorta and travel behind the

Figure 13-20 Major Arteries of the Trunk.

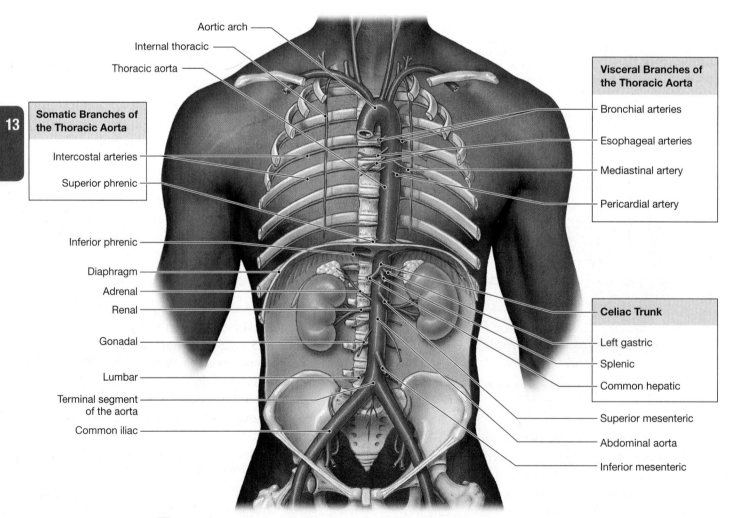

a A diagrammatic view, with most of the thoracic and abdominal organs removed.

Figure 13-20 Major Arteries of the Trunk. (*Continued*)

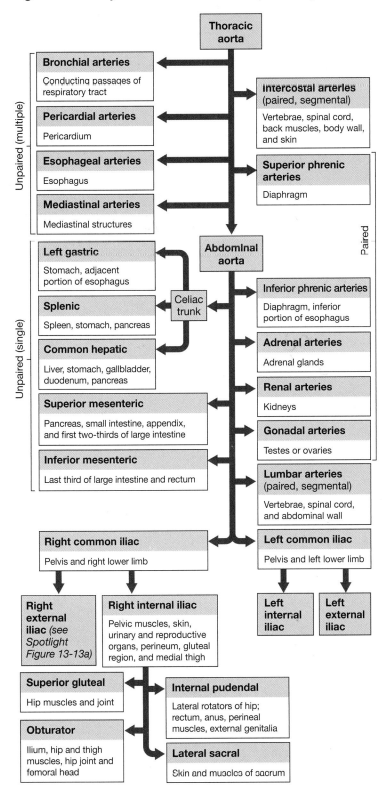

b A flowchart showing major arteries of the trunk.

peritoneal lining to the adrenal glands and kidneys. Small **lumbar arteries** begin on the posterior surface of the aorta and supply the spinal cord and the abdominal wall.

Near the level of vertebra L₄, the abdominal aorta divides to form a pair of muscular arteries. These **common iliac** (IL ē ak) **arteries** carry blood to the pelvis and lower limbs (**Spotlight Figure 13-17a**). As it travels along the inner surface of the ilium, each common iliac artery divides to form an **internal iliac artery**, which supplies smaller arteries of the pelvis, and an **external iliac artery**, which enters the lower limb.

Once in the thigh, the external iliac artery branches, forming the **femoral artery** and the **deep femoral artery**. When it reaches the back of the knee, the femoral artery becomes the **popliteal artery**, which almost immediately branches to form the **anterior tibial**, **posterior tibial**, and **fibular arteries**.

At the ankle, the anterior tibial artery becomes the *dorsalis pedis artery,* and the posterior tibial artery divides in two. These three arteries are connected by two anastomoses. The arrangement produces a *dorsal arch* on the top of the foot and a *plantar arch* on the bottom.

Systemic Veins

Blood from each of the body's tissues and organs returns to the heart by means of a venous network that drains into the right atrium through the superior and inferior venae cavae. **Spotlight Figure 13-17b** illustrates the major vessels of the venous system. Complementary arteries and veins

CLINICAL NOTE

Vasculitis

Vasculitis is an inflammation of a blood vessel. Most vasculitis stems from a variety of rheumatic diseases and syndromes. The inflammatory process is usually segmental, and inflammation within the tunica media of a muscular artery tends to destroy the internal elastic lamina. Necrosis and hypertrophy (enlarging) of the vessel occur, and the vessel wall has a high likelihood of breaching, leaking fibrin and red blood cells into the surrounding tissue. This potentially can lead to partial or total vascular occlusion and subsequent necrosis.

Raynaud's phenomenon is a type of vasculitis that is characterized by episodic ischemia of the fingers or toes as evidenced by digital blanching, cyanosis, and pain. Cold weather or emotional upset have been identified as triggers. Treatment of Raynaud's involves reassurance and having the patient dress warmly and wear gloves. In severe cases, medications that dilate the blood vessels (calcium-channel blockers) are used.

often run side by side. In many cases they even have comparable names. For example, the axillary arteries run alongside the axillary veins. In addition, arteries and veins often travel along with peripheral nerves that have the same names and innervate the same structures.

The Superior Vena Cava

The **superior vena cava (SVC)** receives blood from two regions: the head and neck (**Figure 13-21**), and the upper limbs, shoulders, and chest (**Figure 13-22**).

VENOUS RETURN FROM THE HEAD AND NECK. Small veins in the neural tissue of the brain empty into a network of thin-walled channels called the **dural sinuses**. ⟳ p. 262 The largest, the **superior sagittal sinus**, is located within the fold of dura mater lying between the cerebral hemispheres. Most of the blood leaving the brain passes through one of the dural sinuses and leaves the skull in one of the **internal jugular veins**. These veins descend parallel to the common carotid artery in the neck.

The more superficial **external jugular veins** collect blood from the superficial structures of the head and neck. These veins travel just beneath the skin, and a *jugular venous pulse* can sometimes be detected at the base of the neck. **Vertebral veins** drain the cervical spinal cord and the posterior surface of the skull, descending within the transverse foramina of the cervical vertebrae alongside the vertebral arteries.

VENOUS RETURN FROM THE UPPER LIMBS AND CHEST. The major veins of the upper body are illustrated in **Figure 13-22**. A flowchart indicating the venous tributaries of the SVC is provided in **Figure 13-23** (p. 522). A venous network in the palms collects blood from the digital veins. These vessels drain into the **cephalic vein** and the **basilic vein**. The superficial

Figure 13-21 Major Veins of the Head and Neck. Veins draining the brain and the superficial and deep portions of the head and neck.

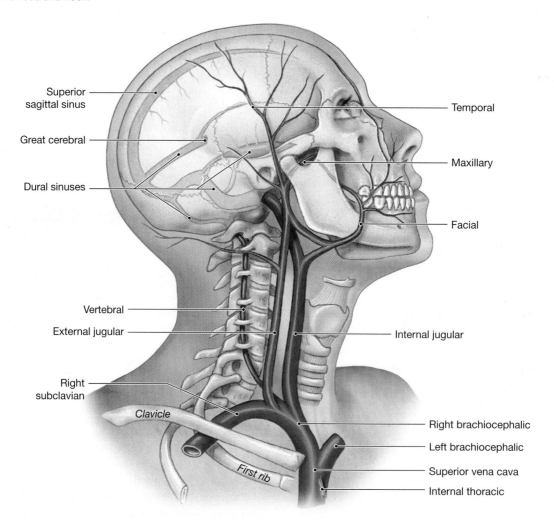

Figure 13-22 The Venous Drainage of the Abdomen and Chest.

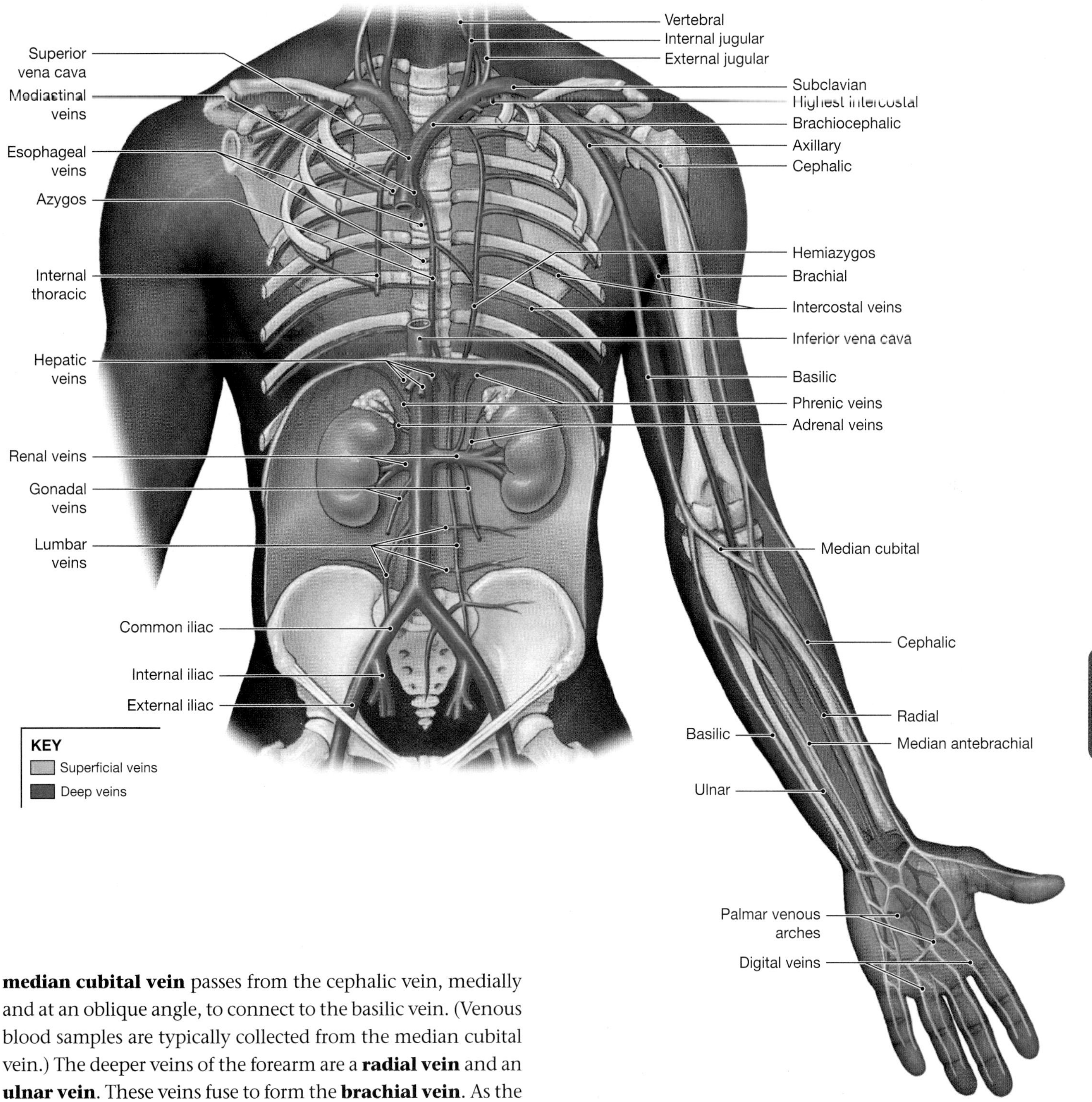
Vertebral
Internal jugular
External jugular
Superior vena cava
Mediastinal veins
Esophageal veins
Azygos
Internal thoracic
Hepatic veins
Renal veins
Gonadal veins
Lumbar veins
Common iliac
Internal iliac
External iliac
KEY
Superficial veins
Deep veins
Subclavian
Highest intercostal
Brachiocephalic
Axillary
Cephalic
Hemiazygos
Brachial
Intercostal veins
Inferior vena cava
Basilic
Phrenic veins
Adrenal veins
Median cubital
Cephalic
Radial
Median antebrachial
Basilic
Ulnar
Palmar venous arches
Digital veins

median cubital vein passes from the cephalic vein, medially and at an oblique angle, to connect to the basilic vein. (Venous blood samples are typically collected from the median cubital vein.) The deeper veins of the forearm are a **radial vein** and an **ulnar vein**. These veins fuse to form the **brachial vein**. As the brachial vein continues toward the trunk, it joins the basilic vein before entering the axilla as the **axillary vein**. The cephalic vein drains into the axillary vein at the shoulder.

The axillary vein then continues into the trunk. At the level of the first rib it becomes the **subclavian vein**. After traveling a short distance inside the thoracic cavity, the subclavian meets and merges with the external and internal jugular veins of that side. This fusion creates the large **brachiocephalic vein**, also known as the *innominate vein*. Near the heart, the two brachiocephalic veins (one from each side of the body) combine to create the SVC. The SVC receives blood from the thoracic body wall through the **azygos** (AZ-ī-gos) **vein** before arriving at the right atrium.

Figure 13-23 A Flowchart of the Tributaries of the Superior and Inferior Venae Cavae.

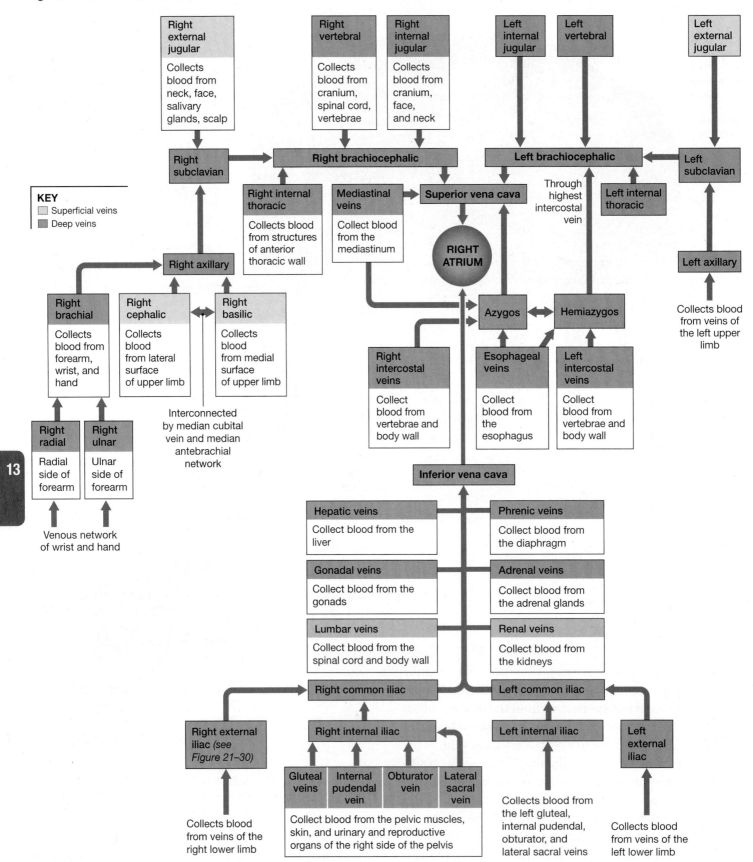

The Inferior Vena Cava

The **IVC** collects most of the venous blood from organs inferior to the diaphragm. (A small amount reaches the SVC through the azygos vein.) A flowchart of the tributaries of the IVC is provided in **Figure 13-23**. The veins of the abdomen are illustrated in **Figure 13-22**. Refer to **Spotlight Figure 13-17b** to see the veins of the lower limbs.

Blood leaving the capillaries in the sole of each foot collects into a network of *plantar veins,* which supply the *plantar venous arch.* The plantar network provides blood to the deep veins of the leg. They are the **anterior tibial vein**, the **posterior tibial vein**, and the **fibular vein**. A *dorsal venous arch* drains blood from capillaries on the superior surface of the foot. This arch is drained by two superficial veins, the **great saphenous vein** (sa-FĒ-nus; *saphenes,* prominent) and the **small saphenous vein**. (Surgeons often use segments of the great saphenous vein, the largest superficial vein, as a bypass vessel during *coronary bypass surgery.*) The plantar arch and the dorsal arch interconnect extensively, so blood flow can easily shift from superficial veins to deep veins.

Behind the knee, the small saphenous, tibial, and fibular veins unite to form the **popliteal vein**. When the popliteal vein reaches the femur, it becomes the **femoral vein**. Before penetrating the abdominal wall, the great saphenous and **deep femoral veins** join the femoral vein. The femoral vein penetrates the body wall and emerges into the pelvic cavity as the **external iliac vein**. As the external iliac travels across the inner surface of the ilium, it is joined by the **internal iliac vein**, which drains the pelvic organs. The resulting **common iliac vein** then meets its counterpart from the opposite side to form the IVC.

Like the aorta, the IVC lies posterior to the abdominopelvic cavity. As it ascends to the heart, it collects blood from several lumbar veins. In addition, the IVC receives blood from the *gonadal, renal, adrenal, phrenic,* and *hepatic veins* before reaching the right atrium (**Figure 13-22**).

CLINICAL NOTE

Peripheral Vascular Conditions

Many peripheral vascular conditions are not considered life threatening but may require prehospital care. They include peripheral arterial atherosclerotic disease, intermittent claudication, deep venous thrombosis, and varicose veins.

Peripheral arterial atherosclerotic disease is a progressive degenerative disease of the medium-sized and large arteries. It affects the aorta and its branches, the brachial and femoral peripheral arteries, and the cerebral arteries. For reasons unknown, it does not affect the coronary arteries. It is a gradual, progressive disease that is often associated with diabetes mellitus. In extreme cases, significant arterial insufficiency may lead to ulcers and gangrene. Occlusion of the peripheral arteries causes chronic and acute ischemia.

In the chronic setting, intermittent claudication (diminished blood flow in exercising muscle) produces pain with exertion. It occurs most commonly with the calf, but can affect any leg muscle. Rest initially relieves this pain. Most patients with intermittent claudication report being able to walk a given distance before leg pain develops. After they rest and the pain resolves, they can resume walking, but as the disease progresses, the pain begins to occur even at rest. The extremity usually appears normal, but pulses will be reduced or absent. As the ischemia worsens, the extremity becomes painful, cold, and numb, and ulceration, gangrene, and necrosis may be present. There usually is no edema. In the acute setting of intermittent claudication, arterial occlusion from an embolus, aneurysm, or thrombosis occurs. The patient experiences a sudden onset of pain, coldness, numbness, and pallor. Pulses are absent distal to the occlusion. Acute occlusion may cause severe ischemia with motor and sensory deficits. Edema is not present.

Deep venous thrombosis is a blood clot in a vein. It most commonly occurs in the larger veins of the thigh and calf, although the subclavian vein is sometimes involved. Predisposing factors include a recent history of trauma, inactivity, pregnancy, or varicose veins. The patient frequently complains of gradually increasing pain and calf tenderness. Often the leg and foot are swollen because of occluded venous drainage. Leg elevation may alleviate the signs and symptoms. In some cases, the patient may be asymptomatic. Gentle palpation of the calf and thigh may reveal tenderness and, on occasion, cord-like clotted veins. Dorsiflexion of the foot may cause *Homan's sign,* which is discomfort behind the knee. This is associated with deep venous thrombosis. The skin may be warm and red. Deep venous thrombosis has traditionally been treated with a blood thinner (heparin) and hospitalization with the affected leg elevated. Heparin must be administered by continuous intravenous infusion, and the patient's coagulation profile must be checked frequently to ensure proper dosing. In many cases, patients are hospitalized at complete bed rest for 7–10 days. With the development of low-molecular-weight heparin (Lovenox), which can be administered by periodic subcutaneous injections, patients with deep venous thrombosis can be treated as out-patients. Patients are instructed to self-administer the drug at home and keep the affected extremity elevated.

Varicose veins are dilated superficial veins, usually in the lower extremities. Predisposing factors include pregnancy, obesity, and genetics. Signs and symptoms include the visible distention of the leg veins, lower leg swelling and discomfort (especially at the end of the day), and skin color and texture changes in the legs and ankles. If the condition is chronic, venous stasis ulcers can develop. Although venous stasis ulcers can rupture, direct pressure usually can control the bleeding, which occasionally is significant. Venous stasis ulcers are usually slow healing and require proper care to prevent additional complications. Treatment of varicose veins primarily involves use of support stockings. Laser therapy and injection of the veins with a sclerosing agent will help improve the legs' cosmetic appearance.

13

The Hepatic Portal System

You may have noticed that the list of veins did not include any names that refer to digestive organs other than the liver. Instead of traveling directly to the IVC, blood leaving the capillaries supplied by the celiac, superior, and inferior mesenteric arteries flows to the liver through the **hepatic portal system** (*porta*, a gate). A blood vessel connecting two capillary beds is called a *portal vessel*, and the network formed is called a *portal system*.

Blood in the hepatic portal vessels is quite different in composition from blood in other systemic veins. That is because it contains substances absorbed by the digestive tract. They include high concentrations of glucose and amino acids, various wastes, and an occasional toxin. The blood within a portal system does not immediately mix with blood in the general circulation because the portal system connects one capillary bed to another. The hepatic portal system delivers blood containing these compounds directly to the liver for storage, metabolic conversion, or excretion. In the process, the liver regulates the concentrations of nutrients in the circulating blood.

Figure 13-24 shows the anatomy of the hepatic portal system. The system begins in the capillaries of the digestive organs. Blood from capillaries along the lower portion of the large intestine enters the **inferior mesenteric vein**. On their way toward the liver, veins from the spleen, the lateral border of the stomach, and the pancreas fuse with the inferior mesenteric, forming the **splenic vein**. The **superior mesenteric vein** also drains the lateral border of the stomach, through

Figure 13-24 The Hepatic Portal System.

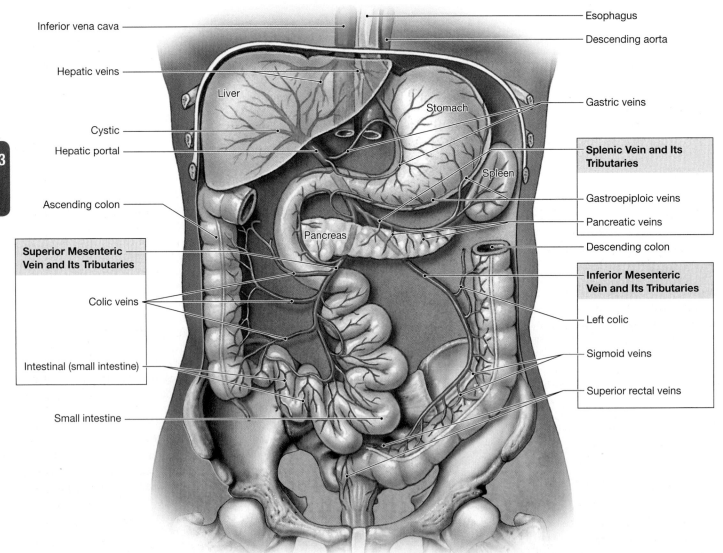

Build Your Knowledge

Recall that the hypothalamus controls the production of hormones in the anterior lobe of the pituitary gland by secreting regulatory hormones (as you saw in **Chapter 10: The Endocrine System**). These hormones first enter a capillary network near the attachment between the hypothalamus and infundibulum. The capillaries unite to form slightly larger vessels called portal vessels that descend to the anterior lobe and then form another capillary network. Together, these portal vessels and two capillary networks make up the hypophyseal portal system. Portal systems ensure that all the blood entering the portal vessels reaches certain target cells before returning to the general circulation. Portal systems are named after their destinations. ⮌**p. 464**

an anastomosis with one of the branches of the splenic vein. In addition, the superior mesenteric collects blood from the entire small intestine and two-thirds of the large intestine. The **hepatic portal vein** forms through the fusion of the superior mesenteric and splenic veins. Of the two, the superior mesenteric normally contributes the greater volume of blood and most of the nutrients. As it proceeds, the hepatic portal vein receives blood from the **gastric veins**, which drain the medial border of the stomach, and the **cystic vein** from the gallbladder. The hepatic portal system ends where the hepatic portal vein empties into the liver capillaries.

After passing through the liver capillaries, blood collects in the hepatic veins, which empty into the IVC. Because blood goes to the liver before returning to the heart, the composition of the blood in the systemic circulation remains relatively stable, regardless of the digestive activities under way.

CHECKPOINT

18. A blockage of which branch of the aortic arch would interfere with blood flow to the left arm?

19. Why would compression of the common carotid arteries cause a person to lose consciousness?

20. Grace is in an automobile accident, and her celiac trunk is ruptured. Which organs will be affected most directly by this injury?

21. Describe the general distribution of major arteries and veins in the neck and limbs. What functional advantage does this distribution provide?

See the blue Answers tab at the back of the book.

13-8 Modifications of fetal and maternal cardiovascular systems promote the exchange of materials until birth

Learning Objective Identify the differences between fetal and adult circulation patterns, and describe the changes in the patterns of blood flow that occur at birth.

The fetal and adult cardiovascular systems have important differences because of their different sources of respiratory and nutritional support. The embryonic lungs are collapsed and nonfunctional. The embryonic digestive tract has nothing to digest. All of the embryo's nutritional and respiratory needs are provided by diffusion across the *placenta*, a structure within the uterine wall where the maternal and fetal circulatory systems are in close contact.

Placental Blood Supply

Circulation in a full-term (9-month-old) fetus is diagrammed in **Figure 13-25a**. The fetus's deoxygenated blood flows to the placenta through a pair of **umbilical arteries**. They arise from the fetus's internal iliac arteries before entering the umbilical cord. At the placenta, fetal blood gives CO_2 and wastes and picks up oxygen and nutrients. Oxygenated blood returns from the placenta in a single **umbilical vein** before reaching the developing liver. Some of the blood flows through capillary networks within the liver. The **ductus venosus** collects blood from the veins of the liver and from the umbilical vein, and empties into the IVC. When the placental connection is broken at birth, blood flow through the umbilical vessels ceases. They soon degenerate.

Fetal Circulation in the Heart and Great Vessels

One of the most interesting aspects of circulatory development reflects the differences between an embryo or fetus and an infant. Throughout embryonic and fetal stages, the lungs are collapsed. Yet right after delivery, the newborn infant must extract oxygen from inhaled air rather than across the placenta.

The interatrial and interventricular septa of the heart develop early in the fetus, but the interatrial partition remains functionally incomplete until birth. The **foramen ovale**, or *interatrial opening*, is associated with a long flap that acts as a valve. Blood can flow freely from the right atrium to the left atrium, but any backflow closes the valve and isolates the two chambers. For this reason, blood entering the heart at the right atrium can

13

Figure 13-25 Fetal Circulation.

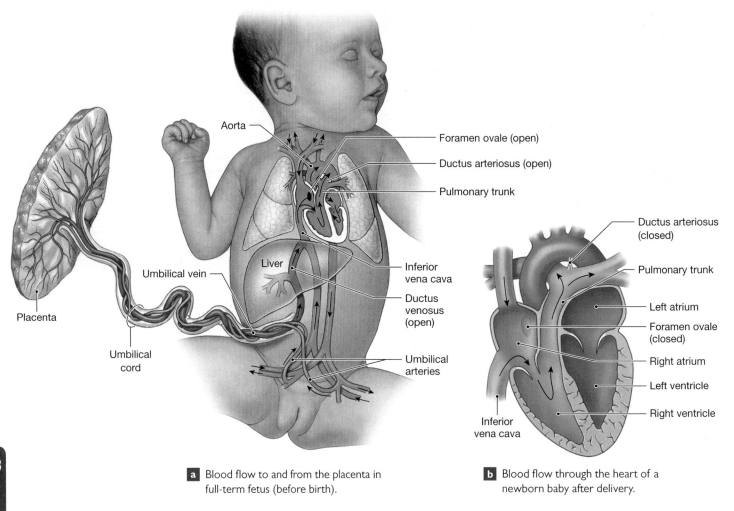

a Blood flow to and from the placenta in full-term fetus (before birth).

b Blood flow through the heart of a newborn baby after delivery.

bypass the pulmonary circuit. A second short-circuit exists between the pulmonary and aortic trunks. This connection, the **ductus arteriosus**, consists of a short, muscular vessel.

With the lungs collapsed, their capillaries are compressed and little blood flows through the lungs. During diastole, blood enters the right atrium and flows into the right ventricle, but it also passes into the left atrium through the foramen ovale. About 25 percent of the blood arriving at the right atrium bypasses the pulmonary circuit in this way. In addition, over 90 percent of the blood leaving the right ventricle passes through the ductus arteriosus and enters the systemic circuit rather than continuing to the lungs.

Circulatory Changes at Birth

At birth, dramatic changes take place. When an infant takes its first breath, the lungs expand, and so do the pulmonary vessels. Within a few seconds, the smooth muscles in the ductus arteriosus contract, isolating the pulmonary and aortic trunks. Blood begins flowing through the pulmonary circuit. As pressures rise in the left atrium, the valvular flap closes the foramen ovale (**Figure 13-25b**). In adults, the interatrial septum bears a shallow depression, the *fossa ovalis*, that marks the site of the foramen ovale (see **Spotlight Figure 12-5**, p. 464). The remnants of the ductus arteriosus persist as a fibrous cord, the *ligamentum arteriosum*.

If the proper cardiovascular changes do not take place at birth or shortly afterward, problems eventually develop. They do so because the heart has to work too hard to provide adequate amounts of oxygenated blood to the systemic circuit. Treatment may involve surgery to close the foramen ovale, the ductus arteriosus, or both. Other congenital heart defects result from abnormal cardiac development or inappropriate connections between the heart and major arteries and veins.

CHECKPOINT

22. Name the three vessels that carry blood to and from the placenta.

23. A blood sample taken from the umbilical cord contains high levels of oxygen and nutrients, and low levels of carbon dioxide and waste products. Is this sample from an umbilical artery or from the umbilical vein? Explain.

24. Name the structures in the fetal circulation that stop functioning at birth. What becomes of these structures?

See the blue Answers tab at the back of the book.

13-9 Aging affects the blood, heart, and blood vessels

Learning Objective Discuss the effects of aging on the cardiovascular system.

The capabilities of the cardiovascular system gradually decline with age. Major changes affect all parts of the cardiovascular system: blood, heart, and vessels.

Age-related changes in blood may include (1) a decreased hematocrit; (2) constriction or blockage of peripheral veins by a stationary blood clot called a *thrombus*, which can become detached, pass through the heart, and become wedged in a small artery (commonly in the lungs) causing *pulmonary embolism*; and (3) the pooling of blood in the veins of the legs because valves are not working effectively.

Age-related changes in the heart include (1) a reduction in maximum cardiac output, (2) changes in the activities of the nodal and conducting cells, (3) a reduction in the elasticity of the cardiac (fibrous) skeleton, (4) progressive atherosclerosis that can restrict coronary circulation, and (5) replacement of damaged cardiac muscle cells by scar tissue.

Age-related changes in blood vessels are often linked to arteriosclerosis, a thickening and toughening of arterial walls. For example, (1) the inelastic walls of arteries become less tolerant of sudden pressure increases, which can lead to a bulge in a weakened arterial wall, or *aneurysm* (AN-ū-rizm). Its rupture may (depending on the vessel) cause a stroke, myocardial infarction, or massive blood loss. Also, (2) calcium salts can be deposited on weakened vascular walls, increasing the risk of a stroke or myocardial infarction. (3) Lipid deposits in the tunica media can form atherosclerotic plaques, and (4) thrombi can form at atherosclerotic plaques.

CHECKPOINT

25. Identify components of the cardiovascular system that are affected by age.

26. Define thrombus.

27. Define aneurysm.

See the blue Answers tab at the back of the book.

CLINICAL NOTE

Vascular Trauma

Injury to the vascular system can interrupt blood flow to the part of the body that is supplied by the artery. Also, some fractures and dislocations can impinge upon nearby arteries, obstructing blood flow; the blood flow often returns when the affected extremity is returned to its anatomical position. Any vascular structure is subject to injury. Laceration of a moderate-sized artery or vein can cause life-threatening hemorrhage. If the vessel is cut cleanly, however, as with a knife, the muscles in the wall of the vessel contract, which constricts the vessel lumen and retracts the end of the severed vessel into the nearby soft tissue. As the muscle is drawn back from the wound, it thickens and further restricts the vessel lumen, which thus restricts blood flow. This, in turn, reduces the rate of blood loss and assists the body's clotting mechanisms. Clean lacerations and amputations therefore do not bleed profusely, but if the vessel is not cleanly lacerated, muscle contraction may actually open the wound, increasing blood flow and loss (**Figure 13-26**).

Traumatic Aneurysm or Rupture of the Aorta

Aortic aneurysm and rupture are extremely life-threatening injuries that result from either blunt or penetrating trauma. The aorta is most commonly injured by blunt trauma and carries an overall mortality of 85–95 percent. It is responsible for 15 percent of all thoracic trauma deaths. Aneurysm and rupture are usually associated with high-speed automobile crashes (most commonly lateral impact) and, in some cases, with high falls. Unlike myocardial rupture, a significant proportion of these victims, possibly as high as 20 percent, will survive the initial insult and aneurysm. Some 30 percent of those initial survivors will die in six hours if not treated; this increases to about 50 percent at 24 hours, and to just under 70 percent by the end of the first week. It is this subset of patients who survive the initial impact and are alive at the scene whom you can most benefit by recognizing their potential injury and then rapidly extricating, packaging, and transporting them to a trauma center.

(Continued)

Figure 13-26 Arterial Laceration. (a) Clean, transverse lacerations cause spasm and contraction of the vessel which slows bleeding. **(b)** In longitudinal lacerations, the muscle fibers can actually hold the wound open, which worsens blood loss.

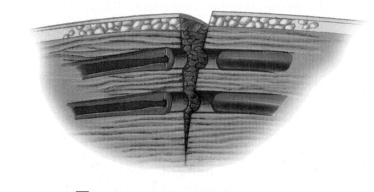

a A clean lateral cut permits the vessel to retract and thicken its wall.

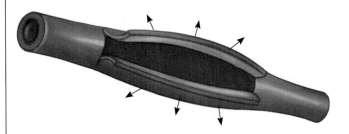

b A longitudinal cut to the vessel causes the wound to open.

The aorta is a large, high-pressure vessel that provides outflow from the left ventricle for distribution to the body. It is relatively fixed at three points as it passes through the thoracic cavity: the aortic annulus, where the aorta joins the heart; the aortic isthmus, where it is joined by the ligamentum arteriosum; and the diaphragm, where it exits the chest. Because of this, the aorta experiences shear forces secondary to severe deceleration of the chest. Traumatic dissecting aneurysm occurs most commonly to the descending aorta and, infrequently, to the ascending aorta. With severe deceleration, shear forces separate the layers of the artery, specifically the interior surface (the *tunica intima*) from the muscle layer (the *tunica media*). This allows blood to enter the area between the layers, and because the blood is under great pressure, it begins to dissect the aortic lining like a bulging inner tube (**Figure 13-27**). The aorta is likely to rupture if it is not surgically repaired.

The patient with aortic rupture will be severely hypotensive, quickly lose all vital signs, and die unless taken immediately to surgery. Dissecting aortic aneurysm progresses more slowly, though the aneurysm may rupture at any moment. The patient will probably have a history of a high fall or severe auto impact and deceleration. Lateral impact is an especially high risk factor for aortic aneurysm. The patient may complain of severe tearing chest pain that may radiate to the back. The patient may have a pulse deficit between the left and right upper extremities and/or reduced pulse strength in the lower extremities. Blood pressure may be high (hypertension) due to stretching of sympathetic nerve fibers in the aorta near the ligamentum arteriosum, or the pressure may be low due to leakage and hypovolemia. Turbulence as the blood exits the heart and passes the disrupted blood vessel wall may create a harsh systolic murmur.

Other Vascular Injuries

Other thoracic vascular structures that can sustain injury during chest trauma are the pulmonary arteries and vena cava. Their injury, and the resulting hemorrhage, may cause significant hemothorax, and possibly lead to hypotension and respiratory insufficiency. The blood may also flow into the mediastinum and compress the great vessels, esophagus, and heart. Penetrating trauma is the primary cause of injury to the pulmonary arteries and vena cava. The patient with pulmonary artery or vena cava injuries will likely have a penetrating wound to the central chest, or elsewhere with a likelihood of central chest involvement. These injuries initially present with the signs and symptoms of hypovolemia and shock and then present with the signs and symptoms of hemothorax or hemomediastinum as those conditions develop.

Figure 13-27 Different Types of Thoracic Aortic Aneurysm. (a) The dissecting aneurysm begins near the aortic valve in the ascending aorta and extends throughout the aorta down to the external iliac arteries. **(b).** Dissecting aneurysm limited to the ascending aorta (as seen in Marfan's syndrome). **(c1).** Dissecting thoracic aortic aneurysm that originates distal to the left subclavian artery. The localized nature of this lesion makes it readily accessible for surgical excision. **(c2)** Dissecting aneurysm that arises distal to the left subclavian artery but extends into the abdominal aorta. Only partial excision is possible.

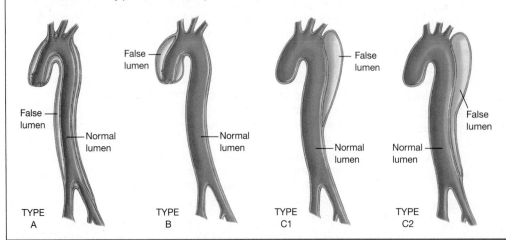

False lumen · Normal lumen — TYPE A

False lumen · Normal lumen — TYPE B

False lumen · Normal lumen — TYPE C1

False lumen · Normal lumen — TYPE C2

13-10 The cardiovascular system is both structurally and functionally linked to all other systems

Learning Objective Give examples of interactions between the cardiovascular system and other body systems.

The section of the chapter on the distribution of blood vessels demonstrated the structural connections between the cardiovascular system and other organ systems. Functionally, the cardiovascular system provides other body systems with oxygen, hormones, nutrients, and white blood cells. It also removes carbon dioxide and metabolic wastes. In addition, circulating blood transfers heat to body tissues.

CHECKPOINT

28. Describe what the cardiovascular system provides for all other body systems.

29. What is the relationship between the skeletal system and the cardiovascular system?

See the blue Answers tab at the back of the book.

Build Your Knowledge

How the CARDIOVASCULAR SYSTEM integrates with the other body systems presented so far on p. 465 reviews the major functional relationships between it and the integumentary, skeletal, muscular, nervous, and endocrine systems.

RELATED CLINICAL TERMS

angiogram: An X-ray of a blood vessel that becomes visible due to a prior injection of dye into the subject's bloodstream.

deep vein thrombosis (DVT): A blood clot in a major vein, usually in the legs. They often occur after extended periods of inactivity, such as long airplane flights. The clot can break free and travel to the lungs as an embolus, where it can cause respiratory distress or respiratory failure.

hypertension: Abnormally high blood pressure; usually defined in adults as blood pressure higher than 140/90.

hypervolemic (hī-per-vō-LĒ-mik): Having an excessive blood volume.

hypovolemic (hī-pō-vō-LĒ-mik): Having a low blood volume.

normotensive: Having normal blood pressure.

orthostatic hypotension: Low blood pressure upon standing, often accompanied by dizziness or fainting; results from a failure of the regulatory processes that increase blood pressure to maintain adequate blood flow to the brain.

phlebitis: Inflammation of a vein.

Raynaud's phenomenon: A condition resulting in the discoloration of the fingers and/or toes when a person is subjected to changes in temperature or to emotional stress.

syncope (SING-kuh-pē)**:** A temporary loss of consciousness due to a sudden drop in blood pressure; fainting.

13

Build Your Knowledge
How the CARDIOVASCULAR SYSTEM integrates with the other body systems presented so far

Integumentary System

- The integumentary system has mast cells that trigger localized changes in blood flow and capillary permeability

- The cardiovascular system delivers immune system cells to injury sites; clotting response seals breaks in skin surface; carries away toxins from sites of infection; provides heat

Skeletal System

- The skeletal system provides calcium needed for normal cardiac muscle contraction; protects blood cells developing in red bone marrow

- The cardiovascular system transports calcium and phosphate for bone deposition; delivers EPO to red bone marrow, parathyroid hormone and calcitonin to osteoblasts and osteoclasts

Nervous System

- The nervous system controls patterns of circulation in peripheral tissues; modifies heart rate and regulates blood pressure; releases antidiuretic hormone (ADH)

- The cardiovascular system has capillaries whose endothelial cells maintain the blood-brain barrier; help generate CSF

Endocrine System

- The endocrine system produces erythropoietin (EPO), which regulates production of RBCs; several hormones increase blood pressure; epinephrine stimulates cardiac muscle, increasing heart rate and force of contraction

- The cardiovascular system distributes hormones throughout the body; the heart secretes atrial natriuretic peptide (ANP)

13

Muscular System

- The muscular system assists venous circulation through skeletal muscle contractions; protects superficial blood vessels, especially in neck and limbs

- The cardiovascular system delivers oxygen and nutrients, removes carbon dioxide, lactic acid, and heat during skeletal muscle activity

Cardiovascular System

The cardiovascular system has blood vessels that provide extensive anatomical connections between it and all the other organ systems. It:
- transports dissolved gases, nutrients, hormones, and metabolic wastes
- regulates pH and ion composition of interstitial fluid
- restricts fluid losses at injury sites
- defends against toxins and pathogens
- stabilizes body temperature

13 Chapter Review

Summary Outline

13-1 Arteries, arterioles, capillaries, venules, and veins differ in size, structure, and function *p. 490*

1. Blood flows through a network of arteries, capillaries, and veins. All chemical and gaseous exchange between the blood and interstitial fluid takes place across **capillary** walls.

2. **Arteries** and **veins** form an internal distribution system, using blood propelled by the heart. Arteries branch repeatedly, decreasing in size until they become **arterioles;** from the arterioles, blood enters the capillary networks. Blood flowing from the capillaries enters small **venules** before entering larger **veins.**

3. The walls of arteries and veins contain three layers: the **tunica intima, tunica media,** and outermost **tunica externa** *(Figure 13-1).*

4. The walls of arteries are usually thicker than the walls of veins. The arterial system includes the large **elastic arteries,** medium-sized **muscular arteries,** and smaller arterioles. As blood proceeds toward the capillaries, the number of vessels increases, but the diameter of the individual vessels decreases and the walls become thinner *(Figure 13-2).*

5. Capillaries are the only blood vessels whose walls permit exchange between blood and interstitial fluid.

6. Capillaries form interconnected networks called **capillary beds.** A **precapillary sphincter** (a band of smooth muscle) adjusts blood flow into each capillary. Blood flow in a capillary changes as **vasomotion** occurs *(Figure 13-3).*

7. Venules collect blood from capillaries and merge into **medium-sized veins** and then **large veins.** The arterial system is a high-pressure system; blood pressure in veins is much lower. **Valves** in veins prevent backflow of blood *(Figure 13-4).*

13-2 Pressure and resistance determine blood flow and affect rates of capillary exchange *p. 495*

8. Blood flows from an area of higher pressure to an area of lower pressure. Its flow rate is proportional to the pressure difference (pressure gradient).

9. For circulation to take place, *circulatory pressure* (the pressure gradient across the systemic circuit) must be greater than *total peripheral resistance* (the resistance of the entire cardiovascular system). For blood to flow into peripheral capillaries, **blood pressure** (arterial pressure) must be greater than the **peripheral resistance** (the resistance of the arterial system). Neural and hormonal control processes regulate blood pressure.

10. The most important determinant of peripheral resistance is arteriole diameter.

11. High arterial pressures overcome peripheral resistance and maintain blood flow through peripheral tissues. **Capillary pressures** are normally low, and small changes in capillary pressure determine the rate of fluid movement into or out of the bloodstream. Venous pressure, normally low, determines venous return and affects cardiac output and peripheral blood flow.

12. Arterial pressure rises in ventricular systole and falls in ventricular diastole. The difference between the **systolic** and **diastolic pressures** is **pulse pressure** *(Figure 13-5).*

13. At the capillaries, solute molecules diffuse across the capillary lining, and water-soluble materials diffuse through small spaces between endothelial cells. Water moves when driven by either capillary hydrostatic pressure (CHP) or blood osmotic pressure (BOP). The direction of water movement is determined by the balance between these two opposing pressures *(Figure 13-6).*

14. Valves, **muscular compression,** and the **respiratory pump** help the relatively low venous pressures propel blood toward the heart *(Figure 13-4).*

13-3 Cardiovascular regulation involves autoregulation, neural processes, and endocrine responses *p. 500*

15. Homeostatic processes ensure that tissue blood flow (*tissue perfusion*) delivers adequate oxygen and nutrients.

16. Blood flow varies with cardiac output, peripheral resistance, and blood pressure.

17. Autoregulation, neural processes, and endocrine processes influence the coordinated regulation of cardiovascular function. Autoregulation involves local factors changing the pattern of blood flow within capillary beds in response to chemical changes in interstitial fluids. Neural processes respond to changes in arterial pressure or blood gas levels. Hormones can assist in both short-term adjustments (changes in cardiac output and peripheral resistance) and long-term adjustments (changes in blood volume that affect cardiac output and gas transport) *(Figure 13-7).*

18. Peripheral resistance is adjusted at the tissues by the dilation or constriction of precapillary sphincters.

19. **Baroreceptor reflexes** respond to the degree of stretch within expandable organs. Baroreceptors are located in the **aortic** and **carotid sinuses** and the right atrium *(Figure 13-9).*

13

20. **Chemoreceptor reflexes** respond to changes in oxygen, carbon dioxide, or pH levels in blood and cerebrospinal fluid. Sympathetic activation leads to stimulation of the *cardioacceleratory* and *vasomotor centers*; parasympathetic activation stimulates the *cardioinhibitory center* (*Figure 13-10*).

21. Short-term endocrine regulation of cardiac output and peripheral resistance is achieved by epinephrine and norepinephrine from the adrenal medullae. Hormones involved in long-term regulation of blood pressure and volume are antidiuretic hormone (ADH), angiotensin II, erythropoietin (EPO), and atrial natriuretic peptide (ANP) (*Figure 13-11*).

22. ANP release is stimulated by an increase in blood pressure. ANP encourages sodium loss and fluid loss, reduces blood pressure, inhibits thirst, and lowers peripheral resistance (*Figure 13-11*).

13-4 The cardiovascular system adapts to physiological stress p. 508

23. During exercise, blood flow to skeletal muscles increases at the expense of circulation to "nonessential" organs, and cardiac output rises. Cardiovascular performance improves with training. Athletes have larger stroke volumes, lower resting heart rates, and greater cardiac reserves than do nonathletes.

24. Blood loss causes an increase in cardiac output, peripheral vasoconstriction, and the secretion of hormones that promote fluid retention and red blood cell production.

13-5 The pulmonary and systemic circuits of the cardiovascular system exhibit three general functional patterns p. 509

25. The peripheral distributions of arteries and veins are generally identical on both sides of the body, except near the heart (*Figure 13-12*).

13-6 In the pulmonary circuit, deoxygenated blood enters the lungs in arteries, and oxygenated blood leaves the lungs in veins p. 510

26. The **pulmonary circuit** includes the **pulmonary trunk,** the **left** and **right pulmonary arteries,** and the **pulmonary veins,** which empty into the left atrium (*Figures 13-12, 13-13*).

13-7 The systemic circuit carries oxygenated blood from the left ventricle to tissues other than the lungs' exchange surfaces, and returns deoxygenated blood to the right atrium p. 512

27. In the **systemic circuit,** the **ascending aorta** gives rise to the coronary circulation. The **aortic arch** communicates with the **descending aorta** (*Spotlight Figure 13-17a; Figures 13-18, 13-19*).

28. Arteries in the neck and limbs are deep beneath the skin. In contrast, two sets of peripheral veins usually occur in those sites, one superficial and one deep. This dual-venous drainage is important for controlling body temperature (*Spotlight Figure 13-17b*).

29. The **superior vena cava (SVC)** receives blood from the head, neck, chest, shoulders, and arms (*Spotlight Figure 13-17b; Figures 13-18 and 13-19*).

30. The **inferior vena cava (IVC)** collects most of the venous blood from organs inferior to the diaphragm (*Figure 13-23*).

31. The **hepatic portal system** directs blood from the other digestive organs to the liver before the blood returns to the heart (*Figure 13-24*).

13-8 Modifications of fetal and maternal cardiovascular systems promote the exchange of materials until birth p. 525

32. The placenta receives deoxygenated blood from the two **umbilical arteries.** Oxygenated blood returns to the fetus through the single **umbilical vein,** which delivers it to the **ductus venosus** in the liver (*Figure 13-25a*).

33. Prior to delivery, blood bypasses the pulmonary circuit by flowing (1) from the right atrium into the left atrium through the **foramen ovale,** and (2) from the pulmonary trunk into the aortic arch through the **ductus arteriosus** (*Figure 13-25b*).

13-9 Aging affects the blood, heart, and blood vessels p. 527

34. Age-related changes in the blood can include (1) a decreased hematocrit, (2) constriction or blockage of peripheral veins by a *thrombus* (stationary blood clot), and (3) pooling of blood in veins of the legs because the valves are not working effectively.

35. Age-related changes in the heart include (1) a reduction in maximum cardiac output, (2) changes in the activities of the nodal and conducting cells, (3) a reduction in the elasticity of the cardiac skeleton, (4) progressive atherosclerosis that can restrict coronary circulation, and (5) replacement of damaged cardiac muscle cells by scar tissue.

36. Age-related changes in blood vessels, often related to arteriosclerosis, include (1) a weakening in the walls of arteries, potentially leading to the formation of an *aneurysm*; (2) the deposition of calcium salts on weakened vascular walls, increasing the risk of stroke or myocardial infarction; (3) lipid deposits in the tunica media forming atherosclerotic plaques; and (4) the formation of thrombi at atherosclerotic plaques.

13-10 The cardiovascular system is both structurally and functionally linked to all other systems p. 529

37. The cardiovascular system has blood vessels that deliver oxygen, nutrients, and hormones to all body systems and carry away carbon dioxide and wastes.

Review Questions

See the blue Answers tab at the back of the book.

Level 1 Reviewing Facts and Terms

Match each item in column A with the most closely related item in column B. Place letters for answers in the spaces provided.

COLUMN A

_____ **1.** Diastolic pressure

_____ **2.** Arterioles

_____ **3.** Hepatic vein

_____ **4.** Renal vein

_____ **5.** Aorta

_____ **6.** Precapillary sphincter

_____ **7.** Medulla oblongata

_____ **8.** Internal iliac artery

_____ **9.** External iliac artery

_____ **10.** Baroreceptors

_____ **11.** Systolic pressure

_____ **12.** Saphenous vein

COLUMN B

a. Drains the liver

b. Largest superficial vein in body

c. Aortic and carotid sinuses

d. Minimum blood pressure

e. Blood supply to leg

f. Blood supply to pelvis

g. Peak blood pressure

h. Vasomotion

i. Largest artery in body

j. Drains the kidney

k. Contains vasomotor center

l. Smallest arterial vessels

13. Identify the major arteries in the following diagram.

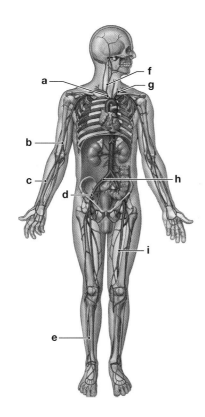

(a) _____   (b) _____
(c) _____   (d) _____
(e) _____   (f) _____
(g) _____   (h) _____
(i) _____

14. Blood vessels that carry blood away from the heart are called
  (a) veins.   **(b)** arterioles.
  (c) venules.   **(d)** arteries.

15. The layer of the arteriole wall that provides the properties of contractility and elasticity is the
  (a) tunica adventitia. **(b)** tunica media.
  (c) tunica intima.   **(d)** tunica externa.

16. The two-way exchange of substances between blood and body cells occurs only through
  (a) arterioles.   **(b)** capillaries.
  (c) venules.   **(d)** a, b, and c are correct.

17. The blood vessels that collect blood from all tissues and organs and return it to the heart are the
  (a) veins.   **(b)** arteries
  (c) capillaries.   **(d)** arterioles.

18. Blood within the veins is prevented from flowing away from the heart because of the presence of
  (a) venous reservoirs. **(b)** muscular walls
  (c) clots.   **(d)** valves.

19. The most important factor in vascular resistance is
  (a) the viscosity of the blood.
  (b) friction between the blood and vessel walls.
  (c) turbulence due to irregular surfaces of blood vessels.
  (d) the length of the blood vessels.

20. In a blood pressure reading of 120/80, the 120 represents _____ and the 80 represents _____.
  (a) diastolic pressure; systolic pressure
  (b) pulse pressure; mean arterial pressure
  (c) systolic pressure; diastolic pressure
  (d) mean arterial pressure; pulse pressure

13

21. Along a capillary, _____ dominates at the arterial end and fluid moves _____; _____ dominates at the venous end and fluid moves _____.
    (a) osmosis, in; filtration, out
    (b) filtration, out; osmosis, in
    (c) filtration, in; osmosis, out
    (d) osmosis, out; filtration, in

22. The two factors that assist the relatively low venous pressures in propelling blood toward the heart are
    (a) ventricular systole and valve closure.
    (b) gravity and vasomotion.
    (c) muscular compression and the respiratory pump.
    (d) atrial and ventricular contractions.

23. Identify the major veins in the following diagram.

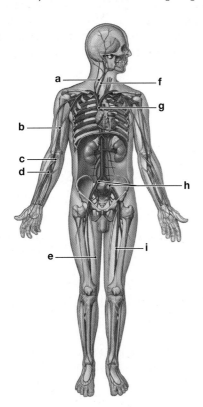

    (a) _____   (b) _____
    (c) _____   (d) _____
    (e) _____   (f) _____
    (g) _____   (h) _____
    (i) _____

24. Arteries of the pulmonary circuit differ from those of the systemic circuit in that they carry
    (a) oxygen and nutrients.
    (b) deoxygenated blood.
    (c) oxygenated blood.
    (d) oxygen, carbon dioxide, and nutrients.

25. The two arteries formed by the division of the brachiocephalic trunk are the
    (a) aorta and internal carotid.
    (b) axillary and brachial.
    (c) external and internal carotid.
    (d) common carotid and subclavian.

26. The unpaired arteries supplying blood to the visceral organs include the
    (a) adrenal, renal, and lumbar arteries.
    (b) iliac, gonadal, and femoral arteries.
    (c) celiac trunk and superior and inferior mesenteric arteries.
    (d) a, b, and c are correct.

27. The artery generally used to feel the pulse at the wrist is the
    (a) ulnar artery.   (b) radial artery.
    (c) fibular artery.   (d) dorsalis artery.

28. The vein that drains the dural sinuses of the brain is the
    (a) cephalic vein.   (b) great saphenous vein.
    (c) internal jugular vein. (d) superior vena cava.

29. The vein that collects most of the venous blood from below the diaphragm is the
    (a) superior vena cava.   (b) great saphenous vein.
    (c) inferior vena cava.   (d) azygos vein.

30. (a) What are the primary forces that cause fluid to move out of a capillary and into the interstitial fluid at its arterial end? (b) What are the primary forces that cause fluid to move into a capillary from the interstitial fluid at its venous end?

31. What two effects result when the baroreceptor response to elevated blood pressure (BP) is triggered?

32. What factors affect the activity of chemoreceptors in the carotid and aortic bodies?

33. What cardiovascular changes occur at birth?

34. What age-related changes take place in the blood, heart, and blood vessels?

Level 2 Reviewing Concepts

35. When dehydration occurs,
    (a) water reabsorption at the kidneys accelerates.
    (b) fluids are reabsorbed from the interstitial fluid.
    (c) blood osmotic pressure increases.
    (d) a, b, and c are correct.

36. Increased CO_2 levels in tissues would promote
    (a) contraction of precapillary sphincters.
    (b) an increase in the pH of the blood.
    (c) relaxation of precapillary sphincters.
    (d) a decrease of blood flow to tissues.

37. Elevated levels of the hormones ADH and angiotensin II will produce
    (a) increased peripheral vasodilation.
    (b) increased peripheral vasoconstriction.
    (c) increased peripheral blood flow.
    (d) increased venous return.

38. Relate the anatomical differences between arteries and veins to their functions.

39. Why do capillaries permit the diffusion of materials, whereas arteries and veins do not?

40. Why is blood flow to the brain relatively continuous and constant?

41. An accident victim displays the following signs and symptoms: hypotension; pale, cool, moist skin; confusion; and disorientation. Identify her condition, and explain why each of these signs and symptoms occurs. If you took her pulse, what would you find?

Level 3 Critical Thinking and Clinical Applications

42. Bob is sitting outside on a warm day and is sweating profusely. His friend Mary wants to practice taking blood pressures, and he agrees to play patient. Mary finds that Bob's blood pressure is elevated, even though he is resting and has lost fluid from sweating. (She reasons that fluid loss should lower blood volume and, thus, blood pressure.) Mary asks you why Bob's blood pressure is high instead of low. What should you tell her?

43. People with allergies frequently take antihistamines and decongestants to relieve their symptoms. (These medications mimic the effects of sympathetic stimulation.) The medications' labels warn that such medications should not be taken by individuals being treated for high blood pressure. Why?

44. Gina awakens suddenly to the sound of her alarm clock. Realizing that she is late for class, she jumps to her feet, feels light-headed, and falls back on her bed. What probably caused this to happen? Why doesn't this always happen?

13

The Lymphatic System and Immunity

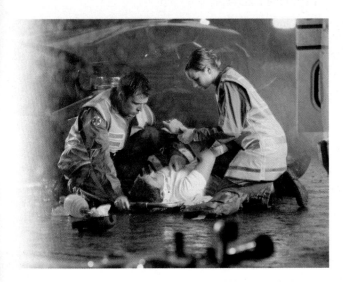

Learning Objectives

These objectives tell you what you should be able to do after completing the chapter. They correspond by number to this chapter's sections.

14-1 Distinguish between innate (nonspecific) defenses and adaptive (specific) defenses.

14-2 Identify the major components of the lymphatic system, and explain the functions of each.

14-3 List the body's innate (nonspecific) defenses and explain how each functions.

14-4 Define adaptive (specific) defenses, identify the forms and properties of immunity, and distinguish between cell-mediated immunity and antibody-mediated (humoral) immunity.

14-5 Discuss the different types of T cells and their roles in the immune response.

14-6 Discuss the processes of B cell sensitization, activation, and differentiation, describe the structure and function of antibodies, and explain the primary and secondary immune responses to antigen exposure.

14-7 List and explain examples of immune disorders and allergies, and discuss the effects of stress on immune function.

14-8 Describe the effects of aging on the lymphatic system and the immune response.

14-9 Give examples of interactions between the lymphatic system and other body systems.

An Introduction to the Lymphatic System and Immunity

We do not live in a completely safe world. The external environment contains a variety of physical hazards—poisonous chemicals, extreme heat, radiation, heavy and/or sharp objects, to name but a few. They can inflict a broad range of injuries, including bumps, cuts, broken bones, and burns. The world is also full of many types of microorganisms that, if allowed to enter into the body, cause some of the most important human diseases. Still other internal processes, such as cancer, can pose extreme, even lethal, danger to the human body.

Many different organs and systems work together to keep us alive and healthy. In this ongoing struggle to maintain health, the *lymphatic system* plays a central role. In this chapter, we discuss the components of the lymphatic system and their interactions.

Build Your Knowledge

Recall that the lymphatic system defends against infection and disease and returns tissue fluids to the bloodstream (as you saw in **Chapter 1: An Introduction to Anatomy and Physiology**). The tissue (interstitial) fluid that is transported by lymphatic vessels is called lymph. Recall also that lymph is a fluid connective tissue. Along the way to the cardiovascular system, lymph is monitored for signs of injury and infection. This recirculation of fluid is essential for homeostasis. ⟳ **pp. 8, 102, 438**

14-1 Anatomical barriers and defense processes make up nonspecific defense, and lymphocytes provide specific defense

Learning Objective Distinguish between innate (nonspecific) and adaptive (specific) defenses.

Our world contains a wide range of viruses, bacteria, fungi, and parasites that cause diseases in humans. Disease-causing organisms are called **pathogens** (*pathos,* disease + *gen,* to produce). Each pathogen has a different mode of life and interacts with the body in a characteristic way. For example, most of the time viruses exist within cells, which they often eventually destroy. (Viruses lack a cellular structure. They consist only of nucleic acid and protein. They can replicate themselves only within a living cell.) Many bacteria multiply in the interstitial fluids. Some of the largest parasites, such as roundworms, burrow through internal organs. And as if that were not enough, we are constantly at risk from renegade cells that have the potential to produce lethal cancers. ⟳ p. 84

The **lymphatic system** includes the cells, tissues, and organs responsible for defending the body. The primary cells of the lymphatic system are *lymphocytes.* ⟳ p. 395 These cells are vital to the body's ability to resist or overcome infection and disease.

Immunity is the ability to resist infection and disease. We have two forms of defense systems that work independently or together to provide immunity. These forms are *innate (nonspecific) defenses* and *adaptive (specific) defenses.*

The body has several anatomical barriers and defense processes that either prevent or slow the entry of infectious organisms, or attack them if they do succeed in gaining entry. These defenses are called *innate* because we are born with them and *nonspecific* because they do not distinguish one potential threat from another.

In contrast, lymphocytes respond to specific threats. If a bacterial pathogen invades peripheral tissues, lymphocytes organize a defense against that particular type of bacterium. For this reason, we say that lymphocytes provide an *adaptive* defense. Defense against specific antigens is known as the **immune response**.

All the cells and tissues involved in the production of immunity are considered part of an *immune system.* The immune system includes parts of the integumentary, skeletal, lymphatic, cardiovascular, respiratory, and digestive systems.

Next we examine the organization of the lymphatic system. Then we will consider the body's nonspecific defenses. Finally, we will see how the lymphatic system interacts with cells and tissues of other systems to defend the body against infection and disease.

CHECKPOINT

1. Define pathogen.
2. Explain the difference between nonspecific defense and specific defense.

See the blue Answers tab at the back of the book.

14-2 Lymphatic vessels, lymphocytes, lymphoid tissues, and lymphoid organs function in body defenses

Learning Objective Identify the major components of the lymphatic system, and explain the functions of each.

The lymphatic system is one of our least familiar organ systems. It includes four components:

1. **Vessels.** A network of **lymphatic vessels**, often called **lymphatics**, begins in peripheral tissues and connects to veins.

2. **Fluid.** A fluid called **lymph** flows through the lymphatic vessels. Lymph resembles plasma but contains a much lower concentration of proteins.

3. **Lymphocytes. Lymphocytes** are specialized cells with an array of specific functions in defending the body.

4. **Lymphoid tissues and organs.** **Lymphoid tissues** are collections of loose connective tissue and lymphocytes in structures called *lymphoid nodules*. The tonsils are an example. **Lymphoid organs** are more complex structures that contain large numbers of lymphocytes and are connected to lymphatic vessels. Examples include the lymph nodes, spleen, and thymus.

Primary lymphoid tissues and organs are sites where lymphocytes are formed and mature. They include the red bone marrow and the thymus gland. Recall that the red bone marrow is also where other defense cells, the monocytes and macrophages, are formed.

Secondary lymphoid tissues and organs are sites where lymphocytes are activated and cloned (produced in large numbers of identical copies). These tissues and organs include the appendix, spleen, lymph nodes, tonsils, and mucosa-associated lymphoid tissue (MALT). **Figure 14-1** provides an overview of the primary vessels, tissues, and organs of the lymphatic system.

Figure 14-1 The Components of the Lymphatic System.

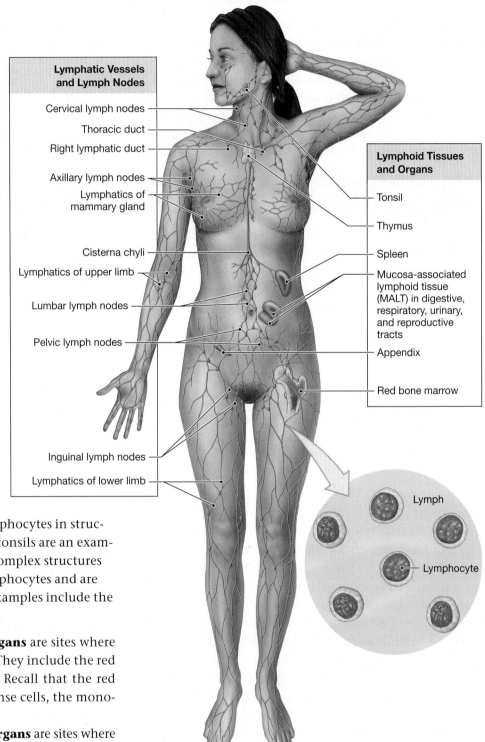

Lymphatic Vessels and Lymph Nodes
- Cervical lymph nodes
- Thoracic duct
- Right lymphatic duct
- Axillary lymph nodes
- Lymphatics of mammary gland
- Cisterna chyli
- Lymphatics of upper limb
- Lumbar lymph nodes
- Pelvic lymph nodes
- Inguinal lymph nodes
- Lymphatics of lower limb

Lymphoid Tissues and Organs
- Tonsil
- Thymus
- Spleen
- Mucosa-associated lymphoid tissue (MALT) in digestive, respiratory, urinary, and reproductive tracts
- Appendix
- Red bone marrow

Lymph

Lymphocyte

Functions of the Lymphatic System

The lymphatic system has three primary functions:

- ***Production, maintenance, and distribution of lymphocytes.*** Lymphocytes are produced in red bone marrow and the thymus. They are stored within lymphoid organs, such as the spleen. Lymphocytes respond to the presence of (1) invading pathogens, such as bacteria or viruses; (2) abnormal body cells, such as virus-infected cells or cancer cells; and (3) foreign proteins, such as the toxins produced by some bacteria. Lymphocytes work to eliminate these threats or render them harmless. They do so through a combination of physical and chemical actions.

- ***Return of fluid and solutes from peripheral tissues to the blood.*** The return of tissue fluids through the lymphatic system maintains normal blood volume and eliminates local variations in the composition of the interstitial fluid. The volume of flow is considerable—roughly 3.6 liters (0.95 gal) per day. A break in a major lymphatic vessel can cause a rapid and potentially fatal decline in blood volume.

- ***Distribution of hormones, nutrients, and waste products from their tissues of origin to the general circulation.*** Substances unable to enter the bloodstream directly may do so by way of lymphatic vessels. For example, lipids absorbed by the digestive tract do not usually enter the bloodstream through capillaries. Instead, they reach the bloodstream only after they have traveled along lymphatic vessels. (We describe this process in Chapter 16.)

Lymphatic Vessels

Lymphatic vessels, or lymphatics, carry lymph from peripheral tissues to the venous system. **Lymphatic capillaries** are the smallest lymphatic vessels. They begin as blind pockets in peripheral tissues (**Figure 14-2a**). Lymphatic capillaries are lined by an endothelium (simple squamous epithelium) with a basement membrane that is incomplete or absent. The endothelial cells are not bound tightly, but they do overlap. The region of overlap acts as a one-way valve. It permits fluids and solutes (including those as large as proteins), along with viruses, bacteria, and cell debris, to enter, but it prevents them from returning to the intercellular spaces.

From lymphatic capillaries, lymph flows into larger lymphatic vessels that lead toward the trunk of the body. The walls of these lymphatics contain layers comparable to those

Figure 14-2 Lymphatic Capillaries.

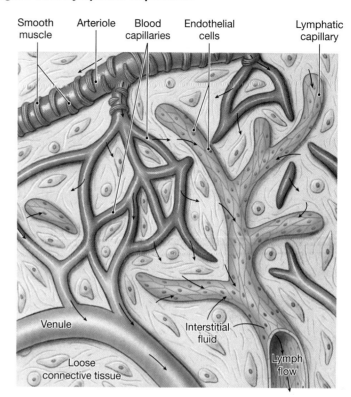

a The interwoven network formed by blood capillaries and lymphatic capillaries. Arrows indicate the movement of fluid out of blood capillaries and the net flow of interstitial fluid and lymph.

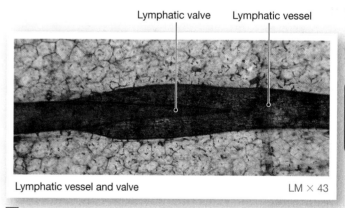

Lymphatic vessel and valve   LM × 43

b Like valves in veins, each lymphatic valve permits movement of fluid in only one direction.

of veins. Like veins, such lymphatic vessels contain valves (**Figure 14-2b**). Pressures within the lymphatic system are extremely low, so the valves are essential to maintaining normal lymph flow. Contractions of skeletal muscles surrounding the lymphatic vessels aid the flow of lymph.

The lymphatic vessels ultimately empty into two large collecting structures called lymphatic ducts (**Figure 14-3**). The **thoracic duct** collects lymph from the lower abdomen, pelvis, and lower limbs, and from the left half of the head,

Figure 14-3 The Lymphatic Ducts and the Venous System.

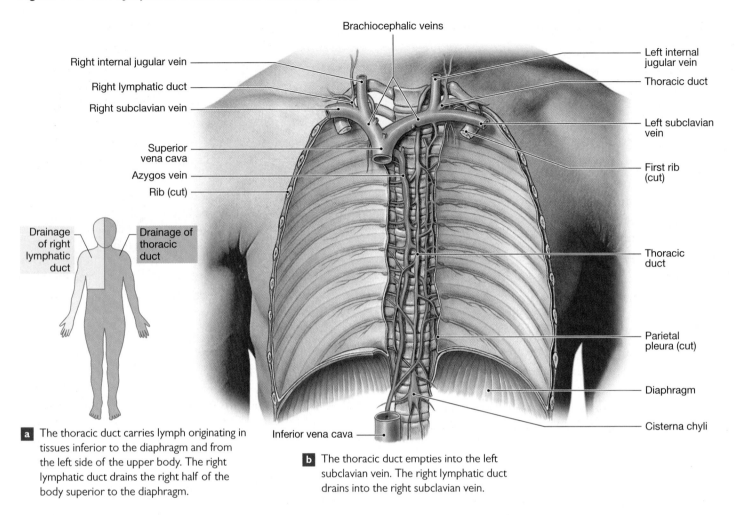

a The thoracic duct carries lymph originating in tissues inferior to the diaphragm and from the left side of the upper body. The right lymphatic duct drains the right half of the body superior to the diaphragm.

b The thoracic duct empties into the left subclavian vein. The right lymphatic duct drains into the right subclavian vein.

neck, and chest. It empties its collected lymph into the venous system near the junction of the left internal jugular vein and the left subclavian vein. The base of the thoracic duct is an expanded, saclike chamber called the **cisterna chyli** (KĪ-lī; *chylos*, juice). The smaller **right lymphatic duct** ends at a comparable location on the right side. It delivers lymph from the right side of the body above the diaphragm. It empties into the right subclavian vein.

Blockage of lymphatic drainage from a limb produces **lymphedema** (limf-e-DĒ-muh). In this condition, interstitial fluids accumulate and the limb gradually becomes swollen and grossly distended.

Lymphocytes

Lymphocytes account for 20–40 percent of circulating white blood cells. ⤴ p. 395 But circulating lymphocytes make up only a small fraction of the total lymphocyte population. Most of the approximately 1 trill (10^{12}) lymphocytes—with a combined weight of over a kilogram (2.2 lb)—are found within lymphoid organs or other tissues. The bloodstream serves as a rapid transport system for lymphocytes moving from one site to another.

Types of Circulating Lymphocytes

Three classes of lymphocytes circulate in the blood: *T cells, B cells,* and *natural killer (NK) cells.* Each has distinctive functions.

T CELLS. Most of the circulating lymphocytes (approximately 80 percent) are **T** (**t**hymus-dependent) **cells.** *Cytotoxic T cells* directly attack foreign cells or virus-infected body cells. These lymphocytes are the primary providers of *cell-mediated immunity,* or *cellular immunity. Helper T cells* stimulate the activities of both T cells and B cells. *Suppressor T cells* inhibit both T cells and B cells. Because they help establish and control the sensitivity of the immune response, helper T cells and suppressor T cells are also called *regulatory T cells.*

B CELLS. **B** (**b**one marrow–derived) **cells** make up 10–15 percent of circulating lymphocytes. Under proper stimulation, B cells differentiate into **plasma cells** that secrete **antibodies**. These antibodies are soluble proteins, also called **immuno-globulins**. ⟳ p. 383 B cells are said to be responsible for *antibody-mediated immunity*. Because antibodies occur in body fluids, antibody-mediated immunity is also known as *humoral* ("liquid") *immunity*. Antibodies bind to specific chemical targets called **antigens**. Most antigens are usually pathogens, parts or products of pathogens, or other foreign compounds. Formation of an antigen–antibody complex starts a chain of events leading to the destruction of the target compound or organism.

NK CELLS. The remaining 5–10 percent of circulating lymphocytes are **NK cells**. NK cells provide innate (nonspecific) immunity. These lymphocytes attack foreign cells, normal cells infected with viruses, and cancer cells that appear in normal tissues. Their continual monitoring of peripheral tissues is known as *immune surveillance.*

The Origin and Circulation of Lymphocytes

Lymphocytes in the blood, bone marrow, spleen, thymus, and peripheral lymphatic tissues are visitors, not residents. All types of lymphocytes move throughout the body. They wander through tissues and then enter a blood vessel or lymphatic vessel for transport to another site. In general, lymphocytes have relatively long life spans. Roughly 80 percent survive for four years. Some last 20 years or more. Throughout your life, you maintain normal lymphocyte populations through the divisions of stem cells in your red bone marrow and lymphoid tissues.

Lymphocyte production and development is called **lymphopoiesis** (lim-fō-poy-Ē-sis). It involves the red bone marrow, thymus, and peripheral lymphoid tissues (**Spotlight Figure 14-4**). As B cells and T cells develop and mature, they gain the ability to respond to the presence of a specific antigen. NK cells gain the ability to respond to a variety of abnormal antigens, allowing them to recognize abnormal cells.

Hematopoietic stem cells (hemocytoblasts) in red bone marrow produce lymphoid stem cells with two different fates. One group remains in the red bone marrow and generates B cells and functional NK cells. The second group of lymphoid stem cells migrates to the thymus. Under the influence of thymic hormones (collectively known as *thymosins*), these cells divide repeatedly to produce large numbers of T cells. These T cells undergo a selection process to ensure that they will not react to the body's own healthy cells and cellular

products. (B cells also undergo a selection process in the red bone marrow with the same results.) As they mature, all three types of lymphocytes enter the bloodstream and migrate to peripheral tissues, including lymphoid tissues and organs, such as the spleen.

The T cells and B cells that migrate from their sites of origin retain the ability to divide and produce daughter cells of the same type. A dividing B cell, for example, produces other B cells, not T cells or NK cells. As we will see, the ability of a specific type of lymphocyte to increase in number is important to the success of the immune response.

Lymphoid Tissues

Lymphoid tissues are loose connective tissues dominated by lymphocytes. In a **lymphoid nodule**, the lymphocytes are densely packed in an area of areolar tissue. In many areas, they form large clusters. Each nodule often contains a pale central region, called a *germinal center*, which contains dividing lymphocytes. A single nodule averages about a millimeter in diameter. Its boundaries are not distinct, because no fibrous capsule surrounds it. As a result, nodule size can increase or decrease, depending on the number of lymphocytes present.

The digestive, respiratory, urinary, and reproductive tracts are open to the external environment. For this reason, they provide a route of entry into the body for potentially harmful organisms and toxins. The epithelia of these systems are protected by a collection of lymphoid tissues called the **MALT**.

MALT associated with the digestive tract plays a particularly important role in defending the body because our food usually contains foreign proteins and often bacteria as well. For example, the **tonsils** are large clusters of lymphoid nodules in the walls of the pharynx. They guard the entrance to the digestive and respiratory tracts (**Figure 14-5**). Five tonsils are usually present: a single *pharyngeal tonsil*, or *adenoid*; a pair of *palatine tonsils*; and a pair of *lingual tonsils*. Aggregates of lymphoid nodules, called *Peyer patches*, also lie beneath the epithelial lining of the small intestine. Another example of MALT is the *appendix*, or *vermiform* ("worm-shaped") *appendix*. The appendix is a blind pouch located near the junction of the small and large intestines. Its walls contain a mass of fused lymphoid nodules.

The lymphocytes in a lymphoid nodule are not always able to destroy bacterial or viral invaders. If pathogens do become established in a lymphoid nodule, an inflammatory response to the infection develops. You are probably familiar with two examples. *Tonsillitis* is the inflammation of one of the tonsils (usually the pharyngeal tonsil). *Appendicitis* is the inflammation of the lymphoid nodules in the appendix.

14

SPOTLIGHT Figure 14-4
ORIGIN AND DISTRIBUTION OF LYMPHOCYTES

Lymphocyte formation, or **lymphopoiesis**, involves the red bone marrow, thymus, and peripheral lymphoid tissues. Of the three, the red bone marrow plays the primary role in the maintenance of normal lymphocyte populations. Hematopoietic stem cells in the red bone marrow produce lymphoid stem cells with two distinct fates.

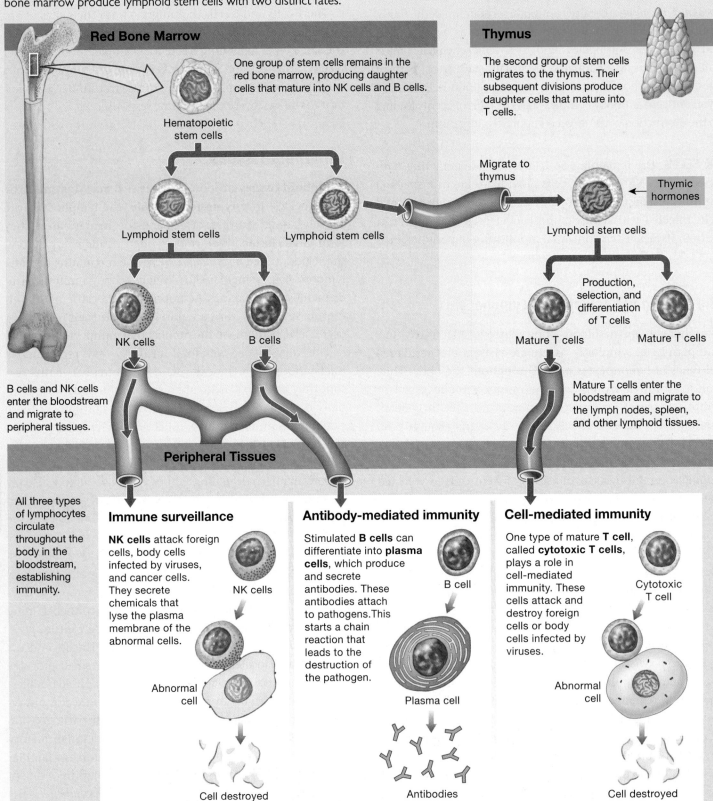

Red Bone Marrow

One group of stem cells remains in the red bone marrow, producing daughter cells that mature into NK cells and B cells.

Hematopoietic stem cells

Lymphoid stem cells

Lymphoid stem cells

NK cells

B cells

B cells and NK cells enter the bloodstream and migrate to peripheral tissues.

Thymus

The second group of stem cells migrates to the thymus. Their subsequent divisions produce daughter cells that mature into T cells.

Migrate to thymus

Thymic hormones

Lymphoid stem cells

Production, selection, and differentiation of T cells

Mature T cells

Mature T cells

Mature T cells enter the bloodstream and migrate to the lymph nodes, spleen, and other lymphoid tissues.

Peripheral Tissues

All three types of lymphocytes circulate throughout the body in the bloodstream, establishing immunity.

Immune surveillance

NK cells attack foreign cells, body cells infected by viruses, and cancer cells. They secrete chemicals that lyse the plasma membrane of the abnormal cells.

NK cells

Abnormal cell

Cell destroyed

Antibody-mediated immunity

Stimulated **B cells** can differentiate into **plasma cells**, which produce and secrete antibodies. These antibodies attach to pathogens. This starts a chain reaction that leads to the destruction of the pathogen.

B cell

Plasma cell

Antibodies

Cell-mediated immunity

One type of mature **T cell**, called **cytotoxic T cells**, plays a role in cell-mediated immunity. These cells attack and destroy foreign cells or body cells infected by viruses.

Cytotoxic T cell

Abnormal cell

Cell destroyed

Figure 14-5 The Tonsils. The tonsils are large clusters of lymphoid nodules in the wall of the pharynx. A single pharyngeal tonsil (the adenoid) lies above the paired palatine and lingual tonsils. Each tonsil contains many germinal centers where lymphocytes divide.

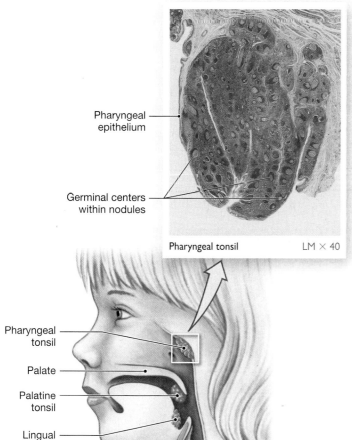

Pharyngeal epithelium

Germinal centers within nodules

Pharyngeal tonsil   LM × 40

Pharyngeal tonsil

Palate

Palatine tonsil

Lingual tonsil

Lymphoid Organs

Lymphoid organs are separated from surrounding tissues by a fibrous connective tissue capsule. Important lymphoid organs include the *lymph nodes*, the *thymus*, and the *spleen*.

Lymph Nodes

Lymph nodes are small, oval lymphoid organs covered by a fibrous capsule. They range in diameter from 1 to 25 mm (up to 1 in.). The greatest number of lymph nodes is located in the neck, armpits, and groin, where they defend us against bacteria and other invaders. **Figure 14-1** shows the general pattern of lymph node distribution in the body.

Two sets of lymphatic vessels are connected to each lymph node (**Figure 14-6**). *Afferent lymphatics* bring lymph to the lymph node from peripheral tissues. *Efferent lymphatics* carry the lymph onward, toward the venous system. A lymph node works like a kitchen water filter. It purifies lymph before it reaches the veins. Within the lymph node, the lymph flows through the subscapular space, cortex, and medullary sinuses. As it passes, at least 99 percent of the antigens present in the arriving lymph are removed by fixed macrophages and branched *dendritic cells*. (We consider their roles in a later section.) As the antigens are removed and processed, T cells and B cells in the lymph node are stimulated, initiating an immune response.

The Thymus

The **thymus** is the site of T cell production and maturation. This pink gland lies in the mediastinum posterior to the sternum (**Figure 14-7a**). The thymus reaches its greatest size (relative to body size) in the first year or two after birth. It grows to its maximum absolute size during puberty, when it weighs between 30 and 40 g (1.06–1.41 oz). Then the thymus gradually decreases in size.

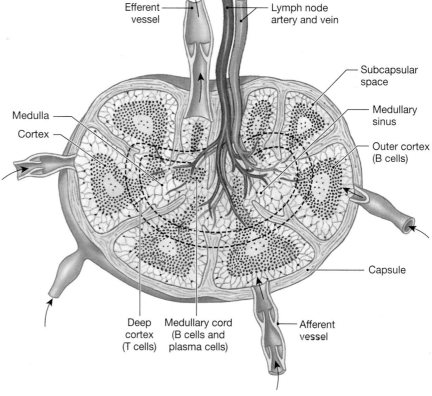

Efferent vessel

Lymph node artery and vein

Subcapsular space

Medulla

Cortex

Medullary sinus

Outer cortex (B cells)

Capsule

Deep cortex (T cells)

Medullary cord (B cells and plasma cells)

Afferent vessel

Figure 14-6 The Structure of a Lymph Node. The arrows indicate the direction of lymph flow. Mature B cells and T cells located in different regions of the cortex and medulla remove antigens from the lymph and initiate immune responses.

Figure 14-7 The Thymus.

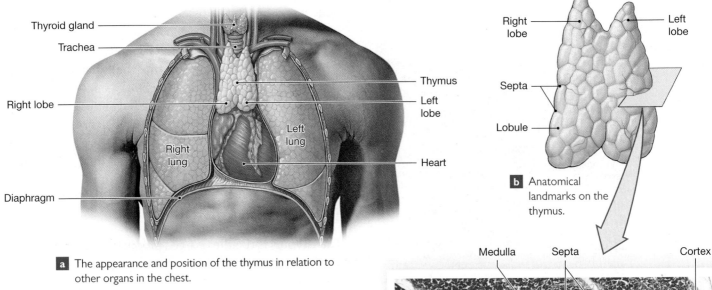

Thyroid gland
Trachea
Right lobe
Diaphragm
Right lung
Left lung
Heart
Thymus
Left lobe

a The appearance and position of the thymus in relation to other organs in the chest.

Right lobe
Left lobe
Septa
Lobule

b Anatomical landmarks on the thymus.

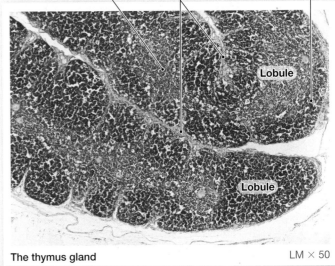

Medulla
Septa
Cortex
Lobule
Lobule

The thymus gland   LM × 50

c Fibrous septa divide the tissue of the thymus into lobules resembling interconnected lymphoid nodules.

CLINICAL NOTE

"Swollen Glands"

Lymph nodes are often called *lymph glands.* "Swollen glands" usually accompany tissue inflammation or infection. Chronic or excessive enlargement of lymph nodes is a sign called *lymph-adenopathy* (lim-fad-e-NOP-a-thē). It may occur in response to bacterial or viral infections, endocrine disorders, or cancer.

Lymphatic capillaries offer little resistance to the entry or passage of cancer cells. For this reason, cancer cells often spread along the lymphatics and become trapped in lymph nodes. An analysis of swollen lymph nodes can provide details on the nature and distribution of cancer cells. Such information aids in choosing appropriate therapies.

Lymphomas are cancers arising from lymphocytes or lymphoid stem cells. They are an important group of cancers of the lymphatic system.

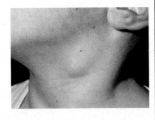

The thymus has two lobes. Each is divided into *lobules* by fibrous partitions, or *septa* (singular, *septum;* a wall) (**Figure 14-7b**). Each lobule consists of an outer cortex and a paler, central *medulla* (**Figure 14-7c**). The cortex contains clusters of lymphocytes surrounded by other cells that secrete the hormones collectively known as thymosins. Thymosins stimulate lymphocyte stem-cell divisions and T cell maturation. After the T cells migrate into the medulla, they leave the thymus in one of the blood vessels in that region.

The Spleen

The adult **spleen** contains the largest collection of lymphoid tissue in the body. It is about 12 cm (5 in.) long and can weigh about 160 g (5.6 oz). Its major function parallels that of the lymph nodes, except that it filters blood instead of lymph. The spleen removes abnormal blood cells and components. It also initiates the responses of B cells and T cells to antigens in the circulating blood. In addition, the spleen stores iron from recycled red blood cells. ⟲ p. 387

The spleen is wedged between the stomach, the left kidney, and the muscular diaphragm. It is attached to the lateral border of the stomach by a broad band of mesentery (**Figure 14-8a**). Splenic blood vessels (the *splenic artery* and *splenic vein*) and lymphatic vessels connect with the spleen

Figure 14-8 The Spleen.

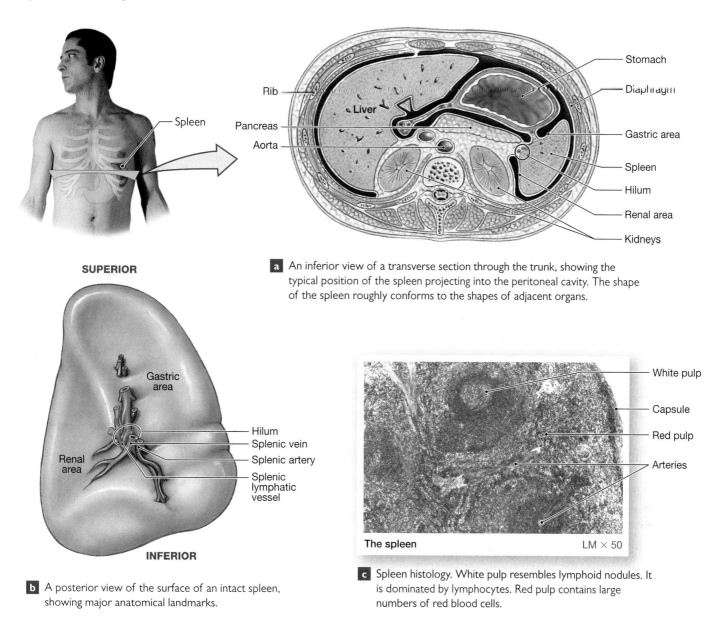

a An inferior view of a transverse section through the trunk, showing the typical position of the spleen projecting into the peritoneal cavity. The shape of the spleen roughly conforms to the shapes of adjacent organs.

b A posterior view of the surface of an intact spleen, showing major anatomical landmarks.

c Spleen histology. White pulp resembles lymphoid nodules. It is dominated by lymphocytes. Red pulp contains large numbers of red blood cells.

The spleen   LM × 50

14

at the *hilum,* a groove at the border between the gastric and renal areas (**Figure 14-8b**). In gross dissection, the spleen normally has a deep red color because of the blood it contains. The cellular components of the spleen are arranged into areas of *red pulp,* which contain large numbers of red blood cells, and areas of *white pulp* resembling lymphoid nodules (**Figure 14-8c**).

After the splenic artery enters the spleen, it branches outward toward the capsule into many smaller arteries that are surrounded by white pulp. Capillaries then discharge the blood into a network of reticular fibers that makes up the red pulp. Blood from the red pulp enters *venous sinusoids* (small vessels lined by macrophages) and then flows into small veins and the

splenic vein. As blood passes through the spleen, macrophages identify and engulf any damaged or infected cells. The presence of lymphocytes nearby ensures that any microorganisms or other abnormal antigens stimulate an immune response.

Roles of the Lymphatic System in Body Defenses

The human body has multiple body defenses. Together, they provide *resistance*—the natural or acquired ability to maintain immunity. We can sort body defenses into two general categories:

1. **Innate (nonspecific) immunity** does not distinguish between one threat and another. The response is the same regardless of the type of invader. These innate

CLINICAL NOTE

Injury to the Spleen

An impact to the left side of the abdomen can distort or damage the spleen. Such injuries are known risks of contact sports, such as football or hockey, and other athletic activities, such as skiing or sledding. Even a seemingly minor blow to the side may rupture the capsule. The result can be serious internal bleeding and eventual circulatory shock. The spleen can also be damaged by infection, inflammation, or invasion by cancer cells.

Depending on the degree of injury, treatment options for a ruptured spleen may range from immediate surgery to allowing time for healing with a period of hospital rest and, if required, blood transfusions. The spleen is very difficult to repair surgically because it is relatively fragile. (Sutures usually tear out before they have been tensed enough to stop the bleeding.) However, surgery for a ruptured spleen can involve stitches (closing the wound with sutures), removing a portion of it, or complete removal. The removal of the spleen is called a *splenectomy* (sple-NEK-to-m). A person without a spleen survives without difficulty but has a greater risk of bacterial infections than do individuals with a functional spleen.

defenses are present at birth. They include *physical barriers, phagocytic cells, immune surveillance, interferons, complement, inflammation,* and *fever.* We discuss all of these defenses shortly. They provide the body with a defensive capability known as **nonspecific resistance**.

2. **Adaptive (specific) immunity** protects against particular threats. For example, an adaptive defense may fight infection by one type of bacterium, but ignore other bacteria and all viruses. Many specific defenses develop after birth as a result of exposure to environmental hazards or infectious agents. Adaptive defenses depend on the activities of specific lymphocytes. B cells and T cells are part of our adaptive defenses, which provide protection known as **specific resistance.**

Innate and adaptive defenses work together. Both are necessary to provide adequate resistance to infection and disease.

CHECKPOINT

3. List the components of the lymphatic system.

4. How would blockage of the thoracic duct affect the flow of lymph?

5. If the thymus gland failed to produce thymic hormones, which population of lymphocytes would be affected?

6. Why do lymph nodes enlarge during some infections?

See the blue Answers tab at the back of the book.

14-3 Innate (nonspecific) defenses respond in a characteristic way regardless of the potential threat

Learning Objective List the body's innate (nonspecific) defenses and explain how each functions.

Innate (nonspecific) defenses deny the entry, or limit the spread within the body, of microorganisms or other environmental hazards. Seven major categories of nonspecific defenses are summarized in **Figure 14-9**.

Physical Barriers

Physical barriers keep hazardous organisms and materials outside the body. To cause trouble, an antigenic substance or a pathogen must enter body tissues. In other words, it must cross an epithelium—either at the skin or across a mucous membrane. The epithelial covering of the skin has a keratin coating, multiple layers of cells, and a network of desmosomes that locks adjacent cells together. ⊃ pp. 93, 124 These barriers provide very effective protection for underlying tissues.

In addition, specialized accessory structures and secretions protect most epithelia. The hairs on most areas of your body provide some protection against mechanical abrasion, especially on the scalp. They often prevent hazardous materials or insects from contacting the skin's surface. The epidermal surface also receives the secretions of sebaceous glands and sweat glands. These secretions flush the surface, washing away microorganisms and chemical agents. The secretions also contain microbe-killing chemicals, destructive enzymes (*lysozymes*), and antibodies.

The epithelia lining the digestive, respiratory, urinary, and reproductive tracts are more delicate, but they are equally well defended. Mucus bathes most surfaces of the digestive tract. The stomach contains a powerful acid that can destroy many potential pathogens. Mucus is swept across the lining of the respiratory tract. Urine flushes the urinary passageways. Glandular secretions flush structures in the reproductive tract. Special enzymes, antibodies, and an acidic pH add to the effectiveness of these secretions.

Phagocytes

Recall that **phagocytes** are cells that can surround and engulf solid objects. They serve as janitors and police in peripheral tissues. They remove cellular debris and

Figure 14-9 The Body's Innate Defenses. Innate (nonspecific) defenses deny pathogens access to the body or destroy them without distinguishing among specific types.

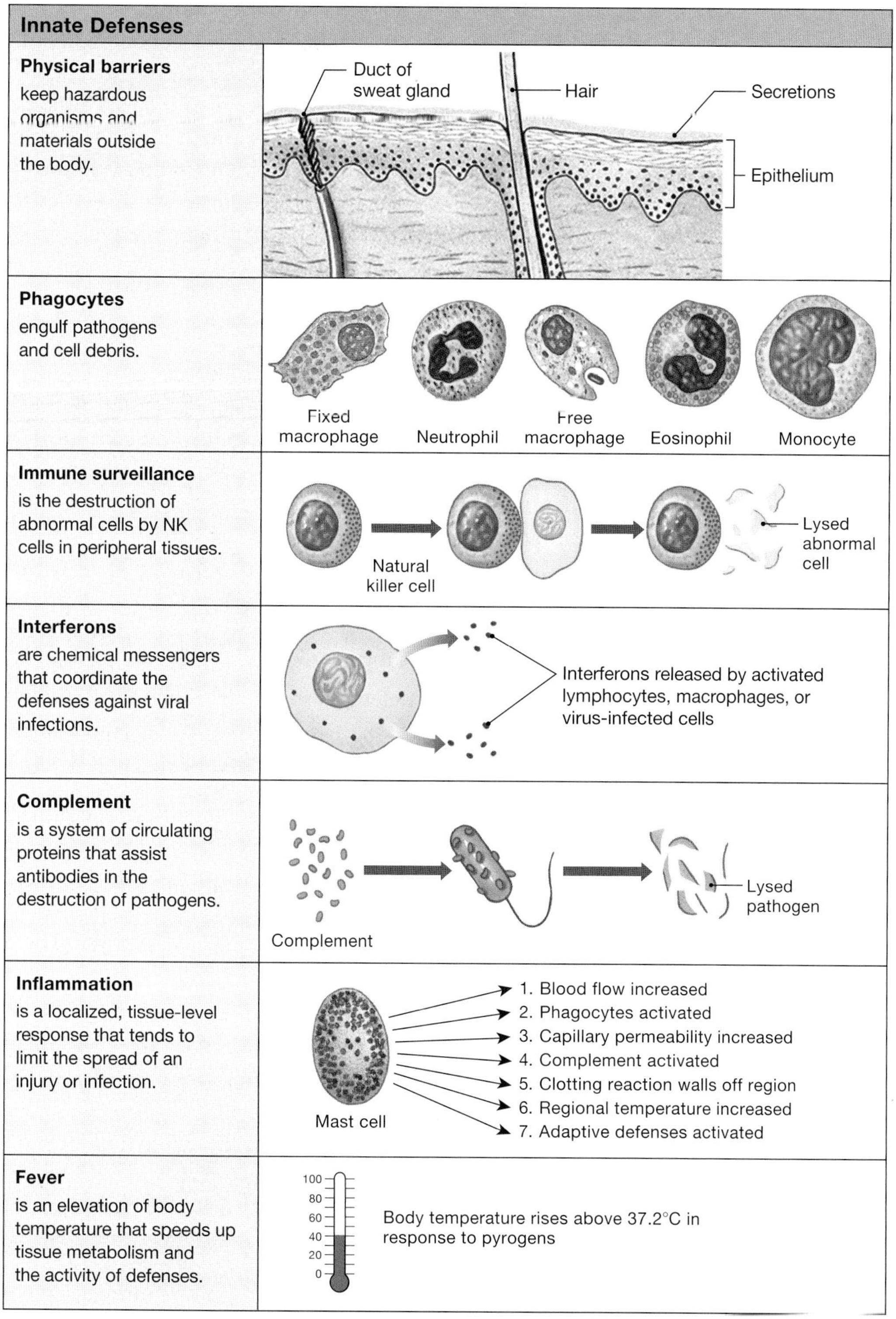

Innate Defenses	
Physical barriers keep hazardous organisms and materials outside the body.	Duct of sweat gland — Hair — Secretions — Epithelium
Phagocytes engulf pathogens and cell debris.	Fixed macrophage, Neutrophil, Free macrophage, Eosinophil, Monocyte
Immune surveillance is the destruction of abnormal cells by NK cells in peripheral tissues.	Natural killer cell — Lysed abnormal cell
Interferons are chemical messengers that coordinate the defenses against viral infections.	Interferons released by activated lymphocytes, macrophages, or virus-infected cells
Complement is a system of circulating proteins that assist antibodies in the destruction of pathogens.	Complement — Lysed pathogen
Inflammation is a localized, tissue-level response that tends to limit the spread of an injury or infection.	Mast cell — 1. Blood flow increased 2. Phagocytes activated 3. Capillary permeability increased 4. Complement activated 5. Clotting reaction walls off region 6. Regional temperature increased 7. Adaptive defenses activated
Fever is an elevation of body temperature that speeds up tissue metabolism and the activity of defenses.	Body temperature rises above 37.2°C in response to pyrogens

classes of phagocytic cells are found in the body: *microphages* and *macrophages.*

Microphages are the neutrophils and eosinophils that normally circulate in the blood. These phagocytic cells leave the bloodstream and enter peripheral tissues subjected to injury or infection. Neutrophils are abundant, mobile, and quick to phagocytize cellular debris or invading bacteria. ⟲ p. 395 Eosinophils are less abundant. They target foreign compounds or pathogens that have been coated with antibodies.

The body also contains several types of **macrophages**—large, actively phagocytic cells derived from circulating monocytes. Almost every tissue in the body shelters resident (fixed) or visiting (free) macrophages. This relatively diffuse collection of phagocytes has been called the **monocyte–macrophage system**, or the *reticuloendothelial system.* In some organs, fixed macrophages have special names. For example, *microglia* are macrophages in the central nervous system. *Kupffer* (KOOP-fer) *cells* are macrophages found in and around blood channels in the liver.

All phagocytic cells function in much the same way, but their targets may differ from one cell type to another. Mobile macrophages and microphages also share a number of other functional characteristics in addition to phagocytosis. All can move through capillary walls by squeezing between adjacent endothelial cells, a process known as *diapedesis* (*dia,* through + *pedesis,* a leaping). They may also be attracted to or repelled by chemicals in the surrounding fluids, a process called **chemotaxis** (*chemo-,* chemistry + *taxis,* arrangement). They are

respond to invasion by foreign compounds or pathogens. Phagocytes represent the "first line of cellular defense," often attacking and removing microorganisms before lymphocytes become aware of their presence. Two general

particularly sensitive to chemicals released by other body cells or by pathogens.

Immune Surveillance

Our immune defenses attack and destroy abnormal cells but generally ignore normal cells in the body's tissues. The constant monitoring of normal tissues is called **immune surveillance**. It primarily involves the lymphocytes known as NK cells. The plasma membrane of an abnormal cell generally contains antigens not found on the membranes of normal cells. NK cells recognize an abnormal cell by detecting those antigens. NK cells are much less selective about their targets than other lymphocytes: They respond to a *variety* of abnormal antigens that may appear on a plasma membrane. When encountering such antigens on a bacterium, a cancer cell, or a cell infected with viruses, NK cells secrete proteins called *perforins*. The perforins kill the abnormal cell by creating large pores in its plasma membrane.

NK cells respond much more rapidly than T cells or B cells upon contact with an abnormal cell. Killing the abnormal cells can slow the spread of a bacterial or viral infection. It may also eliminate cancer cells before they spread to other tissues. Unfortunately, some cancer cells avoid detection, a process called *immunological escape*. Once immunological escape has taken place, cancer cells can multiply and spread without interference by NK cells.

Interferons

Interferons (in-ter-FĒR-onz) are small proteins released by activated lymphocytes, macrophages, and tissue cells infected with viruses. Normal cells exposed to interferon molecules respond by producing *antiviral proteins* that interfere with viral replication inside the cell. In addition to slowing the spread of viral infections, interferons stimulate the activities of macrophages and NK cells. Interferons are examples of **cytokines** (SĪ-tō-kīnz), chemical messengers that tissue cells release to coordinate local activities. Most cytokines act only within one tissue. However, those released by cellular defenders also act as hormones and affect the activities of cells and tissues throughout the body. We discuss their role in the regulation of specific defenses later in the chapter.

The Complement System

Plasma contains over 30 special *complement proteins* that form the **complement system**. The term *complement* refers to the fact that this system adds to or completes the actions of antibodies. Complement proteins interact with one another in chain reactions similar to those of the clotting system. The reaction begins when a particular complement protein binds either to a pair of antibody molecules already attached to a bacterial cell wall or directly to bacterial cell walls. The bound complement protein then interacts with a series of other complement proteins. Complement activation is known to (1) attract phagocytes, (2) stimulate phagocytosis, (3) destroy plasma membranes, and (4) promote inflammation.

Inflammation

Inflammation, or the *inflammatory response*, is a localized tissue response to injury. ↻ p. 116 Inflammation produces local swelling, redness, heat, and pain. Any stimulus that kills cells or damages loose connective tissue can produce inflammation.

Inflammation has several effects:

- The injury is temporarily repaired, and additional pathogens are prevented from entering the wound.
- The spread of pathogens away from the injury is slowed.
- A wide range of defenses are mobilized to overcome the pathogens and aid permanent repairs. The repair process is called *regeneration*.

Mast cells play a key role in inflammation. (Recall that mast cells are small, mobile connective tissue cells. They are often found near blood vessels). ↻ p. 103 **Figure 14-10** summarizes the events of inflammation in the skin. Comparable events occur in almost any tissue subjected to physical damage or to infection.

When stimulated by mechanical stress or chemical changes in the local environment, mast cells release chemicals, including *histamine* and *heparin*, into the interstitial fluid. These chemicals begin the process of inflammation. The histamine makes capillaries more permeable and speeds up blood flow through the area. The combination of abnormal tissue conditions and chemicals released by mast cells stimulates local sensory neurons, producing sensations of pain.

The increased blood flow reddens the area and raises local temperature. These changes increase the rate of enzymatic reactions and speed up the activity of phagocytes. The rise in temperature may also denature foreign proteins or enzymes of invading microorganisms.

Increased vessel permeability allows clotting factors and complement proteins to leave the bloodstream and enter the

Figure 14-10 Events in Inflammation.

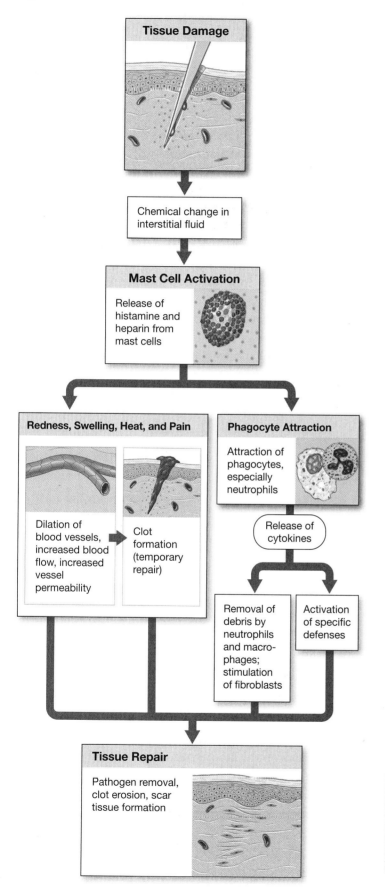

Tissue Damage

↓

Chemical change in interstitial fluid

↓

Mast Cell Activation

Release of histamine and heparin from mast cells

Redness, Swelling, Heat, and Pain

Dilation of blood vessels, increased blood flow, increased vessel permeability → Clot formation (temporary repair)

Phagocyte Attraction

Attraction of phagocytes, especially neutrophils

Release of cytokines

Removal of debris by neutrophils and macrophages; stimulation of fibroblasts

Activation of specific defenses

Tissue Repair

Pathogen removal, clot erosion, scar tissue formation

injured area. Clotting does not take place at the actual site of injury, due to the presence of heparin. However, a clot soon forms around the damaged area. The clot both isolates the region and slows the spread of the chemical or pathogen into healthy tissues. Additionally, the release of histamine stimulates other series of events that activate specific defenses and further pave the way for the repair of the injured tissue.

After an injury, tissue conditions generally become more abnormal before they begin to improve. The tissue destruction that takes place after cells have been injured or destroyed is called **necrosis** (ne-KRŌ-sis). This process begins several hours after the original injury and is due to lysosomal enzymes. Lysosomes break down by autolysis, releasing digestive enzymes that first destroy the injured cells and then attack surrounding tissues. ⌐ p. 72

As local inflammation continues, debris and dead and dying cells collect at the injury site. They form a thick fluid mixture known as **pus**. A buildup of pus in an enclosed tissue space is called an **abscess**.

Fever

Fever is a body temperature greater than 37.2°C (99°F). Recall from Chapter 8 that the hypothalamus contains a temperature-regulating center and acts as the body's thermostat. ⌐ p. 276 Circulating proteins called **pyrogens** (PĪ-rō-jenz; *pyr,* fire + *-gen,* to produce) can reset this thermostat and raise body temperature. Pathogens, bacterial toxins, and antigen–antibody complexes may act as pyrogens or stimulate the release of pyrogens by macrophages.

Within limits, a fever may be beneficial. High body temperatures may inhibit some bacteria and viruses. The most likely beneficial effect is an increase in the rate of metabolism. Cells can move faster (enhancing phagocytosis), and enzymatic reactions proceed more quickly. However, high fevers (over 40°C, or 104°F) can damage many physiological systems. Such high fevers can cause CNS problems, including nausea, disorientation, hallucinations, or convulsions.

CHECKPOINT

7. List the body's innate (nonspecific) defenses.

8. What types of cells would be affected by a decrease in the number of monocyte-forming cells in red bone marrow?

9. A rise in the level of interferon in the body indicates what kind of infection?

10. What effects do pyrogens have in the body?

See the blue Answers tab at the back of the book.

14

CLINICAL NOTE

Fever

It is important to remember that fever is a normal response to infectious diseases. Fever is defined as a temperature 1° or more above the normal. Mild or short-term elevations are common with minor infections. High fevers, with temperatures of 103°F and above, can signal a potentially dangerous infection. Fever, although frightening for parents, can actually be a good thing. It is important to remember that fever is part of the body's way of fighting infections. Thus, not all fevers need to be treated. High fever can make a child uncomfortable and can aggravate problems such as dehydration. Some children who develop high fevers will have febrile seizures. While these are scary for the parents, they are usually self-limited and cause no permanent damage.

If the child is prone to develop febrile seizures or is extremely uncomfortable, fever may be treated with antipyretic medications such as ibuprofen or acetaminophen. Aspirin should never be administered. Sponge baths with tepid water (never with alcohol) can also help lower the child's temperature. With sponging, be sure not to overcool the child; overcooling can cause shivering and shut down the body's cooling mechanisms. The treatment of fever in the prehospital setting is controversial. Always follow local protocols in this regard.

14-4 Adaptive (specific) defenses respond to specific threats and are either cell mediated or antibody mediated

Learning Objective Define adaptive (specific) defenses, identify the forms and properties of immunity, and distinguish between cell-mediated immunity and antibody-mediated (humoral) immunity.

The coordinated activities of T cells and B cells provide adaptive (specific) defenses. These cells respond to the presence of *specific* antigens.

- *T cells* provide a defense against abnormal cells and pathogens inside living cells. This process is called **cell-mediated immunity**, or *cellular immunity.*

- *B cells* provide a defense against antigens and pathogens in body fluids. This process is called **antibody-mediated immunity**, or *humoral immunity.*

Both kinds of immunity are important because they come into play under different circumstances. Activated T cells do not respond to antigens in solution. Antibodies (produced by activated B cells) cannot cross plasma membranes to enter cells. Regardless of whether T cells or B cells are involved, we can categorize immunity into several forms according to when and how it arises in the body (**Figure 14-11**).

Forms of Immunity

As you have seen, we can classify immunity as either innate or adaptive (**Figure 14-11**). **Innate (nonspecific) immunity** is genetically determined and present at birth. It includes the nonspecific defenses previously discussed. **Adaptive (specific) immunity** is not present at birth. Instead, it develops only when you have been exposed to a specific antigen. Adaptive immunity can be active or passive. These forms of immunity can be either naturally acquired or artificially induced.

Active immunity develops after exposure to an antigen. It is a result of the immune response. The immune system is capable of defending against an enormous number of antigens. However, the appropriate defenses are mobilized only after you encounter a particular antigen. In active immunity, the body responds to an antigen by making its own antibody. Active immunity may develop either as a result of natural exposure to an antigen in the environment (naturally acquired active immunity), or from deliberate exposure to an antigen (artificially induced active immunity).

- *Naturally acquired active immunity* is not fully functional at birth. It normally begins to develop after birth. It continues to build as you encounter "new" pathogens or other antigens. This process might be likened to the development of a child's vocabulary: The child begins with a few basic common words and learns new ones as needed.

- *Artificially induced active immunity* stimulates the body to produce antibodies under controlled conditions so that you will be able to overcome natural exposure to the same pathogen in the future. This is the basic principle behind *immunization*, or *vaccination*, to prevent disease. A **vaccine** is a preparation designed to induce an immune response. It contains either a dead or an inactive pathogen, or antigens derived from that pathogen. (Vaccines are given orally or by intramuscular or subcutaneous injection.)

Passive immunity is produced by transferring antibodies to a person from some other source.

- In *naturally acquired passive immunity*, a baby receives antibodies from the mother, either before birth (across the placenta) or in early infancy (through breast milk).

- In *artificially induced passive immunity*, a person receives antibodies to fight infection or prevent disease after exposure to the pathogen. For example, a person recently bitten by a rabid animal receives an injection of antibodies that attack the rabies virus.

Figure 14-11 Forms of Immunity.

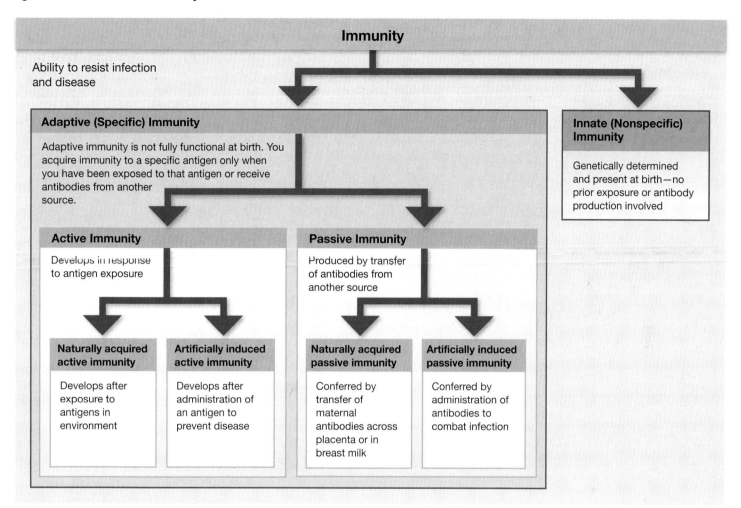

Properties of Adaptive Immunity

Adaptive immunity has four general properties, or characteristics:

1. **Specificity.** A specific defense is activated by a specific antigen. The immune response targets that particular antigen and no others. **Specificity** occurs because the plasma membrane of each T cell and B cell has receptors that will bind only one specific antigen, ignoring all other antigens. Either lymphocyte will inactivate or destroy only that specific antigen, without affecting other antigens or normal tissues.

2. **Versatility.** Millions of antigens in the environment can pose a threat to our health. In the course of a normal lifetime, you only encounter a fraction of that number—perhaps tens of thousands of antigens. Your immune system cannot anticipate which antigens it will encounter. It must be ready to confront *any* antigen

at *any* time. The immune system gets its **versatility** by producing millions of different lymphocyte populations, each with different antigen receptors, as well as through variability in the structure of synthesized antibodies. In this way, the immune system becomes ready to produce appropriate and specific responses to each antigen when exposure occurs.

3. **Memory.** The immune system "remembers" antigens that it encounters. As a result of immunological **memory**, the immune response to a second exposure to an antigen is stronger and lasts longer than the response to the first exposure. During that first response to an antigen, lymphocytes sensitive to its presence divide repeatedly. Two kinds of cells are produced: some that attack the antigen, and others that remain inactive unless they meet the same antigen at a later date. This inactive group is made up of **memory cells** that enable your immune system to "remember" an antigen it has

Figure 14-12 An Overview of the Immune Response.

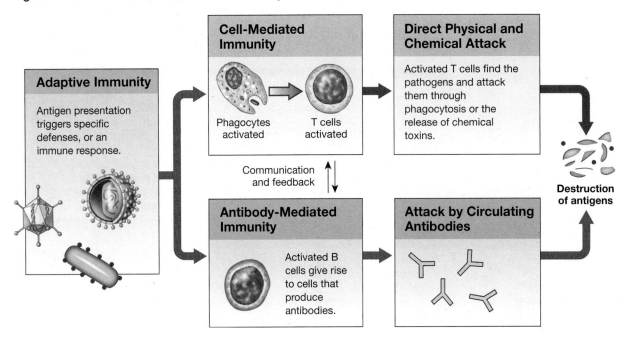

Adaptive Immunity

Antigen presentation triggers specific defenses, or an immune response.

Cell-Mediated Immunity

Phagocytes activated → T cells activated

Communication and feedback

Antibody-Mediated Immunity

Activated B cells give rise to cells that produce antibodies.

Direct Physical and Chemical Attack

Activated T cells find the pathogens and attack them through phagocytosis or the release of chemical toxins.

Attack by Circulating Antibodies

Destruction of antigens

previously encountered, and launch a faster, stronger, and longer-lasting response if such an antigen ever appears again.

4. *Tolerance. The immune system does not respond to all antigens.* The immune response targets foreign cells and compounds, but it generally ignores normal tissues and their antigens. **Tolerance** is said to exist when the immune system does not respond to such antigens. We have tolerance because any B cells or T cells undergoing differentiation (in the red bone marrow and thymus, respectively) are destroyed if they react to normal body antigens. As a result, normal B cells and T cells will ignore normal (or *self*) antigens and will attack foreign (or *nonself*) antigens.

An Overview of the Immune Response

The purpose of the *immune response* (defense against specific antigens) is to inactivate or destroy pathogens, abnormal cells, and foreign molecules (such as toxins). **Figure 14-12** presents an overview of the immune response. When an antigen triggers an immune response, it usually activates both T cells and B cells. T cells are generally activated first, but only after phagocytes have been exposed to the antigen. Once activated, the T cells attack the antigen and stimulate the activation of B cells. The activated B cells mature into cells that produce antibodies. These antibodies in the bloodstream then bind to and attack the antigen.

Build Your Knowledge

Recall that the plasma membrane of a cell contains lipids, proteins, and carbohydrates (as you saw in **Chapter 3: Cell Structure and Function**). Membrane proteins may function as receptors, channels, carriers, enzymes, anchors, and identifiers. Identifiers, or recognition proteins, identify a cell as self or nonself, normal or abnormal, to the immune system. Carbohydrates form complex molecules with lipids or proteins on the outer surface of a plasma membrane. The carbohydrate portion of molecules such as glycoproteins acts as a receptor for extracellular compounds, such as antigens. ⊃ **p. 60**

CHECKPOINT

11. Explain the difference between cell-mediated (cellular) immunity and antibody-mediated (humoral) immunity.

12. Identify the two forms of active immunity and the two forms of passive immunity.

13. List the four general properties of adaptive immunity.

See the blue Answers tab at the back of the book.

14-5 T cells play a role in starting and controlling the immune response

Learning Objective Discuss the different types of T cells and their roles in the immune response.

Before an immune response can begin, T cells must be activated by exposure to an antigen. This activation seldom results from direct interaction between the T cell and the antigen. Foreign substances or pathogens entering a tissue rarely stimulate an immediate immune response.

Antigen Presentation

T cells are activated by antigens bound to glycoprotein receptors in the plasma membrane of other cells. ↪ p. 61 This process is called **antigen presentation**. The structure of these antigen-binding receptors is genetically determined and differs among individuals. The membrane receptors are called *major histocompatibility complex* (*MHC*) *proteins* and are grouped into two classes. An antigen bound to a Class I MHC protein acts like a red flag that in effect tells the immune system "Hey, I'm an abnormal cell—kill me!" An antigen bound to a Class II MHC protein tells the immune system "Hey, this antigen is dangerous—get rid of it!"

Class I MHC proteins are in the plasma membranes of all nucleated cells. These MHC proteins bind and display small peptide molecules (chains of amino acids) that are continuously produced in the cell and exported to the plasma membrane. If the cell is healthy and the peptides are normal (self), T cells ignore them. If the cell contains abnormal (nonself), viral, or bacterial peptides, their appearance in the plasma membrane will activate T cells, leading to destruction of the abnormal cell. The recognition of nonself peptides in transplanted tissue is the primary reason why donated organs are commonly rejected by the recipient. In the case of viruses or bacteria, T cells can be activated by contact with viral or bacterial antigens bound to Class I MHC proteins on the surface of infected cells. The activation of T cells by these antigens results in the destruction of the infected cells.

Class II MHC proteins are found in the membranes of lymphocytes and *antigen-presenting cells* (*APCs*). APCs are specialized for activating T cells to attack foreign cells (including bacteria) and foreign proteins. Among the **APCs** are all the phagocytic cells of the monocyte–macrophage group, including (1) free and fixed macrophages in connective tissues, (2) the Kupffer cells in the liver, and (3) microglia in the central nervous system. ↪ pp. 103, 249 APCs also include the **dendritic cells** in the skin, lymph nodes, and spleen.

Phagocytic APCs engulf and break down pathogens or foreign antigens. Fragments of the foreign antigens are then bound to Class II MHC proteins and displayed on their cell surfaces. T cells that are exposed to an APC membrane containing such an antigen become activated, initiating an immune response.

Dendritic cells remove antigenic materials from their surroundings by phagocytosis and pinocytosis. Their plasma membranes also present antigens bound to class II MHC proteins. More important is that dendritic cells travel with their foreign antigens to lymphocyte-packed lymph nodes. In this way, they differ from macrophages, which do not migrate far from an infection site.

T Cell Activation

How do T cells recognize antigens? Inactive T cells have receptors that can bind either Class I or Class II MHC proteins. The receptors also have binding sites for a specific target antigen. If the MHC protein contains the specific antigen that the T cell is programmed to detect, binding takes place. This process is called **antigen recognition**, because the T cell recognizes that it has found an appropriate target.

Whether a T cell responds to Class I or Class II MHC proteins depends on a type of protein in the T cell's own plasma membrane. The membrane proteins are members of a large group of proteins known as **CD (cluster of differentiation) markers**. Two CD markers important in our discussion are CD8 and CD4. CD8 T cells respond to antigens on Class I MHC proteins. CD4 T cells respond to antigens on Class II MHC proteins.

In order for activation to take place, a T cell must bind to the stimulating cell at a second site. This binding occurs between other membrane proteins, each specific to their cell type (APC or T cell). This *costimulation* confirms that antigen recognition has occurred. It prevents the T cell from mistakenly attacking normal (self) tissues. Costimulation determines whether a T cell will become activated.

Upon activation, T cells divide and differentiate into cells with specific functions in the immune response. The four major cell types are *cytotoxic T cells, helper T cells, memory T cells,* and *suppressor T cells.*

Cytotoxic T Cells

Cytotoxic T (TC) cells, or *killer T cells*, are responsible for cell-mediated immunity. They are CD8 cells and are activated by exposure to antigens bound to Class I MHC proteins (**Figure 14-13**). The activated cells undergo cell divisions that produce more active cytotoxic cells and memory T_C cells. The activated cytotoxic T cells track down and attack the bacteria, fungi, protozoa, or foreign transplanted tissues that contain the target antigen.

A cytotoxic T cell may destroy its target in several ways (**Figure 14-13**):

- By releasing *perforin*, which ruptures the target cell's plasma membrane. ⊃ p. 483

- By secreting *cytokines* that activate genes in the target cell's nucleus that tell the cell to die. This process of genetically programmed cell death is called *apoptosis*. ⊃ p. 82

- By secreting a poisonous *lymphotoxin* (lim-f-TOK-sin), which kills the target cell by disrupting its metabolism.

Helper T Cells

Helper T (T_H) cells have CD4 markers and are activated by exposure to antigens bound to Class II MHC proteins on APCs. Upon activation, they divide to produce both active helper T and memory T_H cells. Activated helper T cells secrete various cytokines that coordinate specific and nonspecific defenses and stimulate both cell-mediated immunity and antibody-mediated immunity. We will learn more about the functions of activated helper T cells in the upcoming section on B cell activation.

Memory T Cells

As previously noted, some of the cells produced following the activation of cytotoxic T cells and helper T cells develop into **memory T cells**. Memory T_C and T_H cells remain "in reserve." If the same antigen appears a second time, these cells will immediately differentiate into cytotoxic T cells and helper T cells, enhancing the speed and effectiveness of the immune response.

Suppressor T Cells

Suppressor T cells have CD8 markers and are activated by exposure to antigens bound to Class I MHC proteins. Activated suppressor T cells suppress the responses of other T cells and of B cells by secreting cytokines called *suppression factors*. Suppression does not take place immediately, because suppressor T cells are activated more slowly than other types of T cells. As a result, suppressor T cells act *after* the initial immune response. In effect, these cells "put on the brakes," limiting the degree of the immune response to a single stimulus.

Figure 14-13 Antigen Recognition and Activation of Cytotoxic T Cells.

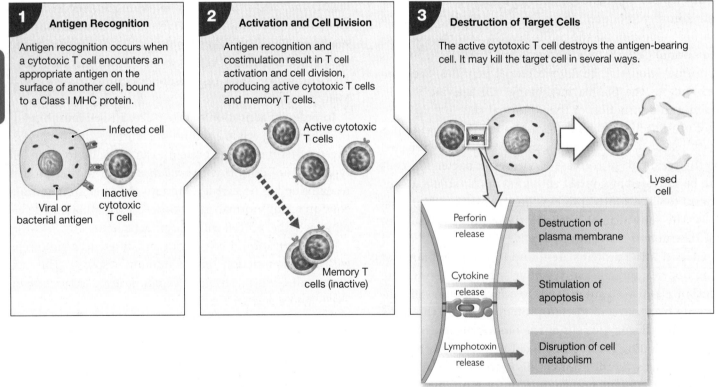

CHECKPOINT

14. Identify the four types of T cells.

15. How can the presence of an abnormal peptide within the cytoplasm of a cell start an immune response?

16. A decrease in the number of cytotoxic T cells would affect which type of immunity?

17. Where are Class I MHC proteins and Class II MHC proteins found?

See the blue Answers tab at the back of the book.

CLINICAL NOTE

Immunology

Overview

The immune system is the principal body system involved in fighting disease. Much of immune system function occurs in the lymphatic system, which consists of the lymphatic vessels, the lymph, and the lymph organs. Its primary functions are the production, maintenance, and distribution of lymphocytes (white blood cells); the return of fluid and solutes from the peripheral tissues to the blood; and the distribution of hormones, nutrients, and waste products from their tissues of origin to the general circulation. Immunity is one of the body's major defense mechanisms. It is provided by the coordinated activities of T cells and B cells, which respond to the presence of specific antigens. T cells provide cellular immunity, while B cells provide humoral immunity.

Physicians who specialize in the immune system disorders are referred to as *allergists* or *allergists/immunologists.* They usually train in general internal medicine or pediatrics and take additional training in allergy and immunology. An immunologist is a scientist (Ph.D., M.D., or D.O.) who specializes in the study of the immune system. A closely related medical discipline is infectious disease. Because infectious disease processes almost always involve the body's immune system, infectious disease specialists often treat immune system disorders. Like an allergist/immunologist, an infectious disease specialist first trains in general internal medicine or pediatrics and then serves a fellowship in infectious disease.

Immunity

The ability of the body's defenses to combat infection with specific responses is called *immunity.* The immune response is a complex cascade of events that occurs following activation by an invading substance, or pathogen. Its goal is the destruction or inactivation of pathogens, abnormal cells, or foreign molecules such as toxins. The body can accomplish this through two mechanisms, cellular immunity and humoral immunity. Cellular immunity involves a direct attack on the foreign substance by specialized cells of the immune system. These cells physically engulf and deactivate or destroy the offending agent. Humoral immunity is much more complicated. Humoral immunity is basically a chemical attack on the invading substance. The principal chemical agents of this attack are *antibodies*, also called *immunoglobulins (Igs)*. Antibodies are a unique class of chemicals that are manufactured by specialized cells of the immune system called B cells. There are five different classes of antibodies: IgA, IgD, IgE, IgG, and IgM.

The humoral immune response begins with exposure of the body to an antigen. An *antigen* is any substance capable of inducing an immune response. Most antigens are proteins. Following exposure to an antigen, antibodies are released from cells of the immune system and attach themselves to the invading substance to facilitate its removal from the body by other cells of the immune system.

The immune system responds differently to a particular antigen depending upon if the body has or has not been exposed previously to that antigen. The initial response to an antigen is called the *primary response.* Following exposure to a new antigen, both the cellular and humoral components of the immune system require several days to respond. Generalized antibodies (IgG and IgM) are first released to help fight the antigen.

At the same time, other components of the immune system begin to develop antibodies specific for the antigen. These cells also develop a memory of the particular antigen. If the body is exposed to the same antigen again, the immune system responds much faster. This is called the *secondary response.* As a part of the secondary response, antibodies specific for the offending antigen are released. Antigen-specific antibodies are much more effective in facilitating removal of the offending antigen than are the generalized antibodies released during the primary response.

Immunity may be either natural or acquired. *Natural immunity*, also called *innate immunity*, is genetically predetermined. It is present at birth and has no relation to previous exposure to a particular antigen. All humans are born with some innate immunity. *Acquired immunity* develops over time and results from exposure to an antigen. The immune system's production of antibodies specific for the antigens to which the body is exposed protects the organism, as subsequent exposure to the same antigen will result in a vigorous immune response. Naturally acquired immunity normally begins to develop after birth and is continually enhanced by exposure to new pathogens and antigens throughout life. For example, a child contracts chicken pox (varicella) at age 18 months. Following the infection, the child's immune system creates antibodies specific for the varicella virus. Repeated exposure to the varicella virus usually will not result in another infection. In fact, it is not unusual for a patient exposed to varicella to develop lifelong immunity to the infection.

Induced active immunity, also called *artificially acquired immunity*, is designed to provide protection from exposure to an antigen at some time in the future (**Table 14–1**). This is achieved

(*continued*)

14

through vaccination and provides relative protection against serious infectious agents. In vaccination, an antigen is injected into the body in order to generate an immune response. This results in the development of antibodies specific for the antigen and provides protection against future infection. Most vaccines contain antigenic proteins from a particular virus or bacterium. Later, when the individual is actually exposed to the pathogen, the immune response will be vigorous and will often be enough to prevent the infection from developing.

An example of a commonly used vaccine is the DPT (diphtheria/pertussis/tetanus) vaccine. This vaccine contains antigenic proteins from the bacteria that cause diphtheria, whooping cough, and tetanus. It is administered at several intervals during the first five years of life and provides protection against infection from these bacteria. Some vaccinations will impart lifelong immunity, while others must be periodically followed with a "booster dose" to ensure continued protection.

Acquired immunity can be either active or passive. Active immunity occurs following exposure to an antigen and results in the production of antibodies specific for the antigen. Most vaccinations result in the development of active immunity. However, it takes some time for a patient to develop specific antibodies. In certain cases, it is necessary to administer antibodies to provide protection until the active immunity can take effect. Passive immunity results from the introduction of antibodies. There are two types of passive immunity. Natural passive immunity occurs when antibodies cross the placental barrier from the mother to the infant to provide protection against embryonic or fetal infections. Induced passive immunity is the administration of antibodies to an individual to help fight infection or prevent diseases.

An example of the clinical use of both active and passive immunity is the regimen used for the prevention of tetanus. Most people from developed countries have received some form of tetanus vaccination during their life. These people typically have some antibodies to tetanus and often need nothing more than a tetanus booster. However, some people have never received any sort of tetanus vaccination. When they seek treatment for a tetanus-prone wound, they must receive prophylaxis for tetanus in addition to care for their wound. This is best achieved by providing both passive and active immunity. To provide immediate protection, the patient is administered antibodies specific for tetanus (tetanus immune globulin [TIG], Hypertet). Then, the patient is also administered a tetanus vaccination (Td or Dt). The TIG provides passive immunity until the body's immune system can respond to the vaccination and develop antibodies specific for tetanus. This should be followed by periodic tetanus boosters until the patient's immunization program is complete.

Immunization

Immunization is the manipulation of the immune system by administering antigens under controlled conditions or by providing antibodies that can combat an existing infection. Active immunization is the process of inducing the immune system to produce specific antibodies through the administration of a *vaccine*. A vaccine is a preparation of antigens derived from a specific pathogen (**Table 14–1**). The vaccine can be given orally or by injection. Most vaccines contain the pathogenic organism. They may contain either the entire organism or just the antigenic proteins found on the organism. Some vaccines may contain the living organism, while others achieve satisfactory results with a dead organism. If a living organism is used, it is usually weakened, or *attenuated*, to lessen the chances of inducing a real infection. Despite attenuation, some vaccines may contain enough of the pathogenic organism to cause mild signs or symptoms. Regardless, the risks of developing a serious illness are quite low compared to those of contracting the disease because of lack of vaccination.

Inactivated, or "killed," vaccines consist of bacterial cell walls or viral protein coats. These vaccines cannot cause the development of even mild disease symptoms. However, they do not induce as strong an immune response as live or attenuated vaccines. Some attenuated vaccines do not induce long-lasting immunity but require periodic booster injections to keep antibody titers at a protective level.

The administration of a vaccine induces the immune system to produce antibodies specific for the antigen or antigens contained within the vaccine. This is a form of active immunity, and protective antibody levels may take several weeks to develop. Immediate protection can, in some cases, be provided by the administration of antibodies. This process, called *passive immunization*, is effective only for certain infections. Antibody preparations may be general or may be specific for a particular disease.

The development of specific antibodies is limited primarily to life-threatening diseases such as tetanus, rabies, diphtheria, and hepatitis that cannot be treated by other methods. Usually, specific passive immunizations are very expensive. General passive immunization involves the injection of various antibodies obtained from the blood donor pool. Referred to as gamma globulin, these agents can provide limited protection until the immune system responds to an administered vaccine.

More and more vaccines are being developed. It is important that emergency personnel be vaccinated against diseases for which they are deemed to be at increased risk. The most important of these is hepatitis B. The hepatitis B vaccine is effective and should be started as soon as possible. It is usually administered in three doses over six months. Hepatitis B vaccine is now a part of most infant immunization programs.

Influenza vaccines are important in the prevention of that disease. However, they must be administered on a yearly basis. Because the influenza viruses often have different antigenic proteins on their surfaces, epidemiologists must try to predict which influenza viruses are going to be a problem in the coming year. They then prepare an influenza vaccine that contains antigenic portions of the predicted influenza viruses. The epidemiologists' predictions are usually accurate, but in some years, inaccurate predictions have resulted in outbreaks of particular strains of influenza.

14-6 B cells respond to antigens by producing specific antibodies

Learning Objective Discuss the processes of B cell sensitization, activation, and differentiation, describe the structure and function of antibodies, and explain the primary and secondary immune responses to antigen exposure.

B cells are responsible for launching a chemical attack on antigens in body fluids. They do so by producing specific antibodies that target specific antigens. B cells do not immediately produce antibodies in response to antigen exposure. They must first undergo sensitization, activation, division, and differentiation into antibody-producing cells (**Figure 14-14**).

Build Your Knowledge

Recall that the plasma proteins in blood include albumins, globulins, and fibrinogen (as you saw in **Chapter 11: The Cardiovascular System: Blood**). Globulins make up about one-third of the plasma proteins. They include antibodies, also called immunoglobulins, and transport proteins. ⊃ **p. 383**

B Cell Sensitization and Activation

The body has millions of populations of B cells. Each B cell carries its own particular antibody molecules in its plasma membrane. If corresponding antigens appear in the interstitial fluid, they interact with these antibodies. When antigen–antibody binding takes place, the B cell prepares for activation by a process called **sensitization**. During sensitization, antigens enter the B cell by endocytosis. They then become displayed on the surface of the B cell, bound to Class II MHC proteins.

The sensitized B cell is now "on standby." It does not become activated until it receives an "OK" from a helper T cell that has become activated to the same antigen. Similar to costimulation in T cells, the need for an activated helper T cell acts like a "safety," thus preventing inappropriate B cell activation.

The activated helper T cell then attaches to the MHC protein–antigen complex of the sensitized B cell, and secretes cytokines. The cytokines have several effects, including promoting B cell activation, stimulating B cell division, and accelerating B cell development into plasma cells.

As **Figure 14-14** shows, the activated B cell divides repeatedly, producing daughter cells that differentiate into

Figure 14-14 The B Cell Response to Antigen Exposure. A B cell is sensitized by exposure to antigens. Once antigens are bound to antibodies in the B cell plasma membrane, the B cell displays those antigens on Class II MHC proteins in its plasma membrane. Activated helper T cells encountering the antigens release cytokines that costimulate the sensitized B cell and trigger its activation. The activated B cell then divides, producing memory B cells and plasma cells that secrete antibodies.

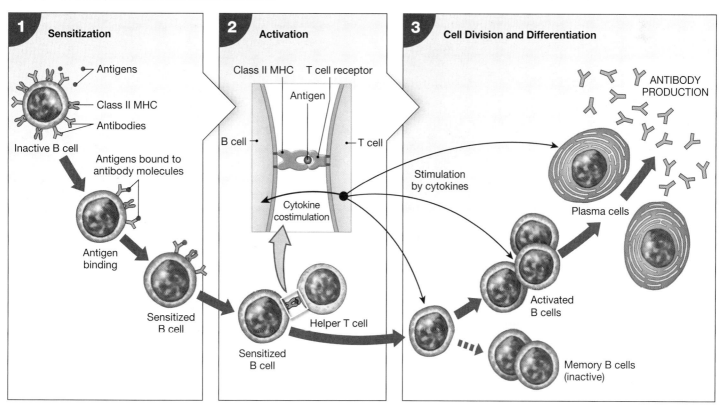

plasma cells and **memory B cells**. The plasma cells synthesize and secrete large quantities of antibodies with the same target as the antibodies on the surface of the sensitized B cell. Memory B cells, like memory T cells, remain in reserve to respond to future exposures to the same antigen. At that time, they respond by differentiating into antibody-secreting plasma cells.

Antibody Structure

An antibody molecule has a Y-shape. It consists of two parallel pairs of polypeptide chains: one pair of long *heavy chains* and one pair of shorter *light chains* (**Figure 14-15a**). Each chain contains *constant* and *variable segments*. The constant segments of the heavy chains form the base of the antibody molecule. B cells produce only five types of constant segments. (These are the basis of the antibody classification scheme described in the following section.)

The specificity of an antibody molecule depends on the structure of the variable segments of the light and heavy chains. The free tips of the two variable segments form the **antigen binding sites** of the antibody molecule. Small differences in the amino acid sequence of the variable segments affect the precise shape of the antigen binding sites. The different shapes of these sites account for the specific differences among the antibodies produced by different B cells. It has been estimated that the approximately 10 trillion B cells of a normal adult can produce 100 million different antibodies.

When an antibody molecule binds to its specific antigen, an **antigen–antibody complex** is formed. Antibodies do not bind to the entire antigen as a whole. Instead, they bind to certain portions of its exposed surface, regions called *antigenic determinant sites* (**Figure 14-15b**). The specificity of that binding depends on the three-dimensional "fit" between the variable segments of the antibody molecule and the corresponding sites of the antigen. A *complete antigen* has at least two antigenic determinant sites, one for each arm of the antibody molecule. Exposure to a complete antigen can lead to B cell sensitization and an immune response. Most environmental antigens have multiple antigenic determinant sites. Entire microorganisms may have thousands.

There are five classes of antibodies, or **immunoglobulins (Igs)**: *IgG, IgM, IgA, IgE,* and *IgD* (**Table 14-1**). Immunoglobulin G, or IgG, is the largest and most diverse class. IgG antibodies are responsible for resistance against many viruses, bacteria, and bacterial toxins. They can also cross the placenta and provide passive immunity to the fetus. Circulating IgM antibodies attack bacteria and also are responsible for the cross-reactions between incompatible blood types. ⊃ p. 392 IgA is present in exocrine secretions, such as mucus, tears, and saliva, and attacks pathogens before they can cross epithelial surfaces and enter the body. IgE that has bound to antigens stimulates basophils and mast cells to release chemicals that stimulate inflammation. IgD is attached to B cells and can be involved in their sensitization.

Figure 14-15 Antibody Structure.

14

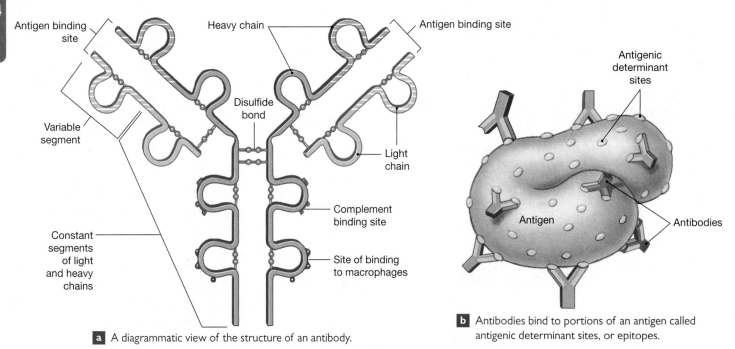

Antigen binding site

Heavy chain

Antigen binding site

Variable segment

Disulfide bond

Antigenic determinant sites

Light chain

Constant segments of light and heavy chains

Complement binding site

Antigen

Antibodies

Site of binding to macrophages

a A diagrammatic view of the structure of an antibody.

b Antibodies bind to portions of an antigen called antigenic determinant sites, or epitopes.

Table 14-1	Classes of Antibodies	
Class	**Function**	**Remarks**
IgG	Responsible for defense against many viruses, bacteria, and bacterial toxins	Largest class (80 percent) of antibodies, with several subtypes; also cross the placenta and provide passive immunity to fetus; anti-Rh antibodies produced by Rh-negative mothers are IgG antibodies that can cross the placenta and attack fetal Rh-positive red blood cells, producing *hemolytic disease of the newborn* ⊃ p. 392
IgM	Anti-A and anti-B forms responsible for cross-reactions between incompatible blood types; other forms attack bacteria insensitive to IgG	First antibody type secreted following initial exposure to antigen; levels decline as IgG production accelerates
IgA	Attacks pathogens before they enter the body tissues	Found in glandular secretions (mucus, tears, and saliva)
IgE	Accelerates inflammation on exposure to antigen	Bound to surfaces of mast cells and basophils and stimulates release of histamine and other inflammatory chemicals; also important in allergic response
IgD	Binds antigens in the extracellular fluid to B cells	Binding can play a role in sensitization of B cells

Antibody Function

The function of antibodies is to eliminate antigens. The formation of an antigen–antibody complex may cause the elimination of antigens in several ways:

1. *Neutralization.* Antibodies can bind to viruses or bacterial toxins, making them incapable of attaching to a cell. This process is called **neutralization**.

2. *Precipitation and Agglutination.* When a large number of antigens are close together, one antibody molecule can bind to antigenic sites on two different antigens. In this way, antibodies can link antigens together and create large complexes. When the antigen is a soluble molecule (such as a bacterial toxin), the complex may then be too large to stay in solution. The complex settles out of body fluids in a process called **precipitation**. When the target antigen is on the surface of a cell, the formation of large complexes is called **agglutination**. The clumping of red blood cells that takes place when incompatible blood types are mixed is an agglutination reaction. ⊃ p. 391

3. *Activation of complement.* Upon binding to an antigen, portions of the antibody molecule change shape, exposing areas of the constant segments that bind complement proteins (**Figure 14-15a**). The bound complement molecules then activate the complement system, destroying the antigen.

4. *Attraction of phagocytes.* Antigens covered with antibodies attract eosinophils, neutrophils, and macrophages. These cells engulf pathogens and destroy cells with foreign or abnormal plasma membranes.

5. *Enhancement of phagocytosis.* A coating of antibodies and complement proteins makes some pathogens with a slick plasma membrane or capsule easier to engulf. The effect is known as *opsonization*.

6. *Stimulation of inflammation.* Antibodies may promote inflammation by stimulating basophils and mast cells. This action can help mobilize nonspecific defenses and slow the spread of the infection to other tissues.

Primary and Secondary Responses to Antigen Exposure

The initial immune response to an antigen is called the **primary response**. When the antigen appears a second time, it triggers a more extensive **secondary response**. The secondary response reflects the presence of large numbers of memory cells that are already "primed" for the arrival of the antigen.

The primary response takes time to develop because the antigen must activate the appropriate B cells, and the B cells must then respond by differentiating into plasma cells (**Figure 14-16**). As plasma cells begin secreting antibodies, the concentration of circulating antibodies undergoes a gradual, sustained rise. The antibody levels in the blood do not peak until one to two weeks after the initial exposure. IgM molecules are the first to appear in the bloodstream, followed by a slow rise in IgG. If the person is no longer exposed to the antigen, the antibody concentrations then decline.

Memory B cells do not differentiate into plasma cells unless they are exposed to the same antigen a second time. If and when that exposure occurs, memory B cells respond right away—faster than the B cells stimulated during the initial exposure. This response is much faster and stronger than the primary response because the numerous memory cells are activated by relatively low levels of antigen. In addition, these cells give rise to plasma cells that secrete massive quantities of antibodies. This antibody secretion is the secondary response to antigen exposure.

Figure 14-16 The Primary and Secondary Immune Responses. The primary response takes about two weeks to develop peak antibody levels, and antibody concentrations do not remain elevated. In the secondary response, antibody concentrations increase very rapidly to levels much higher than those of the primary response. They also remain elevated for an extended period.

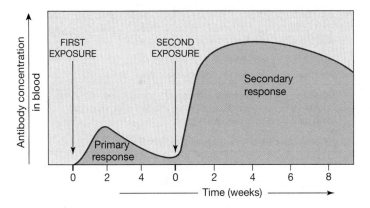

The secondary response produces an immediate rise in IgG concentrations to levels many times higher than those of the primary response. The secondary response appears even if the second exposure takes place years after the first. This is possible because memory cells may survive for 20 years or more.

The relatively slow primary response is much less effective at preventing disease than the more rapid and intense secondary response. Immunization is effective because it stimulates the production of memory B cells under controlled conditions. It is the secondary response that prevents disease.

Summary of the Immune Response

We have now examined the basic cellular and chemical interactions that follow the appearance of a foreign antigen in the body. **Table 14-2** reviews the cells that take part in tissue defenses. **Figure 14-17** provides an integrated view of the immune response and its relationship to innate (nonspecific) defenses.

CLINICAL NOTE

AIDS

Acquired immune deficiency syndrome (AIDS), or late-stage HIV disease, is caused by the human immunodeficiency virus (HIV). HIV is a *retrovirus*, which carries its genetic information in RNA rather than DNA. The virus enters human leukocytes by receptor-mediated endocytosis. ⤴ p. 67 Specifically, the virus binds to CD4, a membrane protein characteristic of helper T cells. HIV also infects several types of antigen-presenting cells, including those of the monocyte–macrophage line. It is the infection of helper T cells that leads to clinical problems.

Cells infected with HIV ultimately die from the infection. The gradual destruction of helper T cells impairs the immune response, because these cells play a central role in coordinating cell-mediated and antibody-mediated responses to antigens. To make matters worse, suppressor T cells are relatively unaffected by the virus. Over time the excess of suppressing factors "turns off" the normal immune response. Circulating antibody levels decline and cell-mediated immunity is reduced. The body is left without defenses against a wide variety of microbial invaders. Microorganisms that ordinarily are harmless can now initiate lethal *opportunistic infections*. The risk of cancer increases because immune surveillance is depressed.

HIV infection takes place through intimate contact with the body fluids of infected persons. The major routes of transmission involve contact with blood, semen, or vaginal secretions, but all body fluids may contain the virus. Most people with AIDS became infected through sexual contact with an HIV-infected person (who may not necessarily show clinical signs of AIDS). The next largest group of infected individuals is intravenous drug users who shared contaminated needles. Relatively few people have become infected with HIV after receiving a transfusion of contaminated blood or blood products. Finally, an increasing number of infants are born with AIDS acquired from infected mothers. HIV may be transmitted during pregnancy, during vaginal childbirth, and by breastfeeding.

AIDS continues to be a public health problem of massive proportions. Current statistics from the Centers for Disease Control and Prevention show that more than 1.2 million people in the United States are infected with HIV. Moreover, nearly 1 in 7 people are not aware that they are infected.

The best defense against AIDS is to abstain from sexual contact or the sharing of needles. All forms of sexual intercourse carry the risk of viral transmission. The use of natural latex (rubber) condoms and synthetic (polyurethane) condoms provides protection from HIV and other viral sexually transmitted diseases. (Natural lambskin condoms are effective in preventing pregnancy, but they do not block the passage of viruses.)

Clinical signs of AIDS may not appear for 5–10 years or more after infection. When they do appear, signs are often mild, consisting of swollen lymph nodes and chronic, but nonfatal, infections. So far as is known, however, AIDS is almost always fatal. Most people infected with the virus eventually die of complications of the disease. (A handful of infected individuals have been able to tolerate the virus without apparent illness for many years.)

Despite intensive efforts, a vaccine has yet to be developed that prevents HIV infection in an uninfected person exposed to the virus. The survival rate for AIDS patients has been steadily increasing. This is because new antiretroviral drugs and drug combinations that slow the progression of the disease are available, and improved antibiotic therapies help combat secondary infections. This combination is extending the life span of patients while the search for more effective treatment continues.

Table 14-2	Cells That Participate in Tissue Defenses
Cell	**Functions**
Neutrophils	Phagocytosis; stimulation of inflammation
Eosinophils	Phagocytosis of antigen–antibody complexes; suppression of inflammation; participation in allergic response
Mast cells and basophils	Stimulation and coordination of inflammation by release of histamine, heparin, prostaglandins
ANTIGEN-PRESENTING CELLS	
Macrophages (free and fixed macrophages, Kupffer cells, microglia, etc.)	Phagocytosis; antigen processing; antigen presentation with Class II MHC proteins; secretion of cytokines, especially interleukins and interferons
Dendritic cells	Phagocytosis and pinocytosis; antigen processing; antigen presentation with Class II MHC proteins
LYMPHOCYTES	
NK cells	Destruction of plasma membranes containing abnormal antigens
Cytotoxic T cells (T_C)	Lysis of plasma membranes containing antigens bound to Class I MHC proteins; secretion of perforin, lymphotoxin, and other cytokines
Helper T cells (T_H)	Secretion of cytokines that stimulate cell-mediated and antibody-mediated immunity; activation of sensitized B cells; enhance nonspecific defenses by attracting macrophages to affected areas
B cells	Differentiation into plasma cells, which secrete antibodies and provide antibody-mediated immunity
Suppressor T cells	Secretion of suppression factors that inhibit the immune response
Memory cells (T_C, T_H, B)	Produced during the activation of T cells and B cells; remain in tissues awaiting reappearance of antigens

Hormones of the Immune System

The body's specific and nonspecific defenses are coordinated by physical interaction and by the release of chemical messengers. An example of physical interaction is the display of antigens by antigen-presenting macrophages. An example of chemical messenger release is the secretion of cytokines by activated helper T cells and other cells involved in the immune response.

Cytokines of the immune response are often classified according to their sources: *lymphokines*, secreted by lymphocytes, and *monokines*, released by active macrophages and other APCs. (These terms are misleading, however, because lymphocytes and macrophages may secrete the same chemical messenger. Cells involved with nonspecific defenses and tissue repair may do the same.) Common groups of cytokines include *interleukins, interferons, tumor necrosis factors, phagocyte regulators*, and *colony-stimulating factors*.

Interleukins (IL) may be the most diverse and important chemical messengers in the immune system. Nearly 20 types of interleukins have been identified. Lymphocytes and macrophages are the primary sources of interleukins. Other cells, such as endothelial cells, fibroblasts, and astrocytes, produce certain interleukins, such as IL-1. Interleukins have widespread effects that include increasing T cell sensitivity to antigens presented by APCs; stimulating B cell activity and antibody production; and enhancing nonspecific defenses, such as inflammation or fever. Some interleukins help suppress immune function and shorten the duration of an immune response.

Interferons make the cell synthesizing them and its neighbors resistant to viral infection, thereby slowing the spread of the virus. In addition to their antiviral activity, interferons attract and stimulate NK cells and macrophages. Interferons are used to treat some cancers.

Tumor necrosis factors (TNFs) slow tumor growth and kill sensitive tumor cells. In addition, TNFs stimulate the production of neutrophils, eosinophils, and basophils; promote eosinophil activity; cause fever; and increase T cell sensitivity to interleukins.

Phagocytic regulators include several cytokines that coordinate the specific and nonspecific defenses by adjusting the activities of phagocytic cells. These cytokines include factors that attract free macrophages and microphages to an area and prevent their premature departure.

Colony-stimulating factors (CSFs) are produced by a wide variety of cells. These cells include active T cells, cells of the monocyte–macrophage group, endothelial cells, and fibroblasts. CSFs stimulate the production of blood cells in the red bone marrow and of lymphocytes in lymphoid tissues and organs. ⟳ p. 389

Figure 14-17 A Summary of the Immune Response and Its Relationship to Innate (Nonspecific) Defenses.

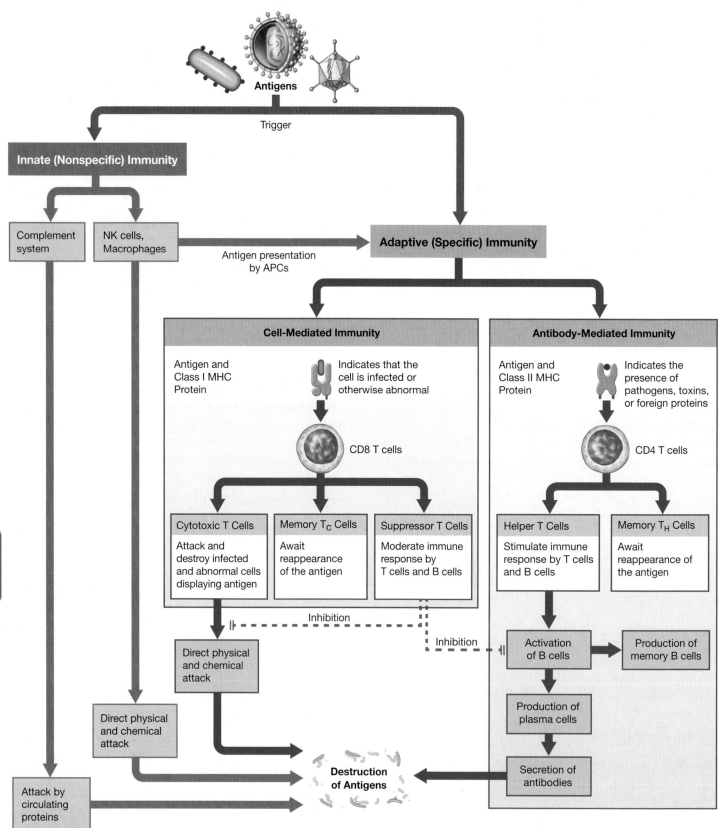

CHECKPOINT

18. Define sensitization.

19. Describe the structure of an antibody.

20. A sample of lymph contains an elevated number of plasma cells. Would you expect the number of antibodies in the blood to be increasing or decreasing? Why?

21. Would the primary response or the secondary response be more affected by a lack of memory B cells for a particular antigen?

See the blue Answers tab at the back of the book.

14-7 Abnormal immune responses result in immune disorders

Learning Objective List and explain examples of immune disorders and allergies, and discuss the effects of stress on immune function.

Immunological competence is the ability to produce a normal immune response after exposure to an antigen. We have already discussed the events in the normal immune response, and its relationship to nonspecific defenses. But what happens when the immune response does not respond as it should?

There are many opportunities for things to go wrong because the immune response is so complex. A variety of clinical conditions result from disorders of immune function. General classes of such disorders include *autoimmune disorders, immunodeficiency diseases,* and *allergies.* Autoimmune disorders and immunodeficiency diseases are relatively rare conditions—clear evidence of the effectiveness of the immune system's control processes. Allergies are far more common (and usually far less dangerous).

Autoimmune Disorders

Autoimmune disorders develop when the immune response mistakenly targets normal body cells and tissues. The immune system usually recognizes but ignores antigens normally found in the body—self-antigens. When the recognition system malfunctions, however, activated B cells make antibodies against normal body cells and tissues. These "misguided" antibodies are called **autoantibodies**. The resulting condition depends on which antigen is attacked. For example, *rheumatoid arthritis* occurs when autoantibodies attack connective tissues around the joints. Type 1 diabetes is caused by autoantibodies that attack cells in the pancreatic islets. ⊃ p. 366

Many autoimmune disorders appear to be cases of mistaken identity. For example, proteins associated with the measles, Epstein-Barr, influenza, and other viruses contain amino acid sequences resembling those of myelin proteins. As a result, antibodies that target these viruses may also attack myelin sheaths. This type of mistake accounts for the neurological complications that sometimes follow a vaccination or viral infection. It also may be responsible for *multiple sclerosis,* a demyelination disorder that may affect the optic nerve, brain, and/or spinal cord. ⊃ p. 251

For unknown reasons, the risk of autoimmune problems increases for people with unusual types of MHC proteins. At least 50 clinical conditions have been linked to specific variations in MHC structure. Examples include psoriasis, rheumatoid arthritis, myasthenia gravis, narcolepsy, Graves disease, Addison's disease, pernicious anemia, systemic lupus erythematosus, and chronic hepatitis.

Immunodeficiency Diseases

In an **immunodeficiency disease**, either the immune system fails to develop normally or the immune response is blocked in some way. Infants born with **severe combined immunodeficiency disease (SCID)** fail to develop either cell- or antibody-mediated immunity. They cannot produce an immune response, so even a mild infection can prove fatal. Total isolation offers protection at great cost, with severe restrictions on lifestyle. Bone marrow transplants and gene-splicing techniques have been used to treat some types of SCID.

AIDS is an immunodeficiency disease (p. 493) that results from a viral infection that targets helper T cells. As the number of helper T cells declines, the normal immune response breaks down.

Allergies

Allergies are inappropriate or excessive immune responses to antigens. The sudden increase in cellular activity or antibody levels can have several unpleasant side effects. For example, neutrophils or cytotoxic T cells may destroy normal cells while attacking the antigen. Or the antigen–antibody complex may trigger a massive inflammatory response. Antigens that set off allergic reactions are often called **allergens**.

14

CLINICAL NOTE

Stress and the Immune Response

One of the first cytokines produced as part of the immune response is *interleukin-1*. It promotes inflammation, but it also stimulates production of adrenocorticotropic hormone by the anterior lobe of the pituitary gland. This hormone in turn leads to the secretion of glucocorticoids by the adrenal cortex. ↻ p. 362 The anti-inflammatory effects of the glucocorticoids may help control the extent of the immune response. In the short term, such suppression is not dangerous.

Chronic stress, however, depresses the immune system and can be a serious threat to health. The long-term secretion of glucocorticoids, as in the resistance phase of the *stress response*, can inhibit the immune response and lower a person's resistance to disease. ↻ p. 371 How does this happen? Glucocorticoids alter the effectiveness of innate and adaptive defenses. Their effects are numerous. They include depressing inflammation, reducing

phagocyte numbers and activity, and inhibiting interleukin production, which depresses the response of lymphocytes.

In another Type I allergy called **anaphylaxis** (an-a-fi-LAK-sis; *ana-,* again + *phylaxis,* protection), a circulating allergen affects mast cells throughout the body. A wide range of signs and symptoms can develop within minutes. Changes in capillary permeability produce swelling and edema in the dermis, and raised welts, or *hives,* appear on the skin. Smooth muscles along the respiratory passageways contract, and the narrowed passages make breathing extremely difficult. In severe cases, an extensive peripheral vasodilation takes place. It produces a drop in blood pressure that can lead to a circulatory collapse. This response is **anaphylactic shock**. ↻ p. 448 The prompt administration of drugs that block the action of histamine, known as **antihistamines** (an-t-HIS-ta-mnz), can prevent many of the signs and symptoms of immediate hypersensitivity.

Four categories of allergies are recognized: *immediate hypersensitivity (Type I)*, *cytotoxic reactions (Type II)*, *immune complex disorders (Type III)*, and *delayed hypersensitivity (Type IV)*. Immediate hypersensitivity is probably the most common type. (We focus on it below.) The cross-reactions that take place after a transfusion of an incompatible blood type are an example of Type II (cytotoxic) reactions. ↻ p. 392 Type III allergies result if phagocytes are not able to rapidly remove circulating antigen–antibody complexes. The presence of these complexes leads to inflammation and tissue damage, especially within blood vessels and the kidneys. Type IV (delayed) hypersensitivity is an inflammatory response that occurs two to three days after exposure to an antigen. An example is the itchy rash that may follow contact with poison ivy or poison oak.

Immediate hypersensitivity is a rapid and especially strong response to an antigen. One common form, *allergic rhinitis*, includes hay fever and environmental allergies. This form may affect 15 percent of the U.S. population. Sensitization to an allergen during the initial exposure leads to the production of large quantities of IgE antibodies. Due to the lag time needed to activate B cells, produce plasma cells, and make antibodies, the first exposure to an allergen does not produce an allergic reaction. Instead, it sets the stage for the next encounter. After sensitization, the IgE antibodies become attached to the plasma membranes of basophils and mast cells throughout the body. When later exposed to the same allergen, these cells are stimulated to release histamine,

heparin, several cytokines, prostaglandins, and other chemicals into the surrounding tissues. As a result, the affected tissues suddenly become inflamed.

The severity of an immediate hypersensitivity allergic reaction depends on the person's sensitivity and the location involved. If allergen exposure takes place at the body surface, the response may be restricted to that area. If the allergen enters the bloodstream, the response could be lethal.

CHECKPOINT

22. Under what circumstances is an autoimmune disorder produced?
23. How does increased stress reduce the effectiveness of the immune response?

See the blue Answers tab at the back of the book.

14-8 The immune response diminishes as we age

Learning Objective Describe the effects of aging on the lymphatic system and the immune response.

As we age, the immune system becomes less effective at fighting disease. T cells become less responsive to antigens, so fewer cytotoxic T cells respond to an infection. This effect may, at least in part, be due to the gradual shrinkage of

CLINICAL NOTE

Manipulating the Immune Response

Advances in our understanding of the immune system and genetic engineering are producing a variety of new therapies. One such therapy involves *monoclonal* (mo-nō-KLŌ-nal) *antibodies*, identical antibodies produced in large quantities in the laboratory by a *clone*, or population of genetically identical cells. One use of monoclonal antibodies is to give passive immunity to patients with a variety of diseases. Another use involves attaching chemotherapy drugs to monoclonal antibodies in order to deliver those drugs to cancer cells.

Genetic engineering can promote active immunity as well. One approach uses gene-splicing techniques. The genes that code for an antigenic protein of a viral or bacterial pathogen are identified, isolated, and inserted into a harmless bacterium that can be grown in the laboratory. As a result, a clone will produce large quantities of pure antigen that can be used to stimulate a primary immune response. Vaccines against hepatitis were developed in this way. A similar strategy may someday be successful in developing vaccines for malaria or AIDS.

the thymus and reduced levels of thymic hormones. With fewer helper T cells as well, B cells are less responsive. As a result, antibody levels rise more slowly after antigen exposure. The net result is an increased susceptibility to viral and bacterial infections. For this reason, vaccinations for acute viral diseases, such as the flu (influenza) and pneumococcal pneumonia, are strongly recommended for elderly individuals.

The increased incidence of cancer in elderly people reflects the fact that immune surveillance declines. As a result, tumor cells are not removed as effectively.

CHECKPOINT

24. Why are elderly people more susceptible to viral and bacterial infections?

25. What may account for the increased incidence of cancer among elderly people?

See the blue Answers tab at the back of the book.

CLINICAL NOTE

Allergies

An *allergic reaction* is an exaggerated response by the immune system to a foreign substance. Allergic reactions can range from mild skin rashes to severe, life-threatening reactions that involve virtually every body system. The most severe type of allergic reaction is called anaphylaxis. Anaphylaxis is a life-threatening emergency that requires prompt recognition and treatment.

The immune system is the principal body system involved in allergic reactions, although other body systems are also affected. These include the cardiovascular system, the respiratory system, the gastrointestinal system, and the nervous system, among others.

An individual's initial exposure, referred to as *sensitization*, results in an immune response. Subsequent exposure induces a much stronger secondary response. Some individuals can become hypersensitive (overly sensitive) to a particular antigen. *Hypersensitivity* is an unexpected and exaggerated reaction to a particular antigen. In many instances, hypersensitivity is used synonymously with the term *allergy*. There are two types of hypersensitivity reactions, delayed and immediate.

Delayed Hypersensitivity

Delayed hypersensitivity results from cellular immunity and therefore does not involve antibodies. It usually occurs in the hours and days following exposure and is the sort of allergy that occurs in normal people. Delayed hypersensitivity most commonly results in a skin rash and is often due to exposure to certain drugs and chemicals. The rash associated with poison ivy is an example of delayed hypersensitivity (**Figure 14–18**).

Immediate Hypersensitivity

When people use the term *allergy*, they usually are referring to immediate hypersensitivity reactions. Examples of immediate

hypersensitivity reactions include hay fever, drug allergies, food allergies, eczema, and asthma. Some individuals have an allergic tendency. This allergic tendency is usually genetic, which means it is passed from parent to child and is characterized by the presence of large quantities of IgE antibodies. Any antigen that causes release of the IgE antibodies is referred to as an *allergen*. Common allergens include:

- Drugs
- Foods and food additives
- Animals
- Insects (Hymenoptera stings) and insect parts
- Fungi and molds
- Radiology contrast materials

Allergens can enter the body through various routes, including oral ingestion, inhalation, topical absorption, injection, and envenomation. The vast majority of anaphylactic reactions result from injection or envenomation.

Parenteral penicillin injections are the most common cause of fatal anaphylactic reactions. Insect stings are the second most frequent cause of fatal anaphylactic reactions. The most frequent offending insects are those in the order *Hymenoptera*. There are three families in this order: fire ants (*Formicoidea*); wasps, yellow jackets, and hornets (*Vespidae*); and honey bees (*Apoidea*). Although these families' venoms all have similar components, each is unique.

Following the body's exposure to a particular allergen, large quantities of IgE antibodies are released. These antibodies attach to the membranes of basophils and mast cells—specialized cells of the immune system containing chemicals that assist in the immune response. When the allergen binds to IgE attached to the basophils and mast cells, those cells release histamine, heparin, and other substances into

14

FIGURE 14–18 Poisonous Plants. Plants of the genus *Toxicodendron* contain the irritative resin urushiol, which causes a cell-mediated reaction and rash. They are: **(a)** poison ivy, **(b)** poison sumac, and **(c)** poison oak.

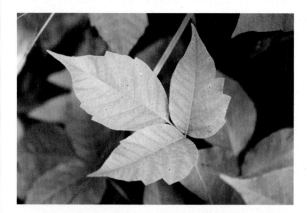

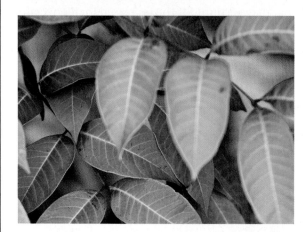

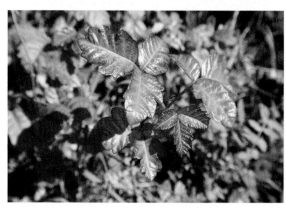

the surrounding tissues. Histamine and other substances are stored in granules found within the basophils and mast cells. (Because of this, basophils and mast cells are often called *granulocytes*.) The process of releasing these substances from the cells, termed *degranulation*, results in what people call an allergic reaction, which can range from very mild to very severe.

The principal chemical mediator of an allergic reaction is *histamine*, which is a potent substance that activates specialized histamine receptors present throughout the body. This causes bronchoconstriction, increased intestinal motility, vasodilation, and increased vascular permeability. Increased vascular permeability causes fluid from the circulatory system to leak into the surrounding tissues. Thus, a common manifestation of severe allergic reactions and anaphylaxis is angioneurotic edema, a marked edema of the skin that usually involves the head, neck, face, and upper airway (**Figure 14–19**).

There are two classes of histamine receptors. H_1 receptors, when stimulated, cause bronchoconstriction and contraction of the intestines. H_2 receptors cause peripheral vasodilation and secretion of gastric acids. The goal of histamine release is to minimize the body's exposure to the antigen. Bronchoconstriction decreases the antigen's possibility of entering through the respiratory tract, while increased gastric acid production helps destroy an ingested antigen. Increased intestinal motility serves to move the antigen quickly through the gastrointestinal system with minimal absorption of the antigen into the body. Vasodilation and capillary permeability help remove the allergen from the circulation, where it has the potential to do the most harm.

FIGURE 14–19 Examples of Angioneurotic Edema. **(a)** Swelling of the face and lips can be severe. **(b)** Marked swelling of the tongue can compromise or obstruct the airway.

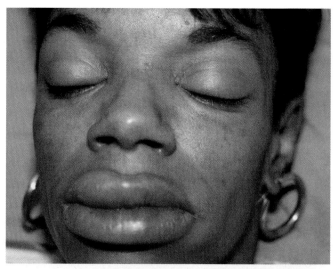

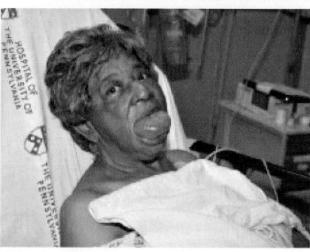

14-9 For all body systems, the lymphatic system provides defenses against infection and returns tissue fluid to the circulation

Learning Objective Give examples of interactions between the lymphatic system and other body systems.

In the first case, thymic hormones and cytokines stimulate TRH production by the hypothalamus, leading to the release of TSH by the pituitary gland. As a result, thyroid hormone levels increase and stimulate cell and tissue metabolism when an immune response is under way.

In the second case, the nervous system can also adjust the sensitivity of the immune response. For example, the PNS innervates dendritic cells in the lymph nodes, spleen, skin, and other APCs. The nerve endings release neurotransmitters that heighten local immune responses. For this reason, some skin conditions, such as *psoriasis*, worsen when a person is under stress. It is also known that a sudden decline in the immune response can take place after even a brief period of emotional distress.

Build Your Knowledge

How the LYMPHATIC SYSTEM integrates with the other body systems presented so far on **p. 499** reviews the major functional relationships between it and the integumentary, skeletal, muscular, nervous, endocrine, and cardiovascular systems. Intense research now focuses on two sets of particularly close relationships. One is between cells involved in the immune response and the endocrine system, and the other is between those cells and the nervous system.

CHECKPOINT

26. Identify the role of the lymphatic system for all body systems.

27. How does the cardiovascular system aid the body's nonspecific and specific defenses?

See the blue Answers tab at the back of the book.

CLINICAL NOTE

Anaphylaxis

The most severe type of allergic reaction is anaphylaxis. Anaphylaxis usually occurs when a specific allergen is injected directly into the circulation. Thus, anaphylaxis is more common following injections of drugs and diagnostic agents and following bee stings (**Table 14–3**). When the allergen enters the circulation, it is rapidly distributed throughout the body. It interacts with both basophils and mast cells, resulting in the massive dumping of histamine and other substances associated with anaphylaxis. The principal body systems affected by anaphylaxis are the cardiovascular system, the respiratory system, the gastrointestinal system, and the skin. Histamine causes widespread peripheral vasodilation as well as increased permeability of the capillaries. In turn, increased capillary permeability results in marked loss of plasma from the circulation. People who sustain anaphylaxis can die from circulatory shock.

Also released from the basophils and mast cells is a substance called *slow-reacting substance of anaphylaxis (SRS-A)*. This substance causes spasm of the bronchial smooth muscle, resulting in an asthma-like attack and occasionally asphyxia. SRS-A potentiates the effects of histamine, especially on the respiratory system.

The signs and symptoms of anaphylaxis typically begin within 30–60 seconds following exposure to the offending allergen. In a small percentage of patients, their onset may be delayed more than an hour. The signs and symptoms of anaphylaxis can vary significantly. The severity of the reaction is often proportional to the speed of onset: reactions that develop very quickly tend to be much more severe. Patients who suffer an anaphylactic reaction often have a sense of impending doom. In addition

to angioneurotic edema that involves the face and neck, laryngeal edema is a frequent complication and can threaten the airway. Initially, laryngeal edema will cause hoarseness, and as the edema worsens, the patient may develop stridor. Finally, this may culminate in complete airway obstruction from either massive laryngeal edema, laryngospasm, oropharyngeal edema, or any combination of these.

The respiratory system is significantly involved in anaphylactic reactions. Initially, the patient will become tachypneic. Later, as lower airway edema and bronchospasm develop, respirations will become labored as evidenced by retractions, accessory muscle usage, and prolonged expiration. Wheezing commonly results from bronchospasm and edema of the smaller airways and may be so pronounced that it can be heard without the aid of a stethoscope. Ultimately, anaphylaxis can result in markedly diminished lung sounds, which reflect decreased air movement and hypoventilation.

The skin is typically involved early in severe allergic reactions and anaphylaxis. Generally, a fine red rash will appear diffusely on the body. As histamine is released, fluid will diffuse from leaky capillaries, which results in urticaria. *Urticaria*, also called *hives*, is a wheal and flare reaction characterized by red raised bumps that may appear and disappear across the body (**Figure 14–20**). As cardiovascular collapse and dyspnea progress, the patient will become diaphoretic. This may, if untreated, progress to cyanosis and pallor.

Histamine's affect on the gastrointestinal system is pronounced. Initially, the patient may note a rumbling sensation in the abdomen as gastrointestinal motility increases. Later, nausea, vomiting, cramping, and diarrhea develop as the body tries to rid itself of the offending allergen.

14

TABLE 14–3	Agents that May Cause Anaphylaxis
Antibiotics and other drugs	
Foreign proteins (e.g., horse serum, streptokinase)	
Foods (nuts, eggs, shrimp)	
Allergen extracts (allergy shots)	
Hymenoptera stings (bees, wasps)	
Hormones (insulin)	
Blood products	
Aspirin	
Nonsteroidal anti-inflammatory drugs (NSAIDs) preservatives (sulfiting agents)	
X-ray contrast media	
Dextran	

Emergency treatment of anaphylaxis includes monitoring the patient with all available devices, including the cardiac monitor, the pulse oximeter, and if the patient is intubated, an end-tidal carbon dioxide detector. As anaphylaxis progresses, the end-tidal carbon dioxide level may climb due to the development of both respiratory and metabolic acidosis, which results in increased carbon dioxide elimination. High concentrations of oxygen should be administered and intravenous fluids should be initiated. Emergency medications used in the treatment of anaphylaxis include oxygen, epinephrine, antihistamines, corticosteroids, and vasopressors. Occasionally, inhaled beta agonists, such as albuterol, may be required. Of these, epinephrine remains the primary treatment.

FIGURE 14–20 Urticaria (Hives) on the Arm.

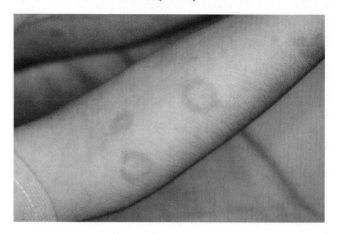

A severe allergic or anaphylactic reaction is a harrowing experience for the patient. Many of the patients you treat will be suffering from forms of allergic reaction less severe than anaphylaxis. An allergic reaction, as contrasted with an anaphylactic reaction, will have a more gradual onset with milder signs and symptoms, and the patient will have a normal mental status. Common manifestations of mild (nonanaphylactic) allergic reactions include itching, rash, and urticaria. Patients with simple itching and nonurticarial rashes may be treated with antihistamines alone. In addition to antihistamines, epinephrine is often necessary for the treatment of urticaria.

Lesser allergic reactions that are not accompanied by hypotension or airway problems can be adequately treated with epinephrine 1:1000 administered subcutaneously or intramuscularly.

14 RELATED CLINICAL TERMS

allograft: Transplant between compatible recipient and donor of the same species.

autograft: A transplant of tissue that is taken from the same person.

bone marrow transplantation: The infusion of bone marrow from a compatible donor after the destruction of the host's marrow by radiation or chemotherapy; a treatment option for acute, late-stage lymphoma.

graft-versus-host disease (GVH): A condition that results when T cells in donor tissues, such as bone marrow, attack the tissues of the recipient.

immunology: The study of the structure and function of the immune system.

immunosuppression: A reduction in the sensitivity of the immune system.

lymphomas: Cancers consisting of abnormal lymphocytes or lymphoid stem cells; examples include *Hodgkin's lymphoma* and *non-Hodgkin lymphoma.*

mononucleosis: A condition resulting from chronic infection by the *Epstein-Barr virus* (*EBV*); signs and symptoms include enlargement of the spleen, fever, sore throat, widespread swelling of lymph nodes, increased numbers of circulating lymphocytes, and the presence of circulating antibodies to the virus.

splenomegaly (splen-ō-MEG-a-lē): Enlargement of the spleen.

systemic lupus erythematosus (LOO-pus e-rith-ē-ma-TŌ-sus) **(SLE):** An autoimmune disorder resulting from a breakdown in the antigen recognition process, leading to the production of antibodies that destroy healthy cells and tissues.

tonsillectomy: The removal of an inflamed tonsil.

tonsillitis: Inflammation of one or more tonsils, typically in response to an infection; signs and symptoms include a sore throat, high fever, and leukocytosis (an elevated white blood cell count).

xenograft: A transplant that is made between two different species.

Build Your Knowledge
How the LYMPHATIC SYSTEM integrates with the other body systems presented so far

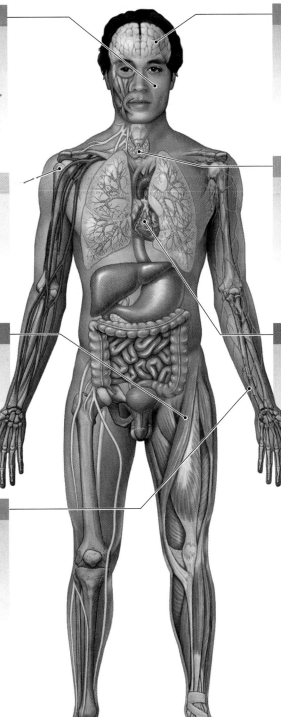

Integumentary System

• The integumentary system provides physical barriers to pathogen entry; dendritic cells in epidermis and macrophages in dermis resist infection and present antigens to trigger the immune response; mast cells trigger inflammation, mobilize cells of lymphatic system

• The lymphatic system provides IgA antibodies for secretion onto integumentary surfaces

Skeletal System

• The skeletal system supports the production of lymphocytes and other cells involved in the immune response in red bone marrow

• The lymphatic system assists in repair of bone after injuries; osteoclasts differentiate from monocyte–macrophage cell line

Muscular System

• The muscular system protects superficial lymph nodes and the lymphatic vessels in the abdominopelvic cavity; muscle contractions help propel lymph along lymphatic vessels

• The lymphatic system assists in repair after injuries

Lymphatic System

The lymphatic system provides adaptive (specific) defenses against infection for all body systems. It
• produces, maintains, and distributes lymphocytes
• returns fluid and solutes from peripheral tissues to the blood
• distributes hormones, nutrients, and waste products from their tissues of origin to the general circulation

Nervous System

• The nervous system has antigen-presenting microglia that stimulate adaptive defenses; glial cells secrete cytokines; innervation stimulates antigen-presenting cells

• The lymphatic system produces cytokines that affect production of CRH and TRH by the hypothalamus

Endocrine System

• The endocrine system produces glucocorticoids that have anti-inflammatory effects; thymosins that stimulate development and maturation of lymphocytes; many hormones that affect immune function

• The lymphatic system secretes thymosins from thymus gland; cytokines affect cells throughout the body

Cardiovascular System

• The cardiovascular system distributes WBCs; carries antibodies that attack pathogens; clotting response helps restrict spread of pathogens; granulocytes and lymphocytes produced in red bone marrow

• The lymphatic system fights infections of cardiovascular organs; returns tissue fluid to circulation

14

14 | Chapter Review

Summary Outline

14-1 Anatomical barriers and defense processes make up nonspecific defense, and lymphocytes provide specific defense p. 537

1. The cells, tissues, and organs of the **lymphatic system** play a central role in the body's defenses against a variety of **pathogens**, or disease-causing organisms.

2. *Lymphocytes*, the primary cells of the lymphatic system, are central to an **immune response** against specific threats to the body. **Immunity** is the ability to resist infection and disease.

14-2 Lymphatic vessels, lymphocytes, lymphoid tissues, and lymphoid organs function in body defenses p. 538

3. The lymphatic system includes a network of **lymphatic vessels** called **lymphatics.** They carry **lymph**, a fluid similar to plasma but with a lower concentration of proteins. **Primary lymphoid tissues and organs** are sites where lymphocytes are formed and mature. **Secondary lymphoid tissues and organs** are sites where lymphocytes are activated and cloned. A series of **lymphoid tissues** and **lymphoid organs** is connected to the lymphatic vessels *(Figure 14-1).*

4. The lymphatic system produces, maintains, and distributes lymphocytes (cells that attack invading organisms, abnormal cells, and foreign proteins). The system also helps maintain blood volume and eliminate local variations in the composition of the interstitial fluid.

5. Lymph flows along a network of lymphatics that originates in the **lymphatic capillaries.** The lymphatic vessels empty into the **thoracic duct** and the **right lymphatic duct** *(Figures 14-1 to 14-3).*

6. The three classes of lymphocytes are **T cells** (**t**hymus-dependent), **B cells** (**b**one marrow–derived), and **natural killer (NK) cells.**

7. *Cytotoxic T cells* attack foreign cells or body cells infected by viruses; they provide *cell-mediated immunity. Regulatory T cells (helper T cells* and *suppressor T cells)* regulate and coordinate the immune response.

8. B cells can differentiate into **plasma cells,** which produce and secrete antibodies that react with specific chemical targets, or **antigens.** Antibodies in body fluids are also called **immunoglobulins.** B cells are responsible for *antibody-mediated immunity,* or *humoral immunity.*

9. NK cells attack foreign cells, normal cells infected with viruses, and cancer cells. They provide a monitoring service called *immune surveillance.*

10. Lymphocytes continuously migrate in and out of the blood through the lymphoid tissues and organs. **Lymphopoiesis** (lymphocyte production and development) involves the red bone marrow, thymus, and peripheral lymphoid tissues *(Spotlight Figure 14-4).*

11. **Lymphoid tissues** are loose connective tissues dominated by lymphocytes. **Mucosa-associated lymphoid tissue (MALT)** protects the epithelia of the digestive, respiratory, urinary, and reproductive tracts. **Tonsils** are clusters of **lymphoid nodules** (lymphoid tissue with densely packed lymphocytes) in the pharynx wall *(Figure 14-5).*

12. Important lymphoid organs include the *lymph nodes,* the *thymus,* and the *spleen.* Lymphoid tissues and organs occur in areas especially vulnerable to invasion by pathogens.

13. **Lymph nodes** are encapsulated masses of lymphoid tissue containing lymphocytes. Lymph nodes monitor and filter the lymph before it drains into the venous system, removing antigens and initiating immune responses *(Figure 14-6).*

14. The **thymus** lies behind the sternum. T cells mature in the thymus *(Figure 14-7).*

15. The adult **spleen** contains the largest mass of lymphoid tissue in the body. *Red pulp* contains large numbers of red blood cells, and *white pulp* resembles lymphoid nodules. The spleen removes antigens and damaged blood cells from the circulation, initiates immune responses, and stores iron from recycled red blood cells *(Figure 14-8).*

16. The lymphatic system is a major component of the body's defenses, which are classified as either (1) **innate (nonspecific) immunity**, which protects without distinguishing one threat from another, and (2) **adaptive (specific) immunity**, which protects against particular threats only.

14-3 Innate (nonspecific) defenses respond in a characteristic way regardless of the potential threat p. 546

17. **Innate** (nonspecific) defenses prevent the approach, deny the entrance, or limit the spread of living or nonliving hazards *(Figure 14-9).*

18. Physical barriers include the skin, mucous membranes, hair, epithelia, and various secretions of the integumentary and digestive systems.

19. **Phagocytes** include **microphages** (neutrophils and eosinophils) and **macrophages** (cells of the *monocyte–macrophage system*).

20. Phagocytes move between cells by *diapedesis*, and they show *chemotaxis* (sensitivity and orientation to chemical stimuli).

21. **Immune surveillance** involves constant monitoring of normal tissues by NK cells sensitive to abnormal antigens on the surfaces of otherwise normal cells. NK cells kill both virus-infected cells and cancer cells displaying tumor-specific surface antigens.

22. **Interferons**—small proteins released by virus-infected cells—trigger the production of antiviral proteins that interfere with viral replication inside other cells. Interferons are *cytokines*, chemical messengers released by tissue cells to coordinate local activities.

23. At least 30 *complement proteins* make up the **complement system**. These proteins interact with each other in chain reactions to destroy target cell membranes, stimulate inflammation, attract phagocytes, and enhance phagocytosis.

24. **Inflammation** represents a coordinated nonspecific response to tissue injury *(Figure 14-10)*.

25. A **fever** (body temperature greater than 37.2°C, or 99°F) can inhibit pathogens and speed up metabolic processes. **Pyrogens** can reset the body's thermostat and raise temperature.

14-4 Adaptive (specific) defenses respond to specific threats and are either cell mediated or antibody mediated *p. 550*

26. **Adaptive** (specific) defenses are provided by T cells and B cells. T cells provide cell-mediated immunity; B cells provide antibody-mediated immunity.

27. Forms of immunity include **innate (nonspecific) immunity** (genetically determined and present at birth) or **adaptive (specific) immunity** (produced by prior exposure to an antigen or antibody production). The two forms of adaptive immunity are **active immunity** (develops following exposure to an antigen) and **passive immunity** (produced by the transfer of antibodies from another source) *(Figure 14-11)*.

28. Adaptive immunity has four general properties: **specificity** (receptors on T cell and B cell membranes bind only to specific antigens); **versatility** (the immune system responds to any of the antigens it encounters); **memory** (memory cells enable the immune system to "remember" previously encountered antigens); and **tolerance** (the ability of the immune system to ignore some antigens, such as those of normal body cells).

29. The purpose of the **immune response** is to inactivate or destroy pathogens, abnormal cells, and foreign molecules. It is triggered by the presence of an antigen and includes cell-mediated and antibody-mediated defenses *(Figure 14-12)*.

14-5 T cells play a role in starting and controlling the immune response *p. 553*

30. **Antigen presentation** takes place when an antigen-MHC protein combination appears in a plasma membrane of a nucleated body cell or **antigen-presenting cell (APC).** Foreign antigens must usually be processed by macrophages or dendritic cells (APCs) and incorporated into their plasma membranes bound to *MHC proteins* before they can activate T cells.

31. T cells respond to antigens bound to Class I and Class II MHC proteins in a process called **antigen recognition.** Activated T cells may differentiate into *cytotoxic T cells, memory T cells, suppressor T cells,* or *helper T cells.*

32. Cell-mediated immunity results from the activation of **CD8** T cells by antigens bound to Class I MHCs. The activated T cells divide to generate **cytotoxic** (or *killer*) **T cells** and **memory T cells.** Activated memory T cells remain in reserve to respond to future exposures to the specific antigen involved *(Figure 14-13)*.

33. **Suppressor T cells** are also CD8 T cells. They act to depress the responses of B cells and other T cells.

34. T cells with **CD4** markers respond to antigens presented by Class II MHC proteins. Activated **helper T cells** secrete cytokines that help coordinate specific and nonspecific defenses, and regulate cell-mediated and antibody-mediated immunity.

14-6 B cells respond to antigens by producing specific antibodies *p. 557*

35. B cells are responsible for antibody-mediated immunity. They must undergo sensitization by a specific antigen before they become activated by helper T cells sensitive to the same antigen.

36. An activated B cell divides and produces plasma cells and **memory B cells.** Plasma cells produce antibodies *(Figure 14-14)*.

37. An antibody molecule consists of two parallel pairs of polypeptide chains containing *fixed segments* and *variable segments (Figure 14-15)*.

38. The binding of an antibody molecule and an antigen forms an **antigen–antibody complex.** Antibodies bind to specific *antigenic determinant sites*.

39. Five classes of antibodies exist in body fluids: (1) **immunoglobulin G (IgG)**, responsible for resistance against many viruses, bacteria, and bacterial toxins; (2) **IgM**, the first antibody class secreted in response to an antigen; (3) **IgA**, found

14

in glandular secretions; (4) **IgE**, which stimulates the release of chemicals that accelerate local inflammation; and (5) **IgD**, found on the surfaces of B cells *(Table 14-1)*.

40. Antibodies can eliminate antigens through **neutralization, precipitation, agglutination,** activation of complement, attraction of phagocytes, enhancement of phagocytosis, and stimulation of inflammation.

41. The antibodies produced by plasma cells upon first exposure to an antigen are the agents of the **primary response.** Maximum antibody levels appear during the **secondary response,** which follows later exposure to the same antigen *(Figure 14-16).*

42. Cytokines are chemical messengers coordinated by the immune system. **Interleukins** increase T cell sensitivity to antigens; stimulate B cell activity, plasma cell formation, and antibody production; and enhance nonspecific defenses.

43. Interferons slow the spread of a virus by making the infected cell's neighbors resistant to viral infections.

44. **Tumor necrosis factors (TNFs)** slow tumor growth and kill tumor cells.

45. Several **phagocytic regulators** adjust the activities of phagocytic cells to coordinate specific and nonspecific defenses.

46. The body's *innate (nonspecific) defenses* and *adaptive (specific) defenses* cooperate to eliminate foreign antigens *(Table 14-2; Figure 14-17).*

14-7 Abnormal immune responses result in immune disorders *p. 563*

47. **Autoimmune disorders** develop when the immune response mistakenly targets normal body cells and tissues.

48. In an **immunodeficiency disease**, the immune system does not develop normally or the immune response is blocked.

49. *Allergies* are inappropriate or excessive immune responses to **allergens** (antigens that trigger allergic reactions). The four types of allergies are *immediate hypersensitivity* (Type I), *cytotoxic reactions* (Type II), *immune complex disorders* (Type III), and *delayed hypersensitivity* (Type IV).

14-8 The immune response diminishes as we age *p. 564*

50. As individuals age, the immune system becomes less effective at combating disease.

14-9 For all body systems, the lymphatic system provides defenses against infection and returns tissue fluid to the circulation *p. 567*

51. The lymphatic system has extensive interactions with the nervous and endocrine systems.

Review Questions

See the blue Answers tab at the back of the book.

Level 1 Reviewing Facts and Terms

Match each item in column A with the most closely related item in column B. Place letters for answers in the spaces provided.

COLUMN A

_____ **1.** Humoral immunity
_____ **2.** Lymphoma
_____ **3.** Complement system
_____ **4.** Microphages
_____ **5.** Macrophages
_____ **6.** Microglia
_____ **7.** Interferon
_____ **8.** Pyrogens
_____ **9.** Innate immunity
_____ **10.** Active immunity
_____ **11.** Passive immunity
_____ **12.** Apoptosis

COLUMN B

a. Induce fever
b. Consists of circulating proteins
c. CNS macrophages
d. Monocytes
e. Genetically programmed cell death
f. Transfers of antibodies
g. Neutrophils, eosinophils
h. Secretion of antibodies
i. Present at birth
j. Cytokine
k. Lymphatic system cancer
l. Exposure to antigen

13. Identify the structures of the lymphatic system in the following diagram.

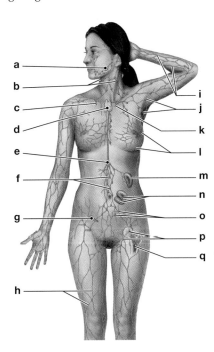

(a) _____	**(b)** _____
(c) _____	**(d)** _____
(e) _____	**(f)** _____
(g) _____	**(h)** _____
(i) _____	**(j)** _____
(k) _____	**(l)** _____
(m) _____	**(n)** _____
(o) _____	**(p)** _____
(q) _____	

14. Lymph collected from the lower abdomen, pelvis, and lower limbs is carried by the
 (a) right lymphatic duct. **(b)** inguinal duct.
 (c) thoracic duct. **(d)** aorta.

15. Lymphocytes responsible for providing cell-mediated immunity are called
 (a) macrophages. **(b)** B cells.
 (c) plasma cells. **(d)** cytotoxic T cells.

16. B cells are responsible for
 (a) cell-mediated immunity. **(b)** immune surveillance.
 (c) antibody-mediated immunity. **(d)** a, b, and c are correct.

17. Lymphoid stem cells that can form all types of lymphocytes occur in the
 (a) bloodstream. **(b)** thymus.
 (c) red bone marrow. **(d)** spleen.

18. Lymphatic vessels are found in all portions of the body except the
 (a) lower limbs. **(b)** central nervous system.
 (c) head and neck region. **(d)** hands and feet.

19. The largest collection of lymphoid tissue in the body is contained in the
 (a) adult spleen. **(b)** adult thymus.
 (c) bone marrow. **(d)** tonsils.

20. Red blood cells that are damaged or defective are removed from the circulation by the
 (a) thymus. **(b)** lymph nodes.
 (c) spleen. **(d)** tonsils.

21. Phagocytes move through capillary walls by squeezing between adjacent endothelial cells, a process known as
 (a) diapedesis. **(b)** chemotaxis.
 (c) adhesion. **(d)** perforation.

22. Perforins are destructive proteins associated with the activity of
 (a) T cells. **(b)** B cells.
 (c) macrophages. **(d)** plasma cells.

23. Complement activation
 (a) stimulates inflammation. **(b)** attracts phagocytes.
 (c) enhances phagocytosis. **(d)** a, b, and c are correct.

24. Inflammation
 (a) aids in temporary repair at an injury site. **(b)** slows the spread of pathogens.
 (c) facilitates permanent repair. **(d)** a, b, and c are correct.

25. CD4 markers are associated with
 (a) cytotoxic cells. **(b)** suppressor cells.
 (c) helper T cells. **(d)** a, b, and c.

26. Which two large collecting vessels are responsible for returning lymph to the veins of the cardiovascular system? What areas of the body does each serve?

27. Give a function for each of the following:
 (a) Cytotoxic T cells **(b)** Helper T cells
 (c) Suppressor T cells **(d)** Plasma cells
 (e) NK cells **(f)** Interferons
 (g) T cells **(h)** B cells
 (i) Interleukins

Level 2 Reviewing Concepts

28. Compared with innate defenses, adaptive defenses
 (a) do not discriminate between one threat and another.
 (b) are always present at birth.
 (c) provide protection against threats on an individual basis.
 (d) deny entry of pathogens to the body.

29. T cells and B cells can be activated only by
 (a) pathogenic microorganisms.
 (b) interleukins, interferons, and colony-stimulating factors.
 (c) cells infected with viruses, bacterial cells, or cancer cells.
 (d) exposure to a specific antigen at a specific site on a plasma membrane.

30. List and explain the four general properties of adaptive immunity.

14

31. In what ways can the formation of an antibody–antigen complex cause elimination of an antigen?

32. What are the effects of complement system activation?

Level 3 Critical Thinking and Clinical Applications

33. Sylvia's grandfather is diagnosed with lung cancer. When his physician takes biopsies of several lymph nodes from neighboring regions of the body, Sylvia wonders why, since his cancer is in his lungs. What would you tell her?

34. Ted finds out that he has been exposed to the measles and is concerned that he might have contracted the disease. His physician takes a blood sample and sends it to a lab to measure antibody levels. The results show an elevated level of IgM antibodies to rubella (German measles) virus but very few IgG antibodies to the virus. Did Ted contract the disease?

14

The Respiratory System

Learning Objectives

These objectives tell you what you should be able to do after completing the chapter. They correspond by number to this chapter's sections.

15-1 Describe the primary functions of the respiratory system, and explain how the respiratory exchange surfaces are protected from debris, pathogens, and other hazards.

15-2 Identify the structures that conduct air to the lungs, and describe their functions.

15-3 Describe the functional anatomy of alveoli, and the superficial anatomy of the lungs.

15-4 Define and compare the processes of external respiration and internal respiration.

15-5 Describe the physical principles governing the movement of air into the lungs and the actions of the respiratory muscles.

15-6 Describe the physical principles governing the diffusion of gases into and out of the blood.

15-7 Describe how oxygen and carbon dioxide are transported in the blood.

15-8 List the factors that influence the rate of respiration, and describe the reflexes that regulate respiration.

15-9 Describe the changes in the respiratory system that occur with aging.

15-10 Give examples of interactions between the respiratory system and other body systems.

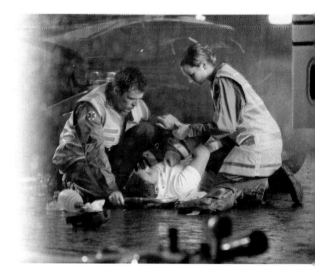

An Introduction to the Respiratory System

When we think of the respiratory system, we generally think of breathing—pulling air into our lungs and pushing it out. However, an efficient respiratory system must do more than move air. Cells need energy for maintenance, growth, defense, and reproduction. Our cells obtain that energy through an aerobic process that requires oxygen and produces carbon dioxide. ↺ p. 73 The respiratory system provides the body's cells with a way to obtain oxygen and get rid of carbon dioxide. An exchange of these gases takes place within the lungs at air-filled pockets called **alveoli** (al-VĒ-ō-lī; singular, *alveolus*). The gas-exchange surfaces of the alveoli are relatively delicate. These surfaces must be very thin for rapid diffusion to take place between the air and the blood.

The cardiovascular system links your interstitial fluids and the exchange surfaces of your lungs. Circulating blood carries oxygen from the lungs to peripheral tissues. Your blood also accepts and transports the carbon dioxide generated by those tissues and delivers it to the lungs.

We begin our discussion of the respiratory system by following air as it travels from outside the body to the alveoli of the lungs. Next we consider the mechanics of breathing—how the actions of respiratory muscles bring air into the lungs. Then we examine the physiology of respiration. This topic includes the process of breathing and the processes of gas exchange and gas transport, both between the air and blood and between the blood and tissues.

Build Your Knowledge

Recall that the respiratory system delivers air to sites in the lungs where gas exchange takes place between air and the bloodstream (as you saw in **Chapter 1: An Introduction to Anatomy and Physiology**). This system also produces sound for communication. ↺ **p. 8**

15-1 The respiratory system, composed of air-conducting and respiratory portions, has several basic functions

Learning Objective Describe the primary functions of the respiratory system, and explain how the respiratory exchange surfaces are protected from debris, pathogens, and other hazards.

The **respiratory system** consists of structures involved in physically moving air into and out of the lungs and in gas exchange.

Functions of the Respiratory System

The respiratory system has five basic functions:

1. Providing a large area for gas exchange between air and circulating blood.

2. Moving air along the respiratory passageways to and from the gas-exchange surfaces of the lungs.

3. Protecting the respiratory surfaces from dehydration, temperature changes, and invading pathogens.

4. Producing sounds for speaking, singing, and other forms of communication.

5. Aiding the sense of smell by the olfactory receptors in the nasal cavity.

Structures of the Respiratory System

On the basis of its anatomical structures, we can divide the respiratory system into upper and lower systems. The **upper respiratory system** consists of the nose, nasal cavity, paranasal sinuses, and pharynx (throat). These structures are the first to filter, warm, and humidify incoming air, protecting the more delicate surfaces of the lower respiratory system. The **lower respiratory system** includes the larynx (voice box); trachea (windpipe); bronchi; and lungs, which contain the bronchioles (air-conducting passageways) and the alveoli (gas-exchange surfaces) (**Figure 15-1**).

The term **respiratory tract** refers to the passageways that carry air to and from the exchange surfaces of the lungs. In functional terms, we can divide the respiratory tract into an upper *conducting portion* and a lower *respiratory portion*. The conducting portion begins at the entrance to the nasal cavity and continues through the pharynx, larynx, trachea, bronchi, and the larger bronchioles. The respiratory portion includes the smallest and most delicate bronchioles and the alveoli within the lungs.

In addition to delivering air to the lungs, the conducting passageways filter, warm, and humidify the air. In this way, they protect the alveoli from debris, pathogens, and environmental extremes. By the time inhaled air reaches the alveoli, most foreign particles and pathogens have been removed.

15

Figure 15-1 The Structures of the Respiratory System.

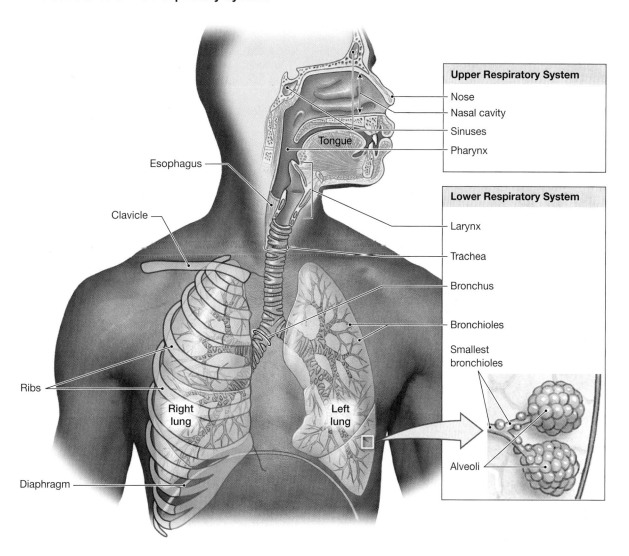

Upper Respiratory System

Nose
Nasal cavity
Sinuses
Pharynx

Lower Respiratory System

Larynx
Trachea
Bronchus
Bronchioles
Smallest bronchioles
Alveoli

Esophagus
Clavicle
Ribs
Right lung
Left lung
Diaphragm
Tongue

Also, the humidity and temperature are within acceptable limits. This "conditioning process" is due to the respiratory mucosa.

The **respiratory mucosa** (mū-KŌ-suh) lines the conducting portion of the respiratory tract. Recall that a *mucosa* is a *mucous membrane*, one of four types of membranes introduced in Chapter 4. It consists of an epithelium and an underlying layer of areolar tissue. ⟳ p. 110 The *respiratory epithelium* of the respiratory mucosa is a ciliated columnar epithelium containing many *mucous cells*. The **lamina propria** (LAM-i-nuh PRŌ-prē-uh) is the underlying areolar layer that supports the epithelium. It contains mucous glands that secrete onto the epithelial surface (**Figure 15-2**).

The exchange surfaces of the respiratory system can be severely damaged if inhaled air is contaminated with debris or pathogens. The ciliated epithelium and the mucous

cells and mucous glands that produce mucus prevent such damage. The mucus bathes the exposed surfaces of the respiratory tract from the nasal cavity to the bronchi. Cilia sweep that mucus and any trapped debris or microorganisms toward the *pharynx*. This process is often called the *mucus*, or *mucociliary, escalator*. The debris and microorganisms can then be swallowed and destroyed by the acids and enzymes of the stomach.

CHECKPOINT

1. Identify the five functions of the respiratory system.
2. List the two anatomical subdivisions of the respiratory system.
3. What membrane lines the conducting portion of the respiratory tract?

See the blue Answers tab at the back of the book.

Figure 15-2 The Respiratory Mucosa.

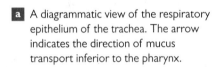

Movement of mucus to pharynx

- Ciliated columnar epithelial cell
- Mucous cell
- Stem cell
- Debris
- Mucous gland
- Mucus layer
- Lamina propria

a A diagrammatic view of the respiratory epithelium of the trachea. The arrow indicates the direction of mucus transport inferior to the pharynx.

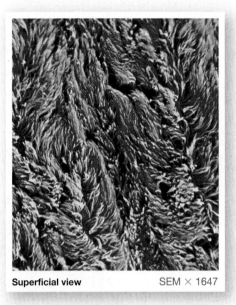

Superficial view   SEM × 1647

b A surface view of the epithelium. The cilia of the epithelial cells form a dense layer that resembles a shag carpet. The movement of these cilia propels mucus across the epithelial surface.

15-2 The nose, pharynx, larynx, trachea, bronchi, and larger bronchioles conduct air into the lungs

Learning Objective Identify the structures that conduct air to the lungs, and describe their functions.

The conducting portion of the respiratory tract begins at the entrance to the nasal cavity. It then continues through the pharynx, larynx, trachea, bronchi, and the larger bronchioles.

The Nose

Air normally enters the respiratory system through the paired **external nares** (NA-rēz), or nostrils. They open into the **nasal cavity** (**Figure 15-3**). The **nasal vestibule** (VES-ti-būl) is the space enclosed by the flexible tissues of the nose. Coarse hairs from the epithelium of the vestibule extend across the nostrils. These hairs guard the nasal cavity from large airborne particles such as sand, dust, and even insects.

The maxillary, nasal, frontal, ethmoid, and sphenoid bones form the lateral and superior walls of the nasal cavity (see **Figure 6-27**, p. 179). The *nasal septum* divides the nasal cavity into left and right sides. The anterior portion of the nasal septum is formed of hyaline cartilage. The bony

posterior septum includes portions of the vomer and the ethmoid bone (see **Figure 6-26**, p. 178). A bony **hard palate**, formed by the palatine and maxillary bones, forms the floor of the nasal cavity and separates the oral and nasal cavities (**Figure 15-3**). A fleshy **soft palate** extends behind the hard palate and underlies the **nasopharynx** (nā-zō-FAR-ingks), or upper part of the throat. The nasal cavity opens into the nasopharynx at the **internal nares**.

The superior, middle, and inferior *nasal conchae* project toward the nasal septum from the lateral walls of the nasal cavity (**Figure 15-3**). Air flowing from the nasal vestibule to the internal nares tends to flow in narrow grooves between adjacent conchae. As the air eddies and swirls like water flowing over rapids, small airborne particles stick to the mucus that coats the lining of the nasal cavity. In addition to promoting filtration, the turbulent flow allows extra time for warming and humidifying the incoming air.

As noted earlier, the nasal cavity is flushed by mucus produced by the *respiratory mucosa*. The respiratory surfaces of the nasal cavity are also cleared by mucus produced in the *paranasal sinuses* (sinuses of the frontal, sphenoid, ethmoid, and paired maxillary and palatine bones) (see **Figure 6-28**, p. 181), and by tears flowing through the nasolacrimal duct (see **Figure 9-8b**, p. 353). Exposure to noxious vapors, large quantities of dust and debris, allergens, or pathogens usually causes mucus production to increase rapidly. As a result, a "runny nose" develops.

15

Figure 15-3 The Nose, Nasal Cavity, and Pharynx. The structures of the nasal cavity and pharynx, as seen in sagittal section with the nasal septum removed.

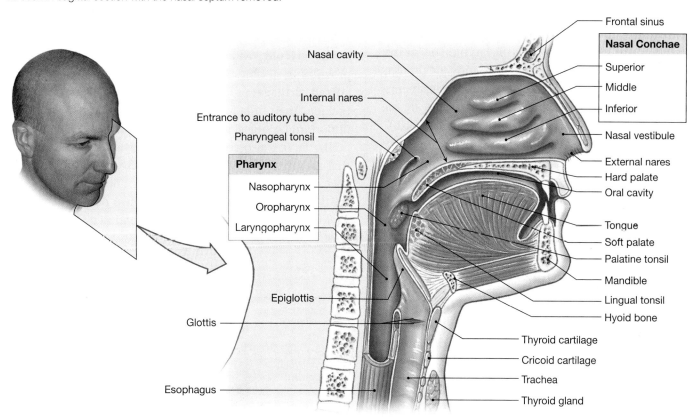

The Pharynx

The **pharynx** (FAR-ingks), or throat, is a chamber shared by the digestive and respiratory systems. It extends between the internal nares and the entrances to the larynx and esophagus. The pharynx has three subdivisions: the nasopharynx, the oropharynx, and the laryngopharynx (**Figure 15-3**).

The **nasopharynx** is connected to the nasal cavity by the internal nares and extends to the posterior edge of the soft palate. The nasopharynx is lined by a typical ciliated respiratory epithelium. The nasopharynx also contains the *pharyngeal tonsil* on its posterior wall and entrances to the *auditory tubes.*

The **oropharynx** extends between the soft palate and the base of the tongue at the level of the hyoid bone. The palatine tonsils lie in the lateral walls of the oropharynx. The narrow **laryngopharynx** (la-rin-gō-FAR-ingks) extends between the level of the hyoid bone and the entrance to the esophagus. Materials entering the digestive tract pass through both the oropharynx and laryngopharynx. Both are lined by a stratified squamous epithelium that can resist abrasion, chemical attack, and invasion by pathogens.

CLINICAL NOTE

Cystic Fibrosis

Cystic fibrosis (CF) is an inherited disease due to a defect of the respiratory mucosa. Mucous cells in the respiratory mucosa of affected individuals produce dense, viscous mucus that cannot be transported by the cilia of the respiratory tract. Mucus transport stops, and mucus blocks the smaller respiratory passageways. The clogged airways make breathing difficult. This inactivation of the normal respiratory defenses leads to frequent bacterial infections. Through the 1950s and until the 1960s, few children with CF lived long enough to enter elementary school. Modern technology and treatment methods have improved survival of many individuals with CF into their 30s and 40s. Death usually results from a massive bacterial infection of the lungs and associated heart failure.

CF is the most common lethal inherited disease affecting individuals of northern European descent. It occurs in 1 birth in 2500. It is less frequent in people of southern European ancestry, in the Ashkenazic Jewish population, and in African Americans. The condition results from a defective gene on chromosome 7.

15

The Larynx

Inhaled air leaves the pharynx and enters the larynx through a narrow opening of the glottis (**Figure 15-3**). The glottis is the vocal apparatus, or "voice box" of the larynx. The **larynx** (LAR-ingks) is a cartilaginous tube that surrounds and protects the glottis. It consists of nine cartilages stabilized by ligaments, skeletal muscles, or both. The three largest cartilages are the *epiglottis, thyroid cartilage*, and *cricoid cartilage* (**Figure 15-4a,b**).

The **epiglottis** (ep-i-GLOT-is) is shaped like a shoehorn and projects superior to the glottis, forming a lid over it. During swallowing, the larynx is elevated, and the elastic epiglottis folds back over the glottis, preventing liquids or solid food from entering the respiratory tract.

The curving **thyroid** (*thyroid*; shield-shaped) **cartilage** forms much of the anterior and lateral surfaces of the larynx. A prominent ridge on the anterior surface of this cartilage forms the "Adam's apple." Inferior to the thyroid cartilage is the **cricoid** (KRĪ-koyd; ring-shaped) **cartilage**, which provides posterior support to the larynx. The thyroid and cricoid cartilages protect the glottis and the entrance to the trachea. Their broad surfaces are sites for the attachment of important laryngeal muscles and ligaments.

The larynx also contains three pairs of smaller cartilages that are supported by the cricoid cartilage. They are the *arytenoid, corniculate,* and *cuneiform cartilages*. Between the thyroid cartilage and these smaller cartilages, two pairs of ligaments, enclosed by folds of epithelium, extend across the larynx.

Figure 15-4 The Anatomy of the Larynx and Vocal Cords.

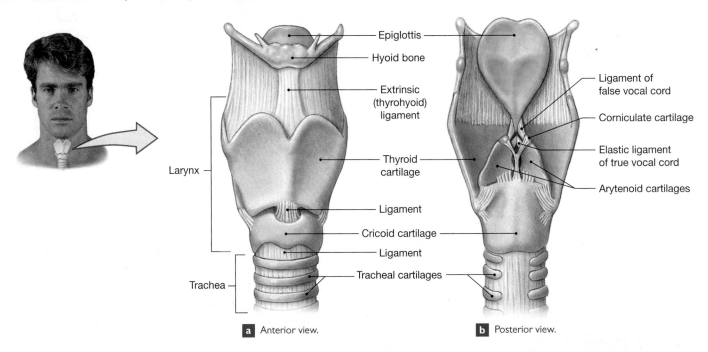

a Anterior view.

b Posterior view.

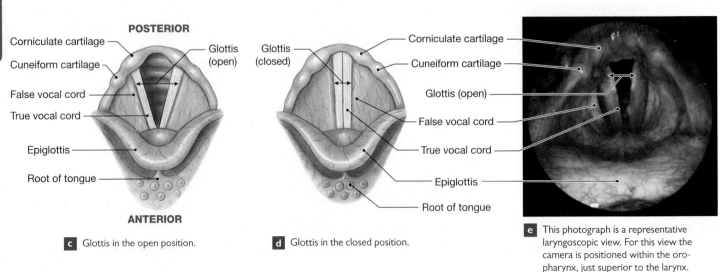

c Glottis in the open position.

d Glottis in the closed position.

e This photograph is a representative laryngoscopic view. For this view the camera is positioned within the oropharynx, just superior to the larynx.

The ligaments of the upper pair are known as the **false vocal cords**. They are relatively inelastic. They help prevent foreign objects from entering the open glottis. They also protect the more delicate, lower pair of folds, the **true vocal cords**. The true vocal cords contain elastic ligaments that extend between the thyroid cartilage and the arytenoid cartilages (**Figure 15-4b**). The elastic true vocal cords are involved in the production of sound. The voice box or **glottis** (GLOT-is) is made up of the true vocal cords and the space between them (**Figure 15-4c,d,e**).

Food or liquids that touch the vocal cords trigger the *coughing reflex*. In a cough, the glottis is kept closed while the chest and abdominal muscles contract, compressing the lungs. When the glottis is opened suddenly, the resulting blast of air through the trachea ejects material blocking the entrance to the glottis.

The Vocal Cords and Sound Production

How do you produce sounds? Air passing through your open glottis vibrates its vocal cords, producing sound waves. The pitch of the sound, like the pitch of a vibrating harp string, depends on the diameter, length, and tension of the vibrating vocal cords. Short, thin strings vibrate rapidly, producing a high-pitched sound. Long, thick strings vibrate more slowly, producing a low-pitched tone. The diameter and length of the vocal cords are directly related to the size of your larynx. Children have small larynxes with slender, short vocal cords, so their voices tend to be high-pitched. At puberty, the larynx of males enlarges more than that of females. Because the vocal cords of adult males are thicker and longer, they produce lower tones than those of adult females. The amount of tension in the vocal cords is controlled by small, intrinsic skeletal muscles of the larynx. These muscles change the position of the arytenoid cartilages. Increased tension in the vocal cords raises the pitch. Decreased tension lowers the pitch.

The distinctive sound of your voice does not depend solely on the sounds produced by the larynx. Further amplification and resonance take place in the pharynx, the oral cavity, the nasal cavity, and the paranasal sinuses. The final production of distinct words further depends on voluntary movements of the tongue, lips, and cheeks.

The Trachea

The **trachea** (TRĀ-kē-uh), or *windpipe*, is a tough, flexible tube. It is about 2.5 cm (1 in.) in diameter and approximately 11 cm (4.25 in.) long (**Figure 15-5a**). The trachea begins at the level of the sixth cervical vertebra, where it attaches to the cricoid cartilage of the larynx. It ends in the mediastinum, at the level of the fifth thoracic vertebra, where it branches to form the right and left primary bronchi.

The trachea contains 15–20 **tracheal cartilages**. They stiffen the tracheal walls and protect the airway. They also prevent the trachea's collapse or overexpansion as pressures change in the respiratory system.

Each tracheal cartilage is C-shaped. The open portion of the "C" faces posteriorly, toward the esophagus (**Figure 15-5b**). Because the cartilages are not continuous, the posterior tracheal wall can easily distort, allowing large masses of food to pass along the esophagus. The ends of each tracheal cartilage are connected by an elastic ligament and the *trachealis muscle*, a band of smooth muscle. The diameter of the trachea is adjusted by the contractions of these muscles, which are under autonomic control. Sympathetic stimulation increases the diameter of the trachea, making it easier to move large volumes of air along the respiratory passageways.

In an emergency, it is common for rescue personnel to place a breathing tube into the trachea (endotracheal intubation). Accidentally inserting the tube too far can cause the tip of the tube to enter the right primary bronchus. This results in only the right lung being effectively ventilated and can lead to hypoxia. Endobronchial intubation results in the absence of breath sounds over the left chest, decreased compliance, and possibly hypoxia. The situation can be remedied by simply withdrawing the tube until bilateral breath sounds return. It is important to frequently reassess tube placement to ensure that dislodgement or endobronchial intubation does not occur.

The Bronchi

The trachea branches within the mediastinum into the **right** and **left primary bronchi** (BRONG-kī) (**Figure 15-5a**). The walls of the primary bronchi resemble the wall of the trachea, including a ciliated epithelium and C-shaped cartilaginous rings. The right primary bronchus supplies the right lung, and the left supplies the left lung. The right primary bronchus is larger in diameter and descends toward the lung at a steeper angle. For these reasons, most foreign objects that enter the trachea find their way into the right primary bronchus rather than the left.

15

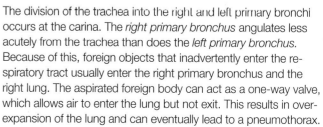

CLINICAL NOTE

Bronchial Angles

The division of the trachea into the right and left primary bronchi occurs at the carina. The *right primary bronchus* angulates less acutely from the trachea than does the *left primary bronchus*. Because of this, foreign objects that inadvertently enter the respiratory tract usually enter the right primary bronchus and the right lung. The aspirated foreign body can act as a one-way valve, which allows air to enter the lung but not exit. This results in overexpansion of the lung and can eventually lead to a pneumothorax.

Figure 15-5 The Anatomy of the Trachea.

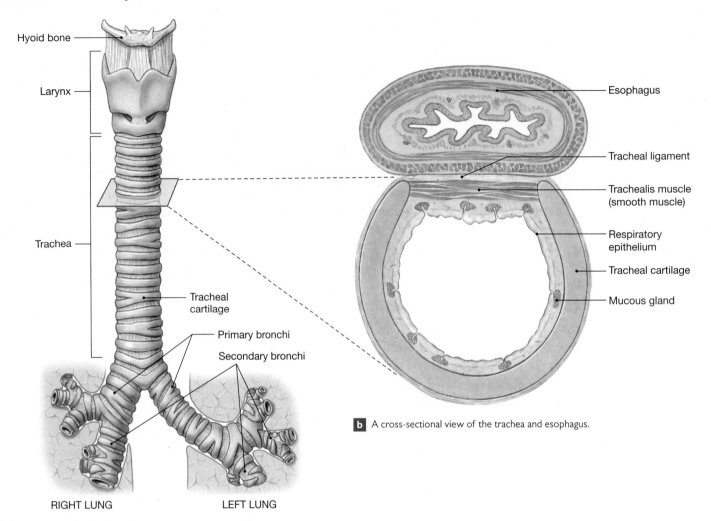

Hyoid bone

Larynx

Trachea

Tracheal cartilage

Primary bronchi

Secondary bronchi

RIGHT LUNG

LEFT LUNG

Esophagus

Tracheal ligament

Trachealis muscle (smooth muscle)

Respiratory epithelium

Tracheal cartilage

Mucous gland

b A cross-sectional view of the trachea and esophagus.

a A diagrammatic anterior view showing the plane of section for part (b).

The primary bronchi and their branches form the *bronchial tree*. **Figure 15-6a** shows the branching pattern of the left primary bronchus as it enters the lung. (The number of branches has been reduced for clarity.) Each primary bronchus gives rise to **secondary bronchi**, which enter the lobes of that lung. In each lung, the secondary bronchi divide to form 9–10 **tertiary bronchi**. Each tertiary bronchus supplies air to a specific region of a lung, called a *bronchopulmonary segment*, where it branches repeatedly into smaller bronchi.

The cartilages of the secondary bronchi are relatively massive, but farther along the branches of the bronchial tree the cartilages become smaller and smaller. When the diameter of the passageway has narrowed to about 1 mm (0.04 in.), cartilages disappear completely. This narrow passage is a **bronchiole**.

The walls of bronchioles are dominated by smooth muscle tissue, whose activity is regulated by the autonomic nervous system. Bronchioles are to respiratory system function as arterioles are to cardiovascular system function. Just as changes to the diameter of arterioles regulate blood flow into capillary beds, changes to the diameter of bronchioles control the resistance to airflow and the distribution of air in the lungs. Sympathetic activation leads to a relaxation of smooth muscles in the walls of bronchioles, causing *bronchodilation*, the enlargement of airway diameter. Parasympathetic stimulation leads to contraction of these smooth muscles and *bronchoconstriction*, a reduction in the diameter of the airway. Extreme bronchoconstriction can almost completely block the passageways, making breathing difficult or impossible. This can occur during an *asthma* (AZ-muh) attack or during allergic reactions in response to inflammation of the bronchioles.

Figure 15-6 The Bronchial Tree and a Lobule of the Lung.

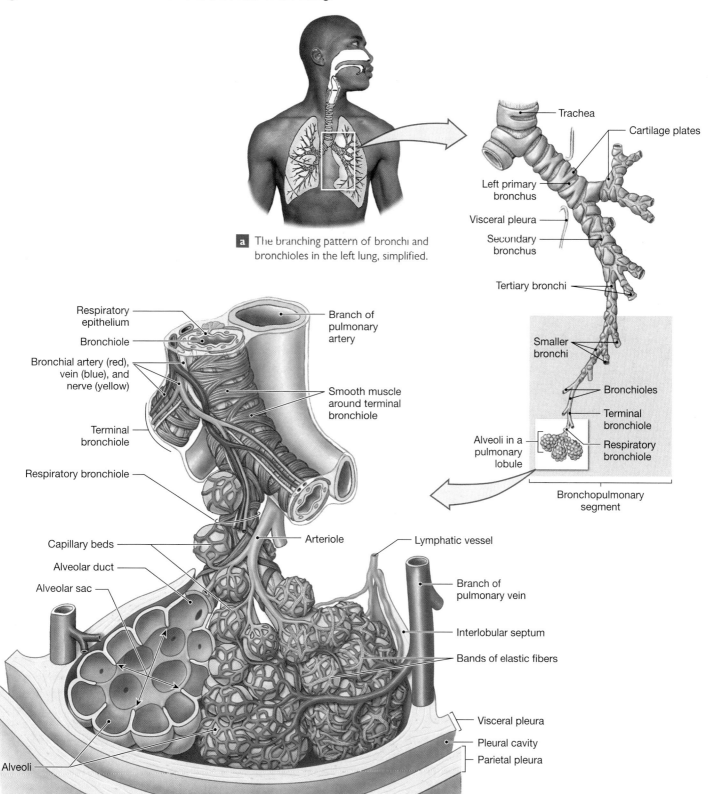

a The branching pattern of bronchi and bronchioles in the left lung, simplified.

Trachea

Cartilage plates

Left primary bronchus

Visceral pleura

Secondary bronchus

Tertiary bronchi

Smaller bronchi

Bronchioles

Terminal bronchiole

Alveoli in a pulmonary lobule

Respiratory bronchiole

Bronchopulmonary segment

Respiratory epithelium

Bronchiole

Bronchial artery (red), vein (blue), and nerve (yellow)

Terminal bronchiole

Respiratory bronchiole

Capillary beds

Alveolar duct

Alveolar sac

Alveoli

Branch of pulmonary artery

Smooth muscle around terminal bronchiole

Arteriole

Lymphatic vessel

Branch of pulmonary vein

Interlobular septum

Bands of elastic fibers

Visceral pleura

Pleural cavity

Parietal pleura

b The structure of a single pulmonary lobule, part of a bronchopulmonary segment.

CLINICAL NOTE

Airway Obstruction

We sometimes breathe in foreign objects. This process is called *aspiration*. Coughing usually expels objects that become lodged in the larynx or trachea. If the person can speak or make a sound, the airway is still open, and no emergency measures should be taken. If the victim can neither breathe or speak, an immediate threat to life exists.

In the *Heimlich* (HĪM-lik) *maneuver*, or *abdominal thrust*, a rescuer applies compression to the abdomen just beneath the diaphragm. This action forcefully elevates the diaphragm and may generate enough pressure to dislodge the blockage. The maneuver must be performed properly to avoid damage to internal organs. Organizations such as the American Red Cross, local fire departments, and other charitable groups periodically hold brief training sessions in the proper performance of the Heimlich maneuver.

If blockage results from a swelling of the epiglottis or tissues surrounding the glottis, a professionally qualified rescuer may insert a curved tube through the pharynx and glottis to permit airflow. This procedure is called *intubation*.

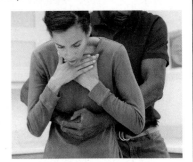

If a tracheal blockage remains, a *tracheostomy* (trā-kē-OS-to-mē; *stoma,* mouth) may be performed. This procedure involves making an incision through the anterior tracheal wall and inserting a tube. The tube bypasses the larynx and permits air to flow directly into the trachea.

CHECKPOINT

4. The surfaces of the nasal cavity are flushed by what materials or fluids?

5. The pharynx is a passageway for which two body systems?

6. When tension in the vocal cords increases, what happens to the pitch of the voice?

7. What is the functional advantage of C-shaped cartilages in the tracheal wall rather than completely circular cartilages?

See the blue Answers tab at the back of the book.

15-3 The smallest bronchioles and the alveoli within the lungs make up the respiratory portion of the respiratory tract

Learning Objective Describe the functional anatomy of alveoli, and the superficial anatomy of the lungs.

The Bronchioles

Bronchioles branch further into the finest conducting passageways, the *terminal bronchioles*. These fine tubes have internal diameters of 0.3–0.5 mm. Each terminal bronchiole supplies air to a lobule of the lung. A **pulmonary lobule** (LOB-l) is a segment of lung tissue that is bounded by connective tissue partitions. Branches of the pulmonary arteries, pulmonary veins, and respiratory passageways supply each lobule (**Figure 15-6b**). Within a lobule, a terminal bronchiole divides to form several *respiratory bronchioles*. These passages are the thinnest branches of the bronchial tree. They deliver air to the gas-exchange surfaces of the lungs.

The Alveolar Ducts and Alveoli

Respiratory bronchioles open into passageways called **alveolar ducts** (**Figure 15-7a**). The ducts end at **alveolar sacs**, common chambers connected to multiple individual alveoli—the exchange surfaces of the lungs. Each lung contains about 150 million alveoli. They give the lung an open, spongy appearance (**Figure 15-7b**).

To meet our metabolic requirements, the alveolar exchange surfaces of the lungs must be very large, equal to approximately 140 square meters—roughly one-half of a tennis court. The alveolar epithelium consists mainly of a simple squamous epithelium (**Figure 15-7c**). The squamous epithelial cells, called *type I pneumocytes*, are unusually thin. Roaming **alveolar macrophages** (*dust cells*) patrol the epithelium. They phagocytize any particles that have reached the alveolar surfaces.

CLINICAL NOTE

Bronchiolitis and Respiratory Synctial Virus Infections

Bronchiolitis, an infection of the smaller airways, is a common disease in children less than 2 years of age. Most cases of bronchiolitis are caused by the *respiratory syncytial virus (RSV)*. It often occurs in epidemics during the midwinter and primarily affects children between the ages of 2 and 6 months. Typically, the child with an RSV infection will develop a runny nose, low-grade fever, and decreased appetite. Then, there will be an increase in the respiratory rate and depth and in the work of breathing. As the disease progresses, there is often a fall in the oxygen saturation, wheezing, and trapping of air within the lungs, which causes hyperexpansion of the chest. Treatment includes intensive monitoring, supplemental oxygen, bronchodilators, and occasionally, ventilatory support. Usually, children develop lifelong immunity following infection.

Figure 15-7 Alveolar Organization.

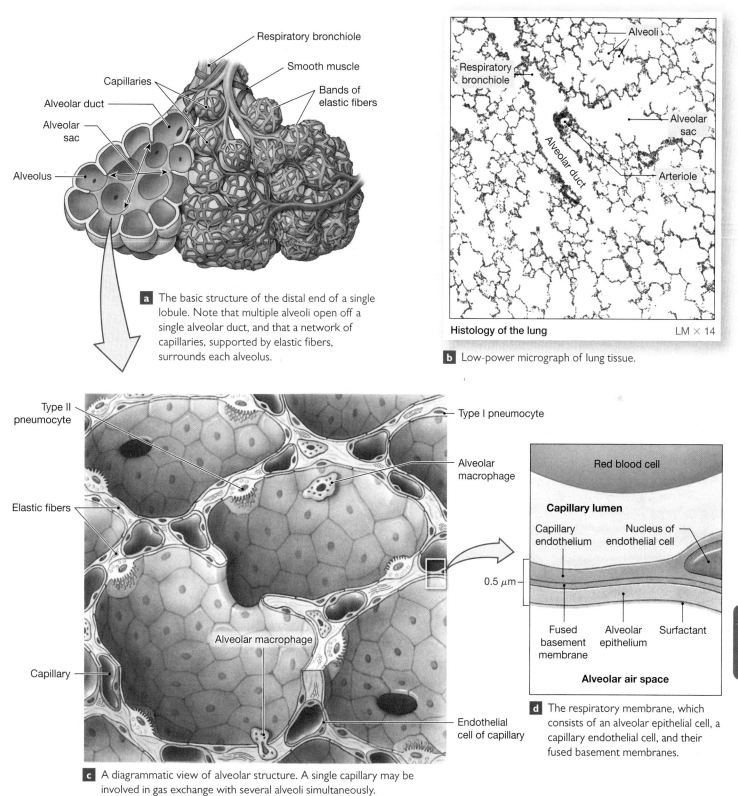

Respiratory bronchiole

Smooth muscle

Capillaries

Bands of elastic fibers

Alveolar duct

Alveolar sac

Alveolus

a The basic structure of the distal end of a single lobule. Note that multiple alveoli open off a single alveolar duct, and that a network of capillaries, supported by elastic fibers, surrounds each alveolus.

Alveoli

Respiratory bronchiole

Alveolar sac

Alveolar duct

Arteriole

Histology of the lung   LM × 14

b Low-power micrograph of lung tissue.

Type II pneumocyte

Type I pneumocyte

Alveolar macrophage

Elastic fibers

Alveolar macrophage

Capillary

Endothelial cell of capillary

Red blood cell

Capillary lumen

Capillary endothelium

Nucleus of endothelial cell

0.5 μm

Fused basement membrane

Alveolar epithelium

Surfactant

Alveolar air space

d The respiratory membrane, which consists of an alveolar epithelial cell, a capillary endothelial cell, and their fused basement membranes.

c A diagrammatic view of alveolar structure. A single capillary may be involved in gas exchange with several alveoli simultaneously.

15

Scattered among the squamous cells are larger **septal cells**, or *type II pneumocytes*. The septal cells produce an oily secretion called **surfactant** (sur-FAK-tant). They secrete surfactant onto the alveolar surfaces, where it forms a superficial coating over a thin layer of water.

Surfactant plays a key role in keeping the alveoli open. It reduces surface tension in the liquid coating the alveolar surfaces. Recall from Chapter 2 that surface tension results from the attraction between water molecules at an air–water boundary. ↻ p. 31 Without surfactant, the surface tension would collapse the thin alveolar walls. When surfactant levels are inadequate (as a result of injury or genetic abnormalities), each inhalation must be forceful enough to pop open the alveoli. An individual with this condition—called **respiratory distress syndrome**—is soon exhausted by the effort required to keep inflating the deflated lungs.

The Respiratory Membrane

Gas exchange takes place across the **respiratory membrane** of the alveoli. The respiratory membrane has three layers (**Figure 15-7d**):

1. *Aveolar epithelium.* Squamous epithelial cells line the alveolus.

2. *Capillary endothelium.* Endothelial cells line an adjacent capillary.

3. *Fused basement membranes.* Lie between the alveolar and endothelial cells.

At the respiratory membrane, only a very short distance separates alveolar air from blood. The total distance can be as little as 0.1 μm, but averages about 0.5 μm. Diffusion across the respiratory membrane proceeds very rapidly because the distance is short and because both oxygen and carbon dioxide molecules are small and lipid soluble. The plasma membranes of the epithelial and endothelial cells do not prevent oxygen and carbon dioxide from moving between blood and alveolar air.

The respiratory exchange surfaces receive blood from arteries of the *pulmonary circuit.* ↻ p. 450 Recall that the pulmonary arteries carry deoxygenated blood. They enter the lungs and branch, following the bronchi and their branches to the lobules. Each lobule receives an arteriole. A network of capillaries surrounds each alveolus directly beneath the

15

CLINICAL NOTE

Pneumonia

Pneumonia is an infection of the lungs and a common medical problem, especially in the aged and those infected with the human immunodeficiency virus (HIV). In fact, pneumonia is one of the leading causes of death in both groups of patients and is the fifth leading overall cause of death in the United States.

Patients with HIV infection and those on immune suppressive therapy (cancer patients) are at high risk of developing pneumonia. In addition, the very young and very old are at higher risk of acquiring pneumonia because of ineffective protective mechanisms. Other risk factors include a history of alcoholism, cigarette smoking, and exposure to cold temperatures.

Pneumonia is a collection of related respiratory diseases caused when a variety of infectious agents invade the lungs. It is crucial to remember the importance of adequate mucous production and the action of respiratory tract cilia in protecting the body against bacterial invasion. When considering which patients are at risk, the unifying concept is that there is a defect in mucous production, ciliary action, or both.

Bacterial and viral pneumonias occur the most frequently, although fungal and other forms of pneumonia do exist. More unusual forms of pneumonia are seen in those patients who are currently or recently have been hospitalized, where they are exposed to a more unusual variety of microorganisms. This is referred to as *hospital-acquired pneumonia.* Cases that develop in the out-of-hospital setting are described as *community-acquired pneumonia.*

The infection begins in one part of the lung and often spreads to nearby alveoli. The infection may ultimately involve the entire lung. As the disease progresses, fluid and inflammatory cells collect in the alveoli, and alveolar collapse may occur. Pneumonia is primarily a ventilation disorder. Occasionally, the infection will extend beyond the lungs into the bloodstream and to more distant sites in the body. This systemic spread may lead to septic shock.

A patient with pneumonia will generally appear ill. He may report a recent history of fever and chills, commonly described as "bed shaking." There is usually a generalized weakness and malaise. The patient will tend to complain of a deep, productive cough and may expel yellow to brown sputum, often streaked with blood. Many cases involve associated pleuritic chest pain; therefore, pneumonia should be considered in any patient who presents complaining of chest pain, especially if accompanied by fever or chills. In pneumonia that involves the lower lobes of the lungs, a patient may complain of nothing more than upper abdominal pain.

In the forms of pneumonia that involve viral, fungal, and rare bacterial causes, the typical symptoms described above are not seen. Instead, these patients may report a nonproductive cough with less prominent lung findings. Systemic symptoms such as headache, malaise, fatigue, muscle aches, sore throat, and abdominal complaints including nausea, vomiting, and diarrhea are more prominent. Fever and chills are not as impressive as in bacterial pneumonia.

alveolar epithelium. After gas exchange takes place, oxygen-rich blood from the alveolar (pulmonary) capillaries passes through the pulmonary venules. This blood then enters the pulmonary veins, which deliver it to the left atrium.

In addition to taking part in gas exchange, the endothelial cells of the alveolar capillaries are the primary source of *angiotensin-converting enzyme (ACE)*. ACE converts circulating angiotensin I to angiotensin II. Angiotensin II plays an important role in regulating blood volume and blood pressure. ⟲ p. 445

How do the tissues of conducting passageways of your lungs get the oxygen and nutrients that they themselves need? This nourishment comes from capillaries supplied by the bronchial arteries, which branch from the thoracic aorta. ⟲ p. 456 The venous blood from these bronchial capillaries then returns to the heart by either the systemic circuit or pulmonary circuit. Most of this venous blood drains into the pulmonary veins, where it dilutes the oxygenated alveolar blood returning to the heart.

Blood pressure in the pulmonary circuit is usually relatively low. Pulmonary artery systolic pressures are 30 mm Hg or less. With pressures that low, pulmonary arteries can easily become blocked by small blood clots, fat masses, or air bubbles. Any drifting masses in the blood are likely to cause problems almost at once because the lungs receive the entire cardiac output. The blockage of a branch of a pulmonary artery will stop blood flow to a group of lobules or alveoli. This condition is called **pulmonary embolism**.

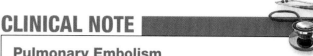

CLINICAL NOTE

Pulmonary Embolism

Pulmonary embolism is a common and potentially deadly disorder that can be extremely difficult to diagnose. It usually arises from the large veins of the leg or pelvis. A blood clot in the leg, referred to as *deep venous thrombosis (DVT),* usually develops over a period of minutes to hours. Prolonged immobilization, such as occurs during hospitalization or a long plane or car ride, has been identified as a risk factor for the development of DVT. Ultimately, the clot breaks loose, travels through the circulatory system, and enters the pulmonary circulation. When it reaches the part of the blood vessel that is smaller than itself, the clot lodges there. Blood flow to the lung is restricted and oxygenation is impaired. Large clots can obstruct a significant portion of the lung and may be rapidly fatal.

The Lungs

The two lungs and the branches of the bronchial tree are shown in **Figure 15-8**. Each of the two **lungs** has distinct **lobes** that are separated by deep fissures. The right lung has three lobes (*superior, middle,* and *inferior*). The left lung has two (*superior* and *inferior*). The bluntly rounded *apex* of each lung extends into the base of the neck above the first rib. The concave base of each lung rests on the superior surface of the diaphragm, the muscular sheet that separates the thoracic and abdominopelvic cavities. The curving

Figure 15-8 The Gross Anatomy of the Lungs.

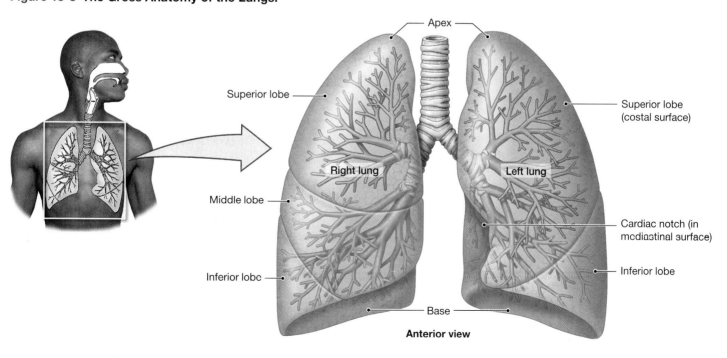

Apex

Superior lobe

Superior lobe (costal surface)

Right lung

Left lung

Middle lobe

Cardiac notch (in mediastinal surface)

Inferior lobe

Inferior lobe

Base

Anterior view

15

costal surface of each lung follows the inner contours of the rib cage. The *mediastinal surfaces* of both lungs have grooves that mark the passage of large blood vessels and indentations of the pericardium. In anterior view, the medial edge of the right lung forms a vertical line, but the medial margin of the left lung is indented at the *cardiac notch*. This notch provides space for the pericardial cavity, which sits to the left of the midline of the body.

The lungs have a light and spongy consistency because most of the actual volume of each lung consists of air-filled passageways and alveoli. Abundant elastic fibers allow the lungs to tolerate large changes in volume.

The Pleural Cavities

The thoracic cavity has the shape of a broad cone. Its walls are the rib cage. Its floor is the muscular diaphragm. Within the thoracic cavity, each lung is surrounded by a single pleural cavity. Each pleural cavity is lined by a serous membrane called the **pleura** (PLOOR-uh). ↻ p. 111 The *parietal pleura* covers the inner surface of the body wall and extends over the diaphragm and mediastinum. The *visceral pleura* covers the outer surfaces of the lungs, extending into the fissures between the lobes (**Figure 15-9**). The two pleural cavities are separated by the mediastinum.

Each pleural cavity actually represents a potential space rather than an open chamber because the parietal and visceral layers are usually in close contact. Both layers secrete a small amount of *pleural fluid*. This slippery fluid reduces friction between the pleural surfaces as you breathe. Pleural fluid is sometimes obtained for diagnostic purposes using a long needle between the ribs. This procedure is called *thoracentesis* (thōr-a-sen-TĒ-sis; *thorac-*, chest + *kentesis*, puncture). The extracted fluid is examined for bacteria, blood cells, and other abnormal components.

If an injury to the chest wall penetrates the parietal pleura or damages the alveoli, the visceral pleura can allow air into the pleural cavity. This condition, called **pneumothorax** (noo-mō-THOR-aks; *pneuma*, air), breaks the fluid bond between the pleurae and allows the lung's elastic fibers to recoil. The result is a collapsed lung, or **atelectasis** (at-e-LEK-ta-sis; *ateles*, imperfect + *ektasis*, expansion). Treatment involves removing as much of the air as possible before sealing the opening. This procedure restores the pleural fluid bond and reinflates the lung. Lung volume can also be reduced if blood accumulates in the pleural cavity. This condition is called **hemothorax**.

CHECKPOINT

8. Trace the path air takes in flowing from the glottis to the respiratory membrane.

9. What would happen to the alveoli if surfactant were not produced?

10. What are the functions of the pleural surfaces?

See the blue Answers tab at the back of the book.

Figure 15-9 Anatomical Relationships in the Thoracic Cavity.

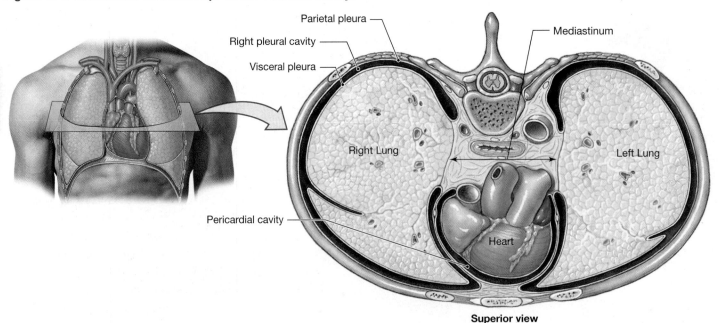

Parietal pleura

Right pleural cavity

Visceral pleura

Mediastinum

Right Lung

Left Lung

Pericardial cavity

Heart

Superior view

CLINICAL NOTE

Tuberculosis

Tuberculosis (too-ber-kū-LŌ-sis), or TB, results from a bacterial infection of the lungs, although other organs may be invaded as well. The bacterium, *Mycobacterium tuberculosis*, may colonize respiratory passageways, interstitial spaces, or alveoli, or a combination of all three. Signs and symptoms vary but generally include coughing and chest pain with fever, night sweats, fatigue, and weight loss.

TB is a major worldwide health problem. In 1900, TB, then known as "consumption," was a leading cause of death. Today, it remains among the most common and serious infectious diseases. An estimated one-third of the world's population is infected with TB. According to the World Health Organization, in 2013, 9 million people were diagnosed with TB and 1.5 million died from the disease. Unlike other deadly infectious diseases, such as AIDS, TB is transmitted through casual contact. By coughing, sneezing, or speaking, an infected individual can send the bacterium into the air in tiny droplets that can be inhaled by other people.

Treatment for TB is complex, because the bacteria are slow growing and can spread to many different tissues, such as the bones, lymphatic system, and meninges. The bacteria can develop resistance to standard antibiotics and require prolonged treatment. As a result, several antibiotic drugs are administered over a period of six to nine months. It is important that individuals take their TB drugs during their full treatment period. Stopping too soon can allow the bacteria still alive to become resistant to two or more antibiotics, making the TB more difficult to treat.

15-4 External respiration and internal respiration allow gas exchange within the body

Learning Objective Define and compare the processes of external respiration and internal respiration.

The general term *respiration* includes two integrated processes: *external respiration* and *internal respiration*. **External respiration** includes all the processes involved in the exchange of oxygen and carbon dioxide between the body's interstitial fluids and the external environment. Its purpose, and the primary function of the respiratory system, is to meet the respiratory demands of cells under various conditions. **Internal respiration** is the absorption of oxygen and the release of carbon dioxide by those cells. (We discuss the cellular pathways involving oxygen use and carbon dioxide release in Chapter 17.)

External respiration has three steps:

1. **Pulmonary ventilation,** or breathing, is the physical movement of air into and out of the lungs.
2. **Gas diffusion** takes place at two sites. One is across the respiratory membrane between alveolar air spaces and alveolar capillaries. The other is across capillary walls between blood and other tissues.
3. **Transport of oxygen and carbon dioxide** takes place between the alveolar capillaries and the capillary beds in other tissues. The bloodstream carries out this step.

Abnormalities in any of these processes will ultimately affect the gas concentrations in the interstitial fluids. As a result, cellular activities will be impacted. If oxygen concentrations decline, the affected tissues will be starved for oxygen. **Hypoxia** (hī-POK-sē-uh), or low tissue oxygen levels, results. It places severe limits on the metabolic activities of the affected area. If the supply of oxygen gets cut off completely, **anoxia** (an-OK-sē-uh), or lack of oxygen, results. Anoxia kills cells very quickly. Much of the damage from strokes and heart attacks results from localized anoxia.

CHECKPOINT

11. Define external respiration and internal respiration.
12. Name the integrated steps involved in external respiration.

See the blue Answers tab at the back of the book.

Patients should also be questioned about the use of smokeless tobacco. Although smokeless tobacco has less impact on the respiratory system than smoke products, it still increases the patient's risk for developing cancers of the mouth and throat.

 Build Your Knowledge

Recall that mitochondria produce about 95 percent of the energy a cell needs to stay alive (as you saw in **Chapter 3: Cell Structure and Function**). The key reactions in mitochondrial activity consume oxygen and generate carbon dioxide. The process of mitochondrial energy production is known as aerobic (*aero-*, air + *bios*, life) metabolism, or *cellular respiration*. This type of respiration differs from both external respiration and internal respiration. ↻ **p. 73**

CLINICAL NOTE

Tension Pneumothorax and Chest Decompression

In certain thoracic emergencies, decompression of the chest by emergency personnel can be life-saving. The most frequently encountered condition that requires pleural decompression is *tension pneumothorax.* With tension pneumothorax, a leak or tear develops in one of the lungs. Air begins to leak into the pleural space, and because it has no way to exit the chest, it begins to accumulate. Eventually, it will start to compress the affected lung, which leads to decreased ventilation and decreased perfusion. If allowed to progress untreated, the expanding mass of air will start to displace the mediastinum away from the injured side. This can decrease ventricular filling, which in turn decreases cardiac output. To prevent continued deterioration, emergency personnel must equalize the pressure in the chest with that of the environment. This will allow removal of the pressurized air mass, reexpansion of the lung, and movement of the mediastinum back to its normal position.

The simplest way to decompress the chest is to place a needle through the chest wall into the pleural space. This procedure is safest at the fifth intercostal space in a midaxillary line or at the second intercostal space in a midclavicular line. Remember that the intercostal neurovascular bundle runs immediately beneath and slightly behind each rib. Accidental puncture of the intercostal artery or vein can cause significant bleeding, and puncture or laceration of the intercostal nerve can cause pain or a loss in sensation to the dermatome it supplies. Because of this, it is important to palpate the rib and insert the needle along the superior border of the rib. The same warning is especially important when placing a thoracostomy tube (chest tube). The incision and tube insertion should be guided across the superior surface of the rib (**Figure 15-10**).

Remember, too, that the pleural pain fibers are located in the parietal pleura and not the visceral pleura. The patient will experience the most pain as the needle exits the chest wall. When placing larger tubes, such as chest tubes, it is important to inject an adequate amount of local anesthetic into the parietal pleura to ensure that the patient is as comfortable as possible.

Figure 15-10

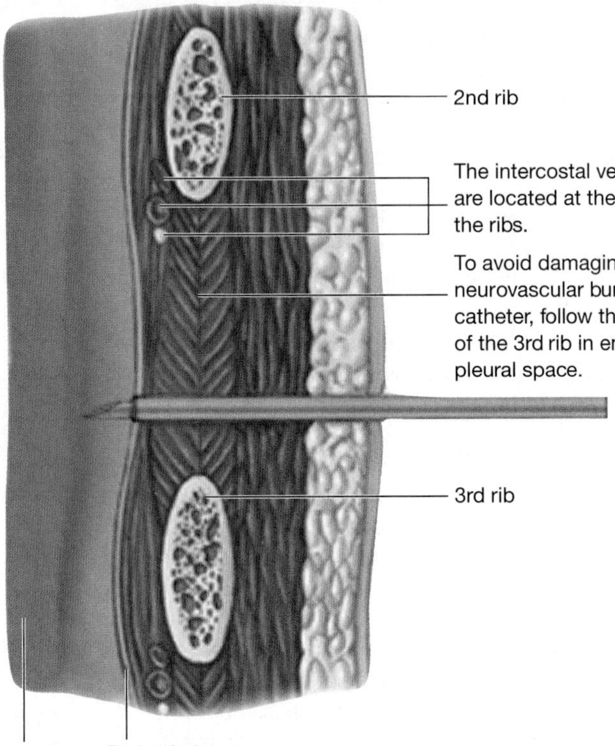

- 2nd rib
- The intercostal vessels and nerves are located at the inferior borders of the ribs.
- To avoid damaging the intercostal neurovascular bundle with needle or catheter, follow the upper border of the 3rd rib in entering the pleural space.
- 3rd rib

Lung   Parietal pleura

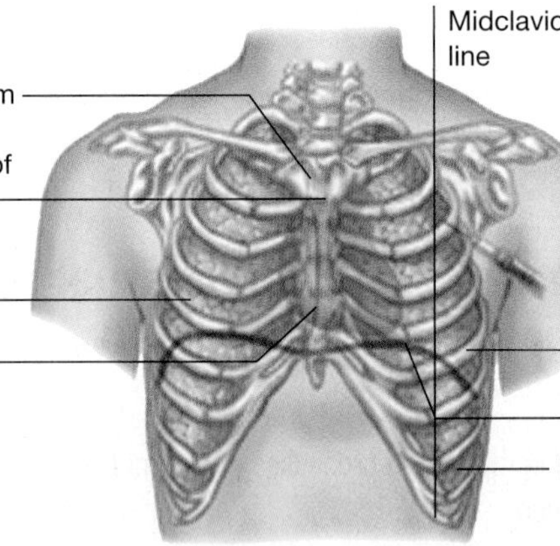

- Sternum
- Angle of Louis
- Lung
- Heart
- Midclavicular line
- Ribs
- Diaphragm
- Pleural space

15-5 Pulmonary ventilation—the exchange of air between the atmosphere and the lungs—involves pressure changes and muscle movement

Learning Objective Describe the physical principles governing the movement of air into the lungs and the actions of the respiratory muscles.

Pulmonary ventilation is the physical movement of air into and out of the respiratory tract. Its primary function is to maintain adequate **alveolar ventilation**, the movement of air into and out of the alveoli. Alveolar ventilation prevents the buildup of carbon dioxide in the alveoli. It also ensures a continuous supply of oxygen for absorption by the bloodstream.

Pressure and Airflow to the Lungs

As we know from television weather reports, air will flow from an area of higher pressure to an area of lower pressure. This difference between the high and low pressures is called

CLINICAL NOTE

Tobacco Abuse

Cigarette smoking and the abuse of tobacco products are significant risk factors for the development of respiratory and cardiovascular illnesses. Always question the patient about cigarette and tobacco usage. Patients will generally underreport it. A better picture of tobacco usage might be obtained from the patient's spouse or another family member.

A patient's cigarette smoking history is generally reported in pack/years. If possible, determine the number of cigarette packs (20 cigarettes/pack) smoked per day and the number of years the patient has smoked. Multiply the number of packs smoked per day by the number of years. For example, a man who has smoked two packs per day for 15 years would have a 30-pack/year smoking history. Medical problems related to smoking, such as emphysema, chronic bronchitis, and lung cancer, usually begin after a patient surpasses a 20-pack/year history, although this can vary significantly. This is an important part of the history and should be determined if the patient's condition allows it.

a *pressure gradient.* Pressure gradients apply both to the movement of atmospheric winds and to the movement of air into and out of the lungs (pulmonary ventilation). In a closed, flexible container (such as a lung), the pressure on a gas (such as air) can be changed by increasing or decreasing the container's volume: As the volume of the container (the lungs) increases, the pressure of the gas (air) decreases. As volume decreases, pressure increases.

The volume of the lungs depends on the volume of the thoracic cavity. As we have seen, only a thin film of pleural fluid separates the parietal and pleural membranes. The two membranes can slide across each other, but they are held together by that fluid film. You can see the same principle when you set a wet glass on a smooth surface. You can slide the glass easily, but when you try to lift it, you feel considerable resistance from this fluid bond. A comparable bond exists between the parietal pleura and the visceral pleura covering the lungs. Due to this bond, the surface of each lung sticks to the inner wall of the chest and to the superior surface of the

CLINICAL NOTE

Respiratory System Interventions

Several emergency interventions are used in the care of respiratory system emergencies. Oftentimes it is necessary to actually take over a patient's breathing until the underlying problem is corrected. This is done with mechanical ventilation, which uses a device to generate a volume of air that can be administered to a patient. Initially, this is done with a bag-valve-mask (BVM) unit, which is a common emergency device that can provide adequate respirations. However, if it is necessary to provide respirations over a prolonged period, a mechanical ventilator is used.

Mechanical Ventilation

Patients who require prolonged ventilation are usually placed on a mechanical ventilator. The mechanical ventilator is a device that provides ventilatory support for patients in respiratory failure.

Mechanical ventilators can be classified as: *pressure-cycled, volume-cycled,* or *time-cycled.* In pressure-cycled ventilators, the inspiratory phase is terminated when a pre-set pressure limit is reached. This type of ventilator works well if the patient's airway compliance remains constant. The airway compliance is the respiratory system's resistance to airflow. The greater the airway resistance, the lower the compliance. Conversely, the less the airway resistance, the greater will be the airway compliance. In the emergency setting, a patient's airway compliance can change. An increase in airway resistance, or a decrease in airway compliance, can cause a decrease in tidal volume. In severe cases, this may lead to hypoventilation. Because of this, most pressure-cycled ventilators have been replaced with volume-cycled ventilators. Pressure-cycled ventilators nonetheless have several distinct advantages. First, they are more compact and can be powered by compressed gas without the need for electrical power. This makes them suitable for ambulance and helicopter usage.

With volume-cycled ventilators, inspiration is terminated when a pre-set tidal volume is reached. The gas is usually delivered from compressible bellows. Most volume-cycled respirators are powered by an external electrical source.

With time-cycled ventilators, inspiration is terminated and expiration begins after a pre-set time has expired. Time-cycled ventilators are like volume-cycled ventilators in that they deliver a fairly constant tidal volume despite changes in the patient's airway compliance. They can also function as pressure-cycled ventilators when the secondary pressure limits are adjusted. Time-cycled ventilators are becoming increasingly popular.

Ventilator Settings

Important ventilator parameters can be controlled on most mechanical ventilators. These include: respiratory rate, tidal volume, inspired oxygen concentration, positive end-expiratory pressure (PEEP), and ventilation mode. The *respiratory rate* is the number of ventilatory cycles per minute. The *tidal volume* is the amount of air delivered during each ventilatory cycle. The tidal volume usually is set initially at 10–15 milliliters per kilogram of ideal body weight. The inspired oxygen concentration, or FiO_2 can also be set. This is usually expressed in percentages or in decimals (i.e., FiO_2 of 0.5 = 50 percent inspired oxygen concentration or FiO_2 of 1.0 = 100 percent inspired oxygen concentration). The *PEEP* is the pressure within the airway at the end of expiration. PEEP is usually expressed in centimeters of water (cm/H_2O) and can be adjusted to meet the patient's needs. Normal PEEP ranges from 0 cm/H_2O to 2 cm/H_2O. Increasing the PEEP improves oxygenation by keeping alveoli open during expiration. It also helps to reexpand any collapsed alveoli, which in turn will help to decrease shunting and improve the PaO_2.

(Continued)

Finally, the ventilatory mode can be set on most ventilators. There are several ventilator modes including:

- *Controlled mechanical ventilation (CMV).* Usually used in situations where the patient is apneic. In CMV mode, the patient is ventilated at the rate set by the operator. The patient cannot breathe between machine breaths.
- *Assist control mode ventilation (ACMV).* With ACMV, the operator sets the minimum rate at which the patient is to be ventilated. If the patient makes no respiratory effort, then only the prescribed number of breaths will be delivered. If the patient tries to breathe, the machine will deliver an extra breath with the same tidal volume as has been set. The amount of negative inspiratory pressure necessary to trigger a ventilation can be adjusted by the operator.
- *Intermittent mandatory ventilation (IMV).* With IMV, as with ACMV, the patient may breathe at a rate faster than set on the ventilator. However, the machine offers no assistance to the patient-generated ventilation, and the patient receives only the tidal volume that is self-generated. This allows medical personnel to determine the rate and depth of the patient's native respiratory efforts.
- *Synchronized intermittent mandatory ventilation (SIMV).* A problem with IMV is that the ventilator sometimes delivers a ventilation just as the patient has completed a spontaneous inspiration. Because of this, SIMV was developed. With SIMV, the mode is the same as IMV except that the ventilator times the machine breaths to fall in a pause between the patient's spontaneous respiratory cycle or to coincide with the initiation of a spontaneous breath.
- *Pressure support ventilation (PSV).* PSV mode was the basic mode used by intermittent positive-pressure breathing machines. When the patient initiates a breath, the machine delivers a constant inspiratory pressure until inspiratory flow drops below 25 percent of the peak level. Thus, the patient determines the rate, and tidal volume is dependent on patient airway compliance. PSV is usually used when weaning a patient from the ventilator.

Prehospital Mechanical Ventilation

Several mechanical ventilators have been developed for use in prehospital care. Most of these are pressure-cycled and powered by compressed oxygen. With most units, the respiratory rate and V_T can be adjusted. With some units, the inspiratory-to-expiratory ratio can be adjusted for use with pediatric patients. Prehospital mechanical ventilators, which are also called *automatic transport* ventilators, are common on EMS units that provide interhospital transport, particularly critical care interhospital transport (**Figure 15-11**). It is important not to become overly reliant on mechanical ventilators. BVM units should be immediately available in case of respiratory failure.

Complications of Mechanical Ventilation

Mechanical ventilation is safe and effective; however, several complications can develop, especially with prolonged mechanical ventilation and use of PEEP. A relatively common complication of ventilator therapy is barotrauma. Pneumothorax is the most common form of barotrauma. Typically, the pneumothorax is simple, but failure to recognize and treat a ventilator-induced pneumothorax can potentially lead to a tension pneumothorax

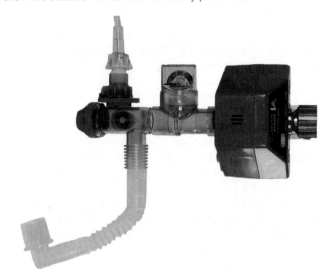

FIGURE 15–11 Prehospital Mechanical Ventilator. New technologies have allowed the development of small, portable ventilators that can be used in out-of-hospital settings. These units allow the selection of several ventilatory parameters.

and cardiovascular collapse. A less common manifestation of barotrauma is pneumoperitoneum. This is often mistaken as a ruptured abdominal viscus and can result in unnecessary surgery. Other complications of mechanical ventilation include diminished cardiac output, pneumonia, and oxygen toxicity.

Positive End-Expiratory Pressure

PEEP, or continuous positive airway pressure (CPAP), can be used to reclaim lost lung volumes and to increase oxygenation. PEEP or CPAP should be considered in cases where decreased pulmonary compliance prevents adequate tidal volumes or when hypoxemia exists despite delivery of 100 percent oxygen.

PEEP and CPAP are usually measured in centimeters of water (cm/H_2O). Initially, a PEEP of 2.5–5.0 cm/H_2O should be tried. This can be slowly increased to 10–15 cm/H_2O. A PEEP of greater than 12–15 cm/H_2O will usually affect cardiac output. PEEP pressures greater than 20 cm/H_2O affect ventricular filling to the point where the benefits of PEEP are not outweighed by the risks. High levels of PEEP result in increased intrathoracic pressure, which decreases venous return to the heart. This reduces ventricular filling and, ultimately, cardiac output. Thus, PEEP should be used with caution in any patient with a head injury, as increased intrathoracic pressure will impair venous return from the brain, and effectively increase intracranial pressure.

Devices are available that allow delivery of CPAP through a tightly fitted facemask. These were initially developed for treatment of obstructive sleep apnea. However, it has been found that use of CPAP can enhance oxygenation and, in many cases, prevent the need for endotracheal intubation. As CPAP devices have become more compact, they are used with increasing frequency in prehospital care.

15

diaphragm. Thus, any expansion or contraction of the thoracic cavity directly affects the volume of the lungs.

Changes in the volume of the thoracic cavity result from movements of the diaphragm and rib cage, as shown in **Spotlight Figure 15-12**:

- *Diaphragm.* The diaphragm forms the floor of the thoracic cavity. When relaxed, the diaphragm is dome shaped. It projects upward into the thoracic cavity, compressing the lungs. When the diaphragm contracts, it flattens, increasing the volume of the thoracic cavity and expanding the lungs. When the diaphragm relaxes, it returns to its original position, which decreases the volume of the thoracic cavity.

- *Rib cage.* Elevating the rib cage increases the volume of the thoracic cavity, because of the way the ribs and the vertebrae articulate. Lowering the rib cage decreases the volume of the thoracic cavity. The external intercostal muscles and accessory muscles (such as the sternocleidomastoid) elevate the rib cage. The internal intercostal muscles and other accessory muscles (such as the rectus abdominis and other abdominal muscles) lower the rib cage.

At the start of a breath, pressures inside and outside the lungs are the same. There is no movement of air (**Spotlight Figure 15-12**). When the diaphragm contracts and the movement of respiratory muscles enlarges the thoracic cavity, the lungs expand. As a result, the pressure inside the lungs decreases. Air now enters the respiratory passageways because the pressure inside the lungs (P_{inside}) is lower than the atmospheric pressure outside ($P_{outside}$) (**Spotlight Figure 15-12**).

During exhalation, downward movement of the rib cage and upward movement of the diaphragm reverse the process and reduce the volume of the lungs. Pressure inside the lungs now exceeds atmospheric pressure. As a result, air moves out of the lungs (**Spotlight Figure 15-12**).

Compliance

The **compliance** of the lungs is the ease with which the lungs stretch and expand. The greater the compliance, the easier it is to fill and empty the lungs. The lower the compliance, the greater is the force required to fill and empty the lungs.

Various disorders affect compliance. For example, compliance increases with the loss of supporting connective tissues due to alveolar damage, as in *emphysema* (see p. 587). Compliance decreases if surfactant production is too low to prevent the alveoli from collapsing on exhalation, as in *respiratory distress syndrome* (see p. 576). Compliance is also decreased when movements of the thoracic cage are limited by arthritis or other skeletal disorders that affect the joints of the ribs or spinal column.

When you are at rest, the muscular activity involved in pulmonary ventilation accounts for 3–5 percent of your resting energy demand. If compliance is reduced, the energy demand increases dramatically. You can become exhausted simply trying to continue breathing.

Modes of Breathing

We use our respiratory muscles in various combinations, depending on the volume of air that must be moved into and out of the system. Respiratory movements are classified as quiet breathing or forced breathing.

In *quiet breathing*, inhalation involves muscular contractions, but exhalation is passive. Inhalation involves the contraction of the primary respiratory muscles—the diaphragm and the external intercostal muscles. Diaphragm contraction normally accounts for around 75 percent of the air movement in normal quiet breathing. The external intercostal muscles account for the remaining 25 percent. These percentages can change, however. For example, pregnant women increasingly rely on movements of the rib cage as the uterus expands and forces abdominal organs against the diaphragm.

In *forced breathing*, both inhalation and exhalation are active. During inhalation, forced breathing involves the accessory respiratory muscles. During exhalation, the internal intercostal muscles and abdominal muscles are used.

Lung Volumes and Capacities

A single breath, or **respiratory cycle**, consists of an inhalation, or *inspiration,* and an exhalation, or *expiration.* The **respiratory rate** is the number of breaths per minute. In normal adults at rest, this rate ranges from 12 to 18 breaths per minute. Children breathe more rapidly. For example, children of 1–5 years of age normally take about 20–30 breaths per minute.

We exchange only a small proportion of the air in our lungs during a single quiet respiratory cycle. This amount of air is called the *tidal volume.* It can be increased by inhaling more vigorously and exhaling more completely.

We can divide the total volume of the lungs into a series of *volumes* and *capacities* (each the sum of various volumes) as shown in **Figure 15-13**:

- The **tidal volume (VT)** is the amount of air you move into or out of your lungs during a single respiratory cycle. It averages about 500 mL in both males and females.

- The **expiratory reserve volume (ERV)** is the amount of air that you can voluntarily expel at the end of a normal, quiet respiratory cycle. With the maximum use of accessory muscles, males can expel about 1000 mL of air. Female ERV averages 700 mL.

15

Pulmonary ventilation, or breathing, is the movement of air into and out of the respiratory system. It occurs by changing the volume of the lungs. Changes in lung volume take place through the contraction of skeletal muscles. The most important respiratory muscles are the diaphragm and the external intercostal muscles.

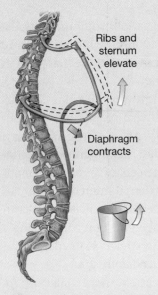

Ribs and sternum elevate

Diaphragm contracts

As the diaphragm is depressed or the ribs are elevated, the volume of the thoracic cavity increases and air moves into the lungs. The outward movement of the ribs as they are elevated resembles the outward swing of a raised bucket handle.

AT REST

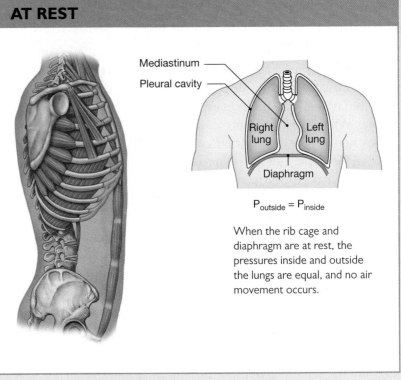

Mediastinum

Pleural cavity

Right lung

Left lung

Diaphragm

$$P_{outside} = P_{inside}$$

When the rib cage and diaphragm are at rest, the pressures inside and outside the lungs are equal, and no air movement occurs.

INHALATION

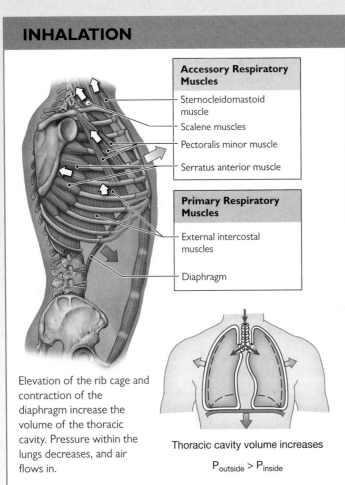

Accessory Respiratory Muscles

Sternocleidomastoid muscle

Scalene muscles

Pectoralis minor muscle

Serratus anterior muscle

Primary Respiratory Muscles

External intercostal muscles

Diaphragm

Elevation of the rib cage and contraction of the diaphragm increase the volume of the thoracic cavity. Pressure within the lungs decreases, and air flows in.

Thoracic cavity volume increases

$$P_{outside} > P_{inside}$$

EXHALATION

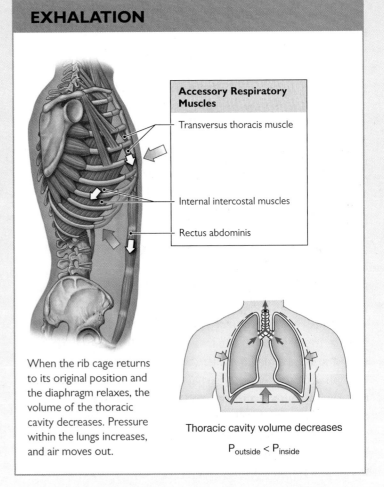

Accessory Respiratory Muscles

Transversus thoracis muscle

Internal intercostal muscles

Rectus abdominis

When the rib cage returns to its original position and the diaphragm relaxes, the volume of the thoracic cavity decreases. Pressure within the lungs increases, and air moves out.

Thoracic cavity volume decreases

$$P_{outside} < P_{inside}$$

Figure 15-13 Pulmonary Volumes and Capacities. The red line indicates the volume of air within the lungs during breathing.

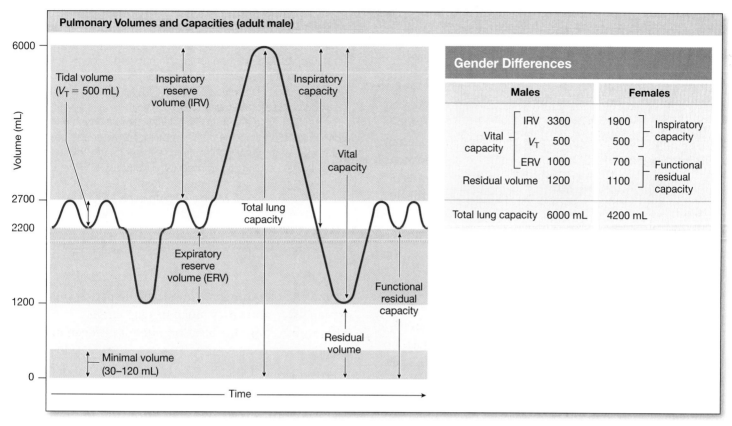

- The **inspiratory reserve volume (IRV)** is the amount of air that you can take in over and above the tidal volume. Because the lungs of males are larger than those of females, the IRV of males averages 3300 mL versus 1900 mL in females.

- The **vital capacity** is the sum of the tidal volume, the ERV, and the IRV. It is the maximum amount of air that you can move into and out of your respiratory system in a single respiratory cycle.

- The **residual volume** is the amount of air that remains in your lungs even after a maximal exhalation. It is typically about 1200 mL in males and 1100 mL in females. Most of this residual volume exists because the lungs are held against the thoracic wall, preventing their elastic fibers from contracting further.

- The **minimal volume** is the amount of air that would remain in your lungs if they were allowed to collapse. The minimal volume ranges from 30 to 120 mL. However, even at minimal volume, some air remains in the lungs, because the surfactant coating the alveolar surfaces prevents their collapse.

Not all of the inhaled air reaches the alveolar exchange surfaces within the lungs. A typical inhalation brings about 500 mL of air into the respiratory system. The first 350 mL travels along the conducting passageways and enters the alveolar spaces, but the last 150 mL never gets farther than the conducting passageways and does not take part in gas exchange with the blood. The total volume of these passageways (150 mL) is known as the *anatomic dead space* of the lungs.

CHECKPOINT

13. Define compliance and identify some factors that affect it.

14. What is tidal volume?

15. Mark breaks a rib that punctures the chest wall on his left side. What do you expect will happen to his left lung as a result?

16. In pneumonia, fluid accumulates in the alveoli of the lungs. How would this accumulation affect vital capacity?

See the blue Answers tab at the back of the book.

15-6 Gas exchange depends on the partial pressures of gases and the diffusion of molecules

Learning Objective Describe the physical principles governing the diffusion of gases into and out of the blood.

During pulmonary ventilation, the alveoli are supplied with oxygen, and carbon dioxide is removed from the bloodstream. The actual process of gas exchange with the external environment takes place between the blood and alveolar air across the respiratory membrane. This process depends on (1) the partial pressures of the gases involved and (2) the diffusion of molecules between a gas and a liquid. ⤶ p. 62

Mixed Gases and Partial Pressures

The air we breathe is a mixture of gases. Nitrogen molecules (N_2) are the most abundant. They account for about 78.6 percent of atmospheric gas molecules. Oxygen molecules (O_2) are the second most abundant. These molecules make up roughly 20.9 percent of air. Most of the remaining 0.5 percent consists of water molecules. Carbon dioxide (CO_2) contributes a mere 0.04 percent.

Atmospheric pressure at sea level is approximately 760 mm Hg. Each of the gases in air contributes to the total atmospheric pressure in proportion to its relative abundance. The pressure contributed by a single gas is the **partial pressure** of that gas, abbreviated as P. All the partial pressures added together equal the total pressure exerted by the gas mixture. For the atmosphere, this relationship can be summarized as:

$$P_{N_2} + P_{O_2} + P_{H_2O} + P_{CO_2} = 760 \text{ mm Hg}$$

We can easily calculate the partial pressure of each gas because we know the individual percentages of each gas in air. For example, the partial pressure of oxygen is 20.9 percent of 760 mm Hg, or approximately 159 mm Hg. The partial pressures of other atmospheric gases are listed in **Table 15-1**.

These values are important because the partial pressure of each gas determines its rate of diffusion between alveolar

air and the bloodstream. Note that the partial pressure of oxygen determines how much oxygen enters solution, but it has no effect on the diffusion rates of nitrogen or carbon dioxide.

Alveolar Air versus Atmospheric Air

As soon as air enters the respiratory tract, its characteristics begin to change. For example, in passing through the nasal cavity, the inhaled air becomes warmer and more humid (the amount of water vapor increases). On reaching the alveoli, the incoming air mixes with air that remained in the alveoli after the previous respiratory cycle. The resulting alveolar gas mixture, thus, contains more carbon dioxide and less oxygen than does atmospheric air.

As noted earlier, the last 150 mL of inhaled air (about 30 percent of the tidal volume) never gets farther than the conducting passageways, the anatomic dead space of the lungs. During the next exhalation, the departing alveolar air mixes with air in the dead space to produce yet another mixture that differs from both atmospheric and alveolar samples. The differences in composition between atmospheric (inhaled) and alveolar air are also given in **Table 15-1**.

CLINICAL NOTE

Pulmonary Function Tests

The efficiency of pulmonary function, especially in obstructive lung disease, can be rapidly determined through *pulse oximeter* and *peak expiratory flow rate (PEFR)* testing. A pulse oximeter is an electronic device that measures the amount of hemoglobin saturated with oxygen. This device is small, easy to use, and quite accurate. PEFR is determined with a *Wright peak expiratory flow meter*. The patient takes a deep breath and blows into the Wright meter. This is repeated twice and the highest reading is recorded. Normal adult PEFR varies from 400 to 600 liters/minute. Any reading less than 400 indicates some degree of airflow obstruction. Peak flow testing should be repeated throughout care in order to determine the degree of improvement.

Table 15-1	Partial Pressures (mm Hg) and Normal Gas Concentrations (%) in Air			
Source of Sample	**Nitrogen (N_2)**	**Oxygen (O_2)**	**Carbon Dioxide (CO_2)**	**Water Vapor (H_2O)**
Inhaled Air (Dry)	597 (78.6%)	159 (20.9%)	0.3 (0.04%)	3.7 (0.5%)
Alveolar Air (Saturated)	573 (75.4%)	100 (13.2%)	40 (5.2%)	47 (6.2%)
Exhaled Air (Saturated)	569 (74.8%)	116 (15.3%)	28 (3.7%)	47 (6.2%)

CLINICAL NOTE

Chronic Respiratory System Diseases

A multitude of problems can arise from the respiratory system. Many of these can develop over weeks or months, while others develop over hours. The following discussion details the more common types of respiratory system problems seen in the emergency setting.

Obstructive Lung Disease

Obstructive lung disease is widespread in our society. The most common obstructive lung diseases encountered in prehospital care are asthma, emphysema, and chronic bronchitis (the last two are often discussed together as chronic obstructive pulmonary disease, or COPD). Asthma afflicts 1–5 percent of the U.S. population, and COPD is found in 25 percent of all adults. Chronic bronchitis alone affects one in five adult males. Patients with COPD have a 50 percent mortality within 10 years of the diagnosis.

Although asthma may have a genetic predisposition, COPD is known to be caused directly by cigarette smoking and environmental toxins. Other factors have been shown to precipitate symptoms in patients who already have obstructive airway disease. Intrinsic factors include stress, upper respiratory infections, and exercise. Extrinsic factors include tobacco smoke, drugs, occupational hazards (chemical fumes, dust, etc.), and allergens such as foods, animal dander, dusts, and molds.

Abnormal ventilation is a common feature of all obstructive lung diseases. This abnormal ventilation is a result of obstruction that occurs primarily in the bronchioles, where several changes occur. One of these changes is bronchospasm (sustained smooth muscle contraction), which may be reversed by beta-adrenergic receptor stimulation. Agents such as terbutaline, albuterol, and epinephrine are used to accomplish this. Increased mucous production by goblet cells that line the respiratory tree also contribute to obstruction. This effect may be worsened by the fact that in many patients the cilia are destroyed, which results in poor clearance of excess mucus. Finally, inflammation of the bronchial passages results in the accumulation of fluid and inflammatory cells. Depending on the underlying cause, some elements of bronchial obstruction are reversible, whereas others are not.

During inspiration, the bronchioles will naturally dilate, allowing air to be drawn into the alveoli. As the patient begins to exhale, the bronchioles constrict. When this natural constriction occurs— in addition to the underlying bronchospasm, increased mucous production, and inflammation in patients with obstructive airway disease—the result is significant air trapping distal to the obstruction. This is one of the hallmarks of obstructive lung disease.

Emphysema

Emphysema results from destruction of the alveolar walls distal to the terminal bronchioles. It is more common in men than in women. The major factor that contributes to emphysema in our society is cigarette smoking. Significant exposure to environmental toxins is another contributing factor.

Continued exposure to noxious substances, such as cigarette smoke, results in the gradual destruction of the walls of the alveoli. This process decreases the alveolar membrane surface area, thus lessening the area available for gas exchange. The progressive loss of the respiratory membrane results in an increased ratio of air to lung tissue. The result is diffusion defects. Additionally, the number of pulmonary capillaries in the lung is decreased, which thus increases resistance to pulmonary blood flow. This condition ultimately causes pulmonary hypertension, which in turn may lead to right-heart failure, cor pulmonale, and death.

Emphysema also causes weakening of the walls of the small bronchioles. When the walls of the alveoli and small bronchioles are destroyed, the lungs lose their capacity to recoil and air becomes trapped in the lungs. Thus, residual volume increases while vital capacity remains relatively normal. The destroyed lung tissue (called *blebs*) results in alveolar collapse. To counteract this effect, patients tend to breathe through pursed lips. This creates continued positive pressure similar to positive end-expiratory pressure and prevents alveolar collapse.

As the disease progresses, the PaO_2 further decreases, which may lead to increased red blood cell production and polycythemia (an excess of red blood cells that results in an abnormally high hematocrit). The $PaCO_2$ also increases and becomes chronically elevated, which forces the body to depend upon hypoxic drive to control respirations. Finally, remember that emphysema is characterized by irreversible airway obstruction.

Patients with emphysema are more susceptible to acute respiratory infections, such as pneumonia, and to cardiac dysrhythmias. Chronic emphysema patients ultimately become dependent on bronchodilators, corticosteroids, and in the final stages, supplemental oxygen.

Chronic Bronchitis

Chronic bronchitis results from an increase in the number of the goblet (mucus-secreting) cells in the respiratory tree. It is characterized by the production of a large quantity of sputum. This often occurs after prolonged exposure to cigarette smoke.

Unlike emphysema, in chronic bronchitis the alveoli are not severely affected and diffusion remains normal. Gas exchange is decreased because alveolar ventilation is lowered, which ultimately results in hypoxia and hypercarbia. Hypoxia may increase red blood cell production, which in turn leads to polycythemia (as occurs in emphysema). Increased $PaCO_2$ levels may lead to irritability, somnolence, decreased intellectual abilities, headaches, and personality changes. Physiologically, an increased $PaCO_2$ causes pulmonary vasoconstriction, which results in pulmonary hypertension and, eventually, cor pulmonale. Unlike emphysema, the vital capacity is decreased, while the residual volume is normal or decreased.

Asthma

Asthma is a common respiratory illness that affects many persons. Although deaths from other respiratory diseases are steadily declining, deaths from asthma have significantly increased during the last decade. Most of the increased asthma

(Continued)

15

deaths have occurred in patients who are 45 years of age or older. In addition, the death rate for black asthmatics has been twice as high as for their white counterparts. Approximately 50 percent of patients who die from asthma do so before reaching the hospital. Thus, EMS personnel are frequently called upon to treat patients suffering an asthma attack. Prompt recognition followed by appropriate treatment can significantly improve the patient's condition and enhance his chance of survival.

Asthma is a chronic inflammatory disorder of the airways. In susceptible individuals, this inflammation causes symptoms usually associated with widespread but variable airflow obstruction. In addition to airflow obstruction, the airway becomes hyperresponsive. The airflow obstruction and hyperresponsiveness are often reversible with treatment. These conditions may also reverse spontaneously.

Asthma may be induced by one of many different factors. These factors, commonly referred to as triggers or inducers, vary from one individual to the next. In allergic individuals, environmental allergens are a major cause of inflammation. These may occur both indoors and outdoors. In addition to allergens, asthma may be triggered by cold air, exercise, foods, irritants, stress, and certain medications. Often, no specific trigger can be identified. Extrinsic triggers tend predominantly to affect children, whereas intrinsic factors trigger asthma in adults.

Within minutes of exposure to the offending trigger, a two-phase reaction occurs. The first phase of the reaction is characterized by the release of chemical mediators such as histamine. These mediators cause contraction of the bronchial smooth muscle and leakage of fluid from peribronchial capillaries. This results in both bronchoconstriction and bronchial edema. These two factors can significantly decrease expiratory air flow and cause the typical asthma attack.

Often, the asthma attack will resolve spontaneously in one to two hours or may be aborted by the use of inhaled bronchodilator medications such as albuterol. However, within six to eight hours after exposure to the trigger, a second reaction occurs. This late phase is characterized by inflammation of the bronchioles as cells of the immune system (eosinophils, neutrophils, and lymphocytes) invade the mucosa of the respiratory tract. This leads to additional edema and swelling of the bronchioles and a further decrease in expiratory airflow.

The second phase reaction will not typically respond to inhaled beta-agonist drugs such as metaproterenol or albuterol. Instead, anti-inflammatory agents such as corticosteroids are often required. It is important to point out that the severe inflammatory changes seen in an acute asthma attack do not develop over a few hours or even a few days. The inflammation will often begin several days or several weeks before the onset of the actual asthma attack. Many asthmatic patients will wait before summoning EMS. The longer the time interval from the onset of the asthma attack until treatment, the less likely it will be that bronchodilator medications will work. Often, after a prolonged asthma attack, the patient may become fatigued. A fatigued patient can quickly develop respiratory failure and subsequently require intubation and mechanical ventilation. Always be prepared to provide airway and respiratory support for the asthmatic.

Status Asthmaticus

Status asthmaticus is a severe, prolonged asthma attack that cannot be broken by repeated doses of bronchodilators. It is a serious medical emergency that requires prompt recognition, treatment, and transport. The patient who suffers from status asthmaticus frequently will have a greatly distended chest from continued air trapping. Breath sounds, and often wheezing, may be absent. The patient is usually exhausted, severely acidotic, and dehydrated. The management of status asthmaticus is basically the same as for asthma. Recognize that respiratory arrest is imminent and be prepared for endotracheal intubation. The patient should be transported immediately with aggressive treatment continued en route.

CLINICAL NOTE

Decompression Sickness

Decompression sickness is a painful condition that develops when a person is exposed to a sudden drop in atmospheric pressure. Nitrogen is the gas responsible for the problems experienced, due to its high partial pressure in air. When the pressure drops, nitrogen comes out of solution and forms bubbles, just as bubbles form when a can of soda is opened. The bubbles may form in joint cavities, in the bloodstream, and in the cerebrospinal fluid. Individuals with decompression sickness typically curl up because of the pain in affected joints. This response accounts for the condition's common name: *the bends*. Decompression sickness most often affects scuba divers who return to the surface too quickly after breathing air under greater than normal pressures while submerged. It can also develop in airline passengers subjected to sudden losses of cabin pressure.

Partial Pressures in the Pulmonary and Systemic Circuits

Figure 15-14 shows the partial pressures of oxygen and carbon dioxide in the pulmonary and systemic circuits. The deoxygenated blood delivered by the pulmonary arteries has a lower PO_2 and a higher PCO_2 than does alveolar air (**Figure 15-14a**). Diffusion between the alveolar air and the pulmonary (alveolar) capillaries then raises the PO_2 of the blood and lowers its PCO_2. By the time the blood enters the pulmonary venules, it has reached equilibrium with the alveolar air. Blood departs the alveoli with a PO_2 of about 100 mm Hg and a PCO_2 of roughly 40 mm Hg.

As this blood enters pulmonary veins, it mixes with blood that flowed through capillaries around the conducting passageways. The blood leaving the conducting passageways carries relatively little oxygen. As a result, the partial pressure of oxygen in the mix of blood in the pulmonary veins

CLINICAL NOTE

Upper Respiratory Infection

Among the most common infections for which patients seek medical attention are those that involve the upper airway and respiratory tract. Although these conditions are rarely life threatening, *upper respiratory infections (URIs)* can make many existing pulmonary diseases worse or lead to direct pulmonary infection. The best defense against the spread of upper respiratory infection is to practice common hygiene such as good hand washing and covering the mouth during coughing and sneezing. Attention to such details is important when caring for patients with underlying pulmonary disease or those who are immunosuppressed (HIV infection, cancer) because URIs are more severe in these populations. Due to the prevalence of such infections, complete protection is impossible.

Remember that the upper airway begins at the nose and mouth, passes through the pharynx, and ends at the larynx. Other related structures are the paranasal sinuses and the eustachian tubes that connect the pharynx and the middle ear. In addition, several collections of lymphoid tissue found in the pharynx (palatine, pharyngeal, and lingual tonsils) produce antibodies and provide immune protection.

Viruses cause the vast majority of URIs. A variety of bacteria may also produce infection of the upper respiratory tract. The most significant is *group A streptococcus*, which is the causative organism in "strep throat" and accounts for up to 30 percent of URIs. These bacteria are also implicated in sinusitis and middle-ear infections. Up to 50 percent of patients who have pharyngitis (inflammation of the pharynx) are not found to have a viral or bacterial cause. Fortunately, most URIs are self-limiting illnesses that resolve after several days of symptoms.

---

drops to 95 mm Hg. This is the in the blood that enters the systemic circuit.

Normal interstitial fluid has a PO_2 of 40 mm Hg and a PCO_2 of 45 mm Hg. As a result, oxygen diffuses out of the capillaries and carbon dioxide diffuses in until the capillary partial pressures are the same as those in the adjacent tissues (**Figure 15-14b**). When the blood returns to the alveolar capillaries, external respiration will replace the oxygen released into the tissues, and the excess CO_2 will be lost.

The major symptoms of URI are dependent upon the portion of the upper respiratory tract that is predominantly affected. Patients with URIs will often have accompanying symptoms such as fever, chills, myalgias (muscle pains), and fatigue. Most upper respiratory infections are treated symptomatically. Acetaminophen or ibuprofen is prescribed for fever, headache, and myalgias. Encourage patients to drink plenty of fluids. Saltwater gargles may be used for throat discomfort. Decongestants and antihistamines may be used to reduce mucous secretion. Encourage patients who are being treated with antibiotics for bacterial causes of URI to continue these agents.

CHECKPOINT

17. True or false: Each gas in a mixture of gases exerts a partial pressure equal to its relative abundance.

18. What happens to air as it passes through the nasal cavity?

19. Compare the oxygen and carbon dioxide content of alveolar air and atmospheric air.

See the blue Answers tab at the back of the book.

15-7 Most O_2 is transported bound to hemoglobin (Hb), and CO_2 is dissolved in plasma, bound to Hb, or transported as bicarbonate ion

Learning Objective Describe how oxygen and carbon dioxide are transported in the blood.

Oxygen and carbon dioxide have limited solubilities (ability to dissolve) in blood plasma. These limits are a problem because peripheral tissues need more oxygen and generate more carbon dioxide than the plasma alone can absorb and transport. Red blood cells (RBCs) solve this problem. They take up dissolved oxygen and carbon dioxide molecules from plasma and bind them (in the case of oxygen) or use them to manufacture soluble compounds (in the case of carbon dioxide). These reactions remove dissolved gases from the blood plasma. As a result, these gases continue to diffuse into the blood and never reach equilibrium.

The important thing about these reactions is that they are both *temporary* and *completely reversible*. When plasma oxygen or carbon dioxide concentrations are high, RBCs remove the excess molecules. When plasma concentrations are falling, RBCs release their stored reserves.

Oxygen Transport

Only about 1.5 percent of the oxygen in arterial blood consists of oxygen molecules in solution. The rest of the oxygen molecules are bound to *hemoglobin (Hb) molecules*. Recall

15

Figure 15-14 An Overview of Respiratory Processes and Partial Pressures in Respiration.

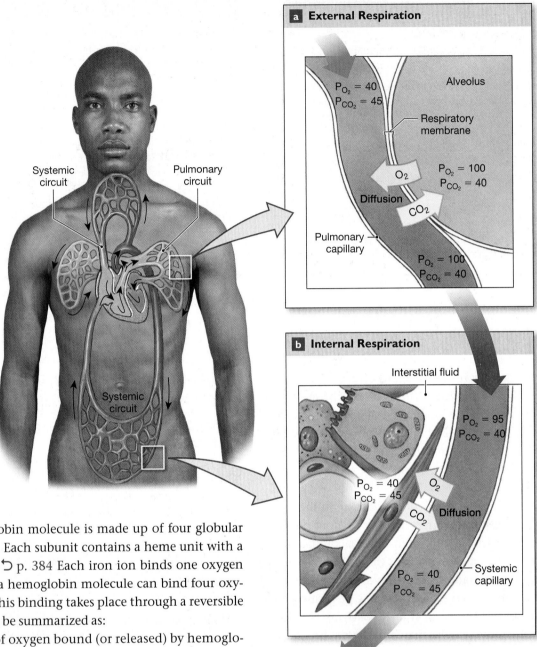

a **External Respiration**

$P_{O_2} = 40$
$P_{CO_2} = 45$

Alveolus

Respiratory membrane

O_2

$P_{O_2} = 100$
$P_{CO_2} = 40$

Diffusion

CO_2

Pulmonary capillary

$P_{O_2} = 100$
$P_{CO_2} = 40$

b **Internal Respiration**

Interstitial fluid

$P_{O_2} = 95$
$P_{CO_2} = 40$

$P_{O_2} = 40$
$P_{CO_2} = 45$

O_2

CO_2

Diffusion

$P_{O_2} = 40$
$P_{CO_2} = 45$

Systemic capillary

Systemic circuit

Pulmonary circuit

Systemic circuit

that the hemoglobin molecule is made up of four globular protein subunits. Each subunit contains a heme unit with a central iron ion. ⊃ p. 384 Each iron ion binds one oxygen molecule. Thus, a hemoglobin molecule can bind four oxygen molecules. This binding takes place through a reversible reaction that can be summarized as:

The amount of oxygen bound (or released) by hemoglobin depends primarily on the P_{O_2} of its surroundings. The lower the oxygen content of a tissue, the more oxygen is released by hemoglobin molecules passing through local capillaries. For example, inactive tissues have little demand for oxygen, and the local P_{O_2} is about 40 mm Hg. Under these conditions, the passing hemoglobin collectively releases about 25 percent of its stored oxygen. In contrast, if the local P_{O_2} of active tissues declines to 15–20 mm Hg (about one-half of the of normal tissue), the passing hemoglobin then collectively releases up to 80 percent of its stored oxygen. In practical terms, this means that active tissues will receive roughly three times as much oxygen as will inactive tissues.

The amount of oxygen released by hemoglobin is also influenced by pH and temperature. Active tissues generate acids that lower the pH of the interstitial fluids. When the pH declines, hemoglobin molecules release their bound oxygen molecules more readily. Hemoglobin also releases more oxygen when body temperature rises.

All three factors (pH, and temperature) are important during maximal exertion. When a skeletal muscle works hard, its temperature rises and the local pH and decline. The combination makes the hemoglobin entering the area release much more oxygen for use by active muscle fibers.

15

Build Your Knowledge

Recall that many important biological reactions are freely reversible (as you saw in **Chapter 2: The Chemical Level of Organization**). A reversible reaction consists of two reactions, synthesis and decomposition, that take place at the same time. At equilibrium, the rates of the two reactions are in balance. As a result, as fast as a molecule is synthesized, another one like it undergoes decomposition. This equilibrium is upset if the concentrations of one or more molecules are changed. When this change takes place, the equilibrium of the reversible reaction will shift so that either more synthesis or more decomposition will occur. ⊃**p. 33**

Without this automatic adjustment, tissue would fall to very low levels almost immediately, and the exertion would end.

Carbon Dioxide Transport

Carbon dioxide is generated by aerobic metabolism in peripheral tissues. Carbon dioxide travels in the bloodstream in three different ways. After entering the blood, a CO_2 molecule either (1) dissolves in the plasma, (2) binds to hemoglobin within RBCs, or (3) is converted to a bicarbonate ion (**Figure 15-15**). All three processes are completely reversible, allowing carbon dioxide to be picked up from body tissues and delivered to the alveoli.

Transport in Plasma

Plasma becomes saturated with carbon dioxide quite rapidly. As a result, only about 7 percent of the carbon dioxide absorbed by peripheral capillaries is transported as dissolved gas molecules. The rest diffuses into RBCs.

Hemoglobin Binding

Once in RBCs, some of the carbon dioxide molecules are bound to the protein "globin" portions of hemoglobin molecules, forming **carbaminohemoglobin** (kar-bām-i-no-hē-mō-GLŌ-bin). Such binding does not interfere with the binding of oxygen to heme units. For this reason, hemoglobin can transport both oxygen and carbon dioxide at the same time. Normally, about 23 percent of the carbon dioxide entering the blood in peripheral tissues is transported as carbaminohemoglobin.

CLINICAL NOTE

Carbon Monoxide Poisoning

Murder victims who die in cars inside a locked garage are common in mystery stories. In real life, entire families are killed each winter by leaky furnaces or space heaters. The cause of death is carbon monoxide (CO) poisoning. The exhaust of automobiles and other petroleum-burning engines, of oil lamps, and of fuel-fired space heaters contains the odorless gas, CO. CO competes with O_2 molecules for the binding sites on heme units. Unfortunately, the CO usually wins. Even at very low partial pressures, it has a much stronger affinity (attraction) for hemoglobin than does oxygen. The attachment of a CO molecule essentially makes that heme unit unavailable for respiratory purposes. If CO molecules make up just 0.1 percent of inhaled air, enough hemoglobin will be affected that survival is impossible without medical assistance. Treatment includes (1) preventing further CO exposure; (2) administering pure oxygen, because at sufficiently high partial pressures the O_2 molecules "bump" the CO from the hemoglobin; and, if necessary, (3) transfusing compatible red blood cells.

Figure 15-15 Carbon Dioxide Transport in Blood.

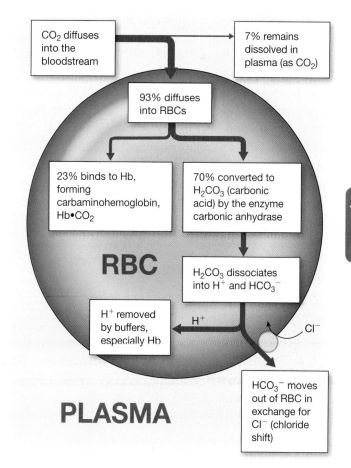

Carbonic Acid Formation and Dissociation

Roughly 70 percent of the carbon dioxide molecules absorbed by blood are ultimately transported in the plasma as bicarbonate ions (HCO_3^-). The bicarbonate ions are not formed directly from carbon dioxide. First, carbon dioxide in RBCs is converted to carbonic acid (H_2CO_3) by the enzyme *carbonic anhydrase*. Each carbonic acid molecule immediately dissociates into a hydrogen ion and a bicarbonate ion. The reactions can be summarized as follows:

The reactions take place very rapidly and are completely reversible. Because most of the carbonic acid formed immediately dissociates into hydrogen ions and bicarbonate, we will ignore the intermediary step and summarize the reaction as follows:

In peripheral capillaries, this reaction rapidly ties up large numbers of carbon dioxide molecules. The equilibrium of this reaction shifts toward the right, because carbon dioxide continues to diffuse out of the interstitial fluids and the hydrogen ions and bicarbonate ions are being continuously removed. Where do they go? Most of the hydrogen ions bind to hemoglobin molecules. This binding prevents their release from the RBCs and a lowering of plasma pH. The bicarbonate ions diffuse into the surrounding plasma. The exit of the bicarbonate ions is matched by the entry of chloride ions from the plasma, thus trading one anion for another. This mass movement of chloride ions into RBCs is known as the *chloride shift.*

When venous blood reaches the alveoli, carbon dioxide diffuses out of the plasma, and the PCO_2 declines. Recall that all of the reactions involved in carbon dioxide transport in RBCs are reversible. Thus, when carbon dioxide diffuses out of the RBCs, the processes shown in **Figure 15-15** proceed in the opposite direction. Hydrogen ions separate from the hemoglobin molecules. Bicarbonate ions diffuse out of the plasma and into the cytoplasm of the RBCs. There they are converted to water and CO_2.

Figure 15-16 summarizes the events by which oxygen and carbon dioxide are transported and exchanged between the respiratory and cardiovascular systems.

CHECKPOINT

20. Identify the three ways that carbon dioxide is transported in the bloodstream.

21. As you exercise, hemoglobin releases more oxygen to active skeletal muscles than it does when the muscles are at rest. Why?

22. How would blockage of the trachea affect blood pH?

See the blue Answers tab at the back of the book.

15-8 Neurons in the medulla oblongata and pons, along with respiratory reflexes, control respiration

Learning Objective List the factors that influence the rate of respiration, and describe the reflexes that regulate respiration.

Cells continuously absorb oxygen from the interstitial fluids and generate carbon dioxide. Under normal conditions, cellular rates of absorption and generation are matched by the rates of delivery and removal at the capillaries. Moreover, those rates are identical to those of oxygen absorption and carbon dioxide removal at the lungs. If these rates become unbalanced, the activities of the cardiovascular and respiratory systems must be adjusted. Homeostatic processes restore equilibrium. They involve (1) changes in blood flow and oxygen delivery under local control and (2) changes in the depth and rate of respiration under the control of the brain's respiratory centers.

The Local Control of Respiration

Both the rate of oxygen delivery at each tissue and the efficiency of oxygen pickup at the lungs are regulated at the local level. If a peripheral tissue becomes more active, the interstitial falls and the rises. These changes increase the difference between partial pressures in the tissues and arriving blood, so more oxygen is delivered and more carbon dioxide is carried away. In addition, rising levels cause smooth muscles in the walls of arterioles in the area to relax, increasing blood flow.

Local adjustments in blood flow, or of airflow into alveoli, also make gas transport more efficient. For example, as blood flows to alveolar capillaries, it is directed to pulmonary lobules with a relatively high PO_2. This takes place because precapillary sphincters in alveolar capillary beds constrict when the local is low. (This response is the opposite of that seen in peripheral tissues. ⊃ p. 434) Also in the lungs, smooth muscles in the walls of bronchioles are sensitive to the PCO_2 of the air they contain. When the PCO_2 increases, the bronchioles dilate, and when the PCO_2 declines, the bronchioles constrict. As a result, airflow is directed to lobules in which the PCO_2 is high.

Control by the Respiratory Centers of the Brain

Respiratory control has both involuntary and voluntary components. Your brain's involuntary respiratory centers (in the medulla oblongata and pons) regulate the respiratory muscles and control the frequency (respiratory rate) and the depth of breathing. These centers respond

Figure 15-16 A Summary of Gas Transport and Exchange. Shown here are the events that occur in oxygen pickup from the alveoli and delivery to peripheral tissues and in carbon dioxide pickup from peripheral tissues and delivery to the alveoli.

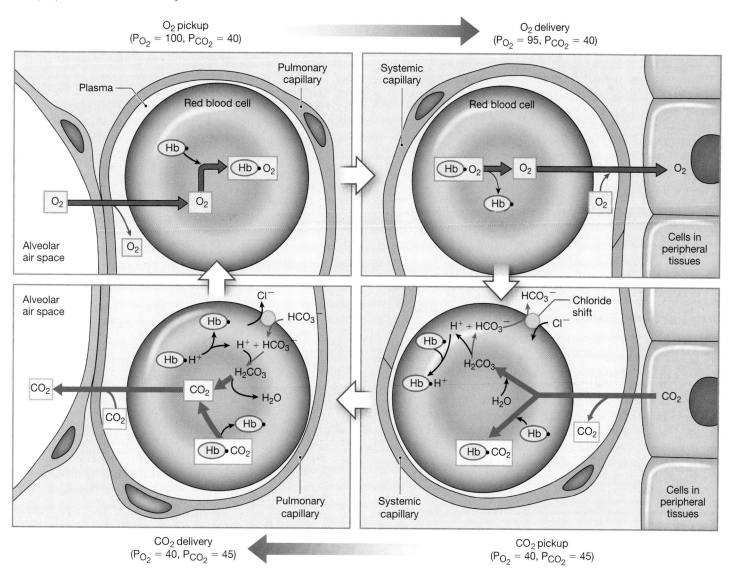

O₂ pickup
($P_{O_2} = 100$, $P_{CO_2} = 40$)

O₂ delivery
($P_{O_2} = 95$, $P_{CO_2} = 40$)

CO₂ delivery
($P_{O_2} = 40$, $P_{CO_2} = 45$)

CO₂ pickup
($P_{O_2} = 40$, $P_{CO_2} = 45$)

CLINICAL NOTE

Pulse Oximetry

The measurement of oxygen levels in the body through *pulse oximetry* has become commonplace in emergency medicine. In fact, the oxygen saturation level, as determined through pulse oximetry, is often referred to as the "fifth vital sign." A pulse oximeter measures the hemoglobin oxygen saturation in peripheral tissues. It is noninvasive, rapidly applied, and easy to operate. Pulse oximetry readings are accurate and continually reflect any changes in peripheral oxygen delivery. In fact, oximetry often detects problems with oxygenation faster than standard physical assessment techniques.

Approximately 98 percent of oxygen is transported to the peripheral tissues bound to hemoglobin. Only 2 percent of oxygen is transported dissolved in the plasma. Normally, there is a fixed

relationship between the partial pressure of oxygen and hemoglobin saturation. However, in certain disease processes, this relationship can be impaired. Pulse oximetry measures only the oxygen bound to hemoglobin.

Peripheral oxygen saturation is measured by placing a probe on a peripheral capillary bed such as the fingertip, toe, or earlobe. In infants, the sensor can be placed on the heel of the foot and secured with tape. The sensor contains two light-emitting diodes (LEDs) and two sensors (photodetectors). One LED emits light at 660 nm (red) and the other emits light at 940 nm (infrared). Photodetectors placed on the opposite side of a capillary bed (such as a fingertip) detect the amount of light transmitted through the capillary bed. The two wavelengths were chosen because one

(Continued)

is absorbed by oxyhemoglobin (hemoglobin with oxygen bound) and the other is absorbed by reduced hemoglobin (hemoglobin without oxygen bound). The amount of light absorbed by these substances is constant with time and does not vary during the cardiac cycle. A small increase in arterial blood flow occurs with each heartbeat, which results in increased light absorption. By comparing the ratio of pulsatile and baseline absorption of light at these two wavelengths, the ratio of oxyhemoglobin to reduced hemoglobin can be calculated (**Figure 15-16**). This figure is the oxygen-saturation percentage or SpO_2.

Pulse oximeters display the SpO_2 and the pulse rate as detected by the sensors. They show the SpO_2 either as a number or as a visual display that also shows the pulse's waveform. The relationship between the SpO_2 and the PaO_2 is very complex. However, the SpO_2 generally correlates with the PaO_2. The greater the PaO_2, the greater will be the oxygen saturation. Since

hemoglobin carries 98 percent of oxygen in the blood while plasma carries only 2 percent, pulse oximetry accurately analyzes peripheral oxygen delivery (**Figure 15-16**).

False readings with pulse oximetry are infrequent. When they do occur, the oximeter often generates an error signal or a blank screen. Causes of false readings include carbon monoxide poisoning, high-intensity lighting, and certain hemoglobin abnormalities. Nail polish, in certain cases, can interfere with oximetry function. This is particularly problematic with blue nail polish, which absorbs light at 960 nm, close to the wavelengths monitored by the oximeter. The absence of a pulse in an extremity also will cause a false reading. In hypovolemia and in severely anemic patients, the pulse oximetry reading can be misleading. While the SpO_2 reading may be normal, the total amount of hemoglobin available to carry oxygen may be so markedly decreased that the patient will remain hypoxic at the cellular level.

CLINICAL NOTE

Arterial Blood Gas Measurements

The partial pressure of the respiratory gases can be determined with an *arterial blood gas (ABG)* measurement. For this, a sample of arterial blood is obtained from the radial, brachial, or femoral artery. The sample is immediately placed into a blood-gas machine and measured. Most blood-gas machines will provide readings of the partial pressure of oxygen (PO_2), the partial pressure of carbon dioxide (PCO_2), the pH, the bicarbonate level (HCO_3^-), and the hemoglobin (Hg). These parameters provide a great deal of information about the efficiency of ventilation and oxygenation and will readily detect acid–base abnormalities. ABGs are an essential tool in the treatment of most severe respiratory disease processes.

to sensory information arriving from the lungs and other portions of the respiratory tract, as well as from a variety of other sites. The voluntary control of respiration reflects activity in the cerebral cortex that affects the output of the respiratory centers or of motor neurons that control respiratory muscles.

The **respiratory centers** are three pairs of nuclei in the reticular formation of the pons and medulla oblongata. The paired **respiratory rhythmicity centers** of the medulla oblongata play a key role in setting the pace for respiration. Each center can be subdivided into a *dorsal respiratory group (DRG)*, which contains an *inspiratory center*, and a *ventral respiratory group (VRG)*, which contains an *expiratory center*. Their output is adjusted by the two pairs of nuclei making up the respiratory centers of the pons. The centers in the pons adjust the respiratory rate and the depth of respiration in response to sensory stimuli, emotional states, or speech patterns.

The Activities of the Respiratory Rhythmicity Centers

Reciprocal inhibition takes place between the neurons involved with inhalation and exhalation. ⊃ p. 284 When the inspiratory neurons are active, the expiratory neurons are inhibited, and vice versa. The pattern of interaction between these groups differs between quiet breathing and forced breathing.

The DRG's inspiratory center functions in every respiratory cycle. It contains neurons that control inspiratory muscles. These muscles are the external intercostal muscles and the diaphragm. During quiet breathing, the neurons gradually increase stimulation of the inspiratory muscles for two seconds. Then the inspiratory center becomes silent for the next three seconds. During that period of inactivity, the inspiratory muscles relax and passive exhalation takes place. The inspiratory center maintains this basic rhythm even in the absence of sensory or regulatory stimuli.

The VRG functions only during forced breathing. It has an expiratory center that contains neurons that control accessory respiratory muscles involved in active exhalation. Its inspiratory center contains neurons involved in maximal inhalation, such as gasping. The relationships between the inspiratory and expiratory centers during quiet breathing and forced breathing are diagrammed in **Figure 15-17**.

Any factor that alters the metabolic or chemical activities of neural tissues can affect the performance of these respiratory centers. For example, elevated body temperature or CNS stimulants (such as amphetamines or caffeine) increase the respiratory rate. Conversely, decreased body temperature or CNS depressants (such as barbiturates or opiates) reduce the respiratory rate. Reflexes triggered by physical or chemical stimuli also strongly influence respiratory activities.

CLINICAL NOTE

Hypoxic Drive

Respiratory drive is controlled primarily by the amount of carbon dioxide in the blood (PCO_2). An increase in the PCO_2 stimulates respirations, while a fall in PCO_2 inhibits respirations. In chronic obstructive pulmonary diseases, such as emphysema or chronic bronchitis, the level of carbon dioxide in the blood gradually rises (hypercapnia). As the disease progresses, the chemoreceptors become accustomed to chronic hypercapnia. When this occurs, the body begins to rely on oxygen levels (PO_2) instead of PCO_2 levels to regulate respirations. This change, referred to as hypoxic drive, occurs only in advanced and severe disease. Administration of supplemental oxygen, which is a routine part of emergency care, can significantly increase PO_2 levels and can inhibit respirations. In severe cases, administration of high levels of supplemental oxygen can cause respiratory arrest.

The Reflex Control of Respiration

Normal breathing takes place automatically without conscious control (**Figure 15-17**). The activities of the respiratory centers are modified by sensory information from mechanoreceptors (such as stretch and pressure receptors) and chemoreceptors. Information from these receptors alters the pattern of respiration. The induced changes are called *respiratory reflexes*.

Mechanoreceptor Reflexes

Mechanoreceptors respond to changes in lung volume or to changes in arterial blood pressure. Several populations of baroreceptors are involved in respiratory function. (See Chapter 9.) ⟳ p. 343

The **inflation reflex** prevents the lungs from overexpanding during forced breathing. The mechanoreceptors involved are stretch receptors that are stimulated when the lungs expand. Sensory fibers leaving the lungs reach the respiratory rhythmicity centers through the vagus nerves. As the volume of the lungs increases, the DRG inspiratory center is gradually inhibited, and the VRG expiratory center is stimulated. Thus, inhalation stops as the lungs near maximum volume, and active exhalation then begins.

The **deflation reflex** normally only functions during forced exhalation. This reflex inhibits the expiratory center and stimulates the inspiratory center when the lungs are deflating. The smaller the volume of the lungs, the greater the inhibition of the expiratory center. Finally, exhalation stops and inhalation begins.

The inflation reflex and the deflation reflex are not involved in normal quiet breathing, but both are important in regulating forced inhalations and exhalations during strenuous exercise. Together, the inflation and deflation reflexes

Figure 15-17 Basic Regulatory Patterns of Respiration.

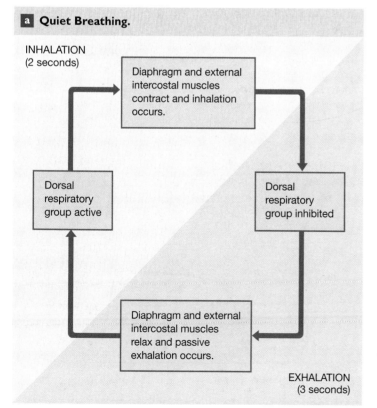

a Quiet Breathing.

INHALATION (2 seconds)

Diaphragm and external intercostal muscles contract and inhalation occurs.

Dorsal respiratory group active

Dorsal respiratory group inhibited

Diaphragm and external intercostal muscles relax and passive exhalation occurs.

EXHALATION (3 seconds)

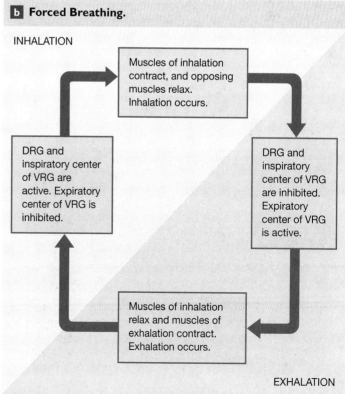

b Forced Breathing.

INHALATION

Muscles of inhalation contract, and opposing muscles relax. Inhalation occurs.

DRG and inspiratory center of VRG are active. Expiratory center of VRG is inhibited.

DRG and inspiratory center of VRG are inhibited. Expiratory center of VRG is active.

Muscles of inhalation relax and muscles of exhalation contract. Exhalation occurs.

EXHALATION

15

are known as the *Hering-Breuer reflexes*, after the physiologists who described them in 1865.

Recall that carotid and aortic baroreceptors affect systemic blood pressure (described in Chapter 13. ⊃ p. 443) The output from these baroreceptors also affects the respiratory centers.

When blood pressure falls, the respiratory rate increases. When blood pressure rises, the respiratory rate declines. This adjustment results from the stimulation or inhibition of the respiratory centers by sensory fibers in the glossopharyngeal (N IX) and vagus (N X) nerves.

CLINICAL NOTE

Capnography

End-tidal carbon dioxide (ETCO$_2$) monitoring is a non-invasive method of measuring the levels of carbon dioxide (CO$_2$) in the exhaled breath. Recordings or displays of exhaled CO$_2$ measurements are called capnography.

Various terms have been applied to capnography, and a review of them may help you to understand the material in this section. These terms include:

- *Capnometry.* Capnometry is the measurement of expired CO$_2$. It typically provides a numeric display of the partial pressure of CO$_2$ (in Torr or mmHg) or the percentage of CO$_2$ present.
- *Capnography.* Capnography is a graphic recording or display of the capnometry reading over time.
- *Capnograph.* A capnograph is a device that measures expired CO$_2$ levels.
- *Capnogram.* A capnogram is the visual representation of the expired CO$_2$ waveform.
- *ETCO$_2$.* ET CO$_2$ is the measurement of the CO$_2$ concentration at the end of expiration (maximum CO$_2$).
- *PETCO$_2$.* PETCO$_2$ is the partial pressure of end-tidal CO$_2$ in a mixed gas solution.
- *PaCO$_2$.* The PaCO$_2$ represents the partial pressure of CO$_2$ in the arterial blood.

CO$_2$ is a normal end product of metabolism and is transported by the venous system to the right side of the heart. It is then pumped from the right ventricle to the pulmonary artery and eventually enters the pulmonary capillaries. There it diffuses into the alveoli and is removed from the body through exhalation. When circulation is normal, ETCO$_2$ levels change with ventilation and are a reliable estimate of the partial pressure of carbon dioxide in the arterial system (PaCO$_2$). Normal ETCO$_2$ is 1–2 mm less than the PaCO$_2$, or approximately

5 percent. A normal PETCO$_2$ is approximately 38 mmHg (0.05×760 mmHg $= 38$ mmHg). When perfusion decreases, as occurs in shock or cardiac arrest, ETCO$_2$ levels reflect pulmonary blood flow and cardiac output, not ventilation.

Decreased ETCO$_2$ levels can be found in shock, cardiac arrest, pulmonary embolism, bronchospasm, and with incomplete airway obstruction (such as mucus plugging). Increased ETCO$_2$ levels are found with hypoventilation, respiratory depression, and hyperthermia. Capnometry provides a non-invasive measure of ETCO$_2$ levels, and provides medical personnel with information about the status of systemic metabolism, circulation, and ventilation (**Figure 15-18**). The use of capnography has become commonplace in the operating room, in the emergency department, and in the prehospital setting (**Figure 15-19**).

When first introduced into prehospital care, ETCO$_2$ monitoring was used exclusively to verify proper endotracheal tube placement in the trachea. The presence of adequate CO$_2$ levels following intubation confirms that the tube is in the trachea through the presence of exhaled CO$_2$. CO$_2$ is detected by using either a colorimetric or an infrared device.

Colorimentric Devices

The colorimetric device is a disposable ETCO$_2$ detector that contains pH-sensitive, chemically-impregnated paper encased within a plastic chamber. It is placed in the airway circuit between the patient and the ventilation device. When the paper is exposed to CO$_2$, hydrogen ions (H$^+$) are generated, which causes a color change in the paper. The color change is reversible and changes breath to breath. A color scale on the device estimates the ETCO$_2$ level. Colorimetric devices cannot detect hypercarbia or hypocarbia (increased or decreased CO$_2$ levels). If gastric contents or acidic drugs (e.g., endotracheal epinephrine) contact the paper in the device, subsequent readings may be unreliable.

FIGURE 15–18 Continuous Waveform Capnography.

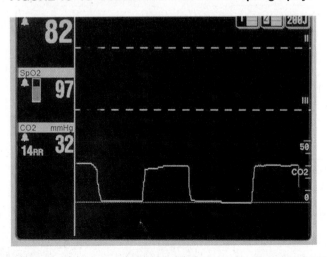

FIGURE 15–19 Normal Capnogram. AB = *Phase I:* late inspiration, early exhalation (no CO$_2$). BC = *Phase II:* appearance of CO$_2$ in exhaled gas. CD = *Phase III:* plateau (constant CO$_2$). D = highest point (ETCO$_2$). DE = *Phase IV:* rapid descent during inspiration. EA = respiratory pause.

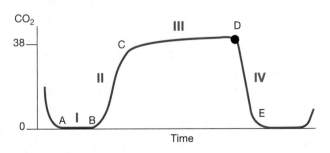

Chemoreceptor Reflexes

Chemoreceptors respond to chemical changes in the blood and cerebrospinal fluid. ⟳ p. 310 Their stimulation leads to an increase in the depth and rate of respiration. Receptors in the carotid bodies (adjacent to the carotid sinus) and the aortic bodies (near the aortic arch) are sensitive to the pH, PCO_2, and PO_2 in arterial blood. Receptors in the medulla oblongata respond to the pH and PCO_2 in cerebrospinal fluid.

Carbon dioxide levels have a much more powerful effect on respiratory activity than do oxygen levels. The reason is that a relatively small increase in arterial PCO_2 stimulates CO_2 receptors, but arterial PO_2 does not usually decline enough to activate oxygen receptors. For this reason, carbon dioxide levels are responsible for regulating respiratory activity under normal conditions. However, when arterial PO_2 does fall, the two types of receptors work together. Carbon dioxide is generated during oxygen consumption, so when O_2 concentrations are falling rapidly, CO_2 levels are usually increasing. For this reason, you cannot hold your breath "until you turn blue." Once the PCO_2 rises to critical levels, you will be forced to take a breath.

The cooperation between the carbon dioxide and oxygen receptors breaks down only under unusual circumstances. For example, you can hold your breath longer than normal by taking deep, full breaths. However, the practice is very dangerous. The danger lies in the fact that the increased ability is due not to extra oxygen, but to the loss of carbon dioxide. If the PCO_2 is reduced enough, breath-holding ability may increase to the point that you become unconscious from oxygen starvation in the brain without ever feeling the urge to breathe.

The chemoreceptors monitoring CO_2 levels are also sensitive to pH. Any condition affecting the pH of blood or cerebrospinal fluid will affect respiratory performance. For example, the rise in lactic acid levels after exercise causes a drop in pH that helps stimulate respiratory activity.

Control by Higher Centers

Higher centers influence respiration through their effects on the respiratory centers of the pons and by the direct control of respiratory muscles. For example, you can voluntarily suppress or exaggerate the contractions of respiratory muscles. This control is necessary during talking or singing. The depth and rate of respiration also change following the activation of centers involved with rage, eating, or sexual arousal. These changes, directed by the limbic system, take place at an involuntary level. **Spotlight Figure 15-20** summarizes the factors involved in the regulation of respiration.

Respiratory Changes at Birth

The respiratory systems of a fetus and a newborn differ in several important ways. Before delivery, pulmonary arterial resistance is high, because the pulmonary vessels are collapsed. The rib cage is compressed, and the lungs and conducting passageways contain only small amounts of fluid and no air.

At birth, the newborn takes a truly heroic first breath through powerful contractions of the diaphragm and the external intercostal muscles. The inhaled air enters the passageways with enough force to overcome surface tension and inflate the bronchial tree and most of the alveoli. The same drop in pressure that pulls air into the lungs pulls blood into the pulmonary circulation. The exhalation that follows fails to empty the lungs completely, because the rib cage does not return to its former, fully compressed state. Cartilages and connective tissues keep the conducting passageways open, and the surfactant covering the alveolar surfaces prevents their collapse. The next breaths complete the inflation of the alveoli.

Pathologists sometimes use these physical changes to determine whether a newborn died before delivery or shortly thereafter. Before the first breath, the lungs are completely filled with amniotic fluid, and extracted lungs will sink if placed in water. After an infant's first breath, even the collapsed lungs contain enough air to keep them afloat.

CHECKPOINT

23. Are peripheral chemoreceptors more or less sensitive to levels of carbon dioxide than they are to levels of oxygen? Why?
24. Strenuous exercise stimulates which set of respiratory reflexes?
25. Little Johnny tells his mother he will hold his breath until he turns blue and dies. Should she worry?

See the blue Answers tab at the back of the book.

15-9 Respiratory performance declines with age

Learning Objective Describe the changes in the respiratory system that occur with aging.

Many factors interact to make the respiratory system less efficient in elderly people. Here are two examples:

1. Chest movements are restricted by several changes. These include arthritic changes in rib joints, decreased

Respiratory Centers and Reflex Controls

Respiratory control involves multiple levels of regulation. Most of the regulatory activities occur outside of our awareness. This illustration shows the locations and relationships between the major respiratory centers in the pons and medulla oblongata and other factors important to the reflex control of respiration. Pathways for conscious control over respiratory muscles are not shown.

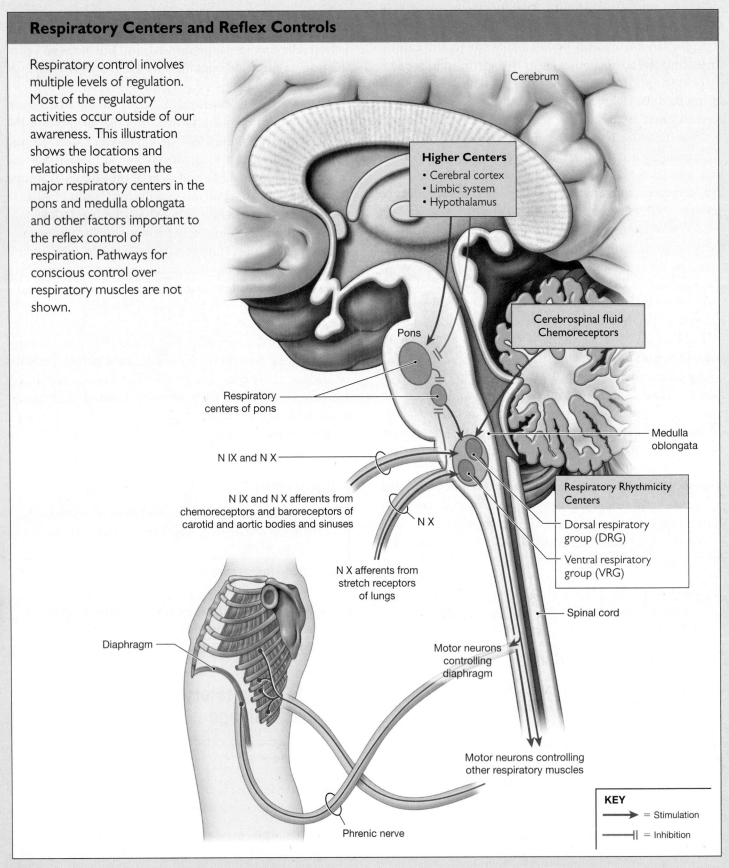

Cerebrum

Higher Centers
• Cerebral cortex
• Limbic system
• Hypothalamus

Pons

Cerebrospinal fluid Chemoreceptors

Respiratory centers of pons

Medulla oblongata

N IX and N X

N IX and N X afferents from chemoreceptors and baroreceptors of carotid and aortic bodies and sinuses

N X

Respiratory Rhythmicity Centers

Dorsal respiratory group (DRG)

Ventral respiratory group (VRG)

N X afferents from stretch receptors of lungs

Spinal cord

Diaphragm

Motor neurons controlling diaphragm

Motor neurons controlling other respiratory muscles

Phrenic nerve

KEY

→ = Stimulation

⊣⊢ = Inhibition

CLINICAL NOTE

Emphysema and Lung Cancer

Emphysema and lung cancer are two relatively common disorders. Both are often associated with cigarette smoking. Emphysema (em-fi-ZĒ-muh) is a chronic, progressive condition. It is characterized by shortness of breath and an inability to tolerate physical exertion. The underlying problem is the destruction of alveolar surfaces and inadequate surface area for gas exchange. In essence, respiratory bronchioles and alveoli no longer function. The alveoli gradually expand, and adjacent alveoli merge to form larger air spaces supported by fibrous tissue without alveolar capillary networks. As connective tissues are eliminated, compliance increases, so air moves into and out of the lungs more easily than before. However, the loss of respiratory surface area restricts oxygen absorption, so the individual becomes short of breath.

Emphysema has been linked to breathing air that contains fine particles or toxic vapors, such as those in cigarette smoke. Genetic factors also predispose individuals to the condition. Some degree of emphysema is a normal consequence of aging. An estimated 66 percent of adult males and 25 percent of adult females have detectable areas of emphysema in their lungs.

Lung cancer, or *bronchopulmonary carcinoma*, is an aggressive class of malignancies originating in the bronchial passageways or alveoli. These cancers affect the epithelial cells that line conducting passageways, mucous glands, or alveoli. Signs and symptoms generally do not appear until tumors restrict airflow or compress adjacent structures. Chest pain, shortness of breath, a cough or a wheeze, and weight loss are common. Treatment programs vary with the cellular organization of the tumor and whether metastasis (cancer cell migration) has taken place. Surgery, radiation therapy, or chemotherapy may be involved.

According to the CDC, more people die from lung cancer than any other type of cancer. In 2011, lung cancer affected an estimated 110,322 men and 97,017 women in the United States. It also accounted for 14 percent of new cancer cases in both men and women and 27 percent of all cancer deaths.

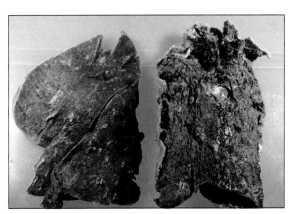

Healthy lung   Smoker's lung

---

flexibility at the costal cartilages, and age-related muscular weakness. (These restrictions counterbalance an increase in compliance of the lungs as elastic tissue deteriorates with age.) Together, the stiffening and reduction in chest movement limit pulmonary ventilation and vital capacity. These changes contribute to the decline in exercise performance and capabilities with increasing age.

2. Some degree of emphysema is normal in people over age 50. The extent varies widely with lifetime exposure to cigarette smoke and other respiratory irritants. Studies comparing nonsmokers and people who have smoked for various lengths of time clearly show the negative effects of smoking on respiratory performance.

CHECKPOINT

26. Describe two age-related changes that combine to reduce the efficiency of the respiratory system.

See the blue Answers tab at the back of the book.

15-10 The respiratory system provides oxygen to, and removes carbon dioxide from, other organ systems

Learning Objective Give examples of interactions between the respiratory system and other body systems.

Refer to Build Your Knowledge: How the RESPIRATORY SYSTEM integrates with the other body systems presented so far on p. 533. It reviews the major functional relationships between this system and the integumentary, skeletal, muscular, nervous, endocrine, cardiovascular, and lymphatic systems. Note that the respiratory system has many structural and functional connections to the cardiovascular system.

CHECKPOINT

27. Identify the key function that the respiratory system provides for all other organ systems presented so far.

28. How does the nervous system support the functions of the respiratory system?

See the blue Answers tab at the back of the book.

15

Build Your Knowledge

How the RESPIRATORY SYSTEM integrates with the other body systems presented so far

Integumentary System

- The integumentary system protects portions of upper respiratory tract; hairs guard entry to external nares

- The respiratory system provides oxygen to nourish tissues and removes carbon dioxide

Endocrine System

- The endocrine system produces epinephrine and norepinephrine, which stimulate respiratory activity and dilate respiratory passageways

- The respiratory system produces angiotensin-converting enzyme (ACE) from capillaries in the lungs. ACE converts angiotensin I to angiotensin II

Skeletal System

- The skeletal system protects the lungs with its axial division; movements of the rib cage are important in breathing

- The respiratory system provides oxygen to skeletal structures and disposes of carbon dioxide

Muscular System

- The muscular system controls the entrances to the respiratory tract; intrinsic laryngeal muscles control airflow through larynx and produce sounds; respiratory muscles change thoracic cavity volume so air moves into and out of lungs

- The respiratory system provides oxygen needed for muscle contractions and disposes of carbon dioxide generated by active muscles

Nervous System

- The nervous system monitors respiratory volume and blood gas levels; controls pace and depth of respiration

- The respiratory system provides oxygen needed for neural activity and disposes of carbon dioxide

Lymphatic System

- The lymphatic system protects against infection with tonsils at entrance to respiratory tract; lymph nodes monitor lymph drainage from lungs and provide specific defenses when infection occurs

- The respiratory system has alveolar macrophages that provide nonspecific defenses; mucous membrane lining the upper respiratory system traps pathogens and protects deeper tissues

Cardiovascular System

- The cardiovascular system circulates the red blood cells that transport oxygen and carbon dioxide between lungs and peripheral tissues

- The respiratory system provides oxygen needed for heart muscle contraction; bicarbonate ions contribute to the buffering capacity of blood; activation of angiotensin II by ACE is important in regulation of blood pressure and blood volume

Respiratory System

The respiratory system provides oxygen and eliminates carbon dioxide for our cells.
It:
- provides a large area for gas exchange between air and circulating blood
- moves air to and from the gas-exchange surfaces of the lungs along the respiratory passageways
- protects the respiratory surfaces from dehydration, temperature changes, and defends against invading pathogens
- produces sounds for speaking, singing, and other forms of communication
- aids the sense of smell by the olfactory receptors in the nasal cavity

15

RELATED CLINICAL TERMS

apnea (AP-nē-uh): The cessation of breathing.

asphyxia: Impaired oxygen–carbon dioxide exchange that results in suffocation.

asthma (AZ-muh): An acute respiratory disorder characterized by unusually sensitive, irritated conducting airways.

bronchitis (brong-KĪ-tis): Inflammation of the bronchial lining.

cardiopulmonary resuscitation (CPR): The application of cycles of compression to the rib cage and mouth-to-mouth breathing to restore cardiovascular and respiratory function.

chronic obstructive pulmonary disease (COPD): A general term describing temporary or permanent lung disease of the bronchial tree; characterized by chronic bronchitis and chronic airway obstruction.

dyspnea (DISP-nē-uh): Difficult or labored breathing.

epistaxis (ep-i-STAK-sis): A nosebleed.

hypercapnia (hī-per-KAP-nē-uh): An abnormally high level of carbon dioxide in the blood.

hypocapnia: An abnormally low level of carbon dioxide in the blood.

influenza: A viral infection of the respiratory tract; "the flu."

pleurisy: Inflammation of the pleurae and secretion of excess amounts of pleural fluid.

sputum: A mixture of saliva and mucus coughed up from the respiratory tract, often as a result of infection.

15 Chapter Review

Summary Outline

An Introduction to the Respiratory System *p. 576*

1. To continue functioning, body cells must obtain oxygen and eliminate carbon dioxide. These processes take place in **alveoli**, air-filled pockets in the lungs.

15-1 The respiratory system, composed of air-conducting and respiratory portions, has several basic functions *p. 576*

2. The functions of the **respiratory system** include (1) providing an area for gas exchange between air and circulating blood; (2) moving air to and from exchange surfaces; (3) protecting exchange surfaces from dehydration, temperature changes, and pathogens; (4) producing sound for speaking; and (5) aiding the stimulation of olfactory (smell) receptors.

3. The respiratory system includes the **upper respiratory system**, composed of the nose, a nasal cavity, paranasal sinuses, and pharynx, and the **lower respiratory system**, which includes the larynx, trachea, bronchi, bronchioles, and alveoli of the lungs *(Figure 15-1).*

4. The **respiratory tract** consists of the conducting passageways that carry air to and from the alveoli.

5. The **respiratory mucosa** (respiratory epithelium and underlying areolar tissue) lines the conducting portion of the respiratory tract *(Figure 15-2).*

15-2 The nose, pharynx, larynx, trachea, bronchi, and larger bronchioles conduct air into the lungs *p. 578*

6. Air normally enters the respiratory system through the **external nares**, which open into the **nasal cavity**. The **nasal vestibule** (entrance) is guarded by hairs that screen out large particles *(Figure 15-3).*

7. The **hard palate** separates the oral and nasal cavities. The **soft palate** separates the superior nasopharynx from the rest of the pharynx. The **internal nares** connect the nasal cavity and nasopharynx *(Figure 15-3).*

8. The **pharynx** (throat) is a chamber shared by the digestive and respiratory systems.

9. Inhaled air passes through the glottis on its way to the lungs. The **larynx** surrounds and protects the glottis, or "voicebox." The **epiglottis** projects into the pharynx. The **glottis** includes the **true vocal cords** and the space between them. Exhaled air passing through the glottis vibrates the true vocal cords and produces sound *(Figure 15-4).*

10. The wall of the **trachea** ("windpipe") contains C-shaped tracheal cartilages, which protect the airway. The posterior tracheal wall can distort to permit large masses of food to pass along the esophagus *(Figure 15-5).*

11. The trachea branches within the mediastinum to form the **right** and **left primary bronchi** *(Figure 15-5).*

12. The primary bronchi, **secondary bronchi**, and their branches form the *bronchial tree*. As the **tertiary bronchi** branch within the lung, the amount of cartilage in their walls decreases, and the amount of smooth muscle increases *(Figure 15-6a).*

15-3 The smallest bronchioles and the alveoli within the lungs make up the respiratory portion of the respiratory tract *p. 584*

13. Each terminal **bronchiole** delivers air to a single pulmonary **lobule.** Within the lobule, the terminal bronchiole branches into *respiratory bronchioles (Figure 15-6b).*

15

14. The respiratory bronchioles open into **alveolar ducts**, which end at **alveolar sacs.** Many alveoli are interconnected at each alveolar sac *(Figure 15-7a,b).*

15. The **respiratory membrane** consists of (1) a simple squamous alveolar epithelium, (2) a capillary endothelium, and (3) their fused basement membranes. The alveolar squamous cells are also called *type I pneumocytes.* **Septal cells** *(type II pneumocytes)* produce **surfactant**, an oily secretion that keeps the alveoli from collapsing. **Alveolar macrophages** engulf foreign particles *(Figure 15-7c,d).*

16. The **lungs** are made up of five **lobes**: three in the right lung and two in the left lung *(Figure 15-8).*

17. Each lung is enclosed by a single pleural cavity lined by a **pleura** (serous membrane) *(Figure 15-9).*

15-4 External respiration and internal respiration allow gas exchange within the body p. 589

18. *Respiration* involves two integrated processes: **external respiration** (the exchange of oxygen and carbon dioxide between interstitial fluid and the external environment) and **internal respiration** (the exchange of oxygen and carbon dioxide between interstitial fluid and cells). If the oxygen content declines, the affected tissues suffer from **hypoxia**; if the oxygen supply is completely shut off, **anoxia** and tissue death result.

19. External respiration includes *pulmonary ventilation*, or breathing (movement of air into and out of the lungs); *gas diffusion* between the alveoli and circulating blood, and between the blood and interstitial fluids; and *transport of oxygen and carbon dioxide* between the alveolar capillaries and capillary beds in other tissues by the bloodstream.

15-5 Pulmonary ventilation—the exchange of air between the atmosphere and the lungs—involves pressure changes and muscle movement p. 590

20. A single breath, or **respiratory cycle**, consists of an inhalation *(inspiration)* and an exhalation *(expiration).*

21. The difference between the pressure inside the respiratory tract and atmospheric pressure determines the direction of airflow *(Spotlight Figure 15-12).*

22. The primary respiratory muscles (the diaphragm and the external intercostal muscles) are involved in *quiet breathing*, in which exhalation is passive. Accessory respiratory muscles become active during the active inhalation and exhalation movements of *forced breathing*, in which exhalation is active *(Spotlight Figure 15-12).*

23. The **vital capacity** includes the **tidal volume** plus the **expiratory reserve volume** and the **inspiratory reserve volume.** The air left in the lungs at the end of maximum expiration is the **residual volume** *(Figure 15-13).*

15-6 Gas exchange depends on the partial pressures of gases and the diffusion of molecules p. 596

24. In a mixed gas, the individual gases exert a pressure proportional to their abundance in the mixture. The pressure contributed by a single gas is its **partial pressure**.

25. Alveolar air and atmospheric air differ in composition. Gas exchange occurs efficiently across the respiratory membrane *(Figure 15-14; Table 15-1).*

15-7 Most O_2 is transported bound to hemoglobin (Hb), and CO_2 is dissolved in plasma, bound to Hb, or transported as bicarbonate ion p. 599

26. Blood entering peripheral capillaries delivers oxygen and takes up carbon dioxide. The transport of oxygen and carbon dioxide in the blood involves reactions that are completely reversible.

27. Over the range of oxygen pressures normally present in the body, a small change in plasma will result in a large change in the amount of oxygen bound or released by hemoglobin.

28. Aerobic metabolism in peripheral tissues generates carbon dioxide. Roughly 7 percent of the CO_2 transported in the blood is dissolved in the plasma; another 23 percent is bound as **carbaminohemoglobin** in RBCs; and 70 percent is converted to carbonic acid, which dissociates into a hydrogen ion and a bicarbonate ion. The bicarbonate ion exits the RBC and enters the plasma *(Figures 15-15, 15-16).*

15-8 Neurons in the medulla oblongata and pons, along with respiratory reflexes, control respiration p. 602

29. Large-scale changes in oxygen demand require the integration of cardiovascular and respiratory responses.

30. Arterioles leading to alveolar capillaries constrict when oxygen is low, and bronchioles dilate when carbon dioxide is high.

31. The **respiratory centers** include three pairs of nuclei in the reticular formation of the pons and medulla oblongata. These nuclei regulate the respiratory muscles and control the respiratory rate and the depth of breathing. The paired **respiratory rhythmicity centers** in the medulla oblongata set the basic pace for respiration. Each center has a *dorsal respiratory group (DRG)*, with an *inspiratory center*, and a *ventral respiratory group (VRG)*, with an *expiratory center* *(Figure 15-17, Spotlight Figure 15-20).*

32. The **inflation reflex** prevents overexpansion of the lungs during forced breathing; the **deflation reflex** stimulates inhalation when the lungs are deflating. Chemoreceptor reflexes respond to changes in the pH, PCO_2, and PO_2 of the blood and cerebrospinal fluid *(Spotlight Figure 15-20).*

33. Conscious and unconscious thought processes can affect respiration by affecting the respiratory centers or the motor neurons controlling respiratory muscles.

15

34. Before delivery, the fetal lungs are fluid filled and collapsed. After the first breath, the alveoli normally remain inflated for the life of the individual.

15-9 Respiratory performance declines with age p. 607

35. The respiratory system is generally less efficient in elderly people because (1) movements of the thoracic cage are restricted by arthritic changes, decreased flexibility of costal cartilages, and age-related muscle weakness, lowering

pulmonary ventilation and vital capacity of the lungs; and (2) some degree of emphysema is normal in elderly people.

15-10 The respiratory system provides oxygen to, and removes carbon dioxide from, other organ systems p. 609

36. The respiratory system has extensive anatomical and physiological connections to the cardiovascular system.

Review Questions
See the blue Answers tab at the back of the book.

Level 1 Reviewing Facts and Terms

Match each item in column A with the most closely related item in column B. Place letters for answers in the spaces provided.

COLUMN A

_____ **1.** Nasopharynx
_____ **2.** Laryngopharynx
_____ **3.** Thyroid cartilage
_____ **4.** Septal cells
_____ **5.** Dust cells
_____ **6.** Parietal pleura
_____ **7.** Visceral pleura
_____ **8.** Hypoxia
_____ **9.** Anoxia
_____ **10.** Collapsed lung
_____ **11.** Inhalation
_____ **12.** Exhalation

COLUMN B

a. No O_2 supply to tissues
b. Alveolar macrophages
c. Produce oily secretion
d. Covers inner surface of thoracic body wall
e. Low O_2 content in tissue fluids
f. Inferior portion of pharynx
g. Inspiration
h. Superior portion of pharynx
i. Adam's apple
j. Covers outer surface of lungs
k. Expiration
l. Atelectasis

13. Identify the structures of the respiratory system in the following figure:

(a) _____
(b) _____
(c) _____
(d) _____
(e) _____
(f) _____
(g) _____
(h) _____
(i) _____

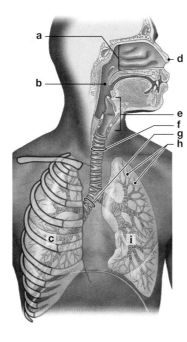

14. Identify the structures in the following figure:

(a) _____
(b) _____
(c) _____
(d) _____
(e) _____

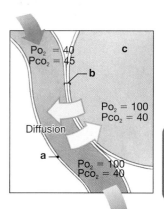

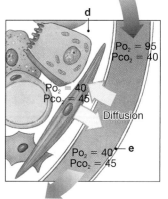

15

Label the pink and light blue arrows in the upper and lower portions of the figure to indicate the directions of the diffusion of oxygen and carbon dioxide.

15. The structure that prevents the entry of liquids or solid food into the respiratory passageways during swallowing is the
    (a) glottis.
    (b) arytenoid cartilage.
    (c) epiglottis.
    (d) thyroid cartilage.

16. The amount of air moved into or out of the lungs during a single respiratory cycle is the
    (a) respiratory rate.
    (b) tidal volume.
    (c) residual volume.
    (d) inspiratory capacity.

Level 2 Reviewing Concepts

17. When the diaphragm contracts, it tenses and moves inferiorly, causing
    (a) an increase in the volume of the thoracic cavity.
    (b) a decrease in the volume of the thoracic cavity.
    (c) decreased pressure on the contents of the abdominopelvic cavity.
    (d) increased pressure in the thoracic cavity.

18. Gas exchange at the respiratory membrane is efficient because
    (a) the differences in partial pressure are substantial.
    (b) the gases are lipid soluble.
    (c) the total surface area is large.
    (d) a, b, and c are correct.

19. What is the functional significance of the decreased amount of cartilage and the increased amount of smooth muscle in the lower respiratory passageways?

20. Why is breathing through the nasal cavity more desirable than breathing through the mouth?

21. How would you justify the statement "The bronchioles are to the respiratory system what the arterioles are to the cardiovascular system"?

Level 3 Critical Thinking and Clinical Applications

22. Individuals who are anemic generally do not exhibit an increase in respiratory rate or tidal volume, even though their blood is not carrying enough oxygen. Why?

23. You spend a winter night at a friend's house. Your friend's home is quite old, and the hot-air furnace lacks a humidifier. When you wake up in the morning, you have a fair amount of nasal congestion and decide you might be coming down with a cold. After you take a steamy shower and drink some juice for breakfast, the nasal congestion disappears. Explain.

15

The Digestive System

Learning Objectives

These Learning Objectives tell you what you should be able to do after completing the chapter. They correspond by number to this chapter's sections.

16-1 Identify the organs of the digestive system, list their major functions, and describe the four layers of the wall of the digestive tract.

16-2 Discuss the anatomy of the oral cavity, and list the functions of its major structures.

16-3 Describe the structures and functions of the pharynx and esophagus, and the key events of the swallowing process.

16-4 Describe the anatomy of the stomach, including its histology, and discuss its roles in digestion and absorption.

16-5 Describe the anatomy of the small intestine, including its histology, and explain the functions and regulation of intestinal secretions.

16-6 Describe the structure and functions of the pancreas, liver, and gallbladder, and explain how their activities are regulated.

16-7 Describe the structure of the large intestine, including its regional specializations, and list its absorptive functions.

16-8 List the nutrients required by the body, describe the chemical digestion of organic nutrients, and discuss the absorption of organic and inorganic nutrients.

16-9 Summarize the effects of aging on the digestive system.

16-10 Give examples of interactions between the digestive system and other body systems presented so far.

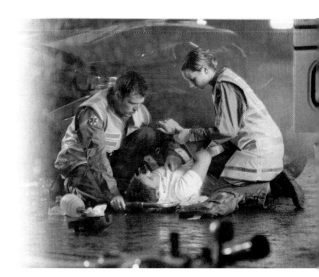

An Introduction to the Digestive System

Few people give any serious thought to the digestive system unless it malfunctions. Still, we spend hours filling and emptying it. We often refer to this system in our everyday language. We "have a gut feeling," "want to chew on" something, or find someone's opinions "hard to swallow." When something does go wrong with the digestive system, even something minor, most people seek immediate relief. For this reason, every hour of television programming contains advertisements for toothpaste and mouthwash, dietary supplements, antacids, and laxatives.

All living organisms must obtain nutrients from their environment to sustain life. These substances serve as raw materials for synthesizing essential compounds (anabolism). They are also broken down to provide the energy that cells need to continue functioning (catabolism). ↺ pp. 31–33, 207–209

In this chapter, we discuss the structure and function of the digestive tract and several digestive glands, notably the liver and pancreas, and the process of digestion.

Build Your Knowledge

Recall that the digestive system processes food and absorbs nutrients (as you saw in **Chapter 1: An Introduction to Anatomy and Physiology**). Nutrients are the substances from food that are necessary for normal physiological functions. They include carbohydrates, proteins, fats, vitamins, minerals, and water. ↺ **pp. 9, 34**

16-1 The digestive system—the digestive tract and accessory organs—performs various food-processing functions

Learning Objective Identify the organs of the digestive system, list their major functions, and describe the four layers of the wall of the digestive tract.

In our bodies, the digestive system provides the fuel that keeps all the body's cells functioning. It also provides the building blocks needed for cell growth and repair. The respiratory system works with the cardiovascular system to supply the oxygen needed to "burn" metabolic fuels (catabolism).

The **digestive system** consists of a muscular tube, the **digestive tract**, and various **accessory organs**. The digestive tract is also called the *gastrointestinal (GI) tract* or *alimentary canal*. It begins with the oral cavity (mouth) and continues through the pharynx (throat), esophagus, stomach, small intestine, and large intestine. It ends at the rectum and anus. These subdivisions of the digestive tract have overlapping functions, but each region has certain areas of specialization and shows distinctive histological specializations.

Accessory digestive organs include the teeth, tongue, and glandular organs such as the salivary glands, liver, and pancreas, as well as the gallbladder, which only has a secretory function. Secretions of the glandular organs and the gallbladder enter ducts that empty into the digestive tract. The major components of the digestive system are shown in **Figure 16-1**.

Functions of the Digestive System

Digestive functions involve six related processes:

1. **Ingestion** takes place when food and drink enter the oral cavity (mouth) of the digestive tract.

2. **Mechanical processing** is the crushing and shearing that makes solid foods easier to propel along the digestive tract. It also increases their surface area, making them more susceptible to attack by enzymes. The tongue and the teeth in the oral cavity begin the process. Swirling, mixing, and churning motions of the stomach and intestines provide mechanical processing after ingestion.

3. **Digestion** refers to the chemical breakdown of food into small organic fragments that can be absorbed by the digestive epithelium.

4. **Secretion** is the release of water, acids, enzymes, and buffers by the epithelium of the digestive tract, glandular organs, and the gallbladder.

5. **Absorption** is the movement of small organic molecules, electrolytes (inorganic ions), vitamins, and water across the digestive epithelium and into the interstitial fluid of the digestive tract.

6. **Excretion** is the removal of waste from the body. Within the digestive tract, waste products from glandular and secretory organs mix with indigestible materials of the digestive process and leave the body. These waste products are ejected from the digestive tract as *feces* through the process of *defecation* (def-e-KĀ-shun).

16

Figure 16-1 The Components of the Digestive System.

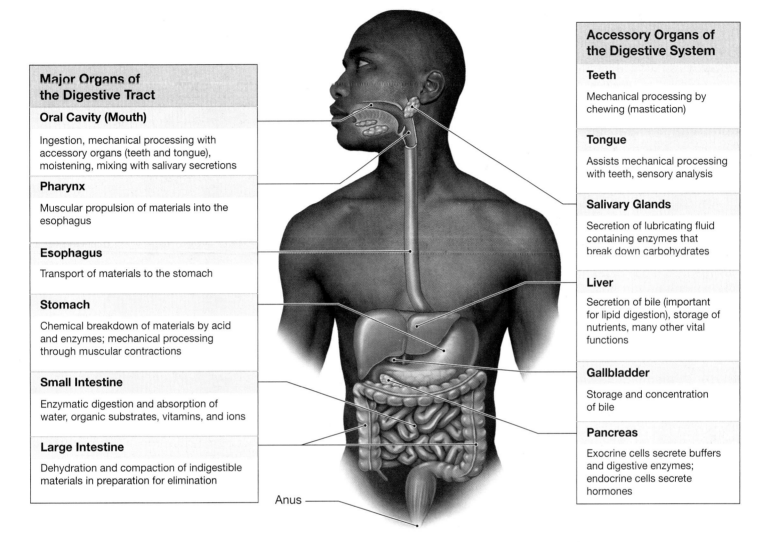

**Major Organs of
the Digestive Tract**

Oral Cavity (Mouth)

Ingestion, mechanical processing with accessory organs (teeth and tongue), moistening, mixing with salivary secretions

Pharynx

Muscular propulsion of materials into the esophagus

Esophagus

Transport of materials to the stomach

Stomach

Chemical breakdown of materials by acid and enzymes; mechanical processing through muscular contractions

Small Intestine

Enzymatic digestion and absorption of water, organic substrates, vitamins, and ions

Large Intestine

Dehydration and compaction of indigestible materials in preparation for elimination

Anus

**Accessory Organs of
the Digestive System**

Teeth

Mechanical processing by chewing (mastication)

Tongue

Assists mechanical processing with teeth, sensory analysis

Salivary Glands

Secretion of lubricating fluid containing enzymes that break down carbohydrates

Liver

Secretion of bile (important for lipid digestion), storage of nutrients, many other vital functions

Gallbladder

Storage and concentration of bile

Pancreas

Exocrine cells secrete buffers and digestive enzymes; endocrine cells secrete hormones

The lining of the digestive tract also plays a defensive role. It protects surrounding tissues from (1) the corrosive effects of digestive acids and enzymes, (2) physical stresses, such as abrasion, and (3) bacteria that either are swallowed with food or reside in the digestive tract. The digestive epithelium and its secretions provide a nonspecific defense against these bacteria. When bacteria reach the underlying tissues, macrophages and other cells of the immune system attack them. ⤴ pp. 481, 487

Histological Organization of the Digestive Tract

The digestive tract has four major layers: the *mucosa*, the *submucosa*, the *muscularis externa*, and the *serosa* (**Figure 16-2**).

The Mucosa

The **mucosa**, or inner lining of the digestive tract, is a *mucous membrane*. ⤴ p. 110 It consists of an epithelium moistened by glandular secretions, called the mucosal epithelium, and an underlying layer of areolar tissue, the *lamina propria*. Along most of the length of the digestive tract, the mucosa has permanent transverse *circular folds*. The folding increases the surface area available for absorption. In the small intestine, the mucosa forms fingerlike projections, called *villi* (*villus*, shaggy hair), that further increase the area for absorption.

The oral cavity, pharynx, esophagus, and anus (where mechanical stresses are most severe) are lined by a stratified squamous epithelium. The remainder of the digestive tract is lined by a simple columnar epithelium, often containing various types of secretory cells. Ducts opening onto the epithelial surfaces carry the secretions of glands located in the lamina propria, in the surrounding submucosa, or within accessory secretory organs.

In most regions of the digestive tract, the outer portion of the mucosa contains a narrow band of smooth muscle and elastic fibers. The circular folds and villi are moved by

Figure 16-2 The Structure of the Digestive Tract. A diagrammatic view of a representative portion of the digestive tract. The features illustrated are typical of the small intestine. The wall of the digestive tract is made up of four layers: the mucosa, submucosa, muscularis externa, and serosa.

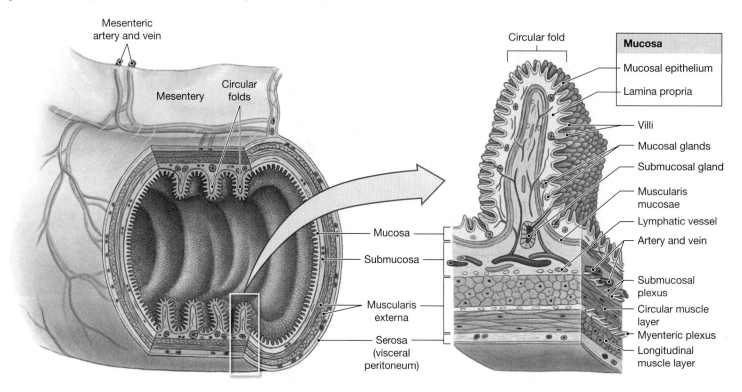

contractions of this layer, called the *muscularis* (mus-kū-LA-ris) *mucosae* (mū-KŌ-sē) (**Figure 16-2**).

The Submucosa

The **submucosa** is a layer of dense irregular connective tissue that binds the mucosa to the muscularis externa. The submucosa contains numerous blood vessels and lymphatic vessels. Along its outer margin, it contains a network of nerve fibers, sensory neurons, and parasympathetic motor neurons. This neural network is the *submucosal plexus*. It is involved in controlling contractions of the smooth muscle in the muscularis mucosae. It is also involved in regulating the secretion of digestive glands.

The Muscularis Externa

The **muscularis externa** is a band of smooth muscle cells arranged in an inner circular layer and an outer longitudinal layer (**Figure 16-2**). Contractions of these layers in various combinations both agitate and propel materials along the digestive tract. Both actions are controlled primarily by another network of nerves, called the *myenteric plexus* (*mys*, muscle + *enteron*, intestine). It lies sandwiched between the circular and longitudinal smooth muscle layers. The myenteric plexus

contains parasympathetic ganglia, sensory neurons, interneurons, and sympathetic postganglionic fibers. Parasympathetic stimulation increases muscular tone and activity. Sympathetic stimulation promotes muscular inhibition and relaxation.

The Serosa

The **serosa**, a serous membrane, covers the muscularis externa along most portions of the digestive tract enclosed by the peritoneal cavity. This *visceral peritoneum* is continuous with the *parietal peritoneum*, which lines the inner surfaces of the body wall. ↻ p. 111 In some areas within the peritoneal cavity, portions of the digestive tract are suspended by **mesenteries** (MEZ-en-ter-ēz). Mesenteries are double sheets of serous membrane composed of the parietal peritoneum and visceral peritoneum. The loose connective tissue sandwiched between the epithelial surfaces of the mesenteries provides a pathway for the blood vessels, nerves, and lymphatic vessels servicing the digestive tract. The mesenteries also stabilize the positions of the attached organs. They prevent the intestines from becoming entangled during digestive movements or sudden changes in body position.

There is no serosa covering the muscularis externa of the oral cavity, pharynx, esophagus, and rectum. Instead, the

16

muscularis externa is surrounded by dense connective tissue with collagen fibers that firmly attaches these regions of the digestive tract to adjacent structures. This fibrous wrapping is called an *adventitia* (ad-ven-TISH-uh).

Build Your Knowledge

Recall that smooth muscle is found within almost every organ, forming sheets, bundles, and sheaths around other tissues (as you saw in **Chapter 7: The Muscular System**). Smooth muscle cells are able to contract over a greater range of lengths than skeletal or cardiac muscle. This ability is important in organs that undergo large changes in volume, such as the stomach. In addition, many smooth muscles are not innervated by motor neurons. Instead, they contract either automatically (in response to pacesetter cells) or in response to environmental or hormonal stimulation. ⊃ **pp. 212, 213**

The Movement of Digestive Materials

Recall that the muscular layers of the digestive tract consist of smooth muscle tissue. *Pacesetter cells* in the smooth muscle of the digestive tract trigger waves of contraction, making rhythmic cycles of activity. The coordinated contractions in the walls of the digestive tract play a vital role in two processes: *peristalsis* (*peri-*, around + *stalsis*, constriction) and *segmentation*. Peristalsis refers to the movement of material along the tract. Segmentation is the mechanical mixing of the material.

The muscularis externa propels materials from one part of the digestive tract to another by means of **peristalsis** (per-i-STAL-sis), waves of muscular contractions that move along

CLINICAL NOTE

Ascites

The peritoneal lining continuously produces peritoneal fluid, which lubricates the opposing parietal and visceral surfaces. Even though about seven liters of fluid is secreted and reabsorbed each day, the volume within the cavity at any moment is very small. Several conditions, including liver disease, kidney disease, and heart failure, can cause an increase in the rate of fluid movement into the peritoneal cavity. The resulting accumulation of fluid creates a characteristic abdominal swelling called *ascites* (a-SĪ-tēz). The distortion of internal organs by the accumulated fluid can result in symptoms such as heartburn, indigestion, and low back pain.

the digestive tract (**Figure 16-3**). During a peristaltic movement, the circular muscles first contract behind the digestive contents, such as a *bolus* (food mass). Then longitudinal muscles contract, shortening adjacent segments of the tract. A wave of contraction in the circular muscles then forces the materials in the desired direction.

Figure 16-3 Peristalsis. Peristalsis propels materials along the length of the digestive tract.

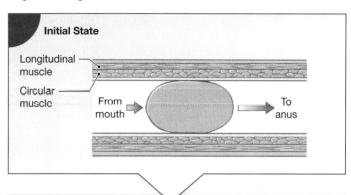
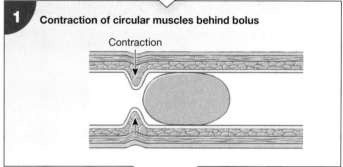
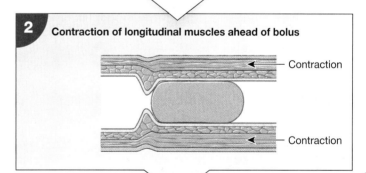
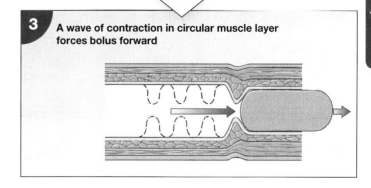

16

Regions of the small intestine also carry out **segmentation**, movements that churn and break up digestive materials. Over time, this action thoroughly mixes the contents with intestinal secretions. Because segmentation movements do not follow a set pattern, they do not propel materials in any particular direction.

CHECKPOINT

1. Identify the organs of the digestive system.

2. List and define the six primary functions of the digestive system.

3. Describe the functions of the mesenteries.

4. Name the layers of the digestive tract from superficial to deep.

5. Which is more efficient in propelling intestinal contents from one place to another—peristalsis or segmentation?

See the blue Answers tab at the back of the book.

16-2 The oral cavity contains the tongue, salivary glands, and teeth, each with specific functions

Learning Objective Discuss the anatomy of the oral cavity, and list the functions of its major structures.

The **oral cavity** (mouth), or **buccal (BUK-ul) cavity**, is the part of the digestive tract that receives food. The oral cavity is lined by the *oral mucosa*, which has a stratified squamous epithelium. The oral cavity (1) senses and analyzes food before swallowing; (2) mechanically processes food through the actions of the teeth, tongue, and surfaces of the palate; (3) lubricates food by mixing it with mucus and salivary gland secretions; and (4) begins limited digestion of carbohydrates and lipids with salivary enzymes.

The boundaries of the oral cavity are shown in **Figure 16-4**. The mucosae of the *cheeks*, or lateral walls of the oral cavity, are supported by pads of fat and the buccinator muscles. Anteriorly, the mucosa of each cheek is continuous with that of the lips, or **labia** (LĀ-bē-uh; singular, *labium*). The **vestibule** is the space between the cheeks (or lips) and the teeth. The **gingivae** (JIN-ji-vē; singular, *gingiva*), or gums, are pink ridges of oral mucosae that surround the bases of the teeth. They cover the tooth-bearing surfaces of the upper and lower jaws.

The **hard palate** and **soft palate** form the roof for the oral cavity. The tongue dominates its floor. The free anterior portion of the tongue is connected to the oral cavity floor by a thin fold of mucous membrane, the **lingual frenulum** (FREN-ū-lum; *frenulum*, a small bridle). The imaginary dividing line between the oral cavity and the oropharynx extends between the base of the tongue and the dangling *uvula* (Ū-vū-luh). The uvula helps prevent food from entering the pharynx too soon.

Figure 16-4 The Oral Cavity.

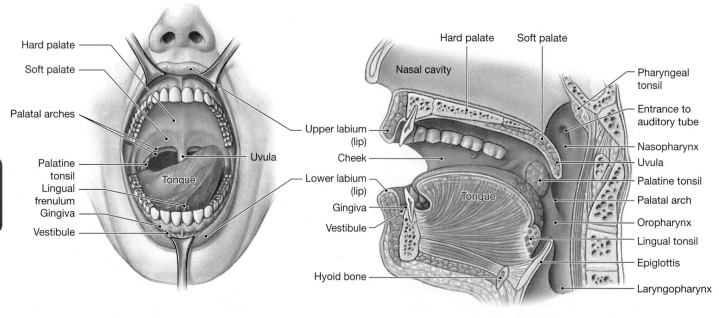

a An anterior view of the oral cavity, as seen through the open mouth.

b Sagittal section of the oral cavity.

The Tongue

The muscular **tongue** manipulates materials inside the mouth and is occasionally used to bring foods (such as ice cream) into the oral cavity. The primary functions of the tongue are (1) mechanical processing by compression, abrasion, and distortion; (2) manipulation to assist in chewing and to prepare food for swallowing; and (3) sensory analysis by touch, temperature, and taste receptors. Small glands under the tongue secrete the enzyme lingual lipase. This enzyme begins lipid digestion in the oral cavity. Most of the tongue lies within the oral cavity, but the base of the tongue extends into the oropharynx. A pair of prominent lateral swellings at the base of the tongue marks the location of the *lingual tonsils*, clusters of lymphoid nodules that help resist infections. ⊃ pp. 476, 478

Salivary Glands

Three pairs of salivary glands secrete into the oral cavity (**Figure 16-5**). On each side, a large **parotid salivary gland** lies under the skin covering the lateral and posterior surface of the mandible. ⊃ p. 160 The **parotid duct** empties into the vestibule at the level of the second upper molar. The **sublingual salivary glands** are located beneath the mucous membrane of the floor of the mouth. Numerous sublingual ducts open along either side of the lingual frenulum. The **submandibular salivary glands** are in the floor of the mouth along the inner surfaces of the mandible.

Figure 16-5 The Salivary Glands. This lateral view shows the relative positions of the salivary glands and ducts on the left side of the head. For clarity, the left ramus and body of the mandible have been removed.

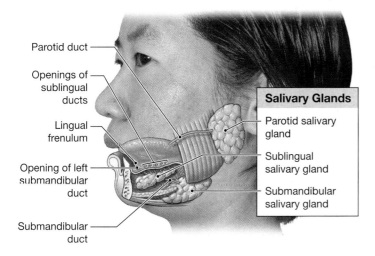

Their ducts open into the mouth behind the teeth on either side of the lingual frenulum.

These salivary glands produce 1.0–1.5 liters of saliva each day. What makes up saliva? Saliva is 99.4 percent water, plus *mucins* and an assortment of ions, buffers, waste products, metabolites, and enzymes. Mucins are glycoproteins that absorb water and form mucus. Buffers in the saliva keep the pH of your mouth near 7. They prevent the buildup of acids produced by bacteria. At mealtimes, large quantities of saliva lubricate the mouth and dissolve chemicals that stimulate the taste buds. Coating the food with slippery mucus reduces friction and makes swallowing possible.

A continuous background level of secretion flushes and cleans the oral surfaces. Salivary antibodies (IgA) and *lysozyme* help control populations of oral bacteria. A reduction or loss of salivary secretions—caused by radiation, emotional distress, certain drugs, sleep, or other factors—triggers a bacterial population explosion. Recurring infections and the progressive erosion of the teeth and gums result.

Each of the salivary glands produces a slightly different kind of saliva. The parotid glands produce a secretion rich in **salivary amylase**, an enzyme that breaks down starches (complex carbohydrates) into smaller molecules that can be absorbed by the digestive tract. Saliva from the submandibular and sublingual salivary glands contains fewer enzymes but more buffers and mucus.

During eating, all three salivary glands increase their rates of secretion. Salivary production may reach 7 mL per minute, with about 70 percent of that volume provided by the submandibular glands. The autonomic nervous system normally controls salivary secretion.

CLINICAL NOTE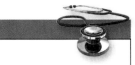

Salivary Gland Disorders

Salivary gland disorders usually cause pain and swelling of the affected gland. Infections of the salivary glands (*siloadenitis*) are the most common disorders and can be either viral or bacterial. Mumps is the most common viral infection and primarily occurs in children. Bacterial infections are seen most frequently in dehydrated or debilitated patients and often result from slowing of the flow of saliva. Stones (*salivary calculi*) can develop in the salivary glands and can block the flow of saliva through the duct, which results in gland enlargement. Treatment includes the use of substances such as hard lemon-drop candy to increase salivary flow.

Figure 16-6 Teeth: Structural Components and Dental Succession.

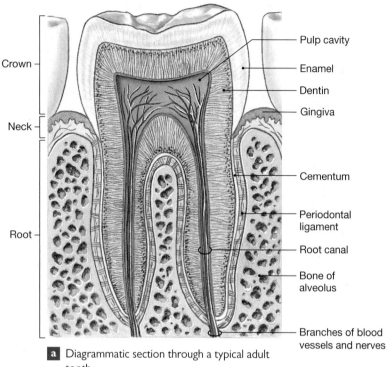

Crown — Neck — Root

— Pulp cavity
— Enamel
— Dentin
— Gingiva

— Cementum

— Periodontal ligament
— Root canal

— Bone of alveolus

— Branches of blood vessels and nerves

a Diagrammatic section through a typical adult tooth.

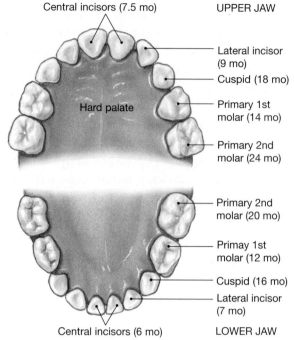

Central incisors (7.5 mo) UPPER JAW

— Lateral incisor (9 mo)
— Cuspid (18 mo)
— Primary 1st molar (14 mo)
— Primary 2nd molar (24 mo)

Hard palate

— Primary 2nd molar (20 mo)
— Primay 1st molar (12 mo)
— Cuspid (16 mo)
— Lateral incisor (7 mo)

Central incisors (6 mo) LOWER JAW

b Primary teeth, with the age at eruption given in months.

Central incisors (7–8 yr)

— Lateral incisor (8–9 yr)
— Cuspid (11–12 yr)
— 1st Premolar (10–11 yr)
— 2nd Premolar (10–12 yr)
— 1st Molar (6–7 yr)
— 2nd Molar (12–13 yr)
— 3rd Molar (17–21 yr)

Upper dental arch

Hard palate

— 3rd Molar (17–21 yr)
— 2nd Molar (11–13 yr)
— 1st Molar (6–7 yr)
— 2nd Premolar (11–12 yr)
— 1st Premolar (10–12 yr)
— Cuspid (9–10 yr)
— Lateral incisor (7–8 yr)

Lower dental arch

Central incisors (6–7 yr)

c Adult teeth, with the age at eruption given in years.

Teeth

Movements of the tongue are important in passing food across the opposing surfaces of the **teeth**. These surfaces carry out chewing, or **mastication** (mas-ti-KĀ-shun), of food. Mastication breaks down tough connective tissues in meat and the plant fibers in vegetables. It also helps saturate the food with salivary secretions.

Figure 16-6a shows the parts of a sectioned tooth. The **neck** of the tooth marks the boundary between the **root** and the **crown**. The crown is the exposed portion of the tooth that projects beyond the gums. A layer of **enamel** covers the crown. Enamel contains a crystalline form of calcium phosphate. Enamel is the hardest biologically manufactured substance. Adequate amounts of calcium, phosphate, and vitamin D_3 during childhood are essential for an enamel coating that is complete and resistant to decay.

Most of each tooth consists of **dentin** (DEN-tin), a mineralized matrix similar to that of bone. Dentin differs from bone in that it does not contain cells. Instead, cytoplasmic processes extend into the dentin from cells within the central **pulp cavity**. The pulp cavity receives blood vessels and nerves through one to four narrow **root canals** at the root (base) of the tooth. The root of each tooth sits within a bony cavity or socket, called the *tooth socket* or *alveolus* (a hollow cavity). Collagen fibers of the **periodontal ligament** (*peri-*,

16

around + *odonto-*, tooth) extend from the dentin of the root to the surrounding bone. A layer of **cementum** (se-MEN-tum) covers the dentin of the root, providing protection and firmly anchoring the periodontal ligament. Cementum is similar in structure to bone, but softer. Where the tooth penetrates the gum surface, epithelial cells form tight attachments to the tooth and prevent bacterial access to the easily eroded cementum of the root.

Tooth decay generally results from the action of bacteria that live in your mouth. Bacteria on the surfaces of the teeth produce a sticky matrix that traps food particles and creates deposits known as *dental plaque*. Over time, this organic matter can calcify and form a hard layer of *tartar*, or *dental calculus*, which can be difficult to remove.

Types of Teeth

A set of adult teeth is shown in **Figure 16-6c**. Each of the four types of teeth has a specific function. **Incisors** (in-SĪ-zerz) are blade-shaped teeth at the front of the mouth. They are useful for clipping or cutting, as when you nip off the tip of a carrot stick. **Cuspids** (KUS-pidz), or *canines*, are conical, with a sharp ridgeline and a pointed tip. They are used for tearing or slashing. You might weaken a tough piece of celery by the clipping action of the incisors and then take advantage of the shearing action provided by the cuspids. **Bicuspids** (bī-KUS-pidz), or *premolars*, and **molars** have flattened crowns with prominent ridges. They are used for crushing, mashing, and grinding. You might shift a tough nut or piece of meat to the premolars and molars for crushing.

Dental Succession

Two sets of teeth form during development. The first to appear are the **deciduous teeth** (dē-SID-ū-us; *deciduus*, falling off), also known as *primary teeth, milk teeth*, or *baby teeth*. Most children have 20 deciduous teeth (**Figure 16-6b**). These teeth are later replaced by the **secondary dentition**, or *permanent dentition* (**Figure 16-6c**), which permit the processing of a wider variety of foods.

As replacement proceeds, the periodontal ligaments and roots of the deciduous teeth erode. The deciduous teeth either fall out or are pushed aside by the **eruption** (emergence) of the secondary teeth. Adult jaws are larger and can accommodate more than 20 teeth. As a person grows up, three additional teeth appear on each side of the upper and lower jaws, bringing the permanent tooth count to 32. The last teeth to appear are the *third molars*, or *wisdom teeth*. Wisdom teeth (or any other teeth) that develop in locations that do not permit their eruption are called *impacted teeth*. Impacted teeth can be surgically removed to prevent abscesses from forming.

CHECKPOINT

6. Name the structures associated with the oral cavity.
7. The oral cavity is lined by which type of epithelium?
8. The digestion of which nutrient would be affected by damage to the parotid salivary glands?
9. Which type of tooth is most useful for chopping off bits of raw vegetables?

See the blue Answers tab at the back of the book.

16-3 The pharynx is a passageway between the oral cavity and the esophagus

Learning Objective Describe the structures and functions of the pharynx and esophagus, and the key events of the swallowing process.

The Pharynx

The **pharynx** (FAR-ingks), or throat, serves as a common passageway for solid food, liquids, and air. (The three major subdivisions of the pharynx were discussed in Chapter 15.) ⤴ p. 509 Food normally passes through the oropharynx and laryngopharynx on its way to the esophagus. Both of these regions of the pharynx have a stratified squamous epithelium similar to that of the oral cavity. The underlying lamina propria contains mucous glands plus the pharyngeal, palatal, and lingual tonsils. The pharyngeal muscles cooperate with muscles of the oral cavity and esophagus to begin the process of swallowing (described shortly). The muscular contractions during swallowing force the food mass into and along the esophagus.

The Esophagus

The **esophagus** (**Figure 16-1**) is a muscular tube that conveys solid food and liquids to the stomach. It is about 25 cm (10 in.) long and about 2 cm (0.75 in.) in diameter. It begins at the pharynx, runs posterior to the trachea in the neck, and passes through the mediastinum in the thoracic cavity. It then enters the abdominopelvic cavity through the *esophageal hiatus* (hī-Ā-tus; a gap or opening), an opening in the diaphragm. Finally it empties into the stomach. In a *diaphragmatic hernia*, or *hiatal* (hī-Ā-tal) *hernia*, abdominal organs slide up into the thoracic cavity through the esophageal hiatus.

The esophagus is lined with a stratified squamous epithelium that resists abrasion, hot or cold temperatures, and chemical attack. The secretions of esophageal mucous glands lubricate this epithelial surface and prevent materials from sticking to it during swallowing. The upper third of its

16

muscularis externa contains skeletal muscle, the lower third contains smooth muscle, and a mixture of each makes up the middle third.

Regions of circular muscle in the superior and inferior ends of the esophagus make up the *upper esophageal sphincter* and the *lower esophageal sphincter*. The lower sphincter is normally in active contraction. This condition prevents the backflow of materials from the stomach into the esophagus.

Swallowing

Swallowing, or **deglutition** (dē-gloo-TISH-un), is a complex process that can be initiated voluntarily but proceeds automatically once it begins. You take conscious control over swallowing when you eat or drink, but swallowing is also controlled at the subconscious level. Before food can be swallowed, it must have the proper texture and consistency. Once food has been shredded or torn by the teeth, moistened with salivary secretions, and "approved" by the taste receptors, the tongue begins compacting the debris into a small mass, or **bolus**.

We can divide the process of swallowing into three phases. The buccal, pharyngeal, and esophageal phases are detailed in **Figure 16-7**. The buccal phase is the only phase of swallowing that we can consciously control.

CLINICAL NOTE

Swallowed Foreign Bodies

Swallowed foreign bodies are a common reason people seek emergency care. Approximately 80 percent of ingested foreign bodies occur in children. Dentures in adults account for the second most frequent type of swallowed foreign body. The presence of dentures impairs the ability to determine how well food is chewed.

Most swallowed foreign bodies pass spontaneously. However, 10–20 percent require some medical intervention. Once an object has passed the pylorus and enters the stomach, it usually passes without further incident. Objects that lodge in the esophagus, however, usually require intervention.

A barium swallow and esophageal X-ray can aid in the diagnosis of an esophageal foreign body. Alternatively, direct examination with a fiber-optic endoscope will confirm the diagnosis.

The type of foreign body present dictates treatment. Food impactions often pass following administration of medications that relax smooth muscle and decrease lower esophageal sphincter pressures. These include glucagon, nifedipine, and nitroglycerin. Sharp objects may require surgical removal. Swallowed batteries are a true emergency, as the alkaline substance in the battery rapidly burns the esophageal mucosa, and thus may result in perforation.

16

Figure 16-7 The Swallowing Process. This sequence, based on a series of X-rays, shows the phases of swallowing and the movement of a bolus from the mouth to the stomach.

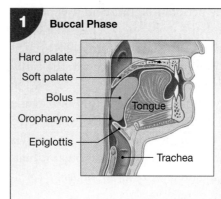

1 Buccal Phase

Hard palate
Soft palate
Bolus
Oropharynx
Epiglottis
Tongue
Trachea

The **buccal phase** begins with the compression of the bolus against the hard palate. Retraction of the tongue then forces the bolus into the oropharynx and assists in elevating the soft palate, thereby sealing off the nasopharynx. Once the bolus enters the oropharynx, reflex responses begin and the bolus is moved toward the stomach.

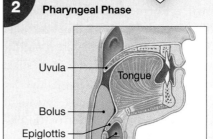

2 Pharyngeal Phase

Uvula
Tongue
Bolus
Epiglottis
Larynx

The **pharyngeal phase** begins as the bolus comes into contact with the palatal arches and the posterior pharyngeal wall. Elevation of the larynx and folding of the epiglottis direct the bolus past the closed glottis. At the same time, the uvula and soft palate block passage back to the nasopharynx.

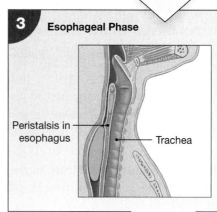

3 Esophageal Phase

Peristalsis in esophagus
Trachea

The **esophageal phase** begins as the contraction of pharyngeal muscles forces the bolus through the entrance to the esophagus. Once in the esophagus, the bolus is pushed toward the stomach by peristalsis.

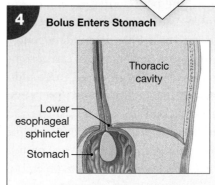

4 Bolus Enters Stomach

Thoracic cavity
Lower esophageal sphincter
Stomach

The approach of the bolus triggers the opening of the lower esophageal sphincter. The bolus then continues into the stomach.

CLINICAL NOTE

Esophagitis and Diaphragmatic (Hiatal) Hernias

A weakened or permanently relaxed lower esophageal sphincter can cause inflammation of the esophagus, or *esophagitis* (ē-sof-a-JĪ-tis), as powerful gastric acids enter the lower esophagus. The esophageal epithelium has few defenses against acids and enzymes, and inflammation, epithelial erosion, and intense discomfort are the result. Occasional incidents of reflux, or backflow, from the stomach are responsible for the symptoms of "heartburn." This relatively common problem supports a multimillion-dollar industry devoted to producing and promoting antacids.

The esophagus and major blood vessels pass from the thoracic cavity to the abdominopelvic cavity through an opening in the diaphragm called the *esophageal hiatus*. In a *diaphragmatic hernia*, or *hiatal* (hī-Ā-tal) *hernia*, abdominal organs slide into the thoracic cavity through the esophageal hiatus. The severity of the condition depends on the location and size of the herniated organ or organs. Hiatal hernias are actually very common, and most go unnoticed. When clinical problems develop, they usually occur because the intruding abdominal organs are exerting pressure on structures or organs in the thoracic cavity.

The involuntary *swallowing reflex* begins when tactile receptors on the palatal arches and uvula are stimulated by the passage of the bolus.

CHECKPOINT

10. Describe the function of the pharynx.

11. What process is occurring when the soft palate and larynx elevate and the glottis closes?

See the blue Answers tab at the back of the book.

16-4 The J-shaped stomach receives food from the esophagus and aids in chemical and mechanical digestion

Learning Objective Describe the anatomy of the stomach, including its histology, and discuss its roles in digestion and absorption.

The **stomach** has four primary functions: (1) storage of ingested food; (2) mechanical breakdown of ingested food; (3) disruption of chemical bonds in food through the action of acids and enzymes; and (4) production of *intrinsic factor*, a compound necessary for the absorption of vitamin B_{12} in the small intestine. Ingested substances mix with secretions of the glands of the stomach. The result is a viscous, highly acidic, soupy mixture of partially digested food called **chyme** (KĪM).

The stomach is a muscular, J-shaped organ. It has four main regions (**Figure 16-8a**). The esophagus connects to the smallest region, the **cardia** (KAR-dē-uh). The bulge of the stomach superior to the cardia is the **fundus** (FUN-dus). The large area between the fundus and the curve of the J is the **body**. The **pylorus** (pi-LOR-us; *pyle*, gate + *ouros*, guard) is the distal part of the J. It connects the stomach with the small intestine. A muscular **pyloric sphincter** regulates the flow of chyme between the stomach and small intestine.

The stomach's volume increases while you eat and then decreases as chyme enters the small intestine. When the stomach is relaxed (empty), the mucosa has prominent longitudinal folds, called **rugae** (ROO-gē; wrinkles). These temporary features let the gastric (*gaster*, stomach) lumen expand. As the stomach expands, the rugae gradually flatten out until, at maximum distension, they almost disappear. (The world record, set in 2013, for eating hot dogs with buns in 10 minutes is 69!) When empty, the stomach resembles a muscular tube with a narrow and constricted lumen. When fully expanded, it can contain 1–1.5 liters of material.

Unlike the two-layered muscularis externa of other parts of the digestive tract, that of the stomach contains three layers. It has a longitudinal layer, a circular layer, and an inner *oblique layer*. The extra layer of smooth muscle strengthens the stomach wall and assists in the mixing and churning essential to forming chyme.

The visceral peritoneum covering the outer surface of the stomach is continuous with a pair of mesenteries. The **greater omentum** (ō-MEN-tum; *omentum*, a fatty skin) extends below the *greater curvature* and forms an enormous pouch that hangs over and protects the abdominal viscera (**Figure 16-8b**). The much smaller **lesser omentum** extends from the *lesser curvature* to the liver.

The Gastric Wall

The stomach is lined by a simple columnar epithelium dominated by mucous cells. This *mucous epithelium* secretes an alkaline mucus that covers and protects epithelial cells from acids, enzymes, and abrasive materials. Shallow depressions, called **gastric pits**, open onto the gastric surface (**Figure 16-8c**). The mucous cells at the base, or *neck*, of each gastric pit actively divide and replace superficial cells of the mucous epithelium

16

Figure 16-8 The Anatomy of the Stomach.

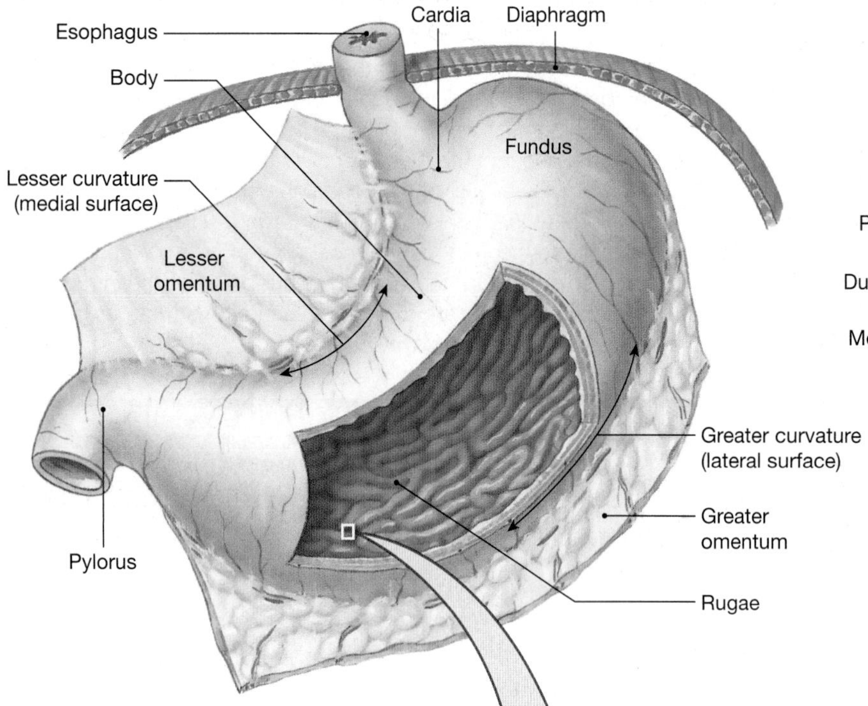

a This anterior view of the stomach shows important superficial landmarks.

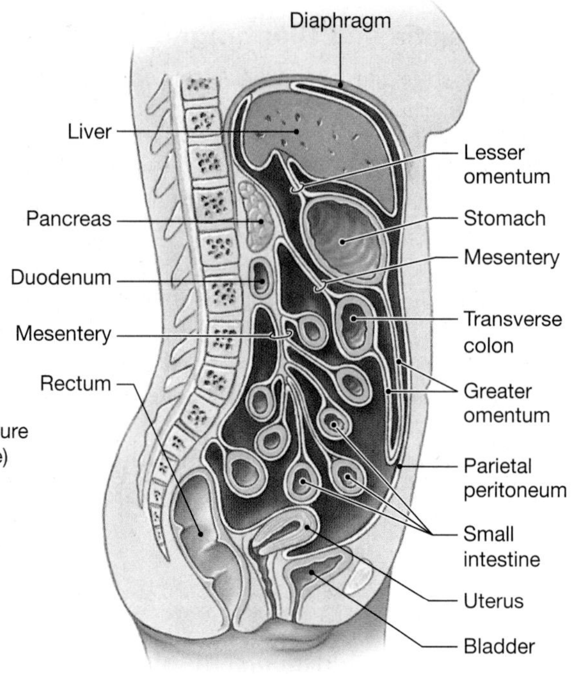

b The stomach is surrounded by the peritoneal cavity. Its position is maintained by the greater and lesser omenta.

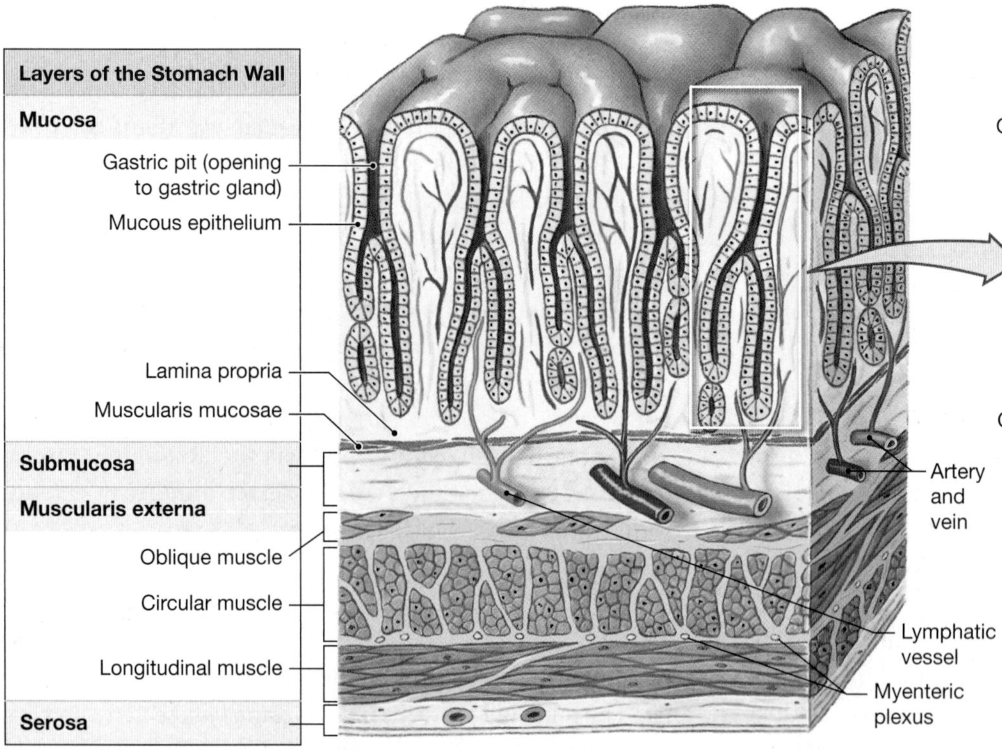

Layers of the Stomach Wall

Mucosa
- Gastric pit (opening to gastric gland)
- Mucous epithelium
- Lamina propria
- Muscularis mucosae

Submucosa

Muscularis externa
- Oblique muscle
- Circular muscle
- Longitudinal muscle

Serosa

c This diagrammatic section shows the organization of the stomach wall.

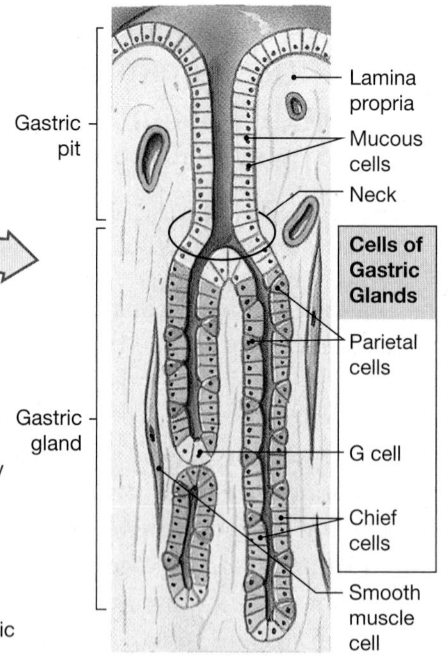

Cells of Gastric Glands

d This diagram of a gastric gland shows the sites of parietal cells and chief cells.

16

shed into the chyme. A typical gastric epithelial cell has a life span of three to seven days.

In the fundus and body of the stomach, each gastric pit is connected with **gastric glands** that extend deep into the underlying lamina propria (**Figure 16-8d**). Gastric glands are dominated by two types of secretory cells: *parietal cells* and *chief cells*. Together, they secrete about 1500 mL of **gastric juice** each day.

Gastric glands within the lower stomach (the *pylorus*) also contain endocrine cells that are involved in regulating gastric activity, as we discuss shortly.

Parietal Cells

Parietal cells secrete intrinsic factor and hydrochloric acid (HCl). **Intrinsic factor** aids the absorption of vitamin B_{12} across the intestinal lining. (Recall from Chapter 11 that this vitamin is needed for normal erythropoiesis.) ⟲ p. 388

HCl lowers the pH of the gastric juice, keeping the stomach contents at a pH of 1.5–2.0. The acidity of gastric juice kills microorganisms, breaks down plant cell walls and connective tissues in meat, and activates enzymes secreted by chief cells.

Chief Cells

Chief cells secrete a protein called **pepsinogen** (pep-SIN–jen) into the stomach lumen. When pepsinogen contacts the HCl released by the parietal cells, it is converted to **pepsin**, a *proteolytic* (protein-digesting) *enzyme*. In newborn infants (but not adults), the stomach produces *rennin* and *gastric lipase*. These enzymes are important for the digestion of milk. Rennin coagulates milk proteins, thus slowing their passage through the stomach and allowing more time for its digestion. Gastric lipase begins the digestion of milk fats.

CLINICAL NOTE

Peptic Ulcers

Peptic ulcers are erosions caused by gastric acid (**Figure 16-9**). They can occur anywhere in the gastrointestinal tract; terminology is based on the portion of the GI tract affected. Duodenal ulcers most frequently occur in the proximal portion of the duodenum; gastric ulcers occur exclusively in the stomach. Overall, peptic ulcers occur in males four times more frequently than in females, and duodenal ulcers occur from two to three times more frequently than do gastric ulcers. Current statistics place the number of peptic ulcers at 4–5 million, with approximately 500,000 new cases diagnosed yearly. Those patients who are more likely to have gastric ulcers are over 50 years old and work in jobs that require physical activity. Their pain usually increases after eating or with a full stomach, and they usually have no pain at night. Duodenal ulcers are more common in patients from 25 to 50 years old who are executives or leaders under high stress. There is also some familial tendency toward duodenal ulcer, which suggests genetic predisposition. Patients with duodenal ulcers commonly have pain at night or whenever their stomach is empty.

Nonsteroidal anti-inflammatory medications (aspirin, Motrin, Advil, Naprosyn), acid-stimulating products (alcohol, nicotine), or *Helicobacter pylori* bacteria are the most common causes of peptic ulcers. To help break down food boluses, the stomach secretes hydrochloric acid. One of the enzymes that control this secretion is pepsinogen. The hydrochloric acid helps to convert pepsinogen into its active form, pepsin. Between them, the pepsin and the hydrochloric acid can make the digestive enzymes very irritating to the GI tract's mucosal lining. Ordinarily, mucous gland secretions protect the stomach's mucosal barrier from these irritants. But when nonsteroidal anti-inflammatory medications, acid stimulators, or *H. pylori* damage the barrier, the

Figure 16-9 Types of Peptic Ulcers.

Peptic ulcers are erosions in the mucosa of the stomach or duodenum. They can erode completely through the wall of the organ, which results in perforation and life-threatening hemorrhage.

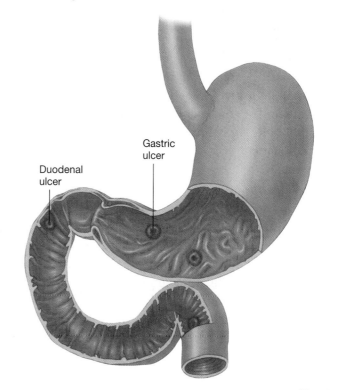

Gastric ulcer

Duodenal ulcer

(Continued)

16

mucosa is exposed to the highly acidic fluid, and peptic ulcers result. Prostaglandin, which is an important locally acting hormone, decreases the stimulation for blood flow through the gastric mucosa, and allows its further destruction.

The recent discovery that *H. pylori* bacteria appear in over 80 percent of gastric and duodenal ulcers has enabled physicians to treat the disease by eliminating its cause with antacids and antibiotics rather than merely treating its symptoms.

A blocked pancreatic duct can also contribute to duodenal ulcers. As chyme passes through the pyloric sphincter from the stomach into the duodenum, the pancreas secretes an alkalotic solution laden with bicarbonate ions that neutralize the acidic hydrogen ions in the chyme. If the pancreatic duct is blocked, however, the acidic chyme can cause ulcerations throughout the intestine. One other cause of duodenal ulcers is Zollinger-Ellison syndrome, in which an acid-secreting tumor provokes the ulcerations.

Acute, severe pain is probably due to a rupture of the ulcer into the peritoneal cavity that causes hemorrhage. Depending on the ulcer's location, the patient may have hematemesis or may have melena. Bouts of nausea and vomiting due to the irritation of the mucosa are common. If the ulcer has eroded through a highly vascular area, massive hemorrhage can occur. Along with the signs of hemorrhage on visual inspection, these patients will appear very ill and have signs of hemodynamic instability, such as pale, cool, and clammy skin, tachycardia, decreased blood pressure, and possibly, altered mental status. Most patients will lie still to decrease the pain. They may have surgical scars from previous ulcer repair. Bowel sounds will usually be absent.

The Regulation of Gastric Activity

The production of acid and enzymes by the stomach mucosa can be (1) controlled by the central nervous system (CNS), (2) regulated by reflexes coordinated in the wall of the stomach, and (3) regulated by hormones of the digestive tract. Regulation of gastric secretion proceeds in three overlapping phases. They are named according to the location of the control center: the cephalic phase, the gastric phase, and the intestinal phase (**Spotlight Figure 16-10**).

1. *Cephalic phase.* The **cephalic phase** of gastric secretion begins when you sense or think of food (**1** in **Spotlight Figure 16-10**). This phase prepares the stomach to receive food. It is directed by different regions of the CNS, including the cerebral cortex and hypothalamus. The neural output proceeds by way of the parasympathetic division of the ANS. The vagus nerves innervate the submucosal plexus of the stomach. Next, postganglionic parasympathetic fibers innervate mucous cells, parietal cells, chief cells, and endocrine cells of the stomach.

2. *Gastric phase.* The **gastric phase** begins when food arrives in the stomach (**2** in **Spotlight Figure 16-10**). The stimulation of stretch receptors in the stomach wall and of chemoreceptors in the mucosa triggers local reflexes controlled by the submucosal and myenteric plexuses. The myenteric plexus stimulates mixing waves in the muscularis externa of the stomach wall. The submucosal plexus stimulates the parietal cells and chief cells. It also stimulates **G cells** in gastric glands within the pylorus to release the hormone **gastrin** into the bloodstream. Proteins, alcohol in small doses, and caffeine are potent stimulators of gastric secretion because they excite the chemoreceptors in the gastric lining. Both parietal and chief cells respond to the presence of gastrin by accelerating their secretory activities. The effect on the parietal cells is the most pronounced, and the pH of the gastric juice drops sharply. This phase may continue for several hours while the acids and enzymes process the ingested materials.

During this period, gastrin also stimulates stomach contractions, which mix the ingested materials with the gastric secretions to form chyme. As mixing proceeds, the contractions begin sweeping down the length of the stomach. Each time the pylorus contracts, a small quantity of chyme squirts through the pyloric sphincter into the small intestine.

CLINICAL NOTE

Gastritis and Peptic Ulcers

Inflammation of the gastric mucosa is called gastritis (gas-TR-tis). It can develop after a person has swallowed drugs, including alcoholic beverages and aspirin. Gastritis is also associated with smoking, severe emotional or physical stress, bacterial infection of the gastric wall, or ingestion of strongly acidic or alkaline chemicals.

Gastritis may lead to ulcer formation. A peptic ulcer develops when the digestive acids and enzymes erode the lining of the stomach or proximal portion of the small intestine (duodenum). The terms gastric ulcer (in the stomach) or duodenal ulcer (in the duodenum of the small intestine) indicate specific locations. Peptic ulcers result from excessive production of acid or inadequate production of the alkaline mucus that protects the epithelium against that acid. It is now known that infection by the bacterium *H. pylori* is responsible for over 80 percent of peptic ulcers. Treatment for ulcers involves the administration of drugs such as *cimetidine* (*Tagamet*) that inhibit gastric acid production, combined with antibiotics if *H. pylori* is present.

Gastric activity is regulated by the central nervous system, by reflexes within the walls of the digestive tract, and by hormones of the digestive tract. Regulation of gastric secretion proceeds in three overlapping phases, named according to the location of the control center.

1 CEPHALIC PHASE

The **cephalic phase** of gastric secretion begins when you see, smell, taste, or think of food. This phase is directed by the parasympathetic division of the autonomic nervous system. It prepares the stomach to receive food. In response to stimulation, the production of gastric juice speeds up, reaching rates of about 500 mL/h, or about 2 cups per hour. This phase generally lasts only minutes.

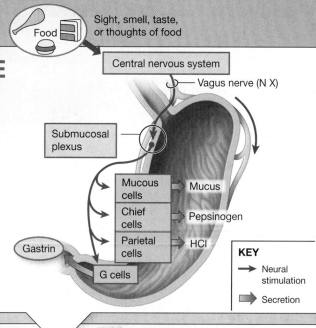

Sight, smell, taste, or thoughts of food

Food

Central nervous system

Vagus nerve (N X)

Submucosal plexus

Mucous cells → Mucus
Chief cells → Pepsinogen
Parietal cells → HCl

Gastrin

G cells

KEY
→ Neural stimulation
⇒ Secretion

2 GASTRIC PHASE

The **gastric phase** begins when food arrives in the stomach. The stimulation of stretch receptors in the stomach wall and of chemoreceptors in the mucosa triggers local reflexes in the submucosal and myenteric plexuses. This results in mixing waves from the muscularis externa, and the secretion of mucus, pepsinogen, and HCl from the cells of the gastric glands.

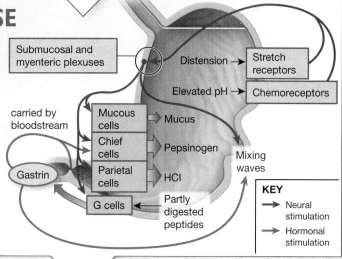

Submucosal and myenteric plexuses

Distension → Stretch receptors
Elevated pH → Chemoreceptors

carried by bloodstream

Mucous cells → Mucus
Chief cells → Pepsinogen
Parietal cells → HCl

Mixing waves

Gastrin

G cells ← Partly digested peptides

KEY
→ Neural stimulation
→ Hormonal stimulation

The *duodenum* (doo-ō-DĒ-num) is the portion of the small intestine closest to the stomach. It plays a key role in controlling digestion because it monitors the contents of the chyme that it receives from the stomach. The duodenum adjusts the activities of the stomach and accessory glands to protect lower (distal) portions of the small intestine.

3 INTESTINAL PHASE

The **intestinal phase** of gastric secretion begins when chyme first enters the duodenum of the small intestine. The function of the intestinal phase is to control the rate of gastric emptying to ensure that the secretory, digestive, and absorptive functions of the small intestine can proceed efficiently.

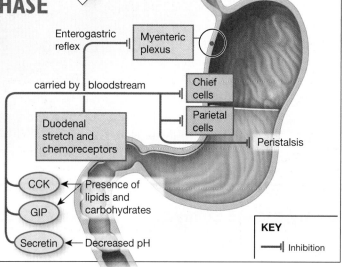

Enterogastric reflex

Myenteric plexus

carried by bloodstream

Chief cells

Parietal cells

Duodenal stretch and chemoreceptors

Peristalsis

CCK ← Presence of lipids and carbohydrates
GIP

Secretin ← Decreased pH

KEY
⊣ Inhibition

CLINICAL NOTE

Stomach Cancer

Stomach (or *gastric*) cancer is one of the most common lethal cancers. The incidence is higher in Japan and Korea, where the typical diet includes large quantities of pickled foods. Because the signs and symptoms can resemble those of gastric ulcers, the condition may not be reported in its early stages. Diagnosis usually involves X-rays of the stomach at various degrees of distension. ⟲ p. 20

The treatment of stomach cancer involves a *gastrectomy* (gas-TREK-to-mē), the surgical removal of part or all of the stomach. The lack of intrinsic factor (produced by the stomach) can be overcome with high daily doses of vitamin B$_{12}$.

3. ***Intestinal phase.*** The **intestinal phase** of gastric secretion begins when chyme first enters the duodenum of the small intestine (❸ in **Spotlight Figure 16-10**). Most of the regulatory controls for this phase (whether neural or endocrine) are inhibitory. By controlling the rate of gastric emptying, they ensure that all functions of the small intestine can proceed efficiently. For example, the movement of chyme temporarily reduces the stimulation of stretch receptors in the stomach wall and increases their stimulation in the wall of the small intestine. This produces the *enterogastric reflex*. This reflex temporarily inhibits neural stimulation of gastrin production and gastric motility, and further movement of chyme. At the same time, the entry of chyme stimulates the release of the intestinal hormones *secretin, cholecystokinin* (*CCK*), and *gastric inhibitory peptide* (*GIP*). The resulting reduced gastric activity gives the small intestine time to adjust to the arriving acids.

Inhibitory reflexes that depress gastric activity are stimulated when the proximal portion of the small intestine becomes too full, too acidic, unduly irritated by chyme, or filled with partially digested proteins, carbohydrates, or fats.

In general, chyme moves into the small intestine at the highest rate when the stomach is greatly distended and the meal contains relatively little protein. A large meal containing small amounts of protein, large amounts of carbohydrates (such as rice or pasta), wine (alcohol), and after-dinner coffee (caffeine) will leave your stomach extremely quickly. Why? This happens because both alcohol and caffeine stimulate gastric secretion and motility.

Digestion in the Stomach

The stomach carries out the preliminary digestion of proteins by pepsin. For a variable period, it allows the digestion of carbohydrates by salivary amylase and of lipids by lingual lipase. These enzymes continue to work until the pH of the stomach contents falls below 4.5. They generally remain active one to two hours after a meal.

As the stomach contents become more fluid and the pH approaches 2.0, pepsin activity increases. Protein disassembly begins. Protein digestion is not completed in the stomach, because time is limited and pepsin attacks only certain peptide bonds. However, pepsin typically breaks down complex proteins into smaller peptide and polypeptide chains before chyme enters the small intestine.

Digestion occurs in the stomach, but nutrients are not absorbed there. Why not? There are four reasons: (1) the epithelial cells are covered by a blanket of alkaline mucus and are not directly exposed to chyme, (2) the epithelial cells lack the specialized transport processes found in cells lining the small intestine, (3) the gastric lining is impermeable to water, and (4) digestion has not been completed by the time chyme leaves the stomach. At this stage, most carbohydrates, lipids, and proteins are only partially broken down.

CHECKPOINT

12. Name the four main regions of the stomach.

13. Discuss the significance of the low pH in the stomach.

14. In a person suffering from chronic gastric ulcers, why might the branches of the vagus nerves serving the stomach be cut in an attempt to provide relief?

See the blue Answers tab at the back of the book.

16-5 The small intestine digests and absorbs nutrients

Learning Objective Describe the anatomy of the small intestine, including its histology, and explain the functions and regulation of intestinal secretions.

The **small intestine** plays a key role in digesting and absorbing nutrients. Ninety percent of nutrient absorption takes place there. (Most of the rest takes place in the large intestine.)

The small intestine is about 6 m (20 ft) long. Its diameter ranges from 4 cm (1.6 in.) at the stomach to about 2.5 cm (1 in.) at the junction with the large intestine. It has three segments: the *duodenum*, the *jejunum*, and the *ileum* (**Figure 16-11a**):

1. The **duodenum** (doo-ō-DĒ-num), 25 cm (10 in.) in length, is the segment closest to the stomach. This portion of the small intestine is the "mixing bowl." It receives chyme from the stomach and digestive secretions from the pancreas and liver. From its connection

Figure 16-11 The Segments of the Small Intestine.

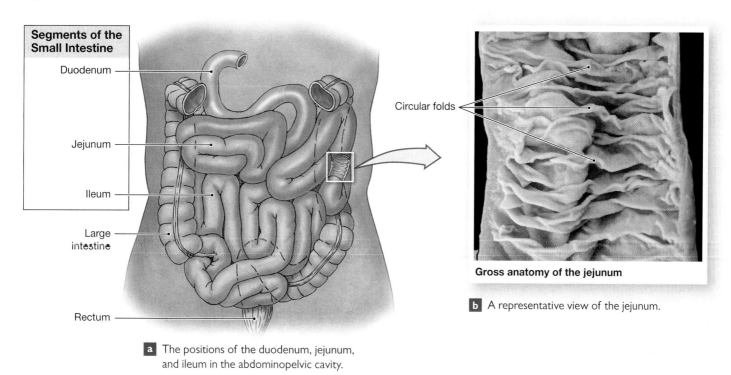

Segments of the Small Intestine
- Duodenum
- Jejunum
- Ileum
- Large intestine
- Rectum

Circular folds

Gross anatomy of the jejunum

b A representative view of the jejunum.

a The positions of the duodenum, jejunum, and ileum in the abdominopelvic cavity.

with the stomach, the duodenum curves in a C that encloses the pancreas. Except for its proximal 2.5 cm (1 in.), the duodenum lies outside the peritoneal cavity (**Figure 16-8b**, p. 548). Organs that lie posterior to the peritoneal cavity are called **retroperitoneal** (*retro*, behind).

2. An abrupt bend marks the boundary between the duodenum and the **jejunum** (je-JOO-num). At this site, the small intestine reenters the peritoneal cavity, supported by a sheet of mesentery. The jejunum is about 2.5 meters (8 ft) long. The bulk of chemical digestion and nutrient absorption takes place in the jejunum. One rather drastic approach to weight control involves surgery to remove a significant portion of the jejunum.

3. The **ileum** (IL-ē-um), the final segment of the small intestine, is also the longest. It averages 3.5 m (12 ft) in length. The ileum ends at the *ileocecal valve*. This sphincter controls the flow of material from the ileum into the *cecum*, the first portion of the large intestine.

The small intestine fills much of the peritoneal cavity. Its position is stabilized by a mesentery attached to the dorsal body wall (**Figure 16-8b**, p. 548). Blood vessels, lymphatic vessels, and nerves run to and from the segments of the small intestine within the connective tissue of the mesentery.

The Intestinal Wall

The intestinal lining bears a series of transverse folds called **circular folds**, or *plicae circulares* (PLĪ-sē sir-kū-LAR-ēz) (**Figure 16-11b**). The circular folds are permanent features. They do not disappear when the small intestine fills.

The mucosa of the small intestine is composed of a multitude of fingerlike projections called **villi** (**Figure 16-12b**). These structures are covered by a simple columnar epithelium carpeted with microvilli (**Figure 16-12c**). Because the microvilli project from the epithelium like the bristles on a brush, these cells are said to have a *brush border* (**Figure 16-12d**).

If the small intestine were a simple tube with smooth walls, it would have a total absorptive area of about 3300 cm^2 (3.6 ft^2). Instead, the mucosa contains roughly 800 circular folds. Each circular fold supports a forest of villi, and each villus is covered by epithelial cells blanketed in microvilli. This arrangement increases the total area for absorption to approximately 2 million cm^2, or more than 2200 ft^2.

Each villus contains a network of capillaries that originate in the submucosa (**Figure 16-12c**). These capillaries carry absorbed nutrients to the hepatic portal circulation for delivery to the liver. ↪ p. 459 In addition to capillaries,

CLINICAL NOTE

Upper Gastrointestinal Bleeding

Upper gastrointestinal (GI) bleeding can be defined as bleeding within the GI tract proximal to the ligament of Treitz, which supports the duodenojejunal junction, which is the point where the first two sections of the small intestine (the duodenum and the jejunum) meet.

Upper GI bleeds account for over 300,000 hospitalizations per year. The mortality rate has remained fairly steady at approximately 10 percent over the past years. Many factors contribute to this high mortality. First, the number of patients who treat their symptoms with home remedies and over-the-counter medications is increasing rapidly. Many of these patients come under medical care only when their disease has caused significant damage, such as large-scale hemorrhage from an ulcerated lesion. Second, the overall age of the population is increasing. The infirmities of age and its greater likelihood of coexisting illnesses, such as hypertension, atherosclerosis, diabetes, and substance abuse (including abuse of medications), make this older population more vulnerable to the effects of upper GI bleeds. The mortality rate is highest in those over 60 years of age. One prevention strategy for the field is to check for such coexisting problems, especially in elderly patients, and to treat accordingly. In particular, look at the history and physical for evidence of tobacco or alcohol use, or both.

The six major identifiable causes of upper GI hemorrhage, in descending order of frequency, are peptic ulcer disease, gastritis, variceal rupture, Mallory-Weiss syndrome (esophageal laceration, usually secondary to vomiting), esophagitis, and duodenitis. Peptic ulcer disease accounts for approximately 50 percent of upper GI bleeds; gastritis accounts for an additional 25 percent. Overall, irritation or erosion of the gastric lining of the stomach causes more than 75 percent of upper GI bleeds. Most cases of upper GI bleeding are chronic irritations or inflammations that cause minimal discomfort and minor hemorrhage. Physicians can manage these conditions on an outpatient basis; however, if a peptic ulcer erodes through the gastric mucosa, if the esophagus is lacerated in Mallory-Weiss syndrome, or if varices (often secondary to alcoholic liver damage) rupture, an acute-onset, life-threatening, and difficult-to-control hemorrhage can result.

Upper GI bleeds may be obvious, or they may be present quite subtly. Most often, patients will complain of some type of abdominal discomfort that ranges from a vague burning sensation to an upset stomach, gas pain, or tearing pain in the upper quadrants. Because blood severely irritates the GI system, most cases present with nausea and vomiting. If the bleeding is in the upper GI tract, the patient may experience hematemesis (bloody vomitus) or, if it passes through the lower GI tract, melena. The partially digested blood will turn the stool black and tarry. For melena to be recognizable, approximately 150 cc of blood must drain into the GI tract and remain there for from five to eight hours. Blood in emesis may be bright red (new, fresh blood) or look like coffee grounds (old, partially digested blood).

Upper GI bleeding may be light or it may be brisk and life threatening. Patients who suffer a rupture of an esophageal varix or a tear or disruption in the esophageal or gastric lining may vomit copious amounts of blood. These hemorrhages can cause the classic signs and symptoms of shock, including alteration in mental status, tachycardia, peripheral vasoconstriction, diaphoresis (sweating that produces pale, cool, clammy skin), and hemodynamic instability. Besides shock, the vomitus itself can compromise the airway, and result in impaired respirations, aspiration, and ultimately, respiratory arrest.

A frequently employed clinical indicator is the tilt test, which indicates if the patient has orthostatic hypotension (a 10-mmHg change in blood pressure or a 20-bpm change in heart rate when the patient rises from supine to standing). Hypotension suggests a decreased circulating volume. The human body can compensate for a circulating volume deficit of approximately 15 percent before clinical indicators such as the tilt test show positive results. Thus, those patients whose systolic blood pressure drops 10 mmHg or whose heart rate increases 20 bpm or more need aggressive fluid resuscitation.

---

each villus contains nerve endings and a lymphatic capillary called a **lacteal** (LAK-tē-ul; *lacteus*, milky). Lacteals transport materials that cannot enter blood capillaries. For example, absorbed fatty acids are carried in protein-lipid packages that are too large to diffuse into the bloodstream. These packets, called *chylomicrons* (*chylos*, juice), reach the venous circulation by way of the thoracic duct of the lymphatic system. The name *lacteal* refers to the pale, milky appearance of lymph that contains large quantities of lipids.

The most important enzymes introduced into the intestinal lumen come from the exposed microvilli of intestinal cells. Brush border enzymes break down materials that come into contact with the brush border. The epithelial cells then absorb the breakdown products. When these cells are shed, they disintegrate within the lumen, releasing both intracellular and brush border enzymes.

At the bases of the villi are entrances to *intestinal glands* (**Figure 16-12b**). Stem cells within the bases of the intestinal glands divide continuously to replenish the intestinal epithelium. Other cells secrete a watery *intestinal juice*. In addition to the intestinal glands, the duodenum contains large *duodenal glands*, or *submucosal glands*, which secrete an alkaline mucus that helps buffer the acids in chyme. Intestinal glands also contain endocrine cells that produce intestinal hormones discussed in a later section.

Figure 16-12 The Intestinal Wall.

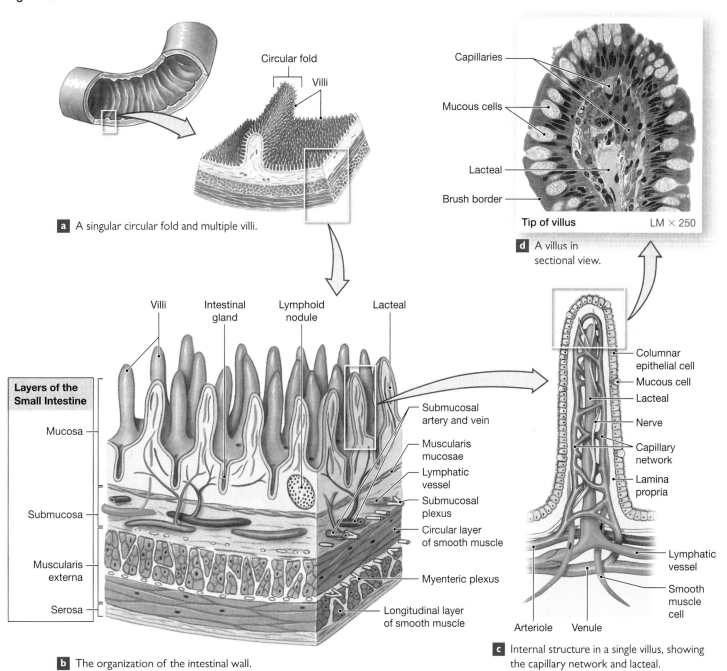

a A singular circular fold and multiple villi.

d A villus in sectional view.

Tip of villus   LM × 250

b The organization of the intestinal wall.

c Internal structure in a single villus, showing the capillary network and lacteal.

Intestinal Movements

After chyme has entered the duodenum, weak peristaltic contractions move it slowly toward the jejunum. These contractions are local reflexes not under CNS control. Their effects are limited to within a few centimeters of the site of the original stimulus.

More elaborate reflexes coordinate activities along the entire length of the small intestine. Distension of the stomach initiates the *gastroenteric* (gas-trō-en-TER-ik) *reflex*. This reflex immediately speeds up glandular secretion and peristaltic activity in all intestinal segments. The increased peristalsis moves materials along the length of the small intestine and empties the duodenum.

The *gastroileal* (gas-trō-IL-ē-al) *reflex* is a response to circulating levels of the hormone gastrin. The entry of food into the stomach triggers the release of gastrin, which relaxes the ileocecal valve at the entrance to the large intestine. With the valve relaxed, peristalsis pushes materials from the ileum into the large intestine. On average, it takes about five hours for ingested food to pass from the duodenum to the end of the ileum. So, the first of the materials to enter the duodenum after breakfast may leave the small intestine during lunch.

Intestinal Secretions

Roughly 1.8 liters of watery **intestinal juice** enters the intestinal lumen each day. Intestinal juice moistens the intestinal contents, helps buffer acids, and keeps both the digestive enzymes and the products of digestion in solution. Much of this fluid arrives by osmosis, as water flows out of the mucosa. The rest is secreted by intestinal glands stimulated by the activation of touch and stretch receptors in the intestinal walls.

Hormonal and CNS controls are important in regulating the secretions of the digestive tract and accessory organs. The duodenum is the focus of these regulatory processes, because it is the first segment of the intestine to receive chyme. Here the acid content of the chyme must be neutralized and the appropriate enzymes added. The duodenal glands protect the duodenal epithelium from gastric acids and enzymes. They increase their secretions in response to local reflexes and also to parasympathetic stimulation carried by the vagus nerves.

As a result of parasympathetic stimulation, the duodenal glands begin secreting during the cephalic phase of gastric secretion, long before chyme reaches the pyloric sphincter. Sympathetic stimulation inhibits their activation, leaving the duodenal lining relatively unprepared for the arrival of the acidic chyme. This is probably why duodenal ulcers can be caused by chronic stress or by other factors that promote sympathetic activation.

Intestinal Hormones

Duodenal endocrine cells produce various peptide hormones that coordinate the secretory activities of the stomach, duodenum, pancreas, and liver. We introduced these hormones in the discussion on the regulation of gastric activity. **Spotlight Figure 16-10** indicates the factors that stimulate their secretion.

Gastrin is secreted by duodenal cells in response to large quantities of incompletely digested proteins. Gastrin promotes increased stomach motility and stimulates the production of acids and enzymes. (Recall that gastrin is

CLINICAL NOTE

Vomiting

Vomiting, also called *emesis*, is a forceful emptying of the stomach and intestinal contents through the mouth. There are several things that can stimulate the vomiting reflex. Locally, distention of the stomach or duodenum can cause vomiting. On a systemic level, vomiting can result from activation of the *chemoreceptor trigger zone* in the medulla of the brain by the neurotransmitter serotonin. Serotonin appears to be released from cells within the intestinal wall and from neurons in the brain stem which then stimulate the vomiting center.

Nausea and retching usually precede vomiting. Nausea is a subjective sensation that is seen with many medical conditions. Increased salivation and an increase in heart rate are often seen. Retching involves contraction of the abdominal muscles and movement of stomach contents into the esophagus, but not into the mouth.

Vomiting usually follows retching. Peristalsis in the duodenum, stomach, and esophagus is reversed. Accompanied by contraction of the abdominal muscles, this results in forceful emptying of the stomach. Medications are available that help alleviate vomiting. Most appear to block serotonin receptors in the chemoreceptor trigger zone.

also secreted by endocrine cells in the distal portion of the stomach.)

Secretin (s-KR-tin) is released when the pH in the duodenum falls as acidic chyme arrives from the stomach. The primary effect of secretin is to increase the secretion of bile and buffers by the liver and pancreas.

Cholecystokinin (k-l-sis-t-K-nin), or **CCK**, is secreted when chyme arrives in the duodenum, especially when it contains lipids and partially digested proteins. CCK also targets the pancreas and gallbladder. In the pancreas, CCK speeds up the production and secretion of all types of digestive enzymes. At the gallbladder, it causes the ejection of *bile* into the duodenum. The presence of either secretin or CCK in high concentrations also reduces gastric motility and the rates of secretions.

GIP is released when fats and carbohydrates (especially glucose) enter the small intestine. GIP inhibits gastric activity and causes the release of insulin from the pancreatic islets.

The functions of the major GI hormones are summarized in **Table 16-1**. Their interactions are diagrammed in **Figure 16-13**.

Hormone	Stimulus	Origin	Target	Effects
Gastrin	Vagus nerve stimulation or arrival of food in the stomach	Stomach	Stomach	Stimulates production of acids and enzymes, increases motility
	Arrival of chyme containing large quantities of undigested proteins	Duodenum	Stomach	Stimulates production of acids and enzymes, increases motility
Secretin	Arrival of chyme in the duodenum	Duodenum	Pancreas	Stimulates production of alkaline buffers
			Stomach	Inhibits gastric secretion and motility
			Liver	Increases rate of bile secretion
Cholecystokinin (CCK)	Arrival of chyme containing lipids and partially digested proteins	Duodenum	Pancreas	Stimulates production of pancreatic enzymes
			Gallbladder	Stimulates contraction of gallbladder
			Duodenum	Causes relaxation of sphincter at base of bile duct
			Stomach	Inhibits gastric secretion and motility
			CNS	May reduce hunger
Gastric inhibitory peptide (GIP)	Arrival of chyme containing large quantities of fats and glucose	Duodenum	Pancreas	Stimulates release of insulin by pancreatic islets
			Stomach	Inhibits gastric secretion and motility

Table 16-1 Important Gastrointestinal Hormones and Their Primary Effects

Figure 16-13 The Activities of Major Digestive Tract Hormones. The primary actions of gastrin, GIP, secretin, and CCK are shown.

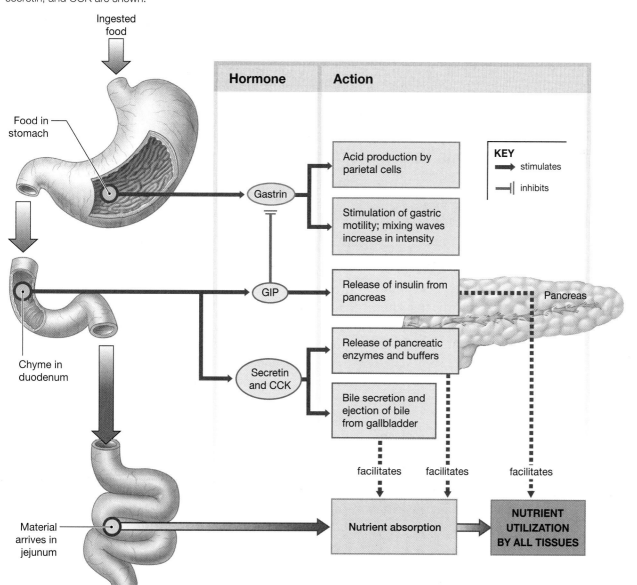

Digestion in the Small Intestine

In the stomach, food becomes saturated with gastric juices and exposed to the digestive effects of a strong acid (HCl) and a proteolytic enzyme (pepsin). Most of the important digestive processes are completed in the small intestine, where the final products of digestion—simple sugars, fatty acids, and amino acids—are absorbed, along with most of the water content. However, the small intestine produces only a few of the enzymes needed to break down the complex materials found in the diet. The liver and pancreas contribute most of the enzymes and buffers, as we discuss next.

CHECKPOINT

15. Which ring of muscle regulates the flow of chyme from the stomach to the small intestine?

16. Name the three segments of the small intestine from proximal to distal.

17. How is the small intestine adapted for the absorption of nutrients?

See the blue Answers tab at the back of the book.

16-6 The pancreas, liver, and gallbladder are accessory organs that assist with the digestive process in the small intestine

Learning Objective Describe the structure and functions of the pancreas, liver, and gallbladder, and explain how their activities are regulated.

The pancreas provides digestive enzymes, as well as buffers that help neutralize chyme. The liver secretes *bile*, a solution stored in the gallbladder for later discharge into the small intestine. Bile contains buffers and *bile salts*, compounds that aid the digestion and absorption of lipids.

The Pancreas

The **pancreas** lies posterior to the stomach. It extends laterally from the duodenum toward the spleen **(Figure 16-14a)**. It is a long, pinkish-gray organ, about 15 cm (6 in.) in length with a weight of around 80 g (3 oz). The surface of the pancreas has a lumpy texture, and its tissue is soft and easily torn. Like the duodenum, the pancreas is retroperitoneal. Only its anterior surface is covered by peritoneum **(Figure 16-8b)**.

Histological Organization of the Pancreas

The pancreas has two distinct functions, one endocrine and the other exocrine. Recall from Chapter 10 that the pancreas contains collections of endocrine cells called **pancreatic islets** that secrete the hormones insulin and glucagon. ⟲ p. 363 However, these cells account for only about 1 percent of the cell population of the pancreas. Exocrine cells and their associated ducts account for the rest. The pancreas is primarily an exocrine organ that produces a mixture of digestive enzymes, water, and buffers called **pancreatic juice**.

The numerous ducts that branch throughout the pancreas end at saclike pouches called **pancreatic acini** (AS-i-nī; singular *acinus*, grape) **(Figure 16-14b)**. The *acinar cells* of these pouches secrete digestive enzymes. The epithelial cells that line the ducts secrete buffers and water that neutralize and dilute the acid in the chyme. The smaller ducts converge to form larger ducts that fuse to form the **pancreatic duct**, which carries these secretions to the duodenum. The pancreatic duct penetrates the duodenal wall with the *common bile duct* from the liver and gallbladder.

Pancreatic enzymes do most of the digestive work in the small intestine. These digestive enzymes are broadly classified according to their intended targets. **Carbohydrases** (kar-bō-HĪ-drā-sez) digest sugars and starches; **lipases** (LĪ-pā-sez) break down lipids; **nucleases** break down nucleic acids (RNA and DNA); and **proteases** (prō-tē-ā-sez) (proteolytic enzymes) break proteins apart.

The Control of Pancreatic Secretion

Each day, the pancreas secretes about 1000 mL (1 qt) of pancreatic juice. The secretions are controlled primarily by hormones from the duodenum.

The duodenum releases secretin when acidic chyme arrives from the stomach. This hormone triggers the pancreas to secrete a watery, alkaline fluid with a pH between 7.5 and 8.8. Among its other components, this secretion contains buffers, primarily *sodium bicarbonate*, that increase the pH of the chyme.

Another duodenal hormone, CCK, stimulates the production and secretion of pancreatic enzymes. The specific enzymes are **pancreatic amylase**, which (like salivary amylase) breaks down carbohydrates; **pancreatic lipase**; a group of nucleases; and several proteases.

Proteases make up about 70 percent of total pancreatic enzyme production. The most abundant proteases are **trypsin** (TRIP-sin), **chymotrypsin** (kī-mō-TRIP-sin), and **carboxypeptidase** (kar-bok-sē-PEP-ti-dās). Together, they break down complex proteins into a mixture of short peptide chains and amino acids.

(1) extract absorbed nutrients or toxins from the blood before they reach the rest of the body and (2) monitor and adjust the circulating levels of organic nutrients. The liver removes and stores excess nutrients. It corrects nutrient deficiencies by mobilizing stored reserves or synthesizing necessary compounds. For example, when blood glucose levels rise, the liver removes glucose and synthesizes the storage compound glycogen. When blood glucose levels fall, the liver breaks down stored glycogen and releases glucose into the circulation. The liver also removes circulating toxins and metabolic wastes for later inactivation or excretion. In addition, it absorbs and stores fat-soluble vitamins (A, D, E, and K).

HEMATOLOGICAL REGULATION. The liver is the largest blood reservoir in the body. It receives about 25 percent of cardiac output. As blood passes through the liver, phagocytic Kupffer cells remove aged or damaged red blood cells, debris, and pathogens. Kupffer cells are antigen-presenting cells that can stimulate an immune response. ⤶ p. 488 Equally important, hepatocytes synthesize the plasma proteins. These molecules determine the osmotic concentration of the blood, transport nutrients, and make up the clotting and complement systems. ⤶ p. 381

THE PRODUCTION AND ROLE OF BILE. Recall that bile is synthesized in the liver and excreted into the lumen of the duodenum. Bile consists mostly of water, ions, *bilirubin* (a pigment derived from hemoglobin), cholesterol, and an assortment of lipids collectively known as **bile salts**. The water and ions in bile help dilute and buffer acids in chyme as it enters the small intestine. Bile salts are synthesized from cholesterol in the liver. They are required for the normal digestion and absorption of fats.

Most dietary lipids are not water soluble. Mechanical processing in the stomach creates large droplets containing various lipids. Pancreatic lipase is not lipid soluble and can interact with lipids only at the surface of the droplet. Large droplets have a lower surface area to volume relationship compared to smaller droplets. As a result, larger droplets have more of their lipids isolated and protected from these digestive enzymes. Bile salts break the droplets apart through a process called **emulsification** (ē-mul-si-fi-KĀ-shun). This process creates tiny droplets with a superficial coating of bile salts. The formation of tiny droplets increases the total surface area available for enzymatic attack. In addition, the layer of bile salts aids the interaction between lipids and lipid-digesting enzymes from the pancreas. (We will return to lipid digestion later.)

CLINICAL NOTE

Portal Hypertension

The portal system is a specialized component of the circulatory system. Veins from the spleen, stomach, pancreas, gallbladder, and intestines do not drain directly into the inferior vena cava, as do the veins from other abdominal organs. Instead, they drain into the portal vein that delivers the blood to the liver. In the liver, blood from the portal circulation mixes with the arterial blood in the hepatic capillaries and is eventually drained from the liver by the hepatic veins. The hepatic veins drain into the inferior vena cava.

Blood in the hepatic portal system contains substances absorbed by the digestive tract. Blood that enters the liver via the portal vein contains greater concentrations of glucose, amino acids, and fats than does blood that leaves the liver via the hepatic vein. The liver regulates the concentration of nutrients, such as glucose or amino acids, in the circulating blood.

The pressure within the portal system is normally 3 mmHg. An increase in portal pressure to at least 10 mmHg is referred to as *portal hypertension*. Portal hypertension is caused by disorders that impede or obstruct blood flow through any part of the portal system or the vena cava.

The obstruction can occur in the liver or in the hepatic veins that drain the liver. The most common cause of portal hypertension is obstruction caused by cirrhosis of the liver. *Cirrhosis* is an irreversible inflammatory disease that disrupts the structure and function of the liver. The most common cause of cirrhosis in the United States is chronic alcohol abuse (**Figure 16-18**). Chronic infectious hepatitis also can cause cirrhosis that results in portal hypertension.

Increased pressure within the portal system causes collateral blood vessels between the portal veins and the systemic veins to open. Blood pressure in the systemic veins is considerably lower than that in the portal system, which enables blood to bypass the obstructed portal vessels. The collateral veins develop in the esophagus, anterior abdominal wall, and rectum. High pressure and increased blood flow are transmitted through these veins from the portal to the systemic venous circulation. Blood that is shunted into the systemic circulation bypasses the liver where toxic metabolic waste products are usually removed. This results in an accumulation of these waste products in the systemic circulation.

(Continued)

16

Figure 16-18 Postmortem Specimens That Compare (a) Normal Liver and (b) Cirrhotic Liver. Note the cirrhotic liver is irregular and smaller than the normal specimen.

Figure 16-19 Esophageal Varices in a Patient with Portal Hypertension Secondary to Alcoholic Cirrhosis.

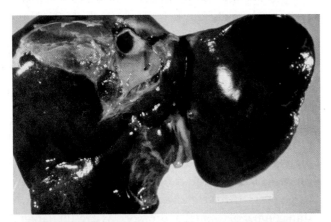

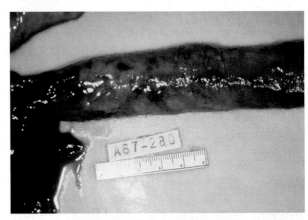

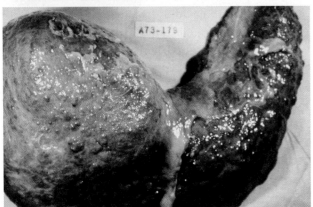

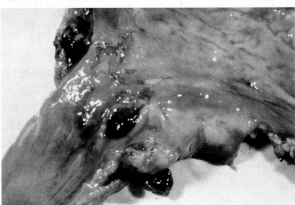

Long-term portal hypertension results in numerous problems that are quite difficult to treat. These include:

- *Varices.* Varices are tortuous, distended collateral veins that develop secondary to long-standing increased portal pressure. They are found in the lower esophagus, upper stomach, and rectum. They are prone to bleeding that can be difficult to control (**Figure 16-19**).
- *Ascites.* Ascites is the accumulation of fluid in the space between the parietal and visceral peritoneum. It is caused by increased pressure in the mesenteric tributaries of the portal vein. Hydrostatic pressure within the veins forces water out of these vessels and into the peritoneal cavity.
- *Splenomegaly.* Splenomegaly, an enlargement of the spleen, results from increased pressure in the splenic vein, which is a branch of the portal vein.
- *Hepatic encephalopathy.* Hepatic encephalopathy is characterized by central nervous system disturbances such as confusion, somnolence, and unconsciousness. Hepatic encephalopathy results from increased amounts of metabolic waste products in the blood, especially ammonia.

Portal hypertension develops over years. The most common clinical manifestation is vomiting of blood from bleeding esophageal varices. Slow, chronic variceal bleeding can cause anemia or melena. Rupture of esophageal varices is painless and can cause massive hemorrhage that is notoriously difficult to control and often fatal. Variceal bleeding can sometimes be controlled by injecting a sclerosing agent into the bleeding varix or banding of the bleeding varix with a fiber-optic esophagogastroduodenoscope. Placing a Sengstaken-Blakemore tube can sometimes control massive hemorrhages. This is a cylindrical balloon with a bulb at the end that is inserted into the distal esophagus and inflated. Inflation of the balloon and the bulb compresses the bleeding varices, slowing or stopping bleeding. Unfortunately, there are numerous, potentially lethal, complications associated with the Sengstaken-Blakemore tube use. Because of this, it is rarely used except as a last resort.

The viable treatment options for portal hypertension are exceedingly limited. Surgical construction of a portacaval shunt (connection of the portal vein to the inferior vena cava) can reduce portal pressure. However, it can cause liver failure or encephalopathy due to reduced hepatic blood flow. In selected cases, liver transplantation can be curative if the disease is not too advanced. Overall, there is no effective, definitive treatment for portal hypertension.

CLINICAL NOTE

Hepatic Abscesses

The liver is the organ most commonly subject to the development of abscesses. Liver abscesses are uncommon, especially in industrialized countries. When they do occur, they most frequently result from parasitic infection. The amoeba *Entamoeba histolytica* is the most common etiological agent, especially in developing countries. Approximately half of all patients with amoebic liver abscess will be asymptomatic. The other half will have low-grade fever, nausea, vomiting, diarrhea, and abdominal pain. The abscesses appear like "anchovy paste" on gross examination. The diagnosis can usually be established by identifying the parasite through stool testing.

In the United States, hepatic abscesses are usually the result of a surgical procedure, especially one that involves the biliary tract and gallbladder. The principle treatment is drainage of the abscess. This may be accomplished through open surgical drainage or placement of a catheter into the abscess.

CLINICAL NOTE

Liver Transplant

Liver transplantation is the replacement of a native, diseased liver with a liver from a brain-dead donor *(allograft)*. This operation allows a patient who otherwise would have died from liver failure to live a relatively full and normal life. The donor liver contains several tissue antigens that can induce an immune response in the recipient. Because of this, the donor and recipient must be checked for tissue antigen compatibility. A good match will decrease the likelihood of *organ rejection.* Patients who receive a liver transplant will be placed on *immuno-suppressive drugs* and will remain on them for the rest of their lives.

Patients with *fulminate liver failure*, regardless of the cause, will die within hours or days if a suitable organ donor cannot be located. In an extreme situation, a liver from a lower animal *(xenograft)*, most commonly a pig, can be used temporarily until a human donor becomes available.

On rare occasions, liver tissue may be harvested from a suitable living donor. Although the procedure is technically more complicated and places a second patient at risk, it is being used with increasing frequency when a suitable donor cannot be found. A lobe of the liver is taken from the donor and placed in the recipient. The liver is unique in that it will regenerate. Thus, in a living donor operation, the livers will grow to normal size in both the donor and the recipient within six to eight weeks.

Table 16-2	**Major Functions of the Liver**
DIGESTIVE AND METABOLIC FUNCTIONS	
Synthesis and secretion of bile	
Storage of glycogen and lipid reserves	
Maintenance of normal blood levels of glucose, amino acids, and fatty acids	
Synthesis and interconversion of nutrient types (e.g., transamination of amino acids or conversion of carbohydrates to lipids)	
Synthesis and release of cholesterol bound to transport proteins	
Inactivation of toxins	
Storage of iron reserves	
Storage of fat-soluble vitamins	
OTHER MAJOR FUNCTIONS	
Synthesis of plasma proteins	
Synthesis of clotting factors	
Synthesis of the inactive hormone angiotensinogen	
Phagocytosis of damaged red blood cells (by Kupffer cells)	
Blood storage (largest blood reservoir in the body)	
Absorption and breakdown of circulating hormones (insulin, epinephrine) and immunoglobulins	
Absorption and inactivation of lipid-soluble drugs	

Table 16-2 provides a summary of the liver's major functions.

The Gallbladder

The **gallbladder** is a hollow, pear-shaped organ that stores and concentrates bile prior to its excretion into the small intestine. This muscular sac lies in a recess in the posterior surface of the liver's right lobe (**Figure 16-17a**). The cystic duct extends from the gallbladder to the point where it unites with the common hepatic duct to form the common bile duct. The common bile duct and the pancreatic duct join and share a passageway that enters the duodenum at the *duodenal papilla* (**Figure 16-17b**). The muscular **hepatopancreatic sphincter** surrounds their shared passageway.

A major function of the gallbladder is *bile storage*. Bile is secreted continuously, roughly 1 liter each day. However, it is released into the duodenum only under the stimulation of the intestinal hormone CCK. In its absence, the hepatopancreatic sphincter remains closed, so bile leaving the liver in the common hepatic duct cannot flow through the common bile duct and into the duodenum. Instead, it enters the cystic duct and is stored within the expandable gallbladder.

16

CLINICAL NOTE

Hepatitis

Hepatitis is an inflammation of the liver and can result from both infectious and noninfectious causes. Medications, toxins, chemicals, and autoimmune disorders may cause *noninfectious hepatitis. Infectious hepatitis* can result from infection with viruses, bacteria, fungi, and parasites. The vast majority of infectious hepatitis cases are viral (**Figure 16-20**).

Several viruses have been identified as causative agents for hepatitis. These include: hepatitis A virus (HAV), hepatitis B virus (HBV), hepatitis C virus (HCV), hepatitis D virus (HDV), hepatitis E virus (HEV), hepatitis F virus (HFV), and hepatitis G virus (HGV). HAV, HBV, and HCV cause more than 90 percent of cases of acute viral hepatitis in the United States. Emergency personnel are at particular risk for exposure to HBV and HCV because of the increased risk of exposure to body fluids. HAV, HBV, HCV, and HDV are the only hepatitis viruses endemic to the United States.

The hepatitis viruses impair liver function by attacking and destroying liver cells. Hepatitis may be either acute or chronic. All hepatitis viruses cause an acute infection. The severity of the infection can vary from asymptomatic to fulminant liver failure. Patients who contract hepatitis A and hepatitis E usually do not develop a chronic infection. However, patients who are infected with hepatitis B, hepatitis C, hepatitis D, and hepatitis G are at risk of developing chronic active hepatitis. Chronic active hepatitis is progressive; it leads to deterioration in liver function and eventually cirrhosis. Many patients will develop hepatocellular cancer. Complications associated with chronic active hepatitis include portal hypertension, ascites, and eventually, hepatic encephalopathy (CNS dysfunction). As liver failure progresses, toxic metabolic waste products are not effectively cleared by the liver and start to accumulate in the blood. Among the more important of these waste products is ammonia. An increase in serum

Figure 16-20 Liver with Marked Inflammation from Hepatitis. Hepatitis can lead to liver failure, and some types can lead to chronic infection that causes cirrhosis and, in some cases, liver cancer.

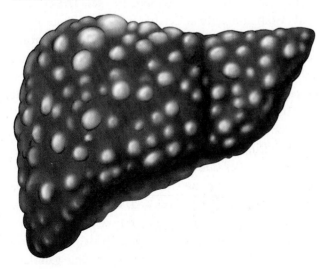

ammonia can cause hepatic encephalopathy which results in disorientation, confusion, somnolence, and eventually unconsciousness. As hepatic encephalopathy worsens, the patient will develop asterixis, which is an involuntary "flapping" of the hands when the patient holds his hands up, flexed at the wrist (such as the motion for stopping traffic).

The signs and symptoms of infectious hepatitis depend on the type of hepatitis involved. Typically, patients will develop a low-grade fever, loss of appetite, and malaise. The skin, sclera, and mucous membranes may become jaundiced (icteric) due to the accumulation of bilirubin in the body. In more severe cases, the patient may develop significant nausea and vomiting that can lead to dehydration as evidenced by tachycardia, dry mucous membranes, and decreased skin turgor. The liver may be diffusely enlarged and tender to palpation.

There are several different types of infectious viral hepatitis depending on the virus involved. These include:

- *Hepatitis A.* Hepatitis A, often called *infectious hepatitis*, is the primary cause of viral hepatitis in the United States. It is transmitted via the fecal-oral route, often through food, water, milk, and shellfish contaminated by fecal wastes. The incubation period is typically two to six weeks. Hepatitis A often occurs in epidemics that can be attributed to a community source such as a restaurant. Hepatitis A is usually a mild, self-limited disease. Infection with HAV confers life-long immunity, and chronic infection with HAV does not occur. A vaccine is available for those deemed to be at increased risk.

- *Hepatitis B.* Hepatitis B, also called *serum hepatitis*, is a major cause of hepatitis worldwide. Hepatitis B is transmitted via blood or other body products, often through mucous membranes. Saliva, serum, and semen have all been demonstrated to be infectious. In addition, HBV can be transmitted perinatally from an infected mother to her unborn child. The incubation period for hepatitis B is considerably longer than for hepatitis A, and ranges from one to six months. Hepatitis B is a serious infection and can develop into a chronic infection. Chronic hepatitis B can lead to cirrhosis of the liver and, eventually, hepatocellular cancer. An effective vaccine against hepatitis B is available and should be administered to emergency personnel.

- *Hepatitis C.* Hepatitis C, formerly referred to as non-A, non-B hepatitis, is a serious infection and the most common cause of chronic viral hepatitis in the United States. Emergency personnel are at increased risk of infection by hepatitis C due to exposure to infected blood or body fluids. The incubation period can range from one to six months. The signs and symptoms of hepatitis C are similar to those of hepatitis B. Approximately 80 percent of those infected with HCV will go on to develop chronic HCV infection. Chronic hepatitis C infection is the leading reason for liver transplantation in the United States. There is no effective vaccine against hepatitis C or post-exposure prophylaxis.

- *Hepatitis D.* Hepatitis D, also called delta hepatitis, is a unique type of hepatitis. It requires the presence of hepatitis B virus in order to replicate. Thus, hepatitis D is often considered to be a coinfection or superinfection of hepatitis B. The transmission of hepatitis D is similar to that for hepatitis B. Patients with both hepatitis B and hepatitis D tend to have a more severe course than those with hepatitis B alone. Hepatitis D tends to lead to chronic infection. A vaccine for hepatitis D is not yet available.

- *Hepatitis E.* Hepatitis E is similar to hepatitis A and is transmitted via the fecal-oral route. The incubation period for hepatitis E ranges from two to nine weeks. Like hepatitis A, the disease is usually self-limited and chronic infection does not occur. Hepatitis E is the most common cause of hepatitis worldwide, but seldom seen in the United States. A vaccine against hepatitis E is not yet available.

- *Hepatitis F.* Hepatitis F is proposed as another hepatitis virus transmitted by the fecal-oral route. A small number of cases have been reported in France. Little else is known about the infection.

- *Hepatitis G.* Hepatitis G virus was identified in 1996 and is associated with both acute and chronic liver disease. The incidence is approximately 0.3 percent of all cases of acute viral hepatitis. Transmission of HGV is blood borne. Chronic infection is common, and occurs in 90–100 percent of infected persons. Much remains to be learned about hepatitis G. A vaccine is not yet available.

Whenever chyme enters the duodenum, CCK is released. Its presence relaxes the hepatopancreatic sphincter and stimulates contractions within the walls of the gallbladder that push bile into the small intestine. The amount of CCK secreted increases if the chyme contains large amounts of fat.

Another function of the gallbladder is *bile modification.* When filled to capacity, the gallbladder contains 40–70 mL of bile. The composition of bile gradually changes as it remains in the gallbladder. Water is absorbed, and the bile salts and other components of bile become increasingly concentrated. If the bile salts become too concentrated, they may precipitate and form *gallstones* that can cause a variety of clinical problems.

CHECKPOINT

18. Does a high-fat meal raise or lower the level of cholecystokinin (CCK) in the blood?

19. The digestion of which nutrient would be most impaired by damage to the exocrine pancreas?

See the blue Answers tab at the back of the book.

CLINICAL NOTE

Biliary Colic and Cholecystitis

Cholecystitis is an inflammation of the gallbladder. Cholelithiasis (the formation of gallstones), which causes 90 percent of cholecystitis cases, occurs in approximately 15 percent of the adult population in the United States, with over one million new cases diagnosed annually. There are two types of gallstones, cholesterol-based and bilirubin-based. Cholesterol-based stones are far more common and are associated with a specific risk profile: obese, middle-aged women with more than one biological child.

Definitive treatment of acute cholecystitis includes antibiotic therapy, laparoscopic surgery, lithotripsy (ultrasound treatment to break up the stones), and surgery if the other, less invasive, therapies fail. With the advent of laparoscopic surgery, mortality has fallen to less then 1 percent, with an overall morbidity of approximately 6 percent.

Cholecystitis caused by gallstones can be chronic or acute (**Figure 16-21**). The liver produces bile, the primary vehicle for removing cholesterol from the body. The bile travels down the common bile duct to empty into the small intestine at the sphincter of Oddi. The sphincter of Oddi opens when chyme exits the stomach through the cardiac sphincter. When the sphincter of Oddi closes, the flow of bile backs up into the gallbladder via the cystic duct. The bile remains in the gallbladder until the sphincter of Oddi opens again.

Figure 16-21 Cholecystitis.
The gallbladder is located immediately under the liver in the right upper abdominal quadrant. Gallstones can enter the cystic duct or the common bile duct. The latter can result in partial or complete obstruction of the duct.

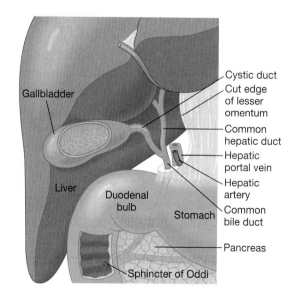

Gallbladder
Cystic duct
Cut edge of lesser omentum
Common hepatic duct
Hepatic portal vein
Hepatic artery
Liver
Duodenal bulb
Stomach
Common bile duct
Pancreas
Sphincter of Oddi

16

(Continued)

The bile can become supersaturated and calculi—stone-like masses based on bilirubin, cholesterol, or both—form. These calculi travel down the cystic duct, and frequently lodge in the common bile duct. When they obstruct the flow of bile, gallbladder inflammation and irritation result. The bile salts subsequently attack the mucosal membrane that lines the gallbladder, which leaves the underlying epithelial tissue without protection. Prostaglandins are also released, which further irritates the epithelial wall. As irritation continues, the inflammation grows; this increases intraluminal pressure and ultimately reduces blood flow to the epithelium.

Other causes of cholecystitis include acalculus cholecystitis (cholecystitis without associated stones) and chronic inflammation caused by bacterial infection. Acalculus cholecystitis usually results from burns, sepsis, diabetes, and multiple organ failure. Chronic cholecystitis that results from a bacterial infection (*Escherichia coli* and enterococci) presents with an inflammatory process similar to cholelithiasis.

An inflamed gallbladder usually causes an acute attack of upper right quadrant abdominal pain. The inflammation can cause an irritation of the diaphragm with referred pain in the right shoulder. If the gallstones are lodged in the cystic duct, the pain may be colicky, due to expansion and contraction of the duct. Often the pain occurs after a meal that is high in fat content because of the secondary release of bile from the gallbladder. The right subcostal region may be tender because of abdominal muscle spasms. Patients may experience extreme pain as the epithelium in the gallbladder erodes away. Sympathetic stimulation because of the pain may cause pale, cool, clammy skin. If peritonitis occurs, the skin may be warm due to increased blood flow to the inflamed peritoneum. Nausea and vomiting are common, due to cystic duct spasm. Many patients will have tenderness under the right costal margin referred to as a positive Murphy's sign.

16-7 The large intestine is divided into three parts with regional specialization

Learning Objective Describe the structure of the large intestine, including its regional specializations, and list its absorptive functions.

The horseshoe-shaped **large intestine** begins at the end of the ileum and ends at the anus. The large intestine lies inferior to the stomach and liver and almost completely frames the small intestine (**Figure 16-22**). The main functions of the large intestine include (1) reabsorption of water and compaction of the intestinal contents into feces, (2) absorption of important vitamins freed by bacterial action, and (3) storage of fecal material prior to defecation.

The large intestine, also called the *large bowel*, has an average length of about 1.5 m (5 ft) and a width of 7.5 cm (3 in.). It can be divided into three parts: (1) the pouchlike *cecum*, the first portion; (2) the *colon*, the largest portion; and (3) the *rectum*, the last 15 cm (6 in.) of the large intestine and the end of the digestive tract.

The Cecum

Material arriving from the ileum first enters an expanded pouch, the **cecum** (SĒ-kum). Compaction begins there. A muscular sphincter, the **ileocecal (il-ē-ō-SĒ-kal) valve**, guards the connection between the ileum and the cecum.

The slender, hollow **appendix**, or *vermiform (vermis,* worm) *appendix*, attaches to the cecum along its posteromedial surface. The appendix is generally about 9 cm (3.5 in.) long, but its size and shape are quite variable. The walls of the appendix are dominated by lymphoid nodules, and it functions primarily as an organ of the lymphatic system. Inflammation of the appendix is known as *appendicitis*.

The Colon

The **colon** has a larger diameter and thinner wall than the small intestine. Major characteristics of the colon are a lack of villi and an abundance of mucous cells. The most striking external feature of the colon is the presence of pouches, or **haustra** (HAWS-truh; singular, *haustrum*). Haustra permit the colon to expand and elongate (**Figure 16-22a**). Three longitudinal bands of smooth muscle—the **teniae coli** (TĒ-nē-ē KŌ-lē; *singular*, tenia)—run along the outer surface of the colon just beneath the serosa. Muscle tone within these bands creates the haustra.

The colon can be divided into four segments. The **ascending colon** begins at the ileocecal valve. It ascends along the right side of the peritoneal cavity until it reaches the inferior margin of the liver. It then turns horizontally, becoming the **transverse colon**. The transverse colon continues toward the left side, passing below the stomach and following the curve of the body wall. Near the spleen, it turns inferiorly to form the **descending colon**. The descending colon continues along the left side until it curves and forms the S-shaped **sigmoid (SIG-moyd;** *sigmeidos,* **the Greek letter** *S*) **colon**. The sigmoid colon empties into the rectum.

Figure 16-22 The Large Intestine.

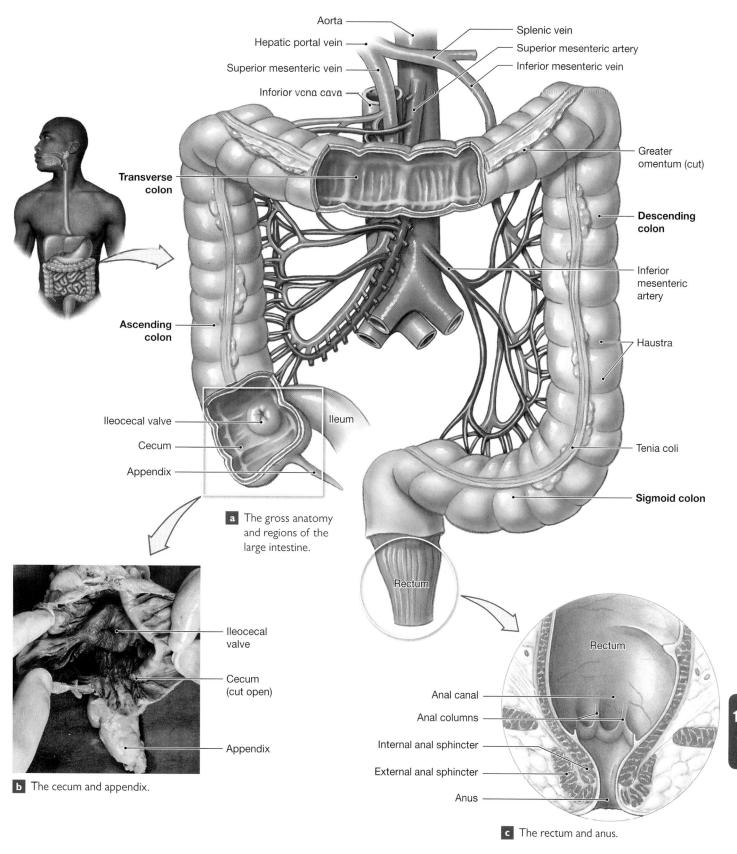

a The gross anatomy and regions of the large intestine.

b The cecum and appendix.

c The rectum and anus.

CLINICAL NOTE

Appendicitis

Appendicitis is an inflammation of the vermiform appendix, which is located at the junction of the small intestine and the large intestine (ileocecal junction). Appendicitis occurs in approximately 10–20 percent of the U.S. population. The maximum incidence occurs in the second and third decades of life and is relatively rare at the extremes of age.

The most common cause of acute appendicitis is obstruction of the lumen of the appendix, usually by fecal material (fecalith). The shape and location of the appendix makes it particularly vulnerable to obstruction by feces or other material, such as food particles or tumor. This inflames the lymphoid tissue and often leads to bacterial infection that subsequently ulcerates the mucosa. The inflammation causes the appendix's internal diameter to expand, which can block blood flow through the appendicular artery and cause thrombosis. With its blood supply cut off, the appendix becomes ischemic, and infarction, tissue necrosis, and gangrene follow. At this point, the walls of the appendix weaken to the point of rupture, spilling the appendiceal contents into the peritoneal cavity. Rupture of the appendix can lead to peritonitis and systemic infection.

The signs and symptoms of appendicitis can vary. Older patients and diabetics tend to have less classical symptoms. Initially, the patient with appendicitis will develop diffuse, colicky abdominal pain, usually associated with nausea and vomiting and low-grade fever. Often the pain is located in the periumbilical region. As the illness progresses, the pain localizes to the right lower quadrant. A common location of appendicitis pain is McBurney's point. McBurney's point is 1.5 to 2 inches above the anterior iliac crest along a direct line from the anterior iliac crest to the umbilicus (**Figure 16-23**). Once the appendix ruptures, the pain becomes diffuse due to the development of peritonitis. Occasionally, the appendix can be affixed to the posterior aspect of the large intestine (cecum). This condition, referred to as retrocecal appendicitis, often causes low-back pain or flank pain instead of pain over McBurney's point. Retrocecal appendicitis can be more difficult to diagnose.

Figure 16-23 McBurney's Point. McBurney's point is located along a line approximately 1½ to 2 inches above the right anterior iliac crest along an imaginary line drawn between the right anterior iliac crest and the umbilicus.

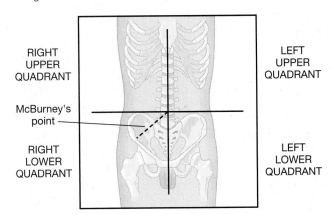

The diagnosis of appendicitis can often be made based on the history and physical examination. Usually, the patient will have an elevated white blood cell count. In uncertain cases, ultrasound examination of the abdomen can aid in diagnosis. Normally, the appendix cannot be seen on ultrasound examination. If seen, then it is highly suggestive of acute appendicitis. Computed tomography of the abdomen is very helpful in confirming the diagnosis of acute appendicitis.

Treatment of appendicitis is surgical removal of the appendix (appendectomy). Today, most appendectomies can be performed using a laparoscope that markedly decreases pain and recovery time. Surgery for appendicitis should be prompt to prevent rupture of the appendix. If appendiceal rupture occurs, the patient often develops bacterial peritonitis. This usually requires a prolonged hospital stay and intravenous antibiotics.

The Rectum

The **rectum** (REK-tum) forms the last 15 cm (6 in.) of the digestive tract (**Figure 16-22c**). It is an expandable organ for the temporary storage of feces. The last portion of the rectum, the **anal canal**, contains small longitudinal folds called *anal columns*. The distal margins of these columns are joined by transverse folds that mark the boundary between the columnar epithelium of the rectum and a stratified squamous epithelium like that found in the oral cavity. Very close to the **anus**, which is the exit of the anal canal, the epidermis becomes keratinized and identical to that on the skin surface.

The circular muscle layer of the muscularis externa in this region forms the **internal anal sphincter**. The smooth muscle cells of this sphincter are not under voluntary control. The **external anal sphincter**, which encircles the anus, consists of skeletal muscle fibers and is under voluntary control.

The Functions of the Large Intestine

The major functions of the large intestine are absorbing a variety of substances and preparing the fecal material for elimination.

CLINICAL NOTE

Hemorrhoids

The *rectum* is drained by the *internal* and *external hemorrhoidal veins*. Swelling of these veins is referred to as *hemorrhoids*. *Internal hemorrhoids* may be asymptomatic or may cause rectal pain, itching, or bright red bleeding (usually with defecation). *External hemorrhoids* tend to thrombose, especially after lifting, and cause severe rectal pain and pressure. Internal hemorrhoids usually respond to rectal creams and analgesics. External hemorrhoids require drainage of the thrombosed hemorrhoid, which usually provides immediate relief.

Absorption in the Large Intestine

The reabsorption of water is an important function of the large intestine. Roughly 1500 mL of watery material enters the colon each day, but only about 200 mL of feces is ejected. To appreciate how efficient our digestion is, consider the average composition of feces: 75 percent water, 5 percent bacteria, and the rest a mixture of indigestible materials, small quantities of inorganic matter, and the remains of intestinal epithelial cells.

In addition to reabsorbing water, the large intestine absorbs a variety of other substances. Examples include useful compounds such as bile salts and vitamins, organic waste products such as bilirubin-derived breakdown products, and various toxins generated by bacterial action.

BILE SALTS. Most of the bile salts entering the large intestine are rapidly absorbed in the cecum. They are then transported to the liver for secretion in bile.

VITAMINS. Vitamins are organic molecules related to lipids and carbohydrates that are essential to many metabolic reactions. Many enzymes require the binding of an additional

CLINICAL NOTE

Colorectal Cancer

Colorectal cancer is relatively common in both men and women. Although colorectal cancer is the third leading cause of cancer-related deaths—an estimated 49,700 colorectal cancer deaths were expected in 2015—the death rate has declined over the past 20 years. The best defense appears to be early detection and prompt treatment. The standard simple screening test involves checking a stool (fecal) sample for blood as part of a routine physical examination.

ion or molecule, called a *cofactor*, before substrates can also bind. *Coenzymes* are nonprotein molecules that function as cofactors, and many vitamins are essential coenzymes.

Bacteria residing within the colon generate three vitamins that supplement our diets:

- *Vitamin K*, a fat-soluble vitamin needed by the liver to synthesize four clotting factors, including prothrombin.

- *Biotin*, a water-soluble vitamin important in glucose metabolism.

- *Vitamin* B_5 (pantothenic acid), a water-soluble vitamin required in the manufacture of steroid hormones and some neurotransmitters.

Vitamin K deficiencies lead to impaired blood clotting. Intestinal bacteria produce roughly half of our daily vitamin K requirements. Deficiencies of biotin or vitamin B_5 are extremely rare after infancy because the intestinal bacteria produce enough to make up for any shortage in the diet.

ORGANIC WASTES. In the large intestine, bacteria convert bilirubin into other products. Some of these are absorbed into the bloodstream and excreted in the urine, producing its yellow color. Others remain in the colon. Upon exposure to oxygen, they are further modified into the pigments that give feces a brown color. (Recall that we discussed the breakdown of heme and its release as bilirubin in the bile in Chapter 11.) ⊃ p. 386

TOXINS. Bacterial action breaks down peptides that remain in the feces. This action generates (1) ammonia; (2) nitrogen-containing compounds that are responsible for the odor of feces; and (3) hydrogen sulfide (H_2S), a gas that produces a "rotten egg" odor. Much of the ammonia and other toxins cross the epithelium of the colon and are absorbed into the hepatic portal circulation. The liver removes these toxins and processes them into relatively nontoxic compounds that are excreted at the kidneys.

Intestinal enzymes do not alter indigestible carbohydrates. They arrive in the colon intact. These polysaccharide molecules are a nutrient source for resident bacteria. The metabolic activities of these bacteria create intestinal gas, or *flatus*. Meals containing large amounts of indigestible carbohydrates (such as beans) stimulate bacterial gas production.

Movements of the Large Intestine

The gastroileal and gastroenteric reflexes move material into the cecum while you eat. Movement from the cecum to the transverse colon is very slow, allowing hours for the

16

reabsorption of water. Powerful peristaltic contractions called *mass movements* take place a few times a day. They move material from the transverse colon through the rest of the large intestine. The normal stimulus is distension of the stomach and duodenum. The commands are over the intestinal nerve plexuses. The contractions force feces into the rectum and produce the conscious urge to defecate.

Defecation

The rectum is usually empty until a powerful peristaltic contraction forces feces out of the sigmoid colon. Distension of the rectal wall then triggers the **defecation reflex**. This reflex involves two positive feedback loops:

1. In the shorter feedback loop, stretch receptors in the rectal walls stimulate a series of increased local peristaltic contractions in the sigmoid colon and rectum. The contractions move feces toward the anus and increase distension of the rectum.

2. The stretch receptors in the rectal walls also stimulate parasympathetic motor neurons in the sacral spinal cord. These neurons stimulate increased peristalsis (mass movements) in the descending colon and sigmoid colon that push feces toward the rectum, further increasing distension there.

The passage of feces through the anal canal requires relaxation of the internal anal sphincter, but when it relaxes, the external sphincter automatically closes. Thus, the actual release of feces requires conscious effort to open the external sphincter voluntarily. Without the conscious commands, peristaltic contractions cease until additional rectal expansion triggers the defecation reflex again.

In addition, other conscious actions can raise intra-abdominal pressures and help to force fecal material out of the rectum. These actions include tensing the abdominal muscles or elevating intra-abdominal pressures by attempting to forcibly exhale with

16

CLINICAL NOTE

Diverticulosis

In diverticulosis (dī-ver-tik-ū-LŌ-sis), pockets called *diverticula* form in the intestinal mucosa, generally in the sigmoid colon. These pockets get forced outward, probably by pressures during defecation. If the pockets push through weak points in the muscularis externa, they form chambers that can become infected and inflamed. The inflammation causes pain and occasional bleeding, a condition known as *diverticulitis* (dī-ver-tik-ū-LĪ-tis). Inflammation of other portions of the colon is called *colitis* (ko-LĪ-tis).

CLINICAL NOTE

Diarrhea and Constipation

Diarrhea (dī-a-RĒ-uh) exists when an individual has frequent, watery bowel movements. Diarrhea results when the mucosa of the colon cannot maintain normal levels of absorption. Bacterial, viral, or protozoan infection of the colon or small intestine can cause acute bouts of diarrhea lasting several days. Severe diarrhea is life threatening due to cumulative fluid and electrolyte losses.

Constipation is infrequent defecation, generally involving dry, hard feces. Constipation occurs when fecal material moves through the colon so slowly that excessive water reabsorption takes place. Constipation can usually be treated by oral administration of stool softeners such as Colace, laxatives, or *cathartics* (ka-THAR-tiks), which promote defecation. These compounds either promote water movement into the feces, add bulk, or irritate the lining of the colon to stimulate peristalsis.

Irritable bowel syndrome is a disorder characterized by diarrhea, constipation, or both.

a closed glottis (called the *Valsalva maneuver*). Such pressures also force blood into the network of veins in the lamina propria and submucosa of the anal canal, causing them to stretch. Repeated bouts of straining to force defecation can cause these veins to be permanently distended, producing *hemorrhoids*.

CHECKPOINT

20. Identify the four segments of the colon.

21. What are some structural differences between the large intestine and the small intestine?

22. A narrowing of the ileocecal valve would hamper movement of chyme between what two organs?

See the blue Answers tab at the back of the book.

16-8 Digestion is the chemical alteration of food that allows the absorption and use of nutrients

Learning Objective List the nutrients required by the body, describe the chemical digestion of organic nutrients, and discuss the absorption of organic and inorganic nutrients.

A balanced diet contains all the ingredients needed to maintain homeostasis. These ingredients include six nutrients: carbohydrates, proteins, lipids, water, electrolytes (minerals), and vitamins. The digestive system handles each one differently. Large organic molecules must be broken down through digestion before absorption can occur. Water, electrolytes, and vitamins can be absorbed without preliminary processing, but special transport processes may be involved.

CLINICAL NOTE

Diverticulitis

Diverticulitis is a relatively common complication of diverticulosis. Diverticulosis is a condition characterized by the presence in the intestine of diverticula, which are small outpouchings of mucosal and submucosal tissue that push through the outermost layer of the intestine, the muscularis. Colonic diverticula are far more common in developed countries such as the United States and increase markedly in prevalence with increased age. They are present in more than half of patients over 60 years of age. Diverticulitis is an inflammation of diverticula secondary to infection. Unlike diverticulosis, it is symptomatic; patients will complain of lower left-sided pain (because most diverticula are in the sigmoid colon); exam and testing will show fever and an increased white blood cell count.

The pathogenesis of an acquired diverticulum is twofold. First, stool passes sluggishly through the colon, a condition associated with the relatively low fiber diets common in developed countries. The colon responds with muscle spasms that increase bulk movement by raising the pressure on the contents inside the colon and pushing the fecal material forward. Second, the outermost layer of colon tissue is made up of fibrous bands of muscle wrapped around one another. Among them are muscles called the *taenia coli*. Nerves and blood vessels enter the colon through small openings within the taenia coli. These openings become weakened with age, and the increased pressure of muscle spasms can cause the inner layers of tissue, the mucosa and submucosa, to herniate through the openings, forming diverticula (**Figure 16-24**).

These diverticula commonly trap small amounts of fecal material, including sunflower seeds, popcorn fragments, okra seeds, sesame seeds, and others. The entrapped feces may allow bacteria other than the normal flora to grow and cause an infection. The problem is compounded when the diverticula become inflamed, and cause diverticulitis. Complications secondary to diverticulitis include possible hemorrhage or larger perforations of the colon wall through which the infected fecal contents can spill into the peritoneal cavity and cause peritonitis.

Figure 16-24 Diverticulum. Diverticula, which are outpouchings of the wall of the colon, can become infected (diverticulitis) or bleed (diverticulosis).

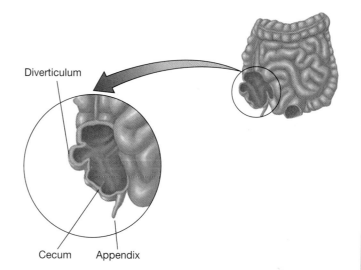

Diverticulum

Cecum   Appendix

The most common presentation of diverticulitis is colicky pain associated with a low-grade fever, nausea and vomiting, and tenderness upon palpation. The pain is usually localized to the lower left side because the sigmoid colon is involved in 95 percent of reported cases. Thus, diverticulitis is often called *left-sided appendicitis*. If the diverticula begin to bleed significantly, the usual signs and symptoms associated with severe lower GI bleeding may be present: cool, clammy skin, tachycardia, and diaphoresis. Bleeding diverticula can also result in bright red and bloody feces (hematochezia) because of their close proximity to the rectum. Patients may additionally complain of the perception that they cannot empty their rectums, even after defecation.

Build Your Knowledge

Recall that a decomposition reaction breaks a molecule into smaller fragments (as you saw in **Chapter 2: The Chemical Level of Organization**). Decomposition reactions involving water are important in breaking down complex molecules in the body. Breaking one of the chemical bonds in a complex molecule by adding a water molecule is called hydrolysis. The components of the water molecule (H and OH) are added to the resulting fragments. ⟳ **p. 33**

The Processing and Absorption of Nutrients

Food contains large organic molecules. Many of them are insoluble. The digestive system first breaks down the physical structure of the ingested material and then disassembles the component molecules into smaller fragments. This disassembly produces small organic molecules that can be released into the bloodstream. Once absorbed by cells, they are used to generate ATP or to build complex carbohydrates, proteins, and lipids.

Foods are usually complex chains of simpler molecules. In a typical dietary carbohydrate, the basic molecules are simple sugars. In a protein, the building blocks are amino acids, and in lipids they are usually fatty acids. Digestive

16

enzymes break the chemical bonds between the component molecules in the process called *hydrolysis*. (The hydrolysis of carbohydrates, lipids, and proteins was detailed in Chapter 2.) ⟲ pp. 38, 40, 43

Digestive enzymes differ in their targets. Carbohydrases break the bonds between sugars. Lipases separate fatty acids from glycerides. Proteases split the linkages between amino acids. Specific enzymes in each class may be even more selective, breaking bonds between specific molecules. For example, a given carbohydrase might ignore all bonds except those connecting two glucose molecules. **Spotlight Figure 16-25** summarizes the chemical events in the digestion of carbohydrates, lipids, and proteins. **Table 16-3** reviews the major digestive enzymes and their functions.

Carbohydrate Digestion and Absorption

Carbohydrate digestion begins in the mouth during mastication, through the action of salivary amylase. This enzyme breaks down complex carbohydrates into smaller fragments, producing a mixture primarily composed of disaccharides (two simple sugars) and trisaccharides (three simple sugars). Salivary amylase continues to digest the starches and glycogen in the meal for an hour or two before stomach acids render it inactive. In the duodenum, the action of pancreatic amylase breaks down the remaining complex carbohydrates.

Brush border enzymes on the surfaces of the intestinal microvilli break disaccharides and trisaccharides into monosaccharides (simple sugars). ⟲ p. 553 The intestinal epithelium then absorbs the resulting simple sugars through carrier-mediated transport processes, such as facilitated diffusion or cotransport. ⟲ p. 65 Glucose uptake, for example, takes place through cotransport with sodium ions. (The sodium ions are then ejected by the sodium–potassium exchange pump.)

Simple sugars entering an intestinal cell diffuse through the cytoplasm and cross the basement membrane by facilitated diffusion to enter the interstitial fluid. They then enter intestinal capillaries for delivery to the hepatic portal vein and liver.

Lipid Digestion and Absorption

Lipid digestion involves lingual lipase from glands of the tongue and pancreatic lipase from the pancreas. Fats, or triglycerides, are the most abundant dietary lipids. (Recall that a triglyceride molecule consists of three fatty acids attached to a single molecule of glycerol. ⟲ p. 41) Triglycerides and other dietary fats are relatively unaffected by conditions in the stomach and enter the duodenum in the form of large lipid droplets.

Recall that bile salts emulsify these drops into tiny droplets that can be more efficiently attacked by pancreatic lipase. This enzyme breaks apart the triglycerides. The resulting mixture of fatty acids and monoglycerides interacts with bile salts to form small lipid-bile salt complexes called **micelles** (mī-SELZ). When a micelle contacts the intestinal epithelium, the enclosed lipids diffuse across the plasma membrane and enter the cytoplasm. The intestinal cells manufacture new triglycerides from the arriving fatty acids and monoglycerides. They are then coated with proteins. This step creates a soluble complex known as a **chylomicron** (kī-lō-MĪ-kron; *chylos*, juice + *mikros*, small). The chylomicrons are secreted by

Table 16-3	Digestive Enzymes and Their Functions		
Enzyme	**Source**	**Target**	**Products**
CARBOHYDRASES			
Amylase	Salivary glands, pancreas	Complex carbohydrates	Disaccharides and trisaccharides
Maltase, sucrase, lactase	Small intestine	Maltose, sucrose, lactose	Monosaccharides
LIPASES			
Lingual lipase	Glands of tongue	Triglycerides	Fatty acids and monoglycerides
Pancreatic lipase	Pancreas	Triglycerides	Fatty acids and monoglycerides
PROTEASES			
Pepsin	Stomach	Proteins, polypeptides	Short polypeptides
Trypsin, chymotrypsin, carboxypeptidase	Pancreas	Proteins, polypeptides	Short peptide chains
Peptidases	Small intestine	Dipeptides, tripeptides	Amino acids
NUCLEASES			
	Pancreas	Nucleic acids	Nitrogenous bases and simple sugars

16

A typical meal contains carbohydrates, proteins, lipids, water, minerals (electrolytes), and vitamins. The digestive system handles each component differently. Large organic molecules must be broken down by digestion before they can be absorbed. Water, minerals, and vitamins can be absorbed without processing, but they may require special transport processes.

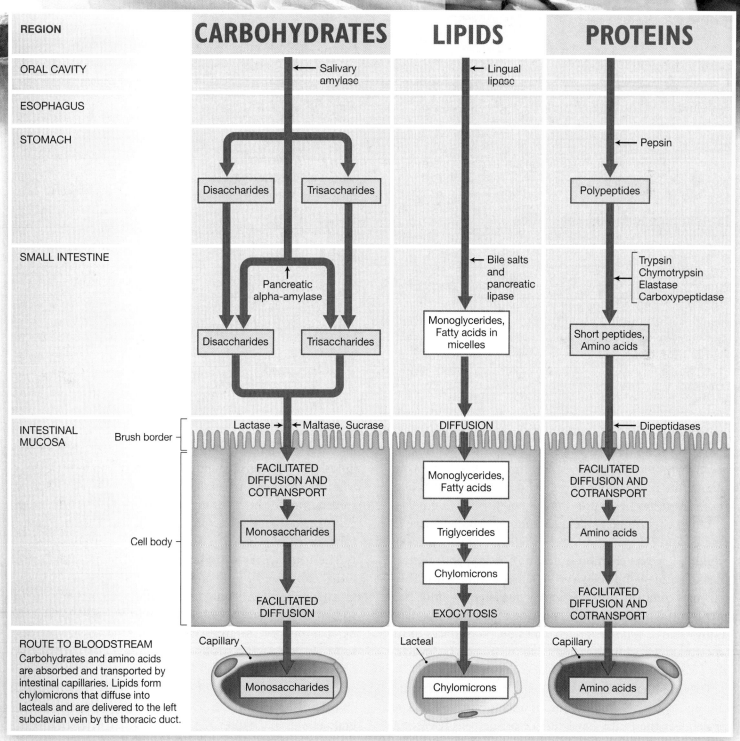

REGION	CARBOHYDRATES	LIPIDS	PROTEINS
ORAL CAVITY	← Salivary amylase	← Lingual lipase	
ESOPHAGUS			
STOMACH	Disaccharides Trisaccharides		← Pepsin Polypeptides
SMALL INTESTINE	↑ Pancreatic alpha-amylase Disaccharides Trisaccharides	← Bile salts and pancreatic lipase Monoglycerides, Fatty acids in micelles	⎡ Trypsin Chymotrypsin Elastase Carboxypeptidase Short peptides, Amino acids
INTESTINAL MUCOSA — Brush border	Lactase → ← Maltase, Sucrase	DIFFUSION	← Dipeptidases
— Cell body	FACILITATED DIFFUSION AND COTRANSPORT Monosaccharides FACILITATED DIFFUSION	Monoglycerides, Fatty acids Triglycerides Chylomicrons EXOCYTOSIS	FACILITATED DIFFUSION AND COTRANSPORT Amino acids FACILITATED DIFFUSION AND COTRANSPORT
ROUTE TO BLOODSTREAM	Capillary Monosaccharides	Lacteal Chylomicrons	Capillary Amino acids

ROUTE TO BLOODSTREAM
Carbohydrates and amino acids are absorbed and transported by intestinal capillaries. Lipids form chylomicrons that diffuse into lacteals and are delivered to the left subclavian vein by the thoracic duct.

CLINICAL NOTE

Lactose Intolerance

Lactose is the primary carbohydrate in milk. The enzyme lactase breaks down lactose. This enzyme performs an essential service throughout infancy and early childhood. If the intestinal mucosa stops producing lactase, the person becomes *lactose intolerant*. After a meal containing milk or other dairy products, such people can experience lower abdominal pain, gas, diarrhea, and vomiting.

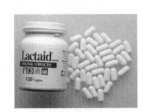

exocytosis into the interstitial fluids. From there, they enter intestinal lacteals through large gaps between adjacent lacteal endothelial cells. From the lacteals they proceed along lymphatic vessels and through the thoracic duct. They enter the bloodstream at the left subclavian vein.

Protein Digestion and Absorption

Proteins have very complex structures, so protein digestion is both complex and time consuming. Protein digestion first requires disrupting the structure of food so that proteolytic enzymes can attack individual protein molecules. This step involves mechanical processing in the oral cavity, through mastication, and chemical processing in the stomach, through the action of HCl.

Exposure of the ingested food to a strongly acid environment breaks down plant cell walls and the connective tissues in animal products. The acid also kills most pathogens. The acidic contents of the stomach provide the proper environment for the activity of pepsin, the proteolytic enzyme secreted by chief cells of the stomach. Pepsin does not complete protein digestion, but it reduces the relatively huge proteins of the chyme into smaller polypeptide fragments.

When chyme enters the duodenum and buffers have increased the pH, pancreatic proteolytic enzymes can begin working. Trypsin, chymotrypsin, and carboxypeptidase each break peptide bonds between different amino acids. These enzymes complete the disassembly of the polypeptide fragments into a mixture of short peptide chains and individual amino acids. *Peptidases* are enzymes on the surfaces of the intestinal microvilli. They complete the process by breaking the peptide chains into individual amino acids.

The intestinal epithelial cells then absorb the amino acids through both facilitated diffusion and cotransport. Carrier proteins at the inner, basal surface of the cells release the absorbed amino acids into the interstitial fluid. Once within the interstitial fluids, most of the amino acids diffuse into intestinal capillaries.

Water and Electrolyte Absorption

Each day, roughly 2000 mL of water enters the digestive tract in food or drink. Salivary, gastric, intestinal, pancreatic, and bile secretions add about 7000 mL. Out of that total of 9000 mL, only about 150 mL is lost in the fecal wastes. This water conservation occurs passively, following osmotic gradients. Recall that in osmosis, water always tends to flow into solutions containing relatively higher concentrations of solutes. ⤴ p. 63

Intestinal epithelial cells are continually absorbing dissolved nutrients and ions. These activities gradually lower the solute concentration of the intestinal contents. As the solute concentration within the intestine decreases, water moves into the surrounding tissues, "following" the solutes and maintaining osmotic equilibrium. The absorption of sodium and chloride ions is the most important factor promoting water movement. Other ions absorbed in smaller quantities are calcium, potassium, magnesium, iodine, bicarbonate, and iron. Calcium absorption takes place under hormonal control, requiring the presence of parathyroid hormone and calcitriol. Regulatory processes governing the absorption or excretion of the other ions are poorly understood.

Absorption of Vitamins

Vitamins are essential organic compounds that are required in very small quantities. ⤴ p. 564 There are two major groups of vitamins: fat-soluble vitamins and water-soluble vitamins.

The four **fat-soluble vitamins**—vitamins A, D, E, and K—enter the duodenum in fat droplets, mixed with dietary lipids. The vitamins remain in association with those lipids when micelles form. The fat-soluble vitamins are then absorbed from the micelles along with the products of lipid digestion. Vitamin K is also produced by the action of resident bacteria in the colon. ⤴ p. 564

The nine **water-soluble vitamins** include the B vitamins, common in milk and meats, and vitamin C, found in citrus fruits. All but one, vitamin B_{12}, are easily absorbed by the digestive epithelium. Vitamin B_{12} cannot be absorbed by the intestinal mucosa unless it is bound to intrinsic factor, a protein secreted by the parietal cells of the stomach. ⤴ p. 549 Bacteria in the intestinal tract are an important source of several water-soluble vitamins. (We consider the functions of vitamins and those of minerals as well in Chapter 17.)

16

CLINICAL NOTE

Emergency Vitamins?

Vitamins are not generally thought of as emergency medications. However, two vitamins play an important role in emergency and critical care: vitamin B₁ and K.

Vitamin B₁, which is commonly referred to as *thiamine*, is important in many of the body's biochemical systems. It is a co-enzyme for the first step of Kreb's cycle and plays an important role in several other metabolic processes. Thiamine deficiency is usually seen in chronic alcoholics and can result in altered mental status and other problems. Because of this, administration of thiamine is often a part of the emergency treatment of patients with altered mental status.

Vitamin K is necessary for blood coagulation. Deficiency can occur in chronic liver disease and causes bleeding. Vitamin K administration stimulates the coagulation system, causing blood clotting. In the United States, all hospital-born babies are pro-phylactically treated with intramuscular vitamin K.

CHECKPOINT

23. What component of food would increase the number of chylomicrons in the lacteals?

24. Removal of the stomach would impair the absorption of which vitamin?

25. Why is it that diarrhea is potentially life threatening but constipation is not?

See the blue Answers tab at the back of the book.

16-9 Many age-related changes affect digestion and absorption

Learning Objective Summarize the effects of aging on the digestive system.

Normal digestion and absorption take place in elderly individuals. However, many changes in the digestive system parallel age-related changes already described for other systems:

- *The division rate of epithelial stem cells declines.* The digestive epithelium becomes more susceptible to damage by abrasion, acids, or enzymes. For this reason, peptic ulcers become more likely. In the mouth, esophagus, and anus, the stratified epithelium becomes thinner and more fragile.

- *Smooth muscle tone decreases.* General GI motility decreases, and peristaltic contractions are weaker. This change slows the rate of intestinal movement and promotes constipation. Sagging and inflammation of the pouches (haustra) in the walls of the colon can occur.

Straining to eliminate compacted feces can stress the less resilient walls of blood vessels, producing hemorrhoids. Weakening of muscular sphincters can lead to esophageal reflux and frequent bouts of "heartburn."

- *The effects of cumulative damage become apparent.* One example is the gradual loss of teeth due to *dental caries* ("cavities") or *gingivitis* (inflammation of the gums). Cumulative damage can involve internal organs as well. Toxins such as alcohol and other injurious chemicals absorbed by the digestive tract are transported to the liver for processing. Liver cells are not immune to these toxic compounds. Chronic exposure can lead to cirrhosis or other liver diseases.

- *Cancer rates increase.* Cancers are most common in organs in which stem cells divide to maintain epithelial cell populations. Rates of colon cancer and stomach cancer rise with age. Oral, esophageal, and pharyngeal cancers are particularly common in older people who smoke.

- *Dehydration is common among the elderly.* One reason is that osmoreceptor sensitivity declines with age.

- *Changes in other systems have direct or indirect effects on the digestive system.* For example, a reduction in bone mass and calcium in the skeleton is associated with erosion of the tooth sockets and eventual tooth loss. The decline in smell and taste sensitivity with age can lead to dietary changes that affect the entire body.

CLINICAL NOTE

Malabsorption Syndromes

Malabsorption is a disorder characterized by abnormal nutrient absorption. The disorder may affect the absorption of only one nutrient or many. A genetic inability to manufacture specific enzymes will result in discrete patterns of malabsorption—*lactose intolerance* is a good example.

Difficulties in the absorption of all classes of compounds will result from damage to the accessory glands or the intestinal mucosa. If the accessory organs are functioning normally but their secretions cannot reach the duodenum, the condition is either *biliary obstruction* (bile duct blockage) or *pancreatic obstruction* (pancreatic duct blockage). Alternatively, the ducts may remain open but the glandular cells are damaged and unable to continue normal secretory activities. Two examples, *pancreatitis* and *cirrhosis*, were noted earlier in the chapter.

Even when fully functional enzymes are in the lumen, absorption will not occur if the mucosa cannot function properly. Mucosal damage due to ischemia (an interruption of the blood supply), radiation exposure (such as from radiation therapy or contaminated food), toxic compounds, or infection will affect absorption and will deplete nutrient and fluid reserves as a result.

16

CHECKPOINT

26. Identify general digestive system changes that occur with aging.

See the blue Answers tab at the back of the book.

16-10 The digestive system is extensively integrated with other body systems

Learning Objective Give examples of interactions between the digestive system and other body systems presented so far.

The digestive system is functionally linked to all other systems. It has extensive anatomical connections to the nervous, cardiovascular, endocrine, and lymphatic systems. We have also seen that the digestive tract is also an endocrine organ that produces a variety of hormones.

Refer to Build Your Knowledge: How the DIGESTIVE SYSTEM integrates with the other body systems presented so far on p. 571. It reviews the major functional relationships between this system and the integumentary, skeletal, muscular, nervous, endocrine, cardiovascular, lymphatic, and respiratory systems. Note that the digestive system has extensive structural and functional connections to the cardiovascular system.

CLINICAL NOTE

Abdominal Pain

Abdominal pain is one of the most frequent reasons people seek emergency care. The cause of abdominal pain can be difficult to determine. Inflammation, distension, or an interruption in blood supply to an organ causes a pain signal to be transmitted to the spinal cord and brain. Hollow organs, such as the stomach, gallbladder, small intestine, and large intestine tend to cause diffuse, poorly localized pain. However, pain from solid organs, such as the liver, pancreas, and kidneys, tends to be more localized. Finally, problems in other parts of the body, such as pneumonia, can cause abdominal pain. This is called *referred pain* and can further complicate the diagnostic workup. The patient with abdominal pain can be a challenge for emergency personnel. A systematic approach and a good knowledge of the pathophysiology of abdominal disorders will help identify the cause.

CHECKPOINT

27. Identify the functional relationships between the digestive system and other body systems presented so far.

28. List the digestive system functions that are related to the cardiovascular system.

See the blue Answers tab at the back of the book.

RELATED CLINICAL TERMS

achalasia (ak-a-LĀ-zē-uh): A condition that results when a bolus cannot reach the stomach due to constriction of the lower esophageal sphincter.

cholecystitis (kō-lē-sis-TĪ-tis): Inflammation of the gallbladder due to a blockage of the cystic duct or common bile duct by gallstones.

cholelithiasis (ko-lē-li-THĪ-a-sis): The presence of gallstones in the gallbladder.

colectomy (ko-LEK-to-mē): The removal of all or a portion of the colon.

colonoscope (ko-LON-o-skōp): A long, flexible, tubular fiber-optic instrument for examining the interior of the colon.

colostomy (ko-LOS-to-mē): The attachment of the cut end of the colon to an opening in the body wall after a colectomy.

esophagitis (ē-sof-a-JĪ-tis): Inflammation of the esophagus.

gastroenteritis (gas-trō-en-ter-Ī-tis): Inflammation of the lining of the stomach and intestine, characterized by vomiting and diarrhea and resulting from bacterial toxins, viral infections, or various poisons.

gastroenterology (gas-trō-en-ter-OL-o-jē): The study of the digestive system and its diseases and disorders.

inflammatory bowel disease (ulcerative colitis): A chronic inflammation of the digestive tract, most commonly affecting the colon.

laparoscopy (lap-a-ROS-ko-pē): The use of a flexible fiber-optic instrument introduced through the abdominal wall to permit direct visualization of the viscera, tissue sampling, and limited surgical procedures.

liver biopsy: A sample of liver tissue, generally taken by inserting a long needle through the anterior abdominal wall.

perforated ulcer: A particularly dangerous ulcer in which gastric acids erode through the wall of the digestive tract, allowing its contents to enter the peritoneal cavity.

periodontal disease: A loosening of the teeth within the bony sockets (alveolar sockets) caused by erosion of the periodontal ligaments by acids produced through bacterial action.

peritonitis (per-i-tō-NĪ-tis): Inflammation of the peritoneal membrane.

polyps (POL-ips): Small growths with a stalk protruding from a mucous membrane that are usually benign.

16

Build Your Knowledge
How the DIGESTIVE SYSTEM integrates with the other body systems presented so far

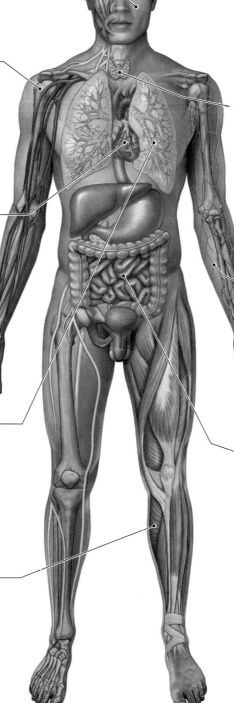

Integumentary System

• The integumentary system provides vitamin D$_3$ needed for the absorption of calcium and phosphorus

• The digestive system provides lipids for storage by adipocytes in hypodermis

Skeletal System

• The skeletal system (axial division and pelvic girdle) supports and protects parts of digestive tract; teeth are used in mechanical processing of food

• The digestive system absorbs calcium and phosphate ions for use in bone matrix; provides lipids for storage in yellow marrow

Cardiovascular System

• The cardiovascular system distributes hormones of the digestive tract; carries nutrients, water, and ions from sites of absorption; delivers nutrients and toxins to liver

• The digestive system absorbs fluid to maintain normal blood volume; absorbs vitamin K; liver excretes heme (as bilirubin), synthesizes blood clotting proteins

Respiratory System

• The respiratory system can assist in defecation by producing increased thoracic and abdominal pressure through contraction of respiratory muscles

• The digestive system produces pressure with digestive organs against the diaphragm that can assist in exhalation and limit inhalation

Muscular System

• The muscular system protects and supports digestive organs in abdominal cavity; controls entrances and exits of digestive tract

• The digestive system regulates blood glucose and fatty acid levels and metabolizes lactate from active muscles with the liver

Nervous System

• The nervous system regulates movement and secretion with the ANS; reflexes coordinate passage of materials along the digestive tract; control over skeletal muscles regulates ingestion and defecation; hypothalamic centers control hunger, satiation, and feeding

• The digestive system provides compounds essential for neurotransmitter synthesis

Endocrine System

• The endocrine system produces epinephrine and norepinephrine that stimulate constriction of sphincters and depress digestive activity; hormones coordinate activity along digestive tract

• The digestive system provides nutrients and substrates to endocrine cells; endocrine cells of pancreas secrete insulin and glucagon; liver produces angiotensinogen

Lymphatic System

• The lymphatic system defends against infection and toxins absorbed from the digestive tract; lymphatic vessels carry absorbed lipids to the general circulation

• The digestive system secretes acids and enzymes that provide innate (nonspecific) defense against pathogens

Digestive System

The digestive system provides organic substrates, vitamins, ions, and water required by all cells. It:
• ingests solid and liquid materials into the body
• mechanically processes solid materials to ease their movement and chemical breakdown in the digestive tract
• digests (chemically breaks down) food into smaller fragments in the digestive tract
• secretes water, acids, enzymes, and buffers into the digestive tract
• absorbs small organic molecules (organic substrates), ions, vitamins, and water across the digestive epithelium
• excretes compacted waste products from the body

16

16 Chapter Review

Summary Outline

16-1 The digestive system—the digestive tract and accessory organs—performs various food-processing functions *p. 616*

1. The digestive system consists of the muscular **digestive tract** and various **accessory organs** (*Figure 16-1*).

2. The digestive tract includes the oral cavity, pharynx, esophagus, stomach, small intestine, large intestine, rectum, and anus. Accessory digestive organs include the teeth, tongue, salivary glands, liver, pancreas, and gallbladder (*Figure 16-1*).

3. Digestive functions include **ingestion, mechanical processing, digestion, secretion, absorption,** and **excretion.**

4. The epithelium and underlying connective tissue, the *lamina propria*, form the **mucosa** (mucous membrane) of the digestive tract. Next, moving deeper, are the **submucosa**, the **muscularis externa**, and the *adventitia*, a layer of dense connective tissue. For viscera projecting into the peritoneal cavity, the muscularis externa is covered by the **serosa**, a serous membrane (*Figure 16-2*).

5. Double sheets of peritoneal membrane called **mesenteries** suspend portions of the digestive tract.

6. The neurons that innervate the smooth muscle of the muscularis externa are not under voluntary control.

7. The muscularis externa propels materials through the digestive tract by means of the contractions of **peristalsis. Segmentation** movements in areas of the small intestine churn digestive materials (*Figure 16-3*).

16-2 The oral cavity contains the tongue, salivary glands, and teeth, each with specific functions *p. 620*

8. The functions of the **oral cavity** are (1) sensory analysis of foods; (2) mechanical processing by the teeth, tongue, and palatal surfaces; (3) lubrication of food by mixing with mucus and salivary secretions; and (4) limited digestion of carbohydrates and lipids.

9. The oral cavity (mouth), or **buccal cavity**, is lined by oral mucosa. The **hard palate** and **soft palate** form its roof, and the tongue forms its floor (*Figure 16-4*).

10. The primary functions of the **tongue** include (1) mechanical processing, (2) manipulation to assist in chewing and swallowing, and (3) sensory analysis.

11. The **parotid, sublingual**, and **submandibular salivary glands** discharge their secretions into the oral cavity. Saliva lubricates the mouth, dissolves chemicals, flushes the oral surfaces, and helps control bacteria (*Figure 16-5*).

12. **Mastication** (chewing) occurs through the contact of the opposing surfaces of the **teeth.** The **periodontal ligament** anchors each tooth in a bony socket. **Dentin** forms the basic structure of a tooth. The **crown** is coated with **enamel**, and the **root** is covered with **cementum** (*Figure 16-6a*).

13. The 20 primary teeth, or **deciduous teeth**, are replaced by the 32 teeth of the **secondary dentition** during development (*Figure 16-6b,c*).

16-3 The pharynx is a passageway between the oral cavity and the esophagus *p. 623*

14. The **pharynx** (throat) serves as a common passageway for solid food, liquids, and air. Pharyngeal muscle contractions during swallowing propel the food mass along the esophagus and into the stomach.

15. The **esophagus** carries solids and liquids from the pharynx to the stomach through an opening in the diaphragm, the *esophageal hiatus*.

16. **Deglutition** (swallowing) can be divided into **buccal, pharyngeal**, and **esophageal phases**. Swallowing begins with the compaction of a **bolus** and its movement into the pharynx, followed by the elevation of the larynx, folding back of the epiglottis, and closure of the glottis. Peristalsis moves the bolus down the esophagus to the *lower esophageal sphincter* (*Figure 16-7*).

16-4 The J-shaped stomach receives food from the esophagus and aids in chemical and mechanical digestion *p. 625*

17. The **stomach** has four major functions: (1) storage of ingested food, (2) mechanical breakdown of food, (3) breakage of chemical bonds by acids and enzymes, and (4) production of intrinsic factor. **Chyme** forms in the stomach as gastric and salivary secretions are mixed with food.

18. The four regions of the stomach are the **cardia, fundus, body**, and **pylorus. The pyloric sphincter** guards the exit out of the stomach. In a relaxed state the stomach lining contains numerous **rugae** (ridges and folds) (*Figure 16-8*).

19. Within the **gastric glands, parietal cells** secrete **intrinsic factor** and hydrochloric acid. **Chief cells** secrete **pepsinogen**, which acids in the gastric lumen convert to the enzyme **pepsin**. Gastric gland **G cells** secrete the hormone **gastrin**.

20. Gastric secretion includes (1) the **cephalic phase**, which prepares the stomach to receive ingested materials; (2) the **gastric phase**, which begins with the arrival of food in the stomach; and (3) the **intestinal phase**, which controls the rate of gastric emptying (*Spotlight Figure 16-10*).

16-5 The small intestine digests and absorbs nutrients *p. 630*

21. The **small intestine** includes the **duodenum**, the **jejunum**, and the **ileum**. A sphincter, the *ileocecal valve*, marks the junction between the small and large intestines (*Figure 16-11*).

22. The intestinal mucosa has transverse **circular folds** and small projections called intestinal **villi**. Both structures increase the surface area for absorption. Each villus contains a lymphatic capillary called a **lacteal** (*Figure 16-12*).

23. Some of the smooth muscle cells in the muscularis externa of the small intestine contract periodically, without stimulation, to produce brief localized peristaltic contractions that slowly move materials along the tract. More extensive peristaltic activities are coordinated by the *gastroenteric* and the *gastroileal reflexes*.

24. Intestinal glands secrete **intestinal juice**, mucus, and hormones. Intestinal juice moistens the chyme, helps buffer acids, and dissolves digestive enzymes and the products of digestion.

25. Intestinal hormones include **gastrin, secretin, cholecystokinin (CCK)**, and **gastric inhibitory peptide (GIP)** (*Figure 16-13; Table 16-1*).

26. Most of the important digestive and absorptive functions occur in the small intestine. Digestive enzymes and buffers are produced by the pancreas and liver.

16-6 The pancreas, liver, and gallbladder are accessory glands that assist with the digestive process in the small intestine *p. 636*

27. The **pancreatic duct** penetrates the wall of the duodenum, where it delivers the secretions of the **pancreas** (*Figure 16-14a*).

28. Exocrine gland ducts branch repeatedly before ending in the **pancreatic acini** (blind pockets) (*Figure 16-14b,c*).

29. The pancreas has both an endocrine function (secreting insulin and glucagon into the blood) and an exocrine function (secreting water, ions, and digestive enzymes into the small intestine). Pancreatic enzymes include **carbohydrases, lipases, nucleases**, and **proteases**.

30. Pancreatic exocrine cells produce a watery **pancreatic juice** in response to hormonal instructions from the duodenum. When chyme arrives in the small intestine, secretin and CCK are released.

31. The release of secretin triggers the pancreatic production of a fluid containing buffers (primarily sodium bicarbonate) that increases the pH of the chyme. CCK stimulates the pancreas to produce and secrete **pancreatic amylase, pancreatic lipase**, nucleases, and several proteolytic enzymes—notably **trypsin, chymotrypsin**, and **carboxypeptidase**.

32. The **liver**, the largest visceral organ in the body, performs over 200 known functions.

33. The liver is made up of four unequally sized lobes: the **left, right, caudate**, and **quadrate lobes** (*Figure 16-15*).

34. The **liver lobule** is the organ's basic functional unit. Blood is supplied to the lobules by branches of the hepatic artery proper and hepatic portal vein. Within the lobules, blood flows past *hepatocytes* through *sinusoids* to the **central vein. Bile canaliculi** carry bile away from the central vein and toward bile ducts (*Figure 16-16*).

35. The bile ducts from each lobule unite to form the **common hepatic duct**, which meets the **cystic duct** to form the **common bile duct**, which empties into the duodenum (*Figure 16-17a*).

36. The liver performs metabolic and hematological regulation, and produces **bile** (*Table 16-2*).

37. The **gallbladder** stores and concentrates bile for release into the duodenum. Stimulation by cholecystokinin (CCK) relaxes the **hepatopancreatic sphincter**, allowing bile to enter the duodenum (*Figure 16-17b*).

16-7 The large intestine is divided into three parts with regional specialization *p. 646*

38. The main functions of the **large intestine** are to (1) reabsorb water and compact the feces, (2) absorb vitamins made by bacteria, and (3) store feces prior to defecation. The large intestine has three parts: the cecum, the colon, and the rectum (*Figure 16-22a*).

39. The **cecum** collects and stores material from the ileum and begins the process of compaction. The **appendix** contains lymphoid tissue and is part of the lymphatic system. It is attached to the cecum.

40. The **colon** has a larger diameter and a thinner wall than the small intestine. It bears **haustra** (pouches) and **teniae coli** (three longitudinal bands of muscle).

41. The **rectum** terminates in the **anal canal**, leading to the **anus** (*Figure 16-22b*).

42. The large intestine reabsorbs water and other substances, such as *vitamins, bile salts, organic wastes*, and *toxins*. Bacteria residing in the large intestine are responsible for intestinal gas, or *flatus*.

43. Distension of the stomach and duodenum stimulates peristalsis, or *mass movements*, of materials from the transverse colon to the rectum. Muscular sphincters control the passage of fecal material to the anus. Distension of the rectal wall triggers the *defecation reflex*. Under normal circumstances, the release of feces cannot occur unless the **external anal sphincter** is voluntarily relaxed.

16

16-8 Digestion is the chemical alteration of food that allows the absorption and use of nutrients *p. 650*

44. The digestive system first breaks down the physical structure of ingested materials, and then digestive enzymes break the component molecules into smaller fragments through a process called *hydrolysis (Spotlight Figure 16-25; Table 16-3).*

45. Amylases break down complex carbohydrates into *disaccharides* and *trisaccharides*. Enzymes at the epithelial surface break these molecules into *monosaccharides* that are absorbed by the intestinal epithelium through facilitated diffusion or cotransport *(Spotlight Figure 16-25).*

46. *Triglycerides* are emulsified into lipid droplets that interact with bile salts to form **micelles**. The fatty acids and monoglycerides resulting from the action of pancreatic lipase diffuse from the micelles across the intestinal epithelium. The intestinal cells then synthesize new triglycerides. These are packaged in **chylomicrons**, which are released into the interstitial fluid for transport to the general circulation by way of the lymphatic system *(Spotlight Figure 16-25).*

47. Protein digestion involves low pH and the enzyme pepsin in the stomach, and various pancreatic proteases in the small intestine. Peptidases liberate amino acids that are absorbed by the intestinal epithelium and released into the interstitial fluids *(Spotlight Figure 16-25).*

48. About 2000 mL of water are ingested each day, and digestive secretions provide another 7000 mL. All but about 150 mL of water is reabsorbed through osmosis.

49. Various processes are responsible for the movement of ions (such as sodium, calcium, chloride, and bicarbonate).

50. The **fat-soluble vitamins** are enclosed within fat droplets and are absorbed with the products of lipid digestion. The **water-soluble vitamins** (except B_{12}) diffuse easily across the digestive epithelium.

16-9 Many age-related changes affect digestion and absorption *p. 655*

51. Age-related digestive system changes include a thinner and more fragile epithelium due to a reduction in epithelial stem cell divisions, weaker peristaltic contractions as smooth muscle tone decreases, the effects of cumulative damage, increased cancer rates, and increased dehydration.

16-10 The digestive system is extensively integrated with other body systems *p. 656*

52. The digestive system has extensive structural and functional connections to the nervous, cardiovascular, endocrine, and lymphatic systems.

Review Questions

See the blue Answers tab at the back of the book.

Level 1 Reviewing Facts and Terms

Match each item in column A with the most closely related item in column B. Place letters for answers in the spaces provided.

COLUMN A

_____ **1.** Pyloric sphincter
_____ **2.** Liver cells
_____ **3.** Intrinsic factor
_____ **4.** Mesentery
_____ **5.** Chief cells
_____ **6.** Palate
_____ **7.** Parietal cells
_____ **8.** Parasympathetic stimulation
_____ **9.** Sympathetic stimulation
_____ **10.** Peristalsis
_____ **11.** Bile salts
_____ **12.** Salivary amylase

COLUMN B

a. Double serous membrane sheet
b. Moves materials along digestive tract
c. Regulates flow of chyme into duodenum
d. Increases muscular activity of digestive tract
e. Starch digestion
f. Inhibits muscular activity of digestive tract
g. Aids vitamin B_{12} absorption
h. Roof of oral cavity
i. Pepsinogen
j. Produce hydrochloric acid
k. Hepatocytes
l. Emulsification of fats

16

13. The enzymatic breakdown of large molecules into their basic building blocks is called
(a) absorption. **(b)** secretion.
(c) mechanical digestion. **(d)** chemical digestion.

14. The activities of the digestive system are regulated by
(a) hormonal processes. **(b)** local processes.
(c) neural processes. **(d)** a, b, and c are correct.

15. The layer of the peritoneum that lines the inner surfaces of the body wall is the
(a) visceral peritoneum. **(b)** parietal peritoneum.
(c) greater omentum. **(d)** lesser omentum.

16. Protein digestion in the stomach results primarily from secretions released by
(a) hepatocytes. **(b)** parietal cells.
(c) chief cells. **(d)** goblet cells.

17. Label the digestive system structures in the following figure.

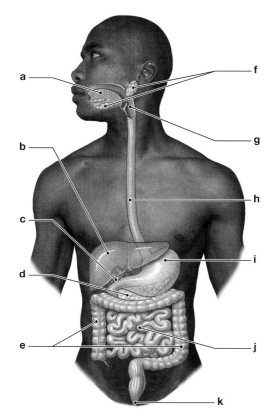

(a) _____	**(b)** _____
(c) _____	**(d)** _____
(e) _____	**(f)** _____
(g) _____	**(h)** _____
(i) _____	**(j)** _____
(k) _____	

18. The part of the gastrointestinal tract that plays the primary role in the digestion and absorption of nutrients is the
(a) large intestine.
(b) small intestine.
(c) stomach.
(d) cecum and colon.

19. The duodenal hormone that stimulates the production and secretion of pancreatic enzymes is
(a) pepsinogen. **(b)** gastrin.
(c) secretin. **(d)** cholecystokinin.

20. The essential service(s) provided by the liver is (are)
(a) metabolic regulation.
(b) hematological regulation.
(c) bile production.
(d) a, b, and c are correct.

21. Label the four layers of the digestive tract in the following figure.

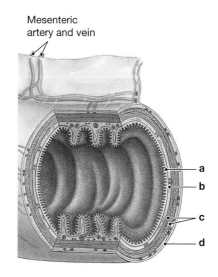

Mesenteric artery and vein

(a) _____	
(b) _____	
(c) _____	
(d) _____	

22. Bile release from the gallbladder into the duodenum occurs only under the stimulation of
(a) cholecystokinin.
(b) secretin.
(c) gastrin.
(d) pepsinogen.

23. The major function(s) of the large intestine is (are)
(a) reabsorption of water and compaction of feces.
(b) absorption of vitamins produced by bacterial action.
(c) storage of fecal material prior to defecation.
(d) a, b, and c are correct.

24. The part of the colon that empties into the rectum is the
(a) ascending colon.
(b) descending colon.
(c) transverse colon.
(d) sigmoid colon.

25. What are the primary digestive functions?

26. What is the function of the transverse (circular) or longitudinal folds in the mucosa of the digestive tract?

27. Describe the layers of the digestive tract, proceeding from superficial (the innermost layer nearest the lumen) to deep (the outermost layer).

28. What are the four primary functions of the oral (buccal) cavity?

16

29. What specific function does each of the four types of teeth perform in the oral cavity?

30. What three segments of the small intestine are involved in the digestion and absorption of food?

31. What are the primary digestive functions of the pancreas, liver, and gallbladder?

32. What are the three major functions of the large intestine?

33. What six age-related changes occur in the digestive system?

Level 2 Reviewing Concepts

34. If the lingual frenulum is too restrictive, an individual
   (a) has difficulty tasting food.
   (b) cannot swallow properly.
   (c) cannot control movements of the tongue.
   (d) cannot eat or speak normally.

35. The gastric phase of secretion is initiated by
   (a) distension of the stomach.
   (b) an increase in the pH of the gastric contents.
   (c) the presence of undigested materials in the stomach.
   (d) a, b, and c are correct.

36. A decrease in pH in the duodenum stimulates the secretion of
   (a) secretin.   **(b)** cholecystokinin.
   (c) gastrin.   **(d)** a, b, and c are correct.

37. Describe how the action and outcome of peristalsis differ from those of segmentation.

38. How does the stomach promote and assist in the digestive process?

39. Describe the events that occur during the three phases of gastric secretion.

Level 3 Critical Thinking and Clinical Applications

40. Some patients with gallstones develop pancreatitis. How could this occur?

41. Barb suffers from Crohn's disease, a regional inflammation of the intestine that is thought to have some genetic basis, although the actual cause remains unknown. When the disease flares up, she experiences abdominal pain, weight loss, and anemia. Which part(s) of the intestine is (are) probably involved, and what might be the causes of her signs and symptoms?

16

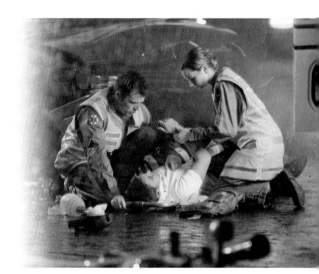

17

Metabolism and Energetics

Learning Objectives

These objectives tell you what you should be able to do after completing the chapter. They correspond by number to this chapter's sections.

17-1 Define metabolism and energetics, and explain why cells need to synthesize new organic molecules.

17-2 Describe the basic steps in glycolysis, the citric acid cycle, and the electron transport system, and summarize the energy yields of glycolysis and cellular respiration.

17-3 Describe the pathways involved in lipid metabolism, and summarize the processes of lipid transport and distribution.

17-4 Discuss protein metabolism and the use of proteins as an energy source.

17-5 Discuss nucleic acid metabolism and the limited use of nucleic acids as an energy source.

17-6 Explain what makes up a balanced diet and why such a diet is important.

17-7 Define metabolic rate, describe the factors involved in determining an individual's BMR, and discuss the homeostatic processes that maintain a constant body temperature.

17-8 Describe the age-related changes in dietary requirements.

An Introduction to Nutrition and Metabolism

The amount and type of nutrients you get from meals can vary widely. Your body builds energy reserves when nutrients, such as carbohydrates or lipids, are abundant. It mobilizes them when nutrients are in short supply. The endocrine and nervous systems adjust and coordinate the metabolic activities of the body's tissues. They also control the storage and mobilization of these energy reserves. In this chapter, we consider what happens to nutrients once they are inside the body.

Build Your Knowledge

Recall that foods are usually complex chains of simpler molecules (as you saw in **Chapter 16: The Digestive System**). In a typical dietary carbohydrate, the basic molecules are simple sugars. In a protein, the building blocks are amino acids. In lipids, they are usually fatty acids. Digestive enzymes, such as carbohydrases, proteases, and lipases, break the chemical bonds of a complex food molecule in the process of hydrolysis. ↺ **p. 566**

17-1 Metabolism refers to all the chemical reactions in the body, and energetics refers to the flow and transformation of energy

Learning Objective Define metabolism and energetics, and explain why cells need to synthesize new organic molecules.

Cells are chemical factories that break down organic molecules to obtain energy. Our cells then use this energy to generate ATP, the body's most important high-energy compound. Chemical reactions within mitochondria provide most of the energy a typical cell needs. ↺ p. 73 To generate energy, cells in the human body must also obtain oxygen and nutrients. Oxygen is absorbed at the lungs. The digestive tract absorbs nutrients. **Nutrients** include essential substances such as water, vitamins, mineral ions, carbohydrates, lipids, and proteins. The cardiovascular system distributes oxygen and nutrients to cells throughout the body.

Mitochondria break down the organic nutrients to provide energy for cell growth, cell division, contraction, secretion, and other functions. Each tissue contains different populations of cells. As a result, the energy and nutrient requirements of any two tissues, such as loose connective tissue and cardiac muscle, can be quite different.

The body's metabolic needs change when cells, tissues, and organs change their levels of activity. Our energy and nutrient requirements can vary from moment to moment (resting versus active), hour to hour (asleep versus awake), and year to year (child versus adult). Understanding energy requirements is part of **energetics**, the study of the flow of energy and its change(s) from one form to another.

The term **metabolism** refers to all the chemical reactions in the body. ↺ p. 31 *Cellular metabolism* refers to the chemical reactions within cells. It provides the energy needed to maintain homeostasis and to perform essential functions. **Figure 17-1** provides an overview of the processes involved in cellular metabolism. Amino acids, lipids, and simple sugars cross the plasma membrane and join the other nutrients already in the cytosol. All the cell's metabolic operations rely on this *nutrient pool* of organic building blocks.

The breakdown of organic molecules is called **catabolism**. This process releases energy that can be used to synthesize ATP or other high-energy compounds. ↺ p. 33 Catabolism proceeds in a series of steps. In general, the first steps take place in the cytosol, where enzymes break down large organic molecules into smaller fragments. Carbohydrates are broken down into short carbon chains. Triglycerides are split into fatty acids and glycerol. Proteins are broken down to individual amino acids.

These preparatory steps produce relatively little ATP. However, further catabolic reactions produce smaller organic molecules that mitochondria can absorb and process. Mitochondrial activity releases significant amounts of energy. As mitochondrial enzymes break the covalent bonds that hold these molecules together, they capture roughly 40 percent of the released energy. The captured energy is used to convert ADP to ATP. ↺ p. 48 The rest escapes as heat that warms the interior of the cell and the surrounding tissues.

Anabolism is the synthesis of new organic molecules. It involves the formation of new chemical bonds. ↺ p. 33 The ATP produced by mitochondria provides energy to support anabolism and other cell functions. Those functions, such as ciliary or cell movement, contraction, active transport, and cell division, vary from one cell to another.

Figure 17-1 Cellular Metabolism. Cells obtain organic molecules from the interstitial fluid and break them down in mitochondria to produce ATP. Only about 40 percent of the energy released through catabolism is captured in ATP. The rest is lost as heat. The ATP generated by catabolism provides energy for all vital cellular activities, including anabolism.

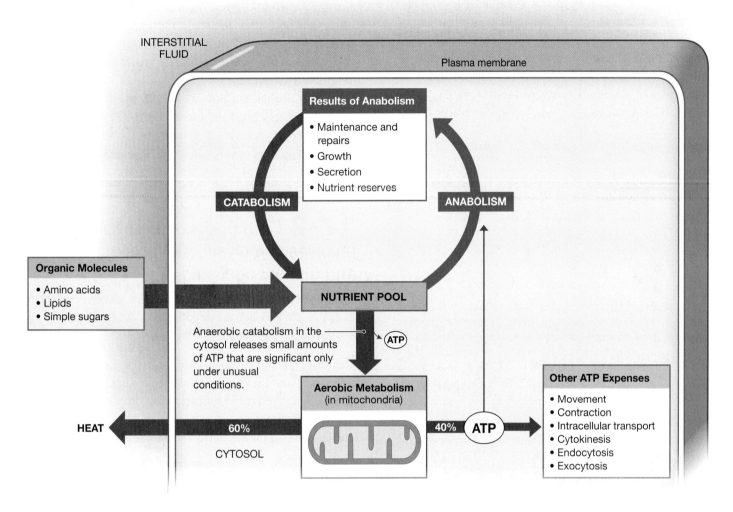

For example, muscle fibers need ATP to provide energy for contraction, and gland cells need ATP to synthesize and transport their secretions.

Cells synthesize new organic components for four basic reasons:

1. ***To carry out structural maintenance and repairs.*** Most structures in the cell are temporary, not permanent. Their removal and replacement are part of the process of **metabolic turnover**.

2. ***To support growth.*** Cells preparing to divide increase in size and synthesize extra proteins and organelles.

3. ***To produce secretions.*** Secretory cells must synthesize their products and deliver them to the interstitial fluid.

4. ***To store nutrient reserves.*** Most cells "prepare for a rainy day"—an emergency, extreme activity, or inadequate nutrient supply in the bloodstream. Cells do so by storing

nutrients in a form that can be mobilized as needed. For example, muscle cells store glucose in the form of glycogen, and fat cells (adipocytes) store fatty acids in triglycerides. Liver cells store both glycogen and triglycerides.

The nutrient pool is the source of organic molecules for both catabolism and anabolism (**Figure 17-1**). Cells tend to conserve materials needed to build new compounds and tend to break down the rest. Cells continuously replace membranes, organelles, enzymes, and structural proteins. These anabolic activities require more amino acids than lipids, and few carbohydrates. Energy-releasing catabolic activities, however, tend to process these organic molecules in the reverse order. In general, when a cell with excess carbohydrates, lipids, and amino acids needs energy, it first breaks down carbohydrates. Lipids are the second choice as an energy source. Amino acids are seldom broken down if other energy sources are available.

17

Mitochondria provide most of the energy that supports cellular operations. In effect, the cell feeds its mitochondria from its nutrient pool, and in return the cell gets the ATP it needs. However, mitochondria are picky eaters: They will accept only specific organic molecules for processing and energy production. Chemical reactions in the cytosol take available organic nutrients and break them into smaller fragments that the mitochondria can use. The mitochondria then break down the fragments further, generating carbon dioxide, water, and ATP. This mitochondrial activity involves two pathways: the *citric acid cycle* and the *electron transport system* (**Figure 17-2**).

CHECKPOINT

1. Define energetics.

2. Define metabolism.

3. Compare catabolism and anabolism.

See the blue Answers tab at the back of the book.

Figure 17-2 Nutrient Use in Cellular Metabolism. Cells use molecules in the nutrient pool to build up reserves and to manufacture cellular structures. Catabolism within mitochondria provides the ATP needed to sustain cell functions. Mitochondria absorb small carbon chains produced by the breakdown of fatty acids, glucose, and amino acids from the nutrient pool. The small carbon chains are broken down further by means of the citric acid cycle and the electron transport system.

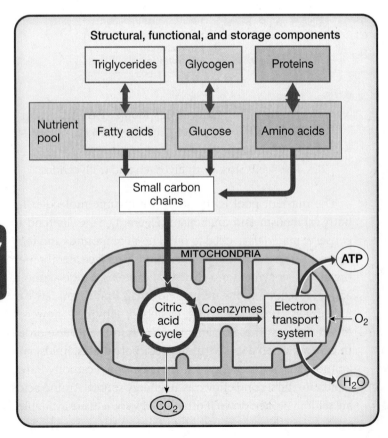

Build Your Knowledge

Recall that the cells in your body generate ATP through anaerobic (non-oxygen-requiring) metabolism in the cytosol and through aerobic (oxygen-requiring) metabolism in mitochondria (as you saw in **Chapter 7: The Muscular System**). The anaerobic breakdown of glucose to pyruvate is called glycolysis. This process generates a small amount of ATP and provides pyruvate molecules that enter mitochondria. The complete breakdown of pyruvate through aerobic metabolism generates most of a body cell's ATP. ⟳ **p. 208**

17-2 Carbohydrate metabolism involves glycolysis, ATP production, and gluconeogenesis

Learning Objective Describe the basic steps in glycolysis, the citric acid cycle, and the electron transport system, and summarize the energy yields of glycolysis and cellular respiration.

Carbohydrates are most familiar to us as sugars and starches. They are important sources of energy. Most cells generate ATP and other high-energy compounds by breaking down carbohydrates, especially glucose. We can summarize the complete reaction sequence as:

$$\underset{\text{glucose}}{C_6H_{12}O_6} + \underset{\text{oxygen}}{6O_2} \longrightarrow \underset{\text{carbon dioxide}}{6CO_2} + \underset{\text{water}}{6H_2O}$$

This overall reaction is called **cellular respiration**. The breakdown of glucose takes place in a series of small steps. Several of these steps release enough energy to support the conversion of ADP to ATP. The complete catabolism of one molecule of glucose provides a typical cell with 30–32 ATP molecules.

Most ATP production occurs inside mitochondria, but the first steps take place in the cytosol. Recall that *glycolysis* breaks down glucose into smaller molecules that mitochondria can absorb and use (see Chapter 7). These reactions are said to be *anaerobic* because glycolysis does not require oxygen. ⟳ p. 207 The subsequent reactions take place within mitochondria. These reactions consume oxygen and are thus *aerobic*. The mitochondrial activity responsible for ATP production is called **aerobic metabolism**. (The terms cellular respiration and aerobic metabolism are often considered interchangeable. However, as we discussed, cellular respiration includes both anaerobic and aerobic reactions.)

Glycolysis

Glycolysis (glī-KOL-i-sis; *glykus*, sweet + *lysis*, a loosening) is the breakdown of glucose to *pyruvic acid*. In this process, a series of enzymatic steps breaks the six-carbon glucose molecule ($C_6H_{12}O_6$) into two three-carbon molecules of pyruvic acid (CH_3—CO—COOH). At the normal pH inside cells, each pyruvic acid molecule loses a hydrogen ion and exists as the negatively charged ion CH_3—CO—COO^-. This ionized form is called **pyruvate**, rather than pyruvic acid.

Glycolysis requires (1) glucose molecules; (2) appropriate cytosolic enzymes; (3) ATP and ADP; and (4) **NAD** (**n**icotinamide **a**denine **d**inucleotide), a coenzyme that removes hydrogen atoms. *Coenzymes* are organic molecules, usually derived from vitamins, that must be present for an enzymatic reaction to occur. ⊃ p. 564 If any of these four participants are missing, glycolysis cannot take place.

The basic steps of glycolysis are summarized in **Figure 17-3**. This reaction sequence yields a net gain of two ATP molecules for each glucose molecule converted to two pyruvate molecules. Two molecules of NADH, another high-energy compound, are also produced.

A few highly specialized cells, such as red blood cells, lack mitochondria and derive all their ATP by glycolysis. Skeletal

Figure 17-3 Glycolysis. Within a cell's cytosol, glycolysis involves a series of enzymatic steps that break down a six-carbon glucose molecule into two three-carbon pyruvate molecules. Each glucose molecule converted to two pyruvate molecules yields a net gain of two ATPs.

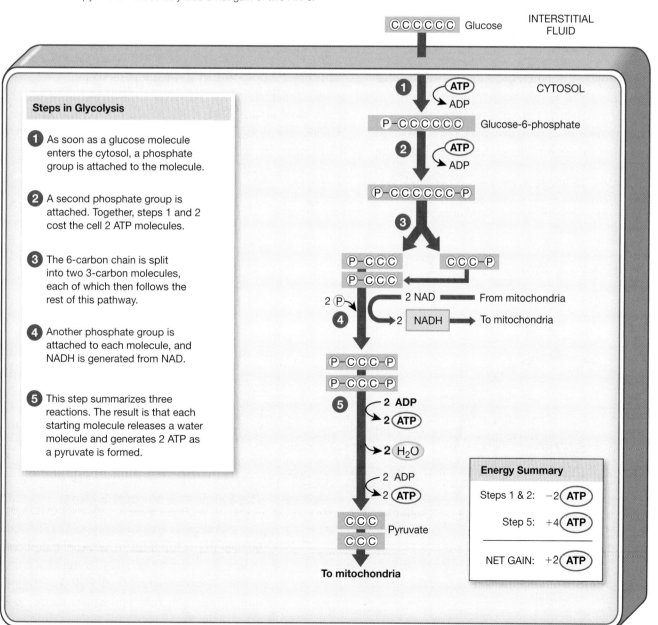

Steps in Glycolysis

1. As soon as a glucose molecule enters the cytosol, a phosphate group is attached to the molecule.

2. A second phosphate group is attached. Together, steps 1 and 2 cost the cell 2 ATP molecules.

3. The 6-carbon chain is split into two 3-carbon molecules, each of which then follows the rest of this pathway.

4. Another phosphate group is attached to each molecule, and NADH is generated from NAD.

5. This step summarizes three reactions. The result is that each starting molecule releases a water molecule and generates 2 ATP as a pyruvate is formed.

Energy Summary

Steps 1 & 2:	−2 **ATP**
Step 5:	+4 **ATP**
NET GAIN:	+2 **ATP**

17

muscle fibers rely on glycolysis for energy production during periods of active contraction. Most cells can survive brief periods of hypoxia (low oxygen levels) by using the small supplies of ATP provided by glycolysis alone. When oxygen is readily available, however, mitochondrial activity provides most of the ATP cells require.

Energy Production within Mitochondria

Glycolysis yields an immediate net gain of two ATP molecules for the cell. However, a great deal of additional energy is still stored in the chemical bonds of pyruvate. The cell's ability to capture that energy depends on the presence of oxygen. If oxygen supplies are adequate, mitochondria will absorb the pyruvate molecules and break them down completely. The hydrogen atoms of pyruvate are removed by coenzymes and are ultimately the source of most of the cell's energy gain. The carbon and oxygen atoms are removed and released as carbon dioxide.

Recall that a double membrane surrounds each mitochondrion. ⊃ p. 73 The outer membrane is permeable to ions and small organic molecules such as pyruvate. Such substances easily enter the intermembrane space between the outer and inner membranes. A carrier protein in the inner membrane transports the pyruvate from the intermembrane space into the mitochondrial matrix.

Once inside the mitochondrion, each pyruvate molecule takes part in a reaction leading to a sequence of enzymatic reactions called the **citric acid cycle** (**Figure 17-4**). This reaction sequence is also known as the *tricarboxylic* (trī-kar-bok-SIL-ik) *acid (TCA) cycle*, and the *Krebs cycle*. We use citric acid cycle as the preferred term, because citric acid is the first substrate of the cycle. The role of the citric acid cycle is to remove hydrogen atoms from organic molecules and transfer them to coenzymes.

The Citric Acid Cycle

In the mitochondrion, a pyruvate molecule takes part in a complex reaction involving NAD and another coenzyme called *coenzyme A* (or *CoA*). This reaction yields one molecule each of carbon dioxide, NADH, and **acetyl-CoA** (AS-e-til-KŌ-ā). Acetyl-CoA consists of a 2-carbon *acetyl group* (CH_3CO) bound to coenzyme A. When the acetyl group is transferred from CoA to a 4-carbon molecule, a 6-carbon molecule called *citric acid* is produced.

As citric acid is produced, CoA is released to bind with another acetyl group. A complete revolution, or turn, of the citric acid cycle removes the two added carbon atoms, regenerating the initial 4-carbon molecule. (This is why this reaction sequence is called a *cycle*.) The two removed carbon atoms become part of two molecules of carbon dioxide (CO_2), a metabolic waste product. The hydrogen atoms of the acetyl group are removed by coenzymes.

The only immediate energy benefit of one revolution of the citric acid cycle is the formation of a single molecule of *GTP* (*guanosine triphosphate*). This high-energy compound is readily converted into ATP. The real value of the citric acid cycle can be seen by following the fate of the hydrogen atoms that are removed by the coenzymes NAD and **FAD** (**f**lavine **ad**enine **d**inucleotide). The two coenzymes form NADH and FADH₂ and transfer the hydrogen atoms to the *electron transport system*.

The Electron Transport System

The **electron transport system (ETS)** is embedded in the inner mitochondrial membrane (**Spotlight Figure 17-5**). The ETS consists of four respiratory protein complexes (I–IV), *coenzyme Q*, and an electron transport chain made up of

Figure 17-4 The Citric Acid Cycle. Within mitochondria, the citric acid cycle breaks down pyruvate molecules produced by glycolysis (and other catabolic pathways). This overview of the citric acid cycle shows the distribution of carbon, hydrogen, and oxygen atoms through one complete turn.

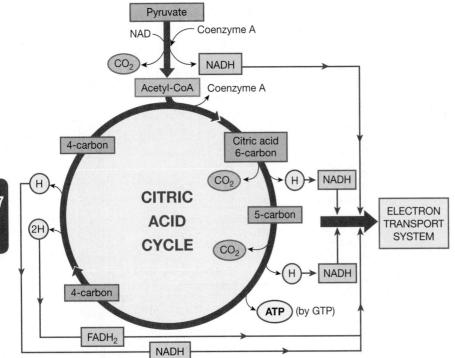

The final step in aerobic ATP production involves the transfer of energy from the high-energy electrons carried by NADH and $FADH_2$ to ATP molecules. This energy transfer occurs in the **electron transport system (ETS)**. The ETS is located in the inner mitochondrial membrane.

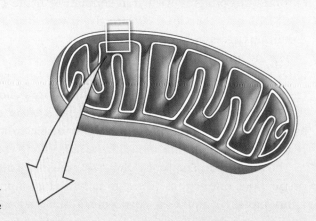

The ETS consists of four respiratory complexes (I–IV), coenzyme Q, and an electron transport chain of cytochrome molecules (*b*, *c*, *a*, and a_3). Except for cytochrome c (*Cyt c*), these molecules are associated with respiratory complexes III and IV. The hydrogen atoms delivered by NADH and $FADH_2$ are first split into electrons (e^-) and protons (H^+). The high-energy electrons are passed along the protein complexes, such that their energy is released in a series of small steps. This energy is used to pump H^+ into the intermembrane space. The result is a H^+ concentration gradient across the inner membrane. This H^+ gradient is used to generate ATP through ATP synthase. The red line with the arrowhead indicates the paths and destination of the electrons.

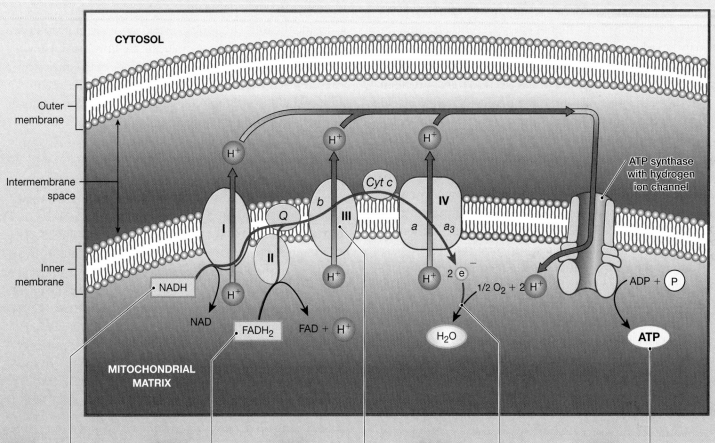

1 The electrons from NADH pass from respiratory complex I to coenzyme Q (Q). The energy released by the electrons is used to pump H^+ from the matrix into the intermembrane space.

2 The electrons from $FADH_2$ are transferred to respiratory complex II and then directly to coenzyme Q.

3 The electrons are transferred from coenzyme Q to respiratory complex III. More electron energy is released and used to pump H^+ into the intermembrane space.

4 The electrons transferred to respiratory complex IV release their remaining energy to pump H^+ into the intermembrane space. The electrons are released into the matrix and combine with oxygen and H^+ to form water molecules.

5 H^+ pass through hydrogen ion channels into the matrix. Their movement provides the energy for the ATP synthase complex to combine ADP and P into ATP.

a series of *cytochrome* molecules (*b, c, a,* and *a*3). The cytochromes are proteins with iron-containing heme groups. The ETS does not produce ATP directly. Instead, it creates the conditions necessary for ATP production.

The hydrogen atoms from the citric acid cycle do not enter the ETS intact. Only their high-energy electrons enter the ETS. Their protons are released into the mitochondrial matrix. The electrons that travel along the ETS release energy as they pass from coenzyme Q and along the electron transport chain of cytochrome molecules.

The red lines in **Spotlight Figure 17-5** show the paths and destinations of electrons. Those from NADH go from respiratory protein complex I to coenzyme Q. The electrons from $FADH_2$ enter the ETS at respiratory protein complex II and are passed to coenzyme Q. As a result, the electrons carried by NADH enter the ETS at a higher energy level than those carried by $FADH_2$. The electrons from both paths are passed from coenzyme Q to respiratory protein complex III, which contains the first cytochrome (*b*) in the electron transport chain. From there, the electrons are shuttled by cytochrome *c* to additional cytochromes within respiratory protein complex IV.

The energy released at each of several steps drives hydrogen ion pumps in respiratory protein complexes I, III, and IV. These pumps move hydrogen ions from the mitochondrial matrix into the intermembrane space (between the two mitochondrial membranes). This pumping creates a large concentration gradient of hydrogen ions across the inner membrane. The concentration gradient provides the energy to convert ADP to ATP.

Despite the concentration gradient, hydrogen ions cannot diffuse into the matrix because they are not lipid soluble. However, hydrogen ion channels in the inner membrane permit H^+ to enter the matrix. These ion channels and attached proteins make up a membrane enzyme called *ATP synthase.* The kinetic energy of the passing hydrogen ions is used to attach a phosphate group to ADP, forming ATP. This overall process is called **chemiosmosis** (kem-ē-oz-MŌ-sis), a term that links the chemical formation of ATP with transport across a membrane. At the end of the ETS, an oxygen atom accepts two electrons from respiratory protein complex IV and combines with two hydrogen ions to form a molecule of water.

The electron transport system is the most important process for generating ATP. It provides roughly 95 percent of the ATP needed to keep our cells alive. Stopping or slowing the rate of mitochondrial activity will usually kill a cell. For example, if the cell's supply of oxygen is cut off, mitochondrial ATP production will cease because the ETS will be unable to pass along its electrons. With the last reaction in the chain stopped, the entire ETS comes to a halt, like a line of cars at a washed-out bridge. When the ETS stops, NADH and $FADH_2$ can't drop off their hydrogen atoms, so the citric acid cycle stops as well. The affected cell quickly dies of energy deprivation. If many cells are affected, the individual may die.

Energy Yield of Glycolysis and Cellular Respiration

For most cells, the main method of generating ATP is the complete reaction pathway, beginning with glucose and ending with carbon dioxide and water. **Figure 17-6** summarizes the process in terms of energy gained:

- During glycolysis in the cytosol, the cell gains two molecules of ATP and two NADH for each glucose molecule broken down to pyruvate.

- Inside the mitochondria, the two pyruvate molecules derived from each glucose molecule are fully broken down in the citric acid cycle. Two revolutions of the citric acid cycle, each yielding a molecule of ATP, provide a gain of two additional molecules of ATP. An additional eight NADH and two $FADH_2$ are also formed.

- For each molecule of glucose broken down, a total of 10 NADH and two $FADH_2$ deliver their high-energy electrons to the electron transport system in the inner mitochondrial membrane. Overall, each NADH yields 2.5 ATP and each $FADH_2$ yields 1.5 ATP. So, the 10 NADH yield 25 ATP and the two $FADH_2$ yield 3 ATP, for a total of 28 ATP. Adding the two ATP generated in glycolysis and the two ATP from the citric acid cycle gives a total of 32 molecules of ATP. That total assumes that the cell expends no energy in transporting the hydrogen atoms from the two NADH formed during glycolysis into a mitochondrion. Because the energy requirements of different transport processes vary, it is estimated that up to two ATP are used to transport the two NADH. Subtracting those two ATP then, leaves us a minimal total of 30 ATP.

Summing up, for each glucose molecule processed, a typical cell gains 30–32 molecules of ATP. *All but two of them are produced within mitochondria.*

Gluconeogenesis (Glucose Synthesis)

Some of the steps in the breakdown of glucose, or glycolysis, are not reversible. For this reason, cells cannot generate glucose simply by using the same enzymes and reversing the steps in glycolysis (**Figure 17-7**). Glycolysis and the production of glucose require different sets of regulatory enzymes. As a result, the two processes are independently regulated.

Figure 17-6 A Summary of the Energy Yield of Aerobic Metabolism. For each glucose molecule brokendown by glycolysis, only two molecules of ATP (net) are produced. However, glycolysis, the formation of acetyl-CoA, and the citric acid cycle all yield coenzyme molecules (NADH or $FADH_2$ molecules). When electrons from these coenzymes pass through the electron transport system, many additional ATP molecules are produced. The citric acid cycle generates an additional two ATP molecules.

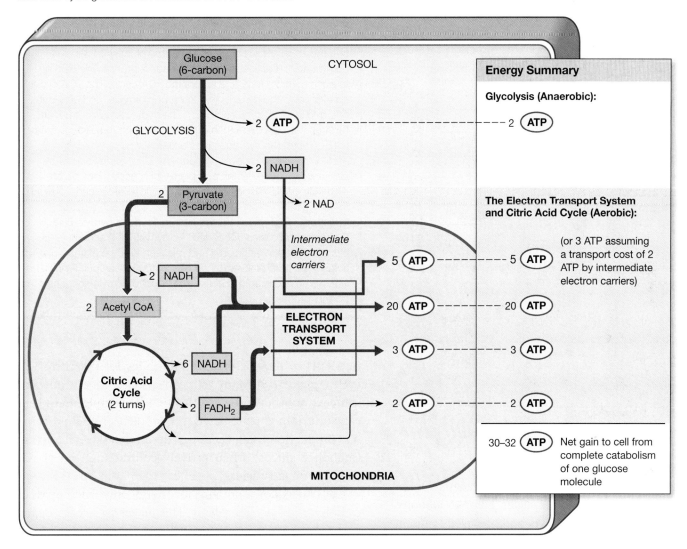

Some three-carbon molecules other than pyruvate can be used to synthesize glucose. For this reason, a cell can create glucose molecules from other carbohydrates, lactate, glycerol, or some amino acids. However, cells cannot use acetyl-CoA to make glucose. This is because the reaction that removes the carbon dioxide molecule (a *decarboxylation*) between pyruvate and acetyl-CoA cannot be reversed.

Gluconeogenesis (gloo-kō-nē-ō-JEN-e-sis; *glykus*, sweet + *neo-*, new + *genesis*, an origin) is the synthesis of glucose from noncarbohydrate precursor molecules, such as lactate (from the dissociation of lactic acid), glycerol (from lipids), or some amino acids (from proteins). Fatty acids and many amino acids cannot be used for gluconeogenesis because their breakdown produces acetyl-CoA.

CLINICAL NOTE

Carbohydrate Loading

Performance in endurance sports improves if muscles have large stores of glycogen. Endurance athletes try to achieve this by eating carbohydrate-rich meals for three days before competing. This practice is called carbohydrate loading. Studies in Sweden, Australia, and South Africa have shown that attempts to deplete carbohydrate stores by exercising to exhaustion before carbohydrate loading—a practice called *carbohydrate depletion/loading*—are less effective than three days of rest or minimal exercise during carbohydrate loading. This less intense approach improves mood and reduces the risks of muscle and kidney damage.

17

Figure 17-7 Carbohydrate Metabolism. This flowchart presents the major pathways of glycolysis and gluconeogenesis. Some amino acids, carbohydrates, lactate, and glycerol can be converted to glucose.

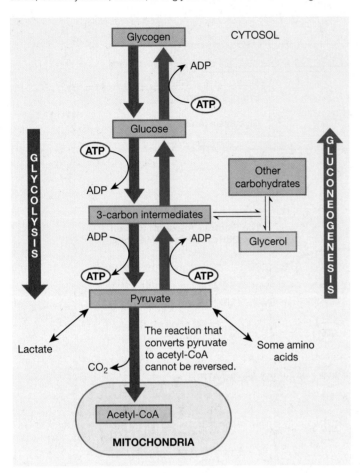

CLINICAL NOTE

Cellular Hypoxia

Oxygen is essential for normal glucose metabolism. Glucose breakdown and energy production begins in the cytosol with glycolysis. Glycolysis, which does not require oxygen, produces two molecules of ATP as it converts the glucose molecule to pyruvic acid. If oxygen supplies are adequate, pyruvic acid enters the mitochondria and enters the TCA cycle. The TCA cycle breaks down the pyruvic acid to carbon dioxide, and generates two additional molecules of ATP. The hydrogen ions removed through the TCA cycle then enter the electron transport system (ETS). There, the hydrogen ions eventually bind with oxygen, and form water. However, through the ETS, 32 molecules of ATP are produced. When completely processed, one glucose molecule yields 36 molecules of ATP. A lack of oxygen, referred to as hypoxia, inhibits or stops the TCA cycle and electron transport, which results in the accumulation of pyruvic acid. Glycolysis continues unheeded. As pyruvic acid accumulates, it is converted to lactic acid and released into the extracellular fluid where it can cause dangerous shifts in body pH. If oxygen is restored, lactic acid is converted back to pyruvic acid and the normal processes resume.

Glucose molecules formed by gluconeogenesis can be used to manufacture other simple sugars, complex carbohydrates, or nucleic acids. In the liver and in skeletal muscle, glucose molecules are stored as **glycogen**. ⟲ p. 39 Glycogen is an important energy reserve that can be broken down when the cell cannot obtain enough glucose from interstitial fluid. Glycogen molecules are large, but glycogen reserves take up very little space because they form compact, insoluble granules.

Alternate Catabolic Pathways

Aerobic metabolism is relatively efficient and capable of generating large amounts of ATP. It is the cornerstone of normal cellular metabolism, but it has one obvious limitation—cells must have adequate supplies of both oxygen and glucose. Cells can survive only for brief periods without oxygen. Low glucose concentrations have a much smaller effect on most cells, because cells can break down other

nutrients to provide organic molecules for the citric acid cycle (**Figure 17-8**). Many cells can switch from one nutrient source to another as the need arises. For example, many cells can shift from glucose-based ATP production to lipid-based ATP production when necessary. Recall that skeletal muscles catabolize glucose when actively contracting, but at rest they rely on fatty acids. ⟲ p. 208

Cells break down proteins for energy only when lipids or carbohydrates are unavailable. This makes sense because the enzymes and organelles that cells need to survive are composed of proteins. Nucleic acids are present only in small amounts, and they are seldom catabolized for energy, even when the cell is dying of acute starvation. This also makes sense, as the DNA in the nucleus determines all the structural and functional characteristics of the cell.

CHECKPOINT

4. What is the primary role of the citric acid cycle in the production of ATP?

5. Hydrogen cyanide gas is a lethal poison that binds to the last cytochrome molecule in the electron transport system. What effect would this have at the cellular level?

6. Define gluconeogenesis.

See the blue Answers tab at the back of the book.

Figure 17-8 Alternate Catabolic Pathways.

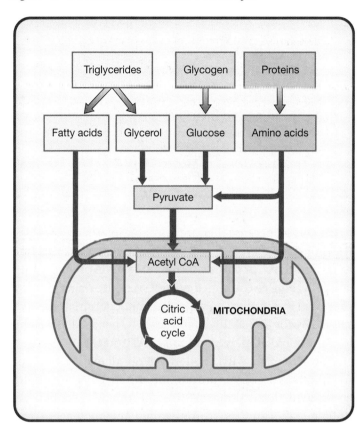

17-3 Lipid metabolism involves lipolysis, beta-oxidation, and the transport and distribution of lipids as lipoproteins and free fatty acids

Learning Objective Describe the pathways involved in lipid metabolism, and summarize the processes of lipid transport and distribution.

Like carbohydrates, lipid molecules contain carbon, hydrogen, and oxygen, but in different proportions. Triglycerides (fats) are the most abundant lipid in the body, so we will focus on their breakdown and synthesis. ⟳ p. 41

Lipid Catabolism

During lipid catabolism, or **lipolysis** (li-POL-i-sis), lipids are broken down into pieces that can be converted to pyruvate or channeled directly into the citric acid cycle (**Figure 17-8**). A triglyceride is first split into its component parts by hydrolysis, yielding one molecule of glycerol and three fatty acid molecules. Enzymes in the cytosol convert glycerol to pyruvate, which then enters the citric acid cycle. The catabolism of fatty acids involves a different set of enzymes that generate acetyl-CoA directly.

CLINICAL NOTE

Complications of Diabetes Mellitus

Diabetes mellitus is a disorder of glucose metabolism. The diabetic under treatment can develop complications that result from an inadequate amount of available glucose *(hypoglycemia)* or an excess amount of available glucose *(hyperglycemia)*. Patients with Type I diabetes require insulin. An excess dose of insulin or inadequate food intake after a standard dose of insulin can cause life-threatening hypoglycemia. Likewise, a lack of insulin or increased food intake with a standard dose of insulin can cause hyperglycemia. Type II diabetics usually do not require insulin. Instead, they are able to manage their blood-sugar levels through diet, exercise, or use of an *oral hypoglycemic agent*. Although much less common, a Type II diabetic can develop hypoglycemia if an excess of oral hypoglycemic medication is taken or if food intake decreases significantly. Like the Type I diabetic, the Type II diabetic can develop hyperglycemia if food intake is increased or if the oral hypoglycemic agent being used does not adequately lower blood-glucose levels.

The extremes of blood sugar can affect many body systems. Prolonged poor control of blood-sugar levels markedly increases the patient's chances of developing many of the long-term complications associated with diabetes. The extremes of blood sugar require prompt treatment by emergency personnel.

- Hypoglycemia. The blood-glucose level at which hypoglycemia occurs varies from individual to individual. However, a blood-glucose level less than 50 mg/dL results in hypoglycemia in most diabetics. Hypoglycemia is a true medical emergency and the most life-threatening complication of diabetes mellitus. The central nervous system (CNS) relies almost exclusively on glucose as its sole source of energy. Thus, an inadequate blood-glucose level can cause CNS injury. The symptoms of hypoglycemia are due to CNS dysfunction. Prompt recognition of hypoglycemia and administration of glucose is essential if CNS injury is to be prevented.

- Hyperglycemia. An abnormal elevation in blood glucose is termed hyperglycemia. Unlike hypoglycemia, which can develop in minutes, hyperglycemia can take hours or even days to develop. In most patients, there is an inadequate level of the insulin necessary for glucose entry into the cells. When glucose entry is impaired, cellular starvation occurs. In addition to its effect on glucose metabolism, insulin is also responsible for the manufacture and storage of lipids (fats) by the body. Inadequate insulin levels cause the breakdown of lipids into glucose, which further increases blood-glucose levels. As a by-product of lipid breakdown, free-fatty acids are converted to ketone bodies. As ketone bodies accumulate, systemic acidosis occurs. The sequence of events results in diabetic ketoacidosis (DKA). In severe DKA, the pH can fall to 7.0 or lower.

  — Diabetic ketoacidosis. Most Type I diabetics develop DKA if their blood-glucose levels are allowed to rise unchecked. The signs and symptoms of DKA are related to the various

(Continued)

17

biochemical derangements described earlier. They include dehydration, hypotension, and reflex tachycardia. As the disease progresses, the patient will develop nausea, vomiting, and abdominal pain. Because of the acidosis, hyperventilation occurs as a compensatory mechanism. The hyperventilation is quite exaggerated and is referred to as *Kussmaul's respiration*. The sweet smell of ketones can sometimes be detected in the patient's breath. Eventually, the patient will develop altered mental status and, in time, unconsciousness. Treatment includes massive intravenous fluid replacement and the administration of insulin.

— Non-ketotic hyperosmolar coma. A certain subset of patients, most of whom have Type II diabetes, will not develop ketones as a complication of hyperglycemia. In these patients, there appears to be enough insulin present to prevent ketone formation. As their blood glucose levels rise, they can develop *non-ketotic hyperosmolar coma (NKHC)*. In NKHC, the blood glucose level can rise to 1000 mg/dL or more. As the glucose is spilled into the urine, the resultant *osmotic diuresis* causes severe dehydration. The *osmolarity* of the blood, which is a measure of concentration of molecules in the blood, climbs significantly. NKHC most commonly occurs in middle-aged or elderly diabetics and is often associated with another disease process such as infection. It typically takes days for NKHC to occur, and the signs and symptoms are similar to those seen in DKA. Kussmaul's respirations are not seen. Treatment is similar to DKA. However, the mortality rate for NHKC is higher than for DKA.

Beta-oxidation is a series of reactions that break the fatty acids down into two-carbon fragments, and generate NADH and $FADH_2$. This process takes place inside mitochondria, so the two-carbon fragments can enter the citric acid cycle immediately as acetyl-CoA. (Some of the two-carbon fragments may combine to form *ketone bodies*, short carbon chains discussed on p. 589.) A cell produces 120 ATP molecules from the breakdown of one 18-carbon fatty acid molecule. This yield is almost 1.3 times the energy obtained from the breakdown of three 6-carbon glucose molecules (90-96 ATP).

Lipids and Energy Production

Lipids are important energy reserves because they can provide large amounts of ATP. Lipids can be stored in compact droplets in the cytosol because they are insoluble in water. However, if the droplets are large, it is difficult for water-soluble enzymes to get at them. For this reason, lipid reserves are more difficult to access than carbohydrate reserves. Also, most lipids are processed inside mitochondria, and mitochondrial activity is limited by the availability of oxygen. The net result is that lipids cannot provide large amounts of ATP quickly.

However, cells with modest energy demands can shift to lipid-based energy production when glucose supplies are limited. Skeletal muscle fibers normally cycle between lipid metabolism and carbohydrate metabolism. At rest (when energy demands are low), these cells break down fatty acids. During activity (when energy demands are high and immediate), skeletal muscle fibers shift to glucose metabolism.

CLINICAL NOTE

Dietary Fats and Cholesterol

Elevated cholesterol levels are associated with the development of *coronary artery disease* ⟳ p. 414 and *atherosclerosis*. ⟳ p. 433 Nutritionists now recommend limiting cholesterol intake to under 300 mg per day—a 40 percent reduction for the average American adult. Yet cholesterol is important. Consider the following points:

• *Cholesterol has many vital functions in the human body.* It is part of all plasma membranes. It waterproofs the epidermis. Cholesterol is also a key constituent of bile, and the precursor of several steroid hormones and one vitamin (D_3). Because cholesterol is so important, the goal of dietary restrictions is *not* to eliminate cholesterol, but to keep cholesterol levels within acceptable limits.

• *The cholesterol in the diet is not the only source of circulating cholesterol.* The human body can manufacture cholesterol from acetyl-CoA obtained during glycolysis or by the breakdown (beta-oxidation) of other lipids. If the diet contains an abundance of saturated fats, excess lipids are broken down to acetyl-CoA and used to make cholesterol. People trying to lower blood cholesterol levels by dietary control must also restrict other lipids—especially saturated fats.

• *Genetic factors affect each person's cholesterol level.* If you reduce your dietary intake of cholesterol, your body will synthesize more to maintain "acceptable" concentrations in the blood. An "acceptable" level depends on your genetic makeup. In virtually all instances, however, dietary restrictions can lower blood cholesterol significantly.

• *Cholesterol levels vary with age and physical condition.* In general, as we age, our cholesterol levels gradually rise. Cholesterol levels are considered unhealthy if they are higher than those of 90 percent of the population in a given age group. For males, this level ranges from 185 mg/dL at age 19 to 250 mg/dL at age 70. For females, the comparable levels are 190 mg/dL and 275 mg/dL, respectively. Everyone should be screened for high cholesterol levels as they age.

17

Lipid Synthesis

Lipogenesis (lip-ō-JEN-e-sis; *lipos*, fat) is the synthesis of lipids. Glycerol is synthesized from an intermediate three-carbon product of glycolysis. The synthesis of most other types of lipids, including steroids and almost all fatty acids, begins with acetyl-CoA. Lipogenesis can use almost any organic molecule because lipids, amino acids, and carbohydrates can be converted to acetyl-CoA.

Body cells cannot *build* every fatty acid they can break down. For example, *linoleic acid* and *linolenic acid* are both 18-carbon unsaturated fatty acids synthesized by plants. They cannot be synthesized in the human body. They are called **essential fatty acids** because they must be included in your diet. These fatty acids are also needed to synthesize prostaglandins and phospholipids in plasma membranes throughout the body.

Lipid Transport and Distribution

Like glucose, lipids are needed throughout the body. All cells use lipids to maintain their plasma membranes. Steroid hormones must reach their target cells in many different tissues. Because most lipids are not soluble in water, special means of transport are required to distribute them around the body. Free fatty acids (FFA) make up a small percentage of the total circulating lipids. Most lipids circulate in the bloodstream as lipoproteins (**Figure 17-9**).

FFA are lipids that can diffuse easily across plasma membranes. A major source of FFA is the breakdown of fat stored in adipose tissue. When released into the blood, the fatty acids bind to albumin, the most abundant plasma protein. Liver cells, cardiac muscle cells, skeletal muscle fibers, and many other body cells can metabolize FFA. They are

Figure 17-9 Lipoproteins and Lipid Transport.

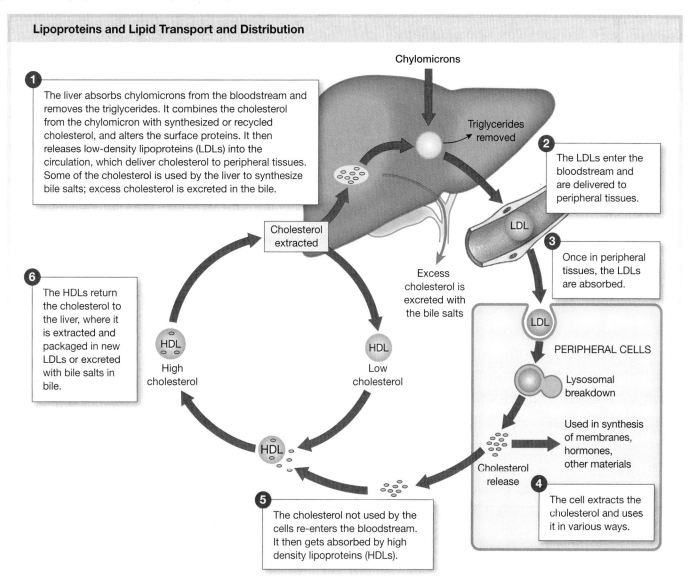

Lipoproteins and Lipid Transport and Distribution

Chylomicrons

1 The liver absorbs chylomicrons from the bloodstream and removes the triglycerides. It combines the cholesterol from the chylomicron with synthesized or recycled cholesterol, and alters the surface proteins. It then releases low-density lipoproteins (LDLs) into the circulation, which deliver cholesterol to peripheral tissues. Some of the cholesterol is used by the liver to synthesize bile salts; excess cholesterol is excreted in the bile.

Triglycerides removed

2 The LDLs enter the bloodstream and are delivered to peripheral tissues.

Cholesterol extracted

LDL

3 Once in peripheral tissues, the LDLs are absorbed.

Excess cholesterol is excreted with the bile salts

LDL

6 The HDLs return the cholesterol to the liver, where it is extracted and packaged in new LDLs or excreted with bile salts in bile.

HDL
High cholesterol

HDL
Low cholesterol

PERIPHERAL CELLS

Lysosomal breakdown

Used in synthesis of membranes, hormones, other materials

Cholesterol release

4 The cell extracts the cholesterol and uses it in various ways.

HDL

5 The cholesterol not used by the cells re-enters the bloodstream. It then gets absorbed by high density lipoproteins (HDLs).

17

an important energy source during periods of starvation, when glucose supplies are limited.

Lipoproteins are lipid–protein complexes that contain triglycerides and cholesterol. An outer coating of phospholipids and proteins makes the entire complex soluble. The exposed proteins bind to specific membrane receptors. This binding determines which cells absorb the associated lipids.

Lipoproteins are classified by size and by their relative proportions of lipid and protein. One group, the *chylomicrons*, is produced by intestinal epithelial cells from the fats in food. ↺ p. 568 They are the largest lipoproteins. About 95 percent of their weight consists of triglycerides. Chylomicrons transport triglycerides absorbed from the intestinal tract to the bloodstream. A capillary wall enzyme breaks down the triglycerides into fatty acids and monoglycerides that are absorbed by skeletal muscle, cardiac muscle, adipose tissue, and the liver.

Two other major groups of lipoproteins are the **low-density lipoproteins (LDLs)** and **high-density lipoproteins (HDLs)**. These lipoproteins are formed in the liver and contain few triglycerides. Their main roles are to shuttle cholesterol between the liver and other tissues. LDLs deliver cholesterol to peripheral tissues. It is often called "bad cholesterol" because LDL cholesterol may end up in arterial plaques. HDLs transport excess cholesterol from peripheral tissues to the liver for storage or excretion in the bile. HDL cholesterol is called "good cholesterol" because it is returning from peripheral tissues and does not cause circulatory problems.

> **CHECKPOINT**
>
> **7.** Define lipolysis and beta-oxidation.
>
> **8.** Why are high-density lipoproteins (HDLs) considered beneficial?
>
> See the blue Answers tab at the back of the book.

17-4 Protein catabolism involves transamination and deamination, and protein synthesis involves amination and transamination

Learning Objective Discuss protein metabolism and the use of proteins as an energy source.

The body can synthesize at least 100,000 different proteins, each with varied functions and structures. Yet each protein contains some combination of the same 20 amino acids. Under normal conditions, cellular proteins are continuously recycled in the cytosol. Peptide bonds are broken, and the resulting free amino acids are used in synthesizing new proteins. ↺ p. 43

If other energy sources are inadequate, mitochondria can generate ATP by breaking down amino acids in the citric acid cycle. Not all amino acids enter the citric acid cycle at the same point, so the ATP benefits vary. However, the average ATP yield is comparable to that of carbohydrate catabolism.

Amino Acid Catabolism

The first step in amino acid catabolism is the removal of the amino group. This step requires a coenzyme derived from **vitamin** B_6 (*pyridoxine*). The amino group is removed in one of two ways.

Transamination (trans-am-i-NĀ-shun) is a process in which one amino acid is formed from another. The process removes the amino group from an amino acid and attaches it to another small carbon chain, creating a "new" amino acid. In this way, a cell can synthesize many of the amino acids needed for protein synthesis. Cells of the liver, skeletal muscles, heart, lung, kidney, and brain are all particularly active in protein synthesis. These cells perform many transaminations.

Deamination (dē-am-i-NĀ-shun) prepares an amino acid for breakdown in the citric acid cycle. Deamination is the removal of an amino group in a reaction that generates an ammonium ion (NH_4^+). Ammonium ions are highly toxic, even in low concentrations. Liver cells are the primary sites of deamination. They have enzymes needed to deal with the problem of ammonium ion generation. Liver cells combine carbon dioxide with ammonium ions to produce **urea**, a relatively harmless, water-soluble compound. It is excreted in the urine.

The fate of the carbon chain remaining after deamination in the liver depends on its structure. The carbon chains of some amino acids can be converted to pyruvate and then used in gluconeogenesis. Other carbon chains are converted to acetyl-CoA and broken down in the citric acid cycle. Still others are converted to **ketone bodies**, metabolic acids that are also produced during lipid catabolism. One example of a ketone body generated in the body is *acetone*, a small molecule that can diffuse into the alveoli of the lungs, giving the breath a distinctive "fruity" odor.

Liver cells do not catabolize ketone bodies. Instead, the ketone bodies diffuse from the liver cells and into the general circulation. Cells in peripheral tissues absorb the ketone bodies and reconvert them into acetyl-CoA for breakdown in the citric acid cycle and the production of ATP. The increased production of ketone bodies during protein and lipid catabolism by the liver results in high ketone body concentrations in body fluids, a condition called **ketosis** (kē-TŌ-sis).

Protein catabolism is not a practical source of quick energy for three reasons:

1. Proteins are more difficult to break apart than are complex carbohydrates or lipids.

2. One of the by-products, ammonium ions, is toxic to cells.

3. Proteins are the most important structural and functional components of any cell. Extensive protein catabolism threatens homeostasis at the cellular and systems levels.

Amino Acids and Protein Synthesis

Your body can synthesize about half of the amino acids needed to build proteins. (The basic process of protein synthesis was detailed in Chapter 3.) ↻ pp. 78–81 There are 10 **essential amino acids**, which must come from the diet. Your body cannot synthesize eight of them (*isoleucine, leucine, lysine, threonine, tryptophan, phenylalanine, valine*, and *methionine*). The other two (*arginine* and *histidine*) can be synthesized, but not in amounts that growing children need.

Other amino acids are called **nonessential amino acids**, because the body can make them on demand. Your body cells can readily synthesize the carbon frameworks for them. Then an amino group can be added by transamination or by **amination**—using an ammonium ion as the reactant.

Protein deficiency diseases develop in people who do not consume adequate amounts of all essential amino acids. All amino acids must be available if protein synthesis is to take place. Every transfer RNA molecule must appear at the active ribosome in the proper sequence, bearing its individual amino acid. If that does not happen, the entire process comes to a halt.

Several inherited metabolic disorders result from an inability to produce specific enzymes involved in amino acid metabolism. People with **phenylketonuria** (fen-il-kē-to-NOO-rē-uh), or **PKU**, cannot convert the amino acid

CLINICAL NOTE

Ketoacidosis

A ketone body is also called a *keto acid* because it dissociates in solution, releasing a hydrogen ion. The appearance of ketone bodies is a threat to blood plasma pH. During even a brief fasting period, production of ketone bodies increases. During prolonged starvation, ketone levels continue to rise. Eventually, the pH-buffering capacities of the blood are exceeded, and a dangerous drop in pH occurs. This acidification of the blood and body tissues is called ketoacidosis (kē-tō-as-i-DŌ-sis). In severe ketoacidosis, pH may fall below 7.05, low enough to disrupt normal tissue activities. Coma, cardiac arrhythmias, and death can result.

In *diabetes mellitus*, most peripheral tissues cannot utilize glucose because of a lack of insulin. ↻ p. 366 Under these circumstances, cells survive by catabolizing lipids and proteins. The result is the production of large numbers of ketone bodies. This condition leads to *diabetic ketoacidosis*, the most common and life-threatening form of ketoacidosis.

phenylalanine to the amino acid tyrosine. This reaction is an essential step in the synthesis of norepinephrine, epinephrine, and melanin. The problem in PKU is a defect in the enzyme phenylalanine hydroxylase. If PKU is not detected in infancy, central nervous system development is inhibited. Severe brain damage results. People with PKU need to follow a diet that limits foods containing phenylalanine. The condition is common enough that a warning is printed on the packaging of products that contain phenylalanine, such as diet drinks.

Figure 17-10 summarizes the major metabolic pathways for lipids, carbohydrates, and proteins. This diagram presents the reactions in a "typical" cell, but no one cell can perform all the anabolic and catabolic operations required by the body as a whole. As cells differentiate during development, each cell type develops its own set of enzymes that determines its metabolic capabilities. With such cellular diversity in the body, homeostasis can be preserved only when the metabolic activities of tissues, organs, and organ systems are coordinated.

17

CHECKPOINT

9. Define transamination and deamination.

10. How would a diet deficient in vitamin B_6 affect protein metabolism?

See the blue Answers tab at the back of the book.

Figure 17-10 A Summary of Catabolic and Anabolic Pathways for Lipids, Carbohydrates, and Proteins. The major catabolic pathways are in red. The major anabolic pathways are in blue.

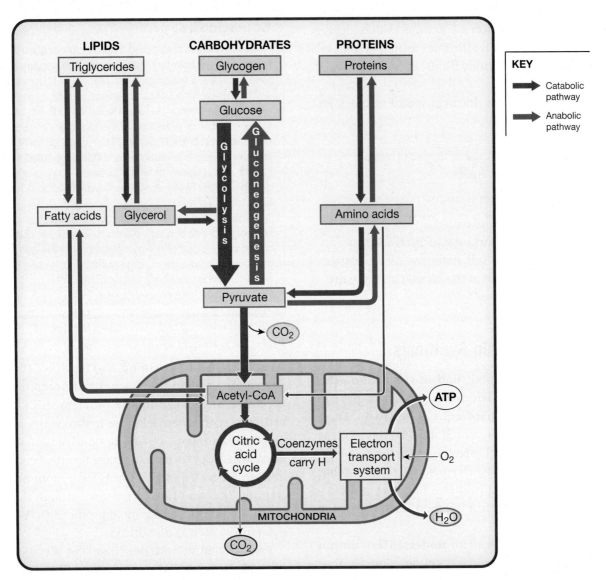

17-5 Nucleic acid catabolism involves RNA, but not DNA

Learning Objective Discuss nucleic acid metabolism and the limited use of nucleic acids as an energy source.

Living cells contain both DNA and RNA. The genetic information contained in nuclear DNA is absolutely essential to the long-term survival of a cell. As a result, DNA is never catabolized for energy, even if the cell is dying of starvation. By contrast, the RNA molecules involved in protein synthesis are broken down and replaced regularly.

RNA Catabolism

In the breakdown of RNA, the molecule is disassembled into individual nucleotides. Most nucleotides are recycled into new nucleic acids, but they can also be broken down to simple sugars and nitrogen bases. When nucleotides are broken down, only the sugars, cytosines, and uracils can enter the citric acid cycle and be used to generate ATP. Adenine and guanine cannot be catabolized. Instead, these nitrogen bases undergo deamination and are excreted as **uric acid**. Like urea, uric acid is a relatively nontoxic waste product, but it is far less soluble than urea. Urea and uric acid are called *nitrogenous wastes*, because they contain nitrogen atoms.

An elevated level of uric acid in the blood is called *hyperuricemia* (hī-per-ū-ri-SĒ-mē-uh). Uric acid saturates body fluids. Although symptoms may not appear immediately, uric acid crystals may begin to form. The condition that then develops is called *gout*. Initially, the joints of the limbs are affected, especially the metatarsal-phalangeal joint of the great toe. Most cases of hyperuricemia and gout are linked to problems with the excretion of uric acid by the kidneys.

Nucleic Acid Synthesis

Most cells synthesize RNA, but DNA synthesis takes place only in cells preparing for mitosis (cell division) or meiosis (gamete production). (We described the process of DNA replication in Chapter 3.) ⤷ p. 82

Messenger RNA (mRNA), transfer RNA (tRNA), and ribosomal RNA (rRNA) are transcribed by different forms of the enzyme RNA polymerase. Messenger RNA is manufactured when specific genes are activated. A strand of mRNA has a life span measured in minutes or hours. Ribosomal RNA and tRNA are more durable than mRNA. For example, the average strand of rRNA lasts just over five days. However, replacement of rRNA and tRNA involves a considerable amount of synthetic activity.

> ### CHECKPOINT
>
> **11.** Why do cells not use DNA as an energy source?
>
> **12.** What are nitrogenous wastes?
>
> **13.** Elevated levels of uric acid in the blood could indicate an increased catabolic rate for which type of macromolecule?
>
> See the blue Answers tab at the back of the book.

17-6 Adequate nutrition is necessary to prevent deficiency disorders and maintain homeostasis

Learning Objective Explain what makes up a balanced diet and why such a diet is important.

Homeostasis can be maintained indefinitely only if the digestive tract absorbs fluids, organic substances, minerals, and vitamins at a rate that keeps pace with cellular demands. The absorption of nutrients from food is called **nutrition**.

The body's requirement for each nutrient varies from day to day and from person to person. *Nutritionists* attempt to analyze a diet in terms of its ability to meet the needs of a specific individual. A **balanced diet** contains all the nutrients needed to maintain homeostasis. Such a diet includes essential amino acids and fatty acids, minerals, vitamins, and substrates for generating energy. In addition, the diet must include enough water to replace losses in urine, feces, and evaporation. A balanced diet prevents **malnutrition**, an unhealthy state resulting from the inadequate or excessive absorption of one or more nutrients.

Food Groups and a Balanced Diet

One way of maintaining good health and preventing malnutrition is to consume a diet based on the ChooseMyPlate plan. To remind Americans to eat a healthful diet, the United States Department of Agriculture created a diagram of a place setting at mealtime called MyPlate (**Figure 17-11**). It shows the proportions of food we should consume from each of the **five basic food groups**: grains (orange), vegetables (green), fruits (red), dairy (blue), and protein (purple). Oils should be used sparingly in addition to the five basic food groups. **Table 17-1** summarizes the benefits of these food groups. (Visit www.choosemyplate.gov for more information.)

Figure 17-11 MyPlate Food Guide. The recommended proportion of each food group at mealtime is indicated by its size on the plate. Foods should be consumed in proportions based on both the food group and the individual's level of activity.

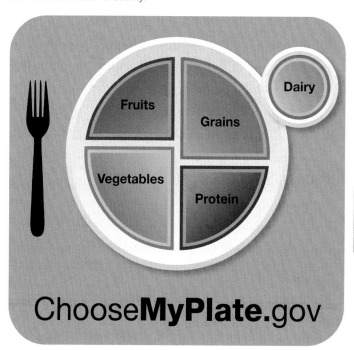

Table 17-1	Basic Food Groups and their Effects on Health	
Nutrient Group	**Provides**	**Health Effects**
Grains (recommended: at least half of the total eaten should be whole grains)	Carbohydrates; vitamins E, thiamine, niacin, folate; calcium; phosphorus; iron; sodium; dietary fiber	Whole grains prevent rapid rise in blood glucose levels, and consequent rapid rise in insulin levels
Vegetables (recommended: especially dark-green and orange vegetables)	Carbohydrates; vitamins A, C, E, folate; dietary fiber; potassium	Reduce risk of cardiovascular disease; protect against colon cancer (folate) and prostate cancer (lycopene in tomatoes)
Fruits (recommended: a variety of fruit each day)	Carbohydrates; vitamins A, C, E, folate; dietary fiber; potassium	Reduce risk of cardiovascular disease; protect against colon cancer (folate)
Dairy (recommended: low-fat or fat-free milk, yogurt, and cheese)	Complete proteins; fats; carbohydrates; calcium; potassium; magnesium; sodium; phosphorus; vitamins A, B_{12}, pantothenic acid, thiamine, riboflavin	Good source of calcium, which strengthens bones; whole milk: high in calories, may cause weight gain; saturated fats correlated with heart disease
Protein (recommended: lean meats, fish, poultry, eggs, dry beans, nuts, legumes)	Complete proteins; fats; calcium; potassium; phosphorus; iron; zinc; vitamins E, thiamine, B_6	Fish and poultry lower risk of heart disease and colon cancer (compared to red meat). Consumption of up to one egg per day does not appear to increase incidence of heart disease; nuts and legumes improve blood cholesterol ratios, lower risk of heart disease and diabetes

It is important that you take in nutrients in sufficient *quantity* (to meet your energy needs) and *quality* (including essential amino acids, fatty acids, vitamins, and minerals). The key is to make intelligent choices about what you eat.

For example, consider the essential amino acids. You must obtain them from your diet. Some foods in the dairy and protein groups—specifically, beef, fish, poultry, eggs, and milk—provide all the essential amino acids in sufficient quantities. They are said to contain **complete proteins**. Many plants also supply adequate *amounts* of protein, but these are **incomplete proteins** because one or more essential amino acids are lacking. People who follow a vegetarian diet, which is largely restricted to the grains, fruits, and vegetables groups (with or without the dairy group), must include a combination of foods that meets all their amino acid requirements. A vegan diet, which avoids all animal products, can be a problem because vitamin B_{12} can be obtained only from animal products, or from fortified cereals or tofu.

Minerals, Vitamins, and Water

Minerals, vitamins, and water are essential components of the diet. The body cannot synthesize minerals. Our cells can generate only a small quantity of water and very few vitamins.

Minerals

Minerals are inorganic ions released through the dissociation of electrolytes, such as sodium chloride. Minerals are important for three reasons:

1. *Ions such as sodium and chloride determine the osmotic concentration of body fluids.* Potassium is important in maintaining the osmotic concentration inside body cells.

2. *Ions in various combinations play major roles in important physiological processes.* As we have seen, these processes include the maintenance of membrane potentials; the construction and maintenance of the skeleton; muscle contraction; the generation of action potentials; the release of neurotransmitters; blood clotting; the transport of respiratory gases; buffer systems; fluid absorption; and waste removal.

Build Your Knowledge

Recall that inorganic compounds are substances that generally do not contain carbon and hydrogen (as you saw in **Chapter 2: The Chemical Level of Organization**). They include small molecules (such as carbon dioxide and water) and ionic compounds. Inorganic compounds held together by ionic bonds undergo dissociation or ionization in water. In this process, ionic bonds are broken as individual ions interact with the positive or negative ends of polar water molecules. ⊃ **pp. 34–35**

Table 17-2	Minerals and Mineral Reserves			
Mineral	**Significance**	**Total Body Content**	**Primary Route of Excretion**	**Recommended Daily Allowance (RDA) in mg**
BULK MINERALS				
Sodium	Major cation in body fluids; essential for normal membrane function	110 g, primarily in body fluids	Urine, sweat, feces	1500
Potassium	Major cation in cytoplasm; essential for normal membrane function	140 g, primarily in cytoplasm	Urine	4700
Chloride	Major anion in body fluids; functions in forming HCl	89 g, primarily in body fluids	Urine, sweat	2300
Calcium	Essential for normal muscle and neuron function, and normal bone structure	1.36 kg, primarily in skeleton	Urine, feces	1000–1200
Phosphorus	In high-energy compounds, nucleic acids, and bone matrix (as phosphate)	744 g, primarily in skeleton	Urine, feces	700
Magnesium	Cofactor of enzymes, required for normal membrane functions	29 g (skeleton, 17 g; cytoplasm and body fluids, 12 g)	Urine	310–400
TRACE MINERALS				
Iron	Component of hemoglobin, myoglobin, cytochromes	3.9 g (1.6 g stored as ferritin or hemosiderin)	Urine (traces)	8–18
Zinc	Cofactor of enzyme systems, notably carbonic anhydrase	2 g	Urine, hair (traces)	8–11
Copper	Required as cofactor for hemoglobin synthesis	127 mg	Urine, feces (traces)	0.9
Manganese	Cofactor for some enzymes	11 mg	Feces, urine (traces)	1.8–2.3

3. *Ions are essential cofactors in a variety of enzymatic reactions.* For example, the enzyme that breaks down ATP (ATPase) in a contracting skeletal muscle requires the presence of calcium and magnesium ions. Another type of ATPase required for the conversion of glucose to pyruvate needs both potassium and magnesium ions.

The major minerals and a summary of their functions are presented in **Table 17-2**. Your body contains reserves of several important minerals. However, the reserves are often small. Chronic dietary deficiencies can lead to various clinical problems. On the other hand, a dietary excess of mineral ions can also prove dangerous.

Vitamins

A **vitamin** (*vita*, life) is an essential organic nutrient that functions as a coenzyme in vital enzymatic reactions. There are two groups: fat-soluble vitamins and water-soluble vitamins.

FAT-SOLUBLE VITAMINS. Vitamins A, D, E, and K are **fat-soluble vitamins**. They dissolve in lipids. They are absorbed primarily from the digestive tract along with the lipid contents of micelles.

The term *vitamin D* refers to a group of steroid-like molecules, including vitamin D_3, or cholecalciferol. ᕐ p. 42 Unlike the other fat-soluble vitamins, which must be absorbed across the digestive tract, vitamin D_3 can usually be synthesized in adequate amounts by skin exposed to sunlight. Current information about the fat-soluble vitamins is summarized in **Table 17-3**.

Fat-soluble vitamins normally diffuse into plasma membranes, including the lipid inclusions in the liver and adipose tissue. As a result, your body contains a significant reserve of these vitamins. For this reason, a dietary insufficiency of fat-soluble vitamins rarely causes the signs and symptoms of **hypovitaminosis** (hī-pō-vī-ta-min-Ō-sis), or *vitamin deficiency disease. Too much* of a vitamin can also have harmful effects. **Hypervitaminosis** (hī-per-vī-ta-min-Ō-sis) occurs when dietary intake exceeds the body's ability to store, use, or excrete a particular vitamin. This condition most often involves one of the fat-soluble vitamins.

WATER-SOLUBLE VITAMINS. Most of the **water-soluble vitamins** are components of coenzymes (**Table 17-4**). For example, NAD is derived from niacin, FAD from vitamin B_2

17

Table 17-3	The Fat-Soluble Vitamins				
Vitamin	**Significance**	**Sources**	**Recommended Daily Allowance (RDA) in mg**	**Effects of Deficiency**	**Effects of Excess**
A	Maintains epithelia; required for synthesis of visual pigments; supports immune system; promotes growth and bone remodeling	Leafy green and yellow vegetables	0.7–0.9	Retarded growth, night blindness, deterioration of epithelial membranes	Liver damage, skin peeling, CNS effects (nausea, anorexia)
D (also known as D_3)	Required for normal bone growth, intestinal calcium and phosphorus absorption, and retention of these ions at the kidneys	Synthesized in skin exposed to sunlight	0.005–0.005*	Rickets, skeletal deterioration	Calcium deposits in many tissues, disrupting functions
E	Prevents breakdown of vitamin A and fatty acids	Meat, milk, vegetables	15	Anemia, other problems suspected	Nausea, stomach cramps, blurred vision, fatigue
K	Essential for liver synthesis of prothrombin and other clotting factors	Vegetables; production by intestinal bacteria	0.09–0.12	Bleeding disorders	Liver dysfunction, jaundice

*Unless exposure to sunlight is inadequate for extended periods and alternative sources (such as fortified milk products) are unavailable.

(riboflavin), and coenzyme A from vitamin B_5 (pantothenic acid). Water-soluble vitamins are rapidly exchanged between the digestive tract and the circulating blood. Excessive amounts are readily excreted in the urine. For this reason, hypervitaminosis involving water-soluble vitamins is relatively uncommon, except among people who take large doses of vitamin supplements.

The bacteria that live in the intestines help prevent deficiency diseases. They produce small amounts of five of the nine water-soluble vitamins, in addition to fat-soluble

Table 17-4	The Water-Soluble Vitamins				
Vitamin	**Significance**	**Sources**	**Recommended Daily Allowance (RDA) in mg**	**Effects of Deficiency**	**Effects of Excess**
B_1 (thiamine)	Coenzyme in many pathways	Milk, meat, bread	1.1–1.2	Muscle weakness, CNS and cardiovascular problems including heart disease; called *beriberi*	Hypotension
B_2 (riboflavin)	Part of FAD	Milk, meat, eggs, cheese	1.1–1.3	Epithelial and mucosal deterioration	Itching, tingling
B_3 (niacin, nicotinic acid)	Part of NAD	Meat, bread, potatoes	14–16	CNS, GI, epithelial, and mucosal deterioration; called *pellagra*	Itching, burning; vasodilation; death after large dose
B_5 (pantothenic acid)	Part of coenzyme A	Milk, meat	10	Delayed growth, CNS disturbances	None reported
B_6 (pyridoxine)	Coenzyme in amino acid and lipid metabolism	Meat, whole grains, vegetables, orange juice, cheese and milk	1.3–1.7	Delayed growth, anemia, convulsions, epithelial changes	CNS alterations, perhaps fatal
B_7 (biotin)	Coenzyme in many pathways	Eggs, meat, vegetables	0.03	Fatigue, muscular pain, nausea, dermatitis	None reported
B_9 (folic acid [synthetic], folate [natural])	Coenzyme in amino acid and nucleic acid metabolisms	Leafy vegetables, some fruits, liver, cereal and bread	0.2–0.4	Delayed growth, anemia, gastrointestinal disorders, developmental abnormalities	Few noted except at massive doses
B_{12} (cobalamin)	Coenzyme in nucleic acid metabolism	Milk, meat	0.0024	Impaired RBC production, causing *pernicious anemia*	Polycythemia (elevated hematocrit)
C (ascorbic acid)	Coenzyme in many pathways	Citrus fruits	75–90; Smokers add 35 mg	Epithelial and mucosal deterioration; called *scurvy*	Kidney stones

17

CLINICAL NOTE

Vitamins

Vitamins are organic compounds needed in small quantities for normal body metabolism. However, they cannot be manufactured by the cells of the body and must be obtained from the diet. Physiological processes that require vitamins include metabolism, growth, development, and tissue repair. The body absorbs most vitamins through the gastrointestinal tract following dietary ingestion. Vitamins are stored in the liver and, to a lesser extent, in the cells. In developed countries, healthy adults usually receive adequate amounts of vitamins and do not need supplements. Vitamin supplements may, however, be indicated for special populations including pregnant and nursing women, patients with absorption disorders, the chronically ill, surgery patients, alcoholics, and the malnourished. Additionally, people on a strict vegetarian diet may need supplemental vitamins.

Vitamins are classified as either fat-soluble or water-soluble (**Tables 17-3** and **17-4**). The liver stores fat-soluble vitamins (A, D, E, and K), so the patient will become deficient only after long periods of inadequate vitamin intake. Vitamin D is unique in that skin produces it with exposure to sunlight. The water-soluble vitamins (C and those in the B complex) must be routinely ingested, as the body does not store them. After short periods of deprivation, patients may begin to experience vitamin deficiency. The B complex vitamins are grouped only because they occur together in foods; otherwise they share no significant characteristics. The individual B vitamins are named for the order in which they were discovered (B_1, B_2, B_6, B_{12}, and so forth). These vitamins also have specific names. For example, B_1 is also known as thiamine, which is a vitamin that plays a key role in carbohydrate metabolism.

CLINICAL NOTE

Beriberi

A deficiency of *thiamine (vitamin B_1)* causes *beriberi.* In developing countries, beriberi is due to consumption of milled (polished) rice. In developed nations, thiamine deficiency is due to inadequate thiamine intake and absorption in chronic alcoholics.

Thiamine deficiency primarily affects the cardiovascular system *(wet beriberi)* and the nervous system *(dry beriberi).* Beriberi heart disease includes peripheral vasodilation, retention of sodium and water that leads to edema, and biventricular myocardial failure. *Acute fulminate cardiovascular beriberi* can end in cardiovascular collapse. Improvement occurs with thiamine replacement.

Two primary nervous system diseases are due to thiamine deficiency. *Wernicke's encephalopathy (WE)*, or cerebral beriberi, causes vomiting, dysfunction of the extraocular muscles, fever, ataxia, and mental deterioration. *Korsakoff's syndrome (KS)*, also called *Korsakoff's psychosis*, is a continuation of WE and includes retrograde amnesia and impaired ability to learn. Thiamine will completely reverse the effects of WE but will only partially reverse the symptoms of KS.

vitamin K. The intestinal epithelium can easily absorb all the water-soluble vitamins except B_{12}. The B_{12} molecule is large. To be absorbed, it must be bound to intrinsic factor from the gastric mucosa, as we discussed in Chapter 16. ↺ p. 549

Water

Daily water requirements average 2500 mL (10 cups), or roughly 40 mL/kg (.08 cup/lb) body weight. The specific requirement varies with environmental conditions and metabolic activities. For example, exercise increases metabolic energy requirements and accelerates water losses due to evaporation and perspiration. The temperature rise accompanying a fever has a similar effect. For each degree (°C) that temperature rises above normal, daily water loss increases by 200 mL. The advice "Drink plenty of fluids" when you are sick has a solid physiological basis.

You obtain most of your daily water ratio by eating or drinking. Food provides roughly 48 percent, and another 40 percent

comes from drinking fluids. A small amount of water—called *metabolic water*—is produced in mitochondria by the electron transport system. ↺ p. 583 Metabolic water amounts to roughly 300 mL of water per day (slightly more than 1 cup), about 12 percent of the average daily water requirement.

Diet and Disease

Diet has a profound influence on our general health. We have already considered the effects of too many and too few nutrients, above-normal or below-normal concentrations of minerals, and hypervitaminosis and hypovitaminosis. More subtle long-term problems can occur when the diet includes the wrong proportions or combinations of nutrients. The average diet in the United States contains too much sodium and too many calories, and lipids—particularly saturated fats—provide too great a proportion of those calories. Such a diet increases the incidence of obesity, heart disease, atherosclerosis, hypertension, and diabetes in the U.S. population.

17

CHECKPOINT

14. Identify the two types of vitamins.

15. What is the difference between foods containing complete proteins and those containing incomplete proteins?

16. How would a decrease in the amount of bile salts in the bile affect the amount of vitamin A in the body?

See the blue Answers tab at the back of the book.

17-7 Metabolic rate is the average caloric expenditure, and thermoregulation involves balancing heat-producing and heat-losing processes

Learning Objective Define metabolic rate, describe the factors involved in determining an individual's BMR, and discuss the homeostatic processes that maintain a constant body temperature.

When chemical bonds are broken, energy is released. Inside cells, some of that energy may be captured as ATP, but much of it is lost to the environment as heat. The unit of energy measurement is the **calorie** (KAL-o-rē) (cal), the amount of energy required to raise the temperature of 1 g of water 1 degree Celsius. One gram of water is not a very practical measure when you are interested in the metabolic operations that keep a 70-kg human alive, so we use the **kilocalorie (kcal)** (KIL-ō-kal-o-rē), or **Calorie** (with a capital C), also known as the "large calorie," instead. One Calorie is the amount of energy needed to raise the temperature of 1 *kilo*gram of water by 1°C. Calorie-counting guides for foods list Calories, not calories.

The Energy Content of Food

How do we know how much energy food contains? In cells, organic molecules combine with oxygen and are broken down to carbon dioxide and water. Oxygen is also consumed when something burns, and this process of combustion can be experimentally observed and measured. A known amount of food is sealed inside a chamber, called a **calorimeter** (kal-ō-RIM-e-ter), which is filled with oxygen and surrounded by a known volume of water. Then the chamber contents are electrically ignited. When the food has completely burned to ash, the number of Calories released can be determined by comparing the water temperatures before and after the test.

Such measurements show that the burning, or catabolism, of lipids releases a considerable amount of energy—roughly 9.46 Calories per gram (Cal/g). In contrast, the catabolism of carbohydrates releases 4.18 Cal/g, and the catabolism of protein releases 4.32 Cal/g. Most foods are mixtures of fats, proteins, and carbohydrates, so the values in a "Calorie counter" vary as a result.

Energy Expenditure: Metabolic Rate

Clinicians can examine your metabolic state and determine how many Calories your body uses. The result can be expressed as Calories per hour, Calories per day, or Calories per unit of body weight per day. What is actually measured is the sum of all the various anabolic and catabolic processes occurring in your body—your **metabolic rate** at that time. Metabolic rate varies with the activity under way. For instance, measurements taken while a person is sprinting are quite different from those taken while a person is sleeping. **Figure 17-12** shows the energy expenditures for various common activities.

To reduce such variations, the testing conditions are standardized so as to determine the **basal metabolic rate (BMR)**. Ideally, the BMR reflects the minimum, resting energy expenditures of an awake, alert person. An average individual has a BMR of 70 Cal per hour, or about 1680 Cal per day. Although the test conditions are standardized, other uncontrollable factors influence the BMR. These factors include age, sex, physical condition, body weight, and genetic differences.

Daily energy expenditures for a given individual vary widely with activity. For example, a person leading a sedentary life may have minimal energy demands, but one hour of swimming can increase the daily caloric requirements by 500 Cal or more. If daily energy intake exceeds the body's total energy demands, the excess energy will be stored, primarily as triglycerides in adipose tissue. If daily caloric expenditures exceed dietary intake, the body's energy reserves will decrease, with a corresponding loss in weight. This relationship explains the importance of both Calorie counting and daily exercise in a weight-control program.

Thermoregulation

The BMR estimates the rate of energy use by the body. Body cells capture only a part of that energy as ATP, and the rest is "lost" as heat. This heat loss serves an important homeostatic purpose. Humans are subject to vast changes in environmental

Figure 17-12 Caloric Expenditures for Various Activities.

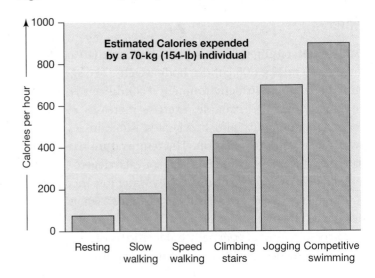

temperatures, but our complex biochemical systems have a major limitation. Our enzymes operate over only a relatively narrow temperature range. Accordingly, our bodies have anatomical and physiological mechanisms that keep body temperatures within acceptable limits, regardless of environmental conditions. This homeostatic process is called **thermoregulation** (*therme*, heat). ⤴ p. 10 Failure to control body temperature can result in serious physiological effects. For example, a body temperature below 36°C (97°F) or above 40°C (104°F) can cause disorientation. A temperature above 42°C (108°F) can cause convulsions and permanent cell damage.

Processes of Heat Transfer

Heat exchange with the environment involves four basic processes: (1) *radiation*, (2) *conduction*, (3) *convection*, and (4) *evaporation* (**Figure 17-13**).

1. ***Radiation.*** Objects warmer than the environment lose heat as infrared radiation. When you feel the sun's heat, you are experiencing radiant heat. Your body loses heat the same way, but in proportionally smaller amounts. More than half of the heat you lose indoors is lost through radiation.

2. ***Conduction.*** Conduction is the direct transfer of energy through physical contact. When you sit on a cold plastic chair in an air-conditioned room, you are immediately aware of this process. Its impact depends on the temperature of the object and the amount of skin area it contacts. Conduction is generally not an effective way of gaining or losing heat.

3. ***Convection.*** Convection is heat loss to the cooler air that moves across the surface of your body. As your body loses

Figure 17-13 Processes of Heat Transfer.

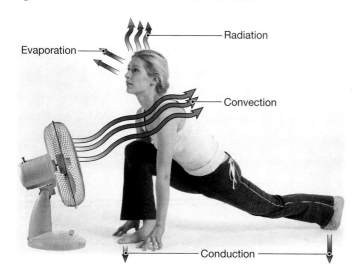

heat to the air next to your skin, that air warms and rises, moving away from the skin surface. Cooler air replaces it, and as this air in turn warms, the pattern repeats. Convection accounts for about 15 percent of the body's heat loss indoors.

4. ***Evaporation.*** When water evaporates, it changes from a liquid to a vapor. Evaporation absorbs energy—roughly 580 calories (0.58 Cal) per gram of water evaporated—and cools the surface on which it occurs. The rate of evaporation at your skin is highly variable. Each hour, 20–25 mL of water crosses epithelia and evaporates from the alveolar surfaces of the lungs and the surface of the skin. This *insensible water loss* remains relatively constant. It accounts for roughly 20 percent of your body's average indoor heat loss. The sweat glands are responsible for *sensible perspiration*. They have a tremendous scope of activity, ranging from virtual inactivity to secretory rates of 2–4 liters (or 2–4 kg) per hour. This rate is equivalent to an entire day's resting water loss in under an hour.

To maintain a constant body temperature, an individual must lose heat as fast as it is generated by metabolic operations. Heat loss and heat gain involve the activities of many different systems. The **heat-loss center** and **heat-gain center** of the hypothalamus coordinate those activities. The heat-loss center adjusts activity through the parasympathetic division of the autonomic nervous system, and the heat-gain center directs its responses through the sympathetic division. The overall effect is to control temperature fluctuations by influencing two events: the rate of heat production and the rate of heat loss to the environment. Changes in behavior, such as moving into the shade or sunlight, or adding or removing clothing, may also support these processes.

PROMOTING HEAT LOSS. When the temperature at the heat-loss center rises above its set point, three responses occur:

1. ***The vasomotor center is inhibited.*** This response causes peripheral blood vessels to dilate, sending warm blood flowing to the surface of the body. The skin takes on a reddish color and rises in temperature. Heat loss through radiation and convection increases.

2. ***Sweat glands are stimulated to increase their secretions.*** The perspiration flows across the skin, and heat loss through evaporation speeds up.

3. ***The respiratory centers are stimulated.*** As a result, the depth of respiration increases. Often, the person begins breathing through the mouth, which enhances heat loss through increased evaporation from the lungs.

17

The efficiency of heat loss by evaporation varies with environmental conditions, especially the "relative humidity" of the air. At 100 percent humidity, the air is saturated. It is holding as much water vapor as it can at that temperature. Under these conditions, cooling by evaporation is ineffective. This is why humid, tropical conditions can be so uncomfortable—people perspire continuously but remain warm and wet.

PROMOTING HEAT GAIN. The function of the heat-gain center of the brain is to prevent **hypothermia** (hī-pō-THER-mē-uh),

or below-normal body temperature. When body temperature falls below acceptable levels, the heat-loss center is inhibited and the heat-gain center is activated. Its activation results in responses that: (1) *conserve body heat* and (2) *promote heat generation.*

Stimulation of the vasomotor center constricts peripheral blood vessels and decreases blood flow to the skin, reducing losses of heat by radiation, convection, and conduction. The skin cools. With blood flow restricted, the skin may take on a bluish or pale coloration. In addition, blood returning

CLINICAL NOTE

Fire-Ground Rehabilitation

Firefighting is one of the most dangerous and physically demanding occupations today. It is common for EMS personnel to establish and staff rehabilitation units on the fire ground. For years, firefighter rehabilitation at the fire scene consisted of coffee and doughnuts provided by volunteer organizations. However, because it has been recognized that stress- and heat-related emergencies are the primary causes of on-duty firefighter deaths, the concept of *Emergency Incident Rehabilitation (EIR)* was developed. Large fires, such as wildfires, can involve hundreds of firefighters from multiple departments. In these situations, multiple rehab/EIR sectors must be established as a functional part of the Incident Command System.

It is important for all fire-ground personnel to report to the Rehab Sector immediately after any of the following activities:

- Strenuous activity such as forcible entry, advancing hose lines, closed space search and rescue, and/or ventilation
- The use and depletion of two self-contained breathing apparatus (SCBA) bottles
- Thirty minutes of operation within a hazardous/dangerous environment
- Failure of an SCBA unit

Incoming personnel should be carefully evaluated including vital signs, breath sounds, examination of skin color and condition, and body core temperature. It is important to try and to determine the firefighters' hydration status. Remember, over 60 percent of body weight is water (**Table 17-5**). Water is the best rehydration agent. Alternatively, water can be mixed with a commercial sport hydration beverage in a 50/50 mixture and administered at about 40°F(4.5°C).

Oral hydration with water is indicated in almost every fire-ground operation, regardless of the season. Large fires, or those that occur during summer months, especially in the South and the Southwest, can cause significant fluid loss. In many cases, firefighting personnel may need several liters of intravenous fluids to restore lost water. There should be established protocols for intravenous hydration in the field. Rehab sector personnel should decide whether a firefighter can return to fire fighting or remain for additional rehabilitation based on protocols (**Figure 17-14**). In addition to hydration, personnel should be provided some form of nutrition while in the rehab sector. Cut fresh fruit, such as apples or oranges, are best. Salty products and salt tablets should not be provided.

Table 17-5	Biochemical Content in Grams of a 70-Kilogram (154-Pound) Man	
CONTENT	**GRAMS**	
Water	41,400	
Fat	12,600	
Protein	12,600	
Carbohydrate	300	
Na	63	
K	150	
Ca	1160	
Mg	21	
Cl	85	
P	670	
S	112	
Fe	3	
L	0.014	

Figure 17-14 Fire-ground Operations. Large fires require multiple rehab sectors. Firefighting personnel should not be released to return to firefighting until cleared by rehab sector personnel.

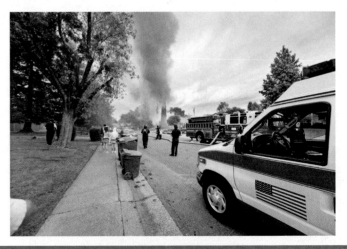

from the limbs is shunted into a network of deep veins that lies beneath an insulating layer of subcutaneous fat. ↺ p. 453 (Under warm conditions, blood flows through a superficial venous network, where heat can be lost.)

In addition to conserving heat, the heat-gain center stimulates two processes that generate heat. In *shivering thermogenesis* (ther-mō-JEN-e-sis), muscle tone is gradually increased until stretch receptors stimulate brief, oscillatory contractions of antagonistic skeletal muscles. The resulting shivering stimulates energy consumption by skeletal muscles, and the generated heat warms the deep vessels to which the blood has been diverted. Shivering can increase the rate of heat generation by as much as 400 percent.

Nonshivering thermogenesis involves the release of hormones that increase the metabolic activity of all tissues. The heat-gain center stimulates the adrenal medullae through the sympathetic division of the autonomic nervous system. As a result, epinephrine is released. It increases both the breakdown of glycogen and glycolysis in the liver and in skeletal muscles, and increases the metabolic rate in most tissues. The heat-gain center also stimulates the release of thyroxine by the thyroid gland, increasing the rate of carbohydrate catabolism and the breakdown of all other nutrients. These effects develop gradually over a period of days to weeks.

CHECKPOINT

17. Compare a pregnant woman's BMR (basal metabolic rate) to her BMR when she is not pregnant.

18. Under what conditions would evaporative cooling of the body be ineffective?

19. What effect would vasoconstriction of peripheral blood vessels have on body temperature on a hot day?

See the blue Answers tab at the back of the book.

17-8 Caloric needs decline with advancing age

Learning Objective Describe the age-related changes in dietary requirements.

Nutritional requirements do not change drastically with age. However, changes in lifestyle, eating habits, and income can affect nutrition and health. The recommended proportions of calories provided by different foods remain the same at all ages. Proteins should provide 11–12 percent of daily caloric intake, carbohydrates 55–60 percent, and fats less than 30 percent.

Caloric *requirements*, however, do change with aging. For each decade after age 50, caloric requirements decrease by 10 percent. These decreases are associated with reductions in metabolic rates, body mass, activity levels, and exercise tolerance.

CLINICAL NOTE

Nutrition and Emergency Medical Services

The job demands and scheduling of emergency medical services (EMS) work make it difficult to eat a balanced diet and obtain adequate exercise. For the most part, EMS work is fairly sedentary. However, at certain times, it can require significant physical exertion and stamina. Because of this, it is essential that emergency personnel eat a balanced diet, obtain moderate aerobic exercise on a regular basis, and maintain normal body weight. Unfortunately, more and more EMS workers can be classified as obese. The definition of obesity varies, but it is generally defined as weighing at least 20 percent or more in excess of your ideal body weight. For example, patients with an ideal body weight of 178 pounds would be considered obese when their weight exceeded 214 pounds. A better measurement of obesity is through determination of the *body mass index (BMI)*. The BMI takes the patient's height into consideration and is calculated by dividing the body weight (in kilograms) by the patient's height (in meters). Many of the health problems associated with obesity begin to cause problems when the person's body weight exceeds 120 percent or more of ideal weight. Low back strain, one of the most common on-the-job injuries in EMS, occurs more frequently in personnel who are overweight.

Unfortunately, a few emergency workers can be classified as being morbidly obese. To be labeled as *morbidly obese*, the individuals must weigh more than two times their ideal body weight. For example, a patient with an ideal body weight of 178 pounds would be considered morbidly obese when their weight exceeds exceeded 356 pounds. People who are morbidly obese have serious risk factors for developing multiple life-threatening problems. Regardless of their overall general health, a morbidly obese person generally cannot perform all of the tasks expected of an EMT or paramedic during the course of routine EMS work.

Many EMS systems have health maintenance programs that identify personnel at risk for illness or injury, including obesity. When employees are identified as being obese, they may be asked to participate in developing a plan that will help them to lose weight and restore them to health. Such plans usually include an exercise regimen, dietary counseling, and wellness education. Physical fitness is more ingrained in the fire service, where most fire-based EMS operations have ongoing fitness programs. Although EMS units roll considerably more often than engine and truck companies, the EMS crew can usually get needed exercise over the course of the day. In busy systems, it may be prudent simply to block out time for exercise with the understanding that an MCI or high system usage would require interruption of exercise regimens.

With age, several factors combine to produce an increased need for calcium. Some degree of osteoporosis is a normal consequence of aging. A sedentary lifestyle contributes to the problem. The rate of bone loss decreases if calcium levels are kept elevated.

Elderly people are also likely to require supplemental vitamin D_3 if they are to absorb the calcium they need. Many elderly people spend most of their time indoors and avoid the sun when outdoors. This behavior slows sun damage to their skin, which is thinner than that of younger people. However, it also halts vitamin D_3 production by the skin. ↻ p. 127 This vitamin is converted to the hormone calcitriol, which stimulates calcium absorption by the small intestine.

Maintaining a healthy diet becomes more difficult with age due to changes in the senses of smell and taste and in the structure of the digestive system. With age, the number and sensitivity of olfactory and gustatory receptors decrease. ↻ p. 338 Food seems less appetizing, so elderly people eat less. The mucosal lining of the digestive tract becomes thinner with age, so nutrient absorption becomes less efficient. Elderly people on fixed budgets may also eat less animal protein, the main source of iron in the diet. Small quantities plus inefficient absorption makes them prone to iron deficiency, which causes anemia.

CHECKPOINT

20. Which changes with aging: nutritional requirements or caloric requirements?

See the blue Answers tab at the back of the book.

RELATED CLINICAL TERMS

anorexia: Persistent loss of appetite.

antipyretic drugs: Drugs administered to control or reduce fever.

eating disorders: Psychological problems that result in inadequate or excessive food consumption. Examples include anorexia nervosa and bulimia.

familial hypercholesterolemia: The most common inherited type of hyperlipidemia (high levels of lipids in the blood). It affects one in every 500 children born, who then present with high LDL levels.

heat exhaustion: A malfunction of thermoregulatory mechanisms caused by excessive fluid loss in perspiration.

heat stroke: A condition in which the thermoregulatory center stops functioning and body temperature rises uncontrollably.

ketonemia (kē-tō-NĒ-mē-uh)**:** Elevated levels of ketone bodies in blood.

ketonuria (kē-tō-NOO-rē-uh)**:** The presence of ketone bodies in urine.

liposuction: The removal of adipose tissue by suction through an inserted tube.

obesity: Body weight more than 20 percent above the ideal weight for a given individual.

pyrexia (pī-REK-sē-uh)**:** A fever; that is, a body temperature greater than 99°F(37.2°C).

17 | Chapter Review

Summary Outline

17-1 Metabolism refers to all the chemical reactions in the body, and energetics refers to the flow and transformation of energy p. 664

1. **Energetics** is the study of the flow of energy and its change(s) from one form to another. Its focus includes understanding a range of energy requirements from cells to the whole body.

2. In general, during *cellular metabolism*, cells break down excess carbohydrates first, then lipids, while conserving amino acids. Only about 40 percent of the energy released through *catabolism* is captured in ATP; the rest is released as heat *(Figure 17-1)*.

3. Cells synthesize new compounds (*anabolism*) to (1) perform structural maintenance and repair, (2) support

growth, (3) produce secretions, and (4) build nutrient reserves.

4. Cells "feed" small organic molecules to their mitochondria; in return, the cells get the ATP they need to perform cellular functions *(Figure 17-2)*.

17-2 Carbohydrate metabolism involves glycolysis, ATP production, and gluconeogenesis p. 666

5. Most cells generate ATP and other high-energy compounds through the breakdown of carbohydrates.

6. **Glycolysis** and **aerobic metabolism** provide most of the ATP used by typical cells. In glycolysis, each molecule of

glucose yields two molecules of pyruvate and two molecules of ATP *(Figure 17-3).*

7. In the presence of oxygen, the pyruvate molecules enter the mitochondria, where they are broken down completely in the **citric acid cycle**. The carbon and oxygen atoms are lost as carbon dioxide, and the hydrogen atoms are passed by *coenzymes* to the *electron transport system (Figure 17-4)*

8. **The electron transport system (ETS)** is embedded in the inner mitochondrial membrane. It is made up of four respiratory protein complexes, coenzyme Q, and *cytochromes* that eventually pass along electrons to oxygen to form water and ATP. Energy released by the passage of the electrons is used to pump H^+ from the matrix to the intermembrane space *(Spotlight Figure 17-5).*

9. ATP is formed through **chemiosmosis**. During this process, H^+ pass from the intermembrane space to the mitochondrial matrix through H^+ channels in the inner membrane. Energy from the movement of the H^+ is used by *ATP synthase* to form ATP from ADP and P *(Spotlight Figure 17-5).*

10. For each glucose molecule processed through glycolysis, the citric acid cycle, and the ETS, a typical cell gains 30–32 ATP molecules *(Figure 17-6).*

11. **Gluconeogenesis**, the synthesis of glucose, enables a cell to manufacture glucose molecules from other carbohydrates, glycerol, or some amino acids. *Glycogen* is an important energy reserve when extracellular glucose is low *(Figure 17-7).*

12. When supplies of glucose are limited, cells can break down other nutrients to provide molecules for the citric acid cycle *(Figure 17-8).*

17-3 Lipid metabolism involves lipolysis, beta-oxidation, and the transport and distribution of lipids as lipoproteins and free fatty acids *p. 673*

13. During **lipolysis** (lipid catabolism), lipids are broken down into pieces that can be converted into pyruvate or channeled into the citric acid cycle.

14. Triglycerides, the most abundant lipids in the body, are split into glycerol and fatty acids. Glycerol enters glycolysis pathways, and fatty acids enter mitochondria.

15. **Beta-oxidation** is the breakdown of fatty acid molecules into two-carbon fragments that can enter the citric acid cycle or be converted to ketone bodies.

16. Lipids cannot provide large amounts of ATP in a short amount of time. However, cells can shift to lipid-based energy production when glucose reserves are limited.

17. In **lipogenesis**, the synthesis of lipids, almost any organic molecule can be used to form glycerol. **Essential fatty acids** cannot be synthesized and must be included in the diet.

18. Lipids circulate as **free fatty acids (FFA)** (fatty acids associated with albumin that can diffuse easily across plasma membranes) or as **lipoproteins** (lipid–protein complexes that contain triglycerides and cholesterol). **Low-density lipoproteins (LDLs)** and **high-density lipoproteins (HDLs)** carry cholesterol between the liver and other tissues *(Figure 17-9).*

17-4 Protein catabolism involves transamination and deamination, and protein synthesis involves amination and transamination *p. 676*

19. If other energy sources are inadequate, mitochondria can break down amino acids. In the mitochondria, the amino group may be removed by *transamination* or *deamination*. The resulting carbon skeleton may enter the citric acid cycle to generate ATP or be converted to ketone bodies.

20. Protein catabolism is impractical as a source of quick energy.

21. The body can synthesize roughly half of the amino acids needed to build proteins. The 10 *essential amino acids* must be acquired through the diet.

22. No one body cell can perform all the anabolic and catabolic operations necessary to support human life. Homeostasis can be preserved only when the metabolic activities of different tissues are coordinated *(Figure 17-10).*

17-5 Nucleic acid catabolism involves RNA, but not DNA *p. 678*

23. DNA in the nucleus is never catabolized for energy. RNA molecules are broken down and replaced regularly; usually they are recycled as new nucleic acids.

17-6 Adequate nutrition is necessary to prevent deficiency disorders and maintain homeostasis *p. 679*

24. **Nutrition** is the absorption of essential nutrients from food. A *balanced diet* contains all the ingredients needed to maintain homeostasis; it prevents **malnutrition**.

25. The five **basic food groups** are grains, vegetables, fruits, dairy, and protein. These are arranged in a mealtime *plate setting* to reflect a recommended daily food consumption *(Figure 17-11, Table 17-1).*

26. **Minerals** act as cofactors in various enzymatic reactions. They also contribute to the osmotic concentration of body fluids, and they play a role in membrane potentials, action potentials, neurotransmitter release, muscle contraction, skeletal construction and maintenance, gas transport, buffer systems, fluid absorption, and waste removal *(Table 17-2).*

27. **Vitamins** are coenzymes in vital enzymatic reactions. They are needed in very small amounts. Vitamins A, D, E, and K are **fat-soluble vitamins**; taken in excess, they can lead to **hypervitaminosis. Water-soluble vitamins** are not stored in the body; a lack of adequate dietary supplies can lead to **hypovitaminosis** (*vitamin deficiency disease*) *(Tables 17-3, 17-4).*

28. Daily water requirements average about 40 mL/kg (.08 cup/lb) body weight. Water is obtained from food, drink, and metabolic generation.

29. A balanced diet can improve a person's general health.

17-7 Metabolic rate is the average caloric expenditure, and thermoregulation involves balancing heat-producing and heat-losing processes *p. 684*

30. The energy content of food is usually expressed as **Calories** per gram (Cal/g). Body cells capture less than half of the energy content of glucose or any other organic nutrient.

31. The catabolism of each gram of lipid releases 9.46°C, about twice the Calories released by the breakdown of the same amount of carbohydrate or protein.

32. The total of all the body's anabolic and catabolic processes over a given period of time is an individual's **metabolic rate**. The **basal metabolic rate (BMR)** is the rate of energy utilization at rest *(Figure 17-12)*.

33. The homeostatic regulation of body temperature is **thermoregulation**. Heat exchange with the environment involves four processes: **radiation, conduction, convection**, and **evaporation** *(Figure 17-13)*.

34. The hypothalamus acts as the body's thermostat, containing the **heat-loss center** and the **heat-gain center**.

35. Responses involved in increasing heat loss include both physiological processes (dilation of superficial blood vessels, increased perspiration, and accelerated respiration) and behavioral adaptations.

36. Body heat may be conserved by reducing blood flow to the skin. Heat can be generated by *shivering thermogenesis* and *nonshivering thermogenesis*.

17-8 Caloric needs decline with advancing age *p. 687*

37. Caloric requirements decrease by 10 percent each decade after age 50. Changes in the senses of smell and taste dull appetite, and changes to the digestive system decrease the efficiency of nutrient absorption from the digestive tract.

Review Questions

See the blue Answers tab at the back of the book.

Level 1 Reviewing Facts and Terms

Match each item in column A with the most closely related item in column B. Place letters for answers in the spaces provided.

COLUMN A

_____ **1.** Glucose formation
_____ **2.** Lipid catabolism
_____ **3.** Synthesis of lipids
_____ **4.** Linoleic acid
_____ **5.** Deamination
_____ **6.** Phenylalanine
_____ **7.** Ketoacidosis
_____ **8.** A, D, E, K
_____ **9.** B complex and vitamin C
_____ **10.** Calorie
_____ **11.** Uric acid
_____ **12.** Hypothermia

COLUMN B

a. Gluconeogenesis
b. Essential amino acid
c. Below-normal body temperature
d. Unit of energy
e. Fat-soluble vitamins
f. Water-soluble vitamins
g. Lipolysis
h. Nitrogenous waste
i. Essential fatty acid
j. Removal of an amino group
k. Decrease in pH
l. Lipogenesis

13. Cells synthesize new organic molecules to
(a) perform structural maintenance and repairs.
(b) support growth.
(c) produce secretions.
(d) a, b, and c are correct.

14. During the complete catabolism of one molecule of glucose, a typical cell gains
(a) 4–6 ATP.   (b) 18–20 ATP.
(c) 30–32 ATP.   (d) 90–96 ATP.

15. The breakdown of glucose to pyruvate is
(a) glycolysis.
(b) gluconeogenesis.
(c) cellular respiration.
(d) beta-oxidation.

16. Glycolysis yields an immediate net gain of _____ molecules for the cell.
(a) 1 ATP   (b) 2 ATP
(c) 4 ATP   (d) 32 ATP

17. The electron transport system yields up to _____ molecules in the complete catabolism of one glucose molecule.
  (a) 2 ATP
  (b) 4 ATP
  (c) 28 ATP
  (d) 32 ATP

18. The synthesis of glucose from simpler molecules is called
  (a) glycolysis.
  (b) lipolysis.
  (c) gluconeogenesis.
  (d) beta-oxidation.

19. Choose from the word bank to label the missing terms in the following diagram of nutrient use in cellular metabolism.

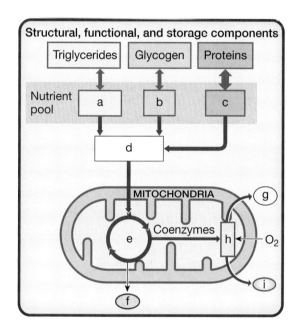

Word Bank: citric acid cycle, amino acids, glucose, electron transport system, fatty acids, ATP, CO$_2$, small carbon chains, H$_2$O.
  (a) _____   (b) _____
  (c) _____   (d) _____
  (e) _____   (f) _____
  (g) _____   (h) _____
  (i) _____

20. The lipoproteins that transport excess cholesterol from peripheral tissues back to the liver for storage or excretion in the bile are the
  (a) chylomicrons.   (b) FFA.
  (c) LDLs.   (d) HDLs.

21. The removal of an amino group in a reaction that generates an ammonium ion is called
  (a) ketoacidosis.
  (b) transamination.
  (c) deamination.
  (d) denaturation.

22. A complete protein contains
  (a) the proper balance of amino acids.
  (b) all the essential amino acids in sufficient quantities.
  (c) a combination of nutrients selected from the food pyramid.
  (d) N compounds produced by the body.

23. All minerals and most vitamins
  (a) are fat soluble.
  (b) cannot be stored by the body.
  (c) cannot be synthesized by the body.
  (d) must be synthesized by the body because they are not present in adequate amounts in the diet.

24. The basal metabolic rate (BMR) represents the
  (a) maximum energy expenditure when exercising.
  (b) minimum, resting energy expenditure of an awake, alert person.
  (c) minimum amount of energy expenditure during light exercise.
  (d) muscular energy expenditure added to the resting energy expenditure.

25. Over half of the heat loss from our bodies is due to
  (a) radiation.   (b) conduction.
  (c) convection.   (d) evaporation.

26. Define the terms metabolism, anabolism, and catabolism.

27. What is a lipoprotein? What are the major groups of lipoproteins, and how do they differ?

28. Why are vitamins and minerals essential components of the diet?

29. What are the energy yields (in Calories per gram) of the catabolism of carbohydrates, lipids, and proteins?

30. What is the basal metabolic rate (BMR)?

31. What four processes are involved in heat transfer?

Level 2 Reviewing Concepts

32. The function of the citric acid cycle is to
  (a) produce energy during periods of active muscle contraction.
  (b) break six-carbon chains into three-carbon fragments.
  (c) prepare the glucose molecule for further reactions.
  (d) remove hydrogen atoms from organic molecules and transfer them to coenzymes.

33. During periods of fasting or starvation, the presence of ketone bodies in the circulation causes
  (a) an increase in blood pH.
  (b) a decrease in blood pH.
  (c) a neutral blood pH.
  (d) diabetes insipidus.

34. Define glycolysis. What substances are required for this process?

35. What substances enter the citric acid cycle, and what substances leave it? Why is it called a cycle?

17

36. How does beta-oxidation function in lipid (triglyceride) catabolism?

37. How can the MyPlate food guide be used as a tool for developing a healthy lifestyle?

38. How is the brain involved in the regulation of body temperature?

39. Articles in popular media sometimes refer to "good cholesterol" and "bad cholesterol." To what types of cholesterol do these terms refer, and what are their functions?

Level 3 Critical Thinking and Clinical Applications

40. Why is a starving individual more susceptible to infectious disease than a well-nourished individual?

41. Charlie has a blood test that shows a normal level of LDLs but an elevated level of HDLs in his blood. Given that his family has a history of cardiovascular disease, he wonders if he should modify his lifestyle. What would you tell him?

18

The Urinary System

Learning Objectives

These objectives tell you what you should be able to do after completing the chapter. They correspond by number to this chapter's sections.

18-1 Identify the organs of the urinary system, and describe the functions of the system.

18-2 Describe the locations and structural features of the kidneys, trace the path of blood flow to, within, and from a kidney, and describe the structure of the nephron.

18-3 Discuss the major functions of each portion of the nephron, and outline the processes involved in urine formation.

18-4 Describe the factors that influence glomerular filtration pressure and the glomerular filtration rate (GFR).

18-5 Describe the structures and functions of the ureters, urinary bladder, and urethra, discuss the control of urination, and describe the micturition reflex.

18-6 Define the terms *fluid balance, electrolyte balance*, and *acid–base balance*, discuss their importance for homeostasis, and describe how water and electrolytes are distributed within the body.

18-7 Explain the basic processes involved in maintaining fluid balance and electrolyte balance.

18-8 Explain the buffering systems that balance the pH of the intracellular and extracellular fluids, and identify the most common threats to acid–base balance.

18-9 Describe the effects of aging on the urinary system.

18-10 Give examples of interactions between the urinary system and other body systems.

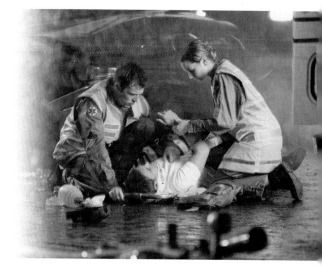

An Introduction to the Urinary System

The human body contains trillions of cells bathed in extracellular fluid. In previous chapters, we compared these cells to factories that burn nutrients to obtain energy. Imagine what would happen if real factories were as close together as cells in the body. Each factory would generate significant quantities of solid and gaseous wastes. Together they would create serious pollution problems.

We do not have such problems in our bodies as long as the activities of the digestive, cardiovascular, respiratory, and urinary systems are coordinated. The digestive tract absorbs nutrients from food and excretes solid wastes. The liver adjusts the nutrient concentration of the circulating blood.

The cardiovascular system delivers these nutrients, plus oxygen from the respiratory system, to peripheral tissues. As blood leaves these tissues, it carries the waste gas carbon dioxide and organic waste products to sites of excretion. The carbon dioxide is eliminated at the lungs (as described in Chapter 15). The urinary system removes most of the organic waste products.

In this chapter, we consider the organization of the urinary system. We describe how the kidneys remove metabolic wastes from the circulation to produce urine. We also examine the roles of fluid balance, electrolyte balance, and acid-base balance in homeostasis.

Build Your Knowledge

Recall that the urinary system eliminates waste products from the blood and controls water balance by regulating the volume of urine produced (as you saw in **Chapter 1: An Introduction to Anatomy and Physiology**). You are already familiar with three examples of waste products—bilirubin-derived pigments, urea, and uric acid—that are excreted by the kidneys. Recall also that the loss of water in urine is important in compensating for high blood pressure and blood volume. ⟲**pp. 9, 386, 589, 591**

18-1 The urinary system—made up of the kidneys, ureters, urinary bladder, and urethra—has three major functions

Learning Objective Identify the organs of the urinary system, and describe the functions of the system.

The **urinary system** has three major functions. They are (1) *excretion*, the removal of organic waste products from body fluids; (2) *elimination*, the discharge of these waste products into the environment; and (3) *homeostatic regulation* of the volume and solute concentration of blood.

The organs of the urinary system include the paired kidneys, paired ureters, urinary bladder, and urethra (**Figure 18-1**). The two **kidneys** perform excretory functions. These organs produce **urine**, a fluid containing water, ions, and small soluble compounds. Urine from the kidneys flows along the **urinary tract**, which consists of paired tubes called **ureters** (ū-RĒ-terz), to the **urinary bladder**, a muscular sac for temporary storage of urine. From the urinary bladder, urine passes through the **urethra** (ū-RĒ-thra) to the exterior.

The urinary bladder and the urethra eliminate urine in a process called **urination** or **micturition** (mik-choo-RISH-un). The muscular urinary bladder contracts to force urine through the urethra and out of the body.

Figure 18-1 The Organs of the Urinary System.

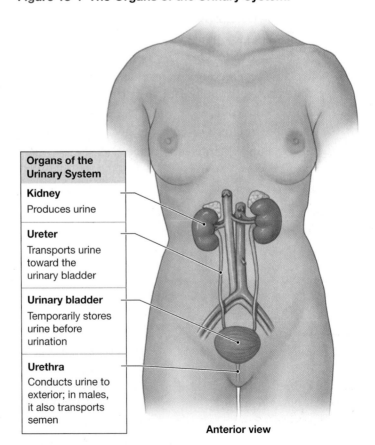

Organs of the Urinary System	
Kidney	Produces urine
Ureter	Transports urine toward the urinary bladder
Urinary bladder	Temporarily stores urine before urination
Urethra	Conducts urine to exterior; in males, it also transports semen

Anterior view

18

The urinary system removes organic wastes generated by the body's cells. It also has several other essential homeostatic functions that are often overlooked. They include

- *Regulating blood volume and blood pressure*, by adjusting how much water is lost in urine, and releasing erythropoietin and renin. ⊃ p. 367

- *Regulating plasma concentrations of sodium, potassium, chloride,* and *other ions*, by controlling how much is lost in the urine. The kidneys also control the concentration of calcium ions through the synthesis of calcitriol. ⊃ p. 367

- *Helping to stabilize blood pH*, by controlling the loss of hydrogen ions (H^+) and bicarbonate ions (HCO_3^-) in urine.

- *Conserving valuable nutrients*, such as glucose and amino acids, by preventing their excretion in urine. The urinary system also excretes organic waste products (especially the nitrogenous wastes *urea* and *uric acid*).

These activities are carefully regulated to keep the composition of the blood within acceptable limits. A disruption of any of these functions has immediate and potentially fatal consequences.

CHECKPOINT

1. Name the three major functions of the urinary system.
2. Identify the organs of the urinary system.
3. Define micturition.

See the blue Answers tab at the back of the book.

18-2 The kidneys are highly vascular organs containing functional units called nephrons, which perform filtration, reabsorption, and secretion

Learning Objective Describe the locations and structural features of the kidneys, trace the path of blood flow to, within, and from a kidney, and describe the structure of the nephron.

The **kidneys** are located on either side of the vertebral column between the last thoracic (T_{12}) and third lumbar (L_3) vertebrae. The right kidney sits slightly lower than the left kidney (**Figure 18-2a**). The superior surface of each kidney is capped by an adrenal gland. The kidneys and adrenal glands lie between the muscles of the dorsal body wall and the peritoneal lining (**Figure 18-2b**). This position is called

Figure 18-2 The Position of the Kidneys.

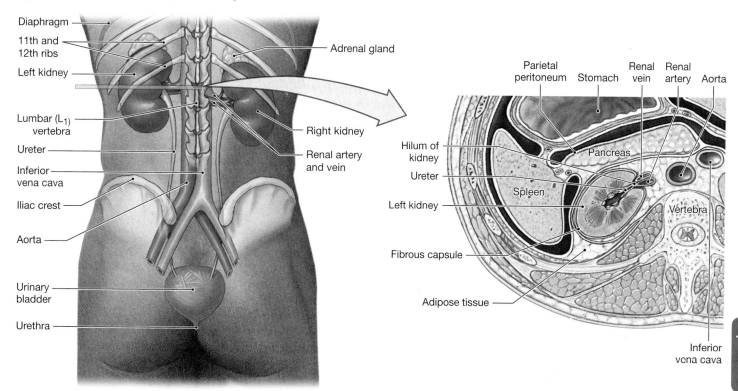

a This posterior view of the trunk shows the positions of the kidneys and other organs of the urinary system.

b A superior view of a section at the level indicated in part (a) shows the kidney's retroperitoneal position.

18

retroperitoneal (re-trō-per-i-tō-NĒ-al; *retro-*, behind) because the organs are behind the peritoneum. ⸠p. 552

The kidneys are held in position within the abdominal cavity by (1) the overlying peritoneum, (2) contact with adjacent organs, and (3) supporting connective tissues. Each kidney is covered by a *fibrous capsule*, surrounded by a cushion of adipose tissue, and anchored to surrounding structures by a dense, fibrous outer layer. Collagen fibers extend from this outer layer to the fibrous capsule. This arrangement of connective tissues helps prevent the jolts and shocks of day-to-day existence from disturbing normal kidney function. Damage to the suspensory fibers of the outer layer may cause the kidney to be displaced and stress attached blood vessels and ureter. This condition is called a *floating kidney*. It is dangerous because the ureters or renal blood vessels may become twisted during movement.

Superficial and Sectional Anatomy of the Kidneys

A typical kidney is reddish-brown. It is about 10 cm (4 in.) long, 5.5 cm (2.2 in.) wide, and 3 cm (1.2 in.) thick in adults. Each kidney weighs about 150 g (5.25 oz). An indentation called the **hilum** is the point of entry for the renal artery and renal nerves. It is also the point of exit for the renal veins and the ureter (**Figure 18-2b**). The **fibrous capsule** covers the surface of the kidney and lines the *renal sinus*, an internal cavity within the kidney. (The adjective *renal* is derived from *ren*, which means "kidney" in Latin.)

The kidney is divided into an outer **renal cortex** and an inner **renal medulla** (**Figure 18-3a,b**). The renal cortex is in contact with the fibrous capsule. The medulla contains 6–18 conical **renal pyramids**. The tip of each pyramid, known as the **renal papilla**, projects into the renal sinus. Bands of the

Figure 18-3 **The Structure of the Kidney.**

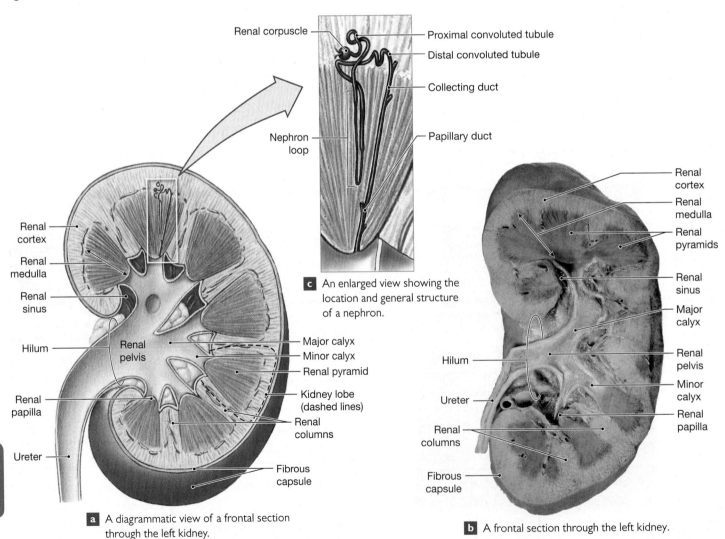

c An enlarged view showing the location and general structure of a nephron.

a A diagrammatic view of a frontal section through the left kidney.

b A frontal section through the left kidney.

renal cortex, called *renal columns*, extend toward the renal sinus between adjacent renal pyramids. A **kidney lobe** consists of a renal pyramid, the overlying layer of renal cortex, and adjacent tissues of the renal columns.

Urine is produced in the kidney lobes. Ducts within each renal papilla discharge urine into a cup-shaped drain, called a **minor calyx** (KĀ-liks; *calyx*, a cup of flowers; plural *calyces*). Four or five minor calyces (KAL-i-sēz) merge to form a **major calyx**. Two or three major calyces combine to form a large, funnel-shaped chamber, the **renal pelvis**. The renal pelvis is connected to the ureter, through which urine drains out of the kidney.

Urine production begins in **nephrons** (NEF-ronz), microscopic tubular structures in the cortex of each kidney lobe (**Figure 18-3c**). Each kidney has roughly 1.25 million nephrons, with a combined length of about 145 km (85 miles).

The Blood Supply to the Kidneys

Because the kidneys function to filter out wastes in the blood and excrete them in the urine, it's not surprising that the kidneys are well supplied with blood. The kidneys receive 20–25 percent of the total cardiac output. In normal, healthy people, about 1200 mL of blood flows through the kidneys each minute—a phenomenal amount of blood for organs with a combined weight of less than 300 g (10.5 oz)!

Kidney blood flow is shown in **Figure 18-4a**. Each kidney receives blood from a **renal artery** that originates from the abdominal aorta. As the renal artery enters the renal sinus, it divides into branches that supply a series of **interlobar arteries** that radiate outward between the renal pyramids. The interlobar arteries supply blood to the **arcuate** (AR-kū-āt) **arteries**, which arch along the boundary between the cortex and medulla. Each arcuate artery gives rise to a number of **cortical radiate arteries**, or *interlobular arteries*, supplying the cortex. **Afferent arterioles** branching from each cortical radiate artery deliver blood to the capillaries supplying individual nephrons (**Figure 18-4b**).

Blood reaches each nephron through an afferent arteriole and leaves in an **efferent arteriole** (**Figure 18-4c,d**). It then travels to the **peritubular capillaries** surrounding the nephron. The peritubular capillaries provide a route for picking up or delivering substances that are reabsorbed or secreted by different portions of the nephron.

The path of blood from the peritubular capillaries differs depending on the location of the nephron. **Cortical nephrons** lie almost entirely within the renal cortex. **Juxtamedullary** (juks-tuh-MED-ū-lar-ē) **nephrons** (*juxta*, near) extend deep within the renal medulla. In juxtamedullary nephrons, the peritubular capillaries are connected to the **vasa recta** (*rectus*, straight)—long, straight capillaries that parallel the nephron loop deep into the renal medulla (**Figure 18-4d**). As we will see later, the juxtamedullary nephrons enable the kidneys to produce concentrated urine.

Blood from the peritubular capillaries and vasa recta enters a network of venules and small veins that converge on the **cortical radiate veins**, or *interlobular veins*. In a mirror image of the arterial distribution, blood continues to converge and empty into the **arcuate** and **interlobar veins**. The interlobar veins drain directly into the **renal vein** (**Figure 18-4a**).

The Nephron

The nephron is the basic functional unit in the kidney. Each nephron consists of two main parts: (1) a *renal corpuscle*, and (2) a *renal tubule*. A renal tubule is about 50 mm (2 in.) in length. The **renal tubule** is composed of two *convoluted* (coiled or twisted) segments separated by a U-shaped tube (**Figure 18-3c**). The convoluted segments are in the cortex. The U-shaped tube extends partially or completely into the medulla.

An Overview of the Nephron and Collecting System

A schematic diagram of a representative nephron is shown in **Figure 18-5**. The nephron begins at the **renal corpuscle** (KOR-pus-ul). This spherical structure consists of the *glomerular* (Bowman's) *capsule*, a cup-shaped chamber that contains a capillary network known as the *glomerulus* (glo-MER-ū-lus; *glomus*, a ball). Each renal corpuscle is about 200 μm (0. 2 mm) in diameter.

As previously described, blood arrives at the glomerulus by way of an *afferent arteriole* and departs in an *efferent arteriole*. In the renal corpuscle, blood pressure forces fluid and dissolved solutes out of the glomerular capillaries and into the surrounding *capsular space*. This process is called *filtration*. ⤷ p. 438 Filtration produces a protein-free solution known as a **filtrate**.

From the renal corpuscle, the filtrate enters the renal tubule. The major segments of the renal tubule are the *proximal convoluted tubule* (PCT), the *nephron loop*, also called the *loop of Henle* (HEN-lē), and the *distal convoluted tubule* (DCT). As the filtrate travels along the renal tubule, it is now called **tubular fluid**, and its composition gradually changes.

Each nephron empties into a *collecting duct*, the start of the **collecting system**. The collecting duct leaves the cortex and descends into the medulla. It carries the tubular fluid from many nephrons toward a *papillary duct* that delivers the fluid, now called *urine*, into the calyces and on to the renal pelvis.

Figure 18-4 The Blood Supply to the Kidneys.

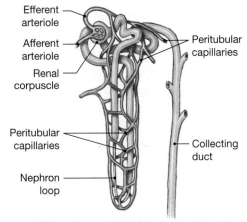

c Further enlargement shows the circulation to a cortical nephron.

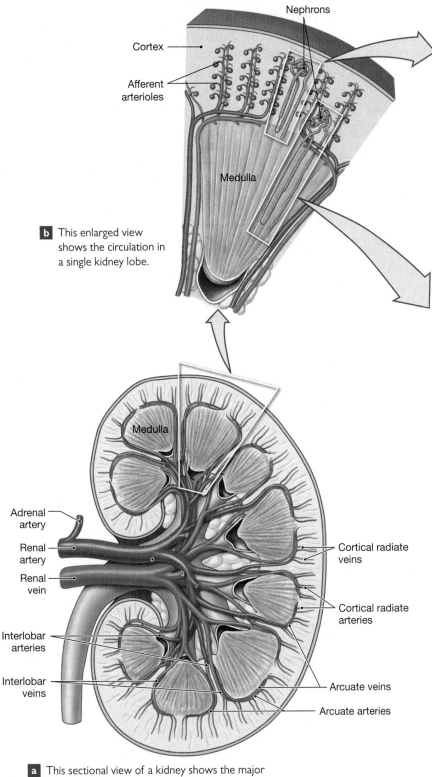

b This enlarged view shows the circulation in a single kidney lobe.

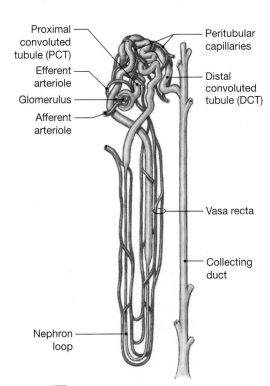

d Further enlargement shows the circulation to a juxtamedullary nephron.

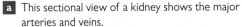

a This sectional view of a kidney shows the major arteries and veins.

Figure 18-5 A Representative Nephron and the Collecting System. This schematic drawing highlights the major structures and functions of each segment of the nephron (purple) and the collecting system (tan).

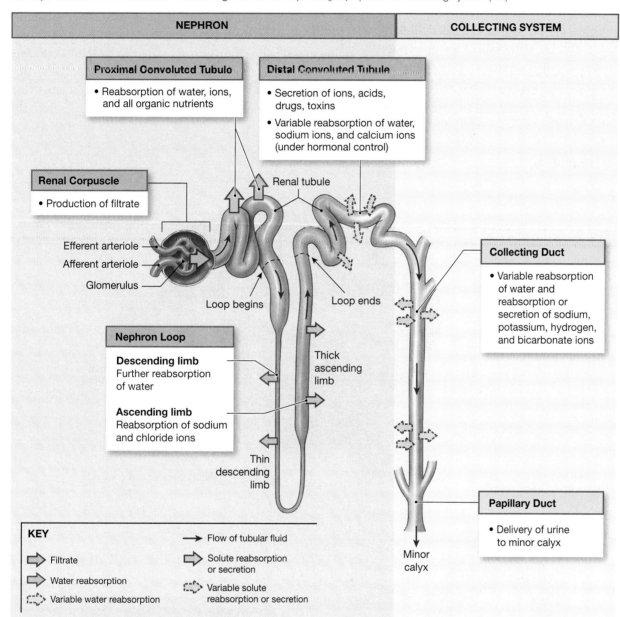

Functions of the Nephron

Urine has a very different composition from the filtrate produced at the renal corpuscle. Each segment of the nephron has a role in converting filtrate to urine (**Figure 18-5**). The renal corpuscle is the site of filtration. The functional advantage of filtration is that it is a passive process and does not require an expenditure of energy. The disadvantage of filtration is that any filter with pores large enough to permit the passage of organic waste products cannot *prevent* the passage of water, ions, and nutrients such as glucose, fatty acids, and amino acids. These substances, along with most of the water, must be reclaimed or they are lost in the urine.

Filtrate leaves the renal corpuscle and enters the renal tubule, which carries out these functions:

- Reabsorbing all the useful organic molecules, or nutrients, from the filtrate.
- Reabsorbing over 90 percent of the water in the filtrate.
- Secreting into the tubular fluid any waste products that were missed by the filtration process.

Additional water and salts will be removed in the collecting system before the urine is released into the minor calyx.

The Renal Corpuscle

A renal corpuscle consists of the capillary network of the **glomerulus** and the **glomerular capsule** (**Figure 18-6a**). The glomerular capsule forms the outer wall of the renal corpuscle and encloses the glomerular capillaries. The glomerulus projects into the glomerular capsule much as the heart projects into the pericardial cavity. A *capsular epithelium* makes up the wall of the capsule. It is continuous with a specialized *visceral epithelium* covering the glomerular capillaries. The two epithelia are separated by the **capsular space**, which receives the filtrate and empties into the renal tubule.

The epithelium covering the capillaries consists of cells called **podocytes** (PŌ-dō-sīts, *podon*, foot) (**Figure 18-6b,c**). Podocytes have long cellular processes, or "feet"—called *pedicels*—that wrap around individual capillaries. A thick basement membrane separates the endothelial cells of the capillaries from the

Figure 18-6 The Renal Corpuscle.

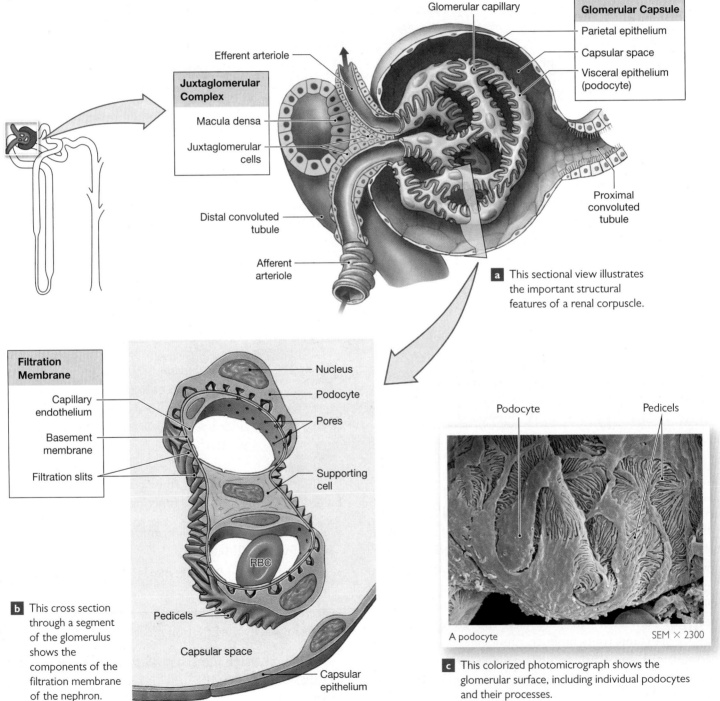

Glomerular capillary

Glomerular Capsule
Parietal epithelium
Capsular space
Visceral epithelium (podocyte)

Juxtaglomerular Complex
Macula densa
Juxtaglomerular cells

Efferent arteriole

Distal convoluted tubule

Afferent arteriole

Proximal convoluted tubule

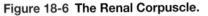

a This sectional view illustrates the important structural features of a renal corpuscle.

Filtration Membrane
Capillary endothelium
Basement membrane
Filtration slits

Nucleus
Podocyte
Pores

Supporting cell

RBC

Pedicels

Capsular space

Capsular epithelium

b This cross section through a segment of the glomerulus shows the components of the filtration membrane of the nephron.

Podocyte   Pedicels

A podocyte   SEM × 2300

c This colorized photomicrograph shows the glomerular surface, including individual podocytes and their processes.

18

podocytes. The glomerular capillaries are said to be *fenestrated* (FEN-e-strā-ted; *fenestra*, a window) because their endothelial cells contain pores (**Figure 18-6b**).

To enter the capsular space, a solute must be small enough to pass through (1) the pores of the endothelial cells, (2) the fibers of the basement membrane, and (3) the *filtration slits* between the slender processes of the podocytes. Together, the fenestrated endothelium, basement membrane, and filtration slits form the **filtration membrane**. The filtration membrane prevents the passage of blood cells and most plasma proteins. It permits the movement of water, metabolic wastes, ions, glucose, fatty acids, amino acids, vitamins, and other solutes into the capsular space. Most of the valuable solutes will be reabsorbed by the PCT.

The Proximal Convoluted Tubule

The filtrate next moves into the first segment of the renal tubule, the **PCT** (**Figure 18-5**). The cells lining the PCT reabsorb organic nutrients, plasma proteins, and ions from the tubular fluid and release them into the interstitial fluid, or *peritubular fluid*, surrounding the renal tubule. The reabsorbed substances in the peritubular fluid eventually reenter the blood. As a result of this transport, the solute concentration of the peritubular fluid increases while that of the tubular fluid decreases. Water then moves out of the tubular fluid by osmosis, reducing the volume of tubular fluid.

The Nephron Loop

The last portion of the PCT bends sharply toward the renal medulla. This turn leads to the **nephron loop**, or *loop of Henle* (**Figure 18-5**). This loop is composed of a *descending limb* and an *ascending limb*. Fluid in the descending limb flows toward the renal pelvis. Fluid in the ascending limb flows toward the renal cortex.

The ascending limb is not permeable to water and solutes, but it actively transports sodium and chloride ions out of the tubular fluid. As a result, the peritubular fluid of the renal medulla contains an unusually high solute concentration. The descending limb is permeable to water, and as it descends into the renal medulla, water moves out of the tubular fluid by osmosis.

The Distal Convoluted Tubule

The ascending limb of the nephron loop ends where it bends and comes in close contact with the glomerulus and its vessels (**Figure 18-3c**). At this point, the **DCT** begins. It passes immediately adjacent to the afferent and efferent arterioles (**Figure 18-6a**).

The DCT is an important site for three vital processes: (1) the active secretion of ions, acids, drugs, and toxins; (2) the selective reabsorption of sodium ions from the tubular fluid; and (3) the selective reabsorption of water, which assists in concentrating the tubular fluid.

The epithelial cells of the DCT closest to the glomerulus are unusually tall, and their nuclei are clustered together. This region is called the *macula densa* (MAK-ū-la DEN-sa) (**Figure 18-6a**). The cells of the macula densa are closely associated with unusual smooth muscle fibers—the *juxtaglomerular* (*juxta*, near) *cells*—in the wall of the afferent arteriole. Together, the macula densa and juxtaglomerular cells form the **juxtaglomerular complex**, an endocrine structure that secretes the hormone erythropoietin and the enzyme renin. These secretions are involved in the regulation of blood volume and blood pressure (see Chapter 10). ⟲ p. 367

The Collecting System

The DCT, the last segment of the nephron, opens into the collecting system, which consists of collecting ducts and papillary ducts (**Figure 18-5**). Each **collecting duct** receives tubular fluid from many nephrons. Several collecting ducts merge to form a **papillary duct**, which delivers urine to a minor calyx. The collecting system does more than transport tubular fluid from the nephrons to the renal pelvis. It also adjusts the fluid's composition and determines the final osmotic concentration and volume of the urine. These adjustments include reabsorbing water, and reabsorbing or secreting sodium, potassium, hydrogen, and bicarbonate ions.

Table 18-1 summarizes the functions of the different regions of the nephron and collecting system.

Table 18-1	The Functions of the Nephron and Collecting System in the Kidney
Region	**Primary Function**
Renal corpuscle	Filtration of plasma to initiate urine formation
Proximal convoluted tubule (PCT)	Reabsorption of ions, organic molecules, vitamins, water
Nephron loop	Descending limb: reabsorption of water from tubular fluid
	Ascending limb: reabsorption of ions; assists in creating the concentration gradient in the renal medulla, enabling the kidney to produce concentrated urine
Distal convoluted tubule (DCT)	Reabsorption of water and sodium ions; secretion of acids, ammonia, and drugs
Collecting duct	Reabsorption of water; reabsorption or secretion of sodium, potassium, bicarbonate, and hydrogen ions
Papillary duct	Conduction of urine to minor calyx

18

CHECKPOINT

4. How does the position of the kidneys differ from that of most other organs in the abdominal region?

5. Why don't plasma proteins pass into the capsular space of the renal corpuscle under normal circumstances?

6. Damage to which part of the nephron would interfere with the hormonal control of blood pressure?

See the blue Answers tab at the back of the book.

18-3 Different portions of the nephron form urine by filtration, reabsorption, and secretion

Learning Objective Discuss the major functions of each portion of the nephron, and outline the processes involved in urine formation.

The primary purpose of **urine** production is to maintain homeostasis by regulating the volume and composition of the blood. This process involves the excretion of dissolved solutes, especially the following three metabolic waste products:

1. **Urea.** Urea is the most abundant organic waste. Your body generates about 21 g (0.74 oz) of urea each day. Most of it is formed during the breakdown of amino acids.

2. **Creatinine.** Creatinine is generated in skeletal muscle tissue through the breakdown of creatine phosphate. Recall that creatine phosphate is a high-energy compound that plays an important role in muscle contraction. ⟲ p. 207 Your body generates roughly 1.8 g (0.06 oz) of creatinine each day.

3. **Uric acid.** Uric acid is a product of the breakdown and recycling of RNA molecules. Your body generates about 480 mg (0.017 oz) of uric acid each day.

These wastes are dissolved in the bloodstream. They can be eliminated only when dissolved in urine. For this reason, their removal involves an unavoidable water loss. The kidneys can minimize this water loss by producing urine with an osmotic concentration more than four times that of blood plasma. If the kidneys could not concentrate the filtrate produced by glomerular filtration, water losses would lead to fatal dehydration within hours. The kidneys also ensure that the excreted urine does not contain potentially useful organic substrates present in blood plasma, such as sugars or amino acids.

Nephron Processes

To carry out its functions, the kidneys rely on three distinct physiological processes (**Figure 18-7**). These processes take place in each nephron and include:

1. **Filtration.** In filtration, blood pressure forces water across the filtration membrane in the renal corpuscle (**Figure 18-7a**). Solute molecules small enough to pass through the membrane are carried by the surrounding water molecules.

2. **Reabsorption.** Reabsorption is the removal of water and solute molecules from the tubular fluid, and their movement across the tubular epithelium and into the peritubular fluid (**Figure 18-7b**). The reabsorbed substances in the peritubular fluid reenter the circulation

Figure 18-7 Physiological Processes of the Nephron.

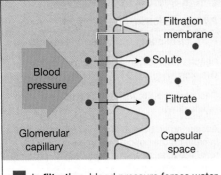

a In **filtration,** blood pressure forces water and solutes across the membranes of the glomerular capillaries and into the capsular space. Solute molecules small enough to pass through the filtration membrane are carried by the surrounding water molecules.

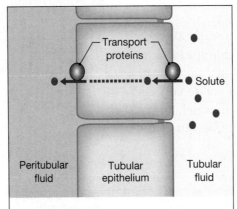

b **Reabsorption** is the removal of water and solutes from the tubular fluid and their movement across the tubular epithelium and into the peritubular fluid.

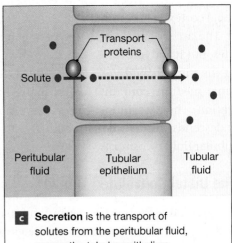

c **Secretion** is the transport of solutes from the peritubular fluid, across the tubular epithelium, and into the tubular fluid.

18

at the peritubular capillaries. Reabsorption takes place after the filtrate has left the renal corpuscle. Filtration is based solely on size, but reabsorption is a selective process. It involves simple diffusion or the activity of carrier proteins in the tubular epithelium. Water reabsorption occurs passively through osmosis.

3. **Secretion.** Secretion is the transport of solutes from the peritubular fluid, across the tubular epithelium, and into the tubular fluid (**Figure 18-7c**). Secretion is necessary because filtration does not force all the dissolved materials out of the blood. Tubular secretion can further lower the plasma concentration of undesirable materials, including many drugs.

Together, these three processes produce a fluid that is very different from other body fluids. **Table 18-2** indicates the efficiency of the renal system by comparing the concentrations of various substances in urine and plasma. The kidneys can continue to work efficiently only so long as filtration, reabsorption, and secretion proceed in proper balance. Any disruption in this balance has immediate and potentially disastrous effects on the composition of the circulating blood. If both kidneys fail to perform their roles, death will occur within a few days unless medical assistance is provided.

As we have seen, all segments of the nephron and collecting system are involved in urine formation. Most regions perform a combination of reabsorption and secretion, but the

balance between these two processes varies from one region to another. As indicated in **Table 18-1**:

- Filtration occurs exclusively in the renal corpuscle, across the glomerular capillary walls.
- Reabsorption of nutrients occurs primarily at the PCT.
- Active secretion occurs primarily at the DCT.
- Regulation of the amounts of water, sodium ions, and potassium ions lost in the urine results from interactions between the nephron loop and the collecting system.

Next, we will take a closer look at events in each of the segments of the nephron and collecting system.

Filtration at the Glomerulus

Blood pressure at the glomerulus tends to force water and solutes out of the bloodstream and into the capsular space. For filtration to occur, this outward force must exceed any opposing pressures, such as the osmotic pressure of the blood. (We introduced the forces acting across capillary walls in Chapter 13. You may find it helpful to review **Figure 13-6**.) ⊃ p. 438 The net force promoting filtration is called the **filtration pressure**. Filtration pressure at the glomerulus is higher than capillary blood pressure elsewhere in the body because of the slight difference in the diameters of afferent and efferent arterioles (**Figure 18-6a**). The diameter of the efferent arteriole is slightly smaller, so it offers more resistance to blood flow than does the afferent arteriole. As a result, blood "backs up" in the afferent arteriole, increasing the blood pressure in the glomerular capillaries.

Filtration pressure is very low (around 10 mm Hg). Kidney filtration will stop if glomerular blood pressure falls significantly. Minor variations in blood pressure are compensated for by reflexive changes in the diameters of the afferent arterioles, the efferent arterioles, and/or the glomerular capillaries. These changes can take place automatically or in response to sympathetic stimulation. More serious declines in systemic blood pressure can reduce or even stop glomerular filtration. As a result, hemorrhage, shock, or dehydration can cause a dangerous or even fatal reduction in kidney function. The kidneys are more sensitive to blood pressure than are other organs, so it is not surprising to find that they control many of the homeostatic processes responsible for regulating blood pressure and blood volume. We consider one example—the renin-angiotensin-aldosterone system—later in this chapter.

Table 18-2	Normal Laboratory Values for Solutes in Urine and Plasma	
Component	Urine	Plasma
IONS (mEq/L)		
Sodium (Na⁺)	40–220	135–145
Potassium (K⁺)	25–100	3.5–5.50
Chloride (Cl⁻)	110–250	100–108
Bicarbonate (HCO₃⁻)	1–9	20–28
METABOLITES AND NUTRIENTS (mg/dL)		
Glucose	0.009	70–110
Lipids	0.002	450–1000
Amino acids	0.188	40
Proteins	0.000	6–8 g/dL
NITROGENOUS WASTES (mg/dL)		
Urea	1800	8–25
Creatinine	150	0.6–1.5
Uric acid	40	2–6
Ammonia	60	<0.1

The Glomerular Filtration Rate

Filtrate production at the glomerulus is called *glomerular filtration*. The **glomerular filtration rate (GFR)** is the amount of filtrate produced in the kidneys each minute. Each kidney contains about 6 square meters—some 64 square feet—of filtration surface and the GFR averages an astounding *125 mL per minute*. This means that almost 20 percent of the fluid delivered to the kidneys by the renal arteries leaves the bloodstream and enters the capsular spaces. In the course of a single day, the glomeruli generate about 180 liters (48 gal) of filtrate, roughly 70 times the total plasma volume. But as the filtrate passes through the renal tubules, over 99 percent of it is reabsorbed.

Tubular reabsorption is obviously an extremely important process! An inability to reclaim the water entering the filtrate, as in *diabetes insipidus*, can quickly cause death by dehydration. (We discussed this condition, caused by inadequate ADH secretion, in Chapter 10.) ⟳ p. 355

Glomerular filtration is the vital first step essential to all kidney functions. Without filtration, waste products are not excreted, pH control is jeopardized, and an important process for regulating blood volume is eliminated. Filtration depends on adequate blood flow to the glomerulus and normal filtration pressures. We discuss the regulatory factors involved in maintaining a stable GFR later in the section on the control of kidney function.

Build Your Knowledge

Recall that cells may move lipid-insoluble substances, such as ions and organic substrates, across their plasma membranes with specialized membrane proteins (as you saw in **Chapter 3: Cell Structure and Function**). This process is called carrier-mediated transport. It may be passive (no ATP required) or active (ATP required). In passive transport, solutes are carried from an area of high concentration to an area of low concentration. Active transport processes may follow or oppose an existing concentration gradient. Recall that the carrier proteins can only bind specific substrates, but may be used over and over again. Many carrier proteins transport one ion or molecule at a time, but some move two solutes at the same time. The two solutes may be moved together in the same direction (into the cell), or in opposite directions (into and out of the cell). ⟳ **pp. 61, 65**

Reabsorption and Secretion along the Renal Tubule

Reabsorption and secretion in the kidney involve a combination of diffusion, osmosis, and carrier-mediated transport. Recall that in carrier-mediated transport, a specific substrate binds to a carrier protein that aids its movement across the plasma membrane. ⟳ p. 65 This movement may or may not require energy from ATP molecules.

Events at the Proximal Convoluted Tubule

The cells of the PCT actively reabsorb organic nutrients, plasma proteins, and ions from the filtrate. The cells then transport them into the peritubular fluid (interstitial fluid) surrounding the renal tubule. Osmotic forces then pull water across the wall of the PCT and into the surrounding peritubular fluid. The reabsorbed materials and water diffuse into peritubular capillaries.

The PCT usually reclaims 60–70 percent of the volume of filtrate produced at the glomerulus, along with virtually all the glucose, amino acids, and other organic nutrients. The PCT also actively reabsorbs ions, including sodium, potassium, calcium, magnesium, bicarbonate, phosphate, and sulfate. The ion pumps involved are individually regulated. They may be influenced by circulating ion or hormone levels. For example, the presence of parathyroid hormone stimulates calcium ion reabsorption. ⟳ p. 360

Reabsorption is the primary function of the PCT. However, a few substances (such as hydrogen ions) can be actively secreted into the tubular fluid. Such active secretion plays an important role in regulating blood pH, a topic we consider in a later section. A few compounds in the tubular fluid, including urea and uric acid, are ignored by the PCT and by other segments of the renal tubule. The concentrations of these waste products gradually rise in the tubular fluid as water and other nutrients are removed.

Events at the Nephron Loop

Approximately 60–70 percent of the volume of the filtrate produced at the glomerulus has been reabsorbed before the tubular fluid reaches the nephron loop. In the process, useful organic molecules and many mineral ions have been reclaimed. The nephron loop reabsorbs more than half of the remaining water, as well as two-thirds of the sodium and chloride ions remaining in the tubular fluid.

The descending and ascending limbs of the nephron loop have different permeability characteristics. The descending limb is permeable to water but not to solutes. For this reason, water can continually flow in or out by osmosis, but solutes cannot cross the tubular epithelium. The ascending limb is impermeable to water. The thin ascending limb is permeable to urea. The thick ascending limb actively pumps sodium and chloride ions out of the tubular fluid and into the surrounding peritubular fluid of the renal medulla.

Over time, a *concentration gradient* is created in the medulla. The highest concentration of solutes (roughly four times that of plasma) occurs near the bend in the nephron loop. Because the descending limb is freely permeable to water, water continually flows out of the tubular fluid and into the peritubular fluid by osmosis. From there, the sodium ions, chloride ions, and water diffuse into the peritubular capillaries and vasa recta and back into circulation.

Roughly half the volume of tubular fluid that enters the nephron loop is reabsorbed in the descending limb. Most of the sodium and chloride ions are removed in the ascending limb. With the loss of the sodium and chloride ions, the solute concentration of the tubular fluid declines to around one-third that of plasma. However, waste products such as urea now make up a significant percentage of the remaining solutes. In essence, most of the water and solutes have been removed, leaving relatively highly concentrated waste products behind.

Events at the Distal Convoluted Tubule and the Collecting System

By the time the tubular fluid reaches the DCT, roughly 80 percent of the water and 85 percent of the solutes have already been reabsorbed. The DCT is connected to a collecting duct that drains into the renal pelvis.

As the tubular fluid passes through the DCT and collecting duct, final adjustments are made in its composition and concentration. Its composition depends on the types of solutes present. Its concentration also depends on the volume of water in which the solutes are dissolved. The DCT and collecting duct are impermeable to solutes. For this reason, changes in tubular fluid composition take place only through active reabsorption or secretion. The primary function of the DCT is active secretion.

Throughout most of the DCT, the tubular cells actively transport sodium ions out of the tubular fluid in exchange for potassium ions or hydrogen ions. The DCT and collecting ducts contain ion pumps that respond to the hormone **aldosterone** from the adrenal cortex. Aldosterone secretion occurs in response to lowered sodium ion concentrations

or elevated potassium ion concentrations in the blood. The higher the aldosterone levels, the more sodium ions are reclaimed, and the more potassium ions are lost.

The amount of water reabsorbed along the DCT and collecting duct is controlled by circulating levels of *anti-diuretic hormone (ADH)*. In the absence of ADH, the DCT and collecting duct are impermeable to water. The higher the level of circulating ADH, the greater the water permeability and its reabsorption. The result is a more concentrated urine. Water moves out of the DCT and collecting duct because in each region the tubular fluid contains fewer solutes than the surrounding interstitial fluid. As previously noted, the tubular fluid arriving at the DCT has a solute concentration only about one-third that of the peritubular fluid in the surrounding cortex. That is because the ascending limb of the nephron loop has removed most of the sodium and chloride ions.

If circulating ADH levels are low, little water reabsorption will take place at the DCT. Virtually all the water reaching the DCT will be lost in the urine (**Figure 18-8a**). If circulating ADH levels are high, the DCT and collecting duct will be very permeable to water (**Figure 18-8b**). In this case, the individual will produce a small quantity of urine with a solute concentration four to five times that of extracellular fluids.

The fluid passing along the collecting duct enters the papillary duct. The papillary duct contains carrier proteins for urea. Urea is transported by facilitated diffusion into the peritubular fluid of the renal medulla. Some of this urea diffuses back into the thin ascending limb. This recycled urea contributes from one-third to one-half of the solutes of the concentration gradient established by the nephron loop.

Normal Urine

The general characteristics of normal urine are listed in **Table 18-3**. However, the composition of the urine excreted each day depends on the metabolic and hormonal events under way. Because the *composition* and *concentration* of the urine vary independently, an individual can produce either a small quantity of concentrated urine or a large quantity of dilute urine and still excrete the same amount of dissolved materials. For this reason, physicians often analyze the urine produced over a 24-hour period rather than testing a single sample. This practice enables them to assess both quantity and composition accurately.

Spotlight Figure 18-9 (pp. 618–619) provides a summary of kidney function. It shows the major steps in the reabsorption of water and the production of concentrated urine.

Figure 18-8 The Effects of ADH on the DCT and Collecting Duct.

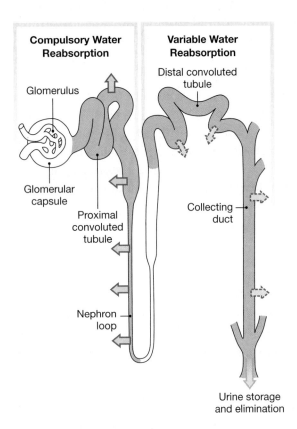

Compulsory Water Reabsorption

Glomerulus

Glomerular capsule

Proximal convoluted tubule

Nephron loop

Variable Water Reabsorption

Distal convoluted tubule

Collecting duct

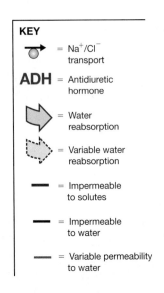

Urine storage and elimination

KEY

$= Na^+/Cl^-$ transport

ADH = Antidiuretic hormone

= Water reabsorption

= Variable water reabsorption

= Impermeable to solutes

= Impermeable to water

= Variable permeability to water

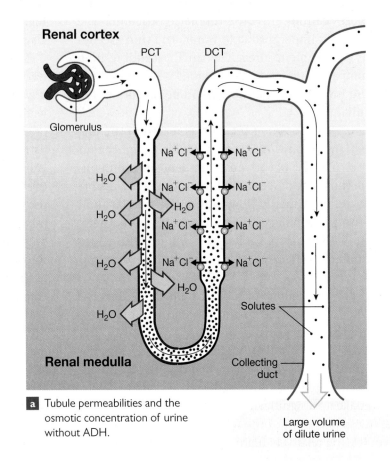

a Tubule permeabilities and the osmotic concentration of urine without ADH.

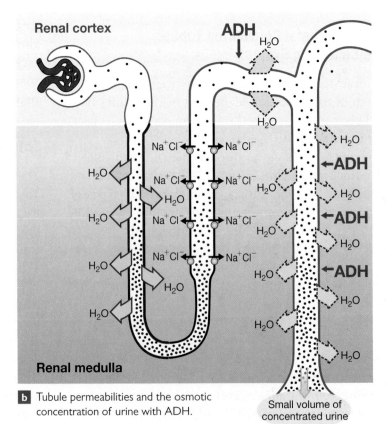

b Tubule permeabilities and the osmotic concentration of urine with ADH.

Table 18-3	General Characteristics of Normal Urine
Characteristic	**Normal range**
pH	4.5–8 (average: 6.0)
Specific gravity (density of urine/density of pure water)	1.003–1.030
Osmotic concentration (Osmolarity) (number of solute particles per liter; for comparison, fresh water ≈ 5 mOsm/L, body fluids ≈ 300 mOsm/L, and seawater ≈ 1000 mOsm/L)	855–1335 mOsm/L
Water content	93–97%
Volume	700–2000 mL/day
Color	Clear yellow
Odor	Varies with composition
Bacterial content	None (sterile)

CHECKPOINT

7. A decrease in blood pressure would have what effect on the GFR?

8. If nephrons lacked a nephron loop, what would be the effect on the volume and solute (osmotic) concentration of the urine produced?

9. What effect would low circulating levels of antidiuretic hormone (ADH) have on urine production?

See the blue Answers tab at the back of the book.

18-4 Normal kidney function depends on a stable GFR

Learning Objective Describe the factors that influence glomerular filtration pressure and the glomerular filtration rate (GFR).

Normal kidney function depends on adequate blood flow. Blood flow is needed to maintain filtration pressures and a stable GFR. Three levels of control regulate GFR: (1) *autoregulation*, or local blood flow regulation; (2) hormonal regulation, started by the kidneys; and (3) autonomic regulation, mostly by the sympathetic division of the autonomic nervous system (ANS).

The Local Regulation of Kidney Function

Autoregulation can compensate for minor variations in blood pressure. Autoregulation takes place through automatic changes in the diameters of afferent arterioles, efferent arterioles, and glomerular capillaries. For example, a reduction in blood flow and in glomerular filtration pressure triggers dilation of the afferent arteriole and glomerular

capillaries, and constriction of the efferent arteriole. This combination keeps glomerular blood pressure and blood flow within normal limits in the short term. As a result, GFRs remain relatively constant. If blood pressure rises, the afferent arteriole walls are stretched. Smooth muscle cells respond by contracting. The resulting reduction in afferent arteriolar diameter decreases glomerular blood flow and keeps the GFR within normal limits.

The Hormonal Control of Kidney Function

Hormonal processes result in long-term adjustments in blood pressure and blood volume that stabilize the GFR. The major hormones involved in regulating kidney function are angiotensin II, ADH, aldosterone, and atrial natriuretic peptide (ANP). (We have discussed these hormones in earlier chapters, so we provide only a brief overview here.) ⤴ p. 445 The secretion of angiotensin II, aldosterone, and ADH is integrated by the *renin-angiotensin-aldosterone system*.

The Renin-Angiotensin-Aldosterone System

Glomerular pressures may remain low because of a decrease in blood volume, a fall in systemic pressures, or a blockage in the renal artery or its tributaries. In response to low glomerular pressures, the juxtaglomerular complex releases the enzyme renin into the circulation. **Renin** converts the inactive *angiotensinogen* to *angiotensin I*. Angiotensin I is then converted to **angiotensin II** by **angiotensin-converting enzyme (ACE)**. This conversion takes place in the lung capillaries. ⤴ p. 516 A general overview of the response of the renin-angiotensin-aldosterone system to a decrease in GFR is diagrammed in **Figure 18-10**. The overall result is increased glomerular pressure.

Angiotensin II acts at peripheral capillary beds, the nephron, adrenal glands, and the CNS. It has these effects:

- *In peripheral capillary beds*, it causes a brief but powerful vasoconstriction. This response raises blood pressure in the renal arteries.

- *At the nephron*, it triggers constriction of the efferent arterioles. This effect raises glomerular pressures and filtration rates.

- *At the adrenal gland*, it stimulates the secretion of aldosterone by the adrenal cortex and of epinephrine (E) and norepinephrine (NE) by the adrenal medulla. A sudden, dramatic increase in systemic blood pressure results. At the kidneys, aldosterone stimulates sodium reabsorption along the DCT and collecting system.

18

SPOTLIGHT Figure 18-9
A SUMMARY OF KIDNEY FUNCTION

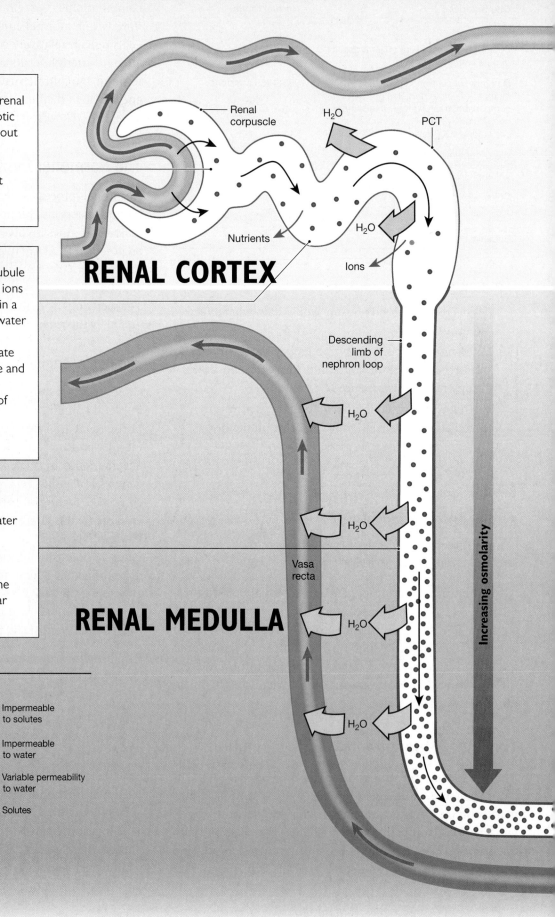

1 The filtrate produced by the renal corpuscle has the same osmotic concentration as plasma—about 300 mOsm/L.
It has the same composition as blood plasma but does not contain plasma proteins.

2 In the proximal convoluted tubule (PCT), the active removal of ions and organic nutrients results in a continuous osmotic flow of water out of the tubular fluid. This decreases the volume of filtrate but keeps the solutions inside and outside the tubule isotonic. Between 60 and 70 percent of the filtrate volume is absorbed here.

3 In the PCT and descending limb of the nephron loop, water moves into the surrounding peritubular fluid. This compulsory reabsorption of water results in a small volume of highly concentrated tubular fluid.

RENAL CORTEX

RENAL MEDULLA

Renal corpuscle

H_2O

PCT

Nutrients

H_2O

Ions

Descending limb of nephron loop

Vasa recta

H_2O

Increasing osmolarity

KEY

= Water reabsorption

= Variable water reabsorption

= Na^+/Cl^- transport

(A) = Aldosterone-regulated pump

(U) = Urea transporter

= Impermeable to solutes

= Impermeable to water

= Variable permeability to water

= Solutes

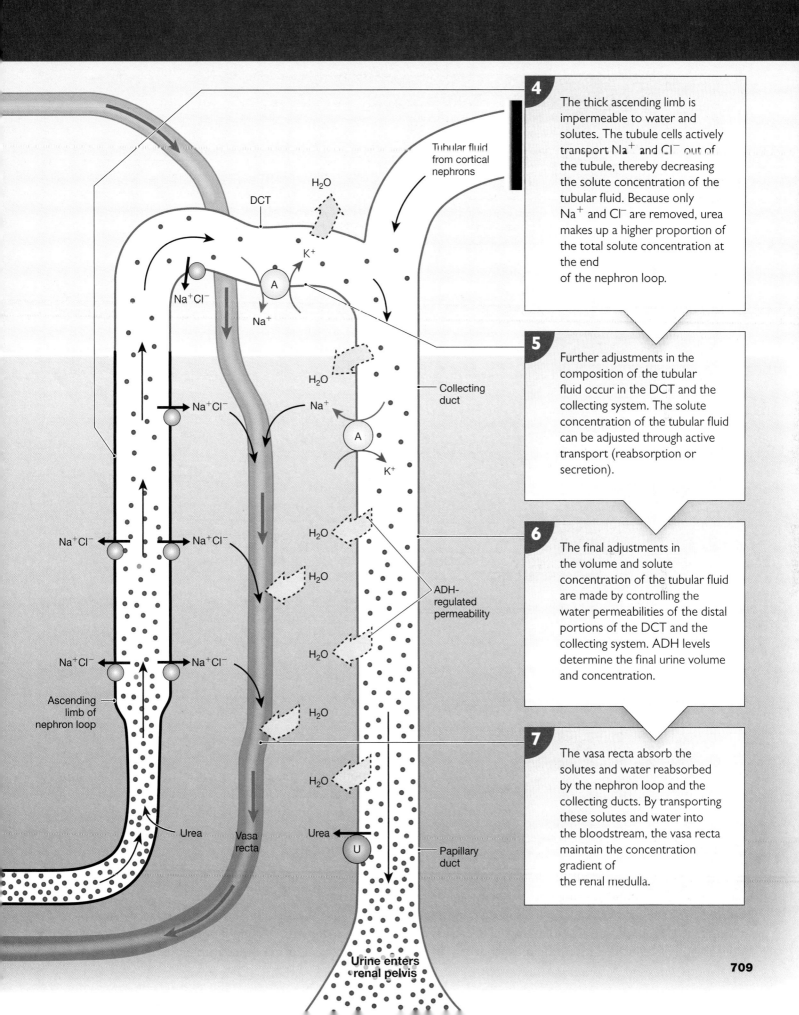

4 The thick ascending limb is impermeable to water and solutes. The tubule cells actively transport Na^+ and Cl^- out of the tubule, thereby decreasing the solute concentration of the tubular fluid. Because only Na^+ and Cl^- are removed, urea makes up a higher proportion of the total solute concentration at the end of the nephron loop.

5 Further adjustments in the composition of the tubular fluid occur in the DCT and the collecting system. The solute concentration of the tubular fluid can be adjusted through active transport (reabsorption or secretion).

6 The final adjustments in the volume and solute concentration of the tubular fluid are made by controlling the water permeabilities of the distal portions of the DCT and the collecting system. ADH levels determine the final urine volume and concentration.

7 The vasa recta absorb the solutes and water reabsorbed by the nephron loop and the collecting ducts. By transporting these solutes and water into the bloodstream, the vasa recta maintain the concentration gradient of the renal medulla.

Tubular fluid from cortical nephrons

DCT

H_2O

K^+

A

Na^+Cl^-

Na^+

Collecting duct

Na^+Cl^-

Na^+

H_2O

A

K^+

Na^+Cl^-

Na^+Cl^-

H_2O

ADH-regulated permeability

H_2O

Na^+Cl^-

Na^+Cl^-

H_2O

Ascending limb of nephron loop

H_2O

Urea

Vasa recta

Urea

U

Papillary duct

Urine enters renal pelvis

Figure 18-10 The Renin-Angiotensin-Aldosterone System and Regulation of GFR.

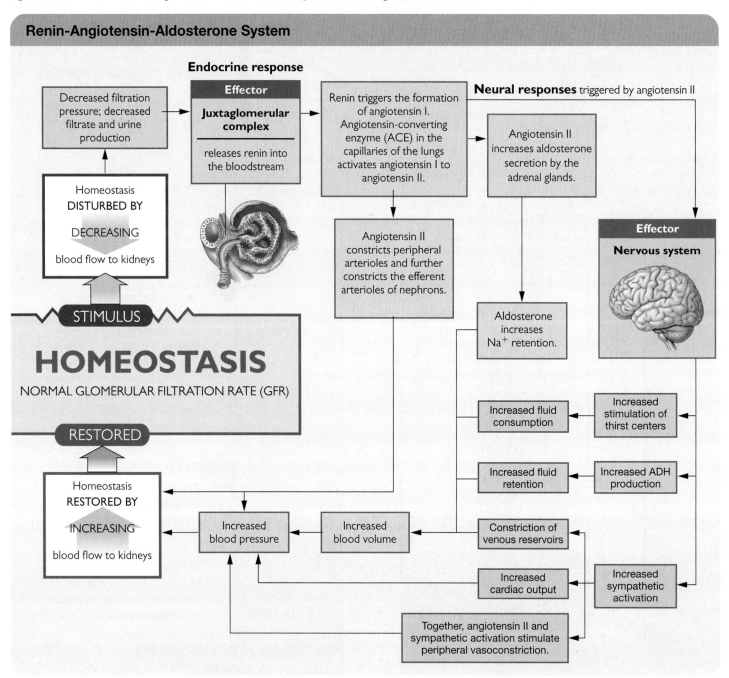

- *In the CNS,* angiotensin II triggers the release of ADH. This hormone, in turn, stimulates the reabsorption of water and sodium ions. It also induces the sensation of thirst.

Antidiuretic Hormone

ADH has two key effects. (1) It increases the water permeability of the DCT and collecting duct, so that water is reabsorbed from the tubular fluid. (2) It also brings on thirst, leading to the intake of water. ADH release takes place both under angiotensin II stimulation, and independently, when

hypothalamic neurons are stimulated. These neurons respond to a reduction in blood pressure or an increase in the solute concentration of the circulating blood.

Aldosterone

Aldosterone stimulates the reabsorption of sodium ions and the secretion of potassium ions along the DCT and collecting duct. Aldosterone secretion primarily takes place (1) under angiotensin II stimulation and (2) in response to a rise in the potassium ion concentration of the blood. ↪ p. 362

CLINICAL NOTE

Acute Kidney Injury (AKI)

Acute kidney injury (AKI), also called acute renal failure, is a dotorioration in renal function over hours or days that causes the accumulation of toxic wastes and causes the loss of internal homeostasis. AKI usually results from a decline in renal blood flow. AKI can result from problems in blood flow to the kidney (prerenal failure), a problem within the kidney itself (intrinsic renal failure), or a problem in urine flow (postrenal failure). Depressed renal blood flow and substances that are toxic to the kidney cause renal cell ischemia and death. Damage to the renal tubules can cause a back leak of glomerular filtrate, which further decreases perfusion pressure. Finally, the sloughing-off of dying cells can obstruct the renal tubules. Recovery depends upon restoration of renal blood flow. In prerenal failure, this involves the replacement of circulating blood volume. Rapid relief of the urinary obstruction in postrenal failure cases will restore glomerular flow as postrenal pressures are reduced. Restoration of renal blood flow and clearance of tubular toxins will aid in correcting intrinsic disease. Once blood supply is restored, the remaining nephrons will increase their filtration rate and eventually hypertrophy. If a critical number of nephrons have been lost, the patient will ultimately deteriorate and develop chronic renal failure that requires hemodialysis.

An all-too-common complication of multiple trauma is the development of acute tubular necrosis. This results from renal ischemia due to prolonged hypotension. If enough nephrons remain functioning, the patient can recover with relatively normal kidney function. If too many nephrons have been lost, then chronic renal failure will eventually develop. Prolonged hypotension due to multiple trauma should be avoided in order to prevent the development of acute tubular necrosis.

CLINICAL NOTE

Hemodialysis

Renal failure (RF) can be either *acute (ARF)* or *chronic (CRF)*. ARF is a sudden drop in urine output to less than half a liter per day. It is not uncommon in the very ill, including the victim of multiple trauma. *Emergency hemodialysis* may be initiated. With hemodialysis, which is the most common type of dialysis, the patient is attached to a machine where his blood comes in contact with a large semipermeable membrane. On the opposite side of the semipermeable membrane is a specialized dialysate solution that is hypo-osmolar for substances that must be removed from the blood. Blood contacts this membrane, and targeted substances diffuse into the dialysate. The net effect of dialysis is the correction of electrolyte abnormalities and blood volume and the removal of toxic substances such as urea or creatinine. For patients who require chronic hemodialysis, a vascular shunt, capable of handling blood flow of 300–400 mL per minute, is placed between a suitable vein and artery for dialysis access. Typically, the patient will dialyze for 2–3 hours, two or three times per week. Prior to the 1960s, dialysis was unavailable and patients with ARF or CRF died.

Atrial Natriuretic Peptide

The actions of ANP oppose those of the renin-angiotensin-aldosterone system (see **Figure 13-10**, ↻ p. 446). Overall, ANP lowers blood volume and blood pressure. Atrial cardiac muscle cells release ANP when blood volume and blood pressure are too high. The actions of ANP that affect the kidneys include (1) a decrease in the rate of sodium ion reabsorption in the DCT, leading to increased sodium ion loss in the urine; (2) dilation of glomerular capillaries, which results in increased glomerular filtration and urinary water loss; and (3) inactivation of the renin-angiotensin-aldosterone system by inhibiting secretion of renin, aldosterone, and ADH. The net result is an accelerated loss of sodium ions and an increase in the volume of urine produced. This combination lowers blood volume and blood pressure.

Sympathetic Activation and Kidney Function

Most autonomic innervation of the kidneys is through the sympathetic division of the ANS. Sympathetic activity mainly serves to shift blood flow away from the kidneys, which lowers the GFR. Sympathetic activation has both direct and indirect effects on kidney function. The direct effect is a powerful constriction of the afferent arterioles, decreasing the GFR and slowing production of filtrate. Triggered by a sudden crisis, such as an acute reduction in blood pressure or a heart attack, sympathetic activation can override the local regulatory processes that act to stabilize the GFR. As the crisis passes and sympathetic activity decreases, the GFR returns to normal.

When the sympathetic division alters the regional pattern of blood circulation, there are often indirect effects on blood flow to the kidneys. For example, the dilation of superficial vessels in warm weather shifts blood away from the kidneys, and glomerular filtration declines temporarily. The effect becomes especially pronounced during strenuous exercise. As blood flow increases to the skin and skeletal muscles, it decreases to the kidneys. At maximal levels of exertion, renal blood flow may be less than one-quarter of normal resting levels.

Such a reduction can create problems for endurance athletes, such as distance swimmers and marathon runners. Metabolic wastes build up during a long event. Protein is commonly lost in the urine because glomerular cells may be damaged by low oxygen levels (hypoxia). If the damage is substantial, blood appears in the urine. Such problems generally disappear within 48 hours. A small number of runners, however, suffer kidney failure (renal failure) and permanent impairment of kidney function.

18

CLINICAL NOTE

Chronic Kidney Disease

Kidney failure, commonly referred to as chronic kidney disease (CKD), occurs when the kidneys become unable to perform the excretory functions needed to maintain homeostasis. Many different conditions can result in renal failure. *Acute kidney injury* occurs when exposure to toxic drugs, renal ischemia, urinary obstruction, or trauma causes a sudden reduction or stoppage of filtration. In *CKD*, kidney function deteriorates gradually, and the associated problems accumulate over time. The condition generally cannot be reversed, only prolonged, and symptoms of acute renal failure eventually develop.

Management of chronic kidney failure typically involves restricting dietary protein, water, and salt intake and reducing caloric intake to a minimum. This combination reduces strain on the urinary system by (1) minimizing the volume of urine produced and (2) preventing the generation of large quantities of nitrogenous wastes. Acidosis—blood plasma pH below 7.35—is a common problem in patients with kidney failure; it can be countered with infusions of bicarbonate ions. If drugs, infusions, and dietary controls cannot stabilize the composition of the blood, more drastic measures are taken, such as dialysis or kidney transplantation.

In *dialysis*, the functions of damaged kidneys are performed by a machine that facilitates diffusion between the patient's blood and a *dialysis fluid* whose composition is carefully regulated. The process, which takes several hours, must be repeated two or three times each week.

In a *kidney transplant*, the kidney of a healthy compatible donor is surgically inserted into the patient's body and connected to the circulatory system. If the surgical procedure is successful, the transplanted kidney(s) can take over all of the normal kidney functions.

CHECKPOINT

10. List the factors that affect the glomerular filtration rate (GFR).

11. What effect would increased aldosterone secretion have on the concentration in urine?

12. What is the effect of sympathetic activation on kidney function?

See the blue Answers tab at the back of the book.

18-5 Urine is transported by the ureters, stored in the bladder, and eliminated through the urethra, aided by the micturition reflex

Learning Objective Describe the structures and functions of the ureters, urinary bladder, and urethra, discuss the control of urination, and describe the micturition reflex.

Filtrate modification and urine production end when the fluid enters the renal pelvis. The ureters, urinary bladder, and urethra make up the *urinary tract*. It transports, stores, and eliminates urine (**Figure 18-11**).

The Ureters

The **ureters** are a pair of muscular tubes that conduct urine from the kidneys to the urinary bladder. This distance is about 30 cm (12 in.) (**Figure 18-1**). Each ureter begins at the funnel-shaped renal pelvis. It ends at the posterior wall of the bladder without entering the peritoneal cavity. The **ureteral openings** within the urinary bladder are slit-like rather than rounded. This shape prevents the backflow of urine into the ureters or kidneys when the urinary bladder contracts.

The wall of each ureter contains three layers. They are an inner transitional epithelium, a middle layer of longitudinal and circular bands of smooth muscle, and an outer connective tissue layer continuous with the renal capsule. About every 30 seconds, a peristaltic contraction begins at the renal pelvis. It sweeps along the ureter, forcing urine toward the urinary bladder.

Solids made of calcium deposits, magnesium salts, or crystals of uric acid may form within the kidney, ureters, or urinary bladder. These solids are called *calculi* (KAL-kū-lī), or *kidney stones*. Their presence results in a painful condition known as *nephrolithiasis* (nef-rō-li-THĪ-uh-sis). Kidney stones not only obstruct the flow of urine but may also reduce or prevent filtration in the affected kidney.

The Urinary Bladder

The **urinary bladder** is a hollow, muscular organ that stores urine prior to urination. Its size varies depending on how distended it is. A full urinary bladder can contain as much as a liter of urine.

18

Figure 18-11 Organs for the Conduction and Storage of Urine.

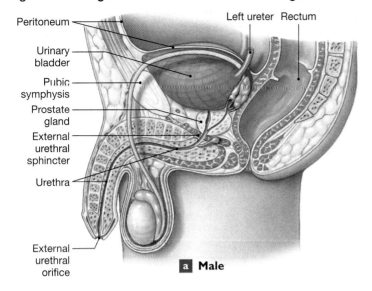

a **Male**

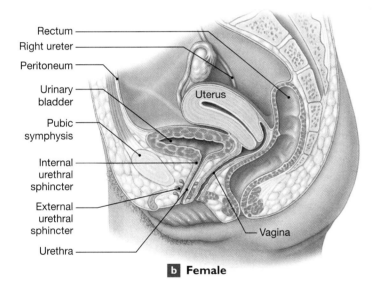

b **Female**

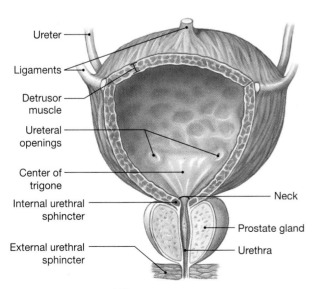

c **Urinary bladder in male**

The urinary bladder lies in the pelvic cavity. Only its superior surface is covered by a layer of peritoneum. It is held in position by peritoneal folds (*umbilical ligaments*) that extend to the umbilicus (navel), and by bands of connective tissue attached to the pelvic and pubic bones. In males, the base of the urinary bladder lies between the rectum and the pubic symphysis (**Figure 18-11a**). In females, the urinary bladder sits inferior to the uterus and anterior to the vagina (**Figure 18-11b**).

The *trigone* (TRĪ-gōn) is a triangular area within the urinary bladder. This area is bounded by the ureteral openings and the entrance to the urethra (**Figure 18-11c**). The urethral entrance lies at the apex of this triangle at the most inferior point in the bladder. The area surrounding the urethral entrance is called the *neck* of the urinary bladder. The neck contains a muscular **internal urethral sphincter**. The smooth muscle of this sphincter provides involuntary control over the discharge of urine from the bladder.

A *transitional epithelium* lines the urinary bladder. This stratified epithelium is continuous with the renal pelvis and the ureters. It can tolerate a considerable amount of stretching (as shown in **Figure 4-5c**). ⟳ p. 99

The bladder wall consists of inner and outer layers of longitudinal smooth muscle with a circular layer between the two. Together, these layers form the powerful **detrusor** (de-TROO-sor) **muscle** of the bladder. Contraction of this muscle compresses the urinary bladder and expels its contents into the urethra.

The Urethra

The **urethra** extends from the neck of the urinary bladder to the exterior of the body. In males, the urethra extends to the external opening, or **external urethral orifice**, at the tip of the penis. This distance may be 18–20 cm (7–8 in.). In females, the urethra is very short. It extends 2.5–3.0 cm (about 1 in.) from the bladder to the exterior (**Figure 18-11b**). The external urethral orifice is near the anterior wall of the vagina. In both sexes, as the urethra passes through the muscular floor of the pelvic cavity, a circular band of skeletal muscle forms the **external urethral sphincter** (**Figure 18-11**). This sphincter consists of skeletal muscle fibers. Its contractions are under voluntary control.

The Micturition Reflex and Urination

As we have seen, peristaltic contractions of the ureters move the urine into the urinary bladder. The **micturition**

18

CLINICAL NOTE

Kidney Stones

Kidney stones, or renal calculi (singular, calculus), represent crystal aggregation in the kidney's collecting system (**Figure 18-12**). This condition is also called *nephrolithiasis* (from Greek *lithos*, stone). Kidney stones affect about 500,000 people each year. Brief hospitalization is common due to the severity of pain as the stone travels from the renal pelvis, through the ureter to the bladder, and is eventually eliminated in urine. If necessary, additional inpatient treatment may include shock-wave lithotripsy, which is a procedure that uses sound waves to break large stones into smaller ones, and other treatment modalities. Overall morbidity and mortality are low, however, unless a complication such as hemorrhage or urinary tract obstruction results.

Kidney stones occur more frequently in the southern and southeastern U.S. which is a region referred to as the Kidney Stone Belt (**Figure 18-13**). North Carolina has more kidney stones per capita than any other state. Several factors appear to be involved in this phenomenon. First, the typical southern diet is high in green vegetables and brewed tea—both of which are high in oxalates, which is a key ingredient for kidney stones. Another factor is the warm climate, which causes increased sweating and increased loss of body fluids. Finally, modern lifestyles often reduce the level of physical activity. Together, these risk factors increase the likelihood of kidney stone development.

Figure 18-12 Kidney Stones. Cross section through a kidney that shows multiple stones, including one "staghorn" stone in the renal pelvis.

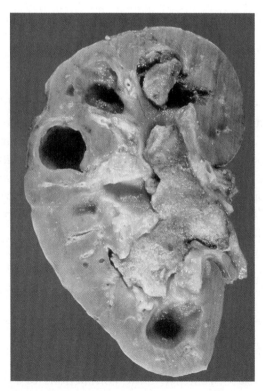

Figure 18-13 The Kidney Stone Belt. The incidence of kidney stones is markedly higher in the southern U.S.

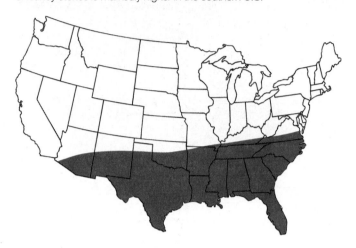

Stones form more commonly in men than women, although the ratio varies for different types of stones with different compositions. Certain stones also occur in familial patterns, which suggests hereditary factors. Another risk factor for calculus formation is immobilization due to surgery or injury, with the latter including immobilization secondary to paraplegia or other paralysis syndromes that involve the absence of motor impulses, sensation, or both. Last, the use of certain medications, including anesthetics, opiates, and psychotropic drugs, increases the risk for stones. Historically, about 60 percent of individuals who have experienced one kidney stone will develop another within seven years. Fortunately, with modern therapy, recurrence can be prevented in more than 95 percent of sufferers.

Stones may form in several metabolic disorders including gout or primary hyperparathyroidism, which produce excessive amounts of uric acid and calcium, respectively. More often, they occur when the general balance between water conservation and dissolution of relatively insoluble substances such as mineral ions and uric acid is lost and excessive amounts of the insolubles aggregate into stones. The problem boils down to "too much insoluble stuff" and "too-concentrated urine," which is a situation that may more likely arise with a change in diet, climate, or physical activity.

Stones that consist of calcium salts (namely calcium oxalate and calcium phosphate) are by far the most common. These compounds are found in 75–85 percent of all stones. Calcium stones are from two to three times more common in men than in women, and the average age at onset is between 20 and 30 years. Their formation frequently runs in families, and anyone who has had a calcium stone is at fairly high risk to form another within two to three years.

Struvite stones (chemically denoted $MgNH_4PO_4$) are also common, and represent about 10–15 percent of all stones. The pathophysiology of struvite stones differs from that of calcium stones. Their formation is associated with chronic urinary tract infection (UTI) or frequent bladder catheterization. The association with bacterial UTI makes struvite stones much more common in women than in men. These stones can grow to fill the renal pelvis, which produces a characteristic "staghorn" appearance on X-rays.

Far less common are stones made of uric acid or cystine. Uric acid stones form more often in men than in women and tend to occur in families; about half of all patients with uric acid stones have gout. Cystine stones are the least common. They are associated with excess levels of the amino acid cystine in filtrate and are probably due at least in part to hereditary factors, as they often run in families.

The largest kidney stone ever reported weighed a fraction under 3 pounds (1.36 kilograms). The smallest stones are the size of grains of sand. Kidney stones come in virtually every color although most are yellow to brown. It is important to try to collect a passed kidney stone for laboratory analysis. Once the chemical composition of the stone has been determined, then prevention strategies can be initiated.

The pain from kidney stones is generally conceded to be among the most painful of human medical conditions. Typically, the patient first notes discomfort as a vague, visceral pain in one flank. Within 30–60 minutes it progresses to an extremely sharp pain that may remain in the flank or migrate downward and anteriorly toward the groin. Migrating pain indicates that the stone has passed into the lowest third of the ureter. Kidney stone pain can be colicky in nature. As a rule, kidney-stone patients cannot lie still. They continuously move or pace due to the unrelenting nature of the pain. Stones that lodge in the lowest part of the ureter, within the bladder wall, often cause characteristic bladder symptoms such as frequency during the day or during the night (nocturia), urgency, and painful urination. Because these latter three symptoms far more frequently suggest bladder infection, making the tentative diagnosis may be difficult, particularly in women. Visible blood in the urine (hematuria) is not uncommon in urine specimens taken during passage of a stone. However, hematuria may be microscopic, which means that it is not visible to the naked eye but can be detected with reagent strips dipped into a urine specimen. Fever, however, is not common unless concomitant infection is present. Whenever kidney stones are suspected, be sure to obtain the patient's personal medical history and family history, because both will often provide useful information.

As mentioned earlier, the patient may be agitated or physically restless; walking sometimes reduces the pain. Vital signs will vary with the level of discomfort experienced by the patient, with highest blood pressure and heart rate associated with the greatest pain. The skin will typically be pale, cool, and clammy. Most patients are nauseated and many vomit because of the severe, unrelenting pain.

Emergency treatment of kidney stones should include hydration and analgesia. Often, the pain is so severe that patients will require large doses of intravenous narcotics for pain control (morphine, meperidine, fentanyl). Virtually all patients with a symptomatic kidney stone will be nauseated or vomiting. Administration of medicine to treat nausea and vomiting will also help to increase the effectiveness of the analgesic medications.

In the hospital, kidney stone patients will usually receive intravenous fluids and parenteral analgesics. The kidney stone can be diagnosed with spiral computerized tomography scanning. Alternatively, physicians can order an intravenous pyelogram, which involves the intravenous administration of a radiopaque contrast dye. The dye collects in the kidneys, which allows the kidneys, ureters, and bladder to be visualized. On occasion, ultrasound can detect a kidney stone.

Many patients will spontaneously pass smaller stones with adequate hydration and analgesia. If the stones do not pass, the urologist can place a stent in the affected ureter and remove the stone with a basket-like device inserted through the cystoscope. Stones that cannot be removed with basket extraction may be treated with other therapies. These include lithotripsy, which uses shock waves to break up stones so that they can pass with little problem. Another technology is lasertripsy, where a laser is threaded through a cystoscope and, once properly positioned, pulverizes the stone. Another available technology is electrohydraulic lithotripsy, where a special probe breaks up small stones with shock waves generated by electricity. The gravel that remains following lithotripsy or lasertripsy easily passes through the ureters into the bladder.

CLINICAL NOTE

Urinary Tract Infections

Urinary tract infections (UTIs) result when bacteria or yeasts (fungi) colonize the urinary tract. The intestinal bacterium *Escherichia coli* is most commonly involved. Women are particularly susceptible to UTIs because the external urethral orifice is so close to the vagina and anus. Sexual intercourse can push bacteria into the urethra. The urinary bladder can also become infected because the urethra is relatively short.

A UTI may produce no symptoms, but it can be detected by the presence of bacteria and blood cells in urine. If the urethral wall becomes inflamed, the condition is termed *urethritis*. Inflammation of the lining of the bladder is called *cystitis*. Many infections, including sexually transmitted diseases such as *gonorrhea*, cause a combination of urethritis and cystitis. These conditions cause painful urination, called *dysuria* (dis–r-uh). The urinary bladder also becomes tender and sensitive to pressure. Despite the discomfort of urination, the person feels the urge to urinate frequently. UTIs generally respond to antibiotics, although reinfections can occur.

In untreated cases, the bacteria may proceed along the ureters to the renal pelvis. Inflammation of the walls of the renal pelvis produces *pyelitis* (pī-e-LĪ-tis). If the bacteria invade the renal cortex and medulla as well, *pyelonephritis* (pī-e-lō-nef-RĪ-tis) results. Its signs and symptoms include a high fever, intense pain on the affected side, vomiting, diarrhea, and blood cells and pus in the urine.

reflex coordinates the process of urination, or micturition (**Figure 18-14**).

As the bladder fills with urine, stretch receptors in the wall of the urinary bladder are stimulated. Afferent sensory fibers in the pelvic nerves carry the resulting impulses to the sacral spinal cord. The increased level of activity in the fibers (1) brings parasympathetic motor neurons in the sacral spinal cord close to threshold and (2) stimulates interneurons that relay sensations to the thalamus, and then, by projection fibers to the cerebral cortex. As a result, you become aware of the fluid pressure within the urinary bladder.

The urge to urinate usually occurs when the bladder contains about 200 mL of urine. As **Figure 18-14** shows,

the micturition reflex begins to function when the stretch receptors have provided adequate stimulation to the parasympathetic preganglionic motor neurons. At this time, the motor neurons stimulate the detrusor muscle in the bladder wall. These commands travel over the pelvic nerves and produce a sustained contraction of the urinary bladder.

This contraction increases fluid pressures inside the bladder. Urine cannot be ejected, however, unless both the internal and external sphincters are relaxed. The external sphincter relaxes under voluntary control. Once that happens, the internal sphincter also relaxes. If the external sphincter does not relax, the internal sphincter remains closed, and the bladder gradually relaxes. A further increase in bladder volume begins the cycle again, usually within an hour. Each increase in urinary volume leads to an increase in stretch receptor stimulation that makes the sensation more acute. Once the volume of the urinary bladder exceeds 500 mL, the micturition reflex may generate enough pressure to force open the internal sphincter. This opening leads to a reflexive relaxation of the external sphincter. Urination takes place despite voluntary opposition or potential inconvenience. At the end of normal micturition, less than 10 mL of urine remains in the bladder.

Figure 18-14 The Micturition Reflex. This diagram illustrates the components of the reflex arc that stimulates smooth muscle contractions in the urinary bladder. Micturition occurs after voluntary relaxation of the external urethral sphincter.

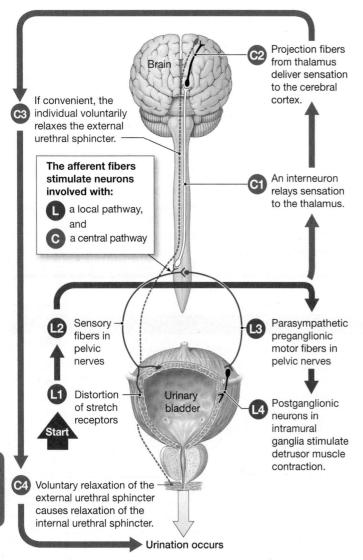

C3 If convenient, the individual voluntarily relaxes the external urethral sphincter.

C2 Projection fibers from thalamus deliver sensation to the cerebral cortex.

Brain

The afferent fibers stimulate neurons involved with:
L a local pathway, and
C a central pathway

C1 An interneuron relays sensation to the thalamus.

L2 Sensory fibers in pelvic nerves

L3 Parasympathetic preganglionic motor fibers in pelvic nerves

L1 Distortion of stretch receptors

Urinary bladder

L4 Postganglionic neurons in intramural ganglia stimulate detrusor muscle contraction.

Start

C4 Voluntary relaxation of the external urethral sphincter causes relaxation of the internal urethral sphincter.

Urination occurs

CLINICAL NOTE

Incontinence

Incontinence (in-KON-ti-nens) is the inability to control urination voluntarily. Infants lack voluntary control over urination because the necessary corticospinal connections have yet to be established. For this reason, "toilet training" before age 2 often involves the parent learning to anticipate the timing of the micturition reflex rather than training the child to exert conscious control.

Trauma to the internal or external urethral sphincter can contribute to incontinence in otherwise normal adults. For example, some new mothers develop *stress urinary incontinence* after childbirth. Pressures caused by a cough or sneeze can overwhelm the sphincter muscles, causing urine to leak out. Incontinence may also develop in older people because of a general loss of muscle tone.

Damage to the CNS, the spinal cord, or the nerves to the bladder or external sphincter may also produce incontinence. For example, incontinence often comes with Alzheimer's disease or spinal cord injury. In most cases, the affected person develops an *automatic bladder*. The micturition reflex remains intact, but voluntary control of the external sphincter is lost, so the person cannot prevent the reflexive emptying of the bladder.

Damage to the pelvic nerves can eliminate the micturition reflex entirely. A catheter must usually be inserted to help discharge the urine.

Build Your Knowledge

Recall that capillaries, unlike other blood vessels, are permeable to small ions, nutrients, organic wastes, dissolved gases, and water (as you saw in **Chapter 13: The Cardiovascular System: Blood Vessels and Circulation**). Two forces, capillary hydrostatic pressure (CHP) and blood osmotic pressure (BOP), are involved in the continual exchange of these materials between the bloodstream and body tissues. At the arterial end of a capillary, CHP is greater than BOP. As a result, fluid is forced out (filtration). Near the venule end of a capillary, BOP is greater than CHP. For this reason, fluid moves into the capillary (reabsorption). Overall, about 3.6 liters (0.95 gal) more fluid leaves the body's capillaries than is absorbed each day. Such capillary exchange plays a key role in homeostasis by maintaining constant communication between blood plasma and interstitial fluid. ⭢ **pp. 434, 438**

CHECKPOINT

13. What is responsible for the movement of urine from the kidneys to the urinary bladder?

14. An obstruction of a ureter by a kidney stone would interfere with the flow of urine between what two structures?

15. Control of the micturition reflex depends on your ability to control which muscle?

See the blue Answers tab at the back of the book.

18-6 Fluid balance, electrolyte balance, and acid–base balance are interrelated and essential to homeostasis

Learning Objective Define the terms *fluid balance, electrolyte balance*, and *acid–base balance*, discuss their importance for homeostasis, and describe how water and electrolytes are distributed within the body.

Few topics have the wide-ranging clinical importance of fluid, electrolyte, and acid–base balance in the body. *Treatment of any serious illness affecting the nervous, cardiovascular, respiratory, urinary, or digestive system must always include steps to restore normal fluid, electrolyte, and acid–base balance.*

Most of your body weight is water. Water accounts for up to 99 percent of the volume of the fluid outside cells. It is an essential ingredient of cytoplasm. All of a cell's operations rely on water as a diffusion medium for the distribution of gases, nutrients, and waste products. If the water content of the body changes, cellular activities are jeopardized. For example, when water content declines too far, proteins denature, enzymes cease functioning, and cells die. To survive, the body must maintain a normal volume and composition in both the **extracellular fluid** or **ECF** (the interstitial fluid, plasma, and other body fluids) and the **intracellular fluid** or **ICF** (the cytosol).

The concentrations of various ions and the pH (hydrogen ion concentration) of the body's water are as important as their absolute quantities. If concentrations of calcium or potassium ions in the ECF become too high, cardiac arrhythmias develop. Death can result. A pH outside the normal range can lead to a variety of dangerous conditions. Low pH is especially dangerous because hydrogen ions break chemical bonds, change the shapes of complex molecules, disrupt cell membranes, and impair tissue functions.

In this section, we consider the dynamics of exchange between the various body fluids, such as blood plasma and interstitial fluid, and between the body and the external environment. Homeostasis of fluid volumes, solute concentrations, and pH involves three interrelated factors:

- *Fluid balance.* You are in **fluid balance** when the amount of water you gain each day is equal to the amount you lose. Maintaining normal fluid balance involves regulating the content and distribution of water in the ECF and ICF. Cells and tissues cannot transport water, but they can transport ions. In this way, they create concentration gradients that are then eliminated by osmosis.

- *Electrolyte balance.* **Electrolytes** are ions released when inorganic compounds dissociate. They are so named because when in solution they can conduct an electrical current. ⭢ p. 37 Each day, your body fluids gain electrolytes from food and drink. Your body fluids also lose electrolytes in urine, sweat, and feces. **Electrolyte balance** exists when there is neither a net gain nor a net loss of any ion in body fluids. Electrolyte balance mainly involves balancing the rates of absorption across the digestive tract with rates of loss at the kidneys.

- *Acid–base balance.* You are in **acid–base balance** when the production of hydrogen ions in your body is equal to their loss. When acid–base balance exists, the pH of body fluids remains within normal limits. ⭢ p. 36 Preventing a reduction in pH is a primary problem because normal metabolic operations generate a variety of acids. The kidneys and lungs play key roles in maintaining the acid–base balance of body fluids.

18

The ECF and the ICF

Figure 18-15a presents an overview of the body makeup of a 70-kg (154-lb) person with a minimum of body fat. The distribution is based on overall average values for males and females aged 18–40 years. Water makes up about 60 percent of the total body weight of an adult male, and 50 percent of that of an adult female (**Figure 18-15b**). This difference between the sexes reflects the relatively larger mass of adipose tissue in adult females, and the greater average muscle mass in adult males. (Adipose tissue is only 10 percent water but skeletal muscle is 75 percent water.)

In both sexes, intracellular fluid contains more of the total body water than does extracellular fluid. Exchange between the ICF and ECF takes place across plasma membranes by osmosis, diffusion, and carrier-mediated transport.

The largest subdivisions of the ECF are the interstitial fluid of peripheral tissues and the plasma of the circulating blood (**Figure 18-15a**). Minor components of the ECF include lymph, cerebrospinal fluid (CSF), synovial fluid, serous fluids (pleural, pericardial, and peritoneal fluids), aqueous humor, perilymph, and endolymph. In clinical situations, it is common practice to estimate that two-thirds of the total body water is in the ICF and one-third in the ECF. This ratio

Figure 18-15 The Composition of the Human Body.

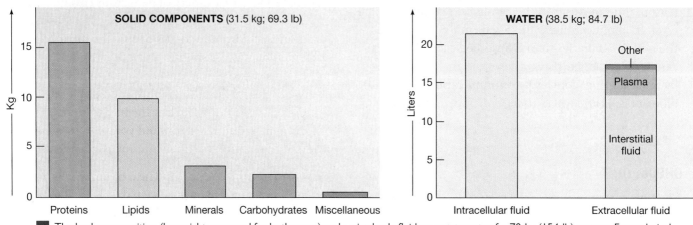

a The body composition (by weight, averaged for both sexes) and major body fluid compartments of a 70-kg (154-lb) person. For technical reasons, it is extremely difficult to determine the precise size of any of these compartments; estimates of their relative sizes vary widely.

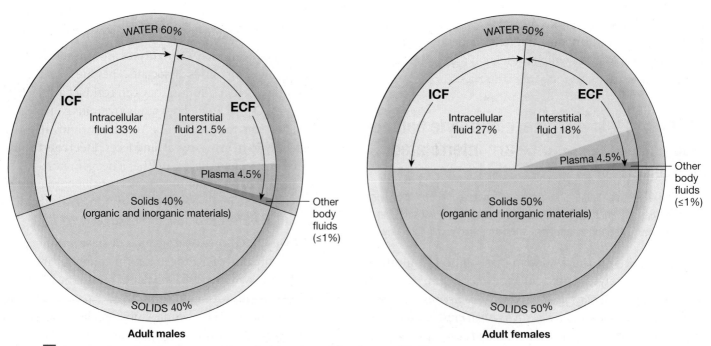

b A comparison of the body compositions of adult males and females, ages 18–40 years.

Figure 18-16 Ions in Body Fluids. Note the differences in the ion concentrations between the plasma and interstitial fluid of the ECF and those in the ICF. (For information concerning the chemical composition of other body fluids, see Appendix.)

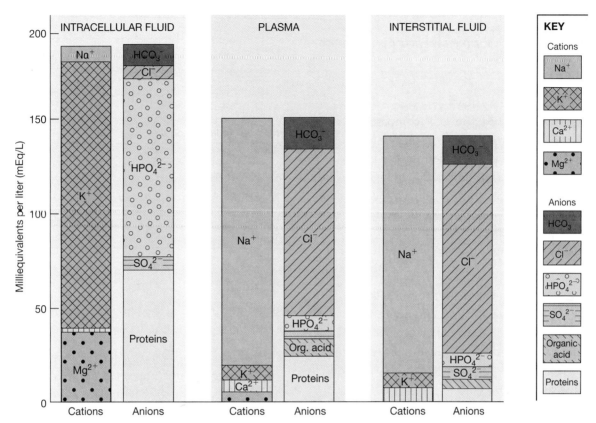

underestimates the real volume of the ECF, because it neglects the water in bone, in many dense connective tissues, and in the minor ECF components. However, these fluid volumes are relatively isolated. Exchange with the rest of the ECF occurs more slowly than does exchange between plasma and other interstitial fluids.

Exchange among the subdivisions of the ECF takes place mainly across the endothelial lining of capillaries. Fluid may also travel from the interstitial spaces to the plasma through lymphatic vessels that drain into the venous system. ⊃ p. 474 The kinds and amounts of dissolved electrolytes, proteins, nutrients, and waste products within each ECF subdivision or component are not the same. However, these variations are relatively minor compared with the major differences *between* the ECF and the ICF.

The ECF and ICF are called **fluid compartments** because they commonly behave as distinct entities. Cells are able to maintain internal environments with a composition that differs from their surroundings. They can do so because of the presence of a plasma membrane and active transport at the membrane surface. The principal ions in the ECF are sodium, chloride, and bicarbonate. The ICF contains an abundance of potassium, magnesium, and phosphate ions, plus large numbers of negatively charged proteins. **Figure 18-16** compares the ICF with the two main subdivisions of the ECF (plasma and interstitial fluid).

Despite these differences in the concentrations of specific substances, the osmotic concentrations of the ICF and ECF are identical. Osmosis eliminates minor differences in concentration almost at once because most plasma membranes are freely permeable to water. The regulation of water balance and electrolyte balance is tightly intertwined because changes in solute concentrations lead to immediate changes in water distribution.

CHECKPOINT

16. Identify the three interrelated processes essential to stabilizing body fluid volumes.

17. List the components of extracellular fluid (ECF) and intracellular fluid (ICF).

See the blue Answers tab at the back of the book.

18

18-7 Blood pressure and osmosis are involved in maintaining fluid and electrolyte balance

Learning Objective Explain the basic processes involved in maintaining fluid balance and electrolyte balance.

Fluid Balance

Water circulates freely within the ECF compartment. At capillary beds throughout the body, capillary blood pressure forces water out of the plasma and into the interstitial spaces. Some of that water is reabsorbed due to higher blood osmotic pressure along the distal portion of the capillary bed. The rest circulates into lymphatic vessels for transport to the venous circulation (see **Figure 13-6**, p. 438).

Fluid also moves continuously among the minor components of the ECF:

1. Water moves back and forth across the epithelial surfaces lining the peritoneal, pleural, and pericardial cavities and through the synovial membranes lining joint capsules. The flow rate is significant. For example, roughly 7 liters (1.8 gal) of peritoneal fluid is produced and reabsorbed each day.

2. Water also moves between the blood and the CSF, between the aqueous humor and vitreous humor of the eye, and between the perilymph and endolymph of the internal ear. The volumes involved in these water movements are small. We will largely ignore them in the discussion that follows.

Table 18-4 indicates the major factors in fluid balance. You lose about 2500 mL of water each day in urine, feces, and *insensible perspiration*—the gradual movement, or evaporation, of water across the epithelia of the skin and respiratory tract. The losses due to *sensible perspiration*—secretion by the sweat glands—varies with the level of activity. In vigorously exercising individuals, the water losses due to sensible perspiration can be considerable, reaching well over 4 liters an hour. ⟳ p. 133 Water losses are normally balanced by the gain of water through eating (40 percent), drinking (48 percent), and metabolic generation (12 percent). *Metabolic generation* of water occurs primarily as a result of mitochondrial ATP production. ⟳ p. 595

Fluid Shifts

Water movement between the ECF and ICF is called a **fluid shift**. Fluid shifts occur relatively rapidly, reaching equilibrium within a period of minutes to hours. These shifts

Table 18-4	Water Balance		
		Daily Input	
Source		**(mL)**	**(%)**
Water content of food		1000	40
Water consumed as liquid		1200	48
Metabolic water produced during catabolism		300	12
Total		2500	100
		Daily Output	
Method of Elimination		**(mL)**	**(%)**
Urination		1200	48
Evaporation at skin		750	30
Evaporation at lungs		400	16
Loss in feces		150	6
Total		2500	100

occur in response to changes in the osmotic concentration, or *osmolarity,* of the extracellular fluid.

- *If the osmotic concentration of the ECF increases, that fluid will become hypertonic with respect to the ICF.* Water will then move from the cells into the ECF until equilibrium is restored.

- *If the osmotic concentration of the ECF decreases, that fluid will become hypotonic with respect to the ICF.* Water will then move from the ECF into the cells, and the ICF volume will increase.

In summary, if the osmolarity of the ECF changes, a fluid shift between the ICF and ECF will tend to oppose the change. The ICF acts as a "water reserve," because the volume of the ICF is much greater than that of the ECF. In effect, instead of a large change in the osmotic concentration of the ECF, smaller changes occur in both the ECF and the ICF.

Electrolyte Balance

As we have noted, you are in electrolyte balance when the rates of gain and loss are equal for each electrolyte in your body. Electrolyte balance is important because:

- *A gain or loss of electrolytes can cause a gain or loss in water.*

- *The concentrations of individual electrolytes affect a variety of cell functions.* We have described many examples of the effects of ions on cell function in earlier chapters. ⟳ pp. 359, 423

Two cations, Na$^+$ and K$^+$, deserve attention because (1) they are major contributors to the osmotic concentrations of the ECF and ICF, respectively, and (2) they directly affect the normal functioning of all cells. Sodium is the main cation within the extracellular fluid. More than 90 percent of the osmotic concentration of the ECF results from the presence of sodium salts, mostly sodium chloride (NaCl) and sodium bicarbonate (NaHCO$_3$). Changes in the osmotic concentration of body fluids usually reflect changes in Na$^+$ concentration. Potassium is the main cation in the intracellular fluid. Extracellular potassium concentrations are normally low. In general:

- *The most common problems involving electrolyte balance are caused by an imbalance between sodium gains and losses.*

- *Problems with potassium balance are less common but significantly more dangerous than those related to sodium balance.*

Sodium Balance

The amount of sodium in the ECF represents a balance between sodium ion absorption at the digestive tract and sodium ion excretion at the kidneys and other sites. The rate of uptake varies directly with the amount included in the diet. Sodium losses take place mainly by excretion in urine and through perspiration. The kidneys are the most important sites for regulating sodium ion losses. In response to circulating aldosterone, the kidneys reabsorb Na$^+$ (which decreases sodium loss). In response to ANP, the kidneys increase the loss of sodium ions. ⤷ pp. 621–622

Whenever the rate of sodium intake or output changes, a corresponding gain or loss of water tends to keep the Na$^+$ concentration constant. For example, eating a heavily salted meal will not raise the sodium ion concentration of body fluids. Why not? As sodium chloride crosses the digestive epithelium, osmosis brings additional water from the digestive tract into the ECF. This is why individuals with high blood pressure are told to restrict their salt intake. When dietary salt is absorbed, "water follows salt," so blood volume—and, thus, blood pressure—increases.

Potassium Balance

Roughly 98 percent of the potassium content of the body is within the ICF. Cells expend energy to recover potassium ions as they diffuse across their plasma membranes and into the ECF. The K$^+$ concentration of the ECF is relatively low. It represents a balance between (1) the rate of gain across the digestive epithelium and (2) the rate of loss in urine.

The rate of gain is proportional to the amount of potassium in the diet. The rate of loss is strongly affected by aldosterone. Urinary potassium losses are controlled through adjustments in the rate of active secretion along the DCTs of a kidney's nephrons. The ion pumps sensitive to aldosterone reabsorb sodium ions from the tubular fluid in exchange for potassium ions from the peritubular (interstitial) fluid. In other words, are secreted into the urine.

High plasma concentrations of potassium ions also stimulate aldosterone secretion directly. When potassium levels rise in the ECF, aldosterone levels increase, and additional potassium ions are lost in the urine. When potassium levels fall in the ECF, aldosterone levels decrease, and potassium ions are conserved.

CHECKPOINT

18. Describe a fluid shift.

19. How would eating a meal high in salt content affect the amount of fluid in the intracellular fluid compartment (ICF)?

20. What effect would being in the desert without water for a day have on the osmotic concentration of your blood plasma?

See the blue Answers tab at the back of the book.

18-8 In acid–base balance, regulation of hydrogen ions in body fluids involves buffer systems and compensation by respiratory and renal processes

Learning Objective Explain the buffering systems that balance the pH of the intracellular and extracellular fluids, and identify the most common threats to acid–base balance.

The pH of your body fluids represents a balance among the acids and bases in solution. The pH of the ECF normally remains within relatively narrow limits, usually 7.35–7.45. Any deviation from the normal range is extremely dangerous. Changes in hydrogen ion concentrations disrupt the stability of cell membranes, alter protein structure, and change the activities of important enzymes. You could not survive for long with a pH below 6.8 or above 7.7.

Acidosis is the physiological state that exists when the pH of blood falls below 7.35. **Alkalosis** exists when the pH exceeds 7.45. These conditions affect virtually all systems. The nervous and cardiovascular systems are particularly sensitive to pH changes. Severe acidosis (pH below 7.0) can be deadly because (1) CNS function deteriorates, and the person becomes comatose; (2) cardiac contractions grow weak and irregular, and signs of heart failure develop; and (3) peripheral vasodilation produces a dramatic drop in blood pressure, and circulatory collapse can occur.

Both acidosis and alkalosis are dangerous. In practice, problems with acidosis are much more common. The reason is that normal cellular activities generate several acids (including carbonic acid).

Acids in the Body

Carbonic acid (H_2CO_3) is an important acid in body fluids. At the lungs, carbonic acid breaks down into carbon dioxide and water. The carbon dioxide then diffuses into the alveoli. In peripheral tissues, carbon dioxide in solution interacts with water to form carbonic acid. The carbonic acid molecules then dissociate into hydrogen ions and bicarbonate ions (see Chapter 15). ↩ p. 526 The complete reaction sequence is

$$\underset{\text{carbon dioxide}}{CO_2} + \underset{\text{water}}{H_2O} \overset{\text{carbonic anhydrase}}{\rightleftharpoons} \underset{\text{carbonic acid}}{H_2CO_3} \rightleftharpoons \underset{\text{hydrogen ion}}{H^+} + \underset{\text{bicarbonate ion}}{HCO_3^-}$$

This reaction occurs spontaneously in body fluids. It takes place much more rapidly in the presence of the enzyme *carbonic anhydrase*. This enzyme is found in many cell types, including red blood cells, liver and kidney cells, and parietal cells of the stomach.

The partial pressure of carbon dioxide (P_{CO_2}) is the most important factor affecting the pH of in body tissues. Most of the carbon dioxide in solution is converted to carbonic acid, and most of the carbonic acid dissociates into hydrogen ions and bicarbonate ions. For this reason, the partial pressure of carbon dioxide (P_{CO_2}) and pH are inversely related, as the seesaw in **Figure 18-17** illustrates. When carbon dioxide concentrations rise, additional hydrogen ions and bicarbonate ions are released, and pH goes down. (Recall that the greater the concentration of hydrogen ions, the lower the pH value.)

Figure 18-17 The Basic Relationship between Carbon Dioxide and Plasma pH. The P_{CO_2} (partial pressure of carbon dioxide) is inversely related to pH.

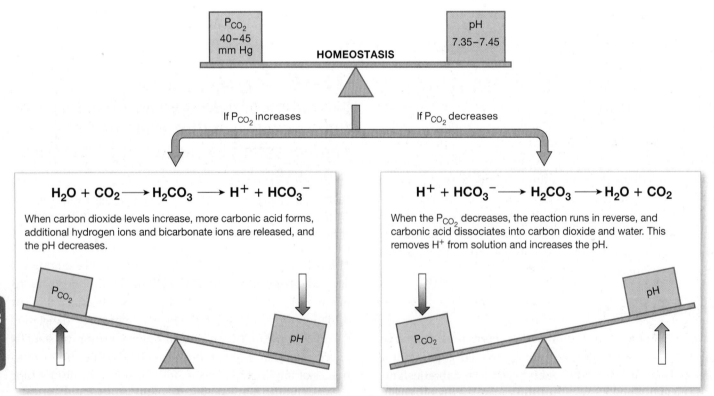

At the alveoli, carbon dioxide diffuses into the atmosphere, the number of hydrogen ions and bicarbonate ions drops, and the pH rises. This process effectively removes hydrogen ions from solution. We will consider it in more detail in the next section.

Organic acids, or metabolic acids, are generated during normal metabolism. Some come from the catabolism of amino acids, carbohydrates, or lipids. One example is lactic acid from the anaerobic metabolism of pyruvate. Another is ketone bodies from the breakdown of fatty acids. Under normal conditions, metabolic acids are recycled or excreted rapidly. For this reason, significant accumulations do not occur.

Buffers and Buffer Systems

The acids produced in normal metabolic operations are temporarily neutralized by buffers and buffer systems in body fluids. *Buffers* are dissolved compounds that can donate or remove hydrogen ions (H^+), thereby stabilizing the pH of a solution (see Chapter 2). ⊃ p. 38 Buffers include *weak acids* that can donate H^+, and *weak bases* that can absorb H^+. A **buffer system** consists of a combination of a weak acid and its dissociation products: a hydrogen ion and an anion.

The body has three major buffer systems: *protein buffer systems*, the *carbonic acid–bicarbonate buffer system*, and the *phosphate buffer system*. They have slightly different characteristics and distributions.

Protein buffer systems contribute to the regulation of pH in the ECF and ICF. Protein buffer systems include proteins and free amino acids. The amino acid side groups of proteins and the side group and structural groups of free amino acids respond to changes in pH by accepting or releasing H^+. If pH climbs, the carboxyl group (—COOH) of the amino acid acts as a weak acid. It dissociates and releases a hydrogen ion. If pH drops, the amino group (—NH_2) can act as a weak base. It can accept an additional hydrogen ion, forming an amino ion (—NH_3^+).

The plasma proteins and hemoglobin in red blood cells contribute to the buffering capabilities of blood. Interstitial fluids contain extracellular protein fibers and dissolved amino acids that also help regulate pH. In the ICF of active cells, structural and other proteins provide an extensive buffering capability. Protein buffering systems help prevent destructive pH changes when cellular metabolism produces metabolic acids, such as lactic acid.

The **carbonic acid–bicarbonate buffer system** is an important buffer system in the ECF. With the exception of red blood cells, your body cells generate carbon dioxide 24 hours a day. As noted earlier, most of the carbon dioxide is converted to carbonic acid, which then dissociates into a hydrogen ion and a bicarbonate ion. The carbonic acid and its dissociation products make up the carbonic acid–bicarbonate buffer system. The carbonic acid acts as a weak acid. The bicarbonate ion acts as a weak base. The net effect of this buffer system is that $CO_2 + H_2O \rightleftharpoons H^+ + HCO_3^-$. If hydrogen ions are removed, they will be replaced through the combining of water with carbon dioxide. If hydrogen ions are added, most will be removed through the formation of carbon dioxide and water.

The primary role of the carbonic acid–bicarbonate buffer system is to prevent pH changes caused by metabolic acids. The hydrogen ions released by the dissociation of these acids combine with bicarbonate ions, producing water and carbon dioxide. The carbon dioxide can then be removed at the lungs. This buffering system can cope with large amounts of acid because body fluids contain an abundance of bicarbonate ions, known as the *bicarbonate reserve*. When hydrogen ions enter the ECF, the bicarbonate ions that combine with them are replaced from the bicarbonate reserve.

The **phosphate buffer system** consists of an anion, *dihydrogen phosphate* ($H_2PO_4^-$), which is a weak acid. This ion and its dissociation products make up the phosphate buffer system:

$$H_2PO_4^- \rightleftharpoons H^+ + HPO_4^{2-}$$
$$\text{dihydrogen phosphate} \quad \text{hydrogen ion} \quad \text{monohydrogen phosphate}$$

In solution, dihydrogen phosphate ($H_2PO_4^-$) reversibly dissociates into a hydrogen ion and monohydrogen phosphate (HPO_4^{2-}). In the ECF, the phosphate buffer system plays only a supporting role in the regulation of pH. The reason is that the concentration of bicarbonate ions far exceeds that of phosphate ions. However, the phosphate buffer system is quite important in buffering the pH of the ICF. There the concentration of phosphate ions is relatively high.

Maintaining Acid–Base Balance

Buffer systems can tie up excess hydrogen ions (H^+), but they provide only a temporary solution to an acid–base imbalance. The hydrogen ions are only made harmless. They have not been eliminated. For homeostasis to be preserved, the captured H^+ must ultimately be removed from body fluids. The problem is that there is a limited supply of buffer molecules. Once a buffer binds a H^+, it cannot bind any more H^+.

18

With the buffer molecules tied up, the capacity of the ECF to absorb more hydrogen ions is reduced. The control of pH is impossible in this case.

Maintaining acid–base balance involves balancing hydrogen ion losses and gains. In this "balancing act," respiratory and renal processes support the buffer systems. They do so by (1) secreting or absorbing hydrogen ions, (2) controlling the excretion of acids and bases, and (3) generating additional buffers. The *combination* of buffer systems and these respiratory and renal processes maintains body pH within narrow limits.

Respiratory Contributions to pH Regulation

Respiratory compensation is a change in the respiratory rate that helps stabilize the pH of the ECF. Respiratory compensation takes place whenever pH exceeds normal limits. Such compensation works because respiratory activity has a direct effect on the carbonic acid–bicarbonate buffer system. Increasing or decreasing the rate of respiration alters pH by lowering or raising the partial pressure of CO_2 (P_{CO_2}). As we have seen, changes in P_{CO_2} directly affect the concentration of hydrogen ions in the plasma. Changes in P_{CO_2} also have an inverse effect on pH. When the P_{CO_2} rises, H^+ concentration increases, and the pH declines. When the P_{CO_2} decreases, H^+ concentration decreases, and the pH increases (**Figure 18-17**).

Changes in the P_{CO_2} have a dominant role in controlling the respiratory rate. (We discussed the processes involved in Chapter 15 ⊃ p. 527.) A rise in P_{CO_2} stimulates

chemoreceptors in the carotid and aortic bodies and within the CNS. This stimulation leads to an increase in the respiratory rate. As the rate of respiration increases, more CO_2 is lost at the lungs, so the P_{CO_2} returns to normal levels. A fall in P_{CO_2} inhibits the chemoreceptors. When the P_{CO_2} of the blood or CSF declines, respiratory activity is then depressed, the breathing rate decreases, and the P_{CO_2} in the extracellular fluids increases.

Renal Contributions to pH Regulation

Renal compensation is a change in the rates of hydrogen ion and bicarbonate ion secretion or reabsorption by the kidneys in response to changes in plasma pH. Under normal conditions, the body generates metabolic acids, which release H^+. The H^+ must then be excreted in the urine to maintain acid–base balance. Glomerular filtration puts hydrogen ions, carbon dioxide, and the other components of the carbonic acid–bicarbonate and phosphate buffer systems into the filtrate. The kidney tubules then modify the pH of the filtrate by secreting hydrogen ions or reabsorbing bicarbonate ions.

Acid–Base Disorders

Together, buffer systems, respiratory compensation, and renal compensation maintain normal acid–base balance. They are usually able to control pH very precisely. As a result,

---

CLINICAL NOTE

Disturbances of Acid–Base Balance

The terms used to describe disturbances of acid–base balance indicate the primary source of the disturbance. *Respiratory acid-base disorders* result from a mismatch between carbon dioxide generation in peripheral tissues and carbon dioxide excretion at the lungs. When a respiratory acid–base disorder is present, the carbon dioxide level of the ECF is abnormal. *Metabolic acid-base disorders* are caused by the generation of metabolic acids or by conditions affecting the concentration of bicarbonate ions in the ECF.

Respiratory compensation alone can often restore normal acid–base balance in people suffering from respiratory disorders. In contrast, compensation processes for metabolic disorders may be able to stabilize pH, but other aspects of acid–base balance (buffer system function, bicarbonate levels, and P_{CO_2}) remain abnormal until the underlying metabolic problem is corrected.

Respiratory Acidosis

Respiratory acidosis develops when the respiratory system is unable to eliminate all the CO_2 generated by peripheral tissues. The primary indication is low plasma pH due to *hypercapnia*, an elevated plasma P_{CO_2}. As carbon dioxide levels climb, hydrogen ion and bicarbonate ion concentrations rise as well. Other buffer systems can tie up some of the hydrogen ions, but once the combined buffering capacity has been exceeded, pH begins to fall rapidly.

Respiratory acidosis represents the most common challenge to acid–base balance. The usual cause is *hypoventilation*, an abnormally low respiratory rate. Because tissues generate carbon dioxide at a rapid rate, even a few minutes of hypoventilation can cause acidosis, reducing the pH of the ECF to as low as 7.0. Under normal circumstances, chemoreceptors monitoring the P_{CO_2} of the plasma and CSF will eliminate the problem by stimulating increases in breathing rate.

Respiratory Alkalosis

Problems with respiratory alkalosis are relatively uncommon. This condition develops when respiratory activity reduces plasma P_{CO_2} to below-normal levels, a condition called *hypocapnia*. Temporary hypocapnia can be produced by *hyperventilation*, when increased respiratory activity leads to a reduction in arterial P_{CO_2}. Continued hyperventilation can elevate pH to levels as high as 8.

This condition usually corrects itself. The reduction in P_{CO_2} removes the stimulation for the chemoreceptors. The urge to breathe then fades until carbon dioxide levels have returned to normal. Respiratory alkalosis caused by hyperventilation seldom persists long enough to cause a clinical emergency.

Metabolic Acidosis

Metabolic acidosis is the second most common type of acid–base imbalance. The most frequent cause is the production of large quantities of metabolic acids such as lactic acid or ketone bodies. Metabolic acidosis can also be caused by an impaired ability to excrete hydrogen ions at the kidneys. Any condition accompanied by severe kidney damage can result in metabolic acidosis.

Compensation for metabolic acidosis usually involves a combination of respiratory and renal processes. Hydrogen ions interacting with bicarbonate ions form carbon dioxide molecules that are eliminated at the lungs. The kidneys excrete additional hydrogen ions into the urine and generate bicarbonate ions that are released into the ECF.

Metabolic Alkalosis

Metabolic alkalosis takes place when bicarbonate ion concentrations become elevated. The bicarbonate ions then interact with hydrogen ions in solution, forming carbonic acid. The reduction in H^+ concentrations produces alkalosis.

Cases of severe metabolic alkalosis are relatively rare. A temporary metabolic alkalosis occurs during meals. At that time, large numbers of bicarbonate ions are released into the ECF during the secretion of HCl by the parietal cells of the stomach. (Hydrogen ions and bicarbonate ions are formed from CO_2 and H_2O within the parietal cells. The bicarbonate ions are released into the blood in exchange for chloride ions.)

Serious metabolic alkalosis may result from bouts of repeated vomiting, because the stomach continues to generate stomach acids to replace those that are lost. As a result, the HCO_3^- concentration of the ECF continues to rise. Compensation for metabolic alkalosis involves a reduction in pulmonary ventilation, coupled with the increased loss of bicarbonates in the urine.

---

the pH of extracellular fluids seldom varies more than 0.1 pH units, from 7.35 to 7.45. When buffering actions are severely stressed, however, pH strays outside these limits. Symptoms of alkalosis or acidosis then appear.

Respiratory acid–base disorders result when abnormal respiratory function causes an extreme rise or fall in CO_2 levels in the ECF. Metabolic acid–base disorders result from the generation of metabolic acids or from conditions affecting the concentration of bicarbonate ions in the ECF.

Table 18-5 summarizes the general causes and treatments of acid–base disorders.

CHECKPOINT

21. Identify the body's three major buffer systems.

22. What effect would a decrease in the pH of body fluids have on the respiratory rate?

23. How would a prolonged fast affect the body's pH?

See the blue Answers tab at the back of the book.

Table 18-5	Acid–Base Disorders		
Disorder	**pH (normal = 7.35–7.45)**	**Remarks**	**Treatment**
Respiratory acidosis	Decreased (below 7.35)	Most common acid–base disorder; generally caused by hypoventilation and CO_2 buildup in tissues and blood	Improve ventilation—in some cases, with bronchodilation and mechanical assistance
Metabolic acidosis	Decreased (below 7.35)	Second most common acid–base disorder; caused by buildup of metabolic acid, impaired H^+ excretion at kidneys, or bicarbonate loss in urine or feces	Administration of bicarbonate (gradual) with other steps as needed to correct primary cause
Respiratory alkalosis	Increased (above 7.45)	Relatively uncommon acid–base disorder; generally caused by hyperventilation and reduction in plasma CO_2 levels	Reduce respiratory rate, allow rise in P_{CO_2}
Metabolic alkalosis	Increased (above 7.45)	Severe cases relatively rare; usually caused by prolonged vomiting and associated acid loss	For pH below 7.55, no treatment; pH above 7.55 may require administration of ammonium chloride

18

18-9 Age-related changes affect kidney function and the micturition reflex

Learning Objective Describe the effects of aging on the urinary system.

In general, aging is associated with an increased incidence of kidney problems. Age-related changes take place in the urinary system, and in aspects of fluid, electrolyte, and acid-base balance. They include

1. *A decrease in the number of functional nephrons.* The total number of nephrons in the kidneys drops 30–40 percent between ages 25 and 85.

2. *A reduction in the GFR.* This reduction results from fewer glomeruli, cumulative damage to the filtration structures in those remaining, and reduced renal blood flow. A reduced GFR and fewer nephrons also reduce the body's ability to regulate pH through renal compensation.

3. *Reduced sensitivity to ADH and aldosterone.* With age, the distal portions of the nephron and collecting system become less responsive to ADH and aldosterone. As the reabsorption of water and sodium ions is reduced, the body's ability to concentrate urine declines. More water is lost in urine.

4. *Problems with the micturition reflex.* Several factors are involved in such problems:
   - The sphincter muscles lose tone and become less effective at voluntarily retaining urine. This leads to incontinence, often involving a slow leakage of urine.
   - The ability to control micturition is often lost after a stroke, Alzheimer's disease, or other CNS problems affecting the cerebral cortex or hypothalamus.
   - In males, *urinary retention* may develop due to enlargement of the prostate gland. Swelling and distortion of surrounding prostate tissues compress the urethra, restricting or preventing the flow of urine.

5. *A gradual decrease of total body water content with age.* Between ages 40 and 60, total body water content declines slightly, to 55 percent for males and 47 percent for females. After age 60, the values decline to roughly 50 percent for males and 45 percent for females. Such decreases result in less dilution of waste products, toxins, and administered drugs, among other effects.

6. *A net loss in body mineral content in many people over age 60 as muscle mass and skeletal mass decrease.* This loss can be prevented, at least in part, by a combination of exercise and increased dietary mineral intake.

7. *Increased incidence of disorders affecting major systems with increasing age.* Most of these disorders have some impact on fluid, electrolyte, and/or acid–base balance.

CHECKPOINT

24. What effect does aging have on the GFR?
25. After age 40, does total body water content increase or decrease?

See the blue Answers tab at the back of the book.

18-10 The urinary system is one of several body systems involved in waste excretion

Learning Objective Give examples of interactions between the urinary system and other body systems.

The urinary system excretes wastes produced by other organ systems. It is not the only organ system involved in excretion. Together, the urinary system and the integumentary, respiratory, and digestive systems are regarded as an anatomically diverse *excretory system*. Each of these body systems performs all the excretory activities that affect the composition of body fluids:

1. *Integumentary system.* Water and electrolyte losses in perspiration can affect the volume and composition of plasma. The effects are most apparent when losses are extreme, such as during peak sweat production. Small amounts of metabolic wastes, including urea, are also eliminated in perspiration.

2. *Respiratory system.* The lungs remove the carbon dioxide generated by cells. Small amounts of other compounds, such as acetone and water, evaporate into the alveoli. They are eliminated when you exhale.

3. *Digestive system.* The liver excretes metabolic waste products in bile. You lose a variable amount of water in feces.

These excretory activities affect the composition of body fluids. The respiratory system, for example, removes carbon dioxide from the body. However, the excretory functions of these systems are not as closely regulated as are those of the kidneys. Normally, the effects of integumentary and digestive excretory activities are minor compared with those of the urinary system.

18

CLINICAL NOTE

Renal Trauma

The renal system is fairly well protected from trauma. Injuries to the genitourinary system occur in only 5 percent or less of all trauma victims. Approximately 10 percent of children with blunt abdominal trauma have renal system injury. Most patients with a kidney injury have other concurrent injuries. The kidneys and ureters are located in the retroperitoneal space and are thus well-protected. The bladder is well-protected by the bony structures of the pelvis. In males, the urethra is more vulnerable to trauma due to the anatomy of the penis. Fortunately, renal system injuries are rarely life threatening and usually do not require immediate intervention.

Trauma to the kidneys and ureters usually results from penetrating trauma such as gunshots or stabbings (**Figure 18-18**). Rapid deceleration forces may cause injury to the renal pedicle or to the vascular structures. The signs and symptoms of urinary system trauma can be subtle. The most common indicator of renal system trauma is blood in the urine (hematuria). This may be gross (readily visible) or microscopic (seen only with a microscope or detected by urine test strips). Trauma to the prostate and urethra can result in blood at the urethral meatus (or on the underwear). Any of these findings warrant further investigation. In the emergency department, a rectal examination should be carried out. A high-riding or floating prostate indicates the need for further studies. After life-threatening problems have been addressed, the urinary system can be studied with contrast X-rays and CT scanning.

Figure 18-18 Renal Trauma. Most cases of renal trauma are due to penetrating injuries. Although this wound is on the anterior abdomen, the right kidney and ureter are lacerated.

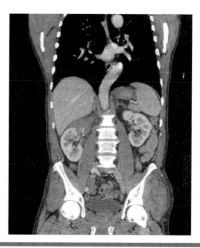

Refer to Build Your Knowledge: How the URINARY SYSTEM integrates with the other body systems presented so far on p. 636. It reviews the major functional relationships between this system and the integumentary, skeletal, muscular, nervous, endocrine, cardiovascular, lymphatic, respiratory, and digestive systems.

CHECKPOINT

26. Name the organ systems that make up the excretory system.

27. Identify the role the urinary system plays for all other body systems.

See the blue Answers tab at the back of the book.

RELATED CLINICAL TERMS

antacid: A substance used to counteract or neutralize stomach acid.

diuretics (dī-ū-RET-iks): Substances that promote fluid loss in urine.

glomerulonephritis (glo-mer-ū-lō-nef-RĪ-tis): Inflammation of the glomeruli (the filtration units of the nephron).

glycosuria (glī-kō-SOO-rē-uh): The presence of glucose in urine.

hematuria: The presence of blood in urine.

hypernatremia: A condition characterized by excess sodium in the blood.

hyponatremia: A condition characterized by lower-than-normal sodium in the blood.

nephritis: Inflammation of the kidneys.

nephrology (ne-FROL-o-jē): The medical specialty concerned with the kidneys and their disorders.

proteinuria: The presence of protein in urine.

pyelogram (PĪ-el-ō-gram): An X-ray image of the kidneys taken after a radiopaque compound has been administered.

urinalysis: A physical and chemical assessment of urine.

urology (ū-ROL-o-jē): Branch of medicine concerned with the urinary system and its disorders, and with the male reproductive tract and its disorders.

18

Build Your Knowledge

How the URINARY SYSTEM integrates with the other body systems presented so far

Integumentary System

- The integumentary system prevents excessive fluid loss through skin surface; produces vitamin D_3, important for the renal production of calcitriol; sweat glands assist in elimination of water and solutes

- The urinary system eliminates nitrogenous wastes; maintains fluid, electrolyte, and acid–base balance of blood that nourishes the skin

Respiratory System

- The respiratory system assists in the regulation of pH by eliminating carbon dioxide

- The urinary system assists in the elimination of carbon dioxide; provides bicarbonate buffers that assist in pH regulation

Cardiovascular System

- The cardiovascular system delivers blood to glomerular capillaries, where filtration occurs; accepts fluids and solutes reabsorbed during urine production

- The urinary system releases renin to elevate blood pressure and erythropoietin (EPO) to accelerate red blood cell production

Skeletal System

- The skeletal system provides some protection for kidneys and ureters with its axial divison; pelvis protects urinary bladder and proximal portion of urethra

- The urinary system conserves calcium and phosphate needed for bone growth

Muscular System

- The muscular system controls urination by closing urethral sphincters. Muscle layers of trunk provide some protection for urinary organs

- The urinary system removes waste products of muscle and protein metabolism; assists in regulation of calcium and phosphate concentrations

Nervous System

- The nervous system adjusts renal blood pressure; monitors distension of urinary bladder and controls urination

- The urinary system eliminates nitrogenous wastes; maintains fluid, electrolyte, and acid–base balance of blood, which is critical for neural function

Endocrine System

- The endocrine system produces aldosterone and ADH, which adjust rates of fluid and electrolyte reabsorption by kidneys

- The urinary system releases renin when local blood pressure drops and erythropoietin (EPO) when renal oxygen levels fall

Lymphatic System

- The lymphatic system provides adaptive (specific) defense against urinary tract infections

- The urinary system eliminates toxins and wastes generated by cellular activities; acid pH of urine provides innate (nonspecific) defense against urinary tract infections

Digestive System

- The digestive system absorbs water needed to excrete wastes at kidneys; absorbs ions needed to maintain normal body fluid concentrations; liver removes bilirubin

- The urinary system excretes toxins absorbed by the digestive epithelium; excretes bilirubin and nitrogenous wastes from the liver; calcitriol production by kidneys aids calcium and phosphate absorption

Urinary System

The urinary system excretes waste products and maintains normal body fluid pH and ion composition.
It
- regulates blood volume and blood pressure
- regulates plasma concentrations of sodium, potassium, chloride, and other ions
- helps to stabilize blood pH
- conserves valuable nutrients

18 Chapter Review

18-1 The urinary system—made up of the kidneys, ureters, urinary bladder, and urethra—has three major functions *p. 694*

1. The three major functions of the **urinary system** are *excretion*, the removal of organic waste products from body fluids; *elimination*, the discharge of these waste products into the environment; and homeostatic regulation of the volume and solute concentration of blood plasma. Other homeostatic functions include regulating blood volume and pressure by adjusting the volume of water lost and releasing hormones, regulating plasma concentrations of ions, helping to stabilize blood pH, and conserving nutrients.

2. The urinary system includes the **kidneys**, the **ureters**, the **urinary bladder**, and the **urethra**. The kidneys produce **urine**, a fluid containing water, ions, and soluble compounds. During **urination** (**micturition**), urine is forced out of the body *(Figure 18-1)*.

18-2 The kidneys are highly vascular organs containing functional units called nephrons, which perform filtration, reabsorption, and secretion *p. 695*

3. The left **kidney** is slightly more superior than the right kidney. Both kidneys lie in a *retroperitoneal* position *(Figure 18-2)*.

4. A fibrous capsule surrounds each kidney. The **hilum** provides entry for the *renal artery* and *renal nerve*, and exit for the *renal vein* and *ureter*.

5. The ureter is continuous with the **renal pelvis**. This chamber branches into two **major calyces**, each connected to four or five **minor calyces**, which enclose the **renal papillae**. Urine production begins in **nephrons** *(Figure 18-3)*.

6. The blood vessels of the kidneys include the **interlobar, arcuate**, and **cortical radiate arteries** and the **interlobar, arcuate**, and **cortical radiate veins**. Blood travels from the **afferent** and **efferent arterioles** to the **peritubular capillaries** and the **vasa recta**. Diffusion occurs between the peritubular capillaries and the vasa recta and the tubule cells of the nephron through the interstitial fluid, or *peritubular fluid*, that surrounds the nephron *(Figure 18-4)*.

7. The **nephron** is the basic functional unit in the kidney. It consists of the *renal corpuscle* and a **renal tubule**, which empties into the **collecting system** through a *collecting duct*. From the renal corpuscle, filtrate travels through the *proximal convoluted tubule*, the *nephron loop*, and the *distal convoluted tubule (Figures 18-3c, 18-5)*.

8. Nephrons are responsible for (1) the production of **filtrate**, (2) the reabsorption of nutrients, and (3) the reabsorption of water and ions.

9. The **renal corpuscle** consists of a knot of intertwined capillaries, called the **glomerulus**, surrounded by the **glomerular capsule** (*Bowman's capsule*). Blood arrives from the *afferent arteriole* and departs in the *efferent arteriole (Figure 18-6)*.

10. At the glomerulus, **podocytes** cover the basement membrane of the capillaries that project into the **capsular space**. The processes of the podocytes are separated by narrow slits *(Figure 18-6)*.

11. The **proximal convoluted tubule (PCT)** actively reabsorbs nutrients, plasma proteins, and electrolytes from the filtrate. These substances are then released into the surrounding peritubular fluid *(Figure 18-5)*.

12. The **nephron loop**, or *loop of Henle*, includes a *descending limb* and an *ascending limb*. The descending limb is permeable to water, so water is reabsorbed. The ascending limb is impermeable to water and solutes but pumps out sodium and chloride ions *(Figure 18-5)*.

13. The ascending limb delivers tubular fluid to the **distal convoluted tubule (DCT)**. The DCT actively secretes ions, toxins, and drugs and reabsorbs sodium ions from the urine. The **juxtaglomerular complex**, which releases renin and erythropoietin, is located at the start of the DCT *(Figure 18-6a)*.

14. The nephron empties tubular fluid into the **collecting system**, consisting of **collecting ducts** and **papillary ducts**. The collecting system makes final adjustments to the urine by reabsorbing water or reabsorbing or secreting various ions.

18-3 Different portions of the nephron form urine by filtration, reabsorption, and secretion *p. 702*

15. The primary purpose in **urine** production is the excretion and elimination of dissolved solutes, principally metabolic waste products such as **urea, creatinine**, and **uric acid**.

16. Nephron processes involve **filtration, reabsorption**, and **secretion** *(Figure 18-7; Tables 18-1, 18-2)*.

17. Glomerular filtration occurs as blood pressure moves fluids across the wall of the glomerular capillaries into the capsular space. The **glomerular filtration rate (GFR)** is the amount of filtrate produced in the kidneys each minute. Any factor that alters the **filtration** (blood) **pressure** will change the GFR and affect kidney function.

18. Declining filtration pressures stimulate the juxtaglomerular complex to release *renin*. The release of renin results in increases in blood volume and blood pressure.

19. The cells of the PCT normally reabsorb 60–70 percent of the volume of the filtrate produced in the renal corpuscle. The PCT reabsorbs nutrients, sodium and other ions, and water from the filtrate and transports them into the peritubular fluid. It also secretes various substances into the tubular fluid.

20. Water and ions are reclaimed from the tubular fluid by the nephron loop. The descending limb reabsorbs water. The thin ascending limb is permeable to urea, and the thick ascending limb pumps out sodium and chloride ions. A concentration gradient in the renal medulla encourages the osmotic flow of water out of the tubular fluid and into the peritubular fluid. As water is lost by osmosis and the volume of tubular fluid decreases, the urea concentration rises.

21. The DCT performs final adjustments by actively secreting or absorbing materials. Sodium ions are actively absorbed in exchange for potassium and hydrogen ions secreted into the tubular fluid. **Aldosterone** increases the rate of sodium reabsorption and potassium secretion.

22. The amount of water in the urine in the collecting ducts is regulated by *antidiuretic hormone (ADH)*. In the absence of ADH, the DCT, collecting tubule, and collecting duct are impermeable to water. The higher the ADH level in circulation, the more water is reabsorbed and the more concentrated the urine *(Figure 18-8)*.

23. More than 99 percent of the filtrate produced each day is reabsorbed before reaching the renal pelvis. Still, normal urine is 93–97 percent water *(Table 18-3)*.

24. Each segment of the nephron and collecting system contributes to the production of urine *(Spotlight Figure 18-9)*.

18-4 Normal kidney function depends on a stable GFR *p. 707*

25. Renal function may be regulated by local, automatic adjustments in glomerular filtration pressures through changes in the diameters of afferent and efferent arterioles.

26. Hormones that regulate kidney function include angiotensin II, aldosterone, ADH, and atrial natriuretic peptide (ANP) *(Figure 18-10)*.

27. Sympathetic activation produces powerful vasoconstriction of afferent arterioles, decreasing the GFR and slowing filtrate production. Sympathetic activation also alters the GFR by changing the regional blood circulation pattern.

18-5 Urine is transported by the ureters, stored in the bladder, and eliminated through the urethra, aided by the micturition reflex *p. 712*

28. Filtrate modification and urine production end when the fluid enters the renal pelvis. The rest of the urinary system is responsible for transporting, storing, and eliminating the urine.

29. The **ureters** extend from the renal pelvis to the urinary bladder. Peristaltic contractions by smooth muscles in the walls of the ureters move the urine *(Figures 18-1, 18-11)*.

30. Internal features of the **urinary bladder**, a distensible sac for urine storage, include the *trigone*, the neck, and the **internal urethral sphincter**. Contraction of the *detrusor muscle* compresses the bladder and expels the urine into the urethra *(Figure 18-11)*.

31. In both sexes, as the urethra passes through the muscular pelvic floor, a circular band of skeletal muscles forms the **external urethral sphincter**, which is under voluntary control *(Figure 18-11)*.

32. The process of **urination** is coordinated by the **micturition reflex**, which is initiated by stretch receptors in the wall of the urinary bladder. Voluntary urination involves coupling this reflex with the voluntary relaxation of the external urethral sphincter, which allows the opening of the internal urethral sphincter *(Figure 18-14)*.

18-6 Fluid balance, electrolyte balance, and acid-base balance are interrelated and essential to homeostasis *p. 717*

33. The maintenance of normal volume and composition in the extracellular and intracellular fluids is vital to life. Three types of homeostasis are involved: *fluid balance, electrolyte balance*, and *acid–base balance*.

34. The **intracellular fluid (ICF)** contains about 60 percent of the total body water; the **extracellular fluid (ECF)** contains the rest. Exchange occurs between the ICF and ECF, but the two **fluid compartments** retain their distinctive characteristics *(Figures 18-15, 18-16)*.

35. Water circulates freely within the ECF compartment.

36. Water losses are normally balanced by gains through eating, drinking, and metabolic generation *(Table 18-4)*.

18-7 Blood pressure and osmosis are involved in maintaining fluid and electrolyte balance *p. 720*

37. Water movement between the ECF and ICF is called a **fluid shift**. If the ECF becomes hypertonic relative to the ICF, water will move from the ICF into the ECF until osmotic equilibrium has been restored. If the ECF becomes hypotonic relative to the ICF, water will move from the ECF into the cells, and the volume of the ICF will increase.

38. Electrolyte balance is important because total electrolyte concentrations affect water balance, and because the levels of individual electrolytes can affect a variety of cell functions. Problems with electrolyte balance generally result from an imbalance between sodium gains and losses. Problems with potassium balance are less common but more dangerous.

39. The rate of sodium uptake across the digestive epithelium is directly related to the amount of sodium in the diet. Sodium losses occur mainly in the urine and through perspiration. Aldosterone stimulates sodium ion reabsorption along the DCT.

18

40. Potassium ion concentrations in the ECF are very low. Potassium excretion increases (1) when sodium ion concentrations decline and (2) as ECF potassium concentrations rise. Aldosterone stimulates potassium ion excretion.

18-8 In acid–base balance, regulation of hydrogen ions in body fluids involves buffer systems and compensation by respiratory and renal processes *p. 721*

41. The pH of normal body fluids ranges from 7.35 to 7.45; variations outside this range produce **acidosis** or **alkalosis**.

42. Carbonic acid is the most important substance affecting the pH of the ECF. In solution, CO_2 reacts with water to form carbonic acid. The dissociation of carbonic acid releases hydrogen ions and bicarbonate ions. An inverse relationship exists between the partial pressure of carbon dioxide (P_{CO_2}) and pH *(Figure 18-17)*.

43. Metabolic acids include products of metabolism such as lactic acid and ketone bodies.

44. A buffer system consists of a weak acid and its anion dissociation product, which acts as a weak base. The three major buffer systems are *protein buffer systems* in the ECF and ICF; the *carbonic acid–bicarbonate buffer system*, most important in the ECF; and the *phosphate buffer system* in the intracellular fluids.

45. In **protein buffer systems**, amino acid side groups of proteins and the side group and structural groups of free amino acids respond to changes in pH by accepting or releasing hydrogen ions. Blood plasma proteins and hemoglobin in red blood cells help prevent drastic changes in pH.

46. The **carbonic acid–bicarbonate buffer system** prevents pH changes due to metabolic acids in the ECF.

47. The **phosphate buffer system** is important in preventing pH changes in the ICF.

48. In **respiratory compensation**, the lungs help regulate pH by affecting the carbonic acid–bicarbonate buffer system; changing the respiratory rate can raise or lower the P_{CO_2} of body fluids, affecting the buffering capacity.

49. In **renal compensation**, the kidneys vary their rates of hydrogen ion secretion and bicarbonate ion reabsorption depending on the pH of extracellular fluids.

50. Respiratory acid–base disorders result when abnormal respiratory function causes an extreme rise or a fall in CO_2 levels. Metabolic acid–base disorders are caused by the formation of metabolic acids or conditions affecting the levels of bicarbonate ions *(Table 18-5)*.

18-9 Age-related changes affect kidney function and the micturition reflex *p. 726*

51. Aging is usually associated with increased kidney problems. Age-related changes in the urinary system include (1) loss of functional nephrons, (2) reduced GFR, (3) reduced sensitivity to ADH and aldosterone, (4) problems with the micturition reflex (urinary retention may develop in men whose prostate gland is inflamed), (5) declining body water content, (6) a loss of mineral content, and (7) disorders affecting either fluid, electrolyte, or acid–base balance.

18-10 The urinary system is one of several body systems involved in waste excretion *p. 726*

52. The urinary system is the major component of the *excretory system* that also includes the integumentary, respiratory, and digestive systems.

Review Questions

See the blue Answers tab at the back of the book.

Level 1 Reviewing Facts and Terms

Match each item in column A with the most closely related item in column B. Place letters for answers in the spaces provided.

COLUMN A

_____ **1.** Urination
_____ **2.** Fibrous capsule
_____ **3.** Hilum
_____ **4.** Renal medulla
_____ **5.** Nephron
_____ **6.** Renal corpuscle
_____ **7.** External urethral sphincter
_____ **8.** Internal urethral sphincter
_____ **9.** Aldosterone
_____ **10.** Podocytes
_____ **11.** Efferent arteriole
_____ **12.** Afferent arteriole
_____ **13.** Vasa recta
_____ **14.** ADH
_____ **15.** ECF
_____ **16.** Sodium
_____ **17.** Potassium

COLUMN B

a. Basic functional unit of the kidney
b. Capillaries around nephron loop
c. Causes sensation of thirst
d. Stimulates sodium reabsorption
e. Voluntary control
f. Filtration slits
g. Covers kidney
h. Blood leaves the glomerulus
i. Dominant cation in ICF
j. Contains the renal pyramids
k. Blood enters the glomerulus
l. Interstitial fluid and plasma
m. Contains glomerulus
n. Exit point for ureter
o. Dominant cation in ECF
p. Involuntary control
q. Micturition

18

18. Identify the different regions of a nephron and the structure into which it empties in the following diagram.

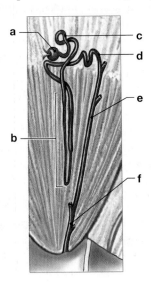

(a) _____ (b) _____
(c) _____ (d) _____
(e) _____ (f) _____

19. The filtrate leaving the glomerular capsule empties into the
(a) distal convoluted tubule.
(b) nephron loop.
(c) proximal convoluted tubule.
(d) collecting duct.

20. The distal convoluted tubule is an important site for
(a) active secretion of ions.
(b) active secretion of acids and other materials.
(c) selective reabsorption of sodium ions from the tubular fluid.
(d) a, b, and c are correct.

21. The endocrine structure that secretes renin and erythropoietin is the
(a) juxtaglomerular complex.
(b) vasa recta.
(c) glomerular capsule.
(d) adrenal gland.

22. The primary purpose of the collecting system is to
(a) transport urine from the bladder to the urethra.
(b) selectively reabsorb sodium ions from tubular fluid.
(c) transport urine from the renal pelvis to the ureters.
(d) make final adjustments to the osmotic concentration and volume of urine.

23. Identify the structures of the kidney in the following diagram.

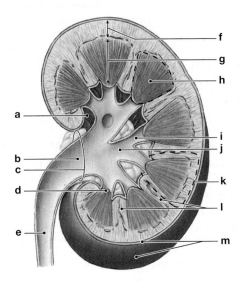

(a) _____ (b) _____
(c) _____ (d) _____
(e) _____ (f) _____
(g) _____ (h) _____
(i) _____ (j) _____
(k) _____ (l) _____
(m) _____

24. A person is in fluid balance when
(a) the ECF and ICF are isotonic.
(b) no fluid movement occurs between compartments.
(c) the amount of water gained each day is equal to the amount lost to the environment.
(d) a, b, and c are correct.

25. The primary components of the extracellular fluid are
(a) lymph and cerebrospinal fluid.
(b) blood plasma and serous fluids.
(c) interstitial fluid and plasma.
(d) a, b, and c are correct.

26. All the homeostatic processes that monitor and adjust the composition of body fluids respond to changes
(a) in the ICF.
(b) in the ECF.
(c) inside the cell.
(d) a, b, and c are correct.

27. The most common problems with electrolyte balance are caused by an imbalance between gains and losses of
    (a) calcium ions.   (b) chloride ions.
    (c) potassium ions.   (d) sodium ions.

28. What is the primary function of the urinary system?

29. What are the structural components of the urinary system?

30. What are fluid shifts? What is their function, and what factors can cause them?

31. What three major hormones affect fluid and electrolyte balance? What are the primary effects of each hormone?

Level 2 Reviewing Concepts

32. The urinary system regulates blood volume and pressure by
    (a) adjusting the volume of water lost in the urine.
    (b) releasing erythropoietin.
    (c) releasing renin.
    (d) a, b, and c are correct.

33. The balance of solute and water reabsorption in the renal medulla is maintained by the
    (a) segmental arterioles and veins.
    (b) interlobar arteries and veins.
    (c) vasa recta.
    (d) arcuate arteries.

34. The higher the plasma concentration of aldosterone, the more efficiently the kidney will
    (a) conserve sodium ions.
    (b) retain potassium ions.
    (c) stimulate urinary water loss.
    (d) secrete greater amounts of ADH.

35. When pure (distilled) water is consumed,
    (a) the ECF becomes hypertonic with respect to the ICF.
    (b) the ECF becomes hypotonic with respect to the ICF.
    (c) the ICF becomes hypotonic with respect to the plasma.
    (d) water moves from the ICF into the ECF.

36. Increasing or decreasing the rate of respiration alters pH by
    (a) lowering or raising the partial pressure of carbon dioxide.
    (b) lowering or raising the partial pressure of oxygen.
    (c) lowering or raising the partial pressure of nitrogen.
    (d) a, b, and c are correct.

37. What interacting controls stabilize the glomerular filtration rate (GFR)?

38. Describe the micturition reflex.

39. Differentiate among fluid balance, electrolyte balance, and acid–base balance, and explain why each is important to homeostasis.

40. Why should a person with a fever drink plenty of fluids?

41. Exercise physiologists recommend that adequate amounts of fluid be ingested before, during, and after exercise. Why is adequate fluid replacement during extensive sweating important?

Level 3 Critical Thinking and Clinical Applications

42. Long-haul truck drivers are on the road for long periods of time between restroom stops. Why might that lead to kidney problems?

43. For the past week, Susan has felt a burning sensation in the area of her urethra when she urinates. She checks her temperature and finds that she has a low-grade fever. What is likely occurring, and what unusual substances are likely to be in her urine?

44. *Mannitol* is a sugar that is filtered but not reabsorbed by the kidneys. What effect would drinking a solution of mannitol have on the volume of urine produced?

18

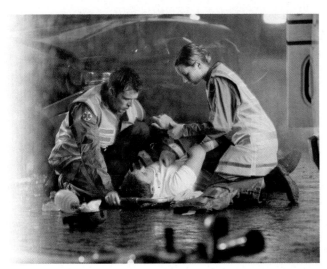

The Reproductive System

Learning Objectives

These objectives tell you what you should be able to do after completing the chapter. They correspond by number to this chapter's sections.

19-1 List the basic structures of the human reproductive system, and summarize the functions of each.

19-2 Describe the structures of the male reproductive system and the roles played by the reproductive tract and accessory glands in producing spermatozoa; describe the composition of semen; and summarize the hormonal processes that regulate male reproductive function.

19-3 Describe the structures of the female reproductive system; explain the process of oogenesis in the ovary; discuss the ovarian and uterine cycles; and summarize the events of the female reproductive cycle.

19-4 Discuss the physiology of sexual intercourse in males and females.

19-5 Describe the reproductive system changes that occur with aging.

19-6 Give examples of interactions between the reproductive system and each of the other body systems.

An Introduction to the Reproductive System

One person's life span lasts only for decades, yet the human species has perpetuated itself for hundreds of thousands of years through the activities of the reproductive system. The entire process of reproduction seems almost magical. Many aboriginal societies did not discover even the basic link between sexual activity and childbirth. They assumed that supernatural forces were responsible for producing new individuals. Our society has a much clearer understanding of the reproductive process, but the events of procreation—the fusion of two reproductive cells, one produced by a man, the other by a woman, which leads to the birth of an infant—still produces a sense of wonder. In this chapter and the next, we will consider this remarkable process.

Build Your Knowledge

Recall that both the male and female reproductive systems produce sex cells and hormones (as you saw in **Chapter 1: An Introduction to Anatomy and Physiology** and **Chapter 3: Cell Structure and Function**). The male produces sperm, and the female produces oocytes—immature ova, or egg cells. The female reproductive system also supports embryonic and fetal development from fertilization to birth. ⮌ **pp. 9, 81**

19-1 Basic reproductive system structures are gonads, ducts, accessory glands and organs, and external genitalia

Learning Objective List the basic structures of the human reproductive system, and summarize the functions of each.

The **reproductive system** ensures the continued existence of the human species. It does so by producing, storing, nourishing, and transporting functional male and female reproductive cells, or **gametes** (GAM-ēts).

The reproductive system includes

- **Gonads** (GŌ-nadz; *gone*, seed generation), or reproductive organs that produce gametes and hormones.

- Ducts that receive and transport the gametes.

- Accessory glands and organs that secrete fluids into the ducts of the reproductive system or other excretory ducts.

- Perineal structures that are collectively known as the **external genitalia** (jen-i-TĀ-lē-uh).

In both males and females, the ducts are connected to chambers and passageways that open to the exterior of the body. The structures involved make up the *reproductive tract*. The male and female reproductive systems are functionally quite different, however.

In adult males, the **testes** (TES-tēz; singular, *testis*), or *testicles*, are male gonads that secrete sex hormones called *androgens* (principally *testosterone*). The testes also produce the male gametes, called **spermatozoa** (sper-ma-tō-ZŌ-uh; singular, *spermatozoon*), or *sperm*. Males produce about one-half billion sperm each day. During *emission*, mature spermatozoa travel along a lengthy duct system, where they are mixed with the secretions of accessory glands. The mixture created is known as **semen** (SĒ-men). During *ejaculation*, semen is expelled from the body.

In adult females, the **ovaries**, or female gonads, release an immature gamete, an **oocyte**. Normally, one oocyte is released per month. This oocyte travels along one of two short *uterine tubes*, which end in the muscular organ called the *uterus* (Ū-ter-us). If a sperm reaches the oocyte and starts the process of *fertilization*, the oocyte matures into an **ovum** (plural, *ova*). A short passageway, the *vagina* (va-JĪ-nuh), connects the uterus with the exterior.

During *sexual intercourse*, ejaculation introduces semen into the vagina. The spermatozoa then ascend the female reproductive tract. If fertilization occurs, the uterus will enclose and support a developing *embryo* as it grows into a *fetus* and prepares for birth.

CHECKPOINT

1. Define gamete.
2. List the basic structures of the reproductive system.
3. Define gonads.

See the blue Answers tab at the back of the book.

19

19-2 Sperm formation (spermatogenesis) occurs in the testes, and hormones from the hypothalamus, pituitary gland, and testes control male reproductive functions

Learning Objective Describe the structures of the male reproductive system and the roles played by the reproductive tract and accessory glands in producing spermatozoa; describe the composition of semen; and summarize the hormonal processes that regulate male reproductive function.

The main structures of the male reproductive system are shown in **Figure 19-1**. Starting from a testis, the spermatozoa travel within the *epididymis* (ep-i-DID-i-mis), the *ductus deferens* (DUK-tus DEF-e-renz), the *ejaculatory* (ē-JAK-ū-la-tō-rē) *duct*, and the *urethra* before leaving the body. This duct system forms the male reproductive tract. Accessory organs secrete their products into the ejaculatory ducts and urethra. These organs include the *seminal* (SEM-i-nal) *glands* (seminal vesicles), the *prostate* (PROS-tāt) *gland*,

and the *bulbo-urethral* (bul-bō-ū-RĒ-thral) *glands*. The external genitalia include the *scrotum* (SKRŌ-tum), which encloses the testes, and the *penis* (PĒ-nis), an erectile organ. The distal portion of the urethra passes through the penis.

The Testes

Each testis has the shape of a flattened egg roughly 5 cm (2 in.) long, 3 cm (1.2 in.) wide, and 2.5 cm (1 in.) thick. Each weighs 10–15 g (0.35–0.53 oz). The testes hang within the **scrotum**, a fleshy pouch anterior to the anus and posterior to the penis.

The scrotum is subdivided into two chambers, or *scrotal cavities*. Each cavity contains a testis. A serous membrane lines the scrotal cavity, reducing friction between the inner surface of the scrotum and the outer surface of the testis.

The scrotum consists of a thin layer of skin. Its dermis contains a layer of smooth muscle, the *dartos* (DAR-tōs) (**Figure 19-2a**). Resting tension in the dartos elevates the

Figure 19-1 The Male Reproductive System. A sagittal section of the male reproductive organs.

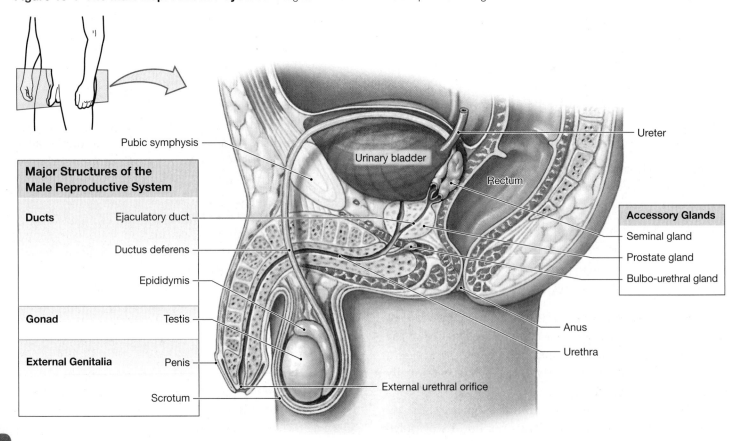

Major Structures of the Male Reproductive System	
Ducts	Ejaculatory duct
	Ductus deferens
	Epididymis
Gonad	Testis
External Genitalia	Penis
	Scrotum

Pubic symphysis

Urinary bladder

Ureter

Rectum

Accessory Glands
Seminal gland
Prostate gland
Bulbo-urethral gland

Anus

Urethra

External urethral orifice

Figure 19-2 The Scrotum, Testes, and Seminiferous Tubules.

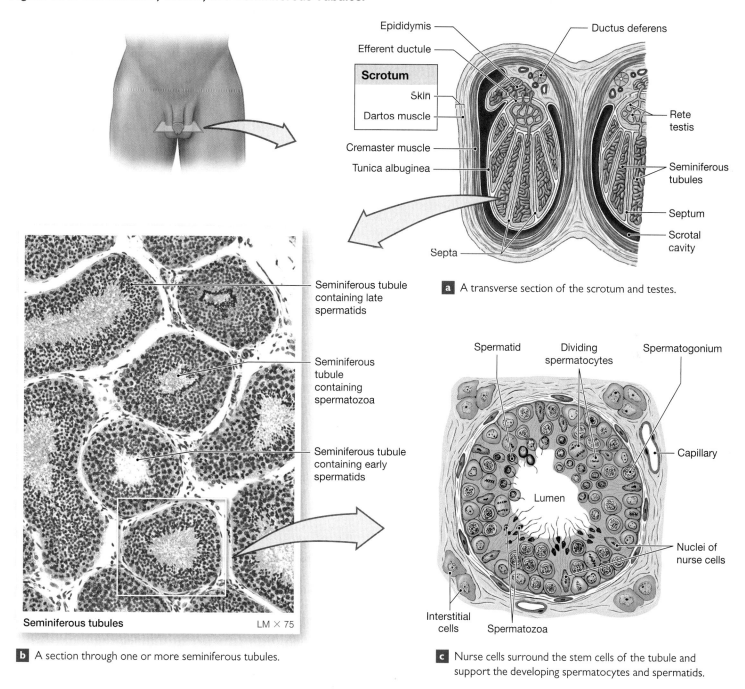

Epididymis — Ductus deferens

Efferent ductule

Scrotum

Skin

Dartos muscle

Cremaster muscle

Tunica albuginea

Rete testis

Seminiferous tubules

Septum

Scrotal cavity

Septa

a A transverse section of the scrotum and testes.

Seminiferous tubule containing late spermatids

Seminiferous tubule containing spermatozoa

Seminiferous tubule containing early spermatids

Seminiferous tubules   LM × 75

b A section through one or more seminiferous tubules.

Spermatid   Dividing spermatocytes   Spermatogonium

Capillary

Lumen

Nuclei of nurse cells

Interstitial cells   Spermatozoa

c Nurse cells surround the stem cells of the tubule and support the developing spermatocytes and spermatids.

testes and causes the characteristic wrinkling of the scrotal surface. A layer of skeletal muscle, the **cremaster** (krē-MAS-ter) **muscle**, lies beneath the dermis. It can contract to pull the testes closer to the body.

Normal sperm development in the testes requires temperatures about 1.1°C (2°F) lower than elsewhere in the body. The cremaster and dartos relax or contract to move the testes away from or toward the body as needed to maintain acceptable testicular temperatures. When air or body temperatures rise, these muscles relax and the testes move away from the body. When the scrotum cools suddenly, as happens during a jump into a cold swimming pool, these muscles contract to pull the testes closer to the body and keep testicular temperatures from falling.

Each testis is wrapped in a tough fibrous capsule, the **tunica albuginea** (TŪ-ni-ka al-bū-JIN-ē-uh). Collagen

19

fibers from this wrapping extend into the testis, forming partitions, or *septa,* that subdivide the testis into roughly 250 *lobules.* Distributed among the lobules are approximately 800 slender, tightly coiled **seminiferous** (sem-i-NIF-er-us) **tubules** (**Figure 19-2b**). Each tubule averages about 80 cm (32 in.) in length. A typical testis contains nearly half a mile of seminiferous tubules. Sperm produced within the seminiferous tubules (by a process discussed shortly) leave the tubules and pass through a maze of passageways known as the **rete** (RĒ-tē; *rete,* a net) **testis**. They then enter 15–20 large *efferent ductules* before entering the epididymis. The epididymis is the first portion of the male reproductive tract (**Figure 19-2a**).

CLINICAL NOTE

Cryptorchidism

During normal development of a male fetus, the testes descend from inside the body cavity and pass through the inguinal canal of the abdominal wall into the scrotum. In cryptorchidism (krip-TOR-ki-dizm; *crypto,* hidden + *orchis,* testis), one or both of the testes have not completed this process (*descent of the testes*) by the time of birth. This condition occurs in about 3 percent of full-term deliveries and about 30 percent of premature births. In most instances, normal descent occurs a few weeks later.

The condition can be surgically corrected if it persists. Corrective measures should be taken before *puberty* (sexual maturation) because a cryptorchid (abdominal) testis will not produce sperm. If both testes are cryptorchid, the male will be *sterile* (*infertile*) and unable to father children. If the testes cannot be moved into the scrotum, they are usually removed. This surgical procedure is called a *bilateral orchiectomy* (or-k-EK-to-m; *ectomy,* excision). About 10 percent of males with uncorrected cryptorchid testes eventually develop testicular cancer.

Most tissue slides show seminiferous tubules in cross section, because the seminiferous tubules are tightly coiled (**Figure 19-2b**). The spaces between the tubules are filled with areolar tissue, numerous blood vessels, and large **interstitial cells** (*Leydig cells*) (**Figure 19-2c**). Interstitial cells produce male sex hormones, or *androgens.* The steroid **testosterone** is the most important androgen. ↪ p. 354

Each seminiferous tubule contains developing sperm cells and **nurse cells**. Nurse cells are also known as *sustentacular* (sus-ten-TAK-ū-lar) (or *Sertoli*) cells. They extend from the perimeter of the tubule to the central lumen (**Figure 19-2c**). Nurse cells nourish the developing sperm cells. Between and adjacent to the nurse cells are the various cells involved in sperm formation, or **spermatogenesis** (sper-ma-tō-JEN-e-sis). In this process, a series of cell divisions ultimately produces sperm cells (spermatozoa). With each successive division, the daughter cells move closer to the lumen.

CLINICAL NOTE

Testicular Cancer

Although cancer of the testicle is relatively rare in men overall, it is the most common cancer in men from 15 to 35 years old. Testicular cancer is highly treatable and usually curable. It is generally divided into seminoma and nonseminoma types for treatment planning because seminomas are more sensitive to radiation therapy. The cure rate for patients with seminoma-type cancers exceeds 90 percent. The cure rate for nonseminoma type cancers approaches 100 percent. Men who have an undescended testicle (cryptorchidism) are at a higher risk of developing cancer of the testicle than those where the testicle has descended properly. This is true even if surgery was performed to place the testicle at the appropriate place in the scrotum.

Treatment of testicular cancer includes surgery, chemotherapy, radiation therapy, and/or bone marrow transplantation. Typically, both testicles are surgically removed. The lymph nodes in the abdomen are often sampled during surgery. Radiation therapy is used to kill cancer cells and shrink tumors. Chemotherapy kills cancer cells that are located outside of the testicle. Autologous bone marrow transplantation is a newer type of treatment. Bone marrow is taken from the patient and treated with drugs to kill any cancer cells. The marrow is then frozen while the patient is given high-dose chemotherapy, either with or without radiation therapy, to destroy all of the remaining marrow. Following this, the marrow that was previously removed and treated is thawed and given back to the patient, which replaces the marrow that was destroyed. The marrow grows and begins to function by producing essential blood cells.

The best treatment for testicular cancer is prevention. The earlier testicular cancer is detected, the better are the chances of obtaining a cure. All men should perform testicular self-examination at least once a month. This is especially important in the 15- to 40-year-old age group. The American Cancer Society and the National Cancer Institute have several tapes and brochures that detail this safe and easy examination.

Spermatogenesis

Spermatogenesis begins at puberty (sexual maturation) and continues until relatively late in life (after age 70). Spermatogenesis involves three processes:

1. **Mitosis.** Spermatogenesis begins with the mitotic divisions of stem cells called **spermatogonia** (sper-ma-tō-GŌ-nē-uh; singular, *spermatogonium*). They are located in the outermost layer of cells in the seminiferous tubules (**Figure 19-2c**). (See Chapter 3 for a review of mitosis and cell division.) ↪ p. 83 Spermatogonia undergo mitosis throughout adult life. One daughter cell from each division remains in place while the other is pushed

Build Your Knowledge

Recall that cell division is essential to growth, development, and the continual replacement of old and damaged cells (as you saw in **Chapter 3: Cell Structure and Function**). Also recall that the life cycle of a cell includes interphase, mitosis, and cytokinesis. Interphase is the time when a cell performs its normal functions between cell divisions. Also during this phase, the cell's chromosomes are duplicated in preparation for cell division. Mitosis refers to the division of a cell's nucleus. In this process, the duplicated chromosomes of the original cell are separated and enclosed in two identical nuclei. Mitosis includes four stages: prophase, metaphase, anaphase, and telophase. Mitosis ensures that each newly formed nucleus contains the same number and kind of chromosomes as the original cell. Cytokinesis follows mitosis. In this process, the cytoplasm of the original cell is divided, forming two identical daughter cells. ⟲**p. 81**

toward the lumen of the seminiferous tubule. The displaced cells differentiate into **spermatocytes** (sper-MA-tō-sīts), which prepare to begin meiosis.

2. **Meiosis.** *Meiosis* (mī-Ō-sis; *meioun*, to make smaller) is a special form of cell division involved in gamete production. In humans, gametes contain 23 chromosomes, half the number in *somatic* (nonreproductive) cells. In

CLINICAL NOTE

Testicular Torsion

Testicular torsion is a major cause of scrotal pain. It occurs when a testicle twists on the spermatic cord. The testicle almost always torses lateral to medial. This usually compromises blood supply to the testicle, which results in severe scrotal and abdominal pain. If emergency surgery is not performed within six hours, the testicle may be lost. Testicular torsion most often occurs at puberty, but can occur at any age. Often there is a history of an athletic event or strenuous physical exercise prior to the onset. The diagnosis is made by physical exam and by scrotal ultrasound. The scrotal ultrasound will detect any interruptions in blood supply to the testicle. Treatment requires surgical exploration and detorsion of the testicle. The urologist will then secure *(pex)* both testicles so that additional torsions cannot occur.

the seminiferous tubules, the meiotic divisions of spermatocytes produce immature gametes called *spermatids* (**Figure 19-2c**).

3. **Spermiogenesis.** In *spermiogenesis*, the small, relatively unspecialized spermatids develop into physically mature spermatozoa, which enter the fluid within the lumen of the seminiferous tubule.

Next we consider these three processes in more detail.

MITOSIS AND MEIOSIS. Mitosis and meiosis differ significantly in terms of the events taking place in the nucleus. **Mitosis** is part of the process of somatic cell division, producing two daughter cells, each with the same number and pairs of chromosomes as the original cell. In humans, each somatic cell contains 23 pairs of chromosomes, or 46 chromosomes. Each pair consists of one paternal chromosome (provided by the father) and one maternal chromosome (provided by the mother) at the time of fertilization. Because daughter cells contain *both* members of each chromosome pair, they are called **diploid** (DIP-loyd; *diplo*, double).

In contrast, **meiosis** involves two cycles of cell division (*meiosis I* and *meiosis II*). We identify the stages within each cycle with I or II, for example, as prophase I, metaphase II, and so on. This process produces four cells, or gametes, each containing 23 individual chromosomes. These cells are called **haploid** (HAP-loyd; *haplo*, single) and contain only one member of each chromosome pair. The fusion of the nuclei of a male haploid gamete and female haploid gamete produces a cell with the normal diploid number of chromosomes (46).

Figure 19-3 illustrates the role of meiosis in spermatogenesis. Each mitotic division of spermatogonia produces two primary spermatocytes. The primary spermatocytes are diploid cells, but they divide by meiosis rather than mitosis. As a primary spermatocyte prepares to begin meiosis, DNA replication occurs within the nucleus, just as it does in a cell preparing to undergo mitosis. As prophase of the first meiotic division (meiosis I) occurs, the chromosomes condense and become visible. As in mitosis, each chromosome consists of two duplicate *chromatids* (KRŌ-ma-tidz).

At this point, the close similarities between meiosis and mitosis end. As prophase I unfolds, similar maternal and paternal chromosomes pair up. This key pairing event is known as **synapsis** (si-NAP-sis). It produces 23 pairs of chromosomes, with each member of the pair consisting of two identical chromatids. A matched set of four chromatids is called a **tetrad** (TET-rad; *tetras*, four). At this time, an exchange of genetic material can take place between the maternal and

Figure 19-3 Spermatogenesis. The events depicted occur within the seminiferous tubules. The fates of three representative chromosomes are shown. Each diploid primary spermatocyte that undergoes meiosis produces four haploid spermatids. Each spermatid then develops into a spermatozoon.

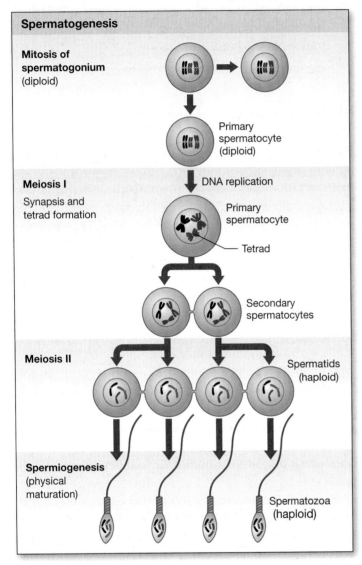

Spermatogenesis

Mitosis of spermatogonium (diploid)

Primary spermatocyte (diploid)

Meiosis I
Synapsis and tetrad formation

DNA replication

Primary spermatocyte

Tetrad

Secondary spermatocytes

Meiosis II

Spermatids (haploid)

Spermiogenesis (physical maturation)

Spermatozoa (haploid)

As anaphase I proceeds, the maternal and paternal chromosomes that had formed a tetrad are randomly distributed. For example, most of the maternal chromosomes may go to one daughter cell, and most of the paternal chromosomes to the other. As a result, telophase I ends with the formation of two daughter cells, each containing a unique combination of maternal and paternal chromosomes. In the testes, the daughter cells produced by meiosis I are called **secondary spermatocytes**.

Every secondary spermatocyte contains 23 chromosomes, each consisting of two duplicate chromatids. The duplicate chromatids will separate during **meiosis II**. The interphase separating meiosis I and meiosis II is very brief. No DNA is replicated during this period. The secondary spermatocyte then enters meiosis II. The completion of meiosis II produces four immature gametes, or **spermatids** (SPER-ma-tidz). They are identical in size and each has 23 chromosomes. In summary, for every diploid primary spermatocyte that enters meiosis, four haploid spermatids are produced (**Figure 19-3**).

SPERMIOGENESIS. In **spermiogenesis**, each spermatid matures into a single **spermatozoon** (sper-ma-tō-ZŌ-on), or sperm cell. The entire process of spermatogenesis, from spermatogonial division to the release of a physically mature spermatozoon, takes approximately 64 days.

Nurse cells play a key role in spermatogenesis and spermiogenesis. Spermatocytes undergoing meiosis and spermatids are not free in the seminiferous tubules. Instead, they are surrounded by the cytoplasm of nurse cells. Because there are no blood vessels inside the seminiferous tubules, all nutrients must diffuse in from the surrounding interstitial fluids. The large nurse cells control the chemical environment inside the seminiferous tubules. They provide nutrients and chemical stimuli that promote the production and differentiation of spermatozoa. They also help regulate spermatogenesis by producing *inhibin* (a hormone introduced in Chapter 10). ↻ p. 368

Anatomy of a Spermatozoon

A sperm cell, or spermatozoon, has four distinct regions: head, neck, middle piece, and tail (**Figure 19-4**). The **head** contains a nucleus filled with densely packed chromosomes. At the tip of the head is the **acrosome** (ak-rō-SŌM), a cap-like compartment containing enzymes essential for fertilization. A short **neck** attaches the head to the **middle piece**. The neck contains both centrioles of the original spermatid. Mitochondria in the middle piece are arranged in a spiral. Mitochondria provide the ATP for moving the tail. The **tail** is

paternal chromatids of a chromosome pair. This exchange, called *crossing-over*, increases genetic variation among offspring. Prophase I ends with the disappearance of the nuclear envelope.

During metaphase I, the tetrads line up along the metaphase plate. As anaphase I begins, the maternal and paternal chromosomes separate and the tetrads break up. This is a major difference between mitosis and meiosis: In mitosis, each daughter cell receives a copy of *every* chromosome, maternal and paternal. In meiosis I, however, each daughter cell receives two copies of *either* the maternal chromosome or the paternal chromosome.

Figure 19-4 Spermatozoon Structure. A spermatozoon measures only 60 μm (0.06 mm) in total length.

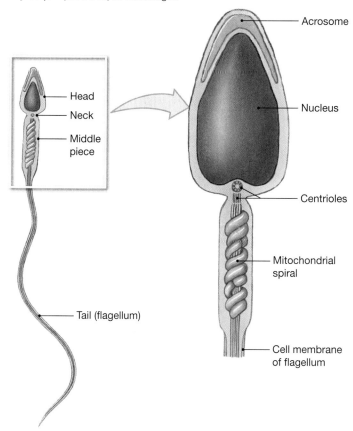

- Head
- Neck
- Middle piece

- Acrosome
- Nucleus
- Centrioles
- Mitochondrial spiral
- Tail (flagellum)
- Cell membrane of flagellum

the only example of a *flagellum* in the human body. Its corkscrew motion moves the sperm cell. ↻ p. 71

Unlike other, less specialized cells, a mature spermatozoon does not have an endoplasmic reticulum, a Golgi apparatus, lysosomes, peroxisomes, and many other intracellular structures. Because a sperm cell contains no glycogen or other energy reserves, it must absorb nutrients (primarily fructose) from the surrounding fluid.

The Male Reproductive Tract

The testes produce physically mature spermatozoa that are not yet capable of fertilizing an oocyte. The other portions of the male reproductive system are responsible for the functional maturation, nourishment, storage, and transport of spermatozoa.

The Epididymis

Late in their development, spermatozoa detach from nurse cells and lie within the lumen of the seminiferous tubule. They have most of the physical characteristics of mature sperm cells, yet they are still functionally immature. They are incapable of coordinated locomotion or fertilization. Fluid currents, created by cilia lining the efferent ducts, transport them into the **epididymis** (plural, *epididymides*) (**Figure 19-1**). The epididymis is the start of the male reproductive tract. It is a coiled tube bound to the posterior of each testis. The epididymides (ep-i-DID-i-mi-dēz) can be felt through the skin of the scrotum. Each epididymis is almost 7 meters (23 ft) long, but it is twisted and coiled so as to take up very little space.

The functions of the epididymis include (1) adjusting the composition of the fluid produced by the seminiferous tubules, (2) acting as a recycling center for damaged spermatozoa, and (3) storing and protecting the maturing spermatozoa. Cells lining the epididymis absorb and break down cellular debris from damaged or abnormal spermatozoa. The resulting products are released into interstitial fluid for pickup by surrounding blood vessels. It takes up to two weeks for a spermatozoon to pass through the epididymis and complete its physical maturation. It then enters the ductus deferens.

Spermatozoa leaving the epididymis are physically mature, but they remain immobile. To become motile (actively swimming) and fully functional, they must undergo **capacitation**. Capacitation occurs after spermatozoa (1) mix with secretions of the seminal glands and (2) are exposed to conditions inside the female reproductive tract. The epididymis secretes a substance that prevents premature capacitation.

The Ductus Deferens

Each **ductus deferens**, or *vas deferens*, is 40–45 cm (16–18 in.) long (**Figure 19-1**). It ascends into the abdominal cavity within the *spermatic cord,* a sheath of connective tissue and muscle that also encloses the blood vessels, nerves, and lymphatics serving the testis. (The passageway through the abdominal musculature is called the *inguinal canal.*)

Inside the abdominal cavity, each ductus deferens passes lateral to the urinary bladder and curves downward past the ureter on its way toward the prostate gland (**Figure 19-5a**). The expanded distal portion of the ductus deferens is called the *ampulla* (am-PUL-uh). Peristaltic contractions in the muscular walls of each ductus deferens propel spermatozoa and fluid along the length of the duct. The ductus deferens also stores spermatozoa in the ampulla for up to several months. During this period, spermatozoa are inactive and have low metabolic rates.

The ampulla of each ductus deferens joins with the duct of the seminal gland to form the *ejaculatory duct,* a relatively

19

Figure 19-5 The Ductus Deferens.

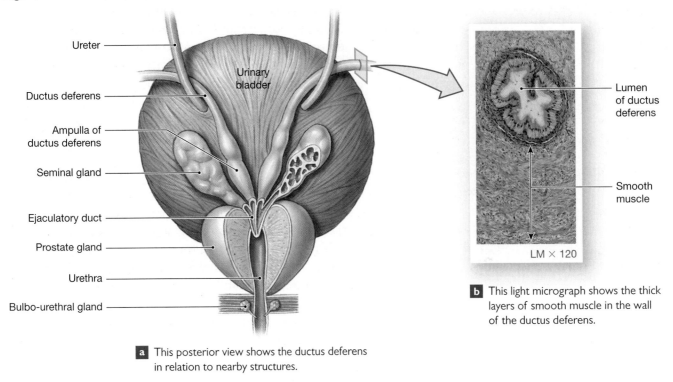

Ureter

Urinary bladder

Ductus deferens

Ampulla of ductus deferens

Seminal gland

Ejaculatory duct

Prostate gland

Urethra

Bulbo-urethral gland

Lumen of ductus deferens

Smooth muscle

LM × 120

b This light micrograph shows the thick layers of smooth muscle in the wall of the ductus deferens.

a This posterior view shows the ductus deferens in relation to nearby structures.

short (2 cm, or less than 1 in.) passageway (**Figure 19-5a**). This duct penetrates the muscular wall of the prostate gland and empties into the urethra near the opening of the ejaculatory duct from the other side.

The Urethra

In males, the urethra extends 18–20 cm (7–8 in.) from the urinary bladder to the tip of the penis (**Figure 19-1**). The male urethra is a passageway for both the urinary and reproductive systems.

The Accessory Glands

The fluids secreted by the seminiferous tubules and the epididymis account for only about 5 percent of the volume of *semen.* The fluid component of semen is a mixture of secretions from the *seminal glands,* the *prostate gland,* and the *bulbo-urethral glands* (**Figure 19-5a**). Primary functions of these glands include (1) activating spermatozoa, (2) providing nutrients spermatozoa need for motility, (3) generating peristaltic contractions that propel spermatozoa and fluids along the reproductive tract, and (4) producing buffers to counteract the acidity of the urethral and vaginal environments.

The Seminal Glands (Seminal Vesicles)

Each **seminal gland**, also called a **seminal vesicle**, is a tubular gland about 15 cm (6 in.) long (**Figures 19-1** and **19-5a**). The body of the gland is coiled and folded into a compact, tapered mass roughly 5 cm by 2.5 cm (2 in. by 1 in.).

The seminal glands are extremely active secretory glands. They contribute about 60 percent of the volume of semen. Their secretions contain (1) fructose, a six-carbon sugar easily metabolized by spermatozoa; (2) prostaglandins, which stimulate smooth muscle contractions along the male and female reproductive tracts; and (3) fibrinogen, which after ejaculation forms a temporary semen clot within the vagina. The slight alkalinity of the secretions helps neutralize acids in secretions of the prostate gland and within the vagina. When mixed with seminal gland secretions, mature but previously inactive spermatozoa undergo the first step of capacitation and begin beating their flagella, becoming highly motile.

The Prostate Gland

The **prostate gland** is a small, muscular, rounded organ, about 4 cm (1.6 in.) in diameter. It surrounds the urethra as it leaves the urinary bladder (**Figure 19-5a**). The *prostatic fluid* it secretes is slightly acidic and makes up 20–30 percent of the volume of semen. In addition to several other compounds, prostatic fluid contains **seminalplasmin** (sem-i-nal-PLAZ-min), a protein with antibiotic properties that may help prevent urinary tract infections in males. These secretions are ejected into the urethra by peristaltic contractions of the muscular prostate wall.

The Bulbo-Urethral Glands

The paired **bulbo-urethral glands**, or *Cowper's glands*, are located at the base of the penis. They are spherical structures almost 10 mm (less than 0.5 in.) in diameter (**Figure 19-5a**). These glands secrete a thick, alkaline mucus that helps neutralize urinary acids that may remain in the urethra and also lubricates the *glans penis*, or tip of the penis.

Semen

Semen (SĒ-men) is the fluid that contains sperm and the secretions of the accessory glands of the male reproductive tract. In a typical *ejaculation* (ē-jak-ū-LĀ-shun), 2–5 mL of semen is expelled from the body. This volume of fluid, called an **ejaculate**, contains three major components:

- *Spermatozoa.* A normal **sperm count** ranges from 20 million to 100 million spermatozoa per milliliter of semen.

- *Seminal fluid.* **Seminal fluid** is the fluid component of semen. It is a mixture of glandular secretions with a distinct ionic and nutrient composition. Of the total volume of seminal fluid, the seminal glands contribute about 60 percent; the prostate, 30 percent; the nurse cells and epididymis, 5 percent; and the bulbo-urethral glands, less than 5 percent.

- *Enzymes.* Several important enzymes are present in seminal fluid. They include (1) a protease that helps dissolve mucus in the vagina; (2) *seminalplasmin*, a prostatic enzyme that kills a variety of bacteria; (3) a prostatic enzyme that causes the semen to clot within a few minutes after ejaculation; and (4) an enzyme that subsequently liquefies the clotted semen.

The External Genitalia

The male external genitalia consist of the scrotum (described earlier on p. 644) and penis. The **penis** is a tubular organ containing the distal portion of the urethra (**Figure 19-1**). It conducts urine to the exterior and introduces semen into the female's vagina during sexual intercourse.

The penis has three main regions (**Figure 19-6a**). The **root** is the fixed portion that attaches the penis to the body wall. The **body (shaft)** is the tubular portion that contains masses of erectile tissue. The **glans penis** is the expanded distal portion surrounding the external urethral opening, or *external urethral orifice.*

The skin overlying the penis resembles that of the scrotum. A fold of skin, called the **prepuce** (PRE-poos), or *foreskin*, surrounds the tip of the penis (**Figure 19-6b**). The prepuce attaches to the relatively narrow neck of the penis and continues over the glans penis. *Preputial glands* in the skin of the neck and inner surface of the prepuce secrete a waxy material called *smegma* (SMEG-ma). Unfortunately, smegma can be an excellent nutrient source for bacteria. Mild inflammation and infections in this region are common, especially if the area is not washed frequently. One way to avoid such problems is *circumcision* (ser-kum-SIZH-un), the surgical removal of the prepuce. In Western societies (especially the United States), this procedure is generally performed shortly after birth. Circumcision lowers the risks of developing urinary tract infections, HIV infection, and penile cancer. The practice remains controversial because it is a surgical procedure with risk of bleeding, infection, and other complications.

Most of the body, or shaft, of the penis consists of three columns of **erectile tissue** (**Figure 19-6c**). Erectile tissue consists of a maze of vascular channels incompletely separated by partitions of elastic connective tissue and smooth muscle. The anterior surface of the flaccid (nonerect) penis covers two cylindrical **corpora cavernosa** (KOR-por-a ka-ver-NŌ-suh). Their bases are bound to the pubis and ischium of the pelvis (**Figure 19-6a**). The corpora cavernosa extend to the glans penis. The relatively slender **corpus spongiosum** (spon-jē-Ō-sum) surrounds the urethra and extends all the way to the tip of the penis, where it forms the glans penis.

CLINICAL NOTE

Prostatitis

Prostatic inflammation, or prostatitis (pros-ta-TĪ-tis), can occur in males of any age but most often afflicts older men. Prostatitis can result from bacterial infections, but it also occurs in the apparent absence of pathogens. Signs and symptoms can resemble those of prostate cancer. Individuals with prostatitis may complain of pain in the lower back, perineum, or rectum, sometimes accompanied by painful urination and the discharge of mucous secretions from the urethral opening. Antibiotic therapy is effective in treating most cases caused by bacterial infection.

Figure 19-6 The Penis.

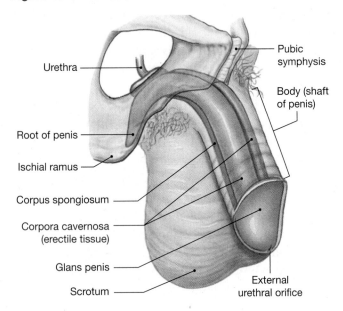

Urethra

Root of penis

Ischial ramus

Corpus spongiosum

Corpora cavernosa
(erectile tissue)

Glans penis

Scrotum

Pubic symphysis

Body (shaft of penis)

External urethral orifice

a An anterior and lateral view of a penis showing the positions of the erectile tissues.

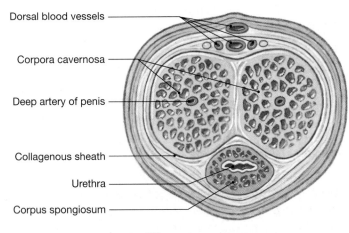

Dorsal blood vessels

Corpora cavernosa

Deep artery of penis

Collagenous sheath

Urethra

Corpus spongiosum

c A sectional view through the penis.

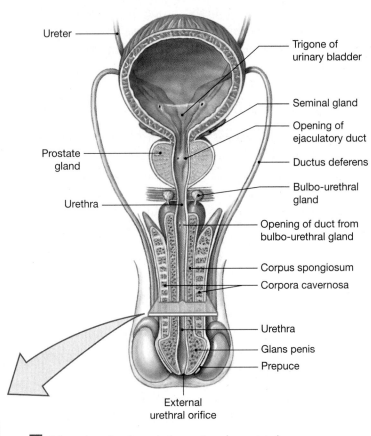

Ureter

Prostate gland

Urethra

Trigone of urinary bladder

Seminal gland

Opening of ejaculatory duct

Ductus deferens

Bulbo-urethral gland

Opening of duct from bulbo-urethral gland

Corpus spongiosum

Corpora cavernosa

Urethra

Glans penis

Prepuce

External urethral orifice

b A frontal section through the penis and associated organs.

CLINICAL NOTE

Male Genital Trauma

The male genitalia are, for the most part, located outside of the body. Despite this, they are rarely injured. The testicles are highly mobile within the scrotum, and the external capsule of the testicle (tunica albuginea) is very tough. These features protect the testes from injury. The most common cause of testicular injury is a direct blow. Most testicular injuries are contusions, although ruptures can occur.

Injuries to the penis can result from several causes. Zippers can trap the penile skin, and cause pain and bleeding. Mineral oil and ice can aid in removing the entrapped skin. In severe cases, a local anesthetic must be injected so that a wire cutter can be used to open the zipper.

Self-inflicted injuries of the penis can range from the common to the bizarre. Vacuum cleaners can cause extensive injury to the glans penis. Blade injuries can cause lacerations or even amputations. Amputation of the penis is best managed by replantation, if possible.

Traumatic rupture of the corpus cavernosum of the penis, which is also called a fracture of the penis, occurs when the erect penis impacts forcibly on a hard object, receives a direct blow, or is subjected to abnormal bending. A cracking sound may be heard. This is usually followed by penile pain, loss of the erection, rapid swelling, discoloration, and deformity. Penile ruptures must be carefully managed surgically to avoid permanent loss of function.

Male reproductive function is regulated by the complex interaction of hormones from the hypothalamus, anterior lobe of the pituitary gland, and the testes. The interaction of positive and negative feedback loops keep testosterone levels within a relatively narrow range until late in life.

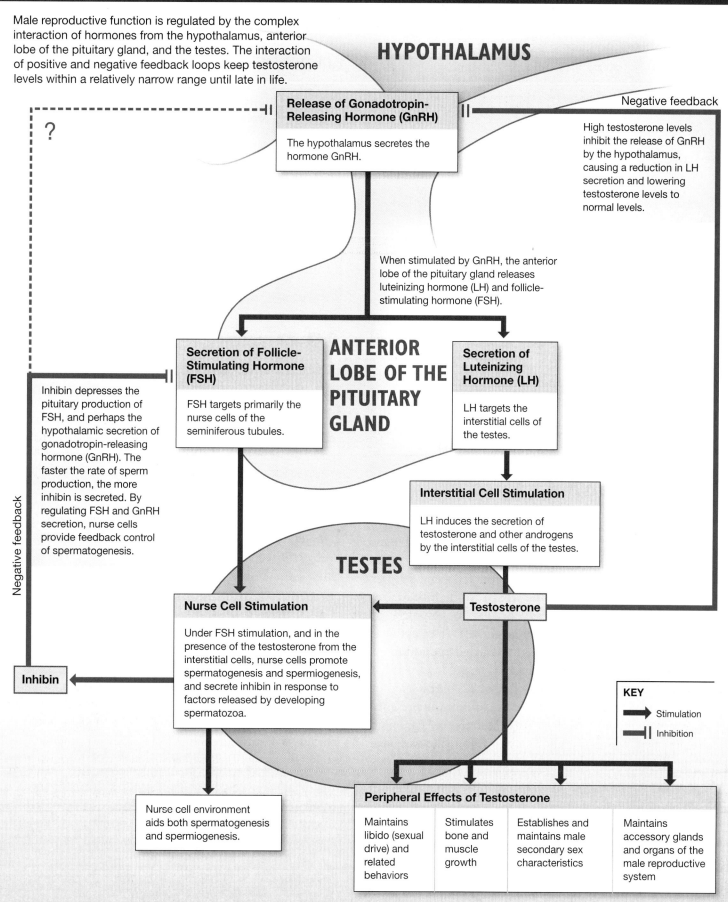

HYPOTHALAMUS

?

Negative feedback

Release of Gonadotropin-Releasing Hormone (GnRH)

The hypothalamus secretes the hormone GnRH.

High testosterone levels inhibit the release of GnRH by the hypothalamus, causing a reduction in LH secretion and lowering testosterone levels to normal levels.

When stimulated by GnRH, the anterior lobe of the pituitary gland releases luteinizing hormone (LH) and follicle-stimulating hormone (FSH).

Secretion of Follicle-Stimulating Hormone (FSH)

FSH targets primarily the nurse cells of the seminiferous tubules.

ANTERIOR LOBE OF THE PITUITARY GLAND

Secretion of Luteinizing Hormone (LH)

LH targets the interstitial cells of the testes.

Inhibin depresses the pituitary production of FSH, and perhaps the hypothalamic secretion of gonadotropin-releasing hormone (GnRH). The faster the rate of sperm production, the more inhibin is secreted. By regulating FSH and GnRH secretion, nurse cells provide feedback control of spermatogenesis.

Interstitial Cell Stimulation

LH induces the secretion of testosterone and other androgens by the interstitial cells of the testes.

Negative feedback

TESTES

Nurse Cell Stimulation

Under FSH stimulation, and in the presence of the testosterone from the interstitial cells, nurse cells promote spermatogenesis and spermiogenesis, and secrete inhibin in response to factors released by developing spermatozoa.

Testosterone

Inhibin

KEY

→ Stimulation

⊣ Inhibition

Nurse cell environment aids both spermatogenesis and spermiogenesis.

Peripheral Effects of Testosterone

Maintains libido (sexual drive) and related behaviors	Stimulates bone and muscle growth	Establishes and maintains male secondary sex characteristics	Maintains accessory glands and organs of the male reproductive system

CLINICAL NOTE

Priapism

Priapism is a prolonged, usually painful, penile erection that is not associated with sexual arousal. In many cases, the cause of priapism is unclear *(idiopathic)*. However, it is associated with sickle cell disease, spinal cord injury, spinal anesthesia, leukemia, and drugs. Most cases of priapism result from intracavernous injection of medications to treat impotence. In high spinal cord injury, priapism can occur if there is unopposed parasympathetic stimulation.

The erection seen in priapism is due to engorgement of the *corpora cavernosa*. The *corpora spongiosum* and the glans are not engorged as with a normal erection. Priapism is a urological emergency. Treatment within hours is necessary to prevent permanent injury.

Little blood flows into the erectile tissue of a flaccid penis. This is because the arterial branches in erectile tissue are constricted and the muscular partitions are tense. During **erection**, the penis stiffens and elevates to an upright position. How does erection occur? The parasympathetic innervation of the penile arteries involves neurons that release nitric oxide (NO) at their axon terminals. In response to NO, the smooth muscles in the arterial walls relax. At that time, the vessels dilate, blood flow increases, and the vascular channels fill with blood.

Hormones and Male Reproductive Function

The hormonal interactions that regulate male reproductive function are diagrammed in **Spotlight Figure 19-7**. (We introduced the major reproductive hormones in Chapter 10.) ↺ p. 367 The anterior lobe of the pituitary gland releases **follicle-stimulating hormone (FSH)** and **luteinizing hormone (LH)**. Their release occurs in response to **gonadotropin-releasing hormone (GnRH)**. This peptide is synthesized in the hypothalamus and carried to the anterior lobe by the hypophyseal portal system.

In males, FSH targets primarily nurse cells of the seminiferous tubules. Under FSH stimulation, and in the presence of testosterone from the interstitial cells, nurse cells promote spermatogenesis and spermiogenesis. LH in males was once called *interstitial cell-stimulating hormone, ICSH*, before it was found to be identical to LH in females. This hormone causes the secretion of testosterone and other androgens by the interstitial cells of the testes.

Testosterone is the most important androgen. It has numerous functions (**Spotlight Figure 19-7**). Testosterone production begins around the seventh week of fetal development

and reaches a peak after six months. The early surge in testosterone levels stimulates the differentiation of the male duct system and accessory organs and affects central nervous system (CNS) development. Testosterone secretion is low at birth. It accelerates markedly at puberty, initiating sexual maturation and the appearance of secondary sex characteristics. In adult males, negative feedback controls the level of testosterone production (**Spotlight Figure 19-7**).

CHECKPOINT

4. List the male reproductive structures.

5. On a warm day, would the cremaster muscle be contracted or relaxed? Why?

6. What happens when arteries within the penis dilate?

7. What effect would low FSH levels have on sperm production?

See the blue Answers tab at the back of the book.

19-3 Ovum production (oogenesis) occurs in the ovaries, and hormones from the pituitary gland and ovaries control female reproductive functions

Learning Objective Describe the structures of the female reproductive system; explain the process of oogenesis in the ovary; discuss the ovarian and uterine cycles; and summarize the events of the female reproductive cycle.

A woman's reproductive system produces sex hormones and gametes. It must also be able to protect and support a developing embryo and nourish a newborn infant. The main organs of the female reproductive system are the *ovaries*, the *uterine tubes*, the *uterus* (womb), the *vagina*, and the external genitalia (**Figure 19-8a**). As in males, a variety of accessory glands release secretions into the reproductive tract.

The Ovaries

The paired ovaries are small, lumpy, almond-shaped organs near the lateral walls of the pelvic cavity (**Figure 19-8b**). The ovaries have three main functions. They (1) produce female gametes, or oocytes; (2) secrete female sex hormones, including *estrogens* and *progesterone*; and (3) secrete inhibin, involved in the feedback control of pituitary FSH production.

A typical **ovary** is a flattened oval that measures approximately 5 cm long, 2.5 cm wide, and 8 mm thick (2 in. × 1 in. × 0.33 in.). It has a pale white or yellowish color. Its consistency resembles cottage cheese or lumpy oatmeal.

Figure 19-8 The Female Reproductive System.

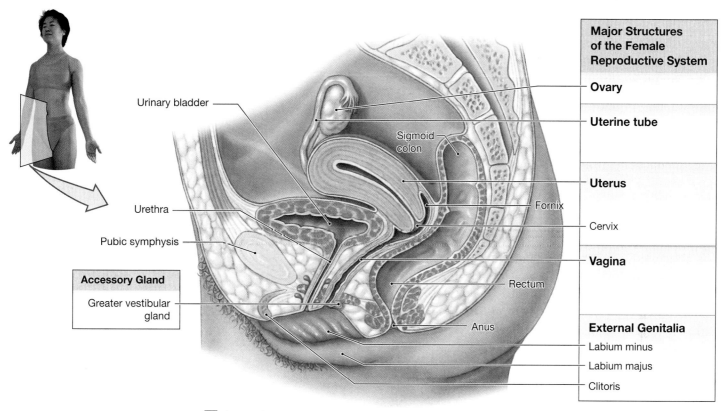

Urinary bladder

Urethra

Pubic symphysis

Accessory Gland

Greater vestibular gland

Sigmoid colon

Fornix

Cervix

Rectum

Anus

Major Structures of the Female Reproductive System

Ovary

Uterine tube

Uterus

Cervix

Vagina

External Genitalia

Labium minus

Labium majus

Clitoris

a A sagittal section showing the female reproductive organs.

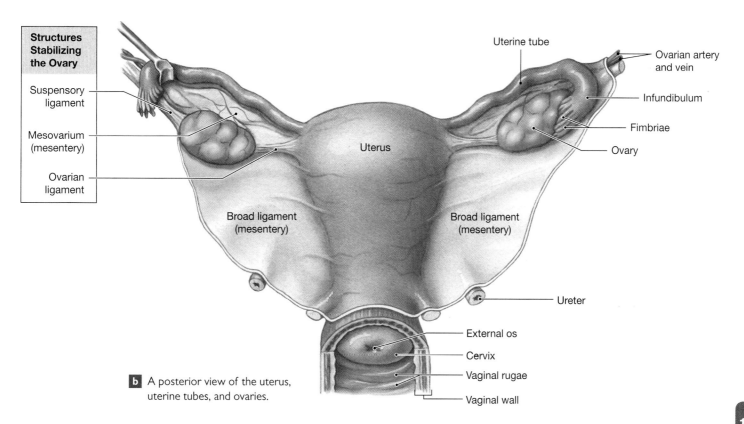

Structures Stabilizing the Ovary

Suspensory ligament

Mesovarium (mesentery)

Ovarian ligament

Broad ligament (mesentery)

Uterus

Uterine tube

Ovarian artery and vein

Infundibulum

Fimbriae

Ovary

Broad ligament (mesentery)

Ureter

External os

Cervix

Vaginal rugae

Vaginal wall

b A posterior view of the uterus, uterine tubes, and ovaries.

19

The position of each ovary is stabilized by a mesentery known as the *broad ligament* and by a pair of supporting ligaments. The mesentery also encloses the uterine tubes and uterus. The ligaments attached to each ovary extend to the uterus (*ovarian ligament*) and pelvic wall (*suspensory ligament*). The suspensory ligament contains the major blood vessels of the ovary: the *ovarian artery* and *ovarian vein*.

Oogenesis

Ovum production, or **oogenesis** (ō-ō-JEN-e-sis; *oon*, egg), begins before a woman's birth. The process accelerates at puberty and ends at *menopause* (*men*, month + *pausis*, cessation). Between puberty and menopause, oogenesis takes place in the ovaries each month, as part of the *ovarian cycle*.

Oogenesis is summarized in **Figure 19-9**. Female reproductive stem cells, called **oogonia** (ō-ō-GŌ-nē-uh), complete their mitotic divisions before birth. Their daughter cells, or **primary oocytes** (Ō-ō-sīts), begin to undergo meiosis between the third and seventh months of fetal development. They proceed as far as prophase of meiosis I. They then remain in that state until the individual reaches puberty. Not all primary oocytes survive until puberty. The ovaries have roughly 2 million at birth, but only about 400,000 at puberty. The rest of the primary oocytes degenerate in a process called *atresia* (a-TRĒ-zē-uh).

The nuclear events of meiosis in the ovary are the same as those in the testis, but the process differs in two important ways:

1. The cytoplasm of the primary oocyte is not evenly distributed during the meiotic divisions. Oogenesis produces one **secondary oocyte** containing most of that cytoplasm, and up to three small nonfunctional **polar bodies** that later disintegrate.

2. The ovary releases a secondary oocyte rather than a mature gamete. The secondary oocyte is suspended in metaphase of meiosis II. The second meiotic division is completed only *after* fertilization.

Follicle Development

Specialized structures called **ovarian follicles** (ō-VAR-ē-an FOL-i-klz) are the sites of both oocyte growth and meiosis I of oogenesis. In the outer portion of each ovary are clusters of primary oocytes, each surrounded by a single layer of *follicle cells*. The combination is known as a **primordial** (prī-MOR-dē-al) **follicle** (❶ in **Figure 19-10**). Beginning at puberty, primordial follicles are continuously activated to join other

Figure 19-9 Oogenesis. In oogenesis, each diploid primary oocyte that undergoes meiosis produces one haploid secondary oocyte plus two or three nonfunctional polar bodies.

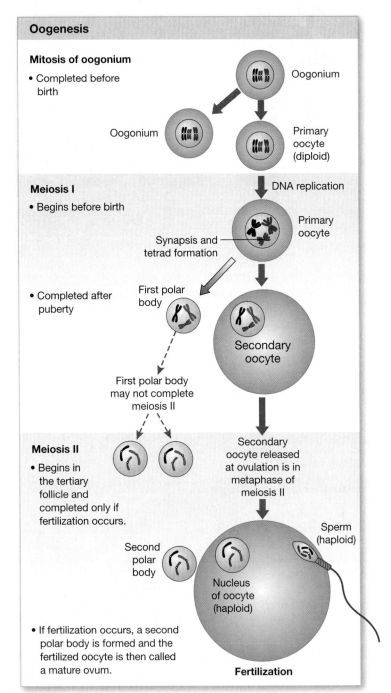

follicles already in development. The activating process is unknown, but local hormones or growth factors in the ovary may be involved. The activated primordial follicle will either eventually mature and be released as a secondary oocyte or degenerate (atresia).

Figure 19-10 Follicle Development and the Ovarian Cycle. The photomicrographs show the changes in a follicle as it develops. Tertiary follicles enter the ovarian cycle. The drawing of the ovary illustrates the sequence and relative sizes of the various stages in the development, ovulation, and degeneration of an ovarian follicle. Follicles do not physically move around the periphery of the ovary.

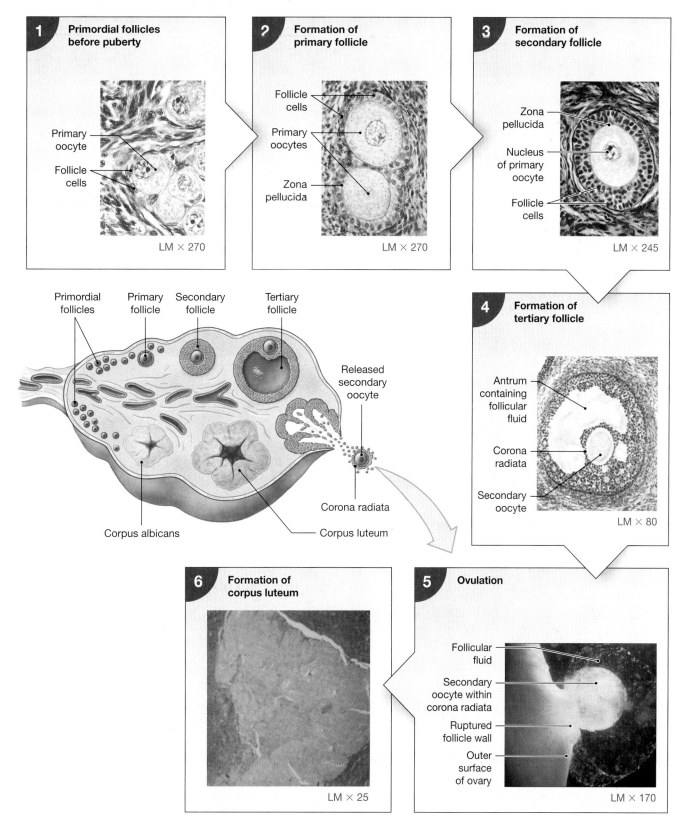

The preliminary steps in follicle development vary in length but may take almost a year to complete. Follicle development begins with the activation of primordial follicles into **primary follicles** (**2** in **Figure 19-10**). The follicle cells enlarge, divide, and form several layers of cells around the growing primary oocyte. The cells begin to produce sex hormones called estrogens. Microvilli from the surrounding follicle cells intermingle with microvilli originating at the surface of the oocyte. This region is called the **zona pellucida** (ZŌ-na pe-LOO-sid-uh; *pellucidus*, translucent). The microvilli increase the surface area available for transferring materials from the follicular cells to the growing oocyte.

Many primordial follicles develop into primary follicles, but only a few primary follicles mature further. This process is apparently under the control of a growth factor produced by the oocyte. The transformation begins as the wall of the follicle thickens. At this stage, the complex is known as a **secondary follicle** (**3** in **Figure 19-10**).

During the next two to three months, the follicle wall continues to grow and the deeper follicular cells begin secreting follicular fluid. This fluid accumulates between the inner and outer cellular layers of the follicle. The secondary follicle as a whole has doubled in size, and is now called a **tertiary follicle**. Tertiary follicles, also called *vesicular follicles*, continue to grow and accumulate follicular fluid.

The Ovarian Cycle

The tertiary follicles are then ready to complete their maturation as part of the 28-day **ovarian cycle**. The ovarian cycle is divided into a **follicular phase**, or *preovulatory phase*, and a **luteal phase**, or *postovulatory phase*. Separated by ovulation, each phase lasts approximately 14 days.

THE FOLLICULAR PHASE. At the start of each ovarian cycle, an ovary contains only a few tertiary follicles destined for further development. Stimulated by FSH, one of these follicles becomes dominant by day 5 of the cycle. It rapidly increases in size as the smaller follicles are resorbed. This tertiary follicle, also called a *mature graafian* (GRAF-ē-an) *follicle*, is roughly 15–20 mm in diameter (**4** in **Figure 19-10**). It is formed by days 10–14 of the ovarian cycle. It creates a bulge in the surface of the ovary. The oocyte and its covering of follicular cells project into the expanded central chamber of the follicle, the **antrum** (AN-trum).

Until this time, the primary oocyte has been suspended in prophase I. As the development of the remaining tertiary follicle ends, rising LH levels prompt the primary oocyte to complete meiosis I. This division produces a secondary oocyte (and a small, nonfunctional polar body; **Figure 19-9**). The secondary oocyte begins meiosis II but stops at metaphase. Meiosis II will not be completed unless fertilization occurs.

Generally, on day 14 of a 28-day ovarian cycle, the secondary oocyte and its surrounding follicular cells lose their connections with the follicular wall and float within the antrum. The follicular cells surrounding the oocyte are now known as the *corona radiata* (ko-RŌ-nuh rā-dē-A-tuh).

OVULATION. At **ovulation** (ōv-ū-LĀ-shun), the tertiary follicle releases the secondary oocyte (**5** in **Figure 19-10**). The distended follicular wall then ruptures, releasing the contents, including the secondary oocyte, into the pelvic cavity. The sticky follicular fluid keeps the corona radiata attached to the surface of the ovary near the ruptured wall of the follicle. Projections of the uterine tube or fluid currents created by its ciliated epithelium sweep the secondary oocyte into the uterine tube.

THE LUTEAL PHASE. The 14-day luteal phase of the ovarian cycle begins at ovulation. The empty follicle collapses. The remaining follicular cells invade the resulting cavity and multiply to create an endocrine structure known as the **corpus luteum** (LOO-tē-um; *lutea*, yellow) (**6** in **Figure 19-10**). The corpus luteum releases progesterone, the main hormone of the luteal phase. Unless fertilization takes place, the corpus luteum begins to degenerate roughly 12 days after ovulation. What remains is scar tissue called the *corpus albicans*. The disintegration of the corpus luteum marks the end of an ovarian cycle. A new ovarian cycle begins with the recruitment of another group of tertiary follicles and the rapid growth and development of one of them into a mature tertiary follicle under the stimulation of FSH.

CLINICAL NOTE

Mittelschmerz

Occasionally, ovulation is accompanied by midcycle abdominal pain known as *mittelschmerz*. It is thought that this pain is related to peritoneal irritation due to follicle rupture or bleeding at the time of ovulation. The unilateral lower quadrant pain is usually self-limited and may be accompanied by midcycle spotting. While some woman may report a low-grade fever, it should be noted that body temperature normally increases at the time of ovulation and remains elevated until the day prior to the onset of the menstrual period. Treatment is symptomatic.

CLINICAL NOTE

Ruptured Ovarian Cysts

Cysts are fluid-filled pockets. When they develop in the ovary, they can rupture and be a source of abdominal pain. When an egg is released from the ovary, a cyst, which is known as a *corpus luteum cyst*, is often left in its place. Occasionally, cysts develop independent of ovulation. When the cysts rupture, a small amount of blood spills into the abdomen. Because blood irritates the peritoneum, it can cause abdominal pain and rebound tenderness. Ovarian cysts may be found during a routine pelvic examination. In the field setting, however, your patient is likely to complain of moderate to severe unilateral abdominal pain, which may radiate to her back. She may also report a history of dyspareunia, irregular bleeding, or a delayed menstrual period. It is not uncommon for patients to rupture ovarian cysts during intercourse or physical activity. This often results in immediate, severe abdominal pain that causes the patient to immediately stop intercourse or other physical activity. Ruptured ovarian cysts may be associated with vaginal bleeding.

The Uterine Tubes

Each **uterine tube** (*Fallopian tube*, or *oviduct*) measures roughly 13 cm (5 in.) in length. The end closest to the ovary forms an expanded funnel, or **infundibulum** (in-fun-DIB-ū-lum; *infundibulum*, a funnel). It has numerous fingerlike projections that extend into the pelvic cavity and drape over the ovary (**Figure 19-8b**). The projections are called **fimbriae** (FIM-brē-ē). The fimbriae and the inner surfaces of the uterine tube are carpeted with cilia that beat toward the uterus.

Oocytes are transported by both ciliary movement and peristaltic contractions in the walls of the uterine tubes. It normally takes three to four days for the oocyte to travel to the uterine cavity. If fertilization is to occur, the secondary oocyte must encounter spermatozoa during the first 12–24 hours of its passage. Unfertilized oocytes degenerate in the uterine tubes or uterus without completing meiosis.

In addition to ciliated cells, the epithelium lining the uterine tubes contains *peg cells* and scattered mucin-secreting cells. The peg cells secrete a fluid that both completes the capacitation of spermatozoa and supplies nutrients to spermatozoa and the developing *pre-embryo* (the cluster of cells produced by initial cell divisions following fertilization).

The Uterus

The **uterus** (Ū-ter-us) protects, nourishes, and removes wastes for the developing *embryo* (weeks 1–8) and *fetus* (week 9 to delivery). In addition, contractions of the muscular uterus are important in ejecting the fetus at birth.

A typical uterus is small and pear-shaped. It is about 7.5 cm (3 in.) long and 5 cm (2 in.) in diameter (**Figure 19-8b**). It weighs 30–40 g (1–1.4 oz). Various ligaments and mesenteries stabilize it. In its normal position, the uterus bends anteriorly near its base (**Figure 19-8a**).

The uterus consists of two regions: the body and the cervix (**Figure 19-11**). The **body** is the largest region. The *fundus* is the rounded portion of the body superior to the attachment of the uterine tubes. Laterally, the body ends at a constriction known as the **isthmus**. The tubular **cervix** (SER-viks) is the inferior portion of the uterus. It projects a short distance into the vagina. There its surface surrounds the **external os** (*os*, an opening or mouth) of the uterus. The cervical canal opens into the **uterine cavity** at the **internal os**.

The uterine wall is made up of an inner **endometrium** (en-dō-MĒ-trē-um) and a muscular **myometrium** (mī-ō-MĒ-trē-um; *myo-*, muscle + *metra*, uterus), covered by the **perimetrium**, a layer of visceral peritoneum (**Figure 19-11**). The endometrium includes the epithelium lining the uterine cavity and the underlying connective tissues. *Uterine glands*, also called *endometrial glands*, open onto the endometrial surface and extend deep into the connective tissue layer almost to the myometrium. The myometrium consists of a thick mass of interwoven smooth muscle cells. In adult women of reproductive age who have not given birth, the uterine wall is about 1.5 cm (0.5 in.) thick.

The endometrium consists of a superficial *functional zone* and a deeper *basilar zone* adjacent to the myometrium. The structure of the basilar layer remains relatively constant over time. In contrast, the functional zone undergoes cyclical changes in response to sex hormone levels. These changes produce the characteristics of the monthly uterine cycle.

CLINICAL NOTE

Endometritis

An infection of the uterine lining called *endometritis* is an occasional complication of miscarriage, childbirth, or gynecological procedures such as dilatation and curettage (D and C). Commonly reported signs and symptoms include mild to severe lower abdominal pain; a bloody, foul-smelling discharge; and fever (101° to 104°F). The onset of symptoms is usually 48–72 hours after the gynecological procedure or miscarriage. These infections often mimic the presentation of PID and can be quite serious if not quickly treated with the appropriate antibiotics. Complications of endometritis may include sterility, sepsis, or even death.

Figure 19-11 The Uterus. A posterior view with the left portion of the uterus, left uterine tube, and left ovary in section.

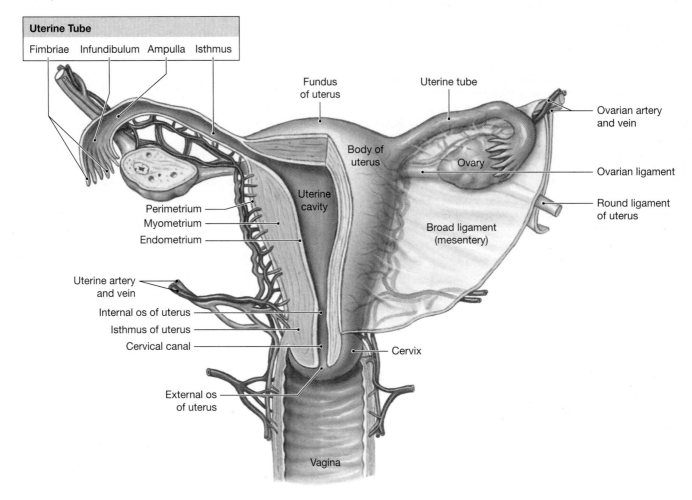

The Uterine Cycle

The **uterine cycle**, or *menstrual* (MEN-stroo-ul) *cycle*, is a repeating series of changes in the structure of the endometrium. The uterine cycle begins with puberty. The first cycle is known as **menarche** (me-NAR-kē). It typically occurs at ages 11–12. The cycles continue until ages 45–55, when **menopause** (MEN-ō-pawz), the last menstrual cycle, occurs. In the interim, the regular menstrual cycles are interrupted only by circumstances such as illness, stress, starvation, or pregnancy.

CLINICAL NOTE

Endometriosis

Endometriosis is a condition in which endometrial tissue is found outside of the uterus. Most commonly it is found in the abdomen and pelvis, although it has been found virtually everywhere in the body, including the central nervous system and lungs. Regardless of its site, the tissue responds to the hormonal changes associated with the menstrual cycle and thus bleeds cyclically. This bleeding causes inflammation, scarring of adjacent tissues, and the subsequent development of adhesions, particularly in the pelvic cavity.

Endometriosis is usually seen in women between the ages of 30 and 40 and is rarely seen in postmenopausal women.

The exact cause is unknown. The most common symptom is dull, cramping pelvic pain that is usually related to menstruation. Dyspareunia and abnormal uterine bleeding are also commonly reported. Painful bowel movements have also been reported when the endometrial tissue has invaded the gastrointestinal tract. Endometriosis is commonly diagnosed when the patient is being evaluated for infertility. Definitive treatment may include medical management with hormones, analgesics, and anti-inflammatory drugs, and/or surgery to remove the excessive endometrial tissue or adhesions from other organs.

CLINICAL NOTE

Pelvic Inflammatory Disease

Probably the most common cause of nontraumatic gynecological pain is pelvic inflammatory disease (PID). PID is an infection of the female reproductive tract that can be caused by bacteria, viruses, or fungi. The organs most commonly involved are the uterus, fallopian tubes, and ovaries. Occasionally the adjoining structures, such as the peritoneum and intestines, also become involved. PID is the most common cause of abdominal pain in women in the child-bearing years, and occurs in one percent of that population. The highest rate of infection occurs in sexually active women ages 15–24. The most common causes of PID are gonorrhea *(Neisseria gonorrhoeae)* or chlamydia *(Chlamydia trachomatis)*, although rarely streptococcus or staphylococcus bacteria may cause it. Commonly, gonorrhea or chlamydia progresses undetected in a female until frank PID develops (**Figure 19–12**).

Predisposing factors include multiple sexual partners, prior history of PID, recent gynecological procedure, or an IUD. Postinfection damage to the fallopian tubes is a common cause for infertility. PID may be either acute or chronic. If it is allowed to progress untreated, sepsis may develop. Additionally, PID

may cause adhesions, in which the pelvic organs "stick together." These adhesions are a common cause of chronic pelvic pain and increase the frequency of infertility and ectopic pregnancies.

While it is possible for a patient with pelvic inflammatory disease to be asymptomatic, most patients with PID complain of abdominal pain. It is often diffuse and located in the lower abdomen. It may be moderate to severe, which occasionally makes distinguishing it from appendicitis difficult. Pain may intensify either before or after the menstrual period. It may also worsen during sexual intercourse (dyspareunia), as movement of the cervix tends to cause increased discomfort. Patients with PID tend to walk with a shuffling gait, since walking often intensifies their pain. In severe cases, fever, chills, nausea, vomiting, or even sepsis may accompany PID. Occasionally, patients have a foul-smelling, often yellow, vaginal discharge, as well as irregular menses. Midcycle bleeding is also common.

The uterine cycle averages 28 days in length, but it can range from 21 to 35 days in healthy individuals. It has three stages: *menses,* the *proliferative phase,* and the *secretory phase.*

CLINICAL NOTE

Menstrual Irregularities

Menstrual irregularities are common. Normal menstrual flow usually lasts less than a week. On the average, about 35 mL (a little more than an ounce) of blood is lost. A disturbance in the menstruation that results in abnormal uterine bleeding is called *dysfunctional uterine bleeding.* It is most commonly associated with a cycle where ovulation has not occurred. The absence of a period is termed amenorrhea. Pregnancy is the most common cause of amenorrhea, although hormonal factors are also frequently implicated. Pelvic pain associated with the onset of menses is called *dysmenorrhea.* Usually, the discomfort begins shortly before the onset of menstruation and ends by the second day. Dysmenorrhea improves in most women with use of oral contraceptives.

MENSES. The uterine cycle begins with the onset of **menses** (MEN-sēz), a period marked by the degeneration of the functional zone of the endometrium. This process is triggered by a decline in progesterone and estrogen levels as the corpus luteum disintegrates. Endometrial arteries constrict, which reduces blood flow to this region. Deprived of oxygen and nutrients, the secretory glands, epithelial cells, and

other tissues of the functional zone begin to die. Eventually the weakened arterial walls rupture, and blood pours into the connective tissues of the functional zone. Blood cells and degenerating tissues break away and enter the uterine cavity, to be lost through the vagina. The shedding of tissue continues until the entire functional zone has been lost. This process is called **menstruation** (men-strū-Ā-shun). It usually lasts one to seven days. About 35–50 mL (1.2 to 1.7 oz) of blood is lost. Painful menstruation, or *dysmenorrhea,* can result from uterine inflammation, myometrial contractions ("cramps"), or conditions involving adjacent pelvic structures.

THE PROLIFERATIVE PHASE. The **proliferative phase** begins in the days after menses. The surviving epithelial cells of the uterine glands multiply and spread across the surface of the endometrium. This repair process is stimulated by rising estrogen levels that accompany the growth of another set of ovarian follicles. By the time ovulation takes place, the functional zone is several millimeters thick, and its new set of uterine glands is secreting a mucus rich in glycogen. In addition, the entire functional zone is filled with small arteries that branch from larger trunks in the myometrium.

THE SECRETORY PHASE. During the **secretory phase** of the uterine cycle, the endometrium prepares for the arrival of a developing embryo. The uterine glands enlarge and increase their rates of secretion. This activity is stimulated by progesterone and estrogens from the corpus luteum. The secretory phase begins at ovulation and lasts as long as the corpus luteum remains intact. Secretory activities peak about 12 days after ovulation. Over the next day or two glandular activity declines, and the uterine cycle ends. A new cycle then begins with the onset of menses and the disintegration of the functional zone.

The Vagina

The **vagina** (va-JĪ-nuh) is an elastic, muscular tube extending between the uterus and the exterior. It opens into the *vestibule*, a space bounded by the external genitalia (**Figure 19-8a**). The vagina is typically 7.5–9 cm (3–3.6 in.) long. Its diameter varies because it is highly distensible. The cervix of the uterus projects into the vagina (**Figure 19-11**). The shallow recess surrounding the cervical protrusion is known as the **fornix** (FOR-niks) (**Figure 19-8a**). The vagina lies parallel to the rectum, and the two are in close contact posteriorly. The urethra extends along the superior wall of the vagina from the urinary bladder to the urethral opening, which opens into the vestibule.

The vaginal walls contain a network of blood vessels and layers of smooth muscle. The lining is moistened by the mucous secretions of the cervical glands and by the movement of water across the permeable epithelium. The **hymen**

(HĪ-men) is an elastic epithelial fold of variable size that partially blocks the entrance to the vagina. An intact hymen is typically stretched or torn during first sexual intercourse, tampon use, pelvic examination, or physical activity. The two *bulbospongiosus muscles* extend along either side of the vaginal entrance. Contractions of the bulbospongiosus muscles constrict the vagina (see **Figure 7-17a**, p. 224). These muscles cover the *vestibular bulbs*, masses of erectile tissue on either side of the vaginal entrance (**Figure 19-12**).

The vagina has three major functions. It (1) serves as a passageway for the elimination of menstrual fluids; (2) receives the penis during sexual intercourse and holds spermatozoa prior to their passage into the uterus; and (3) forms the lower portion of the birth canal, through which the fetus passes during delivery.

The vagina normally contains resident bacteria supported by nutrients in the cervical mucus. The metabolic activity of these bacteria creates an acidic environment, which restricts the growth of many pathogens. Inflammation of the vaginal canal, known as *vaginitis* (vaj-i-NĪ-tis), is typically caused by fungi, bacteria, or parasites. In addition to any discomfort that may result, the condition may reduce fertility by lowering the survival rate of sperm.

Figure 19-12 The Female External Genitalia. The left labium minus has been removed to show erectile tissue (left vestibular bulb) and the left greater vestibular gland.

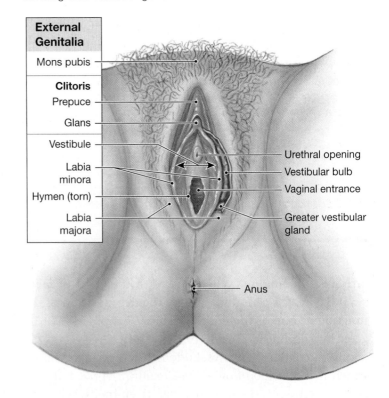

CLINICAL NOTE

Amenorrhea

If menarche does not occur by age 16, or if a woman's normal menstrual cycle becomes interrupted for six months or more, the condition of amenorrhea (ā-men-ō-RĒ-uh) exists. *Primary amenorrhea* is the failure to begin menses. This condition may indicate developmental abnormalities, such as nonfunctional ovaries, the absence of a uterus, or some endocrine or genetic disorder. It can also result from malnutrition: Puberty is delayed if leptin levels are too low. ⊃ p. 368

Severe physical or emotional stresses (such as drastic weight loss, anorexia nervosa, and severe depression or grief) can cause transient *secondary amenorrhea*. In effect, the reproductive system gets "switched off." Amenorrhea has also been observed in marathon runners and other women engaged in rigorous training programs, which may severely reduce body lipid reserves.

The External Genitalia

The area containing the female external genitalia is the **vulva** (VUL-vuh), or *pudendum* (pū-DEN-dum; **Figure 19-12**). The vagina opens into the **vestibule**, a central space bounded by the **labia minora** (LĀ bē uh mi NOR uh; *labia*, lips; sin gular, *labium minus*). The labia minora are covered with smooth, hairless skin. The urethra opens into the vestibule just anterior to the vaginal entrance. Anterior to the urethral opening, the **clitoris** (KLIT-ō-ris) projects into the vestibule. The clitoris is derived from the same embryonic structures as the penis in males. Internally, it contains erectile tissue comparable to the corpora cavernosa of the penis. A small erectile *glans* sits atop it. The vestibular bulbs are erectile tissues along the sides of the vestibule. They are comparable to the corpus spongiosum in the male penis. They engorge with blood during sexual arousal. Extensions of the labia minora encircle the body of the clitoris, forming its *prepuce*, or *hood*.

A variable number of small **lesser vestibular glands** discharge secretions onto the exposed surface of the vestibule, keeping it moist. During sexual arousal, a pair of ducts discharges the secretions of the **greater vestibular glands** into the vestibule near the vaginal entrance (**Figure 19-8**). These mucous glands resemble the bulbo-urethral glands of males.

The mons pubis and labia majora form the outer limits of the vulva. The prominent bulge of the **mons pubis** is created by adipose tissue beneath the skin anterior to the pubic symphysis. Adipose tissue also accumulates in the fleshy **labia majora** (singular, *labium majus*), which encircle and partially conceal the labia minora and vestibular structures.

The Mammary Glands

A newborn cannot yet fend for itself. The infant gains nourishment from the milk secreted by the maternal **mammary glands** (**Figure 19-13**). Milk production, or **lactation** (lak-TĀ-shun), takes place in these glands. In females, the mammary glands are specialized organs of the integumentary system. They are controlled by hormones of the reproductive system and of the *placenta*, a temporary structure that provides the embryo and fetus with nutrients.

Each breast contains a mammary gland within the subcutaneous tissue of the *pectoral fat pad* beneath the skin. Each breast has a **nipple**, a small conical projection where the

Figure 19-13 The Mammary Gland of the Left Breast. Lobes of glandular tissue within each mammary gland are responsible for the production of breast milk.

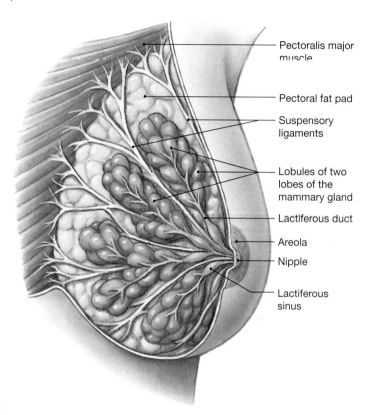

Pectoralis major muscle

Pectoral fat pad

Suspensory ligaments

Lobules of two lobes of the mammary gland

Lactiferous duct

Areola

Nipple

Lactiferous sinus

ducts of the underlying mammary gland open onto the body surface. The reddish-brown skin surrounding each nipple is the **areola** (a-RĒ-ō-luh). Large sebaceous glands beneath the areolar surface give it a grainy texture.

CLINICAL NOTE

Endocrine Effects on the Breast

At puberty, increasing levels of *estrogen* stimulate growth of the breast's *mammary gland*. In pregnancy, the placenta secretes large quantities of estrogens that stimulate growth of the ductal system. Once the ductal system has developed, *progesterone* causes final development of the breasts into milk-secreting glands. While estrogens and progesterone stimulate development of the breasts, they actually inhibit the secretion of milk.

Prolactin causes the production of milk. The prolactin level begins to rise around the fifth week of pregnancy and continues until delivery. When the placenta is delivered, the levels of estrogen and progesterone drop markedly, and the breasts begin to secrete milk. Finally, milk is "let down," or ejected, by the nipples due to stimulation by oxytocin. Suckling of the breast by the baby sends sensory impulses to the hypothalamus, which results in oxytocin secretion.

CLINICAL NOTE

Breast Cancer

Breast cancer is a malignant, metastasizing tumor of the mammary gland. Almost 90 percent of breast cancers begin in the ducts and lobes of the mammary glands. They are called *ductal carcinomas* and *lobular carcinomas*, respectively. If the tumor cells have spread outside of a duct or lobule and into the surrounding tissue, the cancer is called an *invasive ductal* or *lobular carcinoma*. Cancers that have not spread are called *in situ* ("in place"). They are known as *ductal carcinoma in situ* and *lobular carcinoma in situ*.

Breast cancer is the leading cause of death in women between the ages of 35 and 45, but it is most common in women over age 50. An estimated 12 percent of U.S. women will develop breast cancer at some point in their lifetime. Risk factors include (1) a family history of breast cancer, (2) first pregnancy after age 30, and (3) early menarche (first menstrual period) or late menopause (last menstrual period). Breast cancers in males are very rare, but about 400 men die from the disease each year in the United States.

CLINICAL NOTE

Dermoid Cysts

An interesting class of tumors of the female reproductive system is the teratomas. Teratomas are divided into three categories: (1) mature (benign), (2) immature (malignant), and (3) monodermal, or highly specialized. The vast majority of benign teratomas are cystic and are more commonly referred to as *dermoid cysts*. These cysts are lined by skin and are usually filled with a sebaceous cheesy substance. Often, matted hair and teeth can be found within the cyst. The cyst wall arises from stratified squamous epithelium. In more complex cysts, layers of germ cells can give rise to cartilage, bone, thyroid tissue, or organoid formation.

The origination of dermoid tumors has been a matter of fascination for centuries. Some common beliefs blamed witches, night-mares, or adultery with the devil as possible causes. Interestingly, the karyotype of all benign ovarian teratomas is 46,XX (normal human female). Dermoid tumors are usually easily removed, sparing the ovary and uterine tube.

The glandular tissue of a mammary gland consists of separate lobes, each made up of several lobules containing milk glands. Ducts leaving the lobules merge into a single **lactiferous** (lak-TIF-er-us) **duct**. Near the nipple, that forms an expanded chamber called a **lactiferous sinus**. Typically, 15–20 lactiferous sinuses open onto the surface of each nipple.

Dense connective tissue surrounds the duct system and forms partitions between the lobes and lobules. These bands of connective tissue, the *suspensory ligaments of the breast*, originate in the dermis of the overlying skin. A layer of areolar connective tissue separates the mammary gland complex from the underlying pectoralis muscles.

Hormones and the Female Reproductive Cycle

Spotlight Figure 19-14 shows the regulation of female reproduction. As in males, both pituitary and gonadal hormones control the activity of the reproductive system. However, the regulatory pattern in females is much more complicated than in males. In females, circulating hormones must coordinate the ovarian and uterine cycles so that the **female reproductive cycle** results in the proper functioning of all reproductive activities.

Hormones and the Follicular Phase

The **follicular phase** (or *preovulatory phase*) of the ovarian cycle begins each month when FSH from the anterior lobe of the pituitary gland stimulates the rapid growth of a dominant tertiary follicle from a small group of slower-developing tertiary follicles (**Figure 19-10**, p. 656). As the follicle cells enlarge and multiply, they release steroid hormones collectively known as **estrogens**. The most important estrogen is **estradiol** (estra-DĪ-ol). Estrogens have multiple functions. They include (1) stimulating bone and muscle growth; (2) establishing and maintaining female secondary sex characteristics, such as the distributions of body hair and adipose tissue deposits; (3) affecting CNS activity (especially in the hypothalamus, where estrogens increase sexual drive); (4) maintaining functional accessory reproductive glands and organs; and (5) initiating the repair and growth of the endometrium.

Spotlight Figure 19-14 diagrams the hormonal regulation of ovarian activity. Early in the follicular phase, estrogen and inhibin levels are low. The estrogens and inhibin have complementary effects on the secretion of FSH and LH: Low levels of estrogen inhibit LH and FSH secretion. As follicular development proceeds, the levels of circulating estrogens and inhibin rise as the follicular cells increase in number and in secretory activity. As tertiary follicles develop, FSH levels decline due to the negative-feedback effects of inhibin, and estrogen levels continue to rise. Despite the slow decline in FSH concentrations, the combination of estrogens, FSH, and LH continues to support follicular development and maturation.

Estrogen concentrations take a sharp upturn in the second week of the ovarian cycle, with the development of a tertiary follicle as it enlarges in preparation for ovulation. The rapid increase in estrogens leads to the secretion of FSH and LH by acting on the hypothalamus and stimulating the production of GnRH. The pituitary gland also becomes more sensitive to GnRH and contributes to the rise in FSH and LH. At roughly day 10 of the cycle, the effect of estrogen on LH secretion also changes from inhibition to stimulation. At about day 14, estrogen levels peak with the maturation of the tertiary follicle. The high estrogen concentration then triggers a massive release, or surge, of LH from the anterior lobe of the pituitary gland. This LH surge triggers the rupture of the follicular wall and ovulation.

Hormones and the Luteal Phase

The **luteal phase**, or *postovulatory phase*, of the ovarian cycle begins as the high LH levels that triggered ovulation also stimulate the remaining follicular cells to form a corpus luteum. The yellow color of the corpus luteum results from its lipid reserves, which are used to manufacture the steroid hormone **progesterone** (prō-JES-ter-ōn). Progesterone is the principal hormone of the luteal phase. It prepares the uterus for pregnancy by stimulating the growth and development of the blood supply and secretory glands of the endometrium. Progesterone also stimulates metabolic activity and elevates basal body temperature.

LH levels remain elevated for only two days, but that is long enough to stimulate the formation of a functional corpus luteum. Progesterone secretion continues at relatively high levels for the next week. Unless pregnancy occurs, however, the corpus luteum begins to degenerate. Roughly 12 days after ovulation, the corpus luteum becomes non-functional, and progesterone and estrogen levels fall markedly. With this decline, hypothalamic production of GnRH is no longer inhibited and GnRH production increases. The increased secretion of GnRH, in turn, leads to increased FSH production in the anterior lobe of the pituitary gland, and the ovarian cycle begins again.

Hormones and the Uterine Cycle

The declines in progesterone and estrogen levels that accompany the breakdown of the corpus luteum result in menses (**Spotlight Figure 19-14**). The loss of endometrial tissue continues for several days, until rising estrogen levels stimulate the regeneration of the functional zone of the endometrium.

The proliferative phase continues until rising progesterone levels mark the arrival of the secretory phase. The combination of estrogen and progesterone then causes the uterine glands to enlarge and increase their secretions.

CLINICAL NOTE

Infertility

Infertility (*sterility*) is usually defined as an inability to achieve pregnancy after one year of appropriately timed sexual intercourse. Problems with infertility are relatively common. An estimated 10–15 percent of married couples in the United States are infertile, and another 10 percent are unable to have as many children as they desire. It is not surprising that the treatment of infertility has become a major medical industry! Recent advances in our understanding of reproductive physiology offer new solutions to fertility problems as varied as low sperm count, abnormal spermatozoa, inadequate maternal hormone levels, problems with oocyte production or oocyte transport from ovary to uterine tube, blocked uterine tubes, abnormal oocytes, and an abnormal uterine environment. Procedures meant to resolve these difficulties are known as *assisted reproductive technologies*.

Hormones and Body Temperature

At the time of ovulation, the basal body temperature (BBT) declines sharply, making the temperature rise over the following day even more noticeable (**Spotlight Figure 19-14**).

Urine tests that detect LH are available, and testing daily for several days before expected ovulation can detect the LH surges more reliably than the BBT. This information can be very important for individuals who wish to avoid or promote a pregnancy because fertilization typically occurs within a day of ovulation. After that time, oocyte viability and the likelihood of successful pregnancy decrease markedly.

CHECKPOINT

8. Name the structures of the female reproductive system.

9. As the result of infections such as gonorrhea, scar tissue can block both uterine tubes. How would this blockage affect a woman's ability to conceive?

10. What benefit does the acidic pH of the vagina provide?

11. Which layer of the uterus is sloughed off, or shed, during menstruation?

12. Would the blockage of a single lactiferous sinus interfere with delivery of milk to the nipple? Explain.

13. What changes would you expect to observe in the ovarian cycle if the LH surge did not take place?

14. What effect would blockage of progesterone receptors in the uterus have on the endometrium?

15. What event in the uterine cycle occurs when estrogen and progesterone levels decline?

See the blue Answers tab at the back of the book.

The ovarian and uterine cycles must operate on the same time scale to ensure proper reproductive function. If the two cycles are not properly coordinated, infertility results. A female who does not ovulate cannot conceive, even if her uterus is perfectly normal. A female who ovulates normally, but whose uterus is not ready to support an embryo, will also be infertile.

As in males, GnRH from the hypothalamus regulates reproductive function in females. However, in females, GnRH levels change throughout the course of the ovarian cycle.

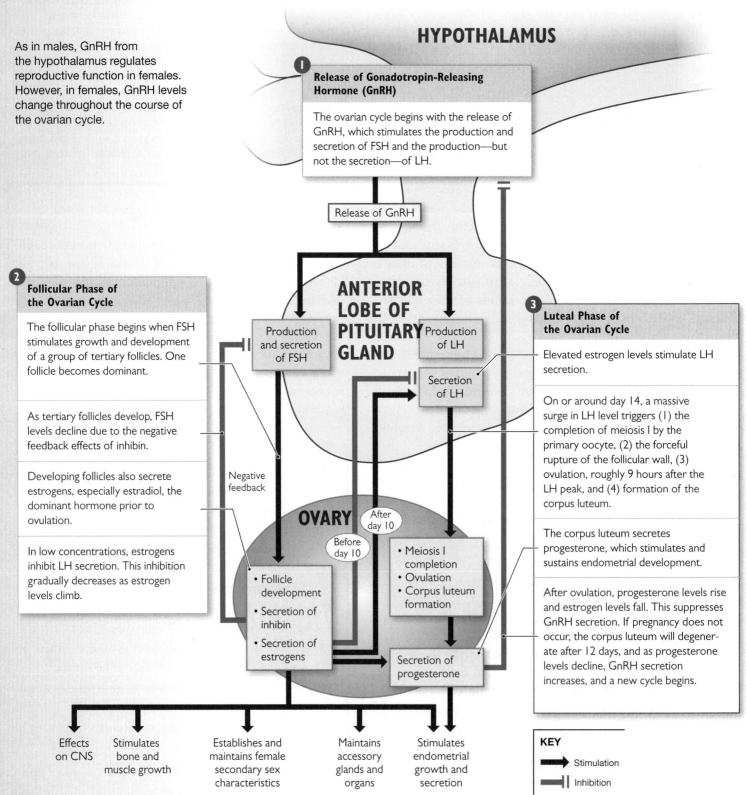

HYPOTHALAMUS

1 **Release of Gonadotropin-Releasing Hormone (GnRH)**

The ovarian cycle begins with the release of GnRH, which stimulates the production and secretion of FSH and the production—but not the secretion—of LH.

Release of GnRH

ANTERIOR LOBE OF PITUITARY GLAND

Production and secretion of FSH

Production of LH

Secretion of LH

2 **Follicular Phase of the Ovarian Cycle**

The follicular phase begins when FSH stimulates growth and development of a group of tertiary follicles. One follicle becomes dominant.

As tertiary follicles develop, FSH levels decline due to the negative feedback effects of inhibin.

Developing follicles also secrete estrogens, especially estradiol, the dominant hormone prior to ovulation.

In low concentrations, estrogens inhibit LH secretion. This inhibition gradually decreases as estrogen levels climb.

Negative feedback

OVARY

After day 10

Before day 10

• Follicle development
• Secretion of inhibin
• Secretion of estrogens

• Meiosis I completion
• Ovulation
• Corpus luteum formation

Secretion of progesterone

3 **Luteal Phase of the Ovarian Cycle**

Elevated estrogen levels stimulate LH secretion.

On or around day 14, a massive surge in LH level triggers (1) the completion of meiosis I by the primary oocyte, (2) the forceful rupture of the follicular wall, (3) ovulation, roughly 9 hours after the LH peak, and (4) formation of the corpus luteum.

The corpus luteum secretes progesterone, which stimulates and sustains endometrial development.

After ovulation, progesterone levels rise and estrogen levels fall. This suppresses GnRH secretion. If pregnancy does not occur, the corpus luteum will degenerate after 12 days, and as progesterone levels decline, GnRH secretion increases, and a new cycle begins.

Effects on CNS

Stimulates bone and muscle growth

Establishes and maintains female secondary sex characteristics

Maintains accessory glands and organs

Stimulates endometrial growth and secretion

KEY

→ Stimulation

⊣ Inhibition

This illustration links together the key events in the ovarian and uterine cycles. The monthly hormonal fluctuations cause physiological changes that affect core body temperature. During the follicular phase—when estrogens are the dominant hormones—the **basal body temperature**, or the resting body temperature measured upon awakening in the morning, is about 0.3°C (0.5°F) lower than it is during the luteal phase, when progesterone dominates.

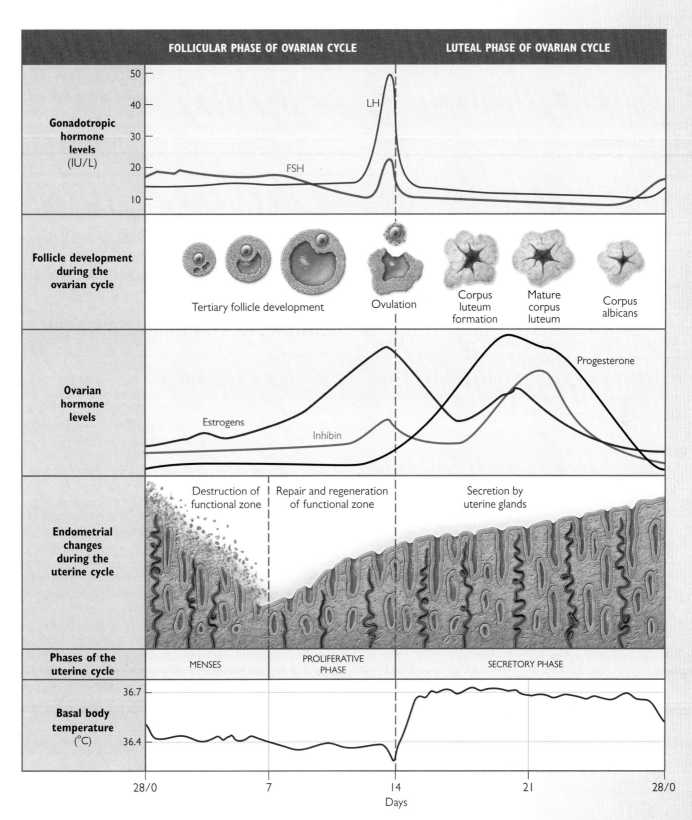

FOLLICULAR PHASE OF OVARIAN CYCLE   **LUTEAL PHASE OF OVARIAN CYCLE**

Gonadotropic hormone levels (IU/L)

50 — 40 — 30 — 20 — 10 —

LH

FSH

Follicle development during the ovarian cycle

Tertiary follicle development   Ovulation   Corpus luteum formation   Mature corpus luteum   Corpus albicans

Ovarian hormone levels

Estrogens   Inhibin   Progesterone

Endometrial changes during the uterine cycle

Destruction of functional zone | Repair and regeneration of functional zone | Secretion by uterine glands

Phases of the uterine cycle

MENSES | PROLIFERATIVE PHASE | SECRETORY PHASE

Basal body temperature (°C)

36.7   36.4

28/0   7   14   21   28/0

Days

759

19-4 The autonomic nervous system influences male and female sexual function

Learning Objective Discuss the physiology of sexual intercourse in males and females.

Sexual intercourse, also known as *coitus* (KŌ-i-tus) or *copulation*, introduces semen into the female reproductive tract.

Male Sexual Function

Male sexual function is coordinated by reflex pathways involving both divisions of the ANS. During sexual **arousal**, erotic thoughts or the stimulation of sensory nerves in the genital region increase the parasympathetic outflow over the pelvic nerves. This outflow leads to erection of the penis (discussed on p. 651). The skin covering the glans penis contains numerous sensory receptors. Erection tenses the skin and increases sensitivity. Subsequent stimulation can initiate secretion from the bulbo-urethral glands, lubricating the urethra and the surface of the glans penis.

During intercourse, the sensory receptors in the penis are rhythmically stimulated. This stimulation eventually results in emission and ejaculation. Emission takes place under sympathetic stimulation. The process begins with peristaltic contractions of the ampulla of the ductus deferens. These contractions push fluid and spermatozoa through the ejaculatory ducts and into the urethra. The seminal glands then begin contracting. Waves of contraction in the prostate gland follow. While these contractions are proceeding, sympathetic commands contract the urinary bladder and close the internal urethral sphincter. These actions prevent semen from entering the bladder.

Ejaculation takes place as powerful, rhythmic contractions appear in the *ischiocavernosus* and *bulbospongiosus* muscles, two superficial skeletal muscles of the pelvic floor. (Their positions are shown in **Figure 7-17b, p. 224.**) Ejaculation is associated with intensely pleasurable sensations, an experience known as male **orgasm** (OR-gazm). Several other physiological changes also occur at this time. They include temporary increases in heart rate and blood pressure.

After ejaculation, blood begins to leave the erectile tissue, and the erection begins to subside. This subsidence is called *detumescence* (dē-tū-MES-ens). It is brought about by the sympathetic nervous system. **Impotence**, or **erectile dysfunction (ED)**, is an inability to achieve or maintain an erection.

CLINICAL NOTE

Sexually Transmitted Diseases

Sexual activity carries with it the risk of infection by a variety of microorganisms. The consequences of such an infection range from merely inconvenient to potentially lethal. Sexually transmitted diseases (STDs), also called sexually transmitted infections, are transferred from person to person during sexual activity, primarily or exclusively by sexual intercourse. At least two dozen bacterial, viral, and fungal infections are currently recognized as STDs. The bacterium *Chlamydia* can cause PID and infertility. AIDS, caused by a virus, is deadly. The incidence of STDs has been increasing in the United States since 1984. An estimated 20 million new cases are diagnosed each year. Almost half are in persons aged 15–24. Poverty, prostitution, intravenous drug use (needle sharing exchanges body fluids), and the appearance of drug-resistant pathogens all contribute to the problem.

Female Sexual Function

The events in female sexual function are largely comparable to those in males. During sexual arousal, parasympathetic activation leads to an engorgement of the erectile

CLINICAL NOTE

Date Rape

Date rape, also called *acquaintance rape*, is defined as forced, unwanted intercourse with a person known by the victim. Sometimes, physical force or threats are used to force the victim to cooperate. In many instances, the victim is given a sedative drug that allows the assailant to carry out the assault.

One of the most frequently used drugs in date rape is the benzodiazepine *flunitrazepam*. Also known as *Rohypnol*, or "roofies," flunitrazepam is used in the short-term management of insomnia and as a sedative-hypnotic and preanesthetic medication. It has pharmacological effects similar to those of diazepam (Valium), although Rohypnol is approximately 10 times more potent. The effects begin within 30 minutes and peak within 2 hours. It has significant amnestic properties, similar to those seen with the sedative midazolam (Versed). Rohypnol is neither manufactured nor sold legally in the United States. It is produced and sold by prescription in Europe and Latin America. It is supplied in 1- and 2-milligram tablets. Rohypnol enters the United States through several routes. It is transported across the Mexican border to Texas and then delivered to other parts of the country. It also enters South Florida from Columbia via international mail services or commercial airlines.

The effects of Rohypnol can be reversed with flumazenil (Romazicon) if needed. Because of Rohypnol's amnestic properties, victims may not even remember the assault. They may wake up in a strange place with their clothing in disarray. Many are too embarrassed to seek help after the assault.

tissues of the clitoris and vestibular bulbs. Secretion from cervical mucous glands and the greater vestibular glands increases for the same reason. Clitoral erection increases the sensitivity of receptors to stimulation. The cervical and vestibular glands lubricate the vaginal walls. A network of blood vessels in the vaginal walls fills with blood at this time. Vaginal surfaces are also moistened by fluid from underlying connective tissues. Parasympathetic stimulation also causes blood vessels at the nipples to become engorged. As a result, the nipples become more sensitive to touch and pressure.

During sexual intercourse, rhythmic contact of the penis with the clitoris and vaginal walls may be reinforced by touch sensations from the breasts and other stimuli (visual, olfactory, and auditory). All this stimulation can lead to orgasm. Female orgasm is accompanied by peristaltic contractions of the uterine and vaginal walls and by rhythmic contractions of the bulbospongiosus and ischiocavernosus muscles. The contractions of these two muscles give rise to the intensely pleasurable sensations of orgasm.

CHECKPOINT

16. List the physiological events of sexual intercourse in both sexes, and note those that occur in males but not in females.

17. An inability to contract the ischiocavernosus and bulbospongiosus muscles would interfere with which part of the sexual response in males?

18. What changes take place in females during sexual arousal as the result of increased parasympathetic stimulation?

See the blue Answers tab at the back of the book.

19-5 With age, decreasing levels of reproductive hormones cause functional changes

Learning Objective Describe the reproductive system changes that occur with aging.

Aging affects all body systems. The reproductive systems of men and women are no exception. These systems become fully functional in both sexes at puberty. After that, the most striking age-related changes in the female reproductive system take place at menopause. Comparable changes in the male reproductive system occur more gradually and over a longer period of time.

Menopause

Menopause is usually defined as the time when ovulation and menstruation cease. Menopause typically takes place at ages 45–55. In the years immediately preceding it, the ovarian and menstrual cycles become irregular. This time period is called *perimenopause*. It normally begins at age 40. A shortage of primordial follicles is the underlying cause of irregular cycles. It has been estimated that almost 7 million potential oocytes are in fetal ovaries after five months of development. The number decreases to about 2 million oocytes at birth. A few hundred thousand remain at puberty. By age 50, there are often no primordial follicles left to respond to FSH. In *premature menopause*, this depletion takes place before age 40.

Menopause is accompanied by a decline in circulating estrogens and progesterone, and a sharp and sustained increase in the production of GnRH, FSH, and LH. The decrease in estrogen levels leads to reductions in the sizes of the uterus and breasts, and thinning of the urethral and vaginal walls. The reduced estrogen concentrations have also been linked to the development of osteoporosis. Presumably, bone is deposited at a slower rate.

A variety of neural effects are also reported. They include "hot flashes," anxiety, and depression. Hot flashes typically begin while estrogen levels are decreasing and cease when estrogen levels reach minimal values. These periods of elevated body temperature are associated with surges in LH production. The hormonal processes involved in other CNS effects of menopause are not well understood. The risks of atherosclerosis and other forms of cardiovascular disease also increase after menopause.

The majority of women have only mild symptoms. Some women, however, have unpleasant symptoms in perimenopause or during or after menopause. For most of these women, hormone replacement therapy involving a combination of estrogens and progestins can control the neural and vascular changes associated with menopause. However, recent studies suggest that taking estrogen-replacement therapy for more than five years increases the risk of heart disease, breast cancer, Alzheimer's disease, blood clots, and stroke.

The Male Climacteric

The male reproductive system changes more gradually than does the female reproductive system. The period of declining reproductive function is known as the **male climacteric**, or *andropause*. It corresponds to perimenopause in women. Levels of circulating testosterone begin to decline between ages 50 and 60, and levels of FSH and LH increase. Sperm production continues. (Men well into their 80s can father children.) Older men experience a gradual reduction in sexual activity. This decrease may be linked to declining testosterone levels. Some clinicians suggest testosterone replacement therapy to enhance libido (sexual drive) in older men, but this may increase the risk of prostate disease.

CHECKPOINT

19. Define menopause.
20. Why does the level of FSH increase and remain high during menopause?
21. What is the male climacteric?

See the blue Answers tab at the back of the book.

19-6 The reproductive system secretes hormones affecting growth and metabolism of all body systems

Learning Objective Give examples of interactions between the reproductive system and each of the other body systems.

Normal human reproduction is a complex process. It involves multiple body systems. The hormones discussed in this chapter play a major role in coordinating reproductive events (**Table 19-1**). Physical factors also play a role.

For example, the male's sperm count must be adequate. The semen must have the correct pH and nutrients. Erection and ejaculation must take place in the proper sequence. The female's ovarian and uterine cycles must be properly coordinated. Ovulation and oocyte transport must take place normally. Her reproductive tract must provide a suitable environment for sperm survival and movement, and for fertilization of the oocyte. For these steps to occur, the digestive, endocrine, nervous, cardiovascular, and urinary systems must all be functioning normally.

Refer to Build Your Knowledge: How the REPRODUCTIVE SYSTEM integrates with the other body systems presented so far on p. 670. It reviews the major functional relationships between this system and the 10 other body systems.

Even when all is normal, and fertilization takes place at the proper time and place, the zygote—a single cell the size of a pinhead—must develop into a full-term fetus that typically weighs about 3 kg (6.6 lb). (In Chapter 20 we will consider the process of development and the mechanisms that determine both body structure and the distinctive characteristics of each individual.)

CHECKPOINT

22. Describe the interactions between the reproductive system and the cardiovascular system.
23. Describe the interaction between the reproductive system and the skeletal system.

See the blue Answers tab at the back of the book.

Table 19-1	Hormones of the Reproductive System		
HORMONE	**SOURCE**	**REGULATION OF SECRETION**	**PRIMARY EFFECTS**
GONADOTROPIN-RELEASING HORMONE (GnRH)	Hypothalamus	*Males:* inhibited by testosterone *Females:* inhibited by estrogens and/or progesterone	Stimulates FSH secretion and LH synthesis in males and females
FOLLICLE-STIMULATING HORMONE (FSH)	Anterior lobe of the pituitary gland	*Males:* stimulated by GnRH, inhibited by inhibin and testosterone *Females:* stimulated by GnRH, inhibited by inhibin, estrogens, and/or progesterone	*Males:* stimulates spermatogenesis and spermiogenesis through effects on nurse cells *Females:* stimulates follicle development, estrogen production, and oocyte maturation
LUTEINIZING HORMONE (LH)	Anterior lobe of pituitary gland	*Males:* stimulated by GnRH *Females:* production stimulated by GnRH and secretion by estrogens	*Males:* stimulates interstitial cells to secrete testosterone *Females:* stimulates ovulation, formation of corpus luteum, and progesterone secretion
ANDROGENS (Primarily Testosterone)	Interstitial cells of testes	Stimulated by LH	Establish and maintain secondary sex characteristics and sexual behavior; promote maturation of spermatozoa; inhibit GnRH secretion
ESTROGENS (Primarily Estradiol)	Follicle cells of ovaries; corpus luteum	Stimulated by FSH	Stimulate LH secretion (at high levels); establish and maintain secondary sex characteristics and behavior; stimulate repair and growth of endometrium; inhibit secretion of GnRH
PROGESTERONE	Corpus luteum	Stimulated by LH	Stimulates endometrial growth and glandular secretion; inhibits GnRH secretion
INHIBIN	Nurse cells of testes and follicle cells of ovaries	Stimulated by factors released by developing sperm (male) and developing follicles (female)	Inhibits secretion of FSH (and possibly GnRH)

CLINICAL NOTE

Birth Control Strategies

For diverse reasons, most U.S. adults practice some form of conception control during their reproductive years. Two out of three U.S. women ages 15–44 use some method of contraception. When the simplest method—sexual abstinence—is unsatisfactory, another means of contraception must be used to avoid unwanted pregnancies. All methods have specific strengths and weaknesses.

Hormonal contraceptives manipulate the female hormonal cycle so that ovulation does not take place. The contraceptive pills produced in the 1950s combined estrogen and progestins (synthetic progesterone) to suppress pituitary GnRH production, so FSH was not released and ovulation did not occur. Most of today's oral contraceptives contain much smaller amounts of estrogen, or only progestins. Current *combination* hormone contraceptives are administered cyclically, using medication for three weeks followed by no medication during week 4. For convenience, monthly injections, weekly skin patches, and insertable vaginal rings are available.

An estimated 200 million women use combination oral contraceptives worldwide. In the United States, 33 percent of women under age 45 use the combination pill to prevent conception. The failure rate for combination oral contraceptives, when used as prescribed, is 0.24 percent over a two-year period. (*Failure* for a birth control method is defined as a pregnancy.) Birth control pills are not risk free. They can worsen problems associated with severe hypertension, diabetes mellitus, epilepsy, gallbladder disease, heart trouble, and acne. Women taking oral contraceptives are also at increased risk for venous thrombosis, strokes, pulmonary embolism, and (for women over 35) heart disease.

Hormonal postcoital contraception, or the emergency "morning after" pill, involves taking either combination estrogen/progestin birth control pills or progestin-only pills within 72 hours of unprotected sexual intercourse. Particularly useful when barrier methods malfunction or coerced intercourse occurs, it reduces expected pregnancy rates by up to 89 percent.

Progestin-only forms of birth control—Depo-Provera and the progestin-only pill ("mini-pill")—are now available. Depo-Provera is injected every three months. It can cause irregular menstruation and temporary amenorrhea. The progestin-only pill is taken daily and may cause irregular uterine cycles. Skipping just one pill may result in pregnancy.

The condom, also called a *prophylactic* or "rubber," covers the glans penis and body of the penis during intercourse. It keeps sperm from reaching the female reproductive tract. Latex condoms also reduce the spread of STDs, such as syphilis, gonorrhea, HPV, and AIDS. The reported condom failure rate varies from 6 to 18 percent.

Vaginal barriers such as the *diaphragm* and *cervical cap* rely on similar principles. A diaphragm, the most popular form of vaginal barrier today, is a dome of latex rubber with a small metal hoop supporting the rim. Before intercourse, the diaphragm is inserted to cover the external os of the uterus, and it

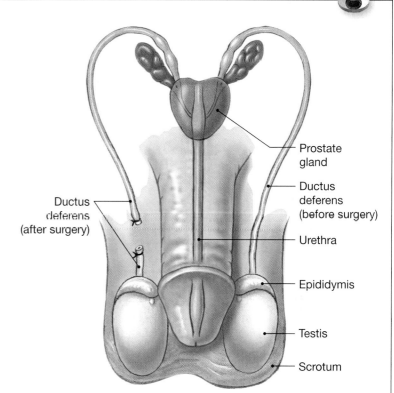

a In a vasectomy, the removal of a 1-cm section of the ductus deferens prevents the passage of sperm cells.

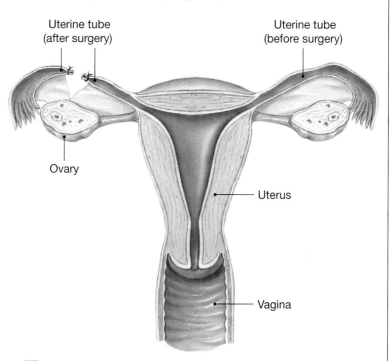

b In a tubal ligation, the removal of a section of the uterine tube prevents the passage of sperm and the movement of an ovum or embryo into the uterus.

(Continued)

19

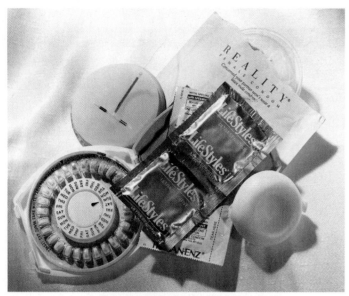

Contraceptive devices

is usually coated with a small amount of spermicidal (sperm-killing) jelly or cream. The failure rate of a properly fitted diaphragm is estimated at 5–6 percent. A *cervical cap* is smaller and lacks the metal rim. It, too, must be fitted carefully, but unlike the diaphragm, it can be left in place for several days. Its failure rate (8 percent) is higher than that for diaphragm use.

An intrauterine device (IUD) consists of a small plastic loop or a T that is inserted into the uterine cavity. The mechanism of action remains uncertain, but IUDs are known to stimulate prostaglandin production in the uterus. The resulting change in the chemical composition of uterine secretions lowers the likelihood of fertilization and *implantation* of the zygote in the uterine lining. (Implantation is discussed in Chapter 20.) In the United States, IUDs are in limited use, but they remain popular in many countries. Failure rate is estimated at 5–6 percent.

The rhythm method involves abstaining from sexual intercourse on the days ovulation might be occurring. The timing is estimated on the basis of previous patterns of menstruation and in some cases by monitoring changes in basal body temperature. The failure rate is very high—almost 25 percent.

Sterilization is a surgical procedure that makes a person unable to provide functional gametes for fertilization. Members of either sex may be sterilized. In a vasectomy (vaz-EK-to-m), a segment of the ductus deferens is removed, making it impossible for sperm to pass from the epididymis to the distal portions of the reproductive tract. The surgery can be performed in a physician's office in a matter of minutes. A 1-cm section of the ductus deferens is removed on each side, and the cut ends are usually tied shut (**a**). In time, scar tissue forms a permanent seal. Alternatively, the cut ends are blocked with silicone plugs that can later be removed in an attempt to restore fertility. After a vasectomy, men have normal sexual function. Sperms continue to develop, but they remain within the epididymis and degenerate. The failure rate for this procedure is 0.08 percent.

The uterine tubes can be blocked through a surgical procedure known as a tubal ligation (**b**). The failure rate is estimated at 0.45 percent. Because the surgery involves entering the abdominopelvic cavity, complications are more likely than with a vasectomy. As in a vasectomy, attempts to restore fertility after a tubal ligation may not be successful. Both vasectomy and tubal ligation contraception should be considered permanent.

Pregnancy is a natural phenomenon, but it has risks. The mortality rate for pregnant women in the United States averages about 8 deaths per 100,000 pregnancies. That average incorporates a broad range. The rate is 7 per 100,000 among women under 20 but 40 per 100,000 for women over 40. Before age 35, the risks associated with contraceptive use are lower than the risks associated with pregnancy. The notable exception involves individuals who take oral contraceptives but also smoke cigarettes. After age 35, the risks of complications associated with oral contraceptive use increase, but the risks of using other methods remains relatively stable. Women over age 35 (smokers) or 40 (nonsmokers) are, therefore, typically advised to seek other forms of contraception.

RELATED CLINICAL TERMS

endometriosis (en-dō-mē-trē-Ō-sis): The growth of endometrial tissue outside the uterus.

genital herpes: A sexually transmitted disease caused by a herpes virus and characterized by painful blisters in the genital region.

gynecology (gī-ne-KOL-o-jē): Branch of medicine that deals with the functions and diseases specific to women and girls affecting the reproductive system.

hysterectomy: The surgical removal of the uterus.

mammography: The use of X-rays to examine breast tissue.

mastectomy: The surgical removal of part or all of a breast, typically as treatment for breast cancer.

oophoritis (ō-of-ō-RĪ-tis): Inflammation of the ovaries.

orchitis (or-KĪ-tis): Inflammation of one or both testicles.

ovarian cancer: A malignancy of the ovaries; the most dangerous reproductive cancer in women.

ovarian cyst: A condition (usually harmless) in which fluid-filled sacs develop in or on the ovary.

prostate cancer: A malignant, metastasizing tumor of the prostate gland; the second most common cancer and the second most common cause of cancer deaths in males.

prostatectomy: The surgical removal of the prostate gland.

salpingitis: Inflammation of a uterine tube.

testicular torsion: A condition in which twisting of the spermatic cord obstructs the blood supply to a testis.

Build Your Knowledge

How the REPRODUCTIVE SYSTEM integrates with the other body systems presented so far

Integumentary System

- The integumentary system covers external genitalia; provides sensations that stimulate sexual behaviors; mammary gland secretions nourish the newborn
- The reproductive system hormones affect the distribution of body hair and subcutaneous fat

Respiratory System

- The respiratory system provides oxygen and removes carbon dioxide generated by tissues of reproductive system and (in pregnant women) by embryonic and fetal tissues
- The reproductive system changes respiratory rate and depth during sexual arousal, under control of the nervous system

Cardiovascular System

- The cardiovascular system distributes reproductive hormones; provides nutrients, oxygen, and waste removal for fetus; local blood pressure changes responsible for physical changes during sexual arousal
- The reproductive system produces estrogens that may help maintain healthy vessels and slow development of atherosclerosis

Digestive System

- The digestive system provides additional nutrients required to support gamete production and (in pregnant women) embryonic and fetal development
- The reproductive system in pregnant women with a developing fetus crowds digestive organs, causes constipation, and increases appetite

Skeletal System

- The skeletal system (pelvic girdle) protects reproductive organs of females, portion of ductus deferens and accessory glands in males
- The reproductive system hormones stimulate bone growth and maintenance, and at puberty accelerate growth and closure of epiphyseal cartilages

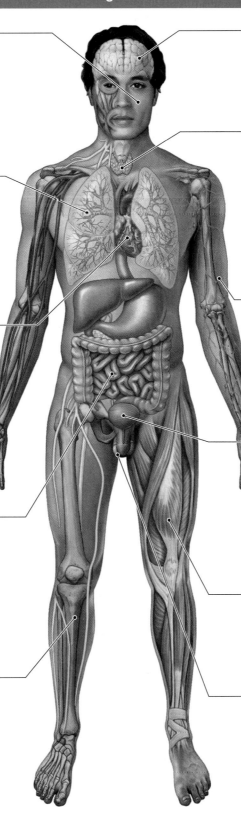

Nervous System

- The nervous system controls sexual behaviors and sexual function
- The reproductive system hormones affect CNS development and sexual behaviors

Endocrine System

- The endocrine system produces hypothalamic regulatory hormones and pituitary hormones that regulate sexual development and function; oxytocin stimulates smooth muscle contractions in uterus and mammary glands
- The reproductive system produces steroid sex hormones and inhibin that inhibit secretory activities of hypothalamus and pituitary gland

Lymphatic System

- The lymphatic system provides IgA for secretions by epithelial glands; assists in repairs and defense against infection
- The reproductive system secretes lysozymes and bactericidal chemicals that provide innate (nonspecific) defense against reproductive tract infections

Urinary System

The urinary system in males carries semen to exterior in urethra; kidneys remove wastes generated by reproductive tissues and (in pregnant women) by a growing embryo and fetus

- The reproductive system secretions may have antibacterial activity that helps prevent urethral infections in males

Muscular System

- The muscular system aids ejaculation of semen from male reproductive tract
- The reproductive system hormone testosterone accelerates skeletal muscle growth

Reproductive System

The reproductive system secretes hormones with effects on growth and metabolism.
It
- produces, stores, nourishes, and transports male and female gametes
- supports the developing embryo and fetus in the uterus

19

19 Chapter Review

Summary Outline

19-1 Basic reproductive system structures are gonads, ducts, accessory glands and organs, and external genitalia *p. 735*

1. The human **reproductive system** produces, stores, nourishes, and transports functional **gametes** (reproductive cells). **Fertilization** is the fusion of male and female gametes.

2. The reproductive system includes **gonads** (**testes** or **ovaries**), ducts, accessory glands and organs, and the **external genitalia**.

3. In males, the testes produce **spermatozoa**, which are expelled from the body in **semen** during *ejaculation*. The ovaries of a sexually mature female produce **oocytes** (immature **ova**) that travel along *uterine tubes* toward the *uterus*. The *vagina* connects the uterus with the exterior of the body.

19-2 Sperm formation (spermatogenesis) occurs in the testes, and hormones from the hypothalamus, pituitary gland, and testes control male reproductive functions *p. 736*

4. In males, the *testes* produce **sperm** cells. The **spermatozoa** travel along the *epididymis*, the *ductus deferens*, the *ejaculatory duct*, and the *urethra* before leaving the body. Accessory organs (*seminal glands, prostate gland,* and *bulbo-urethral glands*) secrete products into the ejaculatory ducts and urethra. The scrotum encloses the testes, and the penis is an erectile organ (*Figure 19-1*).

5. The **testes**, the primary sex organ of males, hang within the **scrotum**. The *dartos* muscle layer gives the scrotum a wrinkled appearance. The **cremaster muscle** pulls the testes closer to the body. The **tunica albuginea** surrounds each testis. Septa subdivide each testis into a series of lobules. **Seminiferous tubules** within each lobule are the sites of sperm production. Between the seminiferous tubules are **interstitial cells,** which secrete sex hormones (*Figure 19-2*).

6. Seminiferous tubules contain **spermatogonia**, stem cells involved in **spermatogenesis**, and **nurse cells**, which sustain and promote the development of spermatozoa (*Figure 19-3*).

7. Each spermatozoon has a **head, middle piece**, and **tail** (*Figure 19-4*).

8. From the testis, the spermatozoa enter the **epididymis**, a long tubule that regulates the composition of the tubular fluid and serves as a recycling center for damaged spermatozoa. Spermatozoa leaving the epididymis are functionally mature, yet immobile.

9. The **ductus deferens**, or *vas deferens*, begins at the epididymis and passes through the inguinal canal within the **spermatic cord**. The junction of the base of the seminal gland and the ampulla of the ductus deferens creates the **ejaculatory duct**, which penetrates the prostate gland and empties into the urethra (*Figure 19-5*).

10. The **urethra** extends from the urinary bladder to the tip of the penis and serves as a passageway for both the urinary and reproductive systems.

11. Each **seminal gland (seminal vesicle)** is an active secretory gland that contributes about 60 percent of the volume of semen. Its secretions contain fructose, which is easily metabolized by spermatozoa. The **prostate gland** secretes fluid that makes up about 30 percent of seminal fluid. Alkaline mucus secreted by the **bulbo-urethral glands** has lubricating properties (*Figure 19-5*).

12. A typical **ejaculation** expels 2–5 mL of semen (an **ejaculate**), which contains 20–100 million sperm per milliliter.

13. The skin overlying the **penis** resembles that of the scrotum. Most of the body of the penis consists of three masses of **erectile tissue**. There are two **corpora cavernosa** and a single **corpus spongiosum**, which surrounds the urethra. Dilation of the erectile tissue with blood produces an **erection** (*Figure 19-6*).

14. Important regulatory hormones of males include **gonadotropin-releasing hormone (GnRH), follicle-stimulating hormone (FSH)**, and **luteinizing hormone (LH)**. Testosterone is the most important *androgen* (*Spotlight Figure 19-7*).

19-3 Ovum production (oogenesis) occurs in the ovaries, and hormones from the pituitary gland and ovaries control female reproductive functions *p. 746*

15. Principal organs of the female reproductive system include the *ovaries, uterine tubes, uterus, vagina,* and *external genitalia* (*Figure 19-8*).

16. The **ovaries** are the primary sex organs of females. Ovaries are the site of **ovum** production, or **oogenesis,** which occurs in **ovarian follicles**. Follicle development proceeds from **primordial follicles** through **primary, secondary**, and **tertiary follicles**. During the **ovarian cycle**, a dominant tertiary follicle forms. At **ovulation**, a secondary oocyte and the attached follicular cells of the **corona radiata** are released through the ruptured ovarian wall (*Figures 19-9, 19-10*).

17. Each **uterine tube** has an **infundibulum**, a funnel that opens into the pelvic cavity. For fertilization to occur, a secondary oocyte must encounter spermatozoa during the first 12–24 hours of its passage from the infundibulum to the uterine cavity (*Figure 19-11*).

18. The **uterus** provides mechanical protection and nutritional support to the developing embryo. It is stabilized by various ligaments and mesenteries. Major anatomical landmarks of the uterus include the **body, cervix, external os, uterine cavity,** and **internal os.** The uterine wall consists of an inner **endometrium**, a muscular **myometrium**, and a superficial **perimetrium** (*Figure 19-11*).

19. A typical 28-day **uterine cycle**, or *menstrual cycle*, begins with the onset of **menses** and the destruction of the *functional zone* of the endometrium. This process of **menstruation** continues from one to seven days.

20. After menses, the **proliferative phase** begins, and the functional zone undergoes repair and thickens. During the **secretory phase**, the uterine glands are active and the uterus is prepared for the arrival of an embryo. Menstrual activity begins at **menarche** and continues until **menopause.**

21. The **vagina** is a muscular tube extending between the uterus and the external genitalia. A thin epithelial fold, the **hymen**, partially blocks the entrance to the vagina.

22. The components of the **vulva** are the **vestibule, labia minora, clitoris, labia majora, mons pubis**, and **lesser** and **greater vestibular glands** (*Figure 19-12*).

23. A newborn infant is nourished by milk secreted by maternal **mammary glands. Lactation** is the process of milk production (*Figure 19-13*).

24. Regulation of the **female reproductive cycle** involves the coordination of the ovarian and uterine cycles by circulating hormones (*Spotlight Figure 19-14*).

25. *Estradiol*, one of the estrogens, is the dominant hormone of the **follicular phase** of the ovarian cycle. Estrogens have multiple functions that affect the activities of many tissues and organs (*Spotlight Figure 19-14*).

26. The hypothalamic secretion of GnRH triggers the pituitary secretion of FSH and the synthesis of LH. FSH initiates follicle development, and activated follicles and ovarian interstitial cells produce estrogens. Ovulation occurs in response to a midcycle surge in LH secretion. **Progesterone** is the main hormone of the **luteal phase** of the ovarian cycle. Changes in estrogen and progesterone levels regulate the uterine, or menstrual, cycle (*Spotlight Figure 19-14*).

19-4 The autonomic nervous system influences male and female sexual function *p. 760*

27. During sexual **arousal** in males, erotic thoughts, sensory stimulation, or both lead to parasympathetic activity that ultimately produces erection. Stimuli accompanying **sexual intercourse** lead to **emission** and **ejaculation**. Strong perineal muscle contractions are associated with **orgasm**.

28. The phases of female sexual function resemble those of the male, with parasympathetic arousal and muscular contractions associated with orgasm.

19-5 With age, decreasing levels of reproductive hormones cause functional changes *p. 761*

29. Menopause (when ovulation and menstruation cease) typically occurs around age 50. Production of GnRH, FSH, and LH rise, while circulating concentrations of estrogen and progesterone decline.

30. During the **male climacteric**, at ages 50–60, circulating testosterone levels decline while levels of FSH and LH rise.

19-6 The reproductive system secretes hormones affecting growth and metabolism of all body systems *p. 762*

31. Hormones play a major role in coordinating reproduction (*Table 19-1*).

32. In addition to the endocrine and reproductive systems, reproduction requires the normal functioning of the digestive, nervous, cardiovascular, and urinary systems.

Review Questions

See the blue Answers tab at the back of the book.

Level 1 Reviewing Facts and Terms

Match each item in column A with the most closely related item in column B. Place letters for answers in the spaces provided.

COLUMN A	COLUMN B
_____ **1.** Gametes	**a.** Production of androgens
_____ **2.** Gonads	**b.** Muscular uterine wall
_____ **3.** Interstitial cells	**c.** Secretions contain fructose
_____ **4.** Seminal glands	**d.** Female erectile tissue
_____ **5.** Prostate gland	**e.** Secretes thick, sticky, alkaline mucus
_____ **6.** Bulbo-urethral glands	
_____ **7.** Prepuce	**f.** Painful menstruation
_____ **8.** Corpus luteum	**g.** Coitus
_____ **9.** Endometrium	**h.** Uterine lining
_____ **10.** Myometrium	**i.** Reproductive cells
_____ **11.** Dysmenorrhea	**j.** First menstrual period
_____ **12.** Menarche	**k.** Milk production
_____ **13.** Clitoris	**l.** Secretes seminalplasmin
_____ **14.** Lactation	**m.** Reproductive organs
_____ **15.** Sexual intercourse	**n.** Foreskin of penis
	o. Secretes progesterone

16. Perineal structures associated with the reproductive system are collectively known as
  (a) gonads.
  (b) sex gametes.
  (c) external genitalia.
  (d) accessory glands.

17. Meiosis in males produces four spermatids, each of which contains
  (a) 23 chromosomes.
  (b) 23 pairs of chromosomes.
  (c) the diploid number of chromosomes.
  (d) 46 pairs of chromosomes.

18. Erection of the penis occurs when
  (a) sympathetic activation of penile arteries occurs.
  (b) arterial branches are constricted and muscular partitions are tense.
  (c) the vascular channels become engorged with blood.
  (d) a, b, and c are correct.

19. In males, the primary target of FSH is the
  (a) nurse cells of the seminiferous tubules.
  (b) interstitial cells of the seminiferous tubules.
  (c) prostate gland.
  (d) epididymis.

20. The ovaries are responsible for
  (a) the production of female gametes.
  (b) the secretion of female sex hormones.
  (c) the secretion of inhibin.
  (d) a, b, and c are correct.

21. Ovum production, or oogenesis, begins
  (a) before birth.
  (b) after birth.
  (c) at puberty.
  (d) after puberty.

22. In females, meiosis is not completed
  (a) until birth.
  (b) until puberty.
  (c) until fertilization occurs.
  (d) until ovulation occurs.

23. Identify the principal structures of the male reproductive system in the following diagram.

(a) _____	**(b)** _____
(c) _____	**(d)** _____
(e) _____	**(f)** _____
(g) _____	**(h)** _____
(i) _____	**(j)** _____

24. Identify the principal structures of the female reproductive system in the following diagram.

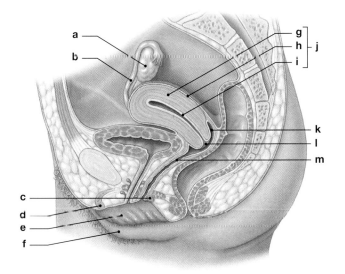

(a) _____   (b) _____
(c) _____   (d) _____
(e) _____   (f) _____
(g) _____   (h) _____
(i) _____   (j) _____
(k) _____   (l) _____
(m) _____

25. If fertilization is to occur, a secondary oocyte must encounter spermatozoa during the first _____ of its passage.
(a) 1–5 hours   (b) 6–11 hours
(c) 12–24 hours   (d) 25–36 hours

26. The part of the endometrium that undergoes cyclical changes in response to variations in sex hormone levels is the
(a) serosa.
(b) basilar zone.
(c) muscular myometrium.
(d) functional zone.

27. A sudden surge in the level of LH causes
(a) the onset of menses.
(b) the rupture of the follicular wall and ovulation.
(c) the beginning of the proliferative phase.
(d) the end of the uterine cycle.

28. At the time of ovulation, basal body temperature
(a) is not affected.
(b) increases noticeably.
(c) declines sharply.
(d) may increase or decrease a few degrees.

29. Identify the reproductive accessory organs and glands in males, and list their functions.

30. What are the primary functions of an epididymis?

31. What are the primary functions of the ovaries?

32. What are the three major functions of the vagina?

Level 2 Reviewing Concepts

33. How does the reproductive system differ functionally from all other organ systems in the body?

34. Define meiosis, and identify the products of this process in both males and females.

35. Using an average uterine cycle of 28 days, describe each of the three phases of the menstrual cycle.

36. Describe the hormonal events associated with the uterine cycle.

37. How does aging affect the reproductive systems of men and women?

Level 3 Critical Thinking and Clinical Applications

38. Diane has peritonitis (inflammation of the peritoneum), which her physician says resulted from a urinary tract infection. Why could this situation occur in females but not in males?

39. In a condition known as endometriosis, endometrial cells are believed to migrate from the body of the uterus into the uterine tubes or by way of the uterine tubes into the peritoneal cavity, where they become established. A major symptom of endometriosis is periodic pain. Why does such pain occur?

40. Female bodybuilders and women with eating disorders such as anorexia nervosa commonly experience amenorrhea. What does this fact suggest about the relation between body fat and menstruation? What effect would amenorrhea have on achieving a successful pregnancy?

19

Development
and Inheritance

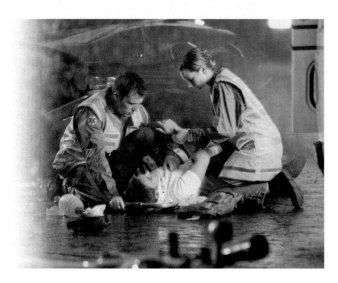

Learning Objectives

These objectives tell you what you should be able to do after completing the chapter. They correspond by number to this chapter's sections.

20-1 Explain the relationship between differentiation and development, and describe the various stages of development.

20-2 Describe the process of fertilization.

20-3 List the three stages of prenatal development, and describe the major events of each.

20-4 Explain how the three germ layers are involved in forming the extraembryonic membranes, and discuss the importance of the placenta as an endocrine organ.

20-5 Describe the interplay between maternal organ systems and the developing fetus, and discuss the structural and functional changes in the uterus during gestation.

20-6 List and discuss the events that occur during labor and delivery.

20-7 Identify the features and physiological changes of the postnatal stages of life.

20-8 Relate the basic principles of genetics to the inheritance of human traits.

An Introduction to Development and Inheritance

The physiological processes that we have studied so far take place fairly quickly. Many last only a fraction of a second, and others may take hours. But some important processes go on for months, years, or decades. A human develops in the womb for nine months, grows to maturity in 15–20 years, and may live the better part of a century. During that time, he or she is always changing. Birth, growth, maturation, aging, and death are all parts of one continuous process. That process does not end with the individual, because humans can pass at least some of their characteristics on to their offspring. Each generation gives rise to a new generation that will repeat the cycle.

In this chapter, we explore how genetic and environmental factors and various physiological processes affect prenatal development and also influence childhood, adolescence, maturity, and aging.

Build Your Knowledge

Recall that male and female gametes (sperm and oocytes) are formed through a special form of cell division called meiosis (as you saw in **Chapter 19: The Reproductive System**). This process involves two cycles of cell division, meiosis I and meiosis II. Meiosis I begins with diploid reproductive stem cells containing 46 chromosomes, composed of 23 pairs. The gametes formed as a result of completing meiosis II are haploid. Each gamete contains 23 individual chromosomes—one member of each of the 23 pairs present in the original reproductive stem cell. In males, spermatozoa formation, or spermatogenesis, results in four haploid sperm cells. In females, ovum production, or oogenesis, produces one secondary oocyte, or immature ovum, in metaphase II. It does not complete meiosis II until fertilization, when it forms a second polar body and becomes a mature ovum. ⮌ **pp. 646, 653**

20-1 Development is a continuous process that occurs from fertilization to maturity

Learning Objective Explain the relationship between differentiation and development, and describe the various stages of development.

Time refuses to stand still. Today's infant will be tomorrow's adult. The gradual change in anatomical structures and physiological characteristics during the period from conception to maturity is called **development**. The changes are truly remarkable. In a mere nine months, a single cell slightly larger than the period at the end of this sentence becomes an individual whose body contains trillions of cells organized into tissues, organs, and organ systems.

The formation of different cell types in this process is called **differentiation**. Differentiation takes place through selective changes in genetic activity. As development proceeds, some genes are turned off and others are turned on. The kinds of genes turned off or on vary from one cell type to another.

Development begins at **fertilization**, or **conception**, when the male and female gametes fuse. We can divide development into several periods. **Embryonic development** includes the events during the first two months after fertilization. The study of these events in the developing organism, or **embryo**, is called **embryology** (em-brē-OL-o-jē).

After two months, the developing embryo becomes a **fetus**. **Fetal development** begins at the start of the ninth week and continues until birth. Together, embryonic development and fetal development are referred to as **prenatal** (*natus*, birth) **development**, the primary focus of this chapter. **Postnatal development** begins at birth and continues to **maturity**, the state of full development or completed growth.

All humans go through the same developmental stages, but differences in genetic makeup produce distinctive individual characteristics. The term **inheritance** or **heredity** refers to the transfer of genetically determined characteristics from generation to generation. The study of the mechanisms of heredity, or *how* those characteristics are transferred, is called **genetics**. In this chapter, we consider basic genetics as it applies to inherited characteristics such as sex, hair color, and various diseases.

20

CHECKPOINT

1. Define differentiation.
2. What event marks the beginning of development?
3. Define inheritance.

See the blue Answers tab at the back of the book.

20-2 Fertilization—the fusion of a secondary oocyte and a spermatozoon—forms a zygote

Learning Objective Describe the process of fertilization.

Fertilization involves the fusion of two haploid gametes, each containing 23 chromosomes. The process produces a *zygote* with 46 chromosomes, the normal diploid number for a *somatic* (nonreproductive) cell.

An Overview of Fertilization

The roles and contributions of the male and female gametes are very different at fertilization. The spermatozoon delivers the paternal (father's) chromosomes to the site of fertilization. It must travel a relatively long distance and is small and streamlined. In contrast, the female oocyte provides all the cellular organelles, nourishment, and genetic programming needed to support development of the embryo for nearly a week after conception. At fertilization, the diameter of the secondary oocyte is more than twice the length of the spermatozoon (**Figure 20-1a**). The ratio of their volumes is even more striking—roughly 2000 to 1.

The sperm deposited in the vagina are already motile, as a result of mixing with secretions of the seminal glands—the first step of *capacitation.* ⤶ p. 649 However, they cannot accomplish fertilization until they have been exposed to conditions in the female reproductive tract. Uterine tube peg cell secretions help with capacitation, but the exact process is not yet known. ⤶ p. 657

Fertilization typically takes place in the upper one-third of a uterine tube within a day after ovulation. It takes sperm between 30 minutes and 2 hours to pass from the vagina to the upper portion of a uterine tube. Of the 200 million spermatozoa in a typical ejaculation, only about 10,000 enter the uterine tube. Fewer than 100 actually reach the secondary oocyte. In general, a male with a sperm count below 20 million per milliliter is sterile because too few sperm survive to reach the oocyte. While it is true that only one sperm fertilizes an oocyte, dozens are required for successful fertilization.

The additional sperm are necessary because, as we will see, a single sperm cannot penetrate the *corona radiata*, the layer of follicle cells that surrounds the oocyte. ⤶ p. 657

Ovulation and Oocyte Activation

Ovulation takes place before the oocyte is completely mature. The secondary oocyte leaving the follicle is in metaphase of the second meiotic division (meiosis II). The cell's metabolic operations have been suspended as it awaits the stimulus for further development. If fertilization does not occur, the oocyte disintegrates without completing meiosis.

Fertilization and the events that follow are diagrammed in **Figure 20-1b**. The corona radiata protects the oocyte as it passes through the ruptured follicular wall and into the infundibulum of a uterine tube. The physical process of fertilization requires that only a single sperm contact the oocyte membrane, but that spermatozoon must first get through the corona radiata. The acrosome of each sperm contains several enzymes, including *hyaluronidase* (hī-uh-lū-RON-i-dās). Hyaluronidase breaks down the bonds between adjacent follicle cells. Dozens of sperm cells must release hyaluronidase before an opening forms between the follicle cells.

No matter how many sperm slip through the resulting gap in the corona radiata, only a single spermatozoon accomplishes fertilization and activates the oocyte (**1**, **Figure 20-1b**). That sperm cell first binds to *sperm receptors* in the zona pellucida, a thick envelope surrounding the oocyte. ⤶ p. 655 This binding triggers the rupture of the acrosome. Hyaluronidase and another proteolytic enzyme digest a path through the zona pellucida to the oocyte membrane. Upon contact, the sperm and oocyte membranes begin to fuse. This step triggers oocyte activation. As the membranes fuse, the entire sperm enters the cytoplasm of the oocyte.

Oocyte activation involves a series of changes in the metabolic activity of the oocyte. Vesicles located just interior to the oocyte membrane undergo exocytosis. They release enzymes that prevent *polyspermy*, or fertilization by more than one sperm. Polyspermy produces a zygote that cannot develop normally. Other important metabolic changes include the completion of meiosis II and a rapid increase in the oocyte's metabolic rate.

After oocyte activation and the completion of meiosis II, the nuclear material remaining within the ovum reorganizes into a *female pronucleus* (**2**, **Figure 20-1b**). At the same time, the nucleus of the spermatozoon swells, becoming the *male pronucleus* (**3**). The male pronucleus and female pronucleus then fuse in a process called **amphimixis** (am-fi-MIK-sis) (**4**).

Figure 20-1 Fertilization.

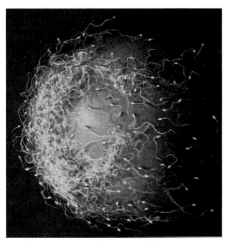

a A secondary oocyte and numerous sperm at the time of fertilization. Notice the difference in size between the gametes.

The cell is now a **zygote** (*zygon*, yoke) that contains the normal diploid number of 46 chromosomes, and fertilization is complete. This is the "moment of conception." The first cleavage division yields two daughter cells (**5**). *Cleavage* is a series of cell divisions that subdivides the cytoplasm of the zygote.

CHECKPOINT

4. What two important roles do the acrosomal enzymes of spermatozoa play prior to fertilization?

5. How many chromosomes are contained within a human zygote?

See the blue Answers tab at the back of the book.

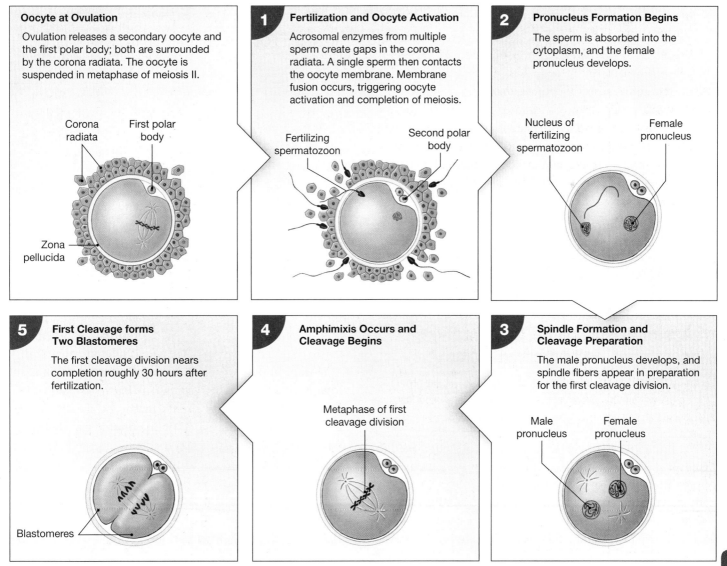

Oocyte at Ovulation

Ovulation releases a secondary oocyte and the first polar body; both are surrounded by the corona radiata. The oocyte is suspended in metaphase of meiosis II.

Corona radiata
First polar body
Zona pellucida

1 Fertilization and Oocyte Activation

Acrosomal enzymes from multiple sperm create gaps in the corona radiata. A single sperm then contacts the oocyte membrane. Membrane fusion occurs, triggering oocyte activation and completion of meiosis.

Fertilizing spermatozoon
Second polar body

2 Pronucleus Formation Begins

The sperm is absorbed into the cytoplasm, and the female pronucleus develops.

Nucleus of fertilizing spermatozoon
Female pronucleus

5 First Cleavage forms Two Blastomeres

The first cleavage division nears completion roughly 30 hours after fertilization.

Blastomeres

4 Amphimixis Occurs and Cleavage Begins

Metaphase of first cleavage division

3 Spindle Formation and Cleavage Preparation

The male pronucleus develops, and spindle fibers appear in preparation for the first cleavage division.

Male pronucleus
Female pronucleus

b Fertilization and the preparations for cleavage.

20-3 Gestation consists of three stages of prenatal development: the first, second, and third trimesters

Learning Objective List the three stages of prenatal development, and describe the major events of each.

During prenatal development, a single cell ultimately forms a 3–4 kg (6.6–8.8 lb) infant. The time spent in prenatal development is known as **gestation** (jes-TĀ-shun), or *pregnancy*. Gestation takes place within the uterus over a period of nine months. Prenatal development is usually divided into three **trimesters**, each lasting three months:

1. The **first trimester** is the period of embryonic and early fetal development. During this period, the beginnings of all major organ systems appear.

2. The **second trimester** is dominated by the development of organs and organ systems. The process nears completion by the end of the sixth month. During this time, body shape and proportions change. By the end of this trimester, the fetus looks distinctively human.

3. The **third trimester** is characterized by rapid fetal growth and deposition of adipose tissue. Early in the third trimester, most of the major organ systems become fully functional. An infant born one month or even two months prematurely has a reasonable chance of survival.

CHECKPOINT

6. Define gestation.

7. Describe the key features of each trimester.

See the blue Answers tab at the back of the book.

20-4 Critical events of the first trimester are cleavage, implantation, placentation, and embryogenesis

Learning Objective Explain how the three germ layers are involved in forming the extraembryonic membranes, and discuss the importance of the placenta as an endocrine organ.

At the moment of conception, a fertilized ovum is a single cell. It is about 0.135 mm (0.005 in.) in diameter and weighs approximately 150 μg. By convention, pregnancies are clinically dated from the last menstrual period (LMP), which is usually two weeks *before* ovulation and conception. At the end of the first trimester (12 weeks from LMP, only 10 developmental weeks), the fetus is almost 5.4 cm (2.13 in.) long and weighs about 14 g (0.5 oz).

Many complex and vital developmental events accompany this increase in size and weight. Perhaps because the events are so complex, it is the most dangerous prenatal stage. Only about 40 percent of conceptions produce embryos that survive the first trimester. For that reason, pregnant women are advised to take great care to avoid drugs, alcohol, tobacco, and other disruptive stresses during this period.

In the sections that follow, we focus on four general processes of the first trimester: *cleavage and blastocyst formation, implantation, placentation,* and *embryogenesis.*

Cleavage and Blastocyst Formation

Cleavage (KLĒV-ij) is a series of cell divisions that begins immediately after fertilization. It produces an ever-increasing number of smaller and smaller daughter cells called **blastomeres** (BLAS-tō-mērz; *blast,* precursor + *meros,* part) (**Figure 20-2**). The first cleavage division produces two daughter cells. Each is half the size of the original zygote. The first division is completed roughly 30 hours after fertilization, and subsequent cleavage divisions occur at intervals of 10–12 hours.

During cleavage, the zygote becomes a *pre-embryo.* After three days of cleavage, the pre-embryo is a solid ball of cells resembling a mulberry (**Figure 20-2**). This stage is called the **morula** (MOR-ū-la; *morula,* mulberry). The morula typically reaches the uterus on day 4.

Over the next two days, the blastomeres form a **blastocyst**, a hollow ball with an inner cavity known as the *blastocoele* (BLAS-tō-sēl; *koiloma,* cavity). The blastomeres are now no longer identical in size and shape. The outer layer of cells separating the outside world from the blastocoele is called the **trophoblast** (TRŌ-fō-blast). As the word trophoblast implies (*trophos,* food + *blast,* precursor), cells in this layer provide food to the developing embryo. A second group of cells, the **inner cell mass**, lies clustered in one portion of the blastocyst. In time, the inner cell mass will form the embryo.

During blastocyst formation, the zona pellucida is shed in a process known as *hatching.* The blastocyst is now freely exposed to the fluid contents of the uterine cavity. This glycogen-rich fluid, secreted by the uterine glands, provides nutrients to the blastocyst. When fully formed, the blastocyst contacts the endometrium, and implantation begins.

Implantation

Implantation (**Figure 20-3**) begins as the blastocyst surface next to the inner cell mass adheres to the uterine lining (day 7, **Figure 20-3**). At the point of contact, the trophoblast cells

Figure 20-2 Cleavage and Blastocyst Formation.

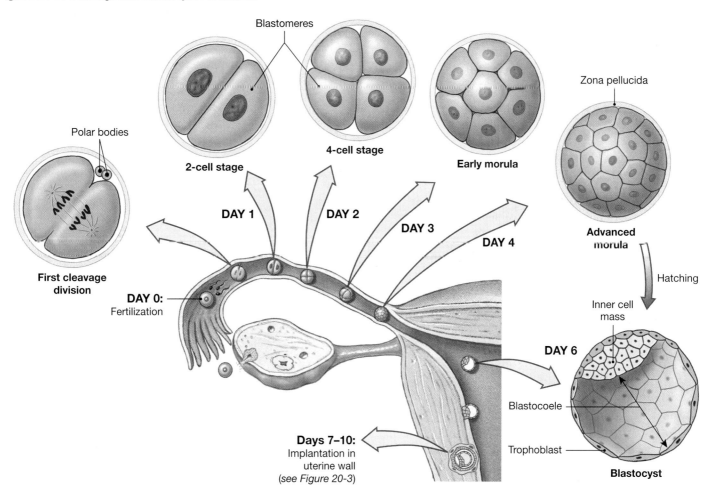

divide rapidly, making the trophoblast several layers thick. The trophoblast cells closest to the interior of the blastocyst remain intact, forming a layer of *cellular trophoblast* (day 8, **Figure 20-3**). Near the uterine wall, the cell membranes separating the trophoblast cells disappear, creating a layer of cytoplasm containing multiple nuclei. This outer layer is called the *syncytial* (sin-SISH-ul) *trophoblast.* It erodes a path through the uterine epithelium by secreting hyaluronidase. At first, this erosion creates a gap in the uterine lining, but the division and migration of uterine epithelial cells soon repair the surface. By day 10, repairs are complete, and the blastocyst no longer contacts the uterine cavity. Further development occurs entirely within the functional zone of the endometrium.

In most cases, implantation occurs in the fundus or elsewhere in the body of the uterus. In an **ectopic pregnancy**, implantation occurs somewhere other than within the uterus, such as in one of the uterine tubes. Approximately 0.6 percent of pregnancies are ectopic pregnancies. They do not produce a viable embryo and can be life-threatening to the mother.

As implantation proceeds, the syncytial trophoblast continues to enlarge into the surrounding endometrium (day 9, **Figure 20-3**). The syncytial trophoblast absorbs nutrients released by the erosion of uterine gland cells. The nutrients then diffuse through the cellular trophoblast to the inner cell mass. These nutrients provide the energy for the early stages of embryo formation. Trophoblast extensions grow around endometrial capillaries. As the capillary walls are destroyed, maternal blood begins to flow through trophoblastic channels known as *lacunae* (*lacuna,* singular). Fingerlike *villi* extend away from the trophoblast into the surrounding endometrium. The villi gradually increase in size and complexity as development proceeds.

Formation of the Amniotic Cavity

By the time of implantation, the inner cell mass has separated from the trophoblast. The separation gradually enlarges, creating a fluid-filled chamber called the **amniotic** (am-nē-OT-ik) **cavity** (day 9, **Figure 20-3**; details from

20

Figure 20-3 Events in Implantation.

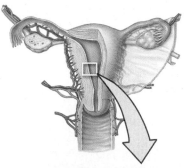

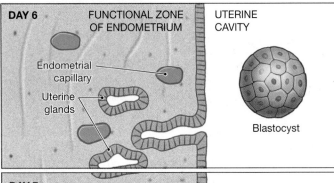

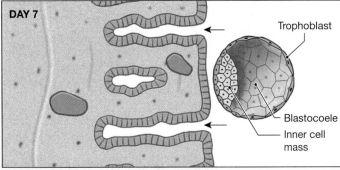

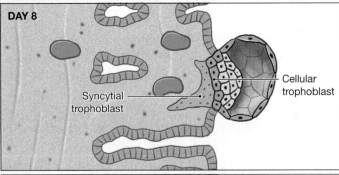

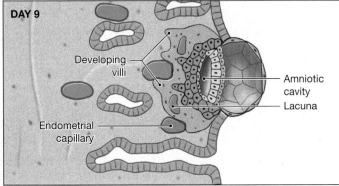

CLINICAL NOTE

Ectopic Pregnancy

The fertilized egg normally is implanted in the endometrial lining of the uterine wall. The term *ectopic pregnancy* refers to the abnormal implantation of the fertilized egg outside of the uterus. Approximately 95 percent of ectopic pregnancies are implanted in the fallopian tube. Occasionally (less than 1 percent), the egg is implanted in the abdominal cavity. Current research indicates that the incidence of ectopic pregnancy is one for every 44 live births. Improved diagnostic technology is credited with an increased incidence, as most are detected between the 2nd and 12th weeks. Ectopic pregnancy accounts for approximately 10 percent of maternal mortality.

Predisposing factors in the development of ectopic pregnancy include scarring of the fallopian tubes due to pelvic inflammatory disease (PID), a previous ectopic pregnancy, or previous pelvic or tubal surgery, such as a tubal ligation. Other factors include endometriosis or use of an intrauterine device (IUD) for birth control.

Ectopic pregnancy most often presents as abdominal pain, which starts as diffuse tenderness and then localizes as a sharp pain in the lower abdominal quadrant on the affected side. This pain is due to rupture of the fallopian tube when the fetus outgrows the available space. The woman often reports that she missed a period or that her LMP occurred 4 to 6 weeks ago, but with decreased menstrual flow that was brownish in color and of shorter duration than usual. As the intra-abdominal bleeding continues, the abdomen becomes rigid and the pain intensifies and is often referred to the shoulder on the affected side. The pain is often accompanied by syncope, vaginal bleeding, and shock.

Assume that any female of childbearing age with lower abdominal pain is experiencing an ectopic pregnancy. Ectopic pregnancy poses a significant life threat to the mother. Surgery is required to resolve the situation.

days 10–12 are shown in **Figure 20-4**). When the amniotic cavity first appears, cells of the inner cell mass are organized into an oval sheet that is two cell layers thick. A superficial layer faces the amniotic cavity and a deeper layer is exposed to the fluid contents of the blastocoele.

Gastrulation and Germ Layer Formation

By day 12, a third layer of cells begins to form between the superficial and deep layers of cells of the inner cell mass through the process of **gastrulation** (gas-troo-LĀ-shun) (day 12, **Figure 20-4**). The superficial layer is called *ectoderm*, the deep layer *endoderm*, and the migrating cells *mesoderm*. Together, the three layers of cells are called *germ layers*. **Table 20-1** lists the contributions each germ layer makes to the body's organ systems.

Figure 20-4 The Inner Cell Mass and Gastrulation.

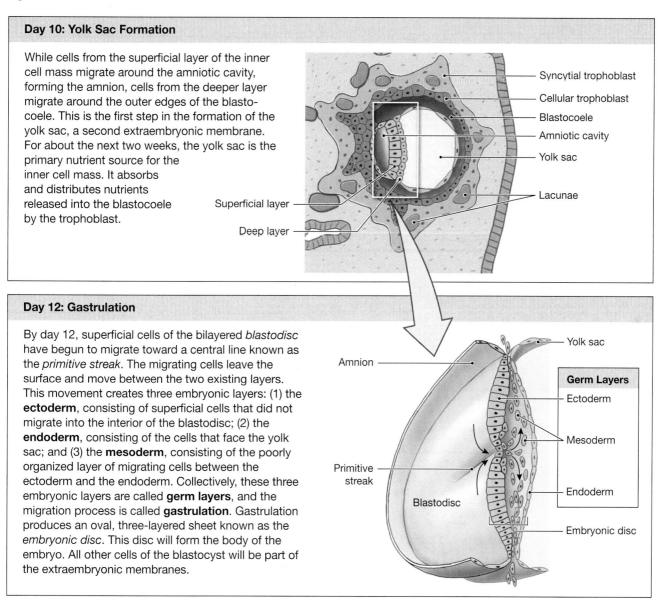

Day 10: Yolk Sac Formation

While cells from the superficial layer of the inner cell mass migrate around the amniotic cavity, forming the amnion, cells from the deeper layer migrate around the outer edges of the blastocoele. This is the first step in the formation of the yolk sac, a second extraembryonic membrane. For about the next two weeks, the yolk sac is the primary nutrient source for the inner cell mass. It absorbs and distributes nutrients released into the blastocoele by the trophoblast.

Syncytial trophoblast
Cellular trophoblast
Blastocoele
Amniotic cavity
Yolk sac
Lacunae
Superficial layer
Deep layer

Day 12: Gastrulation

By day 12, superficial cells of the bilayered *blastodisc* have begun to migrate toward a central line known as the *primitive streak*. The migrating cells leave the surface and move between the two existing layers. This movement creates three embryonic layers: (1) the **ectoderm**, consisting of superficial cells that did not migrate into the interior of the blastodisc; (2) the **endoderm**, consisting of the cells that face the yolk sac; and (3) the **mesoderm**, consisting of the poorly organized layer of migrating cells between the ectoderm and the endoderm. Collectively, these three embryonic layers are called **germ layers**, and the migration process is called **gastrulation**. Gastrulation produces an oval, three-layered sheet known as the *embryonic disc*. This disc will form the body of the embryo. All other cells of the blastocyst will be part of the extraembryonic membranes.

Amnion
Primitive streak
Blastodisc
Yolk sac

Germ Layers
Ectoderm
Mesoderm
Endoderm
Embryonic disc

The Formation of Extraembryonic Membranes

The germ layers also form four **extraembryonic membranes** that support embryonic and fetal development: the *yolk sac*, the *amnion*, the *allantois*, and the *chorion*. **Spotlight Figure 20-5** illustrates and describes the development of these extraembryonic membranes.

YOLK SAC. The first extraembryonic membrane to appear is the **yolk sac**. The yolk sac, already present 10 days after fertilization, forms a pouch within the blastocoele (**Figure 20-4**). As gastrulation proceeds, mesodermal cells migrate around this pouch and complete the formation of the yolk sac (week 2, **Spotlight Figure 20-5**). Blood vessels

soon appear within the mesoderm. The yolk sac becomes an important site of blood cell formation.

AMNION. The **amnion** (AM-nē-on) is composed of both ectoderm and mesoderm. Ectodermal cells first spread over the inner surface of the amniotic cavity and, soon after, mesodermal cells follow and create a second, outer layer. As the embryo and later the fetus enlarges, the amnion continues to expand, increasing the size of the amniotic cavity (week 3, **Spotlight Figure 20-5**). The amnion contains *amniotic fluid*, which surrounds and cushions the developing embryo and fetus (week 10, **Spotlight Figure 20-5**).

20

Table 20-1	Contributions of the Germ Layers to the Body's Organ Systems
ECTODERMAL CONTRIBUTIONS	
Integumentary system: epidermis, hair follicles and hairs, nails, and glands communicating with the skin (sweat glands, mammary glands, and sebaceous glands)	
Skeletal system: pharyngeal cartilages of the embryo develop into portions of sphenoid and hyoid bones, auditory ossicles, and the styloid processes of the temporal bones	
Nervous system: all neural tissue, including brain and spinal cord	
Endocrine system: pituitary gland and the adrenal medullae	
Respiratory system: mucous epithelium of nasal passageways	
Digestive system: mucous epithelium of mouth and anus, salivary glands	
MESODERMAL CONTRIBUTIONS	
Integumentary system: dermis (and hypodermis)	
Skeletal system: all structures except some pharyngeal cartilage derivatives	
Muscular system: all structures	
Endocrine system: adrenal cortex, endocrine tissues of heart, kidneys, and gonads	
Cardiovascular system: all structures	
Lymphatic system: all structures	
Urinary system: the kidneys, including the nephrons and the initial portions of the collecting system	
Reproductive system: the gonads and the adjacent portions of the duct systems	
Miscellaneous: the lining of the pleural, pericardial, and peritoneal cavities and the connective tissues that support all organ systems	
ENDODERMAL CONTRIBUTIONS	
Endocrine system: thymus, thyroid gland, and pancreas	
Respiratory system: respiratory epithelium (except nasal passageways) and associated mucous glands	
Digestive system: mucous epithelium (except mouth and anus), exocrine glands (except salivary glands), liver, and pancreas	
Urinary system: urinary bladder and distal portions of the duct system	
Reproductive system: distal portions of the duct system, stem cells that produce gametes	

THE ALLANTOIS. The **allantois** (a-LAN-tō-is) is a sac of endoderm and mesoderm that extends away from the embryo (week 3, **Spotlight Figure 20-5**). The base of the allantois later gives rise to the urinary bladder. The allantois accumulates some of the small amount of urine produced by the kidneys during embryonic development.

THE CHORION. The **chorion** (KŌ-rē-on) is created as migrating mesodermal cells form a layer beneath the trophoblast, separating it from the blastocoele (weeks 2 and 3, **Spotlight Figure 20-5**). When implantation first occurs, the nutrients absorbed by the trophoblast can easily reach the inner cell mass by diffusion. But as the embryo and trophoblast enlarge, the distance between them increases, and diffusion alone cannot keep pace with the demands of the embryo. Blood vessels now begin to develop within the mesoderm of the chorion, creating a rapid-transit system for nutrients that links the embryo with the trophoblast.

Placentation

The **placenta** is a temporary structure in the uterine wall that provides a site for diffusion between the fetal and maternal circulations. **Placentation** (pla-sen-TĀ-shun), or *placenta formation*, takes place when blood vessels form in the chorion around the periphery of the blastocyst. By week 3 of development, the mesoderm extends along each of the trophoblastic villi, forming *chorionic villi* in contact with maternal tissues (**Spotlight Figure 20-5**). Embryonic blood vessels develop in each villus. Circulation through these chorionic vessels begins early in week 3, when the heart starts beating. These villi continue to enlarge and branch, forming an intricate network within the endometrium. Blood vessels continue to be eroded, and maternal blood flows slowly through the lacunae. Chorionic blood vessels pass close by, and gases and nutrients diffuse between the embryonic and maternal circulations across the trophoblast layers.

At first, the entire blastocyst is surrounded by chorionic villi. The chorion continues to enlarge, expanding like a balloon within the endometrium. By week 4, the embryo, amnion, and yolk sac are suspended within an expansive, fluid-filled chamber. The *body stalk*, the connection between the embryo and the chorion, contains the distal portions of the allantois and blood vessels that carry blood to and from the placenta. The narrow connection between the endoderm of the embryo and the yolk sac is called the *yolk stalk*. As the end of the first trimester approaches, the fetus moves farther away from the placenta. The yolk stalk and body stalk begin to fuse, forming an *umbilical stalk* (week 5, **Spotlight Figure 20-5**). By week 10, the fetus floats free within the amniotic cavity. The fetus remains connected to the placenta by the tubelike **umbilical cord**, which contains the allantois, placental blood vessels, and the yolk stalk (week 10, **Spotlight Figure 20-5**).

Placental Circulation

Figure 20-6 diagrams the circulation at the placenta near the end of the first trimester. Deoxygenated blood flows from the developing embryo or fetus to the placenta through the paired **umbilical arteries**. Oxygenated blood returns to the developing embryo or fetus in a single **umbilical vein**. ↻ p. 462 The chorionic villi provide the surface area for the active and passive exchanges of gases, nutrients, and wastes between the fetal and maternal bloodstreams.

The Endocrine Placenta

In addition to its role in the nutrition of the fetus, the placenta acts as an endocrine organ. Several hormones are synthesized by the syncytial trophoblast and released into the maternal bloodstream. They include *human chorionic gonadotropin, progesterone, estrogens, human placental lactogen, placental prolactin*, and *relaxin*.

Human chorionic (kō-rē-ON-ik)**gonadotropin (hCG)** appears in the maternal bloodstream soon after implantation. Its presence in blood or urine samples is a reliable indication of pregnancy. Home pregnancy tests detect this hormone.

Like luteinizing hormone (LH), hCG maintains the corpus luteum and promotes the continued secretion of progesterone. As a result, the endometrial lining remains perfectly functional, and menses does not occur. Without hCG, the pregnancy ends, because another uterine cycle begins and the functional zone of the endometrium disintegrates.

In the presence of hCG, the corpus luteum persists for three to four months before gradually shrinking. The decline of the corpus luteum does not trigger the return of uterine cycles, because by the end of the first trimester, the placenta is actively secreting both **progesterone** and **estrogens**.

After the first trimester, the placenta produces enough progesterone to maintain the endometrial lining and continue the pregnancy. As the end of the third trimester approaches, estrogen production accelerates. The rising estrogen levels play a role in stimulating labor and delivery.

Human placental lactogen (hPL) and **placental prolactin** help prepare the mammary glands for milk production. The conversion of the mammary glands from resting to active status requires placental hormones (hPL, placental prolactin, estrogen, and progesterone) and several maternal hormones (growth hormone, prolactin, and thyroid hormones).

Relaxin is a hormone secreted by both the placenta and the corpus luteum during pregnancy. Relaxin (1) increases the flexibility of the pubic symphysis, permitting the pelvis to expand during delivery; (2) causes the cervix to dilate, making it easier for the fetus to enter the vaginal canal; and (3) suppresses the release of oxytocin by the hypothalamus and delays the onset of labor contractions.

Embryogenesis

Shortly after gastrulation begins, the body of the embryo begins to separate itself from the rest of the embryonic disc. The body of the embryo and its internal organs start to form. The process of embryo formation is called **embryogenesis** (em-brē-ō-JEN-e-sis). It begins as folding and differential growth of the embryonic disc produce a bulge that projects into the amniotic cavity (**Spotlight Figure 20-5 ❷**). This bulge is known as the *head fold*. Similar movements lead to the formation of a *tail fold* (**Spotlight Figure 20-5 ❸**). By this time, the embryo can be seen to have dorsal and ventral surfaces and left and right sides. The changes in proportions and appearance that occur between week 4 of development and the end of the first trimester are presented in **Figure 20-7**.

The first trimester is a critical period for development. Events during these first 12 weeks establish the basis for **organogenesis**, the process of organ formation. **Table 20-2** includes important developmental milestones, including those during the first trimester.

CHECKPOINT

8. What is the developmental fate of the inner cell mass of the blastocyst?

9. Sue's pregnancy test indicates an elevated level of the hormone hCG (human chorionic gonadotropin). Explain whether she is pregnant or not.

10. What are two important functions of the placenta?

See the blue Answers tab at the back of the book.

20

The germ layers introduced in Figure 20-4 also form four **extraembryonic membranes: (1)** The **yolk sac** (endoderm and mesoderm), **(2)** the **amnion** (ectoderm and mesoderm), **(3)** the **allantois** (endoderm and mesoderm), and **(4)** the **chorion** (mesoderm and trophoblast). These membranes support embryonic and fetal development, but few traces of their existence remain in adults.

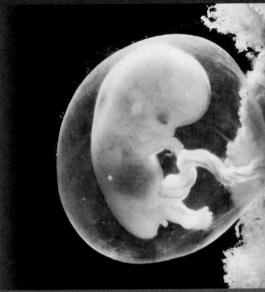

Yolk sac

The yolk sac begins as a layer of cells spreads out around the outer edges of the blastocoele to form a complete pouch. It is the primary nutrient source for early embryonic development, and becomes an important site for blood cell formation.

Amnion

Ectodermal cells spread over the inner surface of the amniotic cavity, soon followed by mesodermal cells. Amniotic fluid is produced, which cushions the developing embryo.

1 Week 2

Migration of mesoderm around the inner surface of the cellular trophoblast forms the chorion. Mesodermal migration around the outside of the amniotic cavity, between the ectodermal cells and the trophoblast, forms the amnion. Mesodermal migration around the endodermal pouch creates the yolk sac.

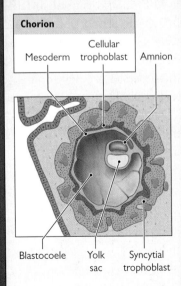

Chorion
Mesoderm — Cellular trophoblast — Amnion

Blastocoele — Yolk sac — Syncytial trophoblast

2 Week 3

The embryonic disc bulges into the amniotic cavity at the head fold. The allantois, an endodermal extension surrounded by mesoderm, extends toward the trophoblast.

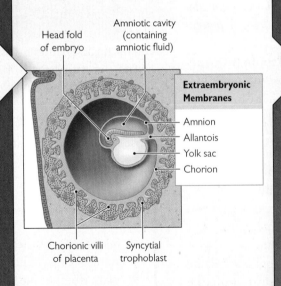

Head fold of embryo — Amniotic cavity (containing amniotic fluid)

Extraembryonic Membranes
— Amnion
— Allantois
— Yolk sac
— Chorion

Chorionic villi of placenta — Syncytial trophoblast

3 Week 4

The embryo now has a head fold and a tail fold. Constriction of the connections between the embryo and the surrounding trophoblast narrows the yolk stalk and body stalk.

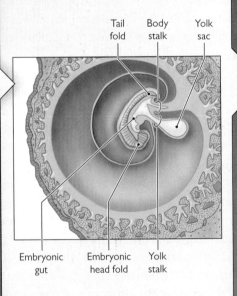

Tail fold — Body stalk — Yolk sac

Embryonic gut — Embryonic head fold — Yolk stalk

Allantois

The allantois begins as an outpocket of the endoderm near the base of the yolk sac. The free endodermal tip then grows toward the wall of the blastocyst, surrounded by a mass of mesodermal cells. The base of the allantois eventually gives rise to the urinary bladder.

Chorion

The mesoderm associated with the allantois spreads around the entire blastocyst, separating the cellular trophoblast from the blastocoele. The appearance of blood vessels in the chorion is the first step in the creation of a functional placenta. By the third week of development, the mesoderm extends along the core of each trophoblastic villus, forming chorionic villi in contact with maternal tissues and blood vessels. These villi continue to enlarge and branch, forming the placenta, the exchange platform between mother and fetus for nutrients, oxygen, and wastes.

4 **Week 5**

The developing embryo and extraembryonic membranes bulge into the uterine cavity. The trophoblast pushing out into the uterine cavity remains covered by endometrium but no longer participates in nutrient absorption and embryo support. The embryo moves away from the placenta, and the body stalk and yolk stalk fuse to form an umbilical stalk.

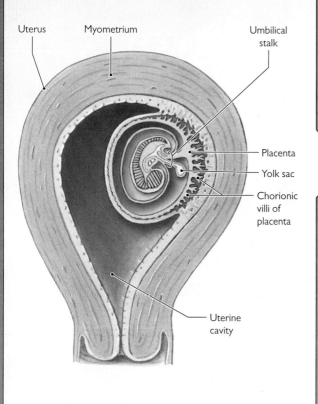

Uterus Myometrium Umbilical stalk

Placenta

Yolk sac

Chorionic villi of placenta

Uterine cavity

5 **Week 10**

The amnion has expanded greatly, filling the uterine cavity. The fetus is connected to the placenta by an elongated umbilical cord that contains a portion of the allantois, blood vessels, and the remnants of the yolk stalk.

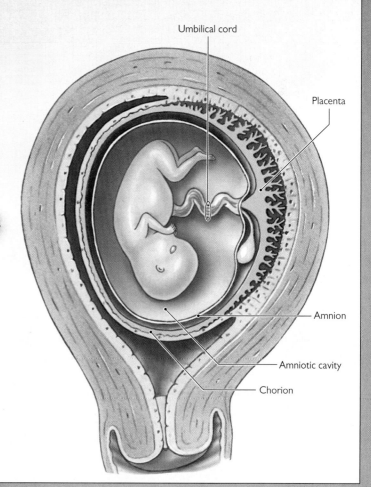

Umbilical cord

Placenta

Amnion

Amniotic cavity

Chorion

Figure 20-6 The Placenta and Placental Circulation. A view of the uterus after the embryo has been removed and the umbilical cord cut. Oxygenated blood flows from the mother into the placenta through ruptured maternal arteries. It then flows around chorionic villi that contain fetal blood vessels. Deoxygenated fetal blood enters the chorionic villi in paired umbilical arteries, and oxygenated blood then leaves in a single umbilical vein. Deoxygenated maternal blood re-enters the mother's venous system through the broken walls of small uterine veins. Note that no mixing of maternal and fetal blood occurs.

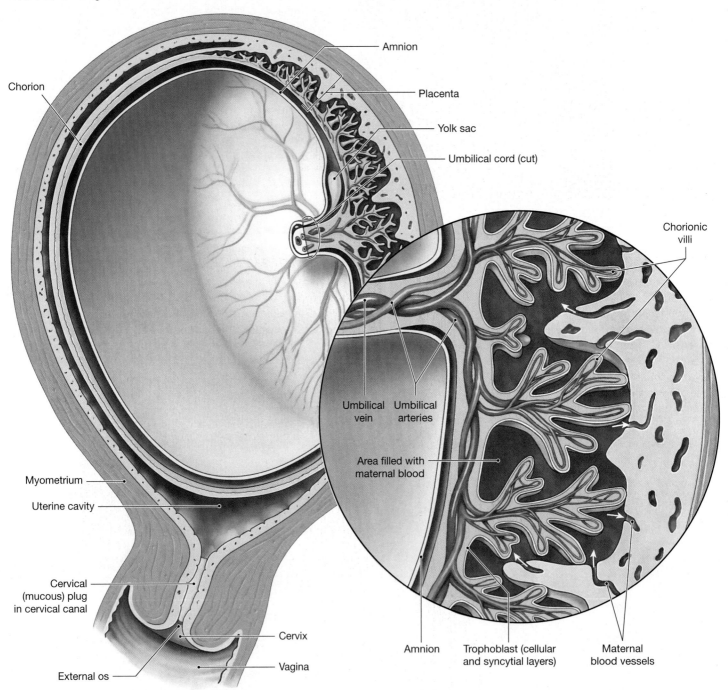

Figure 20-7 Development during the First Trimester.

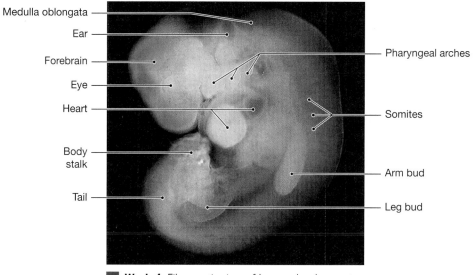

Medulla oblongata

Ear

Forebrain

Eye

Heart

Body stalk

Tail

Pharyngeal arches

Somites

Arm bud

Leg bud

a **Week 4.** Fiber-optic view of human development at week 4 (about 5 mm in size).

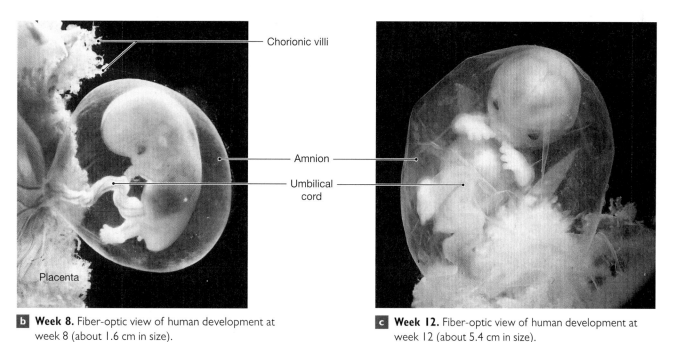

Chorionic villi

Amnion

Umbilical cord

Placenta

b **Week 8.** Fiber-optic view of human development at week 8 (about 1.6 cm in size).

c **Week 12.** Fiber-optic view of human development at week 12 (about 5.4 cm in size).

20-5 During the second and third trimesters, maternal organ systems support the developing fetus, and the uterus undergoes structural and functional changes

Learning Objective Describe the interplay between maternal organ systems and the developing fetus, and discuss the structural and functional changes in the uterus during gestation.

The basic elements of all the major organ systems have formed by the end of the first trimester. Over the next three months, the fetus grows to a weight of about 0.64 kg (1.4 lb). Encircled by the amnion, the fetus grows faster than the surrounding placenta during this second trimester. When the outer surface of the amnion contacts the inner surface of the chorion, these layers fuse. **Figure 20-8a** shows a 4-month-old fetus. **Figure 20-8b** shows a 6-month-old fetus. The changes in body form that occur during the first trimester and part

20

Table 20-2 **An Overview of Prenatal and Early Postnatal Development**

   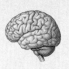

Gestational Age (developmental age plus 2 weeks)(Months)	Size and Weight*	Integumentary System	Skeletal System	Muscular System	Nervous System	Special Sense Organs
1	5 mm (0.2 in.), 0.02 g (0.0007 oz)		(b) Somite formation (paired blocks of mesoderm)	(b) Somite formation	(b) Neural tube formation	(b) Eye and ear formation
2	1.6 cm (0.63 in.), 1.0 g (0.04 oz)	(b) Nail beds, hair follicles, sweat glands	(b) Axial and appendicular cartilage formation	(c) Rudiments of axial musculature	(b) CNS, PNS organization, growth of cerebrum	(b) Taste buds, olfactory epithelium formation
3	5.4 cm (2.13 in.), 14 g (0.05 oz)	(b) Epidermal layers appear	(b) Spreading of ossification centers	(c) Rudiments of appendicular musculature	(c) Basic spinal cord and brain structure	
4	11.6 cm (4.6 in.), 100 g (3.53 oz)	(b) Hair, sebaceous glands formation (c) Sweat glands	(b) Articulations (c) Facial and palatal organization	Movements of fetus can be felt by the mother	(b) Rapid expansion of cerebrum	(c) Basic eye and ear structure (b) Peripheral receptor formation
5	16.4 cm (6.46 in.), 300 g (10.58 oz)	(b) Keratin production, nail production			(b) Myelination of spinal cord	
6	30 cm (11.8 in.), 600 g (1.32 lb)			(c) Perineal muscles	(b) CNS tract formation (c) Layering of cortex	
7	37.6 cm (14.8 in.), 1.005 kg (2.22 lb)	(b) Keratinization, formation of nails, hair				(c) Eyelids open, retinae sensitive to light
8	42.4 cm (16.7 in.), 1.7 kg (3.75 lb)		(b) Epiphyseal cartilage formation			(c) Taste receptors functional
9	47.4 cm (18.66 in.), 3.2 kg (7.05 lb)					
Postnatal Development		Hair changes in consistency and distribution	Formation and growth of epiphyseal cartilages continue	Muscle mass and control increase	Myelination, layering, CNS tract formation continue	

Note: (b) = beginning to form; (c) completed
*From 8 weeks to about 20 weeks, the fetus is measured from crown to rump. From 20 weeks to birth, the length measured is from crown to heel.

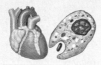 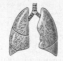

Gestational Age (Months)	Endocrine System	Cardiovascular and Lymphatic Systems	Respiratory System	Digestive System	Urinary System	Reproductive System
1		(b) Heartbeat	(b) Trachea and lung formation	(b) Intestinal tract, liver, and pancreas formation (c) Yolk sac	(c) Allantois	
2	(b) Thymus, thyroid, pituitary, adrenal glands	(c) Basic heart structure, major blood vessels, lymph nodes and ducts (b) Blood formation in liver	(b) Extensive bronchial branching into mediastinum (c) Diaphragm	(b) Intestinal subdivisions, villi, and salivary glands formation	(b) Kidney formation (adult form)	(b) Mammary glands formation
3	(c) Thymus, thyroid gland	(b) Tonsils, blood formation in bone marrow		(c) Gallbladder, pancreas		(b) Formation of gonads, ducts, and genitalia; oogonia in female
4		(b) Migration of lymphocytes to lymphoid organs; blood formation in spleen			(b) Degeneration of embryonic kidneys	
5		(c) Tonsils	(c) Nostrils open	(c) Intestinal subdivisions		
6	(c) Adrenal glands	(c) Spleen, liver, bone marrow	(b) Formation of alveoli	(c) Epithelial organization, glands		
7	(c) Pituitary gland			(c) Intestinal circular folds		(b) Testes descend; primary oocytes in prophase I of meiosis in female
8			Complete pulmonary branching and alveolar formation		(c) Nephron formation	Descent of testes complete at or near time of delivery
9						
Postnatal Development		Cardiovascular changes at birth; immune response gradually becomes operational				

Figure 20-8 The Second and Third Trimesters.

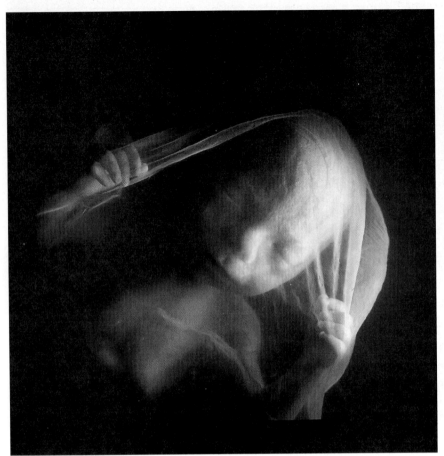

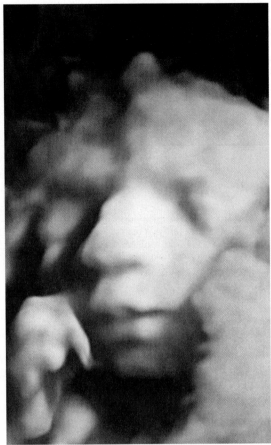

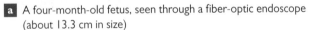

a A four-month-old fetus, seen through a fiber-optic endoscope (about 13.3 cm in size)

b Head of a six-month-old fetus, revealed through ultrasound (about 30 cm in size)

of the second trimester are shown in the upper portion of **Figure 20-8**.

During the third trimester, most of the organ systems become ready to perform their normal functions. The rate of growth starts to slow, but in absolute terms, this trimester sees the greatest weight gain. In the last three months of gestation, the fetus gains about 2.6 kg (5.7 lb), reaching a full-term weight of about 3.2 kg (7 lb). Highlights in organ system development during the second and third trimesters are noted in **Table 20-2** on pp. 784 and 785.

The Effects of Pregnancy on Maternal Systems

The developing fetus is totally dependent on maternal organ systems for nourishment, respiration, and waste removal. The mother must absorb enough oxygen, nutrients, and vitamins for herself *and* her fetus. She must also eliminate all the wastes that are generated. This is not a burden over the beginning weeks of gestation, but the demands placed on the mother become significant as the fetus grows. For the mother to survive under these conditions, maternal systems must make major adjustments. In practical terms, the mother must breathe, eat, and excrete for two. The major changes in maternal systems include the following:

- *Maternal respiratory rate increases and tidal volume increases.* As a result, the mother's lungs deliver the extra oxygen required and remove the excess carbon dioxide the fetus generates.

- *Maternal blood volume increases.* This increase occurs for two reasons. (1) Blood flowing into the placenta reduces the volume in the rest of the systemic circuit. (2) Fetal activity both decreases blood P_{O_2} and increases blood P_{CO_2}. The latter combination stimulates the production of renin and erythropoietin (EPO) by the kidneys, leading to an increase in maternal blood volume (see Figure 13-10, p. 505). By the end of gestation, maternal blood volume has increased by almost 50 percent.

CLINICAL NOTE

TERATOGENICITY

The developing fetus is most vulnerable to birth defects during the first 60 days of pregnancy. The first stage of gestation, *embryogenesis*, begins at conception and continues to day 18. Exposure to a *teratogen* during this time can threaten the entire embryo. (A teratogen is a chemical or disease that causes malformation of a fetus.) The second stage of gestation, *organogenesis*, extends from day 18 to day 60. This is the stage when the fetus is most susceptible to teratogens and when most gross anatomical malformations develop. The third stage, which is the *fetal period*, extends from day 60 to birth. Exposure during this stage can cause abnormal cell growth and differentiation.

- *Maternal requirements for nutrients increase by 10–30 percent.* Pregnant women tend to have increased sensations of hunger because they must nourish both themselves and their fetus.

- *Maternal glomerular filtration rate increases by roughly 50 percent.* This increase corresponds to the increase in blood volume and accelerates the excretion of

metabolic wastes generated by the fetus. Pregnant women need to urinate frequently because the volume of urine produced increases and the weight of the uterus presses down on the urinary bladder.

- *The uterus undergoes a tremendous increase in size.* Structural and functional changes in the expanding uterus are so important that we will discuss them in a separate section.

- *The mammary glands increase in size, and secretory activity begins.* By the end of the sixth month of pregnancy, the mammary glands are fully developed and begin to produce clear secretions that are stored in the duct system of those glands.

Structural and Functional Changes in the Uterus

At the end of gestation, a typical uterus will have grown from 7.5 cm (3 in.) to 30 cm (12 in.) in length, and from 60 g (2 oz) to 1100 g (2.4 lb) in weight. The uterus may then contain 2 liters of fluid, plus fetus and placenta, for a total weight of about 6–7 kg (13–15.4 lb). This remarkable expansion occurs through the

CLINICAL NOTE

Physiologic Changes of Pregnancy

The physiologic changes associated with pregnancy are due to an altered hormonal state, the mechanical effects of the enlarging uterus and its significant vascularity, and the increasing metabolic demands on the maternal system. Paramedics must understand the physiologic changes associated with pregnancy in order to better assess pregnant patients.

- *Reproductive System.* Understandably, the most significant pregnancy-related changes occur in the uterus. In its nonpregnant state, the uterus is a small pear-shaped organ that weighs about 60 g (2 ounces) with a capacity of approximately 10 cc. By the end of pregnancy, its weight has increased to 1000 g (slightly more than 2 pounds), while its capacity is now approximately 5000 mL (**Figure 20–9**). Another notable change is that during pregnancy the vascular system of the uterus contains about one-sixth (16 percent) of the mother's total blood volume. Other changes that occur in the reproductive system include the formation of a mucous plug in the cervix that protects

Figure 20-9 Uterus during Pregnancy. Significant uterine changes are associated with pregnancy. By term, the uterus is the largest organ in the abdomen.

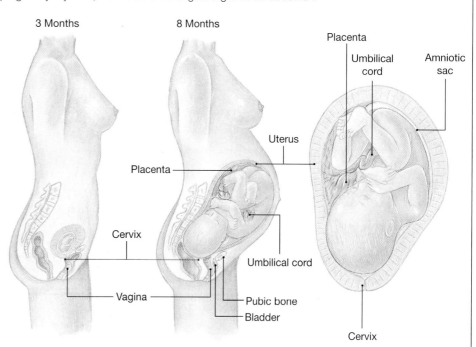

(Continued)

the developing fetus and helps to prevent infection. This plug will be expelled when cervical dilation begins prior to delivery. Estrogen causes the vaginal mucosa to thicken, vaginal secretions to increase, and the connective tissue to loosen to allow for delivery. The breasts enlarge and become more nodular as the mammary glands increase in number and size in preparation for lactation.

- *Respiratory System.* During pregnancy, maternal oxygen demands increase. To meet this need, progesterone causes a decrease in airway resistance. This results in a 20 percent increase in oxygen consumption and a 40 percent increase in tidal volume. There is only a slight increase in respiratory rate. The enlarging uterus pushes up the diaphragm, which results in flaring of the rib margins to maintain intrathoracic volume.

- *Cardiovascular System.* Many changes take place in the cardiovascular system during pregnancy (**Figure 20–10**). Cardiac output increases throughout pregnancy, and peaks at 6–7 liters/minute by the time the fetus is fully developed. The maternal blood volume increases by 45 percent, and although

Figure 20-10 The Hemodynamic Changes Associated with Pregnancy. Pregnancy causes the heart rate to be faster and the blood pressure to be lower. These findings can easily be interpreted as early signs of shock if unaware of the physiological changes of pregnancy.

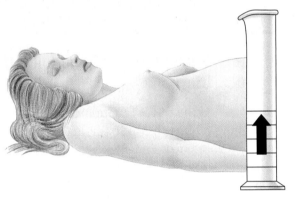

Blood volume usually increases by about 45%. Dilution resulting from the disproportionate increase of plasma volume over the red cell mass is responsible for the so-called "anemia of pregnancy."

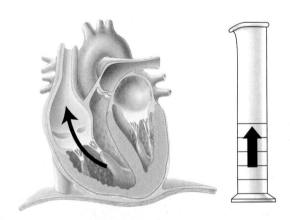

Cardiac output increases by 1.0–1.5 L/min during the 1st trimester, reaches 6–7 L/min by the late 2nd trimester, and is maintained essentially at this level until delivery.

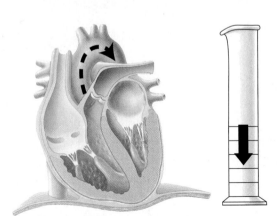

The stroke volume progressively declines to term following a rise early in pregnancy. Heart rate, however, increases by an average of 10–15 beats/min.

both red blood cells and plasma increase, there is slightly more plasma, which results in a relative anemia. To combat this anemia, pregnant women receive supplemental iron to increase the oxygen-carrying capacity of their red blood cells. Due to the increase in blood volume, the pregnant female may suffer an acute blood loss of 30–35 percent without a significant change in vital signs. The maternal heart rate increases by 10–15 beats/minute. Blood pressure decreases slightly during the first two trimesters of pregnancy and then rises to near nonpregnant levels during the third trimester.
- *Gastrointestinal System.* Nausea and vomiting are common in the first trimester of pregnancy as a result of varying hormone levels and changed carbohydrate needs. Peristalsis is slowed, so delayed gastric emptying is likely and bloating or constipation is common. As the uterus enlarges, abdominal organs are compressed, and the resulting compartmentalization of abdominal organs makes assessment difficult.

- *Urinary System.* Renal blood flow increases during pregnancy. The glomerular filtration rate increases by nearly 50 percent in the second trimester and remains elevated throughout the remainder of the pregnancy. As a result, the renal tubular absorption also increases. Occasionally glucosuria (large amounts of sugar in the urine) may result from the kidney's inability to reabsorb all of the glucose being filtered. Glucosuria may be normal or may indicate the development of gestational diabetes. The urinary bladder gets displaced anteriorly and superiorly, which increases the potential for rupture. Urinary frequency is common, particularly in the first and third trimesters, due to uterine compression of the bladder.
- *Musculoskeletal System.* Loosened pelvic joints caused by hormonal influences account for the waddling gait that is often associated with pregnancy. As the uterus enlarges and the mother's center of gravity shifts, posture changes to compensate for anterior growth, which often causes low back pain.

CLINICAL NOTE

Fetal Development

Fetal development begins immediately after fertilization and is quite complex. The time at which fertilization occurs is called *conception.* Since conception occurs approximately 14 days after the first day of the last menstrual period, it is possible to calculate, with fair accuracy, the approximate date the baby should be born. This estimate is usually made during the mother's first prenatal visit. The normal duration of pregnancy is 40 weeks from the first day of the mother's last menstrual period. This is equal to 280 days, which is 10 lunar months, or roughly 9 calendar months. This estimated birth date is commonly called the *due date.* Medically, it is known as the *estimated date of confinement.* Generally, pregnancy is divided into trimesters. Each trimester is approximately 13 weeks, or 3 calendar months, long.

Several different terms are used to describe the stages of fetal development during the course of pregnancy. The pre-embryonic stage covers the first 14 days following conception; the embryonic stage begins at day 15 and ends at approximately 8 weeks; and the fetal stage lasts from 8 weeks of age until delivery. Emergency personnel should be familiar with some of the significant developmental milestones that occur during these three periods (**Table 20–3**). During normal fetal development, the sex of the infant can usually be determined by 16 weeks gestation. By the 20th week, fetal heart tones can be detected by stethoscope. The mother also has generally felt fetal movement. By 24 weeks, the baby may be able to survive if born prematurely. Fetuses born after 28 weeks have an excellent chance of survival. By the 38th week the baby is considered term, or fully developed. Most of the fetus's organ systems develop during the first trimester. Therefore, this is when the fetus is most vulnerable to the development of birth defects.

enlargement of existing cells, especially smooth muscle cells, rather than by an increase in the total number of cells.

The tremendous stretching of the uterus is associated with a gradual increase in the rates of spontaneous smooth muscle contractions in the myometrium. In the early stages of pregnancy, the contractions are weak, painless, and brief. Evidence indicates that progesterone from the placenta has an inhibitory effect on uterine smooth muscle, preventing more extensive and powerful contractions.

After nine months of gestation, several factors interact to produce **labor contractions** in the myometrium of the uterine wall. Once begun, positive feedback ensures that the contractions continue until delivery has been completed. **Figure 20-11** diagrams important placental and fetal factors that initiate labor and delivery.

The actual trigger for the onset of labor may be events in the fetus rather than in the mother. When labor begins, the fetal pituitary gland secretes oxytocin, which is released into the maternal bloodstream at the placenta. This may be the actual trigger for the onset of labor, as it increases myometrial contractions and prostaglandin production, on top of the priming effects of estrogens and maternal oxytocin.

CHECKPOINT

11. List the major changes that take place in maternal systems during pregnancy.

12. Why does a mother's blood volume increase during pregnancy?

13. By what means does the uterus greatly increase in size and weight during pregnancy?

14. Identify three major factors opposing the calming action of progesterone on the uterus.

See the blue Answers tab at the back of the book.

Figure 20-11 Factors Involved in the Initiation of Labor and Delivery.

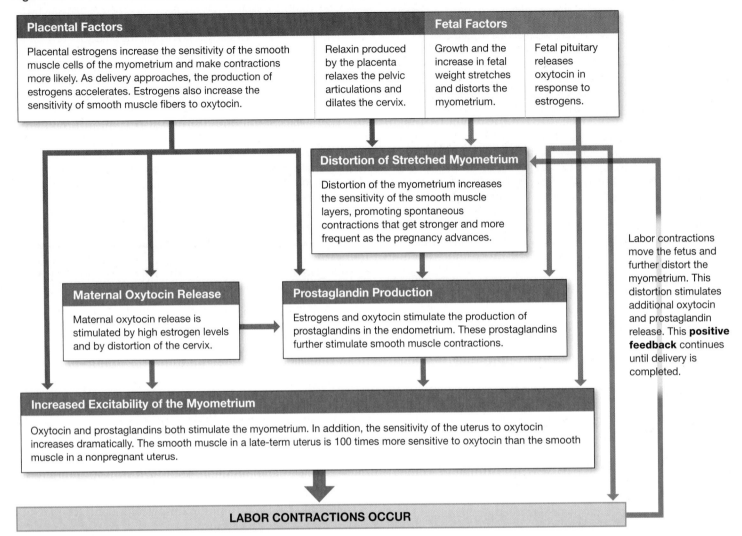

20-6 Labor consists of the dilation, expulsion, and placental stages

Learning Objective List and discuss the events that occur during labor and delivery.

The goal of labor is **parturition** (par-toor-ISH-un), or *childbirth*, the forcible expulsion of the fetus from the uterus. During labor, each uterine contraction begins near the superior portion of the uterus and sweeps in a wave toward the cervix. The contractions are strong and occur at regular intervals. As parturition approaches, the contractions increase in force and frequency, changing the position of the fetus and moving it toward the cervical canal.

The Stages of Labor

Labor consists of three stages: the *dilation stage*, the *expulsion stage*, and the *placental stage* (**Figure 20-12**).

1. The **dilation stage** begins with the onset of labor, as the cervix dilates and the fetus begins to shift toward the cervical canal (❶ in **Figure 20-12**). This stage is highly variable in length but typically lasts eight or more hours. At first, labor contractions last up to one minute and occur once every 10–30 minutes. Their frequency increases steadily. Late in this stage, the amnion usually ruptures. This event is sometimes referred to as the woman having her "water break."

2. The **expulsion stage** begins as the cervix, pushed open by the approaching fetus, dilates completely to about 10 cm (4 in.) (❷ in **Figure 20-12**). In this stage, contractions reach maximum intensity. Expulsion continues until the fetus has emerged from the vagina. In most cases, the expulsion stage lasts less than two hours. The arrival of the newborn into the outside world is **delivery**, or birth.

   If the vaginal canal is too small to permit the passage of the fetus, posing acute danger of perineal tearing, a

Figure 20-12 The Stages of Labor.

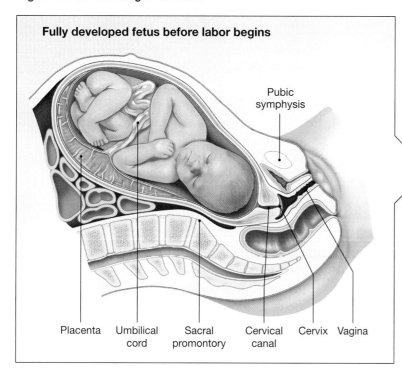

Fully developed fetus before labor begins

Pubic symphysis

Placenta | Umbilical cord | Sacral promontory | Cervical canal | Cervix | Vagina

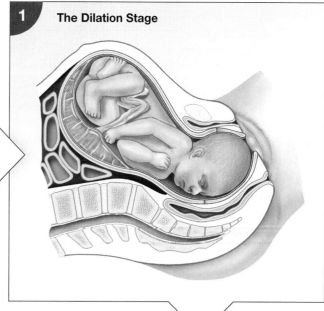

1 **The Dilation Stage**

2 **The Expulsion Stage**

3 **The Placental Stage**

Uterus | Ejection of the placenta

clinician may temporarily enlarge the passageway by performing an **episiotomy** (e-piz-ē-OT-o-mē), an incision through the perineal musculature. After delivery, this surgical cut can be repaired with sutures, a much simpler procedure than suturing the jagged edges associated with an extensive perineal tear.

If complications arise during the dilation or expulsion stage, the infant can be surgically removed by -**cesarean section**, or *"C-section."* In such cases, an incision is made through the abdominal wall, and the uterus is opened just enough to allow passage of the infant's head. Preliminary data released in 2015 from the CDC's National Vital Statistics System showed that cesarean deliveries dropped to 32.2 percent of all live births in 2014, after peaking at 32.9 percent in 2009.

3. During the **placental stage** of labor, muscle tension builds in the walls of the partially empty uterus, which gradually decreases in size (**3** in **Figure 20-12**). This uterine contraction tears the connections between the endometrium and the placenta. In general, within an hour of delivery, the placental stage ends with the ejection of the placenta, or *afterbirth*. The disruption of the placenta is accompanied by a loss of blood. This loss can normally be tolerated without difficulty because maternal blood volume has increased greatly during pregnancy.

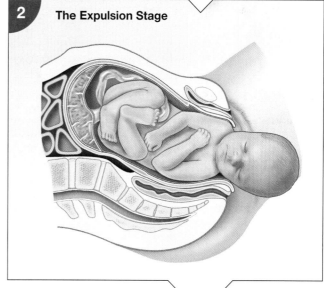
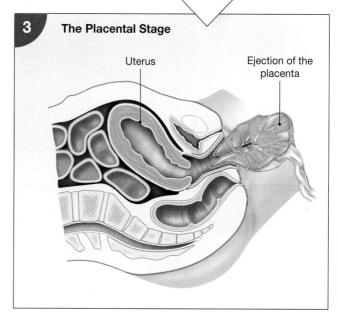

20

Premature Labor

Premature labor occurs when labor contractions begin before the fetus has completed normal development. The newborn's chances of survival are directly related to its body weight at delivery. Even with massive supportive efforts, newborns weighing less than 400 g (14 oz) at birth will not survive, primarily because their respiratory, cardiovascular, and urinary systems are unable to support life. As a result, the dividing line between spontaneous abortion and **immature delivery** is usually set at a body weight of 500 g (17.6 oz), the normal weight near the end of the second trimester.

Most fetuses born at 25–27 weeks of gestation (a birth weight under 600 g or 21.1 oz) die despite intensive neonatal care. Survivors have a high risk of developmental abnormalities. **Premature delivery** usually refers to birth at 28–36 weeks (a birth weight over 1 kg or 2.2 lb). With care, these newborns have a good chance of surviving and developing normally.

Multiple Births

Multiple births (twins, triplets, quadruplets, and so on) can take place for several reasons. The ratio of twin births to single births in the U.S. population is roughly 1:89. "Fraternal twins," or **dizygotic** (dī-zī-GOT-ik) **twins,** develop when two separate oocytes are ovulated and fertilized. Fraternal twins can be of the same or different sexes. About 70 percent of all twins are fraternal.

"Identical twins," or **monozygotic twins**, result either from the separation of blastomeres early in cleavage or from the splitting of the inner cell mass before gastrulation. In either event, the genetic makeup and sex of the pair are identical because both twins formed from the same pair of gametes. Identical twins occur in about 30 percent of all twin births. Triplets and larger multiple births can result from the same processes that produce twins. Taking fertility drugs that stimulate the maturation of abnormally large numbers of follicles can increase the incidence of multiple births.

If the splitting of the blastomeres or of the embryonic disc is not complete, **conjoined** (Siamese) **twins** may develop. These genetically identical twins typically share some skin, a portion of the liver, and perhaps other internal organs as well. When the fusion is minor, the infants can be surgically separated with some success. Most conjoined twins with more extensive fusions fail to survive because their organs cannot support them.

CLINICAL NOTE

Obstetrical Terminology

The field of obstetrics has its own unique terminology. You should be familiar with this terminology, since patient documentation and communications with other health care workers and physicians often require it (**Figure 20–13**).

Figure 20-13 Childbirth. The field of obstetrics has its own unique terminology. Emergency personnel should be familiar with this system, because they must interact with other members of the health care team.

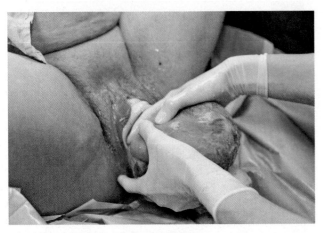

Antepartum	time interval prior to delivery of the fetus
Postpartum	time interval after delivery of the fetus
Prenatal	time interval prior to birth, synonymous with antepartum
Natal	relating to birth or the date of birth
gravidity*	number of times a woman has been pregnant
parity*	number of pregnancies carried to full term
primigravida	woman who is pregnant for the first time
Primipara	woman who has given birth to her first child
multigravida	woman who has been pregnant more than once
nulligravida	woman who has not been pregnant
Multipara	woman who has delivered more than one baby
Nullipara	woman who has yet to deliver her first child
grand multiparity	woman who has delivered at least seven babies
Gestation	period of time for intrauterine fetal development

*Gravidity and parity are expressed in the following shorthand: G_4P_2. The letter G refers to gravidity, and the letter P refers to parity. The woman referred to by "G_4P_2" would have had four pregnancies and two births.

Build Your Knowledge

Recall that the umbilical arteries that carry deoxygenated blood from the fetus to the placenta arise from the fetus's internal iliac arteries (as you saw in **Chapter 13: The Cardiovascular System: Blood Vessels and Circulation**). The umbilical vein carries oxygenated blood from the placenta into the fetus's developing liver. There, the oxygenated blood passes through the ductus venosus, mixes with deoxygenated blood from the liver's network of veins, and then drains into the inferior vena cava.

This blood bypasses the pulmonary circuit due to two fetal circulatory features. Blood from the right atrium either (1) flows directly into the left atrium through the foramen ovale, or interatrial opening, or (2) into the right atrium from where it enters the systemic circuit through a short muscular vessel called the ductus arteriosus. At birth, blood quickly begins to flow in the pulmonary circuit as blood stops flowing in the umbilical vessels, the foramen ovale closes, and the ductus arteriosus degenerates. ⟳**p. 462**

CHECKPOINT

15. Name the three stages of labor.
16. What is the difference between immature delivery and premature delivery?
17. What are the biological terms for fraternal twins and identical twins?

See the blue Answers tab at the back of the book.

20-7 Postnatal stages are the neonatal period, infancy, childhood, adolescence, and maturity, followed by senescence

Learning Objective Identify the features and physiological changes of the postnatal stages of life.

Developmental processes do not stop at delivery. A newborn has few of the anatomical, functional, or physiological characteristics of mature adults. Postnatal development typically includes five **life stages**: (1) *the neonatal* period, (2) *infancy*, (3) *childhood*, (4) *adolescence*, and (5) *maturity* (**Figure 20-14**, p. 692). Each stage has distinctive characteristics and abilities.

The Neonatal Period, Infancy, and Childhood

The **neonatal period** extends from birth to one month of age. **Infancy**, or babyhood, then continues through the first year of life. **Childhood** lasts from infancy until **adolescence**, the period of sexual maturation (puberty) and physical maturation.

Two major events are under way during these developmental stages: (1) the organ systems (except those associated with reproduction) become fully operational and gradually acquire the functional characteristics of adult structures;

and (2) the individual grows rapidly, and body proportions change significantly.

Pediatrics is the medical specialty that focuses on post-natal development from infancy through adolescence. Infants and young children often cannot clearly describe the problems they are experiencing, so pediatricians and parents must be skilled observers. Standardized tests are used to compare developmental progress with average values.

The Neonatal Period

Physiological and anatomical changes take place as a fetus completes the transition to the status of a newborn, or **neonate**. Before delivery, dissolved gases, nutrients, waste products, hormones, and antibodies were transferred across the placenta. At birth, a newborn must come to rely on its own specialized organs and organ systems to carry out respiration, digestion, and excretion. The transition from fetus to neonate can be summarized as follows:

- At birth, the lungs are collapsed and filled with fluid. Filling them with air requires a powerful inhalation. ⟳p. 531

- When the lungs expand, the pattern of cardiovascular circulation changes due to alterations in blood pressure and flow rates. The circulation changes result in separation of the pulmonary and systemic circuits. ⟳p. 462

- Typical neonatal heart rates (120–140 beats per minute) are lower than fetal heart rates (averaging 150 beats per minute). Both neonatal heart rates and respiratory rates (30 breaths per minute) are considerably higher than those of adults.

- Before birth, the digestive system is relatively inactive, but it does accumulate a mixture of bile secretions, mucus, and epithelial cells. This debris, called *meconium*, is excreted in the first few days of life. During that period, the newborn begins to nurse.

Figure 20-14 Growth and Changes in Body Form and Proportion. The views at fetal ages 4, 8, and 16 weeks are presented at actual size. Note that changes in body form and proportion do not stop at birth. For example, the head is proportionally larger at birth than it is during adulthood.

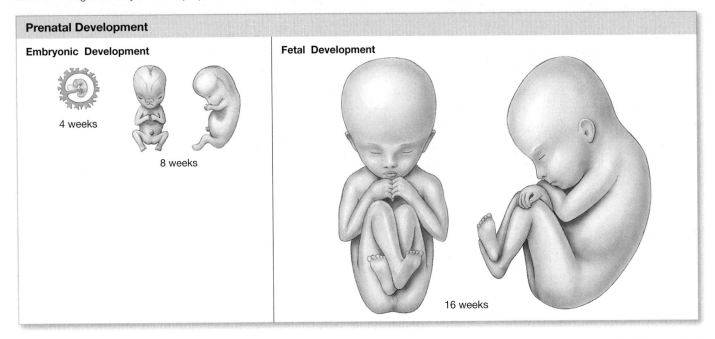

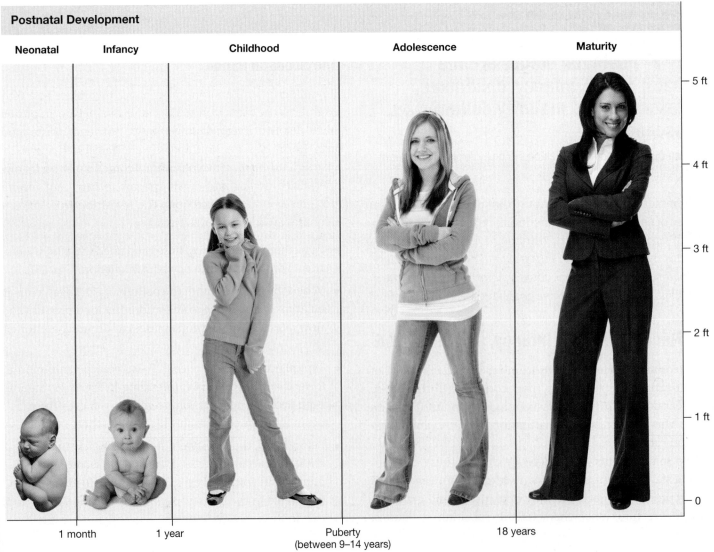

CLINICAL NOTE

Postnatal Development

Developmental processes do not end at delivery. The newborn has few of the anatomical or physiological characteristics of mature adults. In postnatal development, the individual passes through several life stages. These include: *neonatal, infancy, child-hood, adolescence*, and *maturity*. The neonatal period extends from birth to 1 month of age. Infancy is the period from 1 month of age to 2 years of age. Childhood lasts from 2 years of age until the onset of puberty.

Neonates typically lose up to 10 percent of their birth weight as they adjust to extrauterine life. However, this weight is usually recovered within 10 days. Infants should have doubled their birth weight by 5 or 6 months of age. Development occurs in a cephalo-caudal direction: muscle control begins at the head and later spreads toward the lower extremities. The personality begins to develop in early infancy and definite behaviors and characteristics are present by 5–6 months of age (**Figure 20-15**).

It is important for emergency personnel to be familiar with many of the anatomical and physiological differences of children, because they can affect patient care. **Table 20–3** illustrates important anatomical and physiological characteristics of infants and children.

Figure 20-15 Early Infancy. The period from 1 month to 2 years of age is a time of rapid development. The birth weight usually doubles, the infant exhibits improved muscle control, and the personality begins to develop.

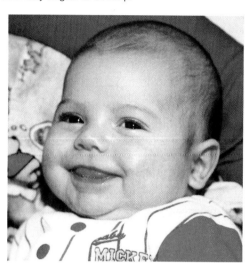

Table 20–3	Anatomical and Physiological Characteristics of Infants and Children
Differences in Infants and Children as Compared to Adults	**Potential Effects that May Impact Assessment and Care**
Tongue proportionately larger	More likely to block airway
Smaller airway structures	More easily blocked
Abundant secretions	Can block the airway
Deciduous (baby) teeth	Easily dislodged; can block the airway
Flat nose and face	Difficult to obtain good face mask seal
Head heavier relative to body and less developed neck structures and muscles	Head may be propelled more forcefully than body, which produces a higher incidence of head injury
Fontanelle and open sutures (soft spots) palpable on top of young infant's head	Bulging fontanelle can be a sign of increased intracranial pressure (but may be normal if infant is crying); shrunken fontanelle may indicate dehydration
Thinner, softer brain tissue	Susceptible to serious brain injury
Head larger in proportion to body	Tips forward when supine; possible flexion of neck, which makes neutral alignment of airway difficult
Shorter, narrower, more elastic (flexible) trachea	Can close off trachea with hyperextension of neck
Short neck	Difficult to stabilize or immobilize
Abdominal breathers	Difficult to evaluate breathing
Faster respiratory rate	Muscles easily fatigued, which causes respiratory distress
Newborns breathe primarily through the nose (obligate nose breathers)	May not automatically open mouth to breathe if nose is blocked; airway more easily blocked
Larger body surface relative to body mass	Prone to hypothermia
Softer bones	More flexible, less easily fractured; traumatic forces may be transmitted to internal organs, and cause injury without fracturing the ribs; lungs easily damaged with trauma
Spleen and liver more exposed	Organ injury likely with significant force to abdomen

- As waste products build up in the arterial blood, the kidneys excrete them. Glomerular filtration is normal, but the neonate's kidneys cannot concentrate urine to any significant degree. As a result, urinary water losses are high. Neonatal fluid requirements are proportionally much greater than those of adults.

- During embryonic and fetal development, the mother's body is at normal body temperature. At birth, the neonate has little ability to control its body temperature. Neonates also lose heat very quickly, because they have a high surface-area-to-volume ratio. To maintain a constant body temperature, their cellular metabolic rates must be high. In fact, the metabolic rate per unit of body weight in neonates is approximately twice that of adults.

LACTATION AND THE MAMMARY GLANDS. By the end of the sixth month of pregnancy, an expectant mother's mammary glands are fully developed. The gland cells begin to secrete **colostrum** (kō-LOS-trum). The newborn ingests it during the first two or three days of life. Colostrum contains more proteins and far less fat than breast milk. Many of the proteins are antibodies that may help the infant ward off infections until its own immune system becomes increasingly functional. As colostrum production drops, the mammary glands convert to milk production. Breast milk consists of water, proteins, amino acids, lipids, sugars, and salts. It also contains large quantities of *lysozymes*, enzymes with antibiotic properties.

Milk becomes available to infants through the **milk let-down reflex** (Figure 20-16). Mammary gland secretion is triggered when the infant begins to suck on the nipple. The stimulation of tactile receptors there leads to the release of oxytocin at the posterior lobe of the pituitary gland. The arrival of circulating oxytocin at the mammary gland then stimulates contractile cells in the walls of the lactiferous ducts and sinuses, resulting in the ejection of milk. The milk let-down reflex continues to function until *weaning* (withdrawing mother's milk), typically one to two years after birth. Milk production stops soon after. The mammary glands gradually return to a resting state.

Infancy and Childhood

The rate of growth is greatest during prenatal development and decreases after delivery. Growth during infancy and childhood takes place under the direction of circulating hormones, notably pituitary growth hormone, adrenal steroids, and thyroid hormones. These hormones affect each tissue and organ in specific ways, depending on the

Figure 20-16 The Milk Let-Down Reflex.

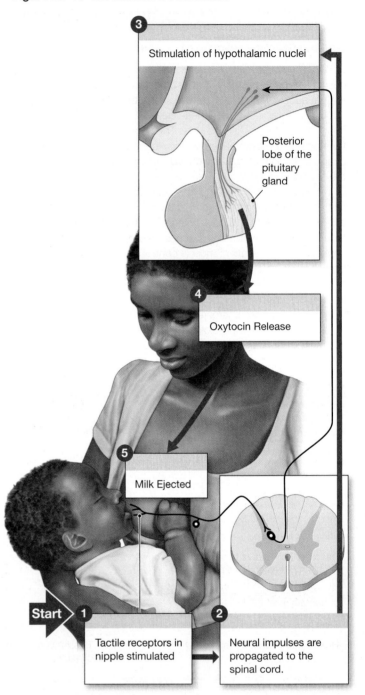

sensitivities of the individual cells. As a result, growth does not occur uniformly, and body proportions gradually change (**Figure 20-14**).

Adolescence and Maturity

Adolescence begins at **puberty**, the period of sexual maturation, and ends when growth is completed. Three major hormonal events interact at the onset of puberty:

1. The hypothalamus increases its production of gonadotropin-releasing hormone (GnRH). Evidence indicates that this increase is dependent on adequate levels of *leptin*, a hormone released by adipose tissues. ⊃ p. 368

2. Endocrine cells in the anterior lobe of the pituitary gland become more sensitive to GnRH, so circulating levels of FSH and LH rise rapidly.

3. Ovarian or testicular cells become more sensitive to FSH and LH. These cells initiate (1) gamete production; (2) the secretion of sex hormones that stimulate the appearance of secondary sex characteristics and behaviors; and (3) a sudden acceleration in the growth rate, ending with closure of the epiphyseal cartilages.

The age at which puberty begins varies. In the United States today, puberty generally begins at about age 12 in boys and at 11 in girls, but the normal ranges are broad (10–15 in boys, 9–14 in girls). The combination of sex hormones, growth hormone, adrenal steroids, and thyroid hormones leads to a sudden acceleration in the growth rate. The timing of the growth spurt varies between the sexes, corresponding to different ages at the onset of puberty. In girls, the growth rate is greatest between ages 10 and 13. Boys grow most rapidly between ages 12 and 15. In both sexes, growth continues at a slower pace until ages 18–21. By that time, most of the epiphyseal cartilages have closed. ⊃ p. 147

The boundary between adolescence and maturity is very hazy, because it has physical, emotional, and behavioral components. Adolescence is often said to be over when growth stops, typically in the late teens or early 20s. The individual is then considered physically mature.

CLINICAL NOTE

Abortion

Abortion, which is the expulsion of the fetus prior to 20 weeks gestation, is the most common cause of bleeding in the first and second trimesters of pregnancy. The terms *abortion* and *miscarriage* can be used interchangeably. Generally, the lay public thinks of *abortion* as termination of pregnancy at maternal request and of miscarriage as an accident of nature. Medically, the term abortion applies to both kinds of fetal loss. Spontaneous abortion, which is the naturally occurring termination of pregnancy that is often called *miscarriage*, is most commonly seen between the 12th and 14th weeks of gestation. It is estimated that 10–20 percent of all pregnancies end in spontaneous abortion. If the pregnancy has not yet been confirmed, the mother often assumes she is merely having a period with unusually heavy flow.

About half of all abortions are due to fetal chromosomal anomalies. Other causes include maternal reproductive system abnormalities, maternal use of drugs, placental defects, or maternal infections. Although many people believe that trauma and psychological stress can cause abortion, research does not support that belief.

Since you will be interacting with other healthcare professionals, you should be familiar with the variety of terms used to describe the classifications of abortion.

- *Complete Abortion.* Abortion in which all of the uterine contents including the fetus and placenta have been expelled.
- *Incomplete Abortion.* Abortion in which some, but not all, fetal tissue has been passed. Incomplete abortions are associated with a high incidence of infection.
- *Threatened Abortion.* Potential abortion characterized by unexplained vaginal bleeding during the first half of pregnancy in which the cervix is slightly open and the fetus remains in the uterus and is still alive. In some cases of threatened abortion, the fetus still can be saved.
- *Inevitable Abortion.* Potential abortion characterized by vaginal bleeding accompanied by severe abdominal cramping and cervical dilatation, in which the fetus has not yet passed from the uterus, but the fetus cannot be saved.

- *Spontaneous Abortion.* Naturally occurring expulsion of the fetus prior to viability, generally as a result of chromosomal abnormalities. Most spontaneous abortions occur before the 12th week of pregnancy. Many occur within two weeks after conception and are mistaken for menstrual periods. Commonly called a miscarriage.
- *Elective Abortion.* Abortion in which the termination of pregnancy is desired and requested by the mother. Elective abortions during the first and second trimesters of pregnancy have been legal in the United States since 1973. Most elective abortions are performed during the first trimester. Some clinics perform second-trimester abortions. Second-trimester abortions have a higher complication rate than first-trimester abortions. Third-trimester elective abortions are generally illegal in this country.
- *Criminal Abortion.* Intentional termination of a pregnancy, under any condition, that is not allowed by law. It is usually the attempt to destroy a fetus by a person who is not licensed or permitted to do so. Criminal abortions are often attempted by amateurs and they are rarely performed in aseptic surroundings.
- *Therapeutic Abortion.* Termination of a pregnancy deemed necessary by a physician, usually to protect maternal health and well-being.
- *Missed Abortion.* Abortion in which fetal death occurs but the fetus is not expelled. This poses a potential threat to the life of the mother if the fetus is retained beyond six weeks.
- *Habitual Abortion.* Spontaneous abortions that occur in three or more consecutive pregnancies.

The patient experiencing an abortion is likely to report crampy abdominal pain and a backache. She is also likely to report vaginal bleeding, which is often accompanied by the passage of clots and tissue. If the abortion was not recent, then frank signs and symptoms of infection may be present. Any tissue or large clots should be retained and given to emergency department personnel. If the abortion occurs during or after the late first trimester, a fetus may be passed.

Physical growth may stop at maturity, but physiological changes continue. The sex-specific differences produced at puberty remain. Further changes take place when sex hormone levels decline at menopause or the male climacteric. ↺ p. 666 All these changes are part of **senescence** (*senesco*, to grow old), or aging, which reduces the individual's functional capabilities. Even without disease or injury, aging-related changes at the molecular level ultimately lead to death.

CHECKPOINT

18. Name the postnatal stages of development.

19. What is the difference between colostrum and breast milk?

20. Increases in the blood levels of GnRH, FSH, LH, and sex hormones mark the onset of which stage of development?

See the blue Answers tab at the back of the book.

20-8 Genes and chromosomes determine patterns of inheritance

Learning Objective Relate the basic principles of genetics to the inheritance of human traits.

Recall that chromosomes contain DNA and proteins, and genes are functional segments of DNA. Each gene carries the information needed to direct the synthesis of a specific polypeptide. We introduced chromosome structure and the functions of genes in Chapter 3. ↺ pp. 76–77 Every nucleated somatic cell in your body carries copies of the original 46 chromosomes present when you were a zygote. Those chromosomes and their genes make up your **genotype** (JĒN-ō-tīp; *geno*, gene + *typos*, mark).

Through development and differentiation, the instructions contained within the genotype are expressed in many ways. No single living cell or tissue makes use of all the information contained within the genotype. For example, in muscle fibers genes are important for excitable membrane formation and contractile protein activity, but a different set of genes is operating in pancreatic islet cells. Collectively, the instructions contained within the genotype determine the anatomical and physiological characteristics that make you a unique person. Those characteristics make up your **phenotype** (FĒ-nō-tīp; *phaino*, to display). The phenotype results from the interaction between the person's genotype and the environment. Specific elements in your phenotype, such as your hair and eye color, skin tone, foot size, or sneezing in response to bright light (photic sneeze reflex) are called phenotypic *traits*, or *characters*.

Your genotype is derived from the genotypes of your parents. Yet you are not an exact copy of either parent. Neither are you an easily identifiable mixture of their characteristics. We begin our discussion of genetics with an overview of the basic patterns of inheritance and their implications. Then we examine the processes that regulate the activities of the genotype during prenatal development.

Patterns of Inheritance

In humans, every somatic cell contains 46 chromosomes arranged in 23 pairs. The sperm contributed one member of each pair, the ovum the other. The two members of each pair are known as **homologous** (hō-MOL-o-gus) **chromosomes**. Twenty-two of those pairs are called **autosomal** (aw-tō-SŌ-mal) **chromosomes**, or *autosomes*. Most of the genes on autosomal chromosomes affect somatic characteristics such as hair color and skin pigmentation. The chromosomes of the 23rd pair are called **sex chromosomes**. One of their functions is to determine whether the individual is genetically male or female. **Figure 20-17** shows the **karyotype** (KAR-ē-ō-tīp; *karyon*, nucleus + *typos*, mark), or entire set of chromosomes, of a normal male.

The two chromosomes in a homologous pair of autosomes have the same structure and carry genes that affect the

Figure 20-17 A Human Male Karyotype. The 23 pairs of somatic cell chromosomes from a normal male.

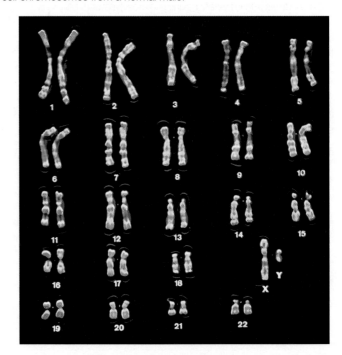

same traits. Suppose one member of the pair contains three genes in a row, with the first gene determining hair color, the second eye color, and the third skin pigmentation. The other member of the pair contains genes that affect the same traits. The genes are in the same positions and sequence along the chromosomes.

The two chromosomes in a pair may not carry the same *form*, or version, of each gene. The various forms of a given gene are called **alleles** (a-LĒLZ; *allelon,* of one another). If both chromosomes in a homologous pair carry the same allele of a particular gene, you are **homozygous** (hō-mō-ZĪ-gus; *homos,* same) for the trait affected by that gene. That allele's trait will be expressed in your phenotype. For example, if you receive a gene for freckles from your father and one for freckles from your mother, you will be homozygous for freckles—and you will have freckles. (In this case, environment also plays a role. That is because exposure to sunlight is necessary to trigger freckle formation.)

The chromosomes of a homologous pair need not carry identical alleles because the two chromosomes have different origins, one from your father and the other from your mother. When you have two different alleles of the same gene, you are **heterozygous** (het-er-ō-ZĪ-gus; *heteros,* other) for the trait determined by that gene. In that case, your phenotype will be determined by the interactions between the corresponding alleles:

- An allele that is **dominant** will be expressed in the phenotype regardless of any conflicting instructions carried by the other allele.

- An allele that is **recessive** will be expressed in the phenotype only if it is present on both chromosomes of a homologous pair. For example, albinism is characterized by an inability to synthesize the yellow-brown pigment *melanin.* ⤿ p. 126 The presence of a single dominant allele results in normal skin coloration. Two recessive alleles must be present to produce albinism.

Predicting Inheritance

Not every allele can be neatly described as dominant or recessive. For the traits listed as dominant in **Table 20-4**, we can predict the characteristics of individuals on the basis of the parents' alleles.

In such calculations, dominant alleles are traditionally represented by capitalized letters, and recessive alleles by lowercase letters. For a given trait, the possible genotypes are *AA* (homozygous dominant), *Aa* (heterozygous), or *aa* (homozygous recessive).

Table 20-4	The Inheritance of Selected Phenotypic Characteristics

DOMINANT TRAITS

One allele determines phenotype; the other is not expressed:
Normal skin pigmentation
Freckles
Brachydactyly (short fingers)
Ability to taste phenylthiocarbamate (PTC)
Free earlobes
Tongue rolling
Nearsightedness
Farsightedness
Color vision
Photic sneeze reflex
Presence of Rh factor on red blood cell membranes

Two different dominant alleles are expressed (codominance):
Type AB blood
Structure of albumins
Structure of hemoglobin molecule

RECESSIVE TRAITS

Albinism
Absence of freckles
Normal digits
Attached earlobes
Inability to roll the tongue into a U-shape
Normal vision
Blond hair
Red hair (expressed only if individual is also homozygous for blond hair)
Lack of A, B surface antigens (Type O blood)

SEX-LINKED TRAITS

Red-green color blindness
Hemophilia

POLYGENIC TRAITS

Skin color
Eye color
Height
Hair colors other than pure blond or red

Each gamete involved in fertilization contributes a single allele for a given trait. That allele must be one of the two contained in all somatic cells in the parent's body. Consider, for example, the offspring of a mother with albinism and a father with normal skin pigmentation. The maternal alleles are abbreviated *aa* because albinism is a homozygous recessive trait. No matter which of her oocytes is fertilized, it will carry the recessive *a* allele. The father has normal pigmentation, a dominant trait. He is therefore either homozygous dominant or heterozygous for this trait, because both *AA* and *Au* will produce the same phenotype—normal skin pigmentation.

A simple box diagram known as a **Punnett square** enables us to predict the probabilities that a given child will

Figure 20-18 Predicting Genotypes and Phenotypes with Punnett Squares.

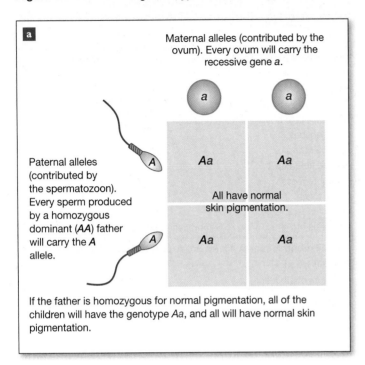

a Maternal alleles (contributed by the ovum). Every ovum will carry the recessive gene *a*.

Paternal alleles (contributed by the spermatozoon). Every sperm produced by a homozygous dominant (*AA*) father will carry the *A* allele.

All have normal skin pigmentation.

If the father is homozygous for normal pigmentation, all of the children will have the genotype *Aa*, and all will have normal skin pigmentation.

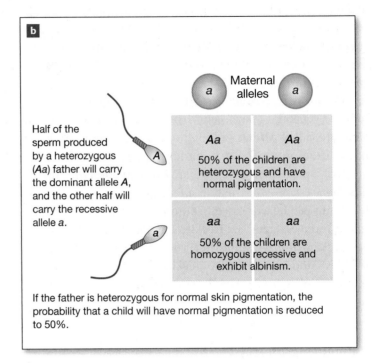

b Maternal alleles

Half of the sperm produced by a heterozygous (*Aa*) father will carry the dominant allele *A*, and the other half will carry the recessive allele *a*.

50% of the children are heterozygous and have normal pigmentation.

50% of the children are homozygous recessive and exhibit albinism.

If the father is heterozygous for normal skin pigmentation, the probability that a child will have normal pigmentation is reduced to 50%.

have particular characteristics. In the Punnett squares in **Figure 20-18**, the two maternal alleles for skin pigmentation are displayed along the horizontal axis, and the two paternal alleles along the vertical axis. The possible combinations of alleles a child can inherit are indicated in the small boxes. **Figure 20-18a** shows the possible offspring of an *aa* mother and an *AA* father. Every child will have the genotype *Aa*, so every child will have normal skin pigmentation. Compare these results with those of **Figure 20-18b**, involving a heterozygous father (*Aa*). The heterozygous male produces two types of gametes, *A* and *a*, and either one may fertilize the oocyte. As a result, the probability is 50 percent that a child of such a father will inherit the genotype *Aa* and so have normal skin pigmentation. The probability of inheriting the genotype *aa*, and thus having the albinism phenotype, is also 50 percent. A Punnett square can also be used to draw certain conclusions about the identity and genotype of a given child's parent. For example, a man with the genotype *AA* cannot be the father of an albino child (*aa*).

In **simple inheritance**, phenotypes are determined by interactions between a single pair of alleles. The frequency of appearance of an inherited disorder resulting from simple inheritance can be predicted using a Punnett square. Although they are rare disorders in terms of overall numbers, more than 1200 inherited conditions are known to reflect the presence of one or two abnormal alleles for a single gene. A partial listing of inherited disorders is given in **Table 20-5**.

In **polygenic inheritance**, phenotypes are determined by interactions among several genes. We cannot predict the presence or absence of these phenotypic traits using a simple Punnett square because the resulting phenotype depends not only on the nature of the alleles but also on how those alleles interact. Many of the developmental disorders responsible for fetal deaths and *congenital* (present at birth) *malformations* result from polygenic inheritance.

Table 20-5	Fairly Common Inherited Disorders
Disorder	**Page in Text**
AUTOSOMAL DOMINANTS	
Marfan's syndrome	p. 104
Huntington's disease	p. 296
AUTOSOMAL RECESSIVES	
Deafness	p. 336
Albinism	p. 126
Sickle cell anemia	p. 386
Cystic fibrosis	p. 509
Phenylketonuria (PKU)	p. 590
SEX-LINKED	
Duchenne muscular dystrophy (DMD)	p. 237
Hemophilia (one form)	p. 399
Red-green color blindness	p. 323

The risks of developing several important adult disorders, including hypertension and coronary artery disease, also fall within this category. In these cases, an individual's genetic composition does not by itself determine the onset of the disease. Instead, the conditions regulated by these genes establish a susceptibility to particular environmental influences. As a result, not every individual with the genetic tendency for a certain condition will actually develop that condition. For this reason, it is difficult to track polygenic conditions through successive generations. However, steps can be taken to prevent a crisis because many inherited polygenic conditions are likely (but not guaranteed) to occur. For example, you can reduce the likelihood of developing hypertension by controlling your diet and fluid volume. You may be able to prevent coronary artery disease by lowering your blood cholesterol levels.

Sex-Linked Inheritance

Sex-linked inheritance involves genes on the sex chromosomes. Unlike the other 22 chromosomal pairs, these chromosomes are not identical in appearance and gene content. There are two types of sex chromosomes: an **X chromosome** and a **Y chromosome**. X chromosomes are considerably larger and have more genes than Y chromosomes. The smaller Y chromosome carries an *SRY gene* not found on the X chromosome. It specifies that an individual with that chromosome will be male. The normal pair of sex chromosomes in males is XY. Females do not have a Y chromosome. Their sex chromosome pair is XX.

All oocytes carry an X chromosome, because the only sex chromosomes females have are X chromosomes. But a sperm may carry either an X chromosome or a Y chromosome. As a Punnett square shows, the ratio of male to female offspring should be 1:1.

The X chromosome also carries genes that affect somatic structures. Genes found on the X chromosome but not on the Y chromosome are called **X-linked**. (The SRY gene that determines "maleness" is an example of a Y-linked gene.) The best-known X-linked traits are associated with noticeable diseases or functional deficits.

The inheritance of color blindness demonstrates the differences between sex-linked and autosomal inheritance. Normal color vision is determined by the presence of a dominant allele, *C,* on the X chromosome (designated X^C). A recessive allele, *c,* on the X chromosome (X^c) results in red–green color blindness. A woman, with her two X chromosomes, can be either homozygous dominant, $X^C X^C$, or heterozygous, $X^C X^c$, and still have normal color vision. She will be unable to distinguish reds from greens only if she carries two recessive alleles,

Figure 20-19 Inheritance of an X-Linked Trait.

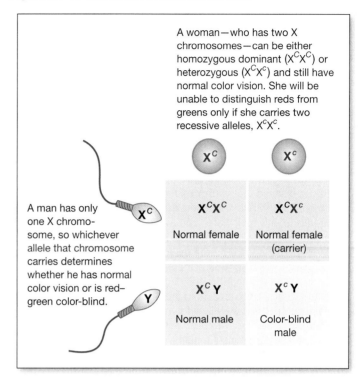

A woman—who has two X chromosomes—can be either homozygous dominant ($X^C X^C$) or heterozygous ($X^C X^c$) and still have normal color vision. She will be unable to distinguish reds from greens only if she carries two recessive alleles, $X^c X^c$.

A man has only one X chromosome, so whichever allele that chromosome carries determines whether he has normal color vision or is red–green color-blind.

$X^C X^C$ Normal female

$X^C X^c$ Normal female (carrier)

$X^C Y$ Normal male

$X^c Y$ Color-blind male

$X^c X^c$. But a male has only one X chromosome, so whichever allele that chromosome carries will determine whether he has normal color vision or is red–green color-blind. The Punnett square in **Figure 20-19** reveals that the sons of a father with normal color vision and a heterozygous (carrier) mother will have a 50 percent chance of being red–green color-blind. Any daughters will have normal color vision.

A number of other clinical disorders involve X-linked traits, including certain forms of hemophilia, diabetes insipidus, and muscular dystrophy. In several instances, advances in molecular genetics techniques have enabled geneticists to locate specific genes on the X chromosome. These techniques provide a relatively direct method of screening for the presence of a particular condition before signs and symptoms appear, and even before birth.

The Human Genome Project and Beyond

The **Human Genome Project (HGP)** was begun in 1990 and completed in 2003. Its goal was to describe the **human genome**—the full set of genetic material (DNA) in our chromosomes.

One of its highlights was the expanded description of roughly 10,000 different single-gene disorders. Most are very rare, but collectively they may affect 1 in every 200 births.

CLINICAL NOTE

Inherited Disorders: Emergency Implications

Inherited diseases are those diseases that are passed from parents to child through the genetic material (DNA). Many diseases are thought to have an inheritable component. It is clear that some disease processes, such as heart disease, diabetes, asthma, and Alzheimer's disease, tend to cluster in families. However, some diseases are inherited directly. While they are somewhat uncommon, several of them develop conditions that require emergency treatment.

- *Marfan's syndrome.* Marfan's syndrome (MS) is a connective tissue disease that is transmitted through autosomal dominant inheritance. MS is characterized by long, thin extremities that are frequently associated with other skeletal changes, reduced vision due to dislocation of the lenses, and aortic aneurysms. Most persons with MS are tall and thin (some historians have suggested that Abraham Lincoln had MS). Dilation and rupture of an aortic aneurysm is the cause of death in many patients with MS and often occurs in the third or fourth decade of life.

- *Huntington's disease.* Huntington's disease (HD), also called *Huntington's chorea,* is a debilitating disease that is transmitted by autosomal dominant patterns. HD develops at about 35–40 years of age and is characterized by progressive dementia and involuntary movements. The disease advances slowly; death occurs, on average, 15–20 years after the onset of symptoms. HD accounts for many of the nursing home admissions of patients in their fourth or fifth decade of life.

- *Sickle cell disease.* Sickle cell disease (SCD) is a group of disorders characterized by the presence of an abnormal form of hemoglobin *(hemoglobin S).* It is inherited in an autosomal recessive pattern. Patients who receive the gene for SCD from only one parent tend to develop *sickle cell trait (SCT).* SCT occurs in 7–13 percent of African Americans. In East Africa, the incidence of SCT may be as high as 45 percent. It appears that SCT may provide protection against lethal forms of malaria. Persons who receive the gene for SCD from both parents develop SCD. SCD causes the red blood cells to *sickle* (assume a crescent shape) due to the abnormal hemoglobin. Sickling causes the clinical signs and symptoms of SCD. Patients with SCD are often frequent visitors to hospital emergency departments as they periodically develop *sickle cell crisis,* where blood flow to small blood vessels in organs such as the bones and spleen become occluded. Sickle cell crisis can be extremely painful, requiring high doses of narcotics to achieve pain control.

- *Cystic fibrosis.* Cystic fibrosis (CF) is an autosomal recessive disease of the exocrine glands that causes production of excess, thick mucus that obstructs the gastrointestinal system and lungs. One of the classic signs of CF is elevated concentrations of sodium chloride in sweat and other secretions. The excess mucus coagulates in the ducts of organs or in the airways, which causes dilation and obstruction. Bronchial obstruction predisposes the patient to the development of lung infection, primarily with *Staphylococcal aureus* and *Pseudomonas aeruginosa.* Often the CF patient becomes permanently colonized with one of these bacteria. Progressive obstruction of the respiratory system eventually leads to respiratory failure. CF also impacts the pancreas, and causes obstruction and destruction of the exocrine glands. The mean life expectancy of the CF patient is about 30 years. The need for medical intervention increases significantly as the patient ages.

- *Muscular dystrophy.* Muscular dystrophy (MD) is a group of disorders that cause degeneration of skeletal muscle fibers. The major type of MD is *pseudohypertrophic MD,* often called *Duchenne's MD,* which causes an abnormality in the intracellular metabolism of the muscle fibers. Duchenne's MD is usually detected in children around 3 years of age. Muscle weakness begins at the pelvic girdle and spreads. Eventually, the pulmonary and cardiovascular systems are affected. Duchenne's MD follows an X-linked recessive pattern and is thought to be caused by a single-gene defect.

- *Hemophilia.* Hemophilia is a disease characterized by abnormal bleeding due to a genetic deficiency in one of the coagulation factors. The most common form of hemophilia is *hemophilia A (classic hemophilia).* It causes a deficiency in factor VII and is inherited as an X-linked recessive disorder that affects males and is transmitted by females. *Hemophilia B,* also called *Christmas disease,* is due to a deficiency in factor IX. It too is an X-linked recessive trait and is clinically indistinguishable from hemophilia A. *Hemophilia C* is an autosomal recessive disease that causes a factor XI deficiency. It occurs equally in males and females. *Von Willebrand disease* is an autosomal dominant trait that causes a defect in factor VIII that differs from the defect caused by hemophilia A. The hemophilias cause bleeding. Spontaneous bleeding into a joint *(hemarthrosis)* is not uncommon and is a frequent reason for hemophiliacs to seek emergency care.

CLINICAL NOTE

Trauma during Pregnancy

Trauma is the number-one killer of pregnant females. Penetrating abdominal trauma alone accounts for as much as 36 percent of overall maternal mortality. Gunshot wounds to the abdomen of the pregnant female also account for fetal mortality rates of between 40 and 70 percent. In blunt trauma, auto collisions are the leading cause of maternal and fetal mortality and morbidity. Proper seat belt placement can significantly reduce injury to the pregnant mother and fetus, while improper placement increases the incidence of both uterine rupture and separation of the placenta from the wall of the uterus. Unrestrained mothers in serious auto collisions are four times more likely to suffer fetal mortality than those who are restrained.

The physiologic changes associated with pregnancy protect both the mother and her abdominal organs. With the increasing size of the uterus, most of the abdominal organs are displaced higher in the abdomen (**Figure 20–20**). This generally protects them unless blunt or penetrating trauma impacts the upper abdomen. If that happens, then the injury may involve numerous organs with increased morbidity and mortality. Direct penetrating injury to the central and lower abdomen of the late-pregnancy mother often spares her from serious injury; the resulting injury, however, often damages the uterus and endangers the fetus.

The female in the later part of her pregnancy is at additional risk of vomiting and possible aspiration. Increasing uterine size increases intra-abdominal pressure, while the hormones of pregnancy relax the cardiac sphincter (the valve that prevents reflux of the stomach contents). The bladder is displaced superiorly early in pregnancy and then becomes more prone to injury and, when injured, bleeds more heavily.

The increasing size and weight of the uterus and its contents have several effects on the mother, especially when trauma strikes. The uterus of a supine patient in late pregnancy may compress the inferior vena cava and reduce the venous return to the heart. This may induce hypotension in the uninjured patient and have severe consequences in the hemorrhaging trauma patient (**Figure 20–20**). The increased intra-abdominal pressure, along with the compression of the inferior vena cava by the gravid uterus, can raise venous pressure in the pelvic region and the lower extremities. This pressure engorges the vessels and increases the rate of venous hemorrhage from pelvic fractures or lower extremity wounds.

The increased maternal vascular volume (up by 45 percent) helps protect the mother from hypovolemia. However, this protection does not extend to the fetus because fetal blood flow is affected well before there are changes in the maternal blood pressure or pulse rate. In fact, changes in maternal blood pressure or heart rate may not become evident until maternal blood loss reaches between 30 and 35 percent. Therefore, it becomes very important to ensure early and aggressive resuscitation of the potentially hypotensive pregnant mother.

In the pregnant female, the thick and muscular uterus contains both the developing fetus and amniotic fluid. This container is strong, and distributes the forces of trauma uniformly to the fetus, which and thereby reduces chances for injury. Significant blunt trauma may cause the uterus to rupture, or penetrating trauma may perforate or tear it. The dangers of severe maternal hemorrhage and disruption of the blood supply to the fetus threaten the lives of the mother and the fetus. The potential release of amniotic fluid into the abdomen is also of great concern. The risk of uterine and fetal injury increases with the length of gestation and is greatest during the third trimester of pregnancy.

If an open wound to the uterus does occur, there may be added risk to the mother, in addition to hemorrhage, if she is Rh negative and the fetus is Rh positive. Penetrating or severe blunt trauma may permit some fetal/maternal blood mixing and lead to compatibility problems. Frank uterine rupture is a rare complication of trauma, but it does occur with severe blunt

Figure 20-20 Expansion of the Gravid Uterus by Weeks.
Note that the other abdominal organs are displaced until the uterus becomes the largest organ in the abdomen.

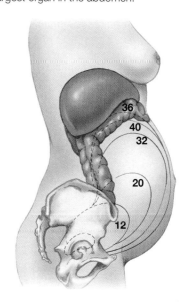

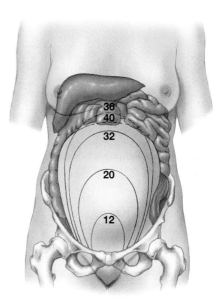

impact, pelvic fracture, and—very infrequently—with stab or shotgun wounds.

Blunt trauma to the uterus may cause the rather inelastic placenta to detach from the very flexible uterine wall. This condition, called *abruptio placentae,* presents a life-threatening risk to both mother and fetus because the separation causes both maternal and fetal hemorrhage (**Figure 20–20**). More frequently than not, this hemorrhage is contained within the uterus and does not extend to the vaginal outlet. Blunt trauma may also cause the premature rupture of the amniotic sac (breaking of the "membranes" or "bag of waters") and may induce an early labor.

Figure 20-21 A Map of Human Chromosomes. This diagram of the chromosomes of a normal male individual shows typical banding patterns and the locations of the genes responsible for specific inherited disorders. The chromosomes are not drawn to scale.

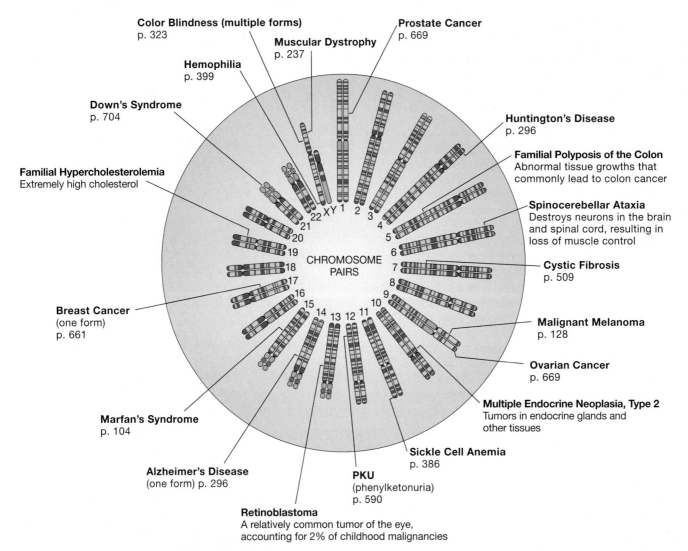

Many of these disorders have been mapped to individual chromosomes. Several examples are included in **Figure 20-21**. Genetic screening and diagnostic tests for abnormal genes are now performed for many of these disorders.

The HGP sequenced the human genome's 3.2 billion base pairs nucleotide by nucleotide, and estimated that it contained 20,000–25,000 protein-coding genes. These genes accounted for only about 2 percent of the entire genome. This led to the assumption that the remaining 98 percent were nonfunctional, or "junk."

It turns out that our genome is not full of useless DNA sequences. Results of a recent, decade-long Encyclopedia of DNA Elements (ENCODE) project have revealed that some 80 percent of the genome is active in one way or another in gene regulation. For example, protein-coding genes are regulated not only by nearby DNA, but also by more distant sequences and by "non-coding" RNA. Non-coding RNA consists of short and long RNA strands that are not translated into protein. Over 18,000 DNA sequences for non-coding RNA have been identified. In addition, ENCODE has documented close to 21,000 protein-coding genes in the human genome.

Our understanding of genetics has recently been extended with the findings that not all of a person's traits are determined solely by their DNA sequences. **Epigenetics** is the study of inherited traits that do not involve a change in a person's genotype or DNA sequences. Epigenetics acts at a level "above" the DNA by externally modifying DNA to turn specific genes "on" or "off." One way this takes place is by marking DNA and its histone proteins with chemical groups that permit or restrict transcription. Non-coding RNAs are another way gene expression can be modified.

Understanding the role of epigenetics in human clinical disorders, disease, and early development is an area of active study. Researchers are piecing together the human *epigenome*, that is, all the chemicals that mark our genome and affect its activities. The epigenetic chemical modifiers are not part of the DNA, but they can be passed on and inherited when cells divide.

The HGP and ENCODE have identified the normal genetic composition of a "typical" human and begun to reveal how our genes are regulated. Yet we all are variations on a basic theme. How do we decide what set of genes to accept as "normal"? Moreover, as we improve our abilities to manipulate our genome, we will face many additional troubling ethical and legal dilemmas. Few people, for example, object to the insertion of a "correct" gene into somatic cells to cure a specific disease. But what if we could insert that modified gene into a gamete and change not only that individual but

all of his or her descendants as well? And what if the goal of manipulating the gene was not to correct or prevent any disorder, but instead to "improve" the individual by increasing his or her intelligence, height, or vision, or by altering some other phenotypic trait? Such difficult questions will not go away. In the years to come, we will have to find answers that are acceptable to us all.

CHECKPOINT

21. Describe the relationship between genotype and phenotype.

22. Define heterozygous.

23. Tongue rolling is an autosomal dominant trait. What would be the phenotype of a person who is heterozygous for this trait?

24. Joe has three daughters and complains that it's his wife's "fault" that he has no sons. Whose "fault" is it?

See the blue Answers tab at the back of the book.

CLINICAL NOTE

Chromosomal Abnormalities and Genetic Analysis

Embryos that have abnormal autosomal chromosomes rarely survive. However, *translocation defects* and *trisomy* are two types of autosomal chromosome abnormalities that do not always result in prenatal death.

In a translocation defect, an exchange takes place between different chromosome pairs. For example, a piece of chromosome 8 may become attached to chromosome 14. The genes moved to their new position may function abnormally, becoming inactive or overactive. In a balanced translocation, where there is no net loss or gain of chromosomal material, an embryo may survive.

In trisomy, a mistake occurs in meiosis. One of the gametes involved in fertilization carries an extra copy of one chromosome. As a result, the zygote then has three copies of this chromosome rather than two. (The nature of the trisomy is indicated by the number of the chromosome involved. For example, individuals with trisomy 13 have three copies of chromosome 13.) Zygotes with extra copies of chromosomes seldom survive. Individuals with trisomy 13 and trisomy 18 may survive until delivery but rarely live longer than a year. The notable exception is trisomy 21.

Trisomy 21, or Down's syndrome, is the most common viable chromosomal abnormality (a). Estimates of its frequency in the U.S. population range from 1.5 to 1.9 per 1000 births. Affected individuals exhibit delayed mental development and have characteristic physical malformations. The degree of developmental disability ranges from moderate to severe. Anatomical

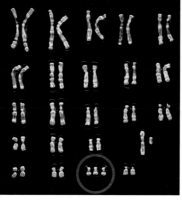

a. Trisomy 21

problems affecting the cardiovascular system often prove fatal during childhood or early adulthood. Some people with Down's syndrome survive to moderate old age, but many develop Alzheimer's disease before age 40.

For unknown reasons, there is a direct correlation between maternal age and the risk of having a child with trisomy 21. For a maternal age below 25, the incidence of Down's syndrome approaches 1 in 2000 births, or 0.05 percent. For maternal ages 30–34, the odds increase to 1 in 900. Over the next decade they go from 1 in 290 to 1 in 46, or more than 2 percent. These statistics are becoming increasingly significant because many women are delaying childbearing until their mid-30s or later.

Abnormal numbers of sex chromosomes do not produce effects as severe as those induced by extra or missing autosomal chromosomes. In Klinefelter syndrome, the individual carries the sex chromosome pattern XXY. The phenotype is male, but the extra X chromosome causes reduced androgen production. As a result, the testes fail to mature. The individuals are sterile, and the breasts are slightly enlarged. The incidence of this condition among newborn males averages 1 in 750 births.

Individuals with Turner's syndrome have only one female sex chromosome. Their sex chromosome complement is represented as XO. This kind of chromosomal deletion is known as monosomy. The incidence of this condition at delivery has been estimated as 1 in 10,000 live births. The condition may not be recognized at birth, because the phenotype is normal female. But maturational changes do not appear at

(Continued)

puberty. The ovaries are nonfunctional, and estrogen production occurs at negligible levels.

Fragile-X syndrome causes developmental disability, abnormal facial development, and enlarged testes in affected males. The cause is an abnormal X chromosome that contains a *genetic stutter*, an abnormal repetition of a single nucleotide triplet. The stutter in some way disrupts the normal functioning of adjacent genes and so produces the signs and symptoms of the disorder.

Many of these conditions can be detected before birth through the analysis of fetal cells. In amniocentesis, a sample of amniotic fluid is removed and the fetal cells it contains are analyzed. This procedure permits the identification of more than 20 congenital conditions, including Down's syndrome. The needle inserted to obtain a fluid sample is guided into position during an ultrasound procedure. ↰ p. 21 Amniocentesis has two major drawbacks:

1. Amniocentesis is performed only when known risk factors are present because the sampling procedure is a potential threat to the health of fetus and mother alike. Examples of risk factors are a family history of specific conditions, or in the case of Down's syndrome, maternal age over 35.

2. Sampling cannot safely be performed until the volume of amniotic fluid is large enough that the fetus will not be injured during the process. The usual time for amniocentesis is at 14–15 weeks of gestation. It may take several weeks to obtain results once samples have been collected, and by that time, an induced or therapeutic abortion may no longer be a viable option.

An alternative procedure is known as chorionic villus sampling (CVS). Cells for analysis are collected from the chorionic villi during the first trimester. CVS carries a slightly higher risk of miscarriage than amniocentesis, but may be preferable because it can be done earlier in gestation.

RELATED CLINICAL TERMS

abruptio placentae (ab-RUP-shē-ō pla-SEN-tē)**:** A tearing away of the placenta from the uterine wall after the fifth gestational month.

Apgar rating: A method of evaluating newborns for developmental problems and neurological damage.

breech birth: A delivery during which the legs or buttocks of the fetus enter the vaginal canal first.

fetal alcohol syndrome (FAS): A neonatal condition resulting from maternal alcohol consumption; characterized by developmental defects typically involving the skeletal, nervous, and/or cardiovascular systems.

geriatrics: A medical specialty concerned with aging and its medical problems.

in vitro fertilization: Fertilization outside the body, generally in a petri dish.

placenta previa: A condition resulting from implantation in or near the cervix, in which the placenta covers the cervix.

preeclampsia: A condition in pregnancy characterized by sudden hypertension, albuminuria (albumin in the urine), and edema of hands, feet, and face. It is the most common complication of pregnancy, affecting about 5 percent of pregnancies.

teratogens (TER-a-tō-jenz)**:** Agents or factors that disrupt normal development by damaging cells, altering chromosome structure, or altering the chemical environment of the embryo.

20 Chapter Review

Summary Outline

20-1 Development is a continuous process that occurs from fertilization to maturity *p. 771*

1. **Development** is the gradual modification of physical and physiological characteristics from **conception** to physical maturity. The creation of different cell types during development is **differentiation.**

2. **Prenatal development** occurs before birth; **postnatal development** begins at birth and continues to maturity, when senescence (aging) begins. **Inheritance, or ¯heredity,** is the transfer of genetically determined characteristics from generation to generation. **Genetics** is the study of the mechanisms of inheritance.

20-2 Fertilization—the fusion of a secondary oocyte and a spermatozoon—forms a zygote *p. 772*

3. **Fertilization** normally occurs in a uterine tube within a day after ovulation. Sperm cannot fertilize an egg until they have undergone **capacitation.**

4. The acrosomal caps of spermatozoa release *hyaluronidase*, an enzyme that separates cells of the *corona radiata*. Another acrosomal enzyme digests the zona pellucida and exposes the oocyte membrane. When a single spermatozoon contacts that membrane, fertilization occurs and **oocyte activation** follows.

5. During activation, the secondary oocyte completes meiosis II, and the penetration of additional sperm is prevented.

6. After activation, the *female pronucleus* and *male pronucleus* fuse in a process called **amphimixis** *(Figure 20-1)*.

20-3 Gestation consists of three stages of prenatal development: the first, second, and third trimesters *p. 774*

7. The nine-month period of **gestation**, or *pregnancy*, can be divided into three **trimesters.**

8. The **first trimester** is the most dangerous period of prenatal development. The processes of *cleavage and blastocyst formation, implantation, placentation*, and *embryogenesis* take place during this critical period.

20-4 Critical events of the first trimester are cleavage, implantation, placentation, and embryogenesis *p. 774*

9. **Cleavage** is a series of cell divisions that subdivide the cytoplasm of the zygote. The zygote becomes a hollow ball of **blastomeres** called a **blastocyst.** The blastocyst consists of an outer **trophoblast** and an **inner cell mass** *(Figure 20-2)*.

10. **Implantation** occurs about seven days after fertilization as the blastocyst adheres to the uterine endometrium *(Figure 20-3)*.

11. As the trophoblast enlarges and spreads, maternal blood flows through open *lacunae*. After **gastrulation**, there is an embryonic disc composed of **endoderm, ectoderm,** and **mesoderm.** It is from these three **germ layers** that the body systems differentiate *(Figure 20-4; Table 20-1)*.

12. Germ layers help form four **extraembryonic membranes:** the *yolk sac, amnion, allantois*, and *chorion (Spotlight Figure 20-5)*.

13. The **yolk sac** is an important site of blood cell formation. The **amnion** encloses fluid that surrounds and cushions the developing embryo. The base of the **allantois** later gives rise to the urinary bladder. Circulation within the vessels of the **chorion** provides a "rapid-transport system" linking the embryo with the trophoblast *(Spotlight Figure 20-5)*.

14. **Placentation** occurs as blood vessels form around the blastocyst and the **placenta** develops. *Chorionic villi* extend outward into the maternal tissues, forming a branching network through which maternal blood flows. As development proceeds, the **umbilical cord** connects the fetus to the placenta *(Figure 20-6)*.

15. The trophoblast synthesizes **human chorionic gonadotropin (hCG)**, estrogens, progesterone, **human placental lactogen (hPL), placental prolactin,** and **relaxin.**

16. The first trimester is critical because events in the first 12 weeks establish the basis for **organogenesis** (organ formation) *(Figure 20-7; Table 20-2)*.

20-5 During the second and third trimesters, maternal organ systems support the developing fetus, and the uterus undergoes structural and functional changes *p. 783*

17. In the **second trimester,** the organ systems increase in complexity. During the **third trimester,** these organ systems become functional *(Figures 20-8, 20-9; Table 20-2)*.

18. The developing fetus is totally dependent on maternal organs for nourishment, respiration, and waste removal. Maternal adaptations include increases in blood volume, respiratory rate, tidal volume, nutrient intake, and glomerular filtration rate.

19. Progesterone produced by the placenta has an inhibitory effect on uterine muscles; its calming action is opposed by estrogens, oxytocin, and prostaglandins. Placental and fetal factors interact to produce **labor contractions** in the uterine wall *(Figure 20-12)*.

20-6 Labor consists of the dilation, expulsion, and placental stages *p. 790*

20. The goal of labor is **parturition,** the forcible expulsion of the fetus from the uterus.

21. Labor can be divided into three stages: the **dilation stage, expulsion stage,** and **placental stage** *(Figure 20-13)*.

22. **Premature labor** results in the delivery of a newborn that has not completed normal development.

23. Twins are either **dizygotic** (fraternal) or **monozygotic** (identical).

20-7 Postnatal stages are the neonatal period, infancy, childhood, adolescence, and maturity, followed by senescence *p. 793*

24. Postnatal development involves a series of five **life stages:** the *neonatal period, infancy, childhood, adolescence*, and *maturity (Figure 20-14)*.

25. The **neonatal period** extends from birth to 1 month of age. **Infancy** then continues to one year of age, and **childhood** lasts until puberty commences. During these stages, major nonreproductive organ systems become fully operational and gradually acquire adult characteristics, and the individual grows rapidly *(Figure 20-14)*.

26. In the transition from fetus to **neonate,** the respiratory, circulatory, digestive, and urinary systems begin functioning independently. The newborn must also begin to perform thermoregulation.

27. Mammary glands produce protein-rich **colostrum** during the neonate's first few days and then convert to milk production. These secretions are released as a result of the *milk let-down reflex (Figure 20-16)*.

28. **Adolescence** begins at **puberty:** (1) The hypothalamus increases its production of GnRH, (2) circulating levels of

20

FSH and LH rise rapidly, and (3) ovarian or testicular cells become more sensitive to FSH and LH. These changes initiate gametogenesis, the production of sex hormones, and a sudden acceleration in growth rate. Adolescence continues until growth is completed.

29. **Maturity,** the end of growth and adolescence, occurs by the early twenties. Postmaturational changes in physiological processes are part of aging, or **senescence.** Aging-related changes ultimately lead to death.

20-8 Genes and chromosomes determine patterns of inheritance *p. 798*

30. Every somatic cell carries copies of the zygote's original 46 chromosomes; these chromosomes and their genes make up the individual's **genotype.** An individual's **phenotype** is his or her anatomical and physiological characteristics. The phenotype results from the interaction between the person's genotype and the environment.

31. Every somatic human cell contains 23 pairs of chromosomes; each pair consists of **homologous chromosomes.** Twenty-two pairs are **autosomal chromosomes.** The chromosomes of the 23rd pair are the **sex chromosomes,** which differ between the sexes *(Figure 20-13).*

32. Chromosomes contain DNA, and genes are functional segments of DNA. The various forms (versions) of a gene are called **alleles.** If both homologous chromosomes carry the same allele of a particular gene, the individual is **homozygous;** if they carry different alleles, the individual is **heterozygous.**

33. Alleles are either **dominant** or **recessive** depending on how their traits are expressed *(Table 20-3).*

34. Combining maternal and paternal alleles in a *Punnett square* helps us to predict the characteristics of offspring *(Figure 20-19).*

35. In **simple inheritance,** phenotypic traits are determined by interactions between a single pair of alleles. **Polygenic inheritance** involves interactions among alleles on several chromosomes *(Table 20-4).*

36. The two types of **sex chromosomes** are an **X chromosome** and a **Y chromosome.** The normal sex chromosome complement of males is XY; that of females is XX. The X chromosome carries **X-linked genes,** which affect somatic structures but have no corresponding alleles on the Y chromosome *(Figure 20-15).*

37. Together the **HGP** and ENCODE have revealed that the human genome contains protein-coding genes, DNA sequences for non-coding RNAs, and epigenetic markings affecting gene expression. Close to 22,000 protein-coding genes have been mapped, including some responsible for inherited disorders *(Figure 20-21; Table 20-4).*

Review Questions

See the blue Answers tab at the back of the book.

Level 1 Reviewing Facts and Terms

Match each item in column A with the most closely related item in column B. Place letters for answers in the spaces provided.

COLUMN A

_____ **1.** Gestation
_____ **2.** Cleavage
_____ **3.** Gastrulation
_____ **4.** Chorionic villi
_____ **5.** Human chorionic gonadotropin
_____ **6.** Birth
_____ **7.** Episiotomy
_____ **8.** Afterbirth
_____ **9.** Senescence
_____ **10.** Neonate
_____ **11.** Phenotype
_____ **12.** Homozygous recessive
_____ **13.** Heterozygous
_____ **14.** Male genotype
_____ **15.** Female genotype
_____ **16.** Trisomy 21

COLUMN B

a. Blastocyst formation
b. Ejection of placenta
c. Germ-layer formation
d. Indication of pregnancy
e. Embryo-maternal circulatory exchange
f. Visible characteristics
g. Time of prenatal development
h. *aa*
i. Down's syndrome
j. Newborn infant
k. *Aa*
l. XY
m. XX
n. Parturition
o. Process of aging
p. Perineal musculature incision

17. The gradual modification of anatomical structures during the period from conception to maturity is
    (a) development.
    (b) differentiation.
    (c) embryogenesis.
    (d) capacitation.

18. Human fertilization involves the fusion of two haploid gametes, producing a zygote containing
    (a) 23 chromosomes.
    (b) 46 chromosomes.
    (c) the normal haploid number of chromosomes.
    (d) 46 pairs of chromosomes.

19. The secondary oocyte leaving the follicle is in
    (a) interphase.
    (b) metaphase of the first meiotic division.
    (c) telophase of the second meiotic division.
    (d) metaphase of the second meiotic division.

20. Identify structures a–e in the following diagram of week 10 of development.

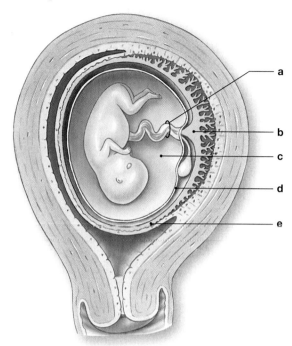

(a) _____ (b) _____
(c) _____ (d) _____
(e) _____

21. The process that establishes the foundation of all major organ systems is
(a) cleavage. (b) implantation.
(c) placentation. (d) embryogenesis.

22. The zygote arrives in the uterine cavity as a
(a) morula. (b) trophoblast.
(c) lacuna. (d) blastomere.

23. The surface that enables active and passive exchange between the fetal and maternal bloodstreams is the
(a) yolk stalk. (b) chorionic villi.
(c) umbilical veins. (d) umbilical arteries.

24. Milk let-down is associated with
(a) events occurring in the uterus.
(b) placental hormonal influences.
(c) circadian rhythms.
(d) reflex action triggered by suckling.

25. If an allele must be present on both the maternal and paternal chromosomes to affect the phenotype, the allele is said to be
(a) dominant. (b) recessive.
(c) complementary. (d) heterozygous.

26. Name the four extraembryonic membranes.

27. Identify the three stages of labor, and describe the events that characterize each stage.

28. Identify the three life stages that occur between birth and approximately age 10. Describe the timing and characteristics of each stage.

Level 2 Reviewing Concepts

29. Relaxin is a hormone that
(a) increases the flexibility of the symphysis pubis.
(b) causes dilation of the cervix.
(c) suppresses the release of oxytocin by the hypothalamus.
(d) a, b, and c are correct.

30. During adolescence, the events that interact to promote increased hormone production and sexual maturation result from activity of the
(a) hypothalamus.
(b) anterior lobe of the pituitary gland.
(c) ovaries and testicular cells.
(d) a, b, and c are correct.

31. In addition to its role in the nutrition of the fetus, what are the primary endocrine functions of the placenta?

32. Discuss the changes that occur in maternal systems during pregnancy, and indicate the functional significance of each change.

33. During labor, what physiological mechanism ensures that uterine contractions continue until delivery has been completed?

34. During the process of labor, what event occurs when the woman has her "water break"?

35. Indicate the nature of the trait and type of inheritance involved in each of the following situations.
(a) Children who exhibit this trait have at least one parent who exhibits the same trait.
(b) Children exhibit this trait even though neither parent does.
(c) The trait is expressed more commonly in sons than in daughters.
(d) Tongue-rolling is expressed equally in both daughters and sons.

36. Explain why more men than women are color-blind. Which type of inheritance is involved?

Level 3 Critical Thinking and Clinical Applications

37. Hemophilia A, a condition in which blood does not clot properly, is a recessive trait located on the X chromosome (X^h). A woman heterozygous for the trait marries a normal male. What is the probability that this couple will have hemophiliac daughters? What is the probability that this couple will have hemophiliac sons?

38. Explain why the normal heart and respiratory rates of neonates are so much higher than those of adults, even though adults are so much larger.

39. Sally gives birth to a baby with a congenital deformity of the stomach. She believes that it is the result of a viral infection she suffered during the third trimester of pregnancy. Is this a possibility? Explain.

20

Answers to Checkpoints and Review Questions

CHAPTER 1

ANSWERS TO CHECKPOINTS

Page 3

1. Metabolism refers to all the chemical operations in the body. Organisms rely on complex chemical reactions to provide the energy for responsiveness, growth, reproduction, and movement.

Page 4

2. Anatomy and physiology are closely related because all specific functions are performed by specific structures. **3.** Histologists specialize in histology, the study of the structure and properties of tissues and the cells that compose tissues. Because histologists must use microscopes to observe cells, they are specialists in microscopic anatomy.

Page 6

4. The major levels of organization from the simplest to the most complex are the following: chemical level —> cellular level —> tissue level —> organ level —> organ system level —> organism level. **5.** The organ systems of the body and their major functions are the integumentary system (protects against environmental hazards, helps control body temperature, and provides sensory information); the skeletal system (provides support, protects tissues, stores minerals, and forms blood cells); the muscular system (provides movement, provides protection and support for other tissues, and produces heat); the nervous system (directs immediate responses to stimuli, usually by coordinating the activities of other organ systems, and provides and interprets sensory information about internal and external conditions); the endocrine system (directs long-term changes in activities of other organ systems); the cardiovascular system (transports cells and dissolved materials, including nutrients, wastes, oxygen, and carbon dioxide); the lymphatic system (defends against infection and disease, and returns tissue fluids to the bloodstream); the respiratory system (delivers air to sites in the lungs where gas exchange can occur between the air and bloodstream, and produces sound for communication); the digestive system (processes food and absorbs nutrients); the urinary system (eliminates waste products from the blood, and controls water balance by regulating the volume of urine produced); and the reproductive system (male produces sex cells [sperm] and hormones, and female produces sex cells [oocytes], hormones, and supports embryonic and fetal development from fertilization to birth). **6.** The endocrine system includes the pituitary gland and directs long-term changes in the activities of other systems.

Page 10

7. Homeostasis refers to the existence of a stable internal environment. **8.** Homeostatic regulation is important because it keeps physiological systems within carefully controlled limits, preventing potentially disruptive changes in the body's internal environment. **9.** When homeostasis fails, organ systems function less efficiently or even malfunction. The result is the state we call disease. If the situation is not corrected, death can result.

Page 13

10. Negative feedback systems provide control over the body's internal conditions—that is, they maintain homeostasis—by counteracting the effects of a stimulus. **11.** Positive feedback is useful in processes that must move quickly to completion, such as blood clotting. It is harmful in situations in which a stable condition must be maintained, because it tends to intensify any departure from the desired condition. Positive feedback in the regulation of body temperature, for example, would cause a slight fever to spiral out of control, with fatal results. For this reason, physiological systems are typically regulated by negative feedback, which tends to oppose any departure from the norm.

Page 15

12. The purpose of anatomical terms is to provide a standardized language and frame of reference for describing the human body. **13.** In the anatomical position, an anterior view displays the body's front, whereas a posterior view displays the back. **11.** The two eyes would be separated by a sagittal section. A midsagittal section would separate them evenly.

Page 19

15. Body cavities protect internal organs and cushion them from movements that occur while walking, running, or jumping. Body cavities also permit organs that they surround to change in size and shape without disrupting the activities of nearby organs. **16.** The thoracic cavity includes the pleural and pericardial cavities, which enclose the lungs and heart respectively. The diaphragm forms the boundary between the superior thoracic cavity and inferior abdominopelvic cavity. The abdominopelvic cavity is subdivided into the superior abdominal cavity and the inferior pelvic cavity. The abdominopelvic cavity contains the peritoneal cavity. **17.** The body cavity inferior to the diaphragm is the abdominopelvic (or peritoneal) cavity.

ANSWERS TO REVIEW QUESTIONS

Level 1: Reviewing Facts and Terms

1. g **2.** d **3.** a **4.** j **5.** b **6.** l **7.** n **8.** f **9.** h **10.** e **11.** c **12.** o **13.** k **14.** i **15.** m **16.** (a) frontal; (b) sagittal; (c) transverse **17.** (a) superior; (b) inferior; (c) posterior or dorsal; (d) anterior or ventral; (e) cranial; (f) caudal; (g) lateral; (h) medial; (i) proximal; (j) distal **18.** c **19.** a **20.** d **21.** c

Level 2: Reviewing Concepts

22. All living things display responsiveness, growth, reproduction, movement, and metabolism. **23.** The levels of organization of your body beginning with atoms are chemical, cellular, tissue, organ, organ system, and organism (you). **24.** Homeostatic regulation refers to adjustments in physiological systems that are responsible for maintaining homeostasis (the existence of a stable internal environment). **25.** In negative feedback, a variation outside normal ranges triggers an automatic response that corrects the situation. In positive feedback, the initial stimulus produces a response that exaggerates the stimulus. **26.** The body is erect, the hands are at the sides with the palms facing forward, and the feet are together. **27.** The stomach. (You would cut the pericardium to access the heart.) **28.** (a) thoracic and abdominopelvic cavities; (b) thoracic cavity; (c) abdominopelvic cavity.

Level 3: Critical Thinking and Clinical Applications

29. When calcitonin is released in response to elevated calcium levels, it brings about a decrease in blood calcium levels, thereby decreasing the stimulus for its own release. **30.** To see a complete view of the medial surface of each half of the brain, midsagittal sections are needed.

CHAPTER 2

ANSWERS TO CHECKPOINTS

Page 28

1. An atom is the smallest stable unit of matter. **2.** The two samples could have different weights if they contain different proportions of hydrogen's three isotopes: hydrogen-1, with a mass of 1; hydrogen-2, with a mass of 2; and hydrogen-3, with a mass of 3.

Page 31

3. A chemical bond is an attractive force acting between two atoms that may be strong enough to hold them together in a molecule or compound. The strongest attractive forces result from the gain, loss, or sharing of electrons. Examples of such chemical bonds are ionic bonds and covalent bonds. **4.** Atoms combine with each other such that their outer electron shells are full. Oxygen atoms do not have a full outer electron shell and so readily combine with many other elements to attain this stable arrangement. Neon does not combine with other elements because it has a full

ANSWERS

outer electron shell. **5.** The atoms in a water molecule are held together by polar covalent bonds. Water molecules are attracted to each other by hydrogen bonds: attractions between a slight negative charge on the oxygen atom of one water molecule and a slight positive charge on a hydrogen atom of another water molecule.

Page 33

6. The molecular formula for glucose, a compound composed of 6 carbon atoms, 12 hydrogen atoms, and 6 oxygen atoms, is $C_6H_{12}O_6$.

Page 34

7. Three types of chemical reactions important to human physiology are decomposition reactions, synthesis reactions, and exchange reactions. In a decomposition reaction, a chemical reaction breaks a molecule into smaller fragments. A synthesis reaction assembles smaller molecules into larger ones. In an exchange reaction, parts of the reacting molecules are shuffled around to produce new products. **8.** Because this reaction involves a large molecule being broken down into two smaller ones, it is a decomposition reaction. **9.** Removing the product of a reversible reaction would keep its concentration lower than the concentrations of the reactants. As a result, the breakdown of the product into reactants would slow down, producing a shift in the equilibrium toward the product. **10.** An enzyme is a special molecule that lowers the activation energy of a chemical reaction, which is the amount of energy required to start the reaction. **11.** Without enzymes, most chemical reactions could proceed in the body only under conditions that cells cannot tolerate (such as high temperatures). By lowering the activation energy, enzymes make it possible for chemical reactions to proceed under conditions compatible with life.

Page 35

12. Inorganic compounds are substances that generally do not contain carbon and hydrogen. (If present, they do not form C—H bonds.) Organic compounds are substances that contain carbon covalently bonded with one or more other elements.

Page 36

13. Specific chemical properties of water that make life possible include its reactivity (it participates in many chemical reactions), its high heat capacity (it absorbs and releases heat slowly), and its ability to dissolve a remarkable number of inorganic and organic substances (its strong polarity enables it to be an excellent solvent). **14.** Heat is an increase in the random motion, or kinetic energy, of molecules, and temperature is a measure of heat. Liquid water resists changes in temperature because hydrogen bonds between water molecules retard molecular motion and must be broken to increase the temperature. Temperature must be quite high before individual water molecules have enough energy to break free of all surrounding hydrogen bonds and become water vapor. **15.** pH is a measure of the concentration of hydrogen ions in solutions, such as body fluids. On the pH scale, 7 represents neutrality, values below 7 indicate acidic solutions, and values above 7 indicate alkaline (basic) solutions. **16.** Fluctuations in pH of body fluids outside the normal range of 7.35 to 7.45 can break chemical bonds, alter the shape of molecules, and affect cell function, thereby harming cells and tissues.

Page 37

17. An acid is a substance whose dissociation in solution releases a hydrogen ion (H^+) and an anion. A base is a substance whose dissociation releases a hydroxide ion (OH^-) or removes a hydrogen ion from the solution. A salt is an ionic compound consisting of a cation other than H^+ and an anion other than OH^-. **18.** Stomach discomfort is commonly the result of excessive stomach acidity ("acid indigestion"). Antacids contain a weak base that neutralizes the excess acid.

Page 41

19. A compound with a C:H:O ratio of 1:2:1 is a carbohydrate. The body uses carbohydrates chiefly as an energy source. **20.** When two monosaccharides undergo a dehydration synthesis reaction, they form a disaccharide.

Page 43

21. Lipids are a diverse group of compounds that include fatty acids, fats (triglycerides), steroids, and phospholipids. They are organic compounds that contain carbon, hydrogen, and oxygen in a ratio that does not approximate 1:2:1. **22.** The most abundant lipid in a sample taken from beneath

the skin would be a triglyceride. **23.** Human cell membranes primarily contain phospholipids, plus small amounts of cholesterol.

Page 47

24. Proteins are organic compounds formed from amino acids, which contain a central carbon atom, a hydrogen atom, an amino group (—NH$_2$), a carboxyl group (—COOH), and an R group, or variable side chain. Proteins function in support, movement, transport, buffering, metabolic regulation, coordination and control, and defense. **25.** The heat of boiling breaks bonds that maintain the protein's three-dimensional shape. The resulting structural change, known as denaturation, affects the ability of the protein molecule to perform its normal biological functions.

Page 49

26. A nucleic acid is a large organic molecule made up of nucleotide subunits containing carbon, hydrogen, oxygen, nitrogen, and phosphorus. Nucleic acids regulate protein synthesis and make up the genetic material in cells. **27.** Both DNA (deoxyribonucleic acid) and RNA (ribonucleic acid) contain nitrogenous bases and phosphate groups, but because this nucleic acid contains the sugar ribose, it is RNA. **28.** Adenosine triphosphate (ATP) is a high-energy compound consisting of adenosine monophosphate (AMP) to which two phosphate groups are attached. The second and third phosphate groups are each attached by a high-energy bond. **29.** Hydrolysis is a decomposition reaction involving water. The hydrolysis of ATP (adenosine triphosphate) yields ADP (adenosine diphosphate) and P (a phosphate group). It also releases energy that is then used for cellular activities.

Page 50

30. Six elements common to organic compounds are carbon (C), hydrogen (H), oxygen (O), nitrogen (N), phosphorus (P), and sulfur (S). **31.** The biochemical building blocks that are components of cells include lipids (forming the cell membrane), proteins (acting as enzymes), nucleic acids (directing the synthesis of cellular proteins), and carbohydrates (providing energy for cellular activities).

ANSWERS TO REVIEW QUESTIONS

Level 1: Reviewing Facts and Terms

1. f **2.** c **3.** i **4.** g **5.** a **6.** l **7.** d **8.** k **9.** b **10.** e **11.** h **12.** j **13.** a.

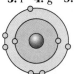

Oxygen atom

b. Two more electrons can fit into the outermost electron shell of an oxygen atom. **14.** a **15.** d **16.** a **17.** Enzymes are specialized protein catalysts that lower the activation energy of chemical reactions. Enzymes speed up chemical reactions but are not used up or changed in the process. **18.** carbon, hydrogen, oxygen, nitrogen, calcium, phosphorus. **19.** carbohydrates, lipids, proteins, nucleic acids **20.** support (structural proteins), movement (contractile proteins), transport (transport proteins), buffering, metabolic regulation, coordination and control, defense **21.** (a) central carbon atom; (b) amino group; (c) R group; (d) carboxyl group.

Level 2: Reviewing Concepts

22. b **23.** d **24.** a **25.** Nonpolar covalent bonds involve equal sharing of electrons, polar covalent bonds involve unequal sharing of electrons, and ionic bonds involve a loss and/or gain of electrons. **26.** A solution with a pH of 7 (such as pure water) is neutral because it contains equal numbers of hydrogen ions and hydroxyl ions. **27.** The pH 2 solution is 10,000 times more acidic than the pH 6 solution—it contains a ten thousand-fold (10^4) increase in the concentration of hydrogen ions (H^+). **28.** A nucleic acid. Carbohydrates and lipids do not contain the element nitrogen. Although both proteins and nucleic acids contain nitrogen, only nucleic acids contain phosphorus.

Level 3: Critical Thinking and Clinical Applications

29. The number of neutrons in an atom is equal to the atomic mass number minus the atomic number. For sulfur, this would be $32 - 16 = 16$ neutrons. Since the atomic number of sulfur is 16, a neutral sulfur atom contains 16 protons and 16 electrons. The electrons would be distributed as follows: 2 in the first level, 8 in the second level, and 6 in the third level. To achieve a full eight electrons in the third level, the sulfur atom could accept two electrons in an ionic bond or share two electrons in a covalent bond. Since hydrogen atoms can share one electron in a covalent bond, the sulfur atom would form two covalent bonds, one with each of two hydrogen atoms. **30.** If a person exhales large amounts of CO_2, the equilibrium of the reactions will shift to the left to replace the lost CO_2. As a result, the level of H^+ in the blood will decrease. A decrease in the amount of H^+ will cause the pH to rise.

CHAPTER 3

ANSWERS TO CHECKPOINTS

Page 59

1. The basic concepts of the cell theory are (1) cells are the building blocks of all plants and animals; (2) cells are the smallest functioning units of life; (3) cells are produced through the division of preexisting cells; and (4) each cell maintains homeostasis. **2.** The study of cells is called cytology.

Page 63

3. The general functions of the plasma membrane include physical isolation, regulation of exchange with the environment, sensitivity to the environment, and structural support. **4.** The phospholipid bilayer of the plasma membrane forms a physical barrier between the cell's internal and external environments. **5.** Channel proteins allow water and small ions to cross the plasma membrane.

Page 68

6. A selectively permeable membrane allows the passage of some substances while restricting the passage of others. It falls between two extremes: impermeable, which allows no substance to pass, and freely permeable, which permits the passage of any substance. **7.** Diffusion is the passive molecular movement of a substance from an area of higher concentration to an area of lower concentration; diffusion proceeds until the concentration gradient is eliminated and equilibrium is reached. **8.** Diffusion is driven by a concentration gradient. The larger the concentration gradient, the faster the rate of diffusion; the smaller the concentration gradient, the slower the rate of diffusion. If the concentration of oxygen in the lungs were to decrease, the concentration gradient between oxygen in the lungs and oxygen in the blood would decrease (as long as the oxygen level of the blood remained constant). Thus, oxygen would diffuse into the blood more slowly. **9.** Osmosis is the diffusion of water across a selectively permeable membrane from one solution to another solution. Movement occurs toward higher solute concentrations because that is where the concentration of water is lower. **10.** Relative to a surrounding hypertonic solution, the contents of a red blood cell are hypotonic; that is, the solute concentration within an RBC is less than that of the solution surrounding it.

Page 74

11. Active transport processes require the expenditure of cellular energy in the form of the high-energy bonds of ATP molecules. Passive transport processes (*diffusion, osmosis,* and *facilitated diffusion*) result in the movement of ions and molecules across the plasma membrane without any energy expenditure by the cell. **12.** An active transport process must be involved because H^+ must be transported from the cells lining the stomach, where H^+ are less concentrated, to the interior of the stomach, where H^+ are more concentrated—that is, against their concentration gradient. **13.** This process is an example of phagocytosis.

Page 79

14. Cytoplasm is the material between the plasma membrane and the nuclear membrane. Cytosol is the fluid portion of the cytoplasm. **15.** The membranous organelles (and their functions) include (1) endoplasmic reticulum = synthesis of secretory products, intracellular storage and transport; (2) rough ER = modification and packaging of newly synthesized proteins; (3) smooth ER = lipid and carbohydrate synthesis; (4) Golgi apparatus = storage, alteration, and packaging of secretory products and lysosomal enzymes; (5) lysosomes = intracellular removal of damaged

organelles or pathogens; (6) mitochondria = production of 95 percent of the ATP required by the cell; (7) peroxisomes = neutralization of toxic compounds. **16.** The fingerlike projections on the surface of intestinal cells are microvilli. They increase the surface area of the intestinal cells so they can absorb nutrients more efficiently. **17.** Cells that lack centrioles are unable to divide. **18.** The SER functions in the synthesis of lipids, including steroids. Cells of the ovaries and testes would be expected to have a great deal of SER because these organs produce large amounts of steroid hormones. **19.** Mitochondria produce energy for the cell in the form of ATP molecules. A large number of mitochondria in a cell would indicate a high demand for energy.

Page 84

20. The nucleus is a cellular organelle that contains DNA, RNA, and proteins. The nuclear envelope is a double membrane that surrounds the nucleus. Nuclear pores allow for chemical communication between the nucleus and the cytosol. **21.** A gene is a portion of a DNA strand that functions as a hereditary unit. Each gene is located at a particular site on a specific chromosome and codes for a specific protein.

Page 85

22. The nucleus controls the cell's activities through DNA, which codes for the production of all of the cell's proteins. Some of these proteins are structural proteins responsible for the cell's shape and other physical characteristics. Other proteins are enzymes that govern cellular metabolism. By ordering or stopping the production of specific enzymes, the nucleus can regulate all of the cell's activities and functions. **23.** A cell lacking RNA polymerase would not be able to transcribe mRNA from DNA. **24.** The deletion of a base from a coding sequence of DNA during transcription would alter the entire mRNA base sequence after the deletion point. This change would result in different codons on the messenger RNA that was transcribed from the affected region. This, in turn, would result in the inclusion of a different series of amino acids into the protein. Almost certainly the protein product would not be functional.

Page 90

25. The biological term for cellular reproduction is *cell division,* and the term for cell death is *apoptosis.* **26.** Interphase is the portion of a cell's life cycle during which the chromosomes are uncoiled and all normal cellular functions except mitosis are under way. The stages of interphase include G_1, S, and G_2. **27.** Mitosis is the essential step in cell division in which a single cell nucleus divides to produce two identical daughter cell nuclei. The four stages of mitosis are prophase, metaphase, anaphase, and telophase. **28.** If spindle fibers failed to form during mitosis, the cell would not be able to separate the chromosomes into two sets. If cytokinesis were to take place, the result would be one cell with two sets of chromosomes, and another cell with none.

Page 91

29. An illness characterized by mutations that disrupt normal control processes and produce potentially malignant cells is termed cancer. **30.** Metastasis is the spread of cancer cells from one organ or tissue to another, leading to the establishment of secondary tumors. **31.** Differentiation is the development of specific cellular characteristics and functions that are different from the original cell. It results from genes in the cells being switched off, restricting the cell's potential functions.

ANSWERS TO REVIEW QUESTIONS

Level 1: Reviewing Facts and Terms

1. e **2.** d **3.** h **4.** a **5.** f **6.** b **7.** g **8.** c **9.** m **10.** k **11.** q
12. i **13.** o **14.** j **15.** l **16.** n **17.** p **18.** b **19.** d **20.** a. isotonic b. hypotonic c. hypertonic **21.** c **22.** d **23.** c **24.** a
25. c **26.** plasma membrane functions: physical isolation, regulation of exchange with the environment, sensitivity, structural support **27.** major transport processes: diffusion, carrier-mediated transport, vesicular transport **28.** ER functions: synthesis of proteins, carbohydrates, and lipids; storage of absorbed molecules; transport of materials; detoxification of drugs or toxins.

Level 2: Reviewing Concepts

29. b **30.** b **31.** c **32.** c

ANSWERS

33.

Facilitated diffusion	Active transport
requires carrier proteins	requires carrier proteins
passive process	active process
no ATP expended	ATP expended
follows concentration gradient	against concentration gradient

34. Cytosol has a high concentration of K^+; interstitial fluid has a high concentration of Na^+. Cytosol also contains a high concentration of suspended proteins, small quantities of carbohydrates, and large reserves of amino acids and lipids. Cytosol may also contain insoluble materials known as inclusions. **35.** In transcription, RNA polymerase uses genetic information to assemble a strand of mRNA. In translation, ribosomes use information carried by the mRNA strand to assemble functional proteins. **36.** Prophase: chromatin condenses and chromosomes become visible; centrioles migrate to opposite ends of the cell and spindle fibers develop; nuclear membrane disintegrates. Metaphase: chromatids attach to spindle fibers and line up along the metaphase plate. Anaphase: chromatids separate and migrate toward opposite ends of the cell. Telophase: the nuclear membrane re-forms; chromosomes disappear as chromatin relaxes; nucleoli reappear. **37.** Cytokinesis is the division of the cytoplasm into two separate daughter cells; it completes cell division.

Level 3: Critical Thinking and Clinical Applications

38. This process is facilitated transport, which requires a carrier molecule but not cellular energy. The energy for the process is provided by the diffusion gradient for the substance being transported. When all the carriers are actively involved in transport, the rate of transport levels out and cannot be increased further. **39.** Solution A must have initially had more solutes than solution B. As a result, water moved by osmosis across the selectively permeable membrane from side B to side A, increasing the fluid level on side A.

CHAPTER 4

ANSWERS TO CHECKPOINTS

Page 97

1. Histology is the study of tissues. **2.** The four basic types of tissues that form all body structures are epithelial, connective, muscle, and neural tissues.

Page 101

3. Epithelial tissue is characterized by closely bound cells, a free surface exposed to the environment or an internal space, attachment to underlying connective tissue by a basement membrane, avascularity (absence of blood vessels), and continual replacement of exposed cells. **4.** Epithelial tissue provides physical protection, controls permeability, provides sensation, and produces specialized secretions. **5.** Epithelial cell junctions include tight junctions, gap junctions, and desmosomes. **6.** The presence of microvilli on the free surface of epithelial cells greatly increases the surface area for absorption or secretion. Cilia function to move materials over the surface of epithelial cells.

Page 108

7. The three cell shapes characteristic of epithelial cells are squamous (flat), cuboidal (cube-like), and columnar (rectangular). **8.** No. A simple squamous epithelium does not provide enough protection against infection, abrasion, and dehydration. The skin surface has a stratified squamous epithelium. **9.** The two primary types of glandular epithelia are endocrine glands and exocrine glands. **10.** Sebaceous glands exhibit holocrine secretion. **11.** This gland is an endocrine gland.

Page 114

12. Functions of connective tissues include (1) supporting, surrounding, protecting, and interconnecting other types of tissue; (2) transporting fluids and dissolved materials; (3) storing energy reserves; and (4) defending the body from invading microorganisms. **13.** The three types of connective tissues are connective tissue proper, fluid connective tissues, and supporting connective tissues. **14.** The connective tissue containing primarily triglycerides is adipose (fat) tissue. **15.** The reduced collagen production resulting from a lack of vitamin C in the diet would cause connective tissue to be weak and prone to damage. **16.** The two connective tissues that contain a fluid matrix are blood

and lymph. **17.** The two types of supporting connective tissue are cartilage and bone. **18.** Cartilage heals slower than bone because it lacks a direct blood supply. As a result, materials needed for repair reach the chondrocytes by the slow process of diffusion from the blood, thus slowing the healing process.

Page 118

19. The four types of tissue membranes found in the body are the cutaneous membrane, mucous membranes, serous membranes, and synovial membranes. **20.** Plasma (cell) membranes are composed of lipid bilayers. Tissue membranes consist of a layer of epithelial tissue and a layer of areolar tissue. **21.** Serous fluid minimizes the friction between the serous membranes that cover the surfaces of organs and the surrounding body cavity. **22.** The lining of the nasal cavity is a mucous membrane.

Page 120

23. The three types of muscle tissue in the body are skeletal muscle, cardiac muscle, and smooth muscle. **24.** Only skeletal muscle tissue is under voluntary control. **25.** Muscle tissue that lacks striations is smooth muscle; both cardiac and skeletal muscles are striated. **26.** The cells are most likely neurons. **27.** Skeletal muscle cells and axons are both called fibers because they are relatively long and slender.

Page 121

28. The two phases in the response to tissue injury are inflammation and regeneration. **29.** Swelling, redness, heat, and pain are the familiar signs and symptoms of inflammation. **30.** Fibrosis is the permanent replacement of normal tissues by fibrous tissue.

Page 123

31. With advancing age, the speed and effectiveness of tissue repair decrease, the rate of energy consumption in general declines, hormonal activity is altered, and other factors contribute to changes in tissue structure and chemical composition.

ANSWERS TO REVIEW QUESTIONS

Level 1: Reviewing Facts and Terms

1. g **2.** d **3.** j **4.** i **5.** a **6.** f **7.** c **8.** e **9.** b **10.** h **11.** l
12. k **13.** (a) simple squamous epithelium; (b) simple cuboidal epithelium; (c) simple columnar epithelium; (d) stratified squamous epithelium; (e) stratified cuboidal epithelium; (f) stratified columnar epithelium. **14.** a **15.** c **16.** d **17.** b **18.** d **19.** c **20.** a **21.** b **22.** b **23.** a **24.** (a) mucous membrane; (b) serous membrane; (c) cutaneous membrane; (d) synovial membrane **25.** Layering in epithelia is either simple or stratified. **26.** Connective tissue contains specialized cells, extracellular protein fibers, and fluid ground substance. **27.** fluid connective tissues: blood and lymph; supporting connective tissues: bone and cartilage **28.** Neural tissue consists of neurons, which propagate, or transmit, electrical impulses, and neuroglia, which include several kinds of supporting cells, some of which play a role in providing nutrients to neurons.

Level 2: Reviewing Concepts

29. a **30.** During holocrine secretion, gland cells become packed with secretory products and then burst, releasing the secretion but killing the cells. The lost gland cells must be replaced by the division of stem cells. **31.** Exocrine secretions are secreted onto a surface or outward through a duct. Endocrine secretions (called hormones) are secreted by ductless glands into surrounding tissues and usually diffuse into the blood for distribution to other parts of the body. **32.** Tight junctions prevent the passage of water or solutes between cells. In the digestive tract, these junctions keep enzymes, acids, and wastes from damaging delicate underlying tissues. **33.** In skin, tight junctions, proteoglycan molecules, and physical interlocking form extensive connections that hold skin cells together, denying the entry of any pathogens present on their free surfaces. If the skin is damaged and the connections are broken, infection can easily occur. **34.** Unlike serous and mucous membranes, cutaneous membranes are thick, relatively waterproof, and usually dry.

Level 3: Critical Thinking and Clinical Applications

35. Animal intestines are specialized for absorption, so you would look for the slide in which a single layer of epithelium lines the cavity. The cells would be cuboidal or columnar and would probably have microvilli (which increase cellular surface area). With the right type of microscope, you could also see tight junctions between the cells. The esophagus receives undigested food, so the slide of it would have a stratified squamous epithelium that protects against mechanical damage or stress. **36.** Step 1: Check for striations. (If striations are present, the tissue is skeletal muscle or cardiac muscle. If striations are absent, the tissue is smooth muscle.) Step 2: Check for the presence of intercalated discs. (If the discs are present, the tissue is cardiac muscle. If they are absent, the tissue is skeletal muscle.)

CHAPTER 5

ANSWERS TO CHECKPOINTS

Page 130

1. Five major functions of the integumentary system include protection, temperature maintenance, synthesis and storage of nutrients, sensory reception, and excretion and secretion.

Page 134

2. The five layers of the epidermis are the stratum basale, stratum spinosum, stratum granulosum, stratum lucidum, and stratum corneum. **3.** Dandruff consists of cells from the stratum corneum. **4.** Sanding the tips of the fingers will not permanently remove fingerprints. The ridges of fingerprints are formed in skin layers that are constantly regenerated, so these ridges will eventually reappear.

Page 135

5. The two pigments in the epidermis are carotene, an orange-yellow pigment, and melanin, a brown, yellow-brown, or black pigment. **6.** When exposed to the ultraviolet radiation in sunlight or tanning lamps, melanocytes in the epidermis (and dermis) synthesize the pigment melanin, darkening the skin. **7.** When skin gets warm, arriving oxygenated blood is diverted to superficial blood vessels to eliminate heat. The oxygenated blood imparts a reddish coloration to the skin.

Page 136

8. In the presence of ultraviolet radiation in sunlight, epidermal cells in the stratum spinosum and stratum basale convert a cholesterol-related steroid into vitamin D_3. **9.** The most common skin cancer is basal cell carcinoma.

Page 137

10. The dermis (a connective tissue layer) lies immediately deep to the epidermis. **11.** The capillaries that supply the epidermis are located in the papillary layer of the dermis, where they follow the contours of the epidermis–dermis boundary.

Page 139

12. The tissue that connects the dermis to underlying tissues is the hypodermis or subcutaneous layer. **13.** The hypodermis is a layer of areolar tissue containing many adipose (fat) cells, which lies below the dermis. It is not considered a part of the integument, but it is important in stabilizing the position of the skin in relation to underlying tissues.

Page 141

14. A typical hair is a keratinous strand produced by epithelial cells of a hair follicle. **15.** Contraction of the arrector pili muscle pulls on the hair follicle, making the hair stand erect. The result is sometimes known as "goose bumps." **16.** Even though hair is a structure derived from the epidermis, the follicles are in the dermis. Where the epidermis and deep dermis are destroyed, new hair will not grow.

Page 143

17. Two types of exocrine glands found in the skin are sebaceous (oil) glands and sweat glands. **18.** Sebaceous secretions (called sebum) lubricate and protect the keratin of the hair shaft, lubricate and condition the surrounding skin, and inhibit bacterial growth. **19.** Deodorants are used to mask the odor of apocrine sweat gland secretions, which contain several kinds of organic compounds that have an odor or produce an odor when metabolized by skin bacteria. **20.** The substance keratin gives nails their strength. **21.** Nail growth occurs at the nail root, an epidermal fold that is not visible from the surface.

Page 149

22. The combination of fibrin clots, fibroblasts, and the extensive network of capillaries in healing tissue is called granulation tissue. **23.** Skin can regenerate effectively even after undergoing considerable damage because stem cells persist in both the epithelial and connective tissue components of skin. When injury occurs, cells of the stratum basale replace epithelial cells while connective tissue stem cells replace cells lost from the dermis.

Page 151

24. As a person ages, the blood supply to the dermis decreases and merocrine sweat glands become less active. These changes make it more difficult for elderly people to cool themselves in hot weather. **25.** With advancing age, melanocyte activity decreases, leading to gray or white hair.

ANSWERS TO REVIEW QUESTIONS

Level 1: Reviewing Facts and Terms

1. f **2.** g **3.** i **4.** j **5.** a **6.** e **7.** b **8.** d **9.** c **10.** h **11.** a **12.** d **13.** (a) epidermis; (b) dermis; (c) papillary layer; (d) reticular layer; (e) hypodermis (subcutaneous layer) **14.** b **15.** c **16.** a **17.** a **18.** (a) hair shaft; (b) sebaceous gland; (c) arrector pili muscle; (d) hair matrix; (e) hair papilla **19.** Carotene and melanin are found in the epidermis. **20.** The dermis is composed of the papillary layer (consists of areolar tissue, and contains capillaries and sensory neurons) and the reticular layer (consists of dense irregular connective tissue and bundles of collagen fibers). Both layers contain blood vessels, lymphatic vessels, and nerve fibers. **21.** Apocrine sweat glands and merocrine sweat glands occur in the skin.

Level 2: Reviewing Concepts

22. a **23.** Fat-soluble drugs are more desirable for transdermal administration because the permeability barrier is composed primarily of lipids surrounding epidermal cells. Water-soluble drugs are not soluble in lipids and have difficulty penetrating the lipid-based barrier. **24.** A tan results from the synthesis of melanin, which helps prevent skin damage by absorbing ultraviolet radiation before it reaches the deep layers of the epidermis and dermis. Melanin accumulates around the nucleus of epidermal cells, absorbing UV light before it can damage nuclear DNA. **25.** The lack of exposure to UV light in sunlight prevents the production of vitamin D_3 from a cholesterol-related steroid in the deepest layers of the epidermis. Thus, vitamin D_3 cannot be modified by the liver and converted into the hormone calcitriol by the kidneys. Calcitriol is essential for the absorption of the calcium and phosphorus needed to form strong bones, so fragile bones result. **26.** Because the hypodermis, or subcutaneous layer, is not highly vascular and lacks major organs, subcutaneous injection reduces the risk of tissue damage. **27.** As a person ages, the dermis becomes thinner and the elastic fiber network decreases in size, weakening the integument and causing loss of resilience.

Level 3: Critical Thinking and Clinical Applications

28. The child probably has a fondness for vegetables high in the yellow-orange pigment carotene, such as sweet potatoes, squash, and carrots. If a child consumes large amounts of carotene, the pigment will be stored in the skin, producing a yellow-orange skin color. **29.** Like most elderly people, Vanessa's grandmother has poor circulation to the skin. As a result, temperature receptors in the skin sense less warmth compared to good circulation. When this sensory information is relayed to the brain, that organ interprets it as coldness, causing Vanessa's grandmother to feel cold. **30.** Using the rule of nines, the right leg is 18% of surface area, the right arm is 9% of surface area, and the back of the trunk is 18% of surface area. Adding these separate values gives a total surface burn area estimate of 45%.

CHAPTER 6

ANSWERS TO CHECKPOINTS

Page 157

1. The five primary functions of the skeletal system are support, storage of minerals and lipids, blood cell production, protection, and leverage.

Page 162

2. The four general shapes of bones are flat, irregular, long, and short. **3.** If the ratio of collagen to calcium in a bone increased, the bone would be weaker (but more flexible).

4. This sample most likely came from the shaft (diaphysis) of a long bone, as concentric layers of bone around a central canal are indicative of osteons, which make up compact bone. The ends (epiphyses) of long bones are primarily spongy (trabecular) bone. **5.** Mature bone cells are known as osteocytes, bone-building cells are called osteoblasts, and osteoclasts are bone-resorbing cells. **6.** When osteoclast activity exceeds osteoblast activity, bone mass decreases, because osteoclasts break down or demineralize bone.

Page 165

7. During intramembranous ossification, fibrous connective tissue is replaced by bone. **8.** An x-ray of the femur (or any long bone) would indicate whether the epiphyseal cartilage, which separates the epiphysis from the diaphysis, is still present. If present, then growth is still occurring. If it is absent, the bone has reached its full length. **9.** Growth continues throughout childhood. At puberty, a growth spurt occurs that is then followed by the closure of the epiphyseal cartilages. The later puberty begins, the taller the child will be at the start of the growth spurt. So, when growth is completed, the individual will be taller than individuals who began puberty earlier. **10.** Pregnant women need large amounts of calcium to support bone growth in the developing fetus. If an expectant mother does not take in enough calcium in her diet, her body will mobilize the calcium reserves of her own skeleton to provide for the needs of the fetus, resulting in weakened bones in the mother, as well as an increased risk of fracture. **11.** Bone remodeling refers to the continuous process whereby old bone is being destroyed by osteoclasts while new bone is being constructed by osteoblasts. **12.** In response to mechanical stress on the arm bones during weight lifting, the bones grow heavier. The arm bones of joggers are lighter because they experience relatively little stress. **13.** Parathyroid hormone (PTH) and calcitriol work together to increase blood calcium levels, whereas calcitonin decreases blood calcium levels. **14.** A closed (simple) fracture is completely internal and there is no break in the skin. An open (compound) fracture projects through the skin. It is more dangerous because of the possibility of infection or uncontrolled bleeding. **15.** Osteopenia is inadequate ossification and is common to the aging process. It results from decreasing osteoblast activity accompanied by normal osteoclast activity. **16.** Osteoporosis is more common in older women because after menopause, levels of estrogens—sex hormones that play an important role in moving calcium into bones—decrease dramatically, making it difficult to replace calcium lost from bones due to normal aging. In men, decreases in sex hormone (androgen) levels occur at later ages.

Page 173

17. A bone marking (surface feature) is an area on the surface of a bone related to a specific function, such as joint formation, muscle attachment, or the passage of nerves and blood vessels. **18.** The axial skeleton includes the skull (8 cranial bones and 14 facial bones); the bones associated with the skull (6 auditory ossicles and the hyoid bone); the bones of the thoracic cage (24 ribs and the sternum); and the vertebral column (26 bones).

Page 187

19. The mastoid and styloid processes are projections on the temporal bones of the skull. **20.** The sella turcica is located in the sphenoid bone. During life, it contains the pituitary gland. **21.** The occipital bone of the cranium (specifically, the occipital condyles) articulates with the vertebral column. **22.** The bones fractured by the ball are the frontal bone (which forms the superior portion of the orbit) and the maxillary and zygomatic bones (which form the inferior portion of the orbit). **23.** The paranasal sinuses lighten some of the heavier skull bones. They contain a mucous epithelium that releases a mucous secretion into the nasal cavities that warms, moistens, and filters particles out of the incoming air. **24.** A fracture of the coronoid process would make it difficult to close the mouth because it would hinder the functioning of muscles that attach to the coronoid process of the mandible (lower jaw). **25.** Because many muscles that move the tongue and the larynx are attached to the hyoid bone, you would expect a person with a fractured hyoid bone to have difficulty moving the tongue, breathing, and swallowing. **26.** The dens is part of the second cervical vertebra, or axis, which is in the neck. **27.** In adults, the five sacral vertebrae fuse to form a single sacrum. **28.** The lumbar vertebrae must support a great deal more weight than do vertebrae that are more superior in the spinal column. The large vertebral bodies allow the weight to be distributed

over a larger area. **29.** True ribs (ribs 1–7) are each attached directly to the sternum by their own costal cartilage. False ribs (ribs 8–12) either do not attach to the sternum (the floating ribs) or attach by means of a shared, common costal cartilage. **30.** Improper compression of the chest during CPR can—and commonly does—result in a fracture of the xiphoid process of the sternum or the ribs.

Page 194

31. By attaching the scapula to the sternum, the clavicle restricts the scapula's range of movement. A broken clavicle thus allows the scapula a greater range of movement (and reduces its stability). **32.** The two rounded projections on either side of the elbow are the lateral and medial epicondyles of the humerus. **33.** The radius is lateral to the ulna when the forearm is in the anatomical position. **34.** The three bones that make up a hip bone are the ilium, the ischium, and the pubis. **35.** The fibula is an important site of attachment for many leg muscles, so its fracture prevents proper muscle function, and moving the leg and walking become difficult and painful. The fibula also helps stabilize the ankle joint. **36.** Cesar has most likely fractured his calcaneus (heel bone).

Page 197

37. The three types of joints as classified by their range of motion are (1) an immovable joint, or synarthrosis; (2) a slightly movable joint, or amphiarthrosis; and (3) a freely movable joint, or diarthrosis. A synarthrosis can be fibrous or cartilaginous, depending on the nature of the connection, or it can be a bony fusion, which develops over time. An amphiarthrosis is either fibrous or cartilaginous, depending on the nature of the connection. A diarthrosis joint is a synovial joint and permits the greatest range of motion. **38.** These are fibrous joints known as sutures.

Page 199

39. (a) Moving the humerus away from the body's longitudinal axis is abduction. (b) Turning the palms forward is supination. (c) Bending the elbow is flexion. **40.** Flexion and extension are associated with hinge joints.

Page 205

41. The tennis player is more likely than the jogger to have subscapular bursitis (inflammation of the bursa) because this bursa is located in the shoulder joint. **42.** Daphne has most likely fractured her ulna. **43.** A complete dislocation of the knee is rare because the joint is stabilized by ligaments on its anterior, posterior, medial, and lateral surfaces, as well as by a pair of ligaments within the joint capsule. **44.** The skeletal system provides structural support for all body systems and stores energy, calcium, and phosphate reserves. The integumentary system synthesizes vitamin D_3, which is essential for calcium and phosphate ion absorption. Calcium and phosphate ions are needed for bone growth and maintenance.

ANSWERS TO REVIEW QUESTIONS

Level 1: Reviewing Facts and Terms

1. i **2.** h **3.** m **4.** l **5.** j **6.** k **7.** f **8.** c **9.** o **10.** b **11.** g **12.** n **13.** d **14.** a **15.** e **16.** b **17.** a **18.** c **19.** b **20.** d **21.** (a) occipital bone; (b) parietal bone; (c) frontal bone; (d) temporal bone; (e) sphenoid bone; (f) ethmoid bone; (g) vomer; (h) mandible; (i) lacrimal bone; (j) nasal bone; (k) zygomatic bone; (l) maxilla (or maxillary bone) **22.** a **23.** a **24.** a **25.** a **26.** b **27.** c **28.** (a) joint capsule; (b) synovial membrane; (c) articular cartilage; (d) joint cavity **29.** d **30.** b **31.** c **32.** In intramembranous ossification, bone develops from fibrous connective tissue. In endochondral ossification, bone develops from a cartilage model. **33.** The hyoid is the only bone in the body that does not articulate with another bone. **34.** The thoracic cage (1) protects the heart, lungs, thymus, and other structures in the thoracic cavity, and (2) serves as an attachment point for muscles involved with respiration, positioning the vertebral column, and moving the pectoral girdles and upper extremities. **35.** The acromion and coracoid processes are parts of the scapula associated with the shoulder joint.

Level 2: Reviewing Concepts

36. The osteons are parallel to the long axis of the shaft, which does not bend when forces are applied to either end. An impact to the side of the shaft can lead to a fracture. **37.** The chondrocytes of the epiphyseal cartilage enlarge and divide, increasing the thickness of the cartilage. On the shaft side, the chondrocytes become ossified, forcing or "chasing" the expanding epiphyseal cartilage away from the shaft. **38.** The lumbar vertebrae have massive bodies and carry a large amount of weight—both causative factors of disc rupture. The cervical vertebrae are more delicate and have small bodies, increasing the possibility of dislocations and fractures compared with other regions of the vertebral column. **39.** The clavicles are small and fragile, so fractures are quite common. Their position also makes them vulnerable to injury and damage. **40.** The pelvic girdle consists of the two hip bones. The pelvis is a composite structure that includes the two hip bones of the appendicular skeleton and the sacrum and coccyx of the axial skeleton. **41.** Articular cartilages resemble hyaline cartilage, but do not have a perichondrium, and their matrix contains more water than do other cartilages. **42.** The slight mobility of the pubic symphysis facilitates childbirth by spreading the pelvis to ease movement of the baby through the birth canal.

Level 3: Critical Thinking and Clinical Applications

43. The fracture might have damaged the epiphyseal cartilage in Yasmin's right leg. Even though the bone healed properly, the damaged leg did not produce as much cartilage as the undamaged leg, producing a shorter bone in the injured leg. **44.** The virus could have been inhaled through the nose and passed into the cranium by way of the cribriform plate of the ethmoid bone. **45.** The large bones of a child's cranium are not yet fused, but connected by areas of connective tissue called fontanelles. By examining the bones, the archaeologist could readily see if sutures had formed. By knowing approximately how long it takes for the various fontanelles to close and by determining their sizes, she could estimate the age of the individual at death. **46.** Frank may have suffered a shoulder dislocation, which is a quite common injury due to the weak nature of the articulation between the scapula and the humerus, or glenohumeral joint. **47.** Ed has a sprained ankle. This condition occurs when ligaments are stretched to the point at which some of the collagen fibers are torn. Stretched ligaments in joints can cause the release of synovial fluid, which results in swelling and pain in the affected area.

CHAPTER 7

ANSWERS TO CHECKPOINTS

Page 213

1. Skeletal muscles produce skeletal movement, maintain body posture and body position, support soft tissues, guard body entrances and exits, and maintain body temperature.

Page 215

2. The epimysium is a dense layer of collagen fibers that surrounds the entire muscle; the perimysium divides the skeletal muscle into a series of compartments, each containing a bundle of muscle fibers called a fascicle; and the endomysium surrounds individual skeletal muscle cells (fibers). **3.** Severing the tendon would prevent the muscle from moving the body part because the muscle would no longer be connected to the bone.

Page 218

4. Sarcomeres, the smallest contractile units of a skeletal muscle cell, are segments of myofibrils. Each sarcomere has dark A bands and light I bands. The A band contains the M line, H band, and the zone of overlap. Each I band contains thin filaments but not thick filaments. Z lines mark the boundaries between adjacent sarcomeres. **5.** Skeletal muscle appears striated when viewed under the microscope because the arrangement of the actin and myosin myofilaments within myofibrils produces a banded appearance. **6.** You would expect to find the greatest concentration of calcium ions in the terminal cisternae of the sarcoplasmic reticulum of a resting skeletal muscle fiber.

Page 222

7. The neuromuscular junction—a specialized intercellular connection between a motor neuron and a muscle cell—enables communication between the nervous system and a skeletal muscle fiber. **8.** A drug that blocks ACh release would prevent muscle contraction. A lack of ACh prevents the generation of an action potential in the sarcolemma, which is necessary for the release of calcium ions from the sarcoplasmic reticulum, and subsequent cross-bridge formation. **9.** If the sarcolemma of a resting skeletal muscle suddenly became permeable to calcium ions, the intracellular concentration of calcium ions would increase, and the muscle would contract.

In addition, because the amount of calcium ions in the sarcoplasm must decline for relaxation to occur, the increased permeability of the sarcolemma to calcium ions might prevent the muscle from relaxing completely.

Page 229

10. The amount of tension produced in a skeletal muscle depends on (1) the frequency of muscle fiber stimulation and (2) the number of muscle fibers activated. **11.** A motor unit with 1500 muscle fibers is most likely from a large muscle involved in powerful, gross movements. Muscles that control fine or precise movements (such as those moving the eye or the fingers) have only a few fibers per motor unit, whereas muscles involved in more powerful contractions (such as those moving the leg) have hundreds of fibers per motor unit. **12.** Yes. A skeletal muscle undergoing an isometric contraction does not shorten, even though tension in the muscle increases. By contrast, in an isotonic contraction, tension remains constant and the muscle shortens.

Page 232

13. Muscle cells continuously synthesize ATP by utilizing creatine phosphate (CP) and metabolizing glycogen and fatty acids. Most cells generate ATP through aerobic metabolism in the mitochondria and through glycolysis in the cytoplasm. **14.** Muscle fatigue is a muscle's reduced ability to contract despite neural stimulation. It may be due to low ATP levels, low pH (lactic acid buildup and dissociation), or other problems. **15.** Oxygen debt is the amount of oxygen required to restore normal, pre-exertion conditions in muscle tissue.

Page 233

16. A sprinter requires large amounts of energy for a relatively short burst of activity. To supply this energy, the sprinter's muscles switch to anaerobic metabolism. Anaerobic metabolism is less efficient in producing energy than aerobic metabolism and produces acidic waste products; this combination contributes to muscle fatigue. By contrast, marathon runners derive most of their energy from aerobic metabolism, which is more efficient and produces fewer waste products than anaerobic metabolism. **17.** Activities that require short periods of strenuous activity produce a greater oxygen debt, because such activities rely heavily on energy production by anaerobic metabolism. Because lifting weights is more strenuous over the short term than swimming laps, which is an aerobic activity, weight lifting would likely produce a greater oxygen debt than would swimming laps. **18.** Individuals who excel at endurance activities have a higher than normal percentage of slow muscle fibers. Slow muscle fibers are better adapted to this type of activity than fast fibers, which are less vascular and fatigue more quickly.

Page 236

19. Intercalated discs enhance cardiac muscle tissue function by tightly binding cardiac muscle fibers, enabling them to "pull together" efficiently. Because intercalated discs also contain gap junctions, ions and small molecules can flow directly between cells. As a result, action potentials generated in one cell spread rapidly to adjacent cells. Thus, all cells contract simultaneously. **20.** Extracellular calcium ions are important for the contraction of cardiac and smooth muscle. In skeletal muscle, calcium ions come from the sarcoplasmic reticulum. **21.** Smooth muscle cells can contract over a relatively large range of resting lengths because their actin and myosin filaments are not as rigidly organized as in skeletal muscle.

Page 239

22. Skeletal muscle names are based on several factors, including location in the body, origin and insertion, action, muscle fascicle orientation, relative position, structural characteristics, muscle shape, number of origins, and size. **23.** The *triceps brachii,* which extends the elbow, is the antagonist of the biceps brachii, which produces flexion at the elbow. **24.** The name *flexor carpi radialis longus* tells you that this muscle is a long muscle (longus) that lies next to the radius (radialis) and flexes (flexor) the wrist (carpus).

Page 248

25. You would likely be chewing; contracting the masseter muscle raises the mandible, whereas relaxing this muscle depresses the mandible. **26.** You would expect the buccinator muscle, which shapes the mouth for blowing, to be well developed in a trumpet player. **27.** Damage to the external intercostal muscles would interfere with the process of breathing. **28.** A blow to the rectus abdominis would cause that muscle to contract forcefully, flexing the torso. In other words, you would "double over."

ANSWERS

Page 256

29. When you shrug your shoulders, you are contracting your levator scapulae muscles. **30.** The rotator cuff muscles are the supraspinatus, infraspinatus, teres minor, and subscapularis. (The acronym SITS is useful in remembering these four muscles.) **31.** Injury to the flexor carpi ulnaris would impair the ability to flex and adduct the wrist.

Page 259

32. A "pulled hamstring" refers to a muscle strain affecting one or more of the three muscles that collectively flex the knee: the biceps femoris, semimembranosus, and semitendinosus muscles. **33.** A torn calcaneal tendon would make plantar flexion difficult because this tendon attaches the soleus and gastrocnemius muscles to the calcaneus (heel bone). **34.** The three functional muscle groups of the lower limb are: (1) muscles that work across the hip joint to move the thigh; (2) muscles that work across the knee joint to move the leg; and (3) muscles that work across the various joints of the foot to move the ankles, feet, and toes. **35.** The sartorius muscle crosses over both the hip and knee joints.

Page 262

36. General age-related effects on skeletal muscles include decreased skeletal muscle fiber diameters, diminished muscle elasticity, decreased tolerance for exercise, and a decreased ability to recover from muscular injuries. **37.** The muscular system generates heat that maintains normal body temperature. **38.** Exercise affects the cardiovascular system by increasing heart rate and dilating blood vessels. With exercise, the rate and depth of respiration increase, and sweat gland secretion increases. The nervous and endocrine systems direct and coordinate the physiological effects of exercise.

ANSWERS TO REVIEW QUESTIONS

Level 1: Reviewing Facts and Terms

1. f **2.** i **3.** d **4.** p **5.** l **6.** c **7.** h **8.** n **9.** b **10.** k **11.** o **12.** a **13.** m **14.** j **15.** g **16.** e **17.** (a) T tubules; (b) terminal cisterna; (c) sarcoplasmic reticulum; (d) triad; (e) sarcolemma; (f) mitochondria; (g) thick filament; (h) thin filament; (i) myofibril **18.** d **19.** (a) supraspinatus; (b) infraspinatus; (c) teres minor **20.** Step 1: calcium ions arrive in the zone of overlap. Step 2: active-site exposure. Step 3: cross-bridge formation. Step 4: pivoting of myosin head (power stroke). Step 5: cross-bridge detachment. Step 6: myosin reactivation (recocking the myosin head) **21.** energy reserves in resting skeletal muscle cells: ATP, creatine phosphate, glycogen. **22.** Aerobic metabolism and glycolysis generate ATP from glucose in muscle cells.

Level 2: Reviewing Concepts

23. b **24.** Acetylcholine released by the motor neuron at the neuromuscular junction changes the permeability of the cell membrane at the motor end plate. The permeability change allows the influx of positive sodium ions, which in turn trigger an electrical event called an action potential. The action potential spreads across the entire surface of the muscle fiber and into the interior along the T tubules. The release of calcium ions from the sarcoplasmic reticulum triggers the start of a contraction. The contraction ends when the ACh has been removed from the synaptic cleft and motor end plate by AChE. **25.** The extra gene copies contained in multiple nuclei speed up the production of enzymes and structural proteins needed to meet the large metabolic requirements of normally contracting skeletal muscle cells. **26.** The spinal column does not need a massive series of flexors because (1) gravity tends to flex the spine (because body weight largely lies anterior to the spinal column) and (2) contractions of many of the large trunk muscles flex the spine. **27.** Voluntary control of urination and defecation is possible because the urethral and anal sphincter muscles are innervated by nerves under conscious control. Voluntary relaxation of the sphincters, which are normally constricted to prevent the passage of urine and feces, allows the passage of wastes. **28.** When the hamstrings are injured, flexion at the knee and extension at the hip are affected.

Level 3: Critical Thinking and Clinical Applications

29. The most obvious sign of organophosphate poisoning is uncontrolled tetanic contractions of skeletal muscles. Organophosphates block the action of the enzyme acetylcholinesterase, so acetylcholine released into the synaptic cleft of the neuromuscular junction would not be inactivated, causing a state of persistent contraction (spastic paralysis). If paralysis affected the muscles of respiration (which is likely), Terry would die of suffocation. **30.** In rigor mortis, the membranes of the dead cells are no longer selectively permeable, and the SR is no longer able to retain calcium ions. As calcium ions enter the cytosol, a sustained contraction develops, making the body extremely stiff. Contraction persists because the dead muscle cells can no longer make the ATP required for cross-bridge detachment from the active sites. Rigor mortis begins a few hours after death and ends after one to six days or when decomposition begins. Decomposition begins when the lysosomal enzymes released by autolysis break down the myofilaments. **31.** Makani should do squatting exercises. Placing a barbell on his shoulders as he does squats will produce better results, because the quadriceps muscles will be working against a greater resistance.

CHAPTER 8

ANSWERS TO CHECKPOINTS

Page 271

1. The two anatomical divisions of the nervous system are the central nervous system (CNS), consisting of the brain and spinal cord, and the peripheral nervous system (PNS), consisting of all neural tissue outside the CNS. **2.** The two functional divisions of the peripheral nervous system are the afferent division, which brings sensory information to the CNS from receptors in peripheral tissues and organs, and the efferent division, which carries motor commands from the CNS to effectors, such as muscles and glands. **3.** Damage to the afferent division of the PNS would affect nerves carrying sensory information to the brain and spinal cord. It would interfere with a person's ability to experience a variety of sensory stimuli.

Page 277

4. Structural components of a typical neuron include a cell body (which contains the nucleus and nucleolus), an axon, dendrites, Nissl bodies, axon hillock, collaterals, and axon terminals. **5.** Unipolar neurons are most likely sensory neurons of the PNS. **6.** CNS neuroglia include ependymal cells, astrocytes, oligodendrocytes, and microglia. **7.** Small phagocytic glial cells called microglia would typically be found in increased numbers in infected (or damaged) areas of the CNS. **8.** In the PNS, neuron cell bodies (gray matter) are located in ganglia and are surrounded by satellite cells.

Page 284

9. If the voltage-gated sodium channels in a neuron's excitable axon membrane were blocked, the neuron would not be able to depolarize because sodium ions could not flow into the cell. **10.** If the extracellular potassium concentration were to decrease, more potassium ions would leave the cell, increasing the electrical gradient across the membrane (the membrane potential). This effect is called hyperpolarization. **11.** The steps in the generation of action potentials are Step 1: depolarization to threshold; Step 2: activation of voltage-gated sodium channels and rapid depolarization; Step 3: inactivation of sodium channels and activation of voltage-gated potassium channels; and Step 4: closing of potassium channels and return to normal permeability. **12.** The axon that carries action potentials at 50 meters per second is myelinated. Myelinated axons propagate action potentials by saltatory propagation at speeds much higher than those by continuous propagation along unmyelinated axons.

Page 284

13. A synapse is the site where a neuron communicates with another cell. It is composed of presynaptic and postsynaptic cells whose plasma membranes are separated by a narrow synaptic cleft. **14.** Blocking calcium channels at the presynaptic terminal of a cholinergic synapse would prevent the influx of calcium ions that triggers the release of acetylcholine. As a result, no communication would occur across the synapse, and the postsynaptic neuron would not be stimulated. **15.** Convergence permits both conscious and subconscious control of the same motor neurons.

Page 289

16. The three meninges surrounding the CNS are the dura mater, arachnoid mater, and pia mater.

Page 292

17. Damage to the ventral root of a spinal nerve, which carries visceral and somatic motor fibers, would interfere with motor function. **18.** You would find poliovirus in the anterior gray horns of the spinal cord, because that is where the cell bodies of somatic motor neurons are located. **19.** All spinal nerves are classified as mixed nerves because they contain both sensory and motor fibers.

Page 309

20. The six regions in the brain and their major functions are (1) the *cerebrum:* conscious thought processes; (2) the *diencephalon:* the thalamic portion contains relay and processing centers for sensory information, and the hypothalamic portion contains centers involved with emotions, autonomic function, and hormone production; (3) the *midbrain:* processes visual and auditory information and generates involuntary motor responses; (4) the *pons* contains tracts and relay centers that connect the brain stem to the cerebellum; (5) the *medulla oblongata* contains major centers concerned with the regulation of autonomic function, such as heart rate, blood pressure, respiration, and digestive activities; and (6) the *cerebellum* adjusts voluntary and involuntary motor activities. **21.** The pituitary gland is attached to the hypothalamus, or the floor of the diencephalon. **22.** If diffusion across the arachnoid granulations decreased, re-entry of cerebrospinal fluid into the bloodstream would be reduced, so the volume of cerebrospinal fluid in the ventricles would increase. **23.** The primary motor cortex is located in the precentral gyrus of the frontal lobes of the cerebrum. **24.** Damage to the temporal lobes of the cerebrum would interfere with the processing of olfactory (smell) and auditory (sound) sensations. **25.** The thalamus acts as a relay point for all ascending sensory information except olfactory information. **26.** Changes in body temperature stimulate the hypothalamus, a portion of the diencephalon. **27.** Damage to the medulla oblongata can have fatal results because, despite its small size, it contains vital reflex centers, including those that control breathing and regulate the heart and blood pressure.

Page 314

28. The abducens nerve (N VI) controls lateral movements of the eyes through the lateral rectus muscles, so individuals with damage to this nerve would be unable to move their eyes laterally (to the side). **29.** Control of the voluntary muscles of the tongue occurs through the hypoglossal nerve (N XII). **30.** Damage to the cervical plexus—or more specifically to the phrenic nerves, which extend to and innervate the diaphragm—would greatly interfere with the ability to breathe (and might even be fatal).

Page 318

31. A reflex is a rapid, automatic response to a specific stimulus. It is important in maintaining homeostasis. **32.** Physicians use stretch reflexes (such as the patellar reflex, or knee-jerk reflex) to test the general condition of the spinal cord, peripheral nerves, and muscles. **33.** Polysynaptic reflexes can produce more complex responses because they include interneurons (between the sensory and motor neurons) that may control several muscle groups simultaneously. In addition, some interneurons may stimulate a muscle group or groups, whereas others may inhibit other muscle groups. **34.** A positive Babinski reflex is abnormal in adults. It indicates possible damage to descending tracts in Tom's spinal cord.

Page 322

35. A tract within the posterior column pathway of the spinal cord carrying information about touch and pressure from the lower part of the body to the brain is being compressed. **36.** The primary motor cortex of the right cerebral hemisphere controls motor function on the left side of the body. **37.** An injury to the superior portion of the motor cortex would affect the ability to control muscles in the hand, arm, and upper portion of the leg.

Page 329

38. The sympathetic division of the autonomic nervous system is responsible for the physiological changes that occur in response to stress and increased activity. **39.** The parasympathetic division is sometimes referred to as "the anabolic system" because parasympathetic stimulation leads to a general increase in the nutrient content of the blood. Cells throughout the body respond to the increase by absorbing the nutrients and using them to support growth and other anabolic activities. **40.** A decrease in sympathetic stimulation would result in reduced airflow because parasympathetic effects would dominate, decreasing the diameter of respiratory airways. **41.** Anxiety or stress causes increased sympathetic stimulation, so a person who is anxious about an impending root canal might exhibit some or all of the following: a dry mouth, increased heart rate, increased blood pressure, increased rate of breathing, cold sweats, an urge to urinate or defecate, change in motility of the digestive tract ("butterflies" in the stomach), and dilated pupils.

Page 330

42. Age-related reduction in brain size and weight results from a decrease in the volume of the cerebral cortex due to the loss of cortical neurons.

Page 334

43. The nervous system controls the actions of the arrector pili muscles and sweat glands of the integumentary system. It also controls skeletal muscle contractions of the muscular system, which, in turn, affects the thickening of bones of the skeletal system.

ANSWERS TO REVIEW QUESTIONS

Level 1: Reviewing Facts and Terms

1. f **2.** g **3.** p **4.** s **5.** m **6.** a **7.** b **8.** j **9.** h **10.** c **11.** d **12.** o **13.** t **14.** q **15.** l **16.** i **17.** n **18.** e **19.** r **20.** k **21.** (a) dendrite; (b) cell body; (c) nucleus; (d) nucleolus; (e) axon hillock; (f) axon; (g) axon terminals **22.** c **23.** a **24.** a **25.** (a) cerebrum; (b) diencephalon; (c) midbrain; (d) pons; (e) medulla oblongata; (f) cerebellum **26.** d **27.** b **28.** b **29.** a **30.** b **31.** c **32.** a **33.** d **34.** The all-or-none principle of action potentials: A given stimulus either triggers a typical action potential, or it does not produce one at all. **35.** N I: olfactory; N II: optic; N III: oculomotor; N IV: trochlear; N V: trigeminal; N VI: abducens; N VII: facial; N VIII: vestibulocochlear; N IX: glossopharyngeal; N X: vagus; N XI: accessory; N XII: hypoglossal **36.** Sympathetic preganglionic fibers emerge from the thoracic and upper lumbar segments (T_1 through L_2) of the spinal cord. Parasympathetic preganglionic fibers emerge from the brain stem and the sacral segments of the spinal cord (craniosacral).

Level 2: Reviewing Concepts

37. d **38.** c **39.** Centers in the medulla oblongata are involved in respiratory and cardiac activity. **40.** Response time in a monosynaptic reflex is faster than in a polysynaptic reflex because with only one synapse, synaptic delay is minimized. In a polysynaptic reflex, total delay is proportional to the number of synapses involved.

41.

Property	Sympathetic	Parasympathetic
Mental alertness	increased	decreased
Metabolic rate	increased	decreased
Digestive/urinary function	inhibited	stimulated
Use of energy reserves	stimulated	inhibited
Respiratory rate	increased	decreased
Heart rate/blood pressure	increased	decreased
Sweat gland activity	stimulated	inhibited

Level 3: Critical Thinking and Clinical Applications

42. Brain tumors do not result from uncontrolled division of neurons, but instead of neuroglial cells, which can divide. In addition, cells of the meningeal membranes can give rise to tumors. **43.** The officer is testing the function of the cerebellum. A person who is under the influence of many drugs, including alcohol, is unable to properly anticipate the range and speed of limb movement because of slow processing and correction by the cerebellum. As a result, an inebriated or intoxicated Bill would have a difficult time performing simple tasks such as walking a straight line or touching his finger to his nose. **44.** Severing the branches of the vagus nerves (N X) helps control stress-induced stomach ulcers by eliminating excessive sympathetic stimulation. Chronic sympathetic stimulation causes constriction of blood vessels, which shuts off the blood supply to the stomach. The reduced blood supply causes cell and tissue death, resulting in ulcers. **45.** The radial nerve is involved in crutch paralysis. **46.** Ramon damaged the femoral nerve. Because this nerve supplies the sensory innervation of the skin on the anteromedial surface of the thigh and medial surfaces of the leg and foot, Ramon may also experience numbness in these regions.

CHAPTER 9

ANSWERS TO CHECKPOINTS

Page 345

1. Adaptation is a decrease in receptor sensitivity or perception after constant stimulation. **2.** Receptor A provides more precise sensory information because it has a smaller receptive field. **3.** The five special senses are smell (olfaction), taste (gustation), vision, balance (equilibrium), and hearing.

Page 349

4. The four types of general sensory receptors (and the stimuli that excite them) are nociceptors (pain), thermoreceptors (temperature), mechanoreceptors (physical distortion), and chemoreceptors (chemical concentration). **5.** The three classes of mechanoreceptors are tactile receptors, baroreceptors, and proprioceptors. **6.** If proprioceptors in your legs could not relay information about limb position and movement to the CNS (especially the cerebellum), your movements would be uncoordinated, and you likely could not walk.

Page 351

7. Olfaction is the sense of smell. It involves olfactory receptor cells in paired olfactory organs responding to chemical stimuli. **8.** Repeated sniffing increases the perception of faint odors by increasing the flow of air and the number of odorant molecules passing over the olfactory epithelium.

Page 353

9. Gustation is the sense of taste, provided by taste receptors responding to chemical stimuli. **10.** Taste receptors are sensitive only to molecules and ions that are in solution. If you dry the surface of your tongue, the salt ions or sugar molecules have no moisture in which to dissolve, so they will not stimulate the taste receptors.

Page 362

11. The first accessory structure of the eye to be affected by inadequate tear production is the conjunctiva. **12.** When the lens becomes more rounded, you are looking at an object close to you. **13.** Malia will likely be unable to see at all. The fovea contains only cones, which need high-intensity light to be stimulated. The dimly lit room contains light that is too weak to stimulate the cones.

Page 369

14. If you were born without cone cells, you would still be able to see—as long as you had functioning rod cells—but you would lack color vision and see in black and white only. **15.** A vitamin A deficiency would reduce the quantity of retinal the body could produce, thereby interfering with night vision (which operates at the body's threshold ability to respond to light).

Page 379

16. If the round window could not move, the vibration of the stapes at the oval window would not move the perilymph, and there would be little or no perception of sound. **17.** Loss of stereocilia from the hair cells of the spiral organ (as a result of constant exposure to loud noises, for instance) would reduce hearing sensitivity and could lead to deafness.

Page 380

18. Because individuals over age 50 experience a decline in the number and sensitivity of taste buds, a given food can be too spicy for children and too bland for the elderly. **19.** With age, the lens loses its elasticity and stiffens, resulting in a flatter lens that cannot be rounded to focus the image of a close-up object on the retina. This condition, called presbyopia, may be corrected with a converging lens.

ANSWERS TO REVIEW QUESTIONS

Level 1: Reviewing Facts and Terms

1. k **2.** c **3.** a **4.** e **5.** f **6.** j **7.** i **8.** b **9.** h **10.** m **11.** g **12.** l **13.** n **14.** d **15.** (a) fibrous layer; (b) cornea; (c) sclera; (d) inner layer, or retina; (e) neural part; (f) pigmented part; (g) vascular layer; (h) iris; (i) ciliary body; (j) choroid **16.** b **17.** d **18.** b **19.** d **20.** b **21.** b **22.** d **23.** a **24.** b **25.** b **26.** b **27.** a **28.** (a) auricle; (b) external acoustic meatus; (c) tympanic membrane; (d) auditory ossicles; (e) semicircular canals; (f) vestibule; (g) auditory tube; (h) cochlea; (i) vestibulocochlear nerve, N VIII **29.** d **30.** The three types of mechanoreceptors

are tactile receptors, baroreceptors, and proprioceptors. **31.** Tactile receptors in skin are (1) free nerve endings: sensitive to touch and pressure; (2) root hair plexuses: monitor distortions and movements across the body surface; (3) tactile discs: detect fine touch and pressure; (4) tactile (Meissner's) corpuscles: detect fine touch and pressure; (5) lamellated (pacinian) corpuscles: sensitive to pulsing or vibrating stimuli (deep pressure); and (6) Ruffini corpuscles: sensitive to pressure and distortion of the skin **32.** (a) The fibrous layer is composed of the sclera and the cornea. (b) The fibrous layer provides mechanical support and some degree of physical protection, serves as attachment sites for the extrinsic eye muscles, and contains structures that assist in focusing. **33.** The vascular layer consists of the iris, ciliary body, and choroid. **34.** Step 1: Sound waves arrive at the tympanic membrane. Step 2: Movement of the tympanic membrane causes displacement of the auditory ossicles. Step 3: Movement of the stapes at the oval window establishes pressure waves in the perilymph of the scala vestibuli. Step 4: The pressure waves distort the basilar membrane on their way to the round window of the scala tympani. Step 5: Vibration of the basilar membrane causes hair cells to vibrate against the tectorial membrane. Step 6: Information about the region and intensity of stimulation is relayed to the CNS over the cochlear branch of cranial nerve VIII.

Level 2: Reviewing Concepts

35. c **36.** c **37.** The general senses include somatic and visceral sensations (temperature, pain, touch, pressure, vibration, and proprioception). The special senses are those whose receptors are confined to the head, and include smell (olfaction), taste (gustation), vision, balance (equilibrium), and hearing. **38.** The CNS receives any stimulus detected by a sensory receptor in the form of action potentials, regardless of the type of stimulus. **39.** An infected sebaceous gland of an eyelash or tarsal gland usually becomes a sty, a painful swelling. **40.** A visual acuity of 20/15 means that Jane is able to see details that would be clear to a "normal" eye only at a distance of 15 feet. Jane's visual acuity is better than 20/20 vision.

Level 3: Critical Thinking and Clinical Applications

41. As you turn to look at your friend, your medial rectus muscles would contract, directing your gaze more medially. In addition, your pupils would constrict and the lenses would become more spherical. **42.** The loud noises from the fireworks have transferred so much energy to the endolymph in the cochlea that the fluid continues to move for a long while. As long as the endolymph is moving, it will vibrate the tectorial membrane and stimulate the hair cells. This stimulation produces the "ringing" sensation that Millie perceives. She finds it difficult to hear normal conversation because the vibrations associated with it are not strong enough to overcome the currents already moving through the endolymph, so the pattern of vibrations is difficult to discern against the background "noise." **43.** The rapid descent in the elevator causes the otoliths of the macula in the saccule of the vestibule to slide upward, producing the sensation of downward vertical acceleration. When the elevator abruptly stops, the otoliths of the macula do not. It takes a few seconds for them to come to rest in the normal position. As long as the otoliths of the macula are displaced, the perception of movement will remain.

CHAPTER 10

ANSWERS TO CHECKPOINTS

Page 388

1. Both the endocrine and nervous systems (1) release chemicals that bind to specific receptors on target cells, (2) share chemical messengers, (3) are primarily regulated by negative feedback processes, and (4) maintain homeostasis by coordinating and regulating the activities of other cells, tissues, organs, and systems.

Page 393

2. A hormone is a chemical messenger that is secreted by one cell and travels through the bloodstream to affect the activities of cells in other parts of the body. **3.** A cell's sensitivity to any hormone is determined by the presence or absence of the receptor molecule specific to that hormone. **4.** A molecule that blocks adenylate cyclase, the enzyme that converts ATP to cAMP, would block the action of any hormone that required cAMP as a second messenger. **5.** Cyclic-AMP is considered a second messenger because it is needed to convert the binding of first messengers—epinephrine, norepinephrine, and peptide hormones, which cannot enter target cells—into some effect on the metabolic activity of the target cell. **6.** The three types of stimuli that control endocrine activity are (1) humoral (changes in the composition of the extracellular fluid), (2) hormonal (changes in the levels of circulating hormones), and (3) neural (the arrival of neurotransmitter at a neuroglandular junction).

Page 398

7. In dehydration, blood osmotic concentration is increased, which would stimulate the posterior lobe of the pituitary gland to release more ADH. **8.** Somatomedins mediate the action of growth hormone. Elevated levels of growth hormone typically accompany elevated levels of somatomedins. **9.** Elevated circulating levels of cortisol inhibit the cells that control the release of ACTH from the pituitary gland, so ACTH levels would decrease. This is an example of negative feedback.

Page 401

10. Hormones of the thyroid gland are thyroxine or tetraiodothyronine (T_4), triiodothyronine (T_3), and calcitonin. **11.** Because an individual who lacks dietary iodine is unable to form the hormone thyroxine, you would expect to see signs and symptoms associated with thyroxine deficiency, such as decreased metabolic rate, decreased body temperature, and an enlarged thyroid gland (goiter). **12.** Most of the thyroid hormone in the blood is bound to transport proteins, forming a large reservoir of thyroxine that would not be depleted until days after the thyroid gland had been removed.

Page 405

13. The hormone secreted by the parathyroid glands is parathyroid hormone (PTH). **14.** Removal of the parathyroid glands would result in decreased blood levels of calcium ions.

Page 409

15. The two regions of the adrenal gland are the cortex and the medulla. The cortex secretes mineralocorticoids (primarily aldosterone), glucocorticoids (mainly cortisol, hydrocortisone, and corticosterone), and androgens. The medulla secretes epinephrine (E) and norepinephrine (NE). **16.** One function of cortisol is to decrease the cellular use of glucose while increasing both the available glucose (by promoting the breakdown of glycogen) and the conversion of amino acids to carbohydrates. Therefore, the net result of elevated cortisol levels would be an elevation of blood glucose.

Page 410

17. Increased amounts of light inhibit the production of melatonin by the pineal gland, which receives neural input through branches of axons making up the visual pathways. **18.** Melatonin may inhibit reproductive functions, protect against free radical damage, and influence circadian rhythms.

Page 412

19. Two important cells of the pancreatic islets (and their hormones) are alpha cells (glucagon) and beta cells (insulin). **20.** Insulin causes skeletal muscle and liver cells to convert glucose to glycogen. **21.** Increased levels of glucagon stimulate the conversion of glycogen to glucose in the liver, which would decrease the amount of glycogen in the liver.

Page 418

22. Two hormones secreted by the kidneys are erythropoietin (EPO) and calcitriol. EPO stimulates red bone marrow cells to produce more red blood cells, which increases the delivery of oxygen to body tissues. Calcitriol stimulates cells lining the digestive tract to absorb calcium and phosphate ions. **23.** Once released into the bloodstream, renin functions as an enzyme, catalyzing a chain reaction that ultimately leads to the formation of the hormone angiotensin II. **24.** Leptin is a hormone released by adipose tissue.

Page 423

25. The hormonal interaction between insulin and glucagon is antagonistic, because the two hormones have opposite effects on their target tissues. **26.** The lack of growth hormone, thyroid hormone, parathyroid hormone, or the gonadal hormones would inhibit the normal formation and development of the skeletal system. **27.** The dominant hormones of the resistance phase of the general adaptation syndrome are the glucocorticoids. They increase blood glucose levels by mobilizing lipid and protein reserves and by stimulating the synthesis and release of glucose

by the liver. **28.** The endocrine system affects the functioning of all other body systems by adjusting metabolic rates and substrate use and by regulating growth and development. **29.** Hormones of the endocrine system adjust muscle metabolism, energy production, and growth; hormones also regulate calcium and phosphate levels, which are critical to normal muscle functioning. For their part, skeletal muscles protect some endocrine organs.

ANSWERS TO REVIEW QUESTIONS

Level 1: Reviewing Facts and Terms

1. h **2.** e **3.** g **4.** l **5.** b **6.** k **7.** c **8.** a **9.** j **10.** i **11.** f **12.** d **13.** (a) hypothalamus; (b) pituitary gland; (c) thyroid gland; (d) thymus; (e) adrenal gland; (f) pineal gland; (g) parathyroid glands; (h) heart; (i) kidney; (j) adipose tissue; (k) digestive tract; (l) pancreatic islets (within pancreas); (m) gonads **14.** d **15.** a **16.** c **17.** d **18.** b **19.** d **20.** c **21.** b **22.** The seven hormones released by the anterior lobe of the pituitary gland are (1) thyroid-stimulating hormones (TSH); (2) adrenocorticotropic hormone (ACTH); (3) follicle-stimulating hormone (FSH); (4) luteinizing hormone (LH); (5) prolactin (PRL); (6) growth hormone (GH); and (7) melanocyte-stimulating hormone (MSH) **23.** The effect of calcitonin is to decrease the Ca^{2+} concentration in body fluids. The effect of parathyroid hormone is to cause an increase in the concentration of Ca^{2+} in body fluids. **24.** (a) The GAS consists of alarm, resistance, and exhaustion phases. (b) Epinephrine is the dominant hormone of the alarm phase. Glucocorticoids are the dominant hormones of the resistance phase.

Level 2: Reviewing Concepts

25. In nervous system communication, the source and destination are quite specific, and the effects are short-lived. In endocrine communication, the effects are slow to appear and often persist for days, and a given hormone can alter the metabolic activities of multiple tissues and organs simultaneously. **26.** Hormones can (1) direct the synthesis of an enzyme (or other protein) that is not already present in the cytoplasm, or (2) turn an existing enzyme "on" or "off" to increase or decrease the rate of synthesis of a particular enzyme or other protein. **27.** The two hormones may (1) have opposing, or antagonistic, effects; (2) have additive or synergistic effects; or (3) have integrative effects by producing different but complementary effects in specific tissues and organs. Additionally, (4) one hormone may have a permissive effect on the other; that is, the first hormone is needed for the second to produce its effect. **28.** Blocking the activity of phosphodiesterase (PDE) would prevent the conversion of cAMP to AMP. This would prolong the effects of hormonal stimulation.

Level 3: Critical Thinking and Clinical Applications

29. Extreme thirst and frequent urination are characteristics of both diabetes insipidus and diabetes mellitus. To distinguish between the two, glucose levels in the blood and urine could be measured. A high glucose concentration would indicate diabetes mellitus. **30.** Julie will likely have elevated blood levels of parathyroid hormone. Because her poor diet does not supply enough calcium for her developing fetus, the fetus removes large amounts of calcium from the maternal blood. The resulting lowered maternal blood calcium levels lead to elevated blood parathyroid hormone levels and increased removal of stored calcium from the maternal skeleton.

CHAPTER 11

ANSWERS TO CHECKPOINTS

Page 431

1. Five major functions of blood are (1) transporting dissolved gases, nutrients, hormones, and metabolic wastes; (2) regulating the pH and ion composition of interstitial fluids; (3) restricting fluid losses at injury sites; (4) defending against toxins and pathogens; and (5) stabilizing body temperature. **2.** Whole blood is composed of plasma and formed elements. **3.** Venipuncture is a common blood sampling technique because superficial veins are easy to locate, the walls of veins are thinner than those of arteries, and the puncture wound seals quickly because blood pressure in veins is relatively low.

Page 434

4. The three major types of plasma proteins are albumins, globulins, and fibrinogen. **5.** A decrease in the amount of plasma proteins in the blood would lower plasma osmotic pressure, reduce the ability to fight infections, and decrease the transport and binding of some ions, hormones, and other molecules.

Page 440

6. Hemoglobin (Hb) is a protein with a complex quaternary structure. It is composed of four globular protein subunits, each bound to a heme molecule, which gives RBCs the ability to transport oxygen in the blood. **7.** After a significant loss of blood, the hematocrit would be reduced. (The hematocrit is the amount of formed elements—mostly red blood cells—as a percentage of the total blood.) **8.** Bilirubin would accumulate in the blood, producing jaundice, because diseases that damage the liver, such as hepatitis or cirrhosis, would impair the liver's ability to excrete bilirubin in the bile. **9.** Keith's hematocrit will increase, because reduced blood flow to the kidneys triggers the release of erythropoietin, which stimulates an increase in erythropoiesis (RBC formation).

Page 444

10. A person with type AB blood lacks both anti-A and anti-B antibodies in the plasma and so can accept type A, type B, type AB, or type O blood. **11.** A person with type A blood cannot safely receive type B blood because the anti-B antibodies in the plasma of the type A recipient would bind to B antigens on the donor's RBCs, causing the transfused RBCs to clump or agglutinate, which could block blood flow to various organs and tissues.

Page 447

12. The five types of white blood cells are neutrophils, eosinophils, basophils, monocytes, and lymphocytes. **13.** An infected cut would contain numerous neutrophils, because these phagocytic WBCs are the first to arrive at the site of an injury. **14.** The WBCs that produce circulating antibodies are lymphocytes. **15.** Basophils respond to an injury by releasing a variety of chemicals, including histamine and heparin. Histamine dilates blood vessels and heparin prevents blood clotting. Basophils also release other chemicals that attract eosinophils and other basophils.

Page 448

16. Platelets are nonnucleated cellular fragments in the blood of mammalian vertebrates, whereas thrombocytes are nucleated platelets found in the blood of vertebrates other than mammals. **17.** Platelet functions include initiating the clotting process and helping to close damaged blood vessels.

Page 453

18. A decreased number of megakaryocytes would impair the clotting process, because fewer megakaryocytes would produce fewer platelets. **19.** The faster extrinsic pathway is initiated by the release of a glycoprotein called tissue factor by damaged endothelial cells or peripheral tissues. The slower intrinsic pathway begins in the bloodstream with the activation of clotting protein proenzymes exposed to damaged collagen fibers and the release of platelet factor by aggregating platelets. **20.** A vitamin K deficiency would reduce the liver's production of clotting factors necessary for normal blood coagulation.

ANSWERS TO REVIEW QUESTIONS

Level 1: Reviewing Facts and Terms

1. f **2.** k **3.** a **4.** l **5.** c **6.** j **7.** e **8.** h **9.** g **10.** b **11.** d **12.** i **13.** c **14.** a **15.** (a) neutrophil; (b) eosinophil; (c) basophil; (d) monocyte; (e) lymphocyte **16.** c **17.** c **18.** d **19.** a **20.** d **21.** d **22.** b **23.** Major types of plasma proteins are (1) albumins, which maintain the osmotic pressure of plasma and are important in transporting triglycerides, fatty acids, and cholesterol; (2) globulins, which (a) bind small ions, hormones, or compounds that might otherwise be filtered out of the blood at the kidneys or have very low solubility in water (transport globulins), or (b) attack foreign proteins and pathogens (immunoglobulins); and (3) fibrinogen, which functions in blood clotting. **24.** (a) anti-B antibodies; (b) anti-A antibodies; (c) neither anti-A nor anti-B antibodies; (d) both anti-A antibodies and anti-B antibodies. **25.** WBCs exhibit (1) amoeboid movement, a gliding movement that moves the cell; (2) emigration (diapedesis), squeezing between adjacent endothelial cells in the capillary wall; (3) positive chemotaxis, the attraction to specific chemical stimuli; and (4) phagocytosis (engulfing particles for neutrophils, eosinophils, and monocytes). **26.** For the common pathway to begin, either the extrinsic or intrinsic pathway must activate Factor X. **27.** An embolus is a drifting blood clot. A thrombus is a blood clot attached to the inner wall of an intact blood vessel.

Level 2: Reviewing Concepts

28. a **29.** d **30.** c **31.** d **32.** Red blood cells are biconcave discs that lack nuclei, ribosomes, and mitochondria, and contain a large amount of the protein hemoglobin.

Level 3: Critical Thinking and Clinical Applications

33. After donating a pint of blood (or after any other blood loss), you would expect to see a substantial increase in the number of reticulocytes. Because there is insufficient time for erythrocytes to mature, the bone marrow releases large numbers of reticulocytes (immature RBCs) in an effort to restore levels of formed elements. **34.** In many cases of kidney disease, the cells responsible for producing erythropoietin (EPO) are either damaged or destroyed. The reduction in EPO levels leads to reduced erythropoiesis and fewer red blood cells, resulting in anemia. **35.** A major function of the spleen is to destroy old, defective, and worn out red blood cells. As the spleen increases in size, so does its capacity to eliminate red blood cells, and this produces anemia. The decreased number of RBCs decreases the body's ability to deliver oxygen to the tissues, so tissue metabolism slows; this accounts for feeling tired and the lack of energy. Because there are fewer RBCs than normal, blood circulating through the skin is not as red, so the person has a pale or whitish skin coloration.

CHAPTER 12

ANSWERS TO CHECKPOINTS

Page 468

1. Damage to the pulmonary semilunar valve on the right side of the heart would affect blood flow into the pulmonary trunk. **2.** Contraction of the papillary muscles (just before the rest of the ventricular myocardium contracts) pulls on the chordae tendineae, which prevents the AV valves from swinging into the atria. **3.** The left ventricle is more muscular than the right ventricle because it must generate enough force to propel blood throughout the body (except the lungs). The right ventricle must generate only enough force to propel blood the few centimeters to the lungs.

Page 478

4. The fact that cardiac muscle cells cannot undergo tetanus—because they have a longer refractory period than skeletal muscle cells—means that they relax long enough so the heart's chambers can refill with blood. **5.** If cells of the SA node did not function, the heart would continue to beat, but at a slower rate, and the AV node would become the pacemaker. **6.** If the impulses from the atria were not delayed at the AV node, they would be conducted through the ventricles so quickly by the bundle branches and Purkinje cells that the ventricles would begin contracting immediately, before the atria had finished contracting. As a result, the ventricles would not be as full of blood as they could be, and the pumping of the heart would not be as efficient, especially during physical activity. **7.** An increase in the size of the QRS complex indicates a larger-than-normal amount of electrical activity during ventricular depolarization. One possible cause is an enlarged heart. Because more cardiac muscle is depolarizing, the size of the electrical event would be greater.

Page 480

8. The alternative term for contraction is systole, and the other term for relaxation is diastole. **9.** No. When pressure in the left ventricle first rises, the heart is contracting but no blood is leaving the heart. During the initial phase of contraction, both the AV and semilunar valves are closed. The increase in pressure results from increased tension as the cardiac muscle contracts. When ventricular pressure exceeds the pressure in the aorta, the aortic semilunar valves are forced open, and blood is rapidly ejected from the ventricle. **10.** "Lubb" is produced by the simultaneous closing of the AV valves and the opening of the semilunar valves. "Dupp" is produced when the semilunar valves close.

Page 485

11. Cardiac output is the amount of blood pumped by the left ventricle in one minute. **12.** Damage to the cardioinhibitory center of the medulla oblongata affects the parasympathetic division of the ANS and would reduce parasympathetic stimulation of the heart. The resulting sympathetic dominance would increase the heart rate. **13.** Stimulating the acetylcholine receptors of the heart lowers heart rate. Given that $CO = HR \times SV$, a reduction in heart rate must produce a reduction in cardiac output (assuming no change in the stroke volume). **14.** According to the Frank–Starling principle, the more the heart muscle is stretched by returning blood (venous return), the more forcefully it will contract (to a point), and the more blood it will eject with each beat (stroke volume). Therefore, increased venous return increases stroke volume (if all other factors are constant). **15.** The heart pumps in proportion to the amount of blood that enters. A heart that beats too rapidly, has too little time to fill completely between beats. Thus, when the heart beats too fast, very little blood leaves the ventricles and enters the circulation, so tissues will suffer damage from an inadequate blood supply.

ANSWERS TO REVIEW QUESTIONS

Level 1: Reviewing Facts and Terms

1. i **2.** e **3.** g **4.** h **5.** a **6.** b **7.** k **8.** l **9.** d **10.** f **11.** c **12.** j **13.** (a) superior vena cava; (b) auricle of right atrium; (c) right ventricle; (d) left ventricle; (e) aortic arch; (f) left pulmonary artery; (g) pulmonary trunk; (h) auricle of left atrium **14.** c **15.** b **16.** d **17.** a **18.** (a) ascending aorta; (b) opening of coronary sinus; (c) right atrium; (d) cusp of right AV (tricuspid) valve; (e) chordae tendineae; (f) right ventricle; (g) pulmonary valve; (h) left pulmonary veins; (i) left atrium; (j) aortic valve; (k) cusp of left AV (mitral or bicuspid) valve; (l) left ventricle; (m) interventricular septum **19.** a **20.** b **21.** c **22.** During ventricular contraction, tension in the papillary muscles pulls against the chordae tendineae, which keep the cusps of the AV valve from swinging into the atrium. This action prevents the backflow, or regurgitation, of blood into the atrium as the ventricle contracts. **23.** The atrioventricular (AV) valves prevent backflow of blood from the ventricles into the atria. The right AV valve is the tricuspid valve, and the left AV valve is the bicuspid (mitral) valve. The pulmonary and aortic semilunar valves prevent the backflow of blood from the pulmonary trunk and aorta into the right and left ventricles. **24.** SA node —> AV node —> AV bundle (bundle of His) —> right and left bundle branches —> Purkinje fibers (into the mass of ventricular muscle tissue) **25.** (a) The cardiac cycle is a complete heartbeat, including a contraction/relaxation period for both atria and ventricles. (b) The cycle begins with atrial systole as the atria contract and push blood into the relaxed ventricles. As the atria relax (atrial diastole), the ventricles contract (ventricular systole), forcing blood through the semilunar valves into the pulmonary trunk and aorta. The ventricles then relax (ventricular diastole). For the rest of the cardiac cycle, both the atria and ventricles are in diastole; passive filling occurs.

Level 2: Reviewing Concepts

26. c **27.** d **28.** a **29.** The right atrium receives blood from the systemic circuit and passes it to the right ventricle, which pumps it into the pulmonary circuit. The left atrium collects blood returning from the lungs and passes it to the left ventricle, which ejects it into the systemic circuit. **30.** The first heart sound ("lubb") marks the start of ventricular contraction and is produced as the AV valves close and the semilunar valves open. The second sound ("dupp") occurs when the semilunar valves close, marking the start of ventricular diastole. Listening to the heart sounds is a simple, effective way to identify certain heart abnormalities. **31.** (a) Sympathetic stimulation causes the release of norepinephrine by postganglionic fibers and the secretion of norepinephrine and epinephrine by the adrenal medullae. These hormones stimulate cardiac muscle cell metabolism and increase contractility (the force of cardiac contraction). (b) Parasympathetic stimulation causes the release of ACh. The primary effect of parasympathetic ACh is inhibition, resulting in a decrease in heart rate and contractility.

Level 3: Critical Thinking and Clinical Applications

32. In this patient, only one of every two action potentials generated by the SA node is reaching the ventricles; thus there are two P waves but only one QRS complex and T wave. This condition frequently results either from damage to the internodal pathways of the atria or problems with the AV node. **33.** Using $CO = HR \times SV$, cardiac output for person A is 4500 mL, and for person B 8550 mL. According to the Frank–Starling principle, in a normal heart CO is directly proportional to venous return, so person B has the greater venous return. Ventricular filling time increases as HR decreases, so person A has the longer ventricular filling time. **34.** Blocking the calcium channels in myocardial cells would lead to a decrease in the force of cardiac contraction. Given that the force of cardiac contraction is directly proportional to stroke volume, you would expect a reduced stroke volume.

CHAPTER 13

ANSWERS TO CHECKPOINTS

Page 495

1. The five general classes of blood vessels are arteries, arterioles, capillaries, venules, and veins. **2.** These blood vessels are veins. Arteries and arterioles have a large amount of smooth muscle tissue in a thick, well-developed tunica media. **3.** The relaxation of precapillary sphincters would increase blood flow through a tissue. **4.** Valves are found in the veins because the very low blood pressure in the venous circulation makes the movement of blood against the force of gravity difficult. Blood flow within peripheral veins depends on the contractions of skeletal muscles to propel the blood, and on valves to prevent blood from backing up.

Page 500

5. The factors that contribute to total peripheral resistance are vascular resistance, vessel length, vessel diameter, blood viscosity, and turbulence. **6.** In a healthy person, blood pressure is greater at the aorta—just leaving the pump (heart)—than at the inferior vena cava. Blood, like other fluids, moves along a pressure gradient from areas of high pressure to areas of low pressure. **7.** While Sally was standing for a period of time, blood pooled in her lower extremities, decreasing venous return to the heart. In turn, cardiac output decreased, so less blood reached her brain, causing light-headedness and fainting. A hot day adds to this effect, because the loss of body water through sweating reduces blood volume.

Page 506

8. Vasodilators increase blood flow locally (that is, through their tissue of origin) by promoting dilation of precapillary sphincters. Vasoconstrictors decrease local blood flow by constricting precapillary sphincters. **9.** Pressure on the common carotid artery would decrease blood pressure at the carotid sinus (the location of the carotid baroreceptors). This decrease would cause the cardioacceleratory center in the medulla oblongata to increase sympathetic stimulation. The result would be an increase in the heart rate. **10.** Renal artery vasoconstriction would decrease both blood pressure and flow at the kidney. In response, the kidney would increase the amount of renin it releases, which in turn would lead to an increase in the level of angiotensin II. The angiotensin II would bring about both increased blood pressure and blood volume.

Page 509

11. Blood pressure increases during exercise because (1) cardiac output increases and (2) resistance in "nonessential" visceral tissues increases. **12.** The immediate problem during hemorrhaging is maintaining adequate blood pressure and peripheral blood flow. The long-term problem is restoring normal blood volume. **13.** Both aldosterone and ADH promote fluid retention and reabsorption at the kidneys, preventing further reductions in blood volume.

Page 510

14. The two circuits of the cardiovascular system are the pulmonary circuit and the systemic circuit. **15.** Three general organizational patterns of blood vessels include (1) nearly identical peripheral distributions of arteries and veins on the body's left and right sides (except near the heart), (2) several names for a single vessel as it crosses specific anatomical boundaries (making accurate anatomical descriptions possible), and (3) the servicing of tissues and organs by several arteries and veins.

Page 512

16. The pulmonary arteries enter the lungs carrying deoxygenated blood. The pulmonary veins leave the lungs carrying oxygenated blood. **17.** Right ventricle —> pulmonary trunk —> left and right pulmonary arteries —> pulmonary arterioles —> alveolar capillaries —> pulmonary venules —> pulmonary veins —> left atrium.

Page 525

18. A blockage of the left subclavian artery would interfere with blood flow to the left arm. **19.** Compression of the common carotid arteries would decrease blood pressure at the carotid sinus and cause a rapid reduction in blood flow to the brain, resulting in a loss of consciousness. An immediate reflexive increase in heart rate and blood pressure would follow. **20.** Rupture of the celiac trunk would most directly affect the stomach, spleen, liver, and pancreas. **21.** Arteries in the neck and limbs are located deep beneath the skin, protected by bones and surrounding soft tissues. Veins in these sites follow two courses, one superficial and one deep. This dual venous drainage helps control body temperature: Blood flow through superficial veins promotes heat loss, and blood flow through deep veins conserves body heat.

Page 527

22. Two umbilical arteries carry blood to the placenta, and one umbilical vein returns blood from the placenta. The umbilical vein drains into the ductus venosus within the fetal liver. (Remember, arteries carry blood away from the heart, and veins carry blood to the heart.) **23.** This blood sample was taken from the umbilical vein, which carries oxygenated, nutrient-rich blood from the placenta to the fetus. **24.** Structures specific to fetal circulation include the two umbilical arteries, an umbilical vein, the ductus venosus, the foramen ovale, and the ductus arteriosus. In the newborn, the foramen ovale closes and persists as the fossa ovalis, a shallow depression. The ductus arteriosus persists as the ligamentum arteriosum, a fibrous cord. The umbilical vessels and ductus venosus persist throughout life as fibrous cords. **25.** Components of the cardiovascular system affected by age include the blood, the heart, and blood vessels. **26.** A thrombus is a stationary blood clot within the lumen of a blood vessel. **27.** An aneurysm is a bulge in a weakened arterial wall resulting from sudden pressure increases.

Page 529

28. The cardiovascular system has blood vessels that provide extensive anatomical connections between it and all the other organ systems. Functionally, it transports dissolved gases, nutrients, hormones, and metabolic wastes; regulates pH and ion composition of interstitial fluid; restricts fluid losses at injury sites; defends against toxins and pathogens; and stabilizes body temperature. **29.** The skeletal system provides calcium needed for normal cardiac muscle contraction, and it protects blood cells developing in the red bone marrow. The cardiovascular system provides calcium and phosphate for bone formation, delivers erythropoietin to red bone marrow, and transports parathyroid hormone and calcitonin to osteoblasts and osteoclasts.

ANSWERS TO REVIEW QUESTIONS

Level 1: Reviewing Facts and Terms

1. d **2.** l **3.** a **4.** j **5.** i **6.** h **7.** k **8.** f **9.** e **10.** c **11.** g **12.** b **13.** (a) brachiocephalic trunk; (b) brachial; (c) radial; (d) external iliac; (e) anterior tibial; (f) right common carotid; (g) left subclavian; (h) right common iliac; (i) femoral **14.** d **15.** b **16.** b **17.** a **18.** d **19.** b **20.** c **21.** b **22.** c **23.** (a) external jugular; (b) brachial; (c) median cubital; (d) radial; (e) great saphenous; (f) internal jugular; (g) superior vena cava; (h) left and right common iliac; (i) femoral **24.** b **25.** d **26.** c **27.** b **28.** c **29.** c **30.** (a) Fluid leaves the capillary at the arterial end primarily in response to hydrostatic pressure. (b) Fluid moves into the capillary at the venous end in response to osmotic pressure. **31.** When elevated BP triggers the baroreceptor response, cardiac output decreases (due to parasympathetic stimulation and inhibition of sympathetic activity) and widespread peripheral vasodilation occurs (due to the inhibition of excitatory neurons in the vasomotor center). **32.** Chemoreceptors in the carotid and aortic bodies are sensitive to changes in CO_2, O_2, or pH levels in blood. **33.** When an infant takes its first breath, the lungs and the pulmonary vessels expand. Smooth muscles in the ductus arteriosus contract, isolating the pulmonary and aortic trunks, and blood begins flowing through the pulmonary circuit. As pressure rises in the left atrium, the valvular flap closes the foramen ovale, completing the separation of the right and left atrial chambers. **34.** Blood: decreased hematocrit, formation of thrombi (stationary blood clots), and valvular malfunction;

Heart: reduction in maximum cardiac output, changes in the activities of the nodal and conducting fibers, reduction in the elasticity of the fibrous skeleton, progressive atherosclerosis, and replacement of damaged cardiac muscle fibers by scar tissue; Blood vessels: progressive inelasticity in arterial walls, deposition of calcium salts on weakened vascular walls, lipid deposits in vessel walls leading to atherosclerotic plaques, and formation of thrombi at atherosclerotic plaques.

Level 2: Reviewing Concepts

35. d **36.** c **37.** b **38.** The thicker walls of arteries contain more smooth muscle and elastic fibers, enabling them to resist the pressure generated by the heart, and to constrict when not expanded by blood pressure. The walls of veins can be thinner because venous pressures are low. **39.** Unlike arteries and veins, capillaries are only one cell thick, and small gaps between adjacent endothelial cells permit the diffusion of water and small solutes into the surrounding interstitial fluid while retaining blood cells and plasma proteins. (Some capillaries also contain pores that permit very rapid exchange of fluids and solutes between the plasma and the interstitial fluid.) **40.** Blood flow to the brain is relatively constant because anastomoses formed from four arteries (left and right internal carotids and basilar artery formed from the joining of the two vertebral arteries) within the cranium ensure that interruption in flow in any one vessel will not compromise the blood supply to the brain. **41.** The accident victim is suffering from shock and acute circulatory crisis. The hypotension results from the loss of blood volume and decreased cardiac output. Her skin is pale and cool due to peripheral vasoconstriction; and the moisture results from the sympathetic activation of sweat glands. Falling blood pressure to the brain causes confusion and disorientation. Her pulse would be rapid and weak, reflecting the heart's response to reduced blood flow and volume.

Level 3: Critical Thinking and Clinical Applications

42. Three factors contribute to Bob's elevated blood pressure: (1) Water loss from sweating increases blood viscosity—resulting from the same number of RBCs in a lower plasma volume—which increases peripheral resistance and contributes to increased blood pressure. (2) Increased blood flow to the skin (to cool Bob's body) increases venous return, which increases stroke volume and cardiac output (Frank–Starling's law of the heart). Increased cardiac output raises blood pressure. (3) The heat stress Bob is experiencing increases sympathetic stimulation (the reason for the sweating), which by elevating heart rate and stroke volume increases cardiac output and blood pressure. **43.** Antihistamines and decongestants not only counteract the symptoms of allergies, they also have the same effects as stimulating the sympathetic nervous system—increases in heart rate, stroke volume, and peripheral resistance—all of which elevate blood pressure. Thus these drugs will aggravate these individuals' hypertension, with potentially hazardous consequences. **44.** When Gina went from lying to standing, gravity caused her blood to move to lower parts of her body away from the heart, decreasing venous return. Decreased venous return lowered blood volume at the end of diastole, which decreased stroke volume and cardiac output. This reduced blood flow to the brain, producing light-headedness and faintness. Normally this does not occur because a rapid drop in blood pressure immediately triggers baroreceptors in the aortic and carotid sinuses to initiate the baroreceptor reflexes. If the expected increase in peripheral resistance by vasoconstriction does not compensate enough for the reduced blood pressure, an increase in heart rate and force of contraction would occur. Normally, these responses occur so quickly that no changes in pressure are noticed after body position is changed.

CHAPTER 14

ANSWERS TO CHECKPOINTS

Page 537

1. A pathogen is any disease-causing organism, such as a virus, bacterium, fungus, or parasite that can thrive inside the body. **2.** Innate (nonspecific) defenses are anatomical barriers and defense processes that slow or prevent the entry of infectious organisms but do not distinguish one potential threat from another. Adaptive (specific) defenses involve an immune response against a specific type of threat.

Page 546

3. Components of the lymphatic system are lymph, lymphatic vessels, lymphocytes, primary lymphoid tissues and organs (red bone marrow and the thymus), and secondary lymphoid tissues and organs (lymph nodes, MALT, tonsils, appendix, and spleen). **4.** Blockage of the thoracic duct would impair the flow of lymph from the body inferior to the diaphragm and from the left side of the body (head and thorax) superior to the diaphragm. The result could be the accumulation of fluid (lymphedema) in the limbs. **5.** A lack of thymic hormones would result in an absence of T lymphocytes. **6.** Lymph nodes enlarge during some infections because lymphocytes and phagocytes in lymph nodes in the affected region multiply to defend against the infectious agent. This increase in the number of cells causes the nodes to become enlarged or swollen.

Page 549

7. The body's innate (nonspecific) defenses include physical barriers, phagocytes, immune surveillance, interferons, complement, inflammation, and fever. **8.** A decrease in the number of monocyte-forming cells in red bone marrow would result in fewer macrophages of all types, including microglia of the CNS, Kupffer cells of the liver, and alveolar macrophages in the lungs. All are derived from monocytes. **9.** A rise in the level of interferon indicates a viral infection. Interferon does not help an infected cell, but "interferes" with the viruses' ability to replicate and infect other cells. **10.** Pyrogens increase body temperature (produce a fever) by stimulating the temperature control area within the hypothalamus.

Page 552

11. In cell-mediated (cellular) immunity, T cells defend against abnormal cells and pathogens inside cells. In antibody-mediated (humoral) immunity, B cells secrete antibodies that defend against antigens and pathogens in body fluids. **12.** The two forms of active immunity are naturally acquired active immunity and artificially induced active immunity; the two forms of passive immunity are naturally acquired passive immunity and artificially induced passive immunity. **13.** The four general properties of adaptive immunity are specificity, versatility, memory, and tolerance.

Page 555

14. The four types of T cells are cytotoxic T cells, helper T cells, memory T cells, and suppressor T cells. **15.** Abnormal peptides within the cytoplasm of a cell become attached to MHC proteins and displayed on the cell's plasma membrane. Recognition of the displayed peptides by T cells starts an immune response. **16.** A decrease in the number of cytotoxic T cells would affect cell-mediated immunity, reducing the effectiveness of cytotoxic T cells in killing foreign cells and virus-infected cells. **17.** Class I MHC proteins are found in the plasma membranes of all nucleated body cells. Class II MHC proteins are found only in the plasma membranes of lymphocytes and antigen-presenting cells (APCs).

Page 563

18. Sensitization is the process by which a B cell becomes able to react with a specific antigen. **19.** An antibody is a Y-shaped molecule that consists of two parallel pairs of polypeptide chains: one pair of heavy chains and one pair of light chains. Each chain contains both constant segments and variable segments. **20.** Plasma cells produce and secrete antibodies, so observing an elevated number of plasma cells would lead us to expect increasing levels of antibodies in the blood. **21.** The secondary response would be more affected by the lack of memory B cells for a particular antigen. The ability to produce a secondary response depends on the presence of memory B cells (and memory T cells) formed during the primary response. The memory cells are held in reserve against future contact with the same antigen.

Page 564

22. An autoimmune disorder is a condition that results when the immune system's sensitivity to normal cells and tissues causes the production of autoantibodies. **23.** Stress can interfere with the immune response by depressing the inflammatory response, reducing the number and activity of phagocytes, and inhibiting interleukin secretion, which depresses the response of lymphocytes.

Page 565

24. Elderly people are more susceptible to viral and bacterial infections because the number of helper T cells declines with age and B cells are less responsive, so antibody levels rise more slowly after antigen exposure. **25.** The increased incidence of cancer among elderly people may reflect the decline of immune surveillance with age, so cancerous cells are not eliminated as effectively.

Page 567

26. The lymphatic system provides adaptive (specific) defenses against infection, performs immune surveillance to eliminate cancer cells, and returns tissue fluid to the circulation. **27.** The cardiovascular system aids the body's nonspecific and specific defenses by distributing white blood cells, transporting antibodies, and restricting the spread of pathogens (through the clotting response).

ANSWERS TO REVIEW QUESTIONS

Level 1: Reviewing Facts and Terms

1. h **2.** k **3.** b **4.** g **5.** d **6.** c **7.** j **8.** a **9.** i **10.** l **11.** f **12.** e **13. (a)** tonsil; **(b)** cervical lymph nodes; **(c)** right lymphatic duct; **(d)** thymus; **(e)** cisterna chyli; **(f)** lumbar lymph nodes; **(g)** appendix; **(h)** lymphatics of lower limb; **(i)** lymphatics of upper limb; **(j)** axillary lymph nodes; **(k)** thoracic duct; **(l)** lymphatics of mammary gland; **(m)** spleen; **(n)** mucosa-associated lymphoid tissue (MALT); **(o)** pelvic lymph nodes; **(p)** inguinal lymph nodes; **(q)** red bone marrow **14.** c **15.** d **16.** c **17.** c **18.** b **19.** a **20.** c **21.** a **22.** a **23.** d **24.** d **25.** c **26.** The thoracic duct collects lymph from the body inferior to the diaphragm and from the left side of the body superior to the diaphragm. The right lymphatic duct collects lymph from the right side of the body superior to the diaphragm. **27. (a)** responsible for cell-mediated immunity, which defends against abnormal cells and pathogens inside living cells; **(b)** stimulate the activation and function of T cells and B cells; (c) inhibit the activation and function of both T cells and B cells; (d) produce and secrete antibodies; (e) recognize and destroy abnormal cells; (f) interfere with viral replication inside cells and stimulate the activities of macrophages and NK cells; (g) provide cell-mediated immunity; (h) provide antibody-mediated immunity, which defends against antigens and pathogenic organisms in the body; (i) enhance nonspecific defenses, increase T cell sensitivity, and stimulate B cell activity

Level 2: Reviewing Concepts

28. c **29.** d **30.** Specificity: Each immune response is triggered by a specific antigen and defends against only that antigen. Versatility: The immune system can differentiate among tens of thousands of antigens it may encounter during an individual's normal lifetime. Memory: The immune response following a second exposure to a given antigen is stronger and lasts longer than the first exposure. Tolerance: Some antigens, such as those on an individual's own normal cells, do not elicit an immune response. **31.** An antigen–antibody complex can eliminate the antigen by neutralization, precipitation and agglutination, activation of complement, attraction of phagocytes, enhancement of phagocytosis by opsonization, and stimulation of inflammation. **32.** Complement system activation destroys target cell plasma membranes, stimulates inflammation, attracts phagocytes, and enhances phagocytosis.

Level 3: Critical Thinking and Clinical Applications

33. Examination of regional lymph nodes for the presence of cancer cells can help the physician determine if the cancer cells have remained localized in the lungs and were discovered at a relatively early stage, or have already spread (or metastasized) through the lymphatic system to establish tumors in other sites of the body. Both the stage of the disease and the sites involved help the physician decide about treatment options. **34.** The presence of an elevated level of IgM antibodies, but very few IgG antibodies, suggests that Ted is in the early stages of a primary response to the rubella measles virus, so he appears to have contracted the disease. The subsequent levels of IgG antibodies will play a crucial role in the eventual control of the disease. (The CDC recommends that children should get two doses of the MMR (measles, mumps, and rubella) vaccine. The first between 12 and 15 months of age and the second between 4 and 6 years of age. The MMR vaccine protects children and adults from all three diseases.)

CHAPTER 15

ANSWERS TO CHECKPOINTS

Page 577

1. The five functions of the respiratory system include providing an extensive surface area for gas exchange between blood and air; moving air to and from gas-exchange surfaces; protecting respiratory surfaces from dehydration, temperature changes, and pathogens; producing sounds; and aiding the sense of smell. **2.** The two anatomical subdivisions of the respiratory system are the upper respiratory system and the lower respiratory system. **3.** The respiratory mucosa lines the conducting portion of the respiratory tract.

Page 584

4. The surfaces of the nasal cavity are swept by mucus (produced by the respiratory mucosa and the paranasal sinuses) and by tears (carried by the nasolacrimal ducts). **5.** The pharynx is a passageway for both air (respiratory system) and food and liquids (digestive system). **6.** Increased tension in the vocal cords raises the pitch of the voice. **7.** The functional advantage of C-shaped tracheal cartilages is that they allow room for the esophagus to expand when food or drink is swallowed.

Page 588

8. Air passing through the glottis flows into the larynx and through the trachea. From there, the air flows into a primary bronchus, which supplies a lung. In the lung, air passes through bronchi, bronchioles, a terminal bronchiole, a respiratory bronchiole, an alveolar duct, an alveolar sac, an alveolus, and ultimately to the respiratory membrane. **9.** Without surfactant, surface tension in the thin layer of liquid that moistens alveolar surfaces would cause the alveoli to collapse. **10.** The pleura is a serous membrane that secretes pleural fluid, which lubricates the opposing parietal and visceral surfaces to prevent friction during breathing.

Page 589

11. External respiration includes all the processes involved in the exchange of oxygen and carbon dioxide between the body's interstitial fluids and the external environment. Internal respiration is the absorption of oxygen and the release of carbon dioxide by the body's cells. **12.** The integrated steps involved in external respiration are pulmonary ventilation (breathing), gas diffusion, and transport of oxygen and carbon dioxide by the bloodstream.

Page 595

13. Compliance is the ease with which the lungs expand. Factors affecting compliance include (a) the connective tissue structure of the lungs, (b) the level of surfactant production, and (c) the mobility of the thoracic cage. **14.** Tidal volume is the amount of air you move into and out of your lungs during a single respiratory cycle under resting conditions—about 500 mL for both males and females. **15.** When the rib penetrates Mark's chest wall, it also penetrates the pleural cavity, allowing atmospheric air to enter, and producing pneumothorax. As a result, the natural elasticity of the lung may cause the lung to collapse, a condition called atelectasis. **16.** The vital capacity would decrease, because the fluid in the alveoli takes up space that would normally be occupied by air.

Page 599

17. True. **18.** Air passing through the nasal cavity becomes warmer and more humid (its content of water vapor increases). **19.** Alveolar air contains less oxygen and more carbon dioxide than atmospheric air.

Page 602

20. Carbon dioxide is transported in the bloodstream dissolved in the plasma, bound to hemoglobin within RBCs, or as bicarbonate ions. **21.** Active skeletal muscles generate more heat than resting muscles, and more acidic waste products that lower the pH of the surrounding fluid. The combination of increased temperature and reduced pH during exercise causes the hemoglobin to release more oxygen than it would when the muscles are at rest. **22.** Blockage of the trachea would lower blood pH by interfering with the body's ability to take in oxygen and eliminate carbon dioxide. Most carbon dioxide is transported in blood as bicarbonate ion formed from the dissociation of carbonic acid. An inability to eliminate carbon dioxide would result in an excess of hydrogen ions, which are also released from the dissociation of carbonic acid. The excess of hydrogen ions would lower blood pH.

Page 607

23. Peripheral chemoreceptors are more sensitive to carbon dioxide levels than to oxygen levels. When carbon dioxide dissolves, it forms carbonic acid, which dissociates and releases hydrogen ions, thereby lowering pH and altering cell or tissue activity. **24.** Strenuous exercise stimulates the inflation and deflation reflexes of the lungs, also known as the Hering-Breuer reflexes. In the inflation reflex, the stimulation of stretch receptors in the lungs inhibits the inspiratory center and stimulates the expiratory center. In contrast, reducing the volume of the lungs initiates the deflation reflex, which inhibits the expiratory center and stimulates the inspiratory center. **25.** Johnny's mother shouldn't worry. While Johnny holds his breath, increasing blood carbon dioxide levels lead to increased stimulation of the inspiratory center, which forces him to breathe again.

Page 609

26. Two age-related changes that reduce the efficiency of the respiratory system are (1) reduced chest movements resulting from arthritic changes in rib joints and stiffening of the costal cartilages and (2) some degree of emphysema stemming from the gradual destruction of alveolar surfaces. **27.** The respiratory system provides oxygen and eliminates carbon dioxide for all body systems. **28.** The nervous system controls the pace and depth of respiration and monitors the respiratory volume of the lungs and levels of blood gases.

ANSWERS TO REVIEW QUESTIONS

Level 1: Reviewing Facts and Terms

1. h **2.** f **3.** i **4.** c **5.** b **6.** d **7.** j **8.** e **9.** a **10.** l **11.** g **12.** k **13.** (a) nasal cavity; (b) pharynx; (c) right lung; (d) nose; (e) larynx; (f) trachea; (g) right bronchus; (h) bronchioles; (i) left lung **14.** (a) pulmonary (alveolar) capillary; (b) respiratory membrane; (c) alveolus; (d) interstitial fluid; (e) systemic capillary. The pink arrows indicate the diffusion of O_2, and the blue arrows diffusion of CO_2. **15.** c **16.** b

Level 2: Reviewing Concepts

17. a **18.** d **19.** Less cartilage and more smooth muscle in the lower respiratory passageways provide greater control of bronchial diameter by smooth muscle, and thus of resistance to air flow. **20.** Breathing through the nasal cavity ensures that inspired air is cleansed, moistened, and warmed. The drier air that enters through the mouth can irritate the trachea, causing throat soreness. **21.** Smooth muscle tissue controls the diameters in both bronchioles and arterioles. Just as vasodilation and vasoconstriction of the arterioles regulate blood flow and distribution, bronchodilation and bronchoconstriction control the amount of resistance to airflow and the distribution of air in the lungs.

Level 3: Critical Thinking and Clinical Applications

22. In anemia, the blood's ability to carry oxygen is decreased due to the lack of functional hemoglobin, red blood cells, or both. Anemia does not interfere with the exchange of carbon dioxide within the alveoli, nor with the amount of oxygen that will dissolve in the plasma. Because chemoreceptors respond to dissolved gases and pH, as long as the pH and the concentrations of dissolved carbon dioxide and oxygen are normal, ventilation patterns should not change significantly. **23.** The air you were breathing while sleeping was so dry that it absorbed more than the normal amount of moisture as it passed through the nasal cavity. The nasal epithelia continued to secrete mucus, but the loss of moisture made the mucus quite viscous, so the cilia had difficulty moving it, causing nasal congestion. After the shower and juice, more moisture was transferred to the mucus, loosening it and making it easier to move—and easing the congestion.

CHAPTER 16

ANSWERS TO CHECKPOINTS

Page 620

1. Organs of the digestive system include the oral cavity (mouth), pharynx (throat), esophagus, stomach, small intestine, large intestine, and accessory organs (teeth, tongue, salivary glands, pancreas, liver, and gallbladder).

2. The six primary functions of the digestive system are (a) ingestion, the eating of food; (b) mechanical processing, the crushing and shearing of food to make it more susceptible to enzymatic attack; (c) digestion, the chemical breakdown of food into smaller products for absorption; (d) secretion, the release of water, acids, and other substances by the epithelium of the digestive tract, glandular organs, and the gallbladder; (e) absorption, the movement of digested materials across the digestive epithelium and into the interstitial fluid of the digestive tract; and (f) excretion, the removal of waste products from the body. **3.** The mesenteries support and stabilize the positions of organs in the abdominopelvic cavity and provide a route for the blood vessels, nerves, and lymphatic vessels associated with the digestive tract. **4.** The layers of the digestive tract, from superficial to deep, are the mucosa, submucosa, muscularis externa, and serosa. **5.** The waves of contractions responsible for peristalsis are more efficient in propelling intestinal contents than segmentation, which is basically a churning action that mixes intestinal contents with digestive fluids.

Page 623

6. Structures associated with the oral cavity include the tongue, salivary glands, and teeth. **7.** The oral cavity is lined by a stratified squamous epithelium. It protects against friction or abrasion by food. **8.** The digestion of carbohydrates would be affected by damage to the parotid salivary glands, because these glands secrete salivary amylase, the enzyme that digests complex carbohydrates (starches). **9.** The incisors are the type of tooth most useful for chopping (or cutting or shearing) pieces of relatively rigid food, such as raw vegetables.

Page 625

10. The pharynx is a passageway that receives food or liquids and passes them on to the esophagus as part of the swallowing process. Air also passes through the pharynx. **11.** The process being described is swallowing (deglutition).

Page 630

12. The four main regions of the stomach are the cardia, fundus, body, and pylorus. **13.** The low pH in the stomach creates an acidic environment that kills most microorganisms ingested with food, denatures proteins and inactivates most enzymes in food, helps break down plant cell walls and meat connective tissue, and activates pepsin. **14.** The vagus nerves contain parasympathetic motor fibers that can stimulate gastric secretions even when the stomach is empty (the cephalic phase of gastric secretion). Cutting the branches of the vagus nerves that supply the stomach would prevent this type of secretion from taking place, and reduce the likelihood of new ulcer formation.

Page 636

15. The pyloric sphincter is the ring of muscle that regulates the flow of chyme into the small intestine. **16.** The three segments of the small intestine from proximal to distal are the duodenum, jejunum, and ileum. **17.** The small intestine has several adaptations that increase its surface area and thus its absorptive capacity for nutrients. Its walls have folds called circular folds (plicae circulares), each of which is covered by fingerlike projections called villi. The epithelial cells covering the villi have an exposed surface covered by small fingerlike projections, the microvilli. In addition, the small intestine has a very rich supply of blood vessels and lymphatic vessels that transport the absorbed nutrients.

Page 645

18. A high-fat meal would increase cholecystokinin (CCK) level in the blood. **19.** Damage to the exocrine pancreas would most impair the digestion of fats (lipids), because that organ is the primary source of lipases. Even though such damage would also reduce carbohydrate and protein digestion, digestive enzymes for these nutrients are also produced by the salivary glands (carbohydrates), the small intestine (carbohydrates and proteins), and the stomach (proteins).

Page 650

20. The four segments of the colon are the ascending colon, transverse colon, descending colon, and sigmoid colon. **21.** The large intestine is larger in diameter than the small intestine, but its relatively thin wall lacks villi, and it has an abundance of mucous glands. **22.** A narrowing of the ileocecal valve would interfere with the flow of chyme from the small intestine to the large intestine.

Page 655

23. Because chylomicrons are formed from the fats digested in a meal, fats would increase the number of chylomicrons in the lacteals. **24.** Removal of the stomach would interfere with the absorption of vitamin B_{12}. Parietal cells of the stomach are the source of intrinsic factor, which is required for the vitamin's absorption. **25.** When someone with diarrhea loses fluid and electrolytes faster than they can be replaced, the resulting dehydration can be fatal. Constipation, although uncomfortable, does not interfere with any major body process. The few toxic waste products that are normally eliminated by defecation can move into the blood and be eliminated by the kidneys.

Page 656

26. General digestive system changes that occur with age include declines in the rates of stem cell divisions (results in ulcers), decreases in smooth muscle tone (causes reduced gastric and intestinal motility), more apparent cumulative damage to other structures or organs, increases in cancer rates, and increases in dehydration (as a result of decreased osmoreceptor sensitivity). **27.** The digestive system absorbs the organic substrates, vitamins, ions, and water needed by cells of all the body's systems. **28.** Digestive system functions related to the cardiovascular system include absorption of water to maintain blood volume, absorption of vitamin K produced by intestinal bacteria (vital to blood clotting), excretion of bilirubin (a breakdown product of the heme portion of hemoglobin) by the liver, and synthesis of blood clotting factors by the liver.

ANSWERS TO REVIEW QUESTIONS

Level 1: Reviewing Facts and Terms

1. c **2.** k **3.** g **4.** a **5.** i **6.** h **7.** j **8.** d **9.** f **10.** b **11.** l **12.** e **13.** d **14.** d **15.** b **16.** c **17.** (a) oral cavity (mouth); (b) liver; (c) gallbladder; (d) pancreas; (e) large intestine; (f) salivary glands; (g) pharynx; (h) esophagus; (i) stomach; (j) small intestine; (k) anus **18.** b **19.** d **20.** d **21.** (a) mucosa; (b) submucosa; (c) muscularis externa; (d) serosa **22.** a **23.** d **24.** d **25.** The primary digestive functions are ingestion, mechanical processing, secretion, digestion, absorption, and excretion. **26.** The transverse (circular) folds increase the surface area available for absorption and the longitudinal folds permit expansion of the lumen after a large meal. **27.** The innermost (superficial) layer, the mucosa, is a mucous membrane consisting of epithelia and the lamina propria (loose connective tissue). The submucosa surrounds the mucosa and contains blood vessels, lymphatic vessels, and neural tissue (the submucosal nerve plexus). The muscularis externa is made up of two layers of smooth muscle tissue—longitudinal and circular, whose contractions agitate and propel materials along the digestive tract—and neural tissue (the myenteric nerve plexus). The outermost (deepest) layer, the serosa, is a serous membrane that protects and supports the digestive tract inside the peritoneal cavity. **28.** The four primary functions of the oral cavity are (1) analysis of material before swallowing; (2) mechanical processing through the actions of the teeth, tongue, and palatal surfaces; (3) lubrication by mixing with mucus and salivary secretions; and (4) limited digestion of carbohydrates and lipids. **29.** Incisors clip or cut; cuspids tear or slash; bicuspids crush, mash, or grind; and molars crush and grind. **30.** The three segments of the small intestine are the duodenum, jejunum, and ileum. **31.** The pancreas produces digestive enzymes as well as buffers that assist in neutralizing acidic chyme. The liver produces bile—a solution that contains additional buffers and bile salts that aid the digestion and absorption of lipids—and the gallbladder stores and concentrates bile. The liver is also responsible for metabolic regulation and is the primary organ involved in regulating the composition of the circulating blood. **32.** The three major functions of the large intestine are (1) reabsorption of water and compaction of chyme into feces, (2) absorption of important vitamins generated by bacterial action, and (3) storage of fecal material prior to defecation. **33.** Age-related changes that occur in the digestive system are (1) the rate of epithelial stem cell division declines, (2) smooth muscle tone decreases, (3) the effects of cumulative damage become apparent, (4) cancer rates increase, (5) dehydration is more common, and (6) changes in other systems have direct or indirect effects on the digestive system.

ANSWERS

Level 2: Reviewing Concepts

34. d **35.** d **36.** a **37.** Peristalsis consists of waves of muscular contractions that move along the length of the digestive tract. During a peristaltic movement, the circular muscles contract behind the digestive contents. The longitudinal muscles contract next, shortening adjacent segments. A wave of contraction in the circular muscles then forces the contents in the desired direction. Segmentation movements churn and fragment the digestive contents, mixing them with intestinal secretions. Because they do not follow a set pattern, segmentation movements do not produce directional movement of materials along the tract. **38.** The stomach performs four major digestive functions: storage of ingested food, mechanical breakdown of ingested food, disruption of chemical bonds in the food through the actions of acids and enzymes, and production of intrinsic factor. **39.** The cephalic phase begins with the sight or thought of food. Directed by the CNS, and transmitted over the parasympathetic division of the ANS, this phase prepares the stomach to receive food. The gastric phase, which begins with the arrival of food in the stomach, is initiated by distension of the stomach, an increase in the pH of the gastric contents, and the presence of undigested materials in the stomach. The intestinal phase begins when chyme starts to enter the small intestine. This phase controls the rate of gastric emptying and ensures that the secretory, digestive, and absorptive functions of the small intestine can proceed efficiently.

Level 3: Critical Thinking and Clinical Applications

40. If a gallstone is small enough, it can pass through the common bile duct and block the pancreatic duct. Enzymes from the pancreas then cannot reach the small intestine. As the enzymes accumulate in the pancreas, they irritate the duct and ultimately the exocrine pancreas, producing pancreatitis. **41.** The small intestine, especially the jejunum and ileum, are likely involved. Barb's abdominal pain results from regional inflammation. Inflamed intestines cannot absorb nutrients. As a result, she is deficient in iron and vitamin B_{12}. Both are necessary for the formation of hemoglobin and red blood cells, and this accounts for her anemia. The reduced absorption of other nutrients accounts for Barb's weight loss.

CHAPTER 17

ANSWERS TO CHECKPOINTS

Page 666

1. Energetics is the study of the flow of energy and its transformation, or change, from one form to another. **2.** Metabolism is all the chemical processes in the body. It includes anabolism and catabolism. **3.** Catabolism is the breakdown of complex organic molecules into simpler components, accompanied by the release of energy. Anabolism is the synthesis of complex organic compounds from simpler molecules and requires an input of energy.

Page 672

4. The primary role of the citric acid cycle is to transfer electrons from organic substrates to coenzymes. These electrons provide energy for the production of ATP by the electron transport system. **5.** The binding of hydrogen cyanide molecules to the final cytochrome of the ETS would prevent the transfer of electrons to oxygen. As a result, cells would be unable to produce ATP in the mitochondria and would die from energy starvation. **6.** Gluconeogenesis is the synthesis of glucose from noncarbohydrate precursor molecules, such as lactate (from the dissociation of lactic acid), glycerol (from lipids), and some amino acids (from proteins).

Page 676

7. Lipolysis is the chemical breakdown of lipids. Beta-oxidation is fatty acid catabolism that produces molecules of acetyl-CoA. **8.** High-density lipoproteins (HDLs) are considered beneficial because they reduce the amount of cholesterol in the bloodstream by transporting it to the liver for storage or for excretion in the bile.

Page 677

9. Transamination is a process in amino acid metabolism and protein synthesis in which an amino group is transferred from one amino acid to form another. Deamination is the removal of an amino group from an amino acid. An ammonium ion is formed in the process and the remaining carbon chain

is broken down to generate ATP. **10.** A diet deficient in vitamin B_6 (pyridoxine), an important coenzyme in deaminating and transaminating amino acids in cells, would interfere with the body's ability to metabolize proteins.

Page 679

11. DNA is never catabolized for energy because the genetic information it contains is essential to the long-term survival of a cell. **12.** Nitrogenous wastes are metabolic waste products that contain nitrogen atoms, such as urea and uric acid. **13.** Elevated blood uric acid levels could indicate increased breakdown of nucleic acids, because uric acid is produced when the nucleotides adenine and guanine are broken down.

Page 683

14. The two types of vitamins are fat-soluble and water-soluble vitamins. **15.** Foods containing complete proteins contain all the essential amino acids in nutritionally required amounts. Foods containing incomplete proteins are deficient in one or more essential amino acids. **16.** A decrease in the amount of bile salts, which are necessary for digesting and absorbing fats and fat-soluble vitamins (including vitamin A), would result in less vitamin A in the body, and perhaps a vitamin A deficiency.

Page 687

17. The BMR of a pregnant woman would be higher than her own BMR when she is not pregnant, due to both the increased metabolism associated with supporting the fetus, and that of the fetus. **18.** Evaporation is ineffective as a cooling process when the relative humidity is high (when the air is holding large amounts of water vapor). **19.** Vasoconstriction of peripheral vessels would decrease blood flow to the skin and thus the amount of heat the body can lose. As a result, body temperature would increase.

Page 688

20. Only caloric requirements change with aging. Caloric requirements generally decrease after age 50 because of associated reductions in metabolic rates, body mass, activity levels, and exercise tolerance.

ANSWERS TO REVIEW QUESTIONS

Level 1: Reviewing Facts and Terms

1. a **2.** g **3.** l **4.** i **5.** j **6.** b **7.** k **8.** e **9.** f **10.** d **11.** h **12.** c **13.** d **14.** c **15.** a **16.** b **17.** c **18.** c **19.** (a) fatty acids; (b) glucose; (c) amino acids; (d) small carbon chains; (e) citric acid cycle; (f) CO_2; (g) ATP; (h) electron transport system; (i) H_2O **20.** d **21.** c **22.** b **23.** c **24.** b **25.** a **26.** Metabolism is all of the chemical reactions occurring in the cells of the body. Anabolism is the set of chemical reactions that convert simple reactant molecules into complex molecules needed for maintenance/repair, growth, and secretion. Catabolism is the breakdown of complex molecules into their building block molecules, resulting in the release of energy for the synthesis of ATP and related molecules. **27.** Lipoproteins are lipid–protein complexes consisting of large insoluble glycerides and cholesterol coated with phospholipids and proteins. The major groups are (a) chylomicrons (the largest lipoproteins), which are 95 percent triglyceride and carry absorbed lipids from the intestinal tract to the circulation; (b) low-density lipoproteins (LDLs), which deliver cholesterol to peripheral tissues (because they can be deposited within arteries, LDLs are also known as "bad cholesterol"); and (c) high-density lipoproteins (HDLs, also called "good cholesterol"), which transport excess cholesterol to the liver for storage or excretion in the bile. **28.** Most vitamins and all minerals are essential (must be provided in the diet) because the body cannot synthesize these nutrients. **29.** Carbohydrates yield 4.18 Cal/g; lipids yield 9.46 Cal/g; and proteins yield 4.32 Cal/g. **30.** The BMR is the minimum, resting energy expenditures of an awake, alert person. **31.** The processes of heat transfer are (a) radiation: heat loss as infrared radiation; (b) conduction: heat loss to surfaces in physical contact; (c) convection: heat loss to the air; and (d) evaporation: heat loss when water evaporates to a gas.

Level 2: Reviewing Concepts

32. d **33.** b **34.** Glycolysis is a series of enzymatic steps that converts glucose to 2 pyruvate molecules plus 4 ATP and 2 NADH molecules. Glycolysis requires glucose, specific cytosolic enzymes, ATP and ADP, inorganic phosphates, and the coenzyme NAD (nicotinamide adenine dinucleotide). **35.** A two-carbon acetyl group (carried by acetyl-CoA) enters the cycle by joining to a four-carbon compound, and CO_2, NADH, ATP, and $FADH_2$ leave it. The citric acid reaction sequence is considered a cycle because the four-carbon starting compound is regenerated at the end. **36.** When a triglyceride is hydrolyzed, glycerol and fatty acids are liberated. The glycerol is converted to pyruvate and enters the citric acid cycle. Beta-oxidation (which occurs inside mitochondria) breaks the fatty acids into two-carbon compounds that also enter the citric acid cycle. **37.** The MyPlate food guide indicates the relative amounts of each of the five basic food groups a person should consume each day to ensure adequate intake of nutrients and calories. **38.** The brain region called the hypothalamus acts as the body's "thermostat" by regulating ANS control (through negative feedback) of such homeostatic processes as sweating and shivering thermogenesis. **39.** These terms refer to lipoproteins in the blood that transport cholesterol. "Good cholesterol" (high-density lipoproteins, or HDLs) transports excess cholesterol to the liver for storage or excretion in the bile. "Bad cholesterol" (low-density lipoproteins, or LDLs) transports cholesterol to peripheral tissues—including, unfortunately, arteries, where the buildup of cholesterol is linked to cardiovascular disease.

Level 3: Critical Thinking and Clinical Applications

40. During starvation, the body must use its fat and protein reserves to supply the energy needed to sustain life. Among the proteins metabolized for energy are antibodies in the blood. The loss of antibodies coupled with a scarcity of amino acids needed to synthesize replacement antibodies, as well as protective molecules such as interferon and complement proteins, renders an individual more susceptible to contracting diseases, and less likely to recover from them. **41.** Based just on the information given, Charlie would appear to be in good health, at least relative to his diet and probable exercise. Problems are associated with elevated levels of LDLs, which carry cholesterol to peripheral tissues and make it available for the formation of atherosclerotic plaques in blood vessels. High levels of HDLs indicate that a considerable amount of cholesterol is being removed from the peripheral tissues and carried to the liver for disposal. You would encourage Charlie not to change, and keep up the good work.

CHAPTER 18

ANSWERS TO CHECKPOINTS

Page 695

1. The major functions of the urinary system include (a) the excretion of organic wastes from body fluids, (b) the elimination of body wastes to the exterior, and (c) the homeostatic regulation of the volume and solute concentration of blood. **2.** The urinary system consists of two kidneys, two ureters, a urinary bladder, and a urethra. **3.** Micturition, or urination, is the elimination of urine from the body.

Page 702

4. The position of the kidneys is unlike most other organs in the abdominal region, because the kidneys are retroperitoneal, and lie behind the peritoneal lining. **5.** Plasma proteins do not normally pass into the capsular space because they are too large to pass through the filtration slits between the processes (pedicels) of the podocytes. **6.** Damage to the juxtaglomerular complex would interfere with the hormonal control of blood pressure.

Page 707

7. A decrease in blood pressure would decrease the GFR by reducing filtration pressure within the glomerulus. **8.** If nephrons lacked nephron loops—the ascending limb of which reabsorbs urea (thin portion) and also pumps Na^+ and Cl^- out of the tubular fluid (thick portion), and the descending limb of which is the site of osmotic flow of water from the tubular fluid—then there could be no concentration gradient in the renal medulla. As a result, less water would be reabsorbed and the production of concentrated urine would not be possible. **9.** Low circulating levels of ADH would result in a larger volume of dilute urine, because little water will be reabsorbed at the DCT and collecting duct.

Page 712

10. The glomerular filtration rate (GFR) depends on the filtration pressure across glomerular capillaries, and is stabilized by interactions among autoregulation (local blood flow regulation), hormonal regulation, and ANS regulation. **11.** Increased aldosterone secretion would increase the K^+

concentration in urine. **12.** Sympathetic activation produces vasoconstriction of the afferent arterioles, which decreases the GFR.

Page 717

13. Peristaltic contractions move urine from the kidneys to the urinary bladder. **14.** An obstruction of a ureter would interfere with the passage of urine from the renal pelvis to the urinary bladder. **15.** Control of the micturition reflex requires the ability to control the external urinary sphincter, a ring of skeletal muscle that acts as a valve.

Page 719

16. The three interrelated processes essential to stabilizing body fluid volume are fluid balance, electrolyte balance, and acid-base balance. **17.** The components of ECF are interstitial fluid, plasma, and other body fluids. The intracellular fluid (ICF) is the cytosol of a cell.

Page 721

18. A fluid shift is a rapid movement of water between the ECF and ICF in response to an osmotic gradient. **19.** Eating a meal high in salt would cause a reduction of fluid in the ICF. Because the ingested salt would temporarily increase the osmolarity of the ECF, water would shift from the ICF to the ECF. **20.** Being in the desert without water, you would lose fluid through perspiration, urine formation, and respiration. As a result, the osmotic concentration of your blood plasma (and other body fluids) would increase.

Page 725

21. The body's three major buffer systems are protein buffer systems, the carbonic acid–bicarbonate buffer system, and the phosphate buffer system. **22.** A decrease in the pH of body fluids would stimulate the respiratory centers in the medulla oblongata to increase the breathing rate. As a result, more CO_2 is eliminated, and pH rises. **23.** In a prolonged fast, catabolism of fatty acids produces acidic ketone bodies, which lower body pH. The eventual result is called ketoacidosis.

Page 726

24. Aging reduces GFR due to a loss of nephrons, cumulative damage to the filtration structures within remaining glomeruli, and reduced blood flow to the kidneys. A reduced GFR and fewer nephrons also reduce the body's ability to regulate pH through renal compensation. **25.** After age 40, total body water content gradually decreases.

Page 727

26. The body's excretory system is made up of the urinary, integumentary, respiratory, and digestive systems. **27.** For all systems, the urinary system excretes waste collected from blood and maintains normal body fluid pH and ion composition.

ANSWERS TO REVIEW QUESTIONS

Level 1: Reviewing Facts and Terms

1. q **2.** g **3.** n **4.** j **5.** a **6.** m **7.** e **8.** p **9.** d **10.** f **11.** h **12.** k **13.** b **14.** c **15.** l **16.** o **17.** i **18.** (a) renal corpuscle; (b) nephron loop; (c) proximal convoluted tubule; (d) distal convoluted tubule; (e) collecting duct; (f) papillary duct **19.** c **20.** d **21.** a **22.** d **23.** (a) renal sinus; (b) renal pelvis; (c) hilum; (d) renal papilla; (e) ureter; (f) renal cortex; (g) renal medulla; (h) renal pyramid; (i) minor calyx; (j) major calyx; (k) kidney lobe; (l) renal columns; (m) fibrous capsule **24.** c **25.** c **26.** b **27.** d **28.** The urinary system excretes waste products generated by cells throughout the body and maintains normal body fluid pH and ion composition. **29.** The urinary system includes the kidneys, ureters, urinary bladder, and urethra. **30.** Fluid shifts are rapid water movements between the ECF and ICF that occur in response to increases or decreases in the osmotic concentration (osmolarity) of the ECF. Such water movements dampen extreme shifts in electrolyte balance. Causes of osmolarity changes include water loss (excessive perspiration, dehydration, vomiting, or diarrhea), water gain (ingestion of pure water, administration of hypotonic solutions through an IV), and changes in electrolyte concentrations (such as sodium). **31.** The three major hormones involved in fluid and electrolyte balance are ADH, which stimulates the thirst center and water conservation at the kidneys; aldosterone, which determines the rate of sodium absorption along the DCT and collecting system; and ANP, which reduces thirst and blocks the release of ADH and aldosterone.

ANSWERS

Level 2: Reviewing Concepts

32. d **33.** c **34.** a **35.** b **36.** a **37.** The controls that stabilize GFR are autoregulation at the local level, hormonal regulation initiated by the kidneys, and autonomic regulation (by the sympathetic division of the ANS). **38.** The micturition reflex typically begins when the bladder contains about 200 mL of urine, at which time stretch receptors provide adequate stimulation to parasympathetic motor neurons. Efferent impulses in the motor neurons travel over the pelvic nerves and generate action potentials in the smooth muscle in the bladder wall, producing a sustained contraction of the urinary bladder. Voluntary relaxation of the external sphincter muscle also relaxes the involuntary internal sphincter muscle allowing urine to pass through the urethra to the exterior. **39.** Fluid balance is a state in which the amount of water gained each day equals the amount lost to the outside. Electrolyte balance exists when there is neither a net gain nor a net loss of any ion in body fluids. Acid-base balance exists when hydrogen ion (H^+) production precisely offsets H^+ losses. These balances are needed to keep fluids, electrolytes, and pH within their relatively narrow normal ranges, for variations outside these ranges can be life threatening. **40.** "Drink plenty of fluids" is physiologically sound advice, because for every degree (°C) body temperature rises above normal, daily water loss increases by 200 mL. **41.** Sweat is usually hypotonic, so loss of a large volume of sweat causes body fluids to become hypertonic. Fluid is lost primarily from the interstitial space, which leads to a reduction in plasma volume and an increase in the hematocrit. Severe dehydration causes blood viscosity to increase substantially, increasing the workload on the heart, and ultimately increasing the probability of heart failure.

Level 3: Critical Thinking and Clinical Applications

42. By resisting the urge to urinate, long-haul truck drivers may not urinate as frequently as they should. The pressure this puts on kidney tissues can lead to tissue death, and ultimately to kidney failure. **43.** The fever and burning sensation suggest that Susan may have a urinary tract infection. Her urine may contain blood cells and bacteria. Because in females the urethra is relatively short, and the urethral orifice is close to the anus and opens near the vagina, bacteria in the anus and vagina can easily reach the urethral orifice (often during sexual intercourse). **44.** Because mannitol is filtered but not reabsorbed, drinking a mannitol solution would lead to an increase in the osmolarity of the tubular fluid. Less water would be reabsorbed, and an increased volume of urine would be produced.

CHAPTER 19

ANSWERS TO CHECKPOINTS

Page 735

1. A gamete is a functional male or female reproductive cell. **2.** Basic structures of the reproductive system are gonads (reproductive organs), ducts (which receive and transport gametes), accessory glands (which secrete fluids), and external genitalia (perineal structures). **3.** Gonads are reproductive organs that produce gametes and hormones.

Page 746

4. Male reproductive structures are the scrotum, testes, epididymides, right and left ductus deferens, ejaculatory duct, urethra, seminal glands (seminal vesicles), prostate gland, bulbo-urethral glands, and penis. **5.** On a warm day, the cremaster muscle (as well as the dartos muscle) would be relaxed so that the scrotum could descend away from the warmth of the body and cool the testes. **6.** When arteries within the penis dilate, the increased blood flow causes the vascular channels within the erectile tissues to fill with blood, producing an erection. **7.** Low FSH levels would lead to low levels of testosterone in the seminiferous tubules, decreasing both the sperm production rate and sperm count.

Page 757

8. Structures of the female reproductive system include the ovaries, uterine tubes, uterus, vagina, and mammary glands. **9.** Blockage of both uterine tubes would eliminate the ability to conceive, resulting in sterility. **10.** The acidic pH of the vagina helps prevent bacterial, fungal, and parasitic infections in this region. **11.** The functional layer of the endometrium sloughs off during menstruation. **12.** Blockage of a single lactiferous sinus

would have little effect on the delivery of milk to the nipple, because each breast generally has 15–20 lactiferous sinuses. **13.** If the LH surge did not take place during an ovarian cycle, ovulation and corpus luteum formation would not occur. **14.** Blockage of progesterone receptors in the uterus would inhibit the development of the endometrium, making the uterus unprepared for pregnancy. **15.** A decline in the levels of estrogen and progesterone signals the beginnings of menses, the end of the uterine cycle.

Page 761

16. The physiological events of sexual intercourse in both sexes are arousal, erection, lubrication, orgasm, and detumescence. Emission and ejaculation are additional phases that occur only in males. **17.** An inability to contract the ischiocavernosus and bulbospongiosus muscles would interfere with a male's ability to ejaculate and to experience orgasm. **18.** Parasympathetic stimulation in females during sexual arousal causes (a) engorgement of the erectile tissue of the clitoris and vestibular bulbs, (b) increased secretion of cervical and vaginal glands, (c) increased blood flow to the wall of the vagina, and (d) engorgement of the blood vessels in the nipples. **19.** Menopause is the time when ovulation and menstruation cease, typically around ages 45–55. **20.** At menopause, circulating levels of estrogens begin to decrease. Estrogen has an inhibitory effect on FSH (and on GnRH). As the level of estrogen decreases, the levels of FSH rise and remain high. **21.** The male climacteric, or andropause, is a period of declining reproductive function in men, typically between ages 50 and 60.

Page 762

22. The cardiovascular system distributes reproductive hormones; provides nutrients, oxygen, and waste removal for the fetus; and produces local blood pressure changes responsible for the physical changes that occur during sexual intercourse. The reproductive system supplies estrogens that may help maintain healthy blood vessels and slow the development of atherosclerosis. **23.** Pelvic bones protect reproductive organs in females, and portions of the ductus deferens and accessory glands in males; sex hormones stimulate growth and maintenance of bone, and accelerate growth and closure of epiphyseal cartilages at puberty.

ANSWERS TO REVIEW QUESTIONS

Level 1: Reviewing Facts and Terms

1. i **2.** m **3.** a **4.** c **5.** l **6.** e **7.** n **8.** o **9.** h **10.** b **11.** f **12.** j **13.** d **14.** k **15.** g **16.** c **17.** a **18.** c **19.** a **20.** d **21.** a **22.** c **23.** (a) urethra; (b) ductus deferens; (c) penis; (d) epididymis; (e) testis; (f) external urethral orifice; (g) scrotum; (h) seminal gland; (i) prostate gland; (j) bulbo-urethral gland **24.** (a) ovary; (b) uterine tube; (c) greater vestibular gland; (d) clitoris; (e) labium minus; (f) labium majus; (g) myometrium; (h) perimetrium; (i) endometrium; (j) uterus; (k) fornix; (l) cervix; (m) vagina **25.** c **26.** d **27.** b **28.** c **29.** The accessory organs and glands in males include the seminal glands, prostate gland, and the bulbo-urethral glands. These structures activate spermatozoa, provide nutrients sperm need for motility, propel sperm and fluids along the reproductive tract, and produce buffers that counteract the acidity of the urethral and vaginal contents. **30.** The epididymis monitors and adjusts the composition of the tubular fluid, acts as a recycling center for damaged spermatozoa, and stores spermatozoa and aids their functional maturation. **31.** The ovaries produce female gametes (oocytes, or immature ova); secrete female sex hormones, including estrogens and progesterone; and secrete inhibin, involved in the feedback control of pituitary FSH production. **32.** The vagina serves as passageway for the elimination of menstrual fluids, receives the penis during sexual intercourse and holds spermatozoa prior to their passage into the uterus, and forms the lower portion of the birth canal through which the fetus passes during delivery.

Level 2: Reviewing Concepts

33. The reproductive system is the only organ system that is not required for the survival of the individual. **34.** Meiosis is the two-step nuclear division resulting in the formation of four haploid cells from one diploid cell. In males, four sperm cells are produced from each diploid cell, whereas in females only one oocyte, or immature ovum, (plus two or three polar bodies) is produced from each diploid cell. **35.** The first phase, menses (days 1–7), is marked by the degeneration and loss of the functional zone of the endometrium; approximately 35–50 mL of blood is lost. In the proliferative phase (end of menses until the beginning of ovulation around day 14), epithelial growth and blood vessel development result in the complete restoration of the functional zone. In the secretory phase (begins at ovulation and persists as long as the corpus luteum remains intact), the combined stimulatory effects of progesterone and estrogens from the corpus luteum cause uterine (endometrial) glands to enlarge and secrete more quickly, preparing the endometrium for the arrival of a developing embryo. **36.** The corpus luteum degenerates, and a decline in progesterone and estrogen levels results in endometrial breakdown (menses). Next, rising FSH, LH, and estrogen levels stimulate the repair and regeneration of the functional zone of the endometrium. During the postovulatory phase, the combination of estrogen and progesterone causes enlargement of the uterine (endometrial) glands and an increase in their secretory activity. **37.** In women, menopause—the time when ovulation and menstruation cease—is accompanied by a sharp and sustained rise in GnRH, FSH, and LH production, while concentrations of circulating estrogens and progesterone decline. Reduced estrogen levels lead to reductions in uterus and breast size, accompanied by a thinning of the urethral and vaginal walls. Reduced estrogen concentrations have also been linked to the development of osteoporosis, presumably because bone deposition proceeds more slowly. During the male climacteric, typically between ages 50 and 60, circulating testosterone levels begin to decline while circulating FSH and LH levels increase. Although sperm production continues in older men, a gradual reduction in sexual activity occurs.

Level 3: Critical Thinking and Clinical Applications

38. Women more frequently experience peritonitis stemming from a urinary tract infection because infectious organisms exiting the urethral orifice can readily enter the nearby vagina. From there, they can then proceed to the uterus, into the uterine tubes, and finally into the peritoneal cavity. No such direct path of entry into the abdominopelvic cavity exists in men. **39.** Regardless of their location, endometrial cells have receptors for and respond to estrogen and progesterone. Under the influence of estrogen at the beginning of the menstrual cycle, any endometrial cells in the peritoneal cavity proliferate and begin to develop glands and blood vessels, which then further develop under the control of progesterone. The dramatic increase in size of this tissue presses on neighboring abdominal tissues and organs, causing periodic painful sensations. **40.** These observations suggest that a certain amount of body fat is necessary for menstrual cycles to occur. The nervous system appears to respond to circulating levels of the adipose tissue hormone leptin; when leptin levels fall below a certain set point, menstruation ceases. Because a woman lacking adequate fat reserves might not be able to have a successful pregnancy, the body prevents pregnancy by shutting down the ovarian cycle, and thus the menstrual cycle. Once sufficient energy reserves become available, the cycles begin again.

CHAPTER 20

ANSWERS TO CHECKPOINTS

Page 772

1. Differentiation is the formation of different types of cells during development. **2.** Development begins at fertilization (conception), that is, with the union of a sperm and an oocyte. **3.** Inheritance refers to the transfer of genetically determined characteristics from one generation to the next.

Page 773

4. Hyaluronidase released from dozens of spermatozoa breaks down the connections between the follicular cells of the corona radiata surrounding the secondary oocyte. Another acrosomal enzyme, released after the binding of a single spermatozoon to the zona pellucida, digests a path through the zona pellucida to the oocyte membrane. **5.** A normal human zygote contains 46 chromosomes.

Page 774

6. Gestation is the period of prenatal development. It consists of three trimesters. **7.** The first trimester is the period of embryonic and early fetal development. The second trimester is a time of organ and organ system development. By the end of this stage, the fetus appears distinctly human.

The third trimester is characterized by rapid fetal growth and the deposition of adipose tissue.

Page 779

8. The inner cell mass of the blastocyst eventually develops into the embryo. **9.** Yes, Sue is pregnant. After fertilization, the developing trophoblast (and later, the placenta) produce and release the hormone hCG. **10.** The placenta (1) supplies the developing fetus with a route for gas exchange, nutrient transfer, and waste elimination, and (2) produces hormones that affect maternal systems.

Page 789

11. The major changes that take place in maternal systems during pregnancy include increases in respiratory rate, tidal volume, blood volume, nutrient requirements, glomerular filtration rate, and size of uterus and mammary glands. **12.** A mother's blood volume increases during pregnancy to compensate for the reduction in maternal blood volume resulting from blood flow through the placenta. **13.** The uterus increases in size and weight during gestation through enlargement of uterine cells, primarily smooth muscle cells of the myometrium. **14.** Three factors opposing the calming action of progesterone on the uterus are increasing estrogen levels, increasing oxytocin levels, and prostaglandin production.

Page 793

15. The three stages of labor are the dilation stage, expulsion stage, and placental stage. **16.** Immature delivery is the birth of a fetus weighing at least 500 g (17.6 oz), which is the normal weight near the end of the second trimester. Premature delivery usually refers to birth at 28–36 weeks at a weight over 1 kg (2.2 lb). **17.** Fraternal twins are dizygotic twins, and identical twins are monozygotic twins.

Page 798

18. The postnatal stages of development are the neonatal period, infancy, childhood, adolescence, and maturity. These stages are followed by senescence, or aging. **19.** Colostrum is produced by the mammary glands from the end of the sixth month of pregnancy until a few days after birth. After that, the glands begin producing breast milk, which contains fewer proteins (including antibodies) and far more fat than colostrum. **20.** Increases in the blood levels of GnRH, FSH, LH, and sex hormones mark the onset of puberty.

Page 805

21. Genotype is a person's genetic makeup. Phenotype is a person's physical and physiological characteristics. It results from the interaction between the person's genotype and the environment.
22. Heterozygous refers to having two different alleles at corresponding sites of a homologous pair of chromosomes. **23.** The phenotype of a person who is heterozygous for tongue rolling—who has one dominant allele and one recessive allele for that trait—would be "tongue roller." **24.** If Joe's lack of sons is anyone's "fault," it's his. The sex of each of his children depends on the genetic makeup of the sperm cell that fertilizes his wife's oocyte. Only males—being XY—can provide a gamete containing a Y chromosome.

ANSWERS TO REVIEW QUESTIONS

Level 1: Reviewing Facts and Terms

1. g **2.** a **3.** c **4.** e **5.** d **6.** n **7.** p **8.** b **9.** o **10.** j **11.** f **12.** h **13.** k **14.** l **15.** m **16.** i **17.** a **18.** b **19.** d **20.** (a) umbilical cord; (b) placenta; (c) amniotic cavity; (d) amnion; (e) chorion **21.** d **22.** a **23.** b **24.** d **25.** b **26.** The four extraembryonic membranes are the yolk sac, amnion, allantois, and chorion. **27.** The first stage of labor, the dilation stage, begins with the onset of labor; the cervix dilates and the fetus begins to shift down the cervical canal. Late in this stage, the amnion usually ruptures. The expulsion stage begins as the cervix dilates completely and continues until the fetus has completely emerged from the vagina (delivery). In the placental stage, the uterus gradually contracts, tearing the connections between the endometrium and the placenta and ejecting the placenta. **28.** During the neonatal period (birth to one month), newborns become relatively self-sufficient and begin to breathe, digest, and excrete for themselves. Heart rates and fluid requirements are higher than those of adults. Neonates have little ability to thermoregulate. During infancy (one month to one year), nonreproductive organ systems become fully operational and start to take on the functional characteristics of adult systems.

During childhood (one year to puberty), children continue to grow, and significant changes in body proportions occur.

Level 2: Reviewing Concepts

29. d **30.** d **31.** The placenta produces human chorionic gonadotropin (hCG), which maintains the integrity of the corpus luteum and promotes the continued secretion of progesterone (keeping the endometrial lining functional); human placental lactogen (hPL) and placental prolactin, which help prepare the mammary glands for milk production; and relaxin, which increases the flexibility of the symphysis pubis, causes dilation of the cervix, and suppresses the release of oxytocin by the hypothalamus, delaying the onset of labor contractions, and, near the end of the third trimester, rising estrogen levels aid in stimulating labor and delivery. **32.** The mother's respiratory rate and tidal volume increase, so that her lungs can meet the fetus's oxygen needs and remove the carbon dioxide it generates. Maternal blood volume increases to compensate for the increased blood flow through the placenta. Nutrient and vitamin requirements climb 10–30 percent in order to nourish the fetus, and glomerular filtration rate increases by about 50 percent, reflecting increased maternal blood volume and the need to excrete fetal metabolic wastes. **33.** Positive feedback ensures that labor contractions continue until delivery is complete. **34.** The event that occurs when a woman has her "water break" during labor is the rupture of the amnion. **35.** The trait and type of inheritance is (a) dominant trait and simple inheritance, (b) recessive trait and simple inheritance, (c) X-linked trait and sex-linked inheritance, and (d) autosomal dominant trait and autosomal inheritance. **36.** More men are color-blind than women because the gene for this trait is on the X chromosome (X-linked). Because men have only one X chromosome, whichever allele is on the X chromosome determines whether a man is color-blind or has normal vision. Women have two X chromosomes, so they will be color-blind only if they are homozygous recessive. This is an example of sex-linked inheritance.

Level 3: Critical Thinking and Clinical Applications

37. None of the couple's daughters will be hemophiliacs, because each will receive a normal allele from her father. There is a 50 percent chance that a son will be hemophiliac because there is a 50 percent chance of receiving either the mother's normal allele or her recessive allele. **38.** Adults' larger body sizes are precisely why their heart and respiratory rates are lower. Because neonates have a high surface-area-to-volume ratio, they lose heat very quickly. To maintain a constant body temperature in the face of this heat loss, cellular metabolic rates must be high. Because cellular metabolism requires oxygen, high metabolic rates require an elevated respiratory rate. Cardiac output must then increase to move blood between the lungs and peripheral tissues. Because stroke volume cannot change much in neonatal hearts, an increase in cardiac output is achieved by increasing heart rate. **39.** The baby's condition is almost certainly not the result of a viral infection or any other event during the third trimester, because all organ systems are fully formed before the end of the second trimester.

ANSWERS

Roles and Responsibilities of Emergency Medical Personnel

A SIGNIFICANT PORTION OF THE EDUCATION of emergency medical personnel occurs in various hospital settings. Because of this, it is important for emergency care providers to understand the roles and responsibilities of other medical personnel as well as their own. The following discussion outlines the health care system and the roles and responsibilities of various health care providers.

The House of Medicine

Medicine is the science and art of diagnosing, treating, and preventing disease and injury. Disease has been one of humanity's greatest problems. Only during the last 100 years has medicine developed weapons to effectively fight disease. Physicians and other health care professionals use clues to identify, or diagnose, a specific disease or injury. This is usually accomplished by taking a medical history, performing a physical examination, and by assessing the results of laboratory tests and imaging exams. After making a diagnosis, physicians choose the best treatment for the patient. Some treatments cure a disease, others only relieve symptoms and do not cure the underlying disease.

Physicians

Physicians are practitioners who diagnose diseases and injuries, administer treatment, and provide advice on ways to stay healthy. The two kinds of physicians in the United States are the doctor of medicine (MD) and the doctor of osteopathic medicine (DO). Both use medicines, surgery, and other standard methods of treating disease. DOs place special emphasis on problems that involve the musculoskeletal system.

Patients may receive care from primary care physicians, specialists, or both. Primary care physicians include general practitioners, family practitioners, general internists, and general pediatricians. Obstetricians/gynecologists are sometimes considered primary care physicians because many women use them as their primary health care providers. Patients usually consult a primary care doctor when they first become ill or injured. Primary care physicians can treat most common disorders, and provide comprehensive care for their patients.

Medical knowledge and technology have advanced so far that no one physician can master the entire field of medicine. Because of this, primary care physicians may refer patients with unusually complicated problems to specialists who have advanced training in a particular disease process or field of medicine. Specialists may even concentrate on one particular area and become subspecialists.

Medical Education

The education of a physician is long and demanding. In the United States, physicians usually complete four years of college before applying to medical school. The actual courses of study that students pursue in college vary, but students must complete a number of science and mathematics classes before applying. Of the 175 medical schools in the United States, 141 award the MD degree and 34 award the DO degree. Entrance to medical or osteopathic school is very competitive. Only students with excellent grades and high scores on the Medical College Admissions Test (MCAT) are accepted. In a recent year, close to 47,000 people applied for admission to medical school, but only 17,000 were accepted. Medical school consists of four years of intense study. Typically, the first two years emphasize basic science education including anatomy, physiology, pharmacology, pathology, microbiology, and much more. First- and second-year medical students are slowly introduced to the practice of medicine through classes in physical examination and through observation of practicing physicians. The last two years of medical school are devoted to learning the clinical sciences and are largely spent in a teaching hospital or clinic. Upon completion of medical school, the physician will be awarded the MD or DO degree. Medical graduates must successfully complete a medical licensure examination. In most states, MDs and DOs take the same exam. However, the physician cannot be licensed until he or she has successfully completed postgraduate training, which was formerly called an *internship*.

Upon graduation, physicians can choose to become primary care physicians or specialist physicians. They learn their chosen area of medicine by completing a residency in that field. Residencies may last from three to six years, depending on the field of study chosen. Residencies in the surgical fields are usually the longest. Some physicians still refer to the first year of residency training as an internship and refer to physicians in their first year of postgraduate training as interns. For the most part, however, physicians in postgraduate residencies are referred to as *residents*. They may also be classified by their year of postgraduate training (i.e., PGY-1, PGY-2). At the completion of residency, physicians take an examination in their chosen field and obtain board certification. Some physicians may choose to further specialize following residency training. In this case, they will enter a fellowship that may last from one to five years. Physicians in fellowship programs are referred to as *fellows*. Cardiothoracic surgeons, for example, must complete four years of college, four years of medical school, six years of surgical residency, and four years of cardiothoracic surgical fellowship. This totals 18 years of education after high school before they practice independently. Upon completion of their fellowship, they will take a board certification examination in their specialty.

In England, Australia, India, and many other foreign countries, students who have been accepted to medical school enter medical school immediately after high school. The medical school program in those countries is six years long. The first two years are similar to regular college courses, although the students begin to have some exposure to clinical medicine. The last four years are similar to U.S. medical schools. At the completion of medical school, students are awarded a bachelor of medicine, bachelor of surgery (MBBS) degree. Following this, they can enter general practice or enter into postgraduate training. The MBBS degree is not recognized in the United States. Thus, when physicians who have the MBBS enter the United States, they are labeled and licensed as MDs and use the MD degree after their name instead of MBBS.

Upon completion of residency and/or fellowship training, physicians enter the independent practice of medicine. Physicians who have completed their postgraduate training are referred to as *attending physicians*. In teaching hospitals, attending physicians supervise and are responsible for all patient care. Medical students report to residents, residents report to fellows, and fellows report to attendings. The level of training can sometimes be determined by the length of the lab coat worn by the physician. By tradition, medical students wear short lab coats (similar in look to a dinner jacket). Residents wear lab coats that extend to halfway down the thigh. Attending physicians wear full lab coats that extend nearly to the knee.

Medical Specialties

There are many different medical specialties. The American Board of Medical Specialties (ABMS), which is the principal accrediting board of MD training programs, recognizes 17 specialties. The American Osteopathic Association (AOA), which is the principal accrediting board of DO training programs, recognizes 18 major medical specialties and numerous subspecialties. A DO may be certified by an ABMS board if he or she completed an MD residency program or by an AOA board if he or she completed a DO residency. Some DOs are certified by both boards. The major medical specialties as recognized by the ABMS are:

- *Allergy and immunology.* Physicians who specialize in allergy and immunology study the diagnosis and treatment of allergic and immunological disorders. The physician must complete a three-year residency in either internal medicine or pediatrics and become board certified in that field. Then, he or she must complete a two-year fellowship in allergy and immunology before becoming board certified.
- *Anesthesiology.* Anesthesiologists are physicians who specialize in providing anesthesia for surgical patients. Many anesthesiologists also specialize in the management of acute and chronic pain. Anesthesiology residencies typically last four years. In addition, anesthesiologists can obtain subspecialty certification in critical care medicine and pain management.
- *Colon and rectal surgery.* Colon and rectal surgeons specialize in surgery of the large intestine and rectum. They must first complete a six-year general surgery residency and become board certified in general surgery. Then, they must complete a one-year fellowship in colon and rectal surgery.
- *Dermatology.* A dermatologist is a physician who specializes in diseases of the skin. Dermatologists must complete a four-year residency. In addition, they can obtain subspecialty certification in dermatopathology and dermatological immunology.

- *Emergency medicine.* Physicians who specialize in emergency medicine train to treat and stabilize emergency injuries and illnesses. Emergency physicians must complete a three- or four-year residency. They can obtain certificates of added qualification in medical toxicology, undersea and hyperbaric medicine, pediatric emergency medicine, and sports medicine through completion of a fellowship.
- *Family practice.* A family practitioner is a primary care physician trained in all aspects of medicine. He or she can manage the majority of problems encountered in general medical practice. Some family practitioners practice uncomplicated obstetrics. The family practice residency program is three years long. In addition, family practitioners can obtain certificates of added qualification in adolescent medicine, geriatric medicine, and sports medicine.
- *Internal medicine.* An internist is a physician who specializes in the diagnosis and treatment of diseases of the adult. Residency training for internal medicine is usually three years. There are 10 subspecialties of internal medicine:

  - *Allergy and immunology.* Allergists must complete a two-year fellowship that emphasizies treatment of allergic and immunological diseases.
  - *Cardiology.* Cardiologists must complete a three-year fellowship that emphasizes the treatment of heart and related disorders. Cardiology is subdivided into clinical cardiac electrophysiology and interventional cardiology.
  - *Endocrinology, diabetes, and metabolism.* Endocrinologists must complete a two-year fellowship that concentrates on diseases of the endocrine system, especially diabetes mellitus.
  - *Gastroenterology.* Gastroenterologists undergo a three-year fellowship that concentrates on diseases of the gastrointestinal system and related organs. Significant emphasis is placed upon obtaining competence at fiber-optic endoscopy of the colon and stomach.
  - *Hematology.* Hematologists complete a two-year fellowship that studies diseases of the blood and related disorders.
  - *Infectious disease.* Physicians interested in infectious disease must complete a two-year fellowship that concentrates on disease spread by infectious agents such as bacteria or viruses.
  - *Medical oncology.* Medical oncologists must complete a two-year fellowship that concentrates on treatment, including chemotherapy, of malignant and similar diseases.
  - *Nephrology.* Nephrologists are physicians who study diseases of the kidneys and genitourinary system. The fellowship program lasts two years.
  - *Pulmonary disease.* Pulmonologists are physicians who complete a two-year fellowship that concentrates on the treatment of diseases of the lungs and respiratory tract.
  - *Rheumatology.* Rheumatologists are physicians who treat diseases of the joints and diseases that are autoimmune in nature. The fellowship program is two years.

In addition to those subspecialties, internists can seek certificates of added qualification in adolescent medicine, critical care medicine, geriatric medicine, and sports medicine.

- *Medical genetics.* Medical geneticists are physicians and scientists who specialize in treating inherited diseases and advising patients about disease possibilities. The residency program is four to five years long.
- *Neurological surgery.* Neurosurgeons specialize in the surgical treatment of injuries and illnesses that involve the brain, spinal cord, or peripheral nerves. Most neurosurgical residencies are five years long.
- *Nuclear medicine.* Nuclear medicine physicians use radioactive and stable substances in the diagnosis and treatment of disease. They must complete a two-year residency.
- *Obstetrics and gynecology.* Physicians who specialize in the treatment of diseases of women are called obstetricians and gynecologists. The residency program is usually four years. Subspecialty certification is available in gynecological oncology, maternal/fetal medicine, and reproductive endocrinology and fertility.
- *Ophthalmology.* Ophthalmologists are physicians who specialize in the medical and surgical treatment of eye disorders. They must complete a four-year residency program before sitting for the board certification exam.
- *Orthopedic surgery.* Surgeons who specialize in the treatment of bone and joint disorders are called orthopedic surgeons. They must complete an accredited orthopedic surgical residency, which usually lasts five to six years. A certificate of added qualification is available in hand surgery (**Figure A1–1**).
- *Otolaryngology.* Physicians who specialize in the medical and surgical treatment of diseases and injuries of the ears, nose, and throat are otolaryngologists. The residency program is five years long.
- *Pathology.* Physicians who specialize in the laboratory study of disease are pathologists. Pathology residencies are at least four years long. Subspecialty certification is available for blood banking/transfusion medicine, chemical pathology, cytopathology, dermatopathology, forensic pathology, hematology, medical microbiology, molecular/genetic pathology, neuropathology, and pediatric pathology.
- *Pediatrics.* Pediatrics is the area of medicine devoted to the care of infants and children. The primary pediatric residency is three years. Subspecialty certification is available in adolescent medicine, pediatric cardiology, pediatric critical care medicine, development/behavioral pediatrics, pediatric emergency medicine, pediatric endocrinology, pediatric gastroenterology, pediatric hematology/oncology, pediatric infectious diseases, neonatal/perinatal medicine, pediatric nephrology, neurodevelopmental disorders, pediatric pulmonology, and pediatric rheumatology.
- *Physical medicine and rehabilitation.* Physiatrists are physicians who have completed a four-year residency in physical medicine and rehabilitation. They concentrate on the assessment and rehabilitation of patients with physical disabilities. Subspecialty certification is available in spinal cord injury medicine, pain management, and pediatric rehabilitation medicine.
- *Plastic surgery.* Plastic surgeons are physicians who perform restorative or cosmetic surgery on the skin and associated structures. Residency training is five to six years. Subspecialty certification is available in hand surgery.
- *Preventative medicine.* Preventative medicine physicians typically will concentrate on aerospace medicine, occupational medicine, or general/preventive medicine. Residency programs are typically four years long. Subspecialty certification is available in undersea and hyperbaric medicine and medical toxicology.
- *Psychiatry and neurology.* Psychiatrists are physicians who specialize in the treatment of behavioral and mental disease. Neurologists treat medical conditions of the nervous system. Psychiatry residencies and neurology residencies are typically four years. Subspecialty certification for psychiatrists is available in addiction medicine, child and adolescent psychiatry, clinical neurophysiology, forensic psychiatry, geriatric psychiatry, and pain management. Neurologists can obtain subspecialty certification in clinical neurophysiology and pain management.
- *Radiology.* Radiology is the specialty of medicine that deals with diagnostic imaging through X-rays, ultrasound, magnetic resonance, and similar technologies. Residency programs are usually four years long. The subspecialties of radiology include diagnostic radiology with special competence in nuclear radiology; certificates of added qualification in

Figure A1–1 An Orthopedist.

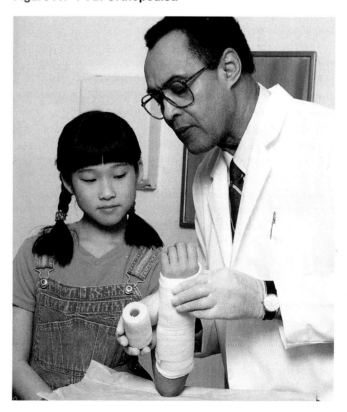

vascular and interventional radiology, neuroradiology, and pediatric radiology.

- *Surgery.* Physicians who provide surgical treatment of injuries and illness are called surgeons. Surgical residency programs are usually six years. The subspecialties of surgery include pediatric surgery, vascular surgery, surgical critical care, and surgery of the hand.
- *Thoracic surgery.* Surgery of the thorax and its contents, including the heart, is the domain of a thoracic surgeon. Thoracic surgery residencies are typically six years long.
- *Urology.* Urology is the surgical treatment of diseases and illnesses of the genitourinary tract. Urologists must complete a six-year residency program.

Osteopathic Medicine

As previously discussed, MDs and DOs are the only complete physicians in the United States. Medicine as practiced by MDs is often referred to as *allopathic medicine*, while that practiced by DOs is called *osteopathic medicine*. Today, the difference between the two disciplines is minimal. DOs obtain additional undergraduate education in the musculoskeletal system and learn to perform osteopathic manipulation. In addition, DOs are trained to treat the "whole patient" instead of some disease entity.

The system of bones and muscles comprises about two-thirds of the body's mass. DOs know that the body's structure plays a critical role in its ability to function. They can use their eyes and hands to identify structural problems and to support the body's natural tendency toward health and self-healing.

Andrew Taylor Still, MD, developed osteopathic medicine in 1874. Dr. Still became dissatisfied with the effectiveness of nineteenth-century medicine after several of his children died of meningitis. He believed that many of the medications of his day were useless or even harmful. In response, he founded a philosophy of medicine based on ideas that dated back to Hippocrates. The philosophy focused on the unity of all body parts. He identified the musculoskeletal system as a key element of health. Recognizing the body's ability to heal itself, he stressed preventive medicine, eating well, and staying fit. He introduced the concept of osteopathic manipulative therapy where problems with the musculoskeletal system were corrected by applying various manual treatment techniques.

Osteopathic medicine was regarded as a cult until the middle of the twentieth century. Because DOs and MDs did not practice together, DOs established a parallel system of osteopathic hospitals where DOs could practice and schools where DOs could train. Following the Vietnam war, during which the United States military commissioned DOs as medical officers, the barriers between MDs and DOs were slowly broken down. Now, DOs have served as surgeon general of the army and as personal physicians for several presidents. Today, DOs and MDs practice together, and in many states, they take the same licensure examination. Unfortunately, because of the demands of medicine today, much of the uniqueness of osteopathic medicine has been lost. Many DOs complete MD residency programs and practice identically to MDs.

Osteopathic medical schools now emphasize primary care, and because of this, approximately 64 percent of all DOs practice in primary care, many in rural areas.

Other Doctoral Health Care Providers

Although DOs and MDs are the only complete physicians in U.S. health care, there are several other doctoral level health care providers. These include dentists, podiatrists, optometrists, psychologists, chiropractors, and naturopaths.

Dentists

Dentists treat problems related to the teeth, gums, and related structures. They look beyond the mouth and treat people as individuals. Many systemic disease processes can be identified by examination of the mouth and teeth. Dentists detect and diagnose disease, provide for the aesthetic appearance of the teeth, provide surgical restoration of the teeth, and provide public information about prevention. Dentists perform surgery related to the mouth and can administer and prescribe medications as needed.

Dental school is four years long. Like medical and osteopathic school, students usually enter dental school after completion of a bachelor's degree, although some enter after two years of college. Dental school admission is highly selective. Students must have good college grades, perform well on the Dental Admissions Test (DAT), and show aptitude toward dentistry. Upon completion of dental school, students are awarded the doctor of dental surgery (DDS) or doctor of dental medicine (DMD) degree. Dentists who desire to practice general dentistry can enter practice after dental school. Those who desire to specialize will enter postgraduate training programs, which usually last two years. The recognized specialties of dentistry include:

- *Dental public health.* The science and art of preventing and controlling dental diseases.
- *Endodontics.* The branch of dentistry that is concerned with the morphology, physiology, and pathology of the human dental pulp and periadicular tissues.
- *Oral and maxillofacial pathology.* The branch of dentistry that deals with the nature, identification, and management of oral and maxillofacial diseases.
- *Oral and maxillofacial surgery.* The specialty of dentistry that includes the diagnosis, surgical and adjunctive treatment of diseases, injuries, and defects that involve the oral and maxillofacial region (also called oral surgeons).
- *Orthodontics and dentofacial orthopedics.* The area of dentistry that corrects the movement and location of teeth and related structures.
- *Pediatric dentistry.* The age-defined specialty of dentistry that is limited to infants and children.
- *Periodontics.* The branch of dentistry that treats the gums and other structures that surround the teeth.

- *Prosthodontics.* The branch of dentistry that pertains to restoration or maintenance of oral functions, comfort, and appearance.
- *Oral and maxillofacial radiology.* Specialty of dentistry that involves imaging of the teeth and associated structures.

General dentists and most specialists are office-based. Some of the surgical specialties of dentistry, such as oral and maxillofacial surgery, are hospital-based. A physician will usually work with the oral surgeon to manage nondental-related problems in hospitalized patients.

Podiatrists

Podiatrists are doctoral health care providers who concentrate on medical and surgical care of the feet. Most students who enter podiatric medical school hold a bachelor's degree. Most podiatric medical schools require that students also write the Medical College Admissions Test (MCAT). Podiatric medical school is four years and similar to medical school, except that the emphasis is on the feet. Upon graduation from podiatric medical school, podiatrists are awarded the doctor of podiatric medicine (DPM) degree. Some will enter general practice and others will complete a one- to two-year residency, often in a teaching hospital. Podiatrists perform surgery on the feet and can prescribe medications for foot and related problems. Podiatrists can obtain specialty certification in podiatric orthopedics, podiatric surgery, or primary podiatric medicine.

Optometrists

Doctors of optometry (ODs) are health care providers who examine, diagnose, treat, and manage diseases and disorders of the visual system, the eye, and associated structures. Optometrists enter optometry school after two to four years of college. Optometry school is four years, and students earn the doctor of optometry (OD) degree upon graduation. Optometrists primarily perform refractive examinations of the eye. In some states, optometrists can prescribe a limited number of medications related to the eye. In other states, they cannot prescribe. Optometrists are often confused with ophthalmologists. Ophthalmologists are MDs or DOs who have completed a four-year residency in the medical and surgical care of the eyes and related structures. Optometrists do not perform surgery.

Psychologists

Psychologists have completed a clinical psychology program and have been awarded the doctor of philosophy (PhD) degree. They provide individual and family counseling for emotional and mental diseases. They also provide diagnostic testing and assessment. Psychologists cannot prescribe medications. The difference between psychiatrists and psychologists is often misunderstood. Psychiatrists are physicians (MD or DO) who have completed a four-year psychiatry residency. They treat emotional and mental illness with multiple modalities including medications. Often, psychiatrists and psychologists work together, with the psychologist providing much of the counseling while the psychiatrist manages medications and other problems.

Chiropractors

Chiropractic is a branch of the healing arts concerned with human health and disease processes. Central to chiropractic is the "vertebral subluxation," a condition in which a vertebra becomes slightly misaligned with an adjacent segment in such a way as to disturb nerve function. The objective of chiropractic is to locate, analyze, and correct vertebral subluxations, usually through spinal manipulation. One criticism of chiropractic is that the vertebral subluxation has never been scientifically proven to exist.

Some chiropractors limit their practice to spinal manipulation for back pain and related problems. Others believe that chiropractic manipulation can treat other conditions by removing impediments to nerve conduction. This is a major source of discord within the chiropractic profession. "Straight" chiropractors limit their practice to treatment of musculoskeletal problems and back pain. They refer patients to medical or osteopathic doctors for problems that are not of a musculoskeletal origin. "Mixer" chiropractors use spinal manipulation, also called chiropractic adjustments, to treat problems outside of the musculoskeletal system such as ear infections, ulcer disease, and gallbladder disease.

Chiropractic was founded in 1878 when Daniel David Palmer, a magnetic healer, applied force to a bump that he detected on the back of a janitor who had recently lost his hearing after working in a cramped, stooped position. As he applied the force, Palmer felt a "pop," and the bump disappeared. Several days later, the janitor's hearing returned and chiropractic was born.

Chiropractic colleges are usually three to four years long. Students usually enter chiropractic school after two years of college. Upon completion of the chiropractic curriculum, they are granted a doctor of chiropractic (DC) degree. They then take a state licensure exam and can begin independent practice. Chiropractors cannot perform surgery or prescribe medication. They can use X-rays for evaluation of the spine and can use various physical therapy modalities. In some states in the United States, chiropractors can refer to themselves as chiropractic physicians.

Spinal manipulation has been found effective for the treatment of mechanical musculoskeletal back pain and similar conditions. Its effectiveness in treating other medical conditions has never been scientifically documented.

Naturopathic Physicians

A relatively new doctoral level health care provider is the naturopathic physician. Naturopathic schools have a four-year program that contains the same basic science courses as traditional medical schools. However, they also study clinical nutrition, acupuncture, homeopathic medicine, botanical medicine, psychology, and counseling. At the completion of their education, students receive a doctor of naturopathic medicine (ND) degree. Naturopathic physicians use holistic and nontoxic approaches to therapy with an emphasis on disease prevention and optimizing wellness. They cannot prescribe medications or practice surgery.

Advanced Practice Providers

With the advent of managed care, a need has arisen to use nonphysicians to assist in primary care roles. These health care providers, often called midlevel practitioners, work with licensed physicians. Physician assistants (PAs), nurse practitioners (NPs), and nurse anesthetists (CRNAs) are the most common midlevel practitioners.

PAs attend physician assistant programs that are usually located in medical schools. They enter after they have completed two years of college. PA school is usually two years long, and some PA programs now offer master's degrees. PAs practice under the direction of a licensed physician. However, the physician does not have to be physically present in the clinic. PAs can specialize in areas of medicine such as family practice, emergency medicine, and pediatrics.

Nurse practitioners are advanced nurses who have completed an approved nurse practitioner program. Nurse practitioners must have a bachelor's degree in nursing and experience as a registered nurse prior to entering NP school. NP school is usually two years long and trains the nurse for practice, usually in a clinic setting. NP programs can specialize in family practice, geriatrics, internal medicine, or pediatrics. NPs work under the direction of a licensed physician. However, the physician does not have to be physically present. NPs often staff rural and public health clinics and can consult with physicians by telephone if needed.

Certified registered nurse anesthetists (CRNAs) are nurses who have completed a two-year program in anesthesia. To enter the program, the nurse must have a bachelor's degree in nursing and several years of clinical nursing experience. Most CRNA programs award a master's degree upon completion. CRNAs work under the supervision of an MD or DO anesthesiologist (although this is being challenged). People often confuse anesthesiologists and anesthetists. Anesthesiologists are MD or DO physicians who have completed a residency program in anesthesiology. Anesthetists are nurses who have completed a nurse anesthesia program.

Nursing

Nurses provide the vast majority of actual patient care in this country. There are two major categories of nurses: registered nurses (RNs) and licensed practical nurses (LPNs). In some states, LPNs are referred to as licensed vocational nurses (LVNs) (**Figure A1–2**).

LPNs undergo an intense one-year program that prepares them to provide bedside nursing care. The first part of the program is classroom-based and includes the basic sciences and nursing science. The latter parts of the class are conducted in the hospital, where the students learn and practice their skills. Upon completion of their training, they receive a certificate and are able to sit for the state licensure examination.

Registered nurses can complete one of three different program types. The shortest is a two-year associate's degree program. In this case, the student completes required prenursing classes, then studies

Figure A1–2 The Nursing Assistant Helps the Nurse Care for the Patient.

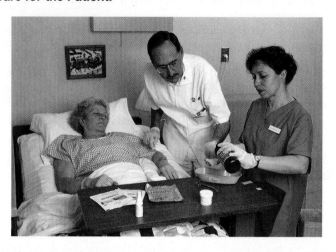

nursing science in the classroom, and finally finishes by learning in the hospital setting. Upon completion of the program, students earn an associate degree in nursing (ADN). Although not common today, some programs still offer a diploma program. This is a three-year program that concentrates on prenursing, classroom, and clinical nursing instruction. Finally, many nursing programs offer a bachelor's degree. The first two years are prenursing courses, and the last two years are classroom and clinical nursing classes. Upon completion, the nurse receives a bachelor of science degree in nursing (BSN).

Graduate courses that lead to a master's of science in nursing (MSN) and a PhD in nursing are available. Many community colleges have begun to offer a paramedic-to-nurse bridge program for paramedics who want to become a nurse. Several programs provide nursing education by correspondence and over the Internet. These programs are popular with EMS personnel because of the difficult work schedules inherent in EMS.

Allied Health Personnel

For one person to be well versed in all aspects of health care is impossible. Because of this, numerous allied health personnel have evolved to assist physicians and nurses in providing patient care. Examples of allied health personnel include

- *Anesthesiologist assistant.* Assists anesthesiologist by preparing equipment and supplies and by monitoring patients.
- *Art therapist.* Provides art therapy as a rehabilitation tool.
- *Athletic trainer.* Provides preventive and field care for various sporting teams and events.
- *Audiologist.* Provides hearing testing and fits hearing aids and similar devices.
- *Blood bank technologist.* Ensures blood is gathered, stored, tested, and administered in a safe and proper manner.
- *Cardiovascular technologist.* Performs cardiovascular diagnostic testing such as electrocardiograms, echo-cardiography, stress testing, and cardiac monitoring.
- *Clinical laboratory science/medical technology.* Staffs the medical laboratory and performs essential testing of body products.

- *Counseling-related occupations.* Provide counseling for mental health, substance abuse, rehabilitation, and similar patients.
- *Cytotechnologist.* Studies and prepares cells and tissues such as Pap smears.
- *Dental assistant.* Chair-side assistant to a dentist in day-to-day practice.
- *Dental hygienist.* Evaluates and cleans teeth in dental office and instructs the patient in preventive dental care.
- *Dental laboratory technician.* Works in dental lab making dentures, crowns, implants, and bridges.
- *Diagnostic medical sonographer.* Performs diagnostic ultrasound, usually in a hospital radiology department.
- *Dietetic technician, dietician.* Instructs patients in dietary health and supervises hospital nutrition programs.
- *Emergency medical technician, paramedic.* Provides advanced emergency care to ill or injured patients.
- *Genetic counselor.* Assists patients and families in regard to diagnosed or possible genetic or hereditary problems.
- *Health information management.* Organizes and controls all patient medical records in hospital or office setting.
- *Histologic technician/histotechnologist.* Prepares tissues for examination by pathologist.
- *Kinesiotherapist.* Assists patients in movement following injury or illness, often working with physical therapists.
- *Medical assistant.* Medical office assistant who provides medical services for a practicing physician or midlevel provider.
- *Music therapist.* Works with other rehabilitative specialists by providing music therapy to rehabilitation and mental health patients.
- *Nuclear medical technologist.* Prepares, administers, and monitors nuclear radioisotopes in a hospital nuclear medicine department.
- *Occupational therapy.* Provides instruction and rehabilitation to patients following injury or illness so they can return to their chosen occupation (**Figure A1–3**).

Figure A1–3 Occupational Therapist.

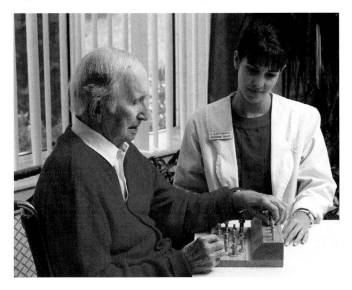

- *Ophthalmic dispensing optician.* Prepares and dispenses eyewear and contact lenses based upon prescription by an optometrist or ophthalmologist.
- *Ophthalmic laboratory technician/technologist.* Technician who prepares prescription lenses in an ophthalmic laboratory.
- *Orthotist.* Prepares braces and similar devices for patients who have had injuries or illnesses.
- *Orthotist and prosthetic technician.* Prepares artificial limbs and other body parts for patients who have undergone amputation or another body changing procedure.
- *Pathologist's assistant.* Assists pathologist in the hospital laboratory and in the autopsy theater.
- *Perfusionist.* Operates cardiac bypass pump for patients undergoing open-heart surgery.
- *Physical therapist/physical therapy assistant.* A physical therapist is a person with a bachelor's or master's degree in physical therapy who prepares and supervises physical rehabilitation for a patient. A physical therapy assistant is a person with an associate's degree who assists a physical therapist in patient care including use of modalities.
- *Radiation therapist/radiographer.* Radiation therapist provides therapeutic radiation therapy to cancer patients. Radiographer or radiological technician performs medical imaging techniques such as X-rays, computed tomography scans, and magnetic resonance imaging scans (**Figure A1–4**).
- *Rehabilitation counselor.* Oversees emotional and mental component of injury or illness rehabilitation (**Figure A1–5**).
- *Respiratory therapist.* Responsible for assessing and providing ordered respiratory procedures for patients. Is also responsible for the preparation and operation of ventilators and all respiratory devices found in a hospital.

Figure A1–4 X-Ray Technician.

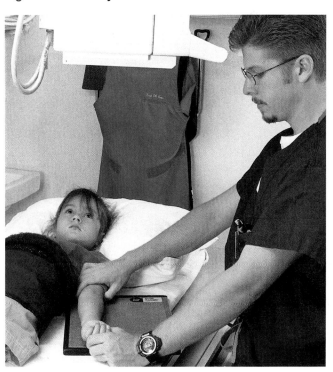

Figure A1–5 Assisting a Patient at Home.

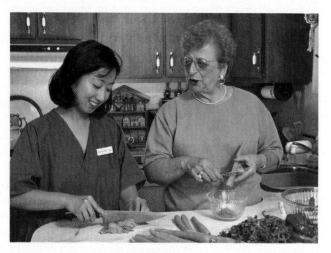

- *Speech-language pathologist.* Assists patients, especially those who have had a stroke or head injury, in learning to speak and communicate.
- *Surgical technologist.* Technologist who works in hospital setting assisting surgeons in performing surgical procedures.
- *Therapeutic recreation specialist.* Instructs and oversees patients' recreation needs, especially those patients who are hospitalized for a prolonged period.

The house of medicine is indeed complex, and this discussion has not covered every aspect of health care provision. However, emergency medical personnel should be familiar with the various health care personnel they will encounter during the course of their hospital rotations, and later as they interact with hospital personnel as members of the emergency medical services system. Remember, emergency medical technicians and paramedics are essential parts of the health care system.

Appendix II   A Periodic Chart of the Elements

The **periodic table** presents the known elements in order of their atomic weights. Each horizontal row represents a single electron shell. The number of elements in that row is determined by the maximum number of electrons that can be stored at that energy level. The element at the left end of each row contains a single electron in its outermost electron shell; the element at the right end of the row has a filled outer electron shell. Organizing the elements in this fashion highlights similarities that reflect the composition of the outer electron shell. These similarities are evident when you examine the vertical columns. All the gases of the rightmost column—helium, neon, argon, krypton, xenon, and radon—have full electron shells; each is a gas at normal atmospheric temperature and pressure, and none reacts readily with other elements. These elements, highlighted in blue, are known as the *noble*, or *inert*, *gases*. In contrast, the elements of the left-most column—lithium, sodium, potassium, and so forth—are silvery, soft metals that are so highly reactive that pure forms cannot be found in nature. The fourth and fifth electron levels can hold 18 electrons. Table inserts are used for the *lanthanide* and *actinide series* to save space, as higher levels can store up to 32 electrons. Elements of particular importance to our discussion of human anatomy and physiology are highlighted in pink.

Atomic number — 1 **H** — Chemical symbol
Hydrogen — Element name
Atomic weight — 1.01

1 **H** Hydrogen 1.01																	2 **He** Helium 4.00
3 **Li** Lithium 6.94	4 **Be** Beryllium 9.01											5 **B** Boron 10.81	6 **C** Carbon 12.01	7 **N** Nitrogen 14.01	8 **O** Oxygen 16.00	9 **F** Fluorine 19.00	10 **Ne** Neon 20.18
11 **Na** Sodium 22.99	12 **Mg** Magnesium 24.31											13 **Al** Aluminum 26.98	14 **Si** Silicon 28.09	15 **P** Phosphorus 30.97	16 **S** Sulfur 32.07	17 **Cl** Chlorine 35.45	18 **Ar** Argon 39.95
19 **K** Potassium 39.10	20 **Ca** Calcium 40.08	21 **Sc** Scandium 44.96	22 **Ti** Titanium 47.88	23 **V** Vanadium 50.94	24 **Cr** Chromium 52.00	25 **Mn** Manganese 54.94	26 **Fe** Iron 55.85	27 **Co** Cobalt 58.93	28 **Ni** Nickel 58.69	29 **Cu** Copper 63.55	30 **Zn** Zinc 65.39	31 **Ga** Gallium 69.72	32 **Ge** Germanium 72.61	33 **As** Arsenic 74.92	34 **Se** Selenium 78.96	35 **Br** Bromine 79.90	36 **Kr** Krypton 83.80
37 **Rb** Rubidium 85.47	38 **Sr** Strontium 87.62	39 **Y** Yttrium 88.91	40 **Zr** Zirconium 91.22	41 **Nb** Niobium 92.91	42 **Mo** Molybdenum 95.94	43 **Tc** Technetium (98)	44 **Ru** Ruthenium 101.07	45 **Rh** Rhodium 102.91	46 **Pd** Palladium 106.42	47 **Ag** Silver 107.87	48 **Cd** Cadmium 112.41	49 **In** Indium 114.82	50 **Sn** Tin 118.71	51 **Sb** Antimony 121.76	52 **Te** Tellurium 127.60	53 **I** Iodine 126.90	54 **Xe** Xenon 131.29
55 **Cs** Cesium 132.91	56 **Ba** Barium 137.33	57 **La** Lanthanum 138.91 *	72 **Hf** Hafnium 178.49	73 **Ta** Tantalum 180.95	74 **W** Tungsten 183.85	75 **Re** Rhenium 186.21	76 **Os** Osmium 190.2	77 **Ir** Iridium 192.22	78 **Pt** Platinum 195.08	79 **Au** Gold 196.97	80 **Hg** Mercury 200.59	81 **Tl** Thallium 204.38	82 **Pb** Lead 207.2	83 **Bi** Bismuth 208.98	84 **Po** Polonium (209)	85 **At** Astatine (210)	86 **Rn** Radon (222)
87 **Fr** Francium (223)	88 **Ra** Radium 226.03	89 **Ac** Actinium 227.03 †	104 **Db** Dubnium (261)	105 **Jl** Joliotium (262)	106 **Rf** Rutherfordium (263)	107 **Bh** Bohrium (262)	108 **Hn** Hahnium (265)	109 **Mt** Meitnerium (266)	110 Unnamed (269)	111 Unnamed (272)	112 Unnamed (272)						

Lanthanide series	58 **Ce** Cerium 140.12	59 **Pr** Praseodymium 140.91	60 **Nd** Neodymium 144.24	61 **Pm** Promethium (145)	62 **Sm** Samarium 150.36	63 **Eu** Europium 151.96	64 **Gd** Gadolinium 157.25	65 **Tb** Terbium 158.93	66 **Dy** Dysprosium 162.50	67 **Ho** Holmium 164.93	68 **Er** Erbium 167.26	69 **Tm** Thulium 168.93	70 **Yb** Ytterbium 173.04	71 **Lu** Lutetium 174.97
Actinide series	90 **Th** Thorium 232.04	91 **Pa** Protactinium 231.04	92 **U** Uranium 238.03	93 **Np** Neptunium 237.05	94 **Pu** Plutonium (244)	95 **Am** Americium (243)	96 **Cm** Curium (247)	97 **Bk** Berkelium (247)	98 **Cf** Californium (251)	99 **Es** Einsteinium (252)	100 **Fm** Fermium (257)	101 **Md** Mendelevium (258)	102 **No** Nobelium (259)	103 **Lr** Lawrencium (260)

Weights and Measures

Accurate descriptions of physical objects would be impossible without a precise method of reporting the pertinent data. Dimensions such as length and width are reported in standardized units of measurement, such as inches or centimeters. These values can be used to calculate the **volume** of an object, which is a measurement of the amount of space the object fills. **Mass** is another important physical property. The mass of an object is determined by the amount of matter the object contains; on Earth the mass of an object determines the object's weight.

In the United States, length and width are typically described in inches, feet, or yards; volumes in pints, quarts, or gallons; and weights in ounces, pounds, or tons. These are units of the **U.S. system** of measurement. **Table A3–1** summarizes terms used in the U.S. system. For reference purposes, this table also includes a definition of the "household units," which are popular in recipes. The U.S. system can be very difficult to work with because there is no logical relationship between the various units. For example, there are 12 inches in a foot, 3 feet in a yard, and 1760 yards in a mile. Without a clear pattern of organization, converting feet to inches or miles to feet can be confusing and time-consuming. The relationships among ounces, pints, quarts, and gallons are no more logical than those among ounces, pounds, and tons.

In contrast, the **metric system** has a logical organization based on powers of 10, as indicated in **Table A3–2**. For example, a **meter** (**m**) is the basic unit for the measurement of size. For measuring larger objects, data can be reported in **dekameters** (*deka*, ten), **hectometers** (*hekaton*, hundred), or **kilometers** (**km**; *chilioi*, thousand); for smaller objects, data can be reported in **decimeters** (0.1 m; *decem*, ten), **centimeters** (**cm** = 0.01 m; *centum*, hundred), **millimeters** (**mm** = 0.001 m; *mille*, thousand), and so forth. In the metric system, the same prefixes are used to report weights, based on the **gram** (**g**), and volumes, based on the **liter** (**L**).

This text reports data in metric units, usually with U.S. equivalents. Use this opportunity to become familiar with the metric system because most technical sources report data only in metric units, and most of the world outside the United States uses the metric system exclusively. Conversion factors are included in **Table A3–2**.

The U.S. and metric systems also differ in their methods of reporting temperatures: in the United States, temperatures are usually reported in degrees Fahrenheit (°F), whereas scientific literature and individuals in most other countries report temperature in degrees centigrade or degrees Celsius (°C). The relationship between temperatures in degrees Fahrenheit and those in degrees centigrade is indicated in **Table A3–2**.

The following illustration spans the entire range of measurements that we consider in this book. Gross anatomy traditionally deals with structural organization as seen with the naked eye or with a simple hand lens. A microscope can provide higher levels of magnification and reveal finer details. Before the 1950s, most information was provided by *light microscopy*. A photograph taken through a light microscope is called a **light micrograph** (**LM**). Light microscopy can magnify cellular structures about 1000 times and show details as fine as 0.25 μm. The symbol **μm** stands for **micrometer**; 1 μm = 0.001 mm, or 0.00004 inches. With a light microscope, we can identify cell types, such as muscle cells or neurons, and see large structures within a cell. Because individual

Table A3–1	The U.S. System of Measurement		
Physical Property	Unit	Relationship to Other U.S. Units	Relationship to Household Units
Length	Inch (in.)	1 in. = 0.083 ft	
	Foot (ft)	1 ft = 12 in.	
		= 0.33 yd	
	Yard (yd)	1 yd = 36 in.	
		= 3 ft	
	Mile (mi)	1 mi = 5280 ft	
		= 1760 yd	
Volume	Fluidram (fl dr)	1 fl dr = 0.125 fl oz	
	Fluid ounce (fl oz)	1 fl oz = 8 fl dr	= 6 teaspoons (tsp)
		= 0.0625 pt	= 2 tablespoons (tbsp)
	Pint (pt)	1 pt = 128 fl dr	= 32 tbsp
		= 16 fl oz	= 2 cups (c)
		= 0.5 qt	
	Quart (qt)	1 qt = 256 fl dr	= 4c
		= 32 fl oz	
		= 2 pt	
		= 0.25 gal	
	Gallon (gal)	1 gal = 128 fl oz	
		= 8 pt	
		= 4 qt	
Mass	Grain (gr)	1 gr = 0.002 oz	
	Dram (dr)	1 dr = 27.3 gr	
		= 0.063 oz	
	Ounce (oz)	1 oz = 437.5 gr	
		= 16 dr	
	Pound (lb)	1 lb = 7000 gr	
		= 256 dr	
		= 16 oz	
	Ton (t)	1 t = 2000 lb	

Table A3–2 — The Metric System of Measurement

Physical Property	Unit	Relationship to Standard Metric Units	Conversion to U.S. Units	
Length	Nanometer (nm)	1 nm = 0.000000001 m (10^{-9})	= 4 ∞ 10^{-8} in.	25,400,000 nm = 1 in.
	Micrometer (μm)	1 μm = 0.000001 m (10^{-6})	= 4 ∞ 10^{-5} in.	25,400 μm = 1 in.
	Millimeter (mm)	1 mm = 0.001 m (10^{-3})	= 0.0394 in.	25.4 mm = 1 in.
	Centimeter (cm)	1 cm = 0.01 m (10^{-2})	= 0.394 in.	2.54 cm = 1 in.
	Decimeter (dm)	1 dm = 0.1 m (10^{-1})	= 3.94 in.	0.254 dm = 1 in.
	Meter (m)	Standard unit of length	= 39.4 in.	0.0254 m = 1 in.
			= 3.28 ft	0.3048 m = 1 ft
			= 1.09 yd	0.914 m = 1 yd
	Dekameter (dam)	1 dam = 10 m		
	Hectometer (hm)	1 hm = 100 m		
	Kilometer (km)	1 km = 1000 m	= 3280 ft	
			= 1093 yd	
			= 0.62 mi	1.609 km = 1 mi
Volume	Microliter (μL)	1 μL = 0.000001 L (10^{-6}) = 1 cubic millimeter (mm^3)		
	Milliliter (mL)	1 mL = 0.001 L (10^{-3}) = 1 cubic centimeter (cm^3 or cc)	= 0.03 fl oz	5 mL = 1 tsp
				15 mL = 1 tbsp
				30 mL = 1 fl oz
	Centiliter (cL)	1 cL = 0.01 L (10^{-2})	= 0.34 fl oz	3 cL = 1 fl oz
	Deciliter (dL)	1 dL = 0.1 L (10^{-1})	= 3.38 fl oz	0.29 dL = 1 fl oz
	Liter (L)	Standard unit of volume	= 33.8 fl oz	0.0295 L = 1 fl oz
			= 2.11 pt	0.473 L = 1 pt
			= 1.06 qt	0.946 L = 1 qt
Mass	Picogram (pg)	1 pg = 0.000000000001 g (10^{-12})		
	Nanogram (ng)	1 ng = 0.000000001 g (10^{-9})	= 0.000000015 gr	66,666,666 ng = 1 gr
	Microgram (μg)	1 μg = 0.000001 g (10^{-6})	= 0.000015 gr	66,666 μg = 1 gr
	Milligram (mg)	1 mg = 0.001 g (10^{-3})	= 0.015 gr	66.7 mg = 1 gr
	Centigram (cg)	1 cg = 0.01 g (10^{-2})	= 0.15 gr	6.67 cg = 1 gr
	Decigram (dg)	1 dg = 0.1 g (10^{-1})	= 1.5 gr	0.667 dg = 1 gr
	Gram (g)	Standard unit of mass	= 0.035 oz	28.4 g = 1 oz
			= 0.0022 lb	454 g = 1 lb
	Dekagram (dag)	1 dag = 10 g		
	Hectogram (hg)	1 hg = 100 g		
	Kilogram (kg)	1 kg = 1000 g	= 2.2 lb	0.454 kg = 1 lb
	Metric ton (mt)	1 mt = 1000 kg	= 1.1 t	
			= 2205 lb	0.907 mt = 1 t

Temperature	Centigrade	Fahrenheit
Freezing point of pure water	0°	32°
Normal body temperature	36.8°	98.6°
Boiling point of pure water	100°	212°
Conversion	°C → °F: °F = (1.8 × °C) + 32	°F → °C: °C = (°F − 32) × 0.56

cells are relatively transparent, thin sections cut through a cell are treated with dyes that stain specific structures, which makes them easier to see.

Although special staining techniques can show the general distribution of proteins, lipids, carbohydrates, and nucleic acids in a cell, many fine details of intracellular structure remained a mystery until investigators began using *electron microscopy*. This technique uses a focused beam of electrons, rather than a beam of light, to examine cell structure. In *transmission electron microscopy*, electrons pass through an ultrathin section to strike a photographic plate. The result is a **transmission electron micrograph (TEM)**. Transmission electron microscopy shows the fine structure of cell membranes and intracellular structures. In *scanning electron microscopy*, electrons bouncing off exposed surfaces create a **scanning electron micrograph (SEM)**. Although it cannot achieve as much magnification as transmission microscopy, scanning microscopy provides a three-dimensional perspective of cell structure.

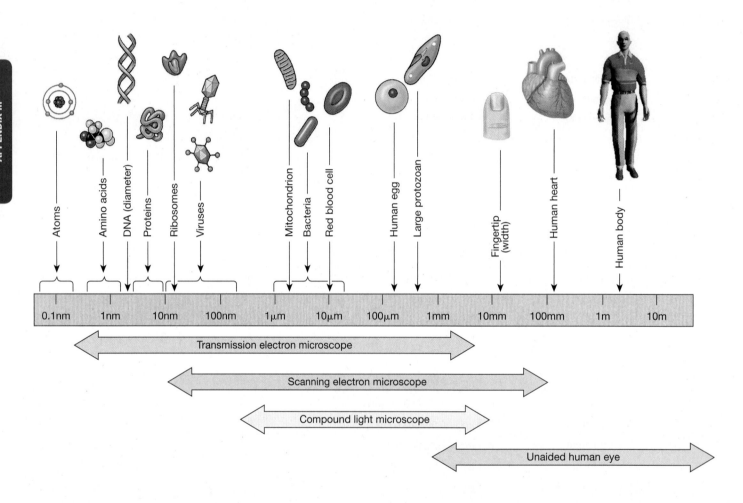

Appendix IV Normal Physiological Values

Tables A4–1 and 4–2 present normal averages or ranges for the chemical composition of body fluids. These values are approximations rather than absolute values, because test results vary from laboratory to laboratory due to differences in procedures, equipment, normal solutions, and so forth. Sources used in the preparation of these tables are indicated on p. 785. Blanks in the tabular data appear where data are not available.

Table A4–1	The Chemistry of Blood, Cerebrospinal Fluid, and Urine		
	Normal Ranges		
Test	**Blood**	**CSF**	**Urine**
pH	S: 7.38–7.44	7.31–7.34	4.5–8.0
OSMOLARITY (MOSM/L)	S: 280–295	292–297	855–1335
ELECTROLYTES	(mEq/L unless noted)		(urinary loss per 24-hour period[a])
Bicarbonate	P: 21–28	20–24	
Calcium	S: 4.5–5.3	2.1–3.0	6.5–16.5 mEq
Chloride	S: 100–108	116–122	120–240 mEq
Iron	S: 50–150 μg/L	23–52 μg/L	40–150 μg
Magnesium	S: 1.5–2.5	2–2.5	4.9–16.5 mEq
Phosphorus	S: 1.8–2.6	1.2–2.0	0.8–2 g
Potassium	P: 3.8–5.0	2.7–3.9	35–80 mEq
Sodium	P: 136–142	137–145	120–220 mEq
Sulfate	S: 0.2–1.3		1.07–1.3 g
METABOLITES	(mg/dL unless noted)		(urinary loss per 24-hour period[b])
Amino acids	P/S: 2.3–5.0	10.0–14.7	41–133 mg
Ammonia	P: 20–150 μg/dL	25–80 μg/dL	340–1200 mg
Bilirubin	S: 0.5–1.0	<0.2	0.02–1.9 mg
Creatinine	P/S: 0.6–1.2	0.5–1.9	1.01–2.5
Glucose	P/S: 70–110	40–70	16–132 mg
Ketone bodies	S: 0.3–2.0	1.3–1.6	10–100 mg
Lactic acid	WB: 5–20[c]	10–20	100–600 mg
Lipids (total)	S: 400–1000	0.8–1.7	0–31.8 mg
Cholesterol (total)	S: 150–300	0.2–0.8	1.2–3.8 mg
Triglycerides	S: 40–150	0–0.9	
Urea	P/S: 23–43	13.8–36.4	12.6–28.6
Uric acid	S: 2.0–7.0	0.2–0.3	80–976 mg
PROTEINS	(g/dL)	(mg/dL)	(urinary loss per 24-hour period[b])
Total	S: 6.0–7.8	2.0–4.5	47–76.2 mg
Albumin	S: 3.2–4.5	10.6–32.4	10–100 mg
Globulins (total)	S: 2.3–3.5	2.8–15.5	7.3 mg (average)
Immunoglobulins	S: 1.0–2.2	1.1–1.7	3.1 mg (average)
Fibrinogen	P: 0.2–0.4	0.65 (average)	

S = serum, P = plasma, WB = whole blood.
[a]Because urinary output averages just over 1 liter per day, these electrolyte values are comparable to mEq/L.
[b]Because urinary metabolite and protein data approximate mg/L or g/L, they must be divided by 10 for comparison with CSF or blood concentrations.
[c]Venous blood sample.

Table A4–2 The Composition of Minor Body Fluids

Test	Perilymph	Endolymph	Normal Averages or Ranges			
			Synovial Fluid	Sweat	Saliva	Semen
pH			7.4	4–6.8	6.4[a]	7.19
SPECIFIC GRAVITY			1.008–1.015	1.001–1.008	1.007	1.028
ELECTROLYTES (mEq/L)						
Potassium	5.5–6.3	140–160	4.0	4.3–14.2	21	31.3
Sodium	143–150	12–16	136.1	0–104	14[a]	117
Calcium	1.3–1.6	0.05	2.3–4.7	0.2–6	3	12.4
Magnesium	1.7	0.02		0.03–4	0.6	11.5
Bicarbonate	17.8–18.6	20.4–21.4	19.3–30.6		6[a]	24
Chloride	121.5	107.1	107.1	34.3	17	42.8
PROTEINS (mg/dL)						
Total	200	150	1.72 g/dL	7.7	386[b]	4.5 g/dL
METABOLITES (mg/dL)						
Amino acids				47.6	40	1.26 g/dL
Glucose	104		70–110	3.0	11	224 (fructose)
Urea				26–122	20	72
Lipids (total)	12		20.9	c	25–500[d]	188

[a]Increases under salivary stimulation.
[b]Primarily alpha-amylase, with some lysozymes.
[c]Not present in eccrine secretions.
[d]Cholesterol.

Index

A

A band, 217, 218
Abdominal aorta, 517
Abdominal aortic aneurysm, 512–513
Abdominal cavity, 19
Abdominal pain, 656
Abdominal reflex, 317
Abdominopelvic cavity: Portion of the ventral body cavity that contains abdominal and pelvic subdivision, 19
Abdominopelvic quadrants, 13
Abdominopelvic regions, 13
Abducens nerve, 310
Abduction: Movement away from the midline, 197–198
Abnormal hemoglobin, 436
Abnormal hemostasis, 450
Abortion, 797
Abrasion, 144
Abruptio placentae, 803, 806
Abscess, 549
Absence seizures, 306
Absorption: The active or passive uptake of gases, fluids, or solutes, 651–655
Accessory nerve, 312
Accommodation: Alteration in the curvature of the lens to focus an image on the retina, 361
Acetabulum: Fossa on lateral aspect of pelvis that accommodates the head of the femur, 191
Acetylcholine (ACh): Chemical neurotransmitter in the brain and PNS; dominant neurotransmitter in the PNS, released at neuromuscular junctions and synapses of the parasympathetic division, 218, 219, 285, 286, 328
Acetylcholinesterase (AChE): Enzyme found in the synaptic cleft, bound to the postsynaptic membrane, and in tissue fluids; breaks down and inactivates ACh molecules, 218, 286, 328
Acid: A compound whose dissociation in solution releases a hydrogen ion and an anion; an acid solution has a pH below 7.0 and contains an excess of hydrogen ions, 36–37
Acid-base balance, 38, 39, 717–719
Acid-base disorders, 724–725
Acidic, 36
Acidosis: An abnormal physiological state characterized by a plasma pH below 7.38, 712, 722
ACMV, 592
Acquaintance rape, 760
Acquired immunity, 555, 556
Acromegaly, 422
Acromion, 187, 188
Acrosome: A caplike compartment containing enzymes essential for fertilization, 740
ACTH. *See* Adrenocorticotropic hormone (ACTH)

Actin: Protein component of microfilaments; form thin filaments in skeletal muscles and produce contractions of all muscles through interaction with thick (myosin) filaments, 75
Action potential: A conducted change in the membrane potential of excitable cells, initiated by a change in the membrane permeability to sodium ions, 284
Activation, 34
Active immunity, 550, 551
Active processes, 64
Active transport: The ATP-dependent absorption or excretion of solutes across a cell membrane, 69–72
Acute arterial occlusion, 518
Acute coronary syndrome, 236, 469–470, 471
Acute glaucoma, 369
Acute myocardial infarction (AMI), 469
Acute renal failure (ARF), 711
Acute tubular necrosis, 711
Adaptation, 345
Adaptive immunity, 546
Addison's disease, 408, 409
Adduction: Movement toward the axis or midline of the body as viewed in the anatomical position, 192, 197, 198
Adductor brevis, 258
Adductor longus, 258
Adductor magnus, 256, 258
Adenine: One of the nitrogenous bases in the nucleic acids RNA and DNA, 48
Adenosine diphosphate (ADP): Adenosine with two phosphate groups attached, 49
Adenosine monophosphate (AMP): A nucleotide consisting of adenosine plus a phosphate group also known as adenosine phosphate, 49
Adenosine triphosphate (ATP): A high-energy compound consisting of adenosine with three phosphate groups attached; the third is attached by a high-energy bond, 49, 229–232
Adenylate cyclase: An enzyme bound to the inner surfaces of cell membranes that can convert ATP to cyclic-AMP; also called adenyl cyclase or adenylyl cyclase, 390
ADH. *See* Antidiuretic hormone (ADH)
Adipocytes, 109
Adipose tissue: Loose connective tissue dominated by adipocytes, 111, 112, 418
Adolescence, 793
ADP: Adenosine with two phosphate groups attached, 49
Adrenal cortex: Superficial portion of adrenal gland that produces steroid hormones, 389, 406–408

Adrenal glands: Small endocrine glands secreting hormones, located superior to each kidney, 406–409
Adrenal insufficiency, 407, 408–409
Adrenal medulla: Core of the adrenal gland; a modified sympathetic ganglion that secretes hormones into the blood following sympathetic activation, 323, 325, 408
Adrenergic: A synaptic terminal that releases norepinephrine when stimulated, 286
Adrenergic receptors, 325
Adrenocorticotropic hormone (ACTH): Hormone that stimulates the production and secretion of glucocorticoids by the adrenal cortex; released by the anterior pituitary, 395
Adult-onset diabetes, 413
Advanced practice providers (APPs), APP-6
Adventitia: Superficial layer of connective tissue surrounding an internal organ; fibers are continuous with those of surrounding tissues, providing support and stabilization, 619
AEDs, 475
Aerobic endurance, 233
Aerobic metabolism: The complete breakdown of organic substrates into carbon dioxide and water; a process that yields large amounts of ATP but requires mitochondria and oxygen, 79, 230, 666
Afferent arteriole: An arteriole that carries blood to a glomerulus of the kidney, 697
Afferent division, 270
Agglutination: Aggregation of red blood cells due to interactions between surface agglutinogens and plasma agglutinins, 442, 559
Aging
  cancer, 123
  digestive system, 655
  hormones, 420–423
  immune response, 564–565
  nervous system, 329–330
  nutritional requirements, 687–688
  reproductive system, 761–762
  respiratory system, 607–609
  senses, 379–380
  skeletal system, 165
  tissues, 123
  urinary system, 726
Agonist: A muscle responsible for a specific movement, 239
Agranulocytes, 444
AIDS, 560
Albinism: Absence of pigment in hair and skin caused by inability of melanocytes to produce melanin, 134
Albumin, 67, 431

Aldosterone: A mineralocorticoid produced by the adrenal cortex; stimulates sodium and water conservation at the kidneys; secreted in response to the presence of angiotensin II, 406, 705, 710
Alkaline, 36
Alkalosis: Condition characterized by a plasma pH of greater than 7.45 and associated with relative deficiency of hydrogen ions or an excess of bicarbonate ions, 722
All-or-none principle, 279
Allantois: One of the four extraembryonic membranes; it provides blood vessels to the chorion and is, therefore, essential to placenta formation; the proximal portion becomes the urinary bladder; the distal portion becomes part of the umbilical cord, 738, 777, 778
Alleles: Alternate forms of a particular gene, 799
Allergen: An antigenic compound that produces a hypersensitivity response, 563
Allergies, 563–564, 565–566
Allergy and immunology, APP-2
Allied health personnel, APP-6–APP-8
Allopathic medicine, APP-4
Alpha cells: Cells in the pancreatic islets that secrete glucagon, 410
Alpha waves, 304
Alternate catabolic pathways, 672
Alveolar ducts, 584
Alveolar macrophages, 584
Alveolar organization, 585
Alveolar ventilation, 590
Alveoli: Blind pockets at the end of the respiratory tree, lined by a simple squamous epithelium and surrounded by a capillary network; site of gas exchange with the blood, 512, 576, 584, 585
Alzheimer's disease, 330, 331
Amenorrhea, 754
AMI, 469
Amination, 677
Amino acids: Organic compounds whose chemical structure can be summarized as, 43, 44–45, 654, 665
Amnesia, 305
Amniocentesis, 107
Amnion: One of the four extra-embryonic membranes; surrounds the developing embryo/fetus, 777
Amniotic cavity, 775–776
AMP: A nucleotide consisting of adenosine plus a phosphate group also known as adenosine phosphate, 49
Amphiarthrosis: An articulation that permits a small degree of independent movement, 195
Amphimixis: The fusion of male and female pronuclei following fertilization, 772

INDEX

Base: A compound whose dissociation releases a hydroxide ion (OH⁻) or removes a hydrogen ion from the solution, 37

Basement membrane: A layer of filaments and fibers that attach an epithelium to the underlying connective tissue, 98

Basic, 36

Basilar artery, 517

Basilar membrane: Membrane that supports the organ of Corti and separates the cochlear duct from the tympanic duct in the inner ear, 375

Basilic vein, 520

Basophils: Circulating granulocytes (WBCs) similar in size and function to tissue mast cells, 446

Behavior, 420

Benign tumor, 90

Beriberi, 683

Berry aneurysms, 331

Beta cells: Cells of the pancreatic islets that secrete insulin in response to elevated blood sugar concentrations, 410

Beta waves, 304

Beta-oxidation: A series of reactions that break the fatty acids down into two-carbon fragments, and generate NADH and FADH2, 674

Biceps brachii, 252

Biceps femoris, 256

Biceps reflex, 317

Bicuspid: A premolar tooth, 623

Bicuspid valve: The left AV valve; also known as the mitral valve, 463

BIG IO device, 159

Bilateral orchiectomy, 738

Bile: Exocrine secretion of the liver that is stored in the gallbladder and ejected into the duodenum, 636

Bile canaliculi, 640, 659

Bile salts: Steroid derivatives in the bile, responsible for the emulsification of ingested lipids, 636

Biliary colic, 645

Biliary obstruction, 655

Bilirubin: A pigment that is the by-product of hemoglobin catabolism, 436

Biliverdin, 436

Biology, 2

Biotin, 649, 682

Bipolar neurons, 273

Birth control pills, 763

Birth control strategies, 763–764

Bladder: A muscular sac that distends as fluid is stored, and whose contraction ejects the fluid at an appropriate time; used alone, the term usually refers to the urinary bladder, 694

Blastocyst: An early stage in the developing embryo, consisting of an outer trophoblast and an inner cell mass, 774

Blastomeres, 773, 774

Bleaching, 366

Blood, 429–455, 720
    blood type, 440–444
    clotting process, 448
    collection and analysis, 431
    formed elements, 431–433
    functions and characteristics, 430–431

    hemostasis, 448–453
    laboratory values, APP-3
    plasma, 432
    platelets, 433
    red blood cells, 433, 434–440
    white blood cells, 433, 439, 444–447

Blood banking and transfusion, 451

Blood clot: A network of fibrin fibers and trapped blood cells, 449–453

Blood compatibility, 443

Blood flow, 496–497

Blood osmotic pressure (BOP), 499

Blood pressure: A force exerted against the vascular walls by the blood, as the result of the push exerted by cardiac contraction and the elasticity of the vessel walls; usually measured along one of the muscular arteries, with systolic pressure measured during ventricular systole, diastolic pressure during ventricular diastole, 491, 496

Blood transfusion, 444, 452

Blood volume reflexes, 481

Blunt chest trauma, 110

Blunt eye trauma, 368

Blunt myocardial injury, 481

BMR. See Basal metabolic rate (BMR)

BNP, 236, 417

Body cavities, 15–19

Body defenses. See Lymphatic system and immunity

Bone, 114, 157–162. See also Skeletal system

Bone Injection Gun (BIG) IO device, 159

Bone markings (surface feature): is an area on the surface of a bone with a specific function, 173, 174

Bone marrow, 158

Bony labyrinth, 371

BOP, 498, 499

Botulism, 219, 229

Bovine spongiform encephalopathy (BSE), 291

Bowman's capsule, 697

Brachial artery, 516

Brachial plexus: Network formed by branches of spinal nerves en route to innervating the upper limb, 312, 313

Brachial vein, 521

Brachialis, 255

Brachiocephalic trunk, 513

Brachiocephalic vein, 521

Brachioradialis, 255

Bradycardia, 475

Brain, 296–309
    association areas, 301
    basal nuclei, 305–306
    cerebellum, 308–309
    cerebral hemispheres, 300
    cerebral processing centers, 302–303
    cerebrum, 299–306
    CSF, 298–299
    diencephalon, 306–307
    epithalamus, 296, 307
    hemispheric lateralization, 302, 303
    hypothalamus, 296, 307
    limbic system, 306
    medulla oblongata, 309
    memory, 304–305
    midbrain, 307–308
    pons, 308
    thalamus, 307

    ventricles, 298–300

Brain abscess, 291

Brain natriuretic peptide (BNP), 417

Brain waves, 304

Breast cancer, 756

Breathing, 593

Broca's area: The speech center of the brain, usually found on the neural cortex of the left cerebral hemisphere, 303

Bronchial tree: The trachea, bronchi, and bronchioles, 582, 583

Bronchioles, 582

Bronchiolitis, 584

Bronchoconstriction, 582

Bronchodilation: Dilation of the bronchial passages; can be caused by sympathetic stimulation, 582

Bronchus (bronchi): One of the branches of the bronchial tree between the trachea and bronchioles, 581–582

Brown-Séquard syndrome, 296

Brudzinski's sign, 290

BSE, 291

Buccinator, 241, 243

Buffer system, 723

Buffer: A compound that stabilizes the pH of a solution by removing or releasing hydrogen ions, 37, 723

Bulbospongiosus, 248

Bulbo-urethral glands: Mucous glands at the base of the penis that secrete into the penile urethra; also called Cowper's glands, 736, 743

Bundle of His: Specialized conducting cells in the interventricular septum that carry the contracting stimulus from the AV node to the bundle branches and thence to the Purkinje fibers; also called AV bundle, 473

Burns, 147–149

Burr holes, 289

Bursae, 196

Bursitis, 202

C

C cells, 400–401

C-type natriuretic peptide (CNP), 417

CABG, 471

Calcaneus: The heelbone, the largest of the tarsal bones, 193

Calcification: The deposition of calcium salts within a tissue, 162

Calcitonin: Hormone secreted by C cells of the thyroid when calcium ion concentrations are abnormally high; restores homeostasis by increasing the rate of bone deposition and the renal rate of calcium loss, 173, 392

Calcitriol, 164, 173, 405, 412

Calcium, 27, 165, 217, 681

Calcium ion concentrations, 401, 402

Calcium stones, 714

Calorie: The amount of heat required to raise the temperature of one gram of water 1°C, 684

Calorigenic effect, 399

Calorimeter, 684

cAMP, 390

CAMs, 99

Canaliculi: Microscopic passageways between cells; bile canaliculi carry bile to bile ducts in the liver; in bone, canaliculi permit the diffusion of nutrients and wastes to and from osteocytes, 114

Cancer: Illness characterized by mutations leading to the uncontrolled growth and replication of the affected cells, 90
    aging, 123
    breast, 756
    cell division, 86
    colon, 646
    lung, 609
    rectal, 649
    skin, 135
    stomach, 630
    testicular, 738

Capacitation, 741, 772

Capillaries, 490

Capillary bed, 494

Capillary blood pressure, 509

Capillary exchange, 498–499

Capillary hydrostatic pressure (CHP), 499

Capillary physiology, 499

Capillary pressure, 498–499

Capitulum: A small, elevated articular process; used to refer to the rounded distal surface of the humerus that articulates with the radial head, 189

Capnogram, 606

Capnograph, 606

Capnography, 606

Capnometry, 606

Carbohydrate: Organic compound containing carbon, hydrogen, and oxygen in a 1:2:1 ratio, 41, 50

Carbohydrate digestion, 652

Carbohydrate loading, 671

Carbohydrate metabolism, 666–672

Carbon, 27

Carbon dioxide: a compound produced by the decarboxylation reactions of aerobic metabolism, 35, 722–723

Carbon dioxide transport, 601–602

Carbon monoxide (CO), 601

Carbon monoxide poisoning, 601

Carbonic acid, 722

Carbonic acid-bicarbonate buffer system, 723, 724

Cardiac arrhythmias, 478

Cardiac center, 484

Cardiac cycle: One complete heartbeat, including atrial and ventricular systole and diastole, 478

Cardiac muscle cells, 460

Cardiac muscle tissue, 118–120, 233–234

Cardiac output (CO): The amount of blood ejected by the left ventricle each minute; normally about 5 liters, 481–484

Cardiac skeleton, 465

Cardiac veins, 463

Cardiogenic shock, 509

Cardiology, APP-2

Cardiovascular centers: Poorly localized centers in the reticular formation of the medulla of the brain; includes cardioacceleratory, cardioinhibitory, and vasomotor centers, 309

Cochlear duct: Membranous tube within the cochlea that is filled with endolymph and contains the organ of Corti, 372, 375

Codon: A sequence of three nitrogenous bases along an mRNA strand that will specify the location of a single amino acid in a peptide chain, 84

Collagen fibers, 110, 136

Collateral ganglia, 325

Collecting duct, 697

Collecting system, 697, 699

Colle's fracture, 167

Colloid osmotic pressure, 67

Colloids, 67, 72

Colon: The large intestine, 646

Colon and rectal surgery, APP-2

Colon cancer, 655

Colony-stimulating factors (CSFs), 447, 561

Colorectal cancer, 649

Colorimetric devices, 606

Colostrum, 796

Columnar epithelium, 102

Comminuted fracture, 167

Common iliac arteries, 512

Common iliac vein, 523

Common pathway: In the clotting response, the events that begin with the appearance of prothrombinase and end with the formation of a clot, 449

Commotio cordis, 481

Community-acquired pneumonia, 586

Compact bone: Dense bone containing parallel osteons, 158

Complement system, 548

Complementary base pairs, 49

Complete abortion, 797

Complete proteins, 680

Complete tetanus, 223

Complete transection, 295

Compound: A molecule containing two or more elements in a specific combination, 28

Compression, 223

Compression fractures, 185

Concentration gradient: Regional differences in the concentration of a particular substance, 64

Conception, 771

Condensation, 33

Condom, 763

Conducting cells, 473

Conducting system, 473–475

Conduction, 685

Condylar process, 181

Cone: Retinal photoreceptor responsible for color vision, 357, 364

Congenital hypothyroidism, 422

Congestive heart failure, 499

Conjoined (Siamese) twins, 792

Conjunctiva: A layer of stratified squamous epithelium that covers the inner surfaces of the lids and the anterior surface of the eye to the edges of the cornea, 354

Conjunctival abrasion, 368

Conjunctival injuries, 368

Conjunctivitis, 354

Connective tissue fibers, 110

Connective tissue proper, 108, 109–112

Connective tissues: One of the four primary tissue types; provides a structural framework for the body that stabilizes the relative positions of the other tissue types; includes connective tissue proper, cartilage, bone, and blood; always has cell products, cells, and ground substance, 108–114

classifying connective tissues, 108

connective tissue proper, 108, 109–110

fluid, 112–113

supporting, 109, 113–114

Constipation, 650

Continuous positive airway pressure (CPAP), 592

Continuous propagation, 282

Contractile cells, 471–473

Contrecoup injury, 332

Control center, 6

Control of room temperature, 10

Controlled mechanical ventilation (CMV), 592

Convection, 685

Convergence: In the nervous system, the term indicates that the axons from several neurons innervate a single neuron; most common along motor pathways, 287

COPD, 597

Copper, 681

Coracobrachialis, 252

Coracoid process: A hook-shaped process of the scapula that projects above the anterior surface of the capsule of the shoulder joint, 188

Cord compression, 295

Cord concussion, 295

Cord contusion, 295

Cord hemorrhage, 295

Cord lacerations, 295

Cornea: Transparent portion of the fibrous tunic of the anterior surface of the eye, 354, 355

Corneal injuries, 368

Cornified, 133

Coronal plane, 14

Coronal suture, 176

Coronary arteries, 467

Coronary arteriography, 469, 485

Coronary artery bypass grafting (CABG), 471

Coronary artery disease, 468–471

Coronary circulation, 458, 467

Coronary sinus, 463, 468

Coronary sulcus, 459

Coronoid fossa, 189

Coronoid process, 189

Corpora cavernosa, 743

Corpus luteum: Progestin-secreting mass of follicle cells that develops in the ovary after ovulation, 749

Corpus spongiosum, 743

Cortex: Outer layer or portion of an organ, 140

Cortical nephrons, 697

Corticospinal pathway, 318, 320

Corticosteroids: A steroid hormone produced by the adrenal cortex, 406

Corticosterone, 406

Cortisol: One of the corticosteroids secreted by the adrenal cortex; a glucocorticoid, 406

Cortisone, 406

Costal cartilages, 186

Cotransport: Membrane transport of a nutrient, such as glucose, in company with the movement of an ion, usually sodium; transport requires a carrier protein but does not involve direct ATP expenditure and can occur regardless of the concentration gradient for the nutrient, 69

Coughing reflex, 581

Counter-transport, 69

Coup injury, 332

Covalent bond: A chemical bond between atoms that involves the sharing of electrons, 30

Cowper's glands, 703

Coxal bone, 190, 191

CP. *See* Creatine phosphate (CP)

CPAP, 592

CPK, 229

Cranial, 16

Cranial cavity, 175

Cranial-facial disjunction, 171

Cranial nerves: The twelve peripheral nerves originating at the brain, 310–312

Cranium, 174

Creatine kinase (CK), 236

Creatine phosphate (CP): A high-energy compound present in muscle cells; during muscular activity, the phosphate group is donated to ADP, regenerating ATP, 229

Creatine phosphokinase (CPK), 229

Creatinine: A breakdown product of creatine metabolism, 702

Crenation: Cellular shrinkage due to an osmotic movement of water out of the cytoplasm, 66

Creutzfeldt-Jakob Disease (CJD), 291

Cribriform plate: Portion of the ethmoid bone of the skull that contains the foramina used by the axons of olfactory receptors en route to the olfactory bulbs of the cerebrum, 180

Cricoid cartilage: Ring-shaped cartilage forming the inferior margin of the larynx, 580

Criminal abortion, 797

Crista ampullaris: Hair cells attached to the wall of the ampulla form a raised structure, 374

Crista galli, 180

CRNAs, APP-6

Cross-bridge: Myosin head that projects from the surface of a thick filament and that can bind to an active site of a thin filament in the presence of calcium ions, 217–218

Crossing-over, 740

Crush injury, 145

Cryptorchidism, 738

Crystalloids, 70–72

CSF. *See* Cerebrospinal fluid (CSF)

CSFs, 561

CT scan, 20

Cuboidal epithelium, 102

Cushing's disease, 422

Cushing's syndrome, 408–409

Cuspids, 623

Cutaneous membrane: The epidermis and papillary layer of the dermis, 118, 129

Cuticle: Layer of dead, cornified cells surrounding the shaft of a hair; for nails, 140

CVA, 331–332

Cyanosis: Bluish coloration of the skin due to the presence of deoxygenated blood in vessels near the body surface, 135

Cystic fibrosis (CF), 575, 579, 802

Cystic vein, 525

Cysticercosis, 291

Cytokines, 548, 549

Cytokinesis: The cytoplasmic movement that separates two daughter cells at the completion of mitosis, 89

Cytology, 3, 58

Cytoplasm: The material between the cell membrane and the nuclear membrane, 74–79

Cytosine: One of the nitrogenous base components of nucleic acids, 48

Cytoskeleton: A network of microtubules and microfilaments in the cytoplasm, 75

Cytosol: The fluid portion of the cytoplasm, 75

Cytotoxic T cells: Lymphocytes involved in call-mediated immunity that kill target cells by direct contact or through the secretion of lymphotoxins; also called killer T cells, 540, 553–554

D

D_5W, 70, 71

DAI, 333

Date rape, 760

Daughter chromosomes, 89

DCIS, 756

DCT. *See* Distal convoluted tubule (DCT)

Deamination, 676

Deciduous teeth, 623

Decomposition reaction: A chemical reaction that breaks a molecule into smaller fragments, 31–33

Decompression of the chest, 590

Decompression sickness, 598

Deep, 16

Deep femoral artery, 519

Deep femoral vein, 523

Deep venous thrombosis, 453, 587

Defecation: The elimination of fecal wastes, 650

Defecation reflex, 650

Defibrillation, 471, 475

Deflation reflex, 605

Degenerative joint disease (DJD), 197

Degloving avulsion, 145

Dehydration: A reduction in the water content of the body that threatens homeostasis, 67

Dehydration synthesis: The joining of two molecules associated with the removal of a water molecule, 33

Delayed hypersensitivity, 565

Delivery, 790

Delta receptors, 347

Delta waves, 304, 347

Deltoid, 250, 252

INDEX

Electron transport system (ETS): The cytochrome system responsible for most of the energy production in cells; a complex bound to the inner mitochondrial membrane, 668–670

Element: All of the atoms with the same atomic number, 26

Elevation: Movement in a superior, or upward, direction, 199

Ellipsoidal joints, 201

Embolectomy, 518

Embolus: An air bubble, fat globule, or blood clot drifting in the bloodstream, 450

Embryo: Developmental stage beginning at fertilization and ending at the start of the third developmental month, 751

Embryogenesis, 779

Embryology: The study of embryonic development, focusing on the first 2 months after fertilization, 771

Embryonic development, 771

Emergency cardiac care (ECC), 478

Emergency incident rehabilitation (EIR), 686

Emergency medical services. *See* EMS

Emergency medicine, APP-2

Emmetropia, 363

Emphysema, 593, 597, 609

EMS
   nutrition, 687
   obesity, 112
   physical demands, 246
   stress, 420

Enamel: Crystalline material similar in mineral composition to bone, but harder and without osteocytes, that covers the exposed surfaces of the teeth, 622

Encephalitis, 291

Encyclopedia of DNA Elements (ENCODE), 804

Endergonic, 34

Endocardium: The simple squamous epithelium that lines the heart and is continuous with the endothelium of the great vessels, 460, 462

Endochondral ossification: The conversion of a cartilaginous model to bone; the characteristic mode of formation for skeletal elements other than the bones of the cranium, the clavicles, and sesamoid bones, 162–164

Endocrine disorders, 422

Endocrine emergencies, 392

Endocrine pancreas, 410

Endocrine secretions, 99

Endocrine system, 8, 386–427
   adipose tissue, 418
   adrenal glands, 406–408
   aging, 420–423
   behavior, 420
   emergencies/system disorders, 392
   endocrine regulation, 392–393
   gonads, 417–418
   growth, 419
   heart, 415–417
   hormonal action, 389–392
   intercellular communication in homeostasis, 387–388
   intestines, 412
   kidneys, 412–415

   pancreas, 410–412
   parathyroid glands, 405
   pineal gland, 409–410
   pituitary gland, 394–398
   stress, 420
   thymus, 417
   thyroid gland, 398–401

Endocrinology diabetes and metabolism, APP-2

Endocytosis: The movement of relatively large volumes of extracellular material into the cytoplasm via the formation of a membranous vesicle at the cell surface; includes pinocytosis and phagocytosis, 72–73

Endoderm: One of the three primary germ layers; the layer on the undersurface of the embryonic disc that gives rise to the epithelia and glands of the digestive system, the respiratory system, and portions of the urinary system, 776, 777

Endolymph: Fluid contents of the membranous labyrinth (the saccule, utricle, semicircular canals, and cochlear duct) of the inner ear, 371

Endometriosis, 752

Endometrium: The mucous membrane lining the uterus, 751

Endomysium: A delicate network of connective tissue fibers that surrounds individual muscle cells, 214

Endoplasmic reticulum (ER): A network of membranous channels in the cytoplasm of a cell that function in intracellular transport, synthesis, storage, packaging, and secretion, 76, 77

Endosteum, 160

End-tidal CO_2 ($ETCO_2$), 606

Energy, 31

Energy concepts, 31

Enzyme: A protein that catalyzes a specific biochemical reaction, 34, 47, 63

Eosinophil: A granulocyte (WBC) with a lobed nucleus and red-staining granules; participates in the immune response and is especially important during allergic reactions, 446

Ependyma: Layer of cells lining the ventricles and central canal of the CNS, 274, 275

Ependymal cells, 274, 275

Epicardium: Serous membrane covering the outer surface of the heart; also called visceral pericardium, 459, 462

Epicranial aponeurosis, 242

Epicranium, 242

Epidermal ridges, 131

Epidermis: The epithelium covering the surface of the skin, 130–134

Epididymis: Coiled duct that connects the rete testis to the ductus deferens; site of functional maturation of spermatozoa, 736, 741

Epidural block, 288

Epidural hematoma, 289, 333

Epidural hemorrhage, 289

Epidural space: Space between the spinal dura mater and the walls of the vertebral foramen; contains blood vessels and adipose tissue; a frequent site of injection for regional anesthesia, 288

Epiglottis: Blade-shaped flap of tissue, reinforced by cartilage, that is attached to the dorsal and superior surface of the thyroid cartilage; it folds over the entrance to the larynx during swallowing, 580

Epilepsy, 306

Epimysium: A dense layer of collagen fibers that surrounds a skeletal muscle and is continuous with the tendons/aponeuroses of the muscle and with the perimysium, 214

Epinephrine, 407

Epiphyseal closure, 164

Epiphyseal line, 164

Epiphyses: The head of a long bone, 158

Episiotomy, 791

Epithalamus, 296, 307

Epithelia: One of the four primary tissue types; a layer of cells that forms a superficial covering or an internal lining of a body cavity or vessel, 97

Epithelial tissue, 97–101
   basement membrane, 100–101
   classifying epithelia, 102–104
   epithelial renewal and repair, 101
   epithelial surface, 99–100
   functions, 97–98
   glandular epithelia, 104–107
   intercellular connections, 99

EPO. *See* Erythropoietin (EPO)

Eponychium, 143

EPS, 321

Epsilon receptors, 347

Equilibrium, 33, 372–375

ER. *See* Endoplasmic reticulum (ER)

Erectile dysfunction (ED): an inability to achieve or maintain an erection, 760

Erector spinae, 244

ERV, 593

Erythroblasts, 438

Erythropoiesis: The formation of red blood cells, 434, 438–440

Erythropoietin (EPO): Hormone released by kidney tissues exposed to low oxygen concentrations; stimulates erythropoiesis in bone marrow, 412, 419, 434, 438, 506

Esophagitis, 625

Esophagus: A muscular tube that connects the pharynx to the stomach, 617

Essential amino acids: Amino acids that cannot be synthesized in the body in adequate amounts and must be obtained from the diet, 677

Essential fatty acids: Fatty acids that cannot be synthesized in the body and must be obtained from the diet, 675

Estradiol, 756

Estrogens: A class of steroid sex hormones that includes estradiol, 417, 418, 746, 757, 761, 762

Ether, 52

Ethmoid bone, 180

Ethmoidal sinuses, 180

ETS. *See* Electron transport system (ETS)

Evaporation: Movement of molecules from the liquid to the gaseous state, 685

Eversion: A turning outward, 199

Exanthems, 138

Excessive coagulation, 450

Exchange pump, 69

Exchange reaction, 33

Exercise, 508–509

Exergonic, 34

Exfoliative cytology, 107

Exocrine glands: A gland that secretes onto the body surface or into a passageway connected to the exterior, 107

Exocrine secretions, 104

Exocytosis: The ejection of cytoplasmic materials by fusion of a membranous vesicle with the cell membrane, 73–74

Expiratory reserve volume (ERV), 593

Expulsion stage, 790

Extension: An increase in the angle between two articulating bones; the opposite of flexion, 197

Extensor carpi radialis, 255, 256

Extensor carpi ulnaris, 255, 256

Extensor digitorum, 255

Extensor digitorum longus, 261

Extensor hallucis longus, 261

External anal sphincter, 248, 648

External callus, 166

External carotid artery, 517

External ear: The pinna, external acoustic canal, and tympanum, 370–371

External hemorrhoids, 649

External iliac vein, 523

External intercostals, 248

External jugular veins, 520

External nares: The nostrils; the external openings into the nasal cavity, 578

External oblique, 248

External receptors, 273

External respiration, 589

External urethral sphincter, 248, 713

Extracellular fluid (ECF): All body fluid other than that contained within cells; includes plasma and interstitial fluid, 59, 60, 717

Extraembryonic membranes: The yolk sac, amnion, chorion, and allantois, 777–778, 780

Extrapyramidal motor syndromes, 321

Extrinsic eye muscles, 354, 355

Extrinsic pathway: Clotting pathway that begins with damage to blood vessels or surrounding tissues and ends with the activation of Factor X, forming prothrombinase, 449, 450

Eye, 353–359
   accessory structures, 353–354
   accommodation, 361–362
   aqueous humor, 359
   emergencies, 368–369
   image formation, 362
   lens, 359–360
   light refraction, 361–362
   optic disc, 359
   retina, 357–359
   visual pathway, 366–369
   visual physiology, 362–369

INDEX

Glossopharyngeal nerve: Cranial nerve IX, 312

Glottis: The passage from the pharynx to the larynx, 581

Glucagon: Hormone secreted by the alpha cells of the pancreatic islets; elevates blood glucose concentrations, 410

Glucocorticoids (GCs): Hormones secreted by the adrenal cortex to modify glucose metabolism; cortisol, cortisone, and corticosterone are important examples, 406–408

Gluconeogenesis: The synthesis of glucose from protein or lipid precursors, 670–672

Glucose: A six-carbon sugar, the preferred energy source for most cells and the only energy source for neurons under normal conditions, 39

Gluteal nerves, 313

Gluteus maximus, 258

Gluteus medius, 258

Gluteus minimus, 258

Glycerol, 43

Glycogen: A polysaccharide that represents an important energy reserve; a polymer consisting of a long chain of glucose molecules, 41, 672

Glycolysis: The anaerobic cytoplasmic breakdown of glucose into lactic acid by way of pyruvic acid, with a net gain of two ATP, 230–231, 667–668

GnRH, 745, 746, 758

Goiter, 422

Golgi apparatus: Cellular organelle consisting of a series of membranous plates that gives rise to lysosomes and secretory vesicles, 77–78

Gomphosis, 195

Gonadal arteries, 519

Gonadotropin-releasing hormone (GnRH): Hypothalamic releasing hormone that causes the secretion of FSH and LH by the anterior pituitary gland, 745, 746, 758

Gonadotropins, 395

Gonads: Organs that produce gametes and hormones, 417–428

Gracilis, 258

Graded potentials, 279

Grand mal seizures, 306

Granulation tissue, 145

Granulocytes: White blood cells containing granules visible with the light microscope; includes eosinophils, basophils, and neutrophils; also called granular leukocytes, 444

Graves' disease, 403

Gray matter: Areas in the CNS dominated by neuron bodies, glial cells, and unmyelinated axons, 272, 275, 292

Great saphenous vein, 523

Greater omentum: A large fold of the dorsal mesentery of the stomach that hangs in front of the intestines, 625

Greater trochanter, 192, 193

Greater tubercle, 188

Greenstick fracture, 167

Gross anatomy: The study of the structural features of the human body without the aid of a microscope, 3

Ground substance, 110

Growth, 419

Growth hormone (GH): Anterior pituitary hormone that stimulates tissue growth and anabolism when nutrients are abundant and restricts tissue glucose dependence when nutrients are in short supply, 397

Growth-plate injuries, 169–170

Guanine: One of the nitrogenous bases found in nucleic acids, 48

Gustatory cortex, 301

Gustatory receptors, 352

H

H_1 receptors, 566

H_2 receptors, 566

Habitual abortion, 797

Hair: A keratinous strand produced by epithelial cells of the hair follicle, 139–141

Hair cells: Sensory cells of the inner ear, 370, 372

Hair color, 140–141

Hair follicle: An accessory structure of the integument; a tube, lined by a stratified squamous epithelium, that begins at the surface of the skin and ends at the hair papilla, 139

Hair loss, 140

Hair papilla, 139

Hair root: A thickened, conical structure consisting of a connective tissue papilla and the overlying matrix; a layer of epithelial cells that produces the hair shaft, 140

Hair shaft, 140

Hallux, 194

Hamstrings, 256, 258

Haploid: Possessing half the normal number of chromosomes; a characteristic of gametes, 739

Hard palate: The bony roof of the oral cavity, formed by the maxillary and palatine bones, 578, 620

Haversian canal, 160

Haversian system, 160

hCG. *See* Human chorionic gonadotropin (hCG)

HDLs, 675, 676

HDN, 443

Headache, 321–322

Hearing, 375

deficits, 378

Heart, 415, 457–486. *See also* Cardiovascular system

anatomical figures, 459, 461

blood supply, 467–468

cardiac cycle, 478–480

cardiac muscle cells, 460

cardiac output, 481–484

conducting system, 473–475

connective tissue, 461

contractile cells, 471–473

coronary artery disease, 468–471

ECC, 478

ECG, 470–471, 476–477

fibrous skeleton, 465

hormones, 481

internal anatomy and blood flow, 464

sounds, 480

valves, 465

ventricles, 458

wall, 459–460, 462

Heart attack, 236

Heart rate, 501

Heart sounds, 480

Heart wall, 459–460, 462

Heartbeat, 468–478

Heat-gain center, 685

Heat-loss center, 685

Helper T cells: Lymphocytes whose secretions and other activities coordinate the cellular and humoral immune responses, 540, 554

Hematocrit: Percentage of the volume of whole blood contributed by cells; also called packed cell volume (PCV) or volume of packed red cells (VPRC), 432

Hematology, APP-2

Hematopoietic stem cells (HSC), 438

Heme: A special organic compound containing a central iron atom that can reversibly bind oxygen molecules; a component of the hemoglobin molecule, 435

Hemidesmosomes, 99

Hemispheric lateralization, 303

Hemocytoblasts, 438, 541

Hemoglobin: Protein composed of four globular subunits, each bound to a single molecule of heme; the protein found in red blood cells that gives them the ability to transport oxygen in the blood, 434

Hemoglobin recycling, 436–438

Hemoglobinuria, 436

Hemolysis: Breakdown (lysis) of red blood cells, 66

Hemolytic disease of the newborn (HDN), 443

Hemophilia, 450–451, 799

Hemopoiesis: Blood cell formation and differentiation, 432

Hemorrhage: Blood loss, 508

Hemorrhagic strokes, 331

Hemorrhoids, 649

Hemostasis, 448–449

Hemothorax, 588

Heparin, 446

Hepatic abscesses, 643

Hepatic portal system, 524–525

Hepatic portal vein: Vessel that carries blood between the intestinal capillaries and the sinusoids of the liver, 525

Hepatitis A, 644

Hepatitis B, 644

Hepatitis C, 644

Hepatitis D, 644–645

Hepatitis E, 645

Hepatitis F, 645

Hepatitis G, 645

Hepatocyte: A liver cell, 639

Hepatopancreatic sphincter, 643

Hernia, 245

Herniated disc, 200

Herpes zoster, 138

Hespan, 72

Hetastarch, 72

Heterozygous: Possessing two different alleles at corresponding locations on a chromosome pair; a heterozygous individual's phenotype may be determined by one or both alleles, 799

hGH, 397

Hiatal hernia, 245, 625

High-density lipoprotein (HDL): A lipoprotein with a relatively small lipid content, thought to be responsible for the movement of cholesterol from peripheral tissues to the liver, 676

High-energy bonds, 49

High-energy compounds, 49, 52

Hilum: A localized region where blood vessels, lymphatics, nerves, and/ or other anatomical structures are attached to an organ, 696

Hinge joints, 201, 203

Hip fractures, 171, 172, 192

Hip joint, 203–204

Hirsutism, 141

Histamine: Chemical released by stimulated mast cells or basophils to initiate or enhance an inflammatory response, 548

Histology: The study of tissues, 3, 97

Histones, 82

HIV, 560

Holocrine secretion, 106

Homan's sign, 523

Homeostasis: The maintenance of a relatively constant internal environment, 6

Homeostatic regulation, 6

Homologous chromosomes: The members of a chromosome pair, each containing the same gene loci, 798

Homozygous: Having the same allele for a particular character on two homologous chromosomes, 799

Hormonal contraceptives, 763

Hormones: Compound secreted by one cell that travel through the circulatory system to affect the activities of cells in another portion of the body, 43, 44

athletic performance, 419

body temperature, 757

cardiovascular regulation, 506

defined, 387

endocrine system (*see* Endocrine system)

female reproductive cycle, 756–757, 762

immune system, 561–563

intestinal, 633–634

kidney function, 707–711

male reproductive system, 746, 762

placental, 778–779

Hospital-acquired pneumonia, 586

hPL. *See* Human placental lactogen (hPL)

Human chorionic gonadotropin (hCG): Placental hormone that maintains the corpus luteum for the first three months of pregnancy, 779

Human Genome Project, 801–805

Human growth hormone (hGH), 397

Human physiology, 4

Human placental lactogen (hPL): Placental hormone that stimulates the functional development of the mammary glands, 779

Humerus, 188

Huntington's disease: An inherited disease marked by a progressive deterioration of mental abilities and by motor disturbances, 800, 802

Hyaline cartilage, 114, 115

Hydrocephalus, 390

Hydrogen, 27

Hydrogen bond: Weak interaction between the hydrogen atom on one molecule and a negatively charged portion of another molecule, 30–31

Hydrogen ions, 37

Hydrolysis: The breakage of a chemical bond through the addition of a water molecule; the reverse of dehydration synthesis, 31–32, 652

Hydrophilic, 62

Hydrophobic, 62

Hydrostatic pressure, 66

Hyoid bone, 181

Hyperadrenalism, 408–409

Hyperextension, 197

Hyperglycemia, 673

Hyperopia, 363

Hyperpolarization, 278

Hypertension, 497

Hypertonic solutions, 68, 70

Hypertrophy: Increase in the size of tissue without cell division, 233

Hyphema, 360, 368

Hypodermis, 137

Hypoglossal nerve, 311, 312

Hypoglycemia, 409, 414, 673

Hypogonadism, 396

Hypophyseal portal system: Network of vessels that carry blood from capillaries in the hypothalamus to capillaries in the anterior pituitary (hypophysis), 394

Hypophysis: The anterior pituitary, 394

Hypothalamus: The floor of the diencephalon; region of the brain containing centers involved with the unconscious regulation of visceral functions, emotions, drives, and the coordination of neural and endocrine functions, 296, 389, 393

Hypothyroidism, 402

Hypotonic solutions, 68, 70

Hypovolemic shock, 509

Hypoxia: Low tissue oxygen concentrations, 438, 589

Hypoxic drive, 605

I

I band, 217, 218

IACD, 475

ICF, 717

ICH, 333

IgA, 559

IgD, 559

IgE, 559

IGFs, 397

IgG, 559

IgM, 559

IH, 393

IL. *See* Interleukins (IL)

Ileum: The last 2.5 m of the small intestine, 631

Iliocostalis, 244

Ilium: The largest of the three bones whose fusion creates a coxa, 190

Immediate hypersensitivity, 564, 565

Immune disorders, 563–564

Immune response, 564

Immunity, 555–556. *See also* Lymphatic system and immunity

Immunization: Developing immunity by the deliberate exposure to antigens under conditions that prevent the development of illness but stimulate the production of memory B cells, 550, 556

Immunodeficiency disease, 563

Immunoglobulin: A circulating antibody, 433, 541, 558

Immunological escape, 548

Impacted fracture, 171

Implantation: The erosion of a blastocyst into the uterine wall, 764, 774–776

Implanted automatic cardioverter-defibrillator (IACD), 475

IMV, 592

Inadequate coagulation, 450–451

Incisional hernia, 245

Incisors, 623

Incomplete abortion, 797

Incomplete proteins, 680

Incomplete tetanus, 223

Incontinence, 716

Incus: The central auditory ossicle, situated between the malleus and the stapes in the middle ear cavity, 371

Inevitable abortion, 797

Infectious disease, APP-2

Inferior, 15, 16

Inferior mesenteric artery, 518

Inferior mesenteric vein, 524

Inferior nasal conchae, 180

Inferior vena cava: The vein that carries blood from the parts of the body below the heart to the right auricle, 463, 523

Infertility, 757

Inflammation: A nonspecific defense mechanism that operates at the tissue level, characterized by swelling, redness, warmth, pain, and some loss of function, 120, 547

Inflation reflex: A reflex mediated by the vagus nerve that prevents overexpansion of the lungs, 605

Infra-orbital foramen, 180

Infraspinatus, 252

Infraspinous fossa, 188

Infundibulum: A tapering, funnel-shaped structure; in the nervous system, the connection between the pituitary gland and the hypothalamus; in the uterine tube, the entrance bounded by fimbriae that receives the oocytes at ovulation, 751

Ingestion: The introduction of materials into the digestive tract via the mouth, 616

Inguinal hernia: The area near the junction of the trunk and the thighs that contains the external genitalia, 245

Inheritance, 771

Inherited disorders, 802

Inhibin: A hormone produced by the sustentacular cells that inhibits the pituitary secretion of FSH, 396, 417, 740, 762

Inhibiting hormone (IH), 393

Innate immunity, 545, 555

Inner cell mass: Cells of the blastocyst that will form the body of the embryo, 774, 777

Inorganic compounds, 34–35

Inspiratory reserve volume (IRV): The maximum amount of air that can be drawn into the lungs over and above the normal tidal volume, 595

Insula, 300

Insulin: Hormone secreted by the beta cells of the pancreatic islets; causes a reduction in plasma glucose concentrations, 408, 410

Insulin-like growth factors (IGFs), 397

Insulin shock, 414

Integumentary system, 7, 128–154

  aging, 149–151

  burns, 147–149

  dermis, 136–137

  epidermis, 130–134

  functions, 129

  hair, 139–141

  limb replantation, 146–147

  nail, 143

  sebaceous glands, 141–142

  skin cancer, 136

  skin color, 134–135

  skin diseases, 138

  skin repair, 151

  soft-tissue wounds, 145–146

  sweat glands, 142–143

Interatrial septum, 463, 464

Intercalated discs: Regions where adjacent cardiocytes interlock and where gap junctions permit the movement of ions and action potentials between the cells, 234, 460

Intercellular cement: A combination of protein and carbohydrate molecules, especially hyaluronic acid, between adjacent epithelial cells, 99

Interferons: Peptides released by virus-infected cells, especially lymphocytes, that make other cells more resistant to viral infection and slow viral replication, 547, 548, 561

Interleukins (IL): Peptides released by activated monocytes and lymphocytes that assist in the coordination of the cellular and humoral immune responses, 561

Interlobar arteries, 697

Interlobular arteries, 697

Interlobular veins, 697

Intermittent mandatory ventilation (IMV), 592

Internal anal sphincter, 648

Internal callus, 166

Internal carotid artery, 517

Internal ear, 371–372

Internal hemorrhoids, 649

Internal iliac artery, 519

Internal iliac vein, 523

Internal intercostals, 246

Internal jugular veins, 520

Internal medicine, APP-2

Internal nares: The entrance to the nasopharynx from the nasal cavity, 578

Internal oblique, 248

Internal receptors: Sensory receptors monitoring the functions and status of internal organs and systems, 273

Internal respiration, 589

Internal thoracic artery, 516

Internal urethral sphincter, 713

Interneuron: An association neuron; neurons inside the CNS that are interposed between sensory and motor neurons, 273

Internship, APP-1

Interphase: Stage in the life of a cell during which the chromosomes are uncoiled and all normal cellular functions except mitosis are underway, 87–88

Interstitial cells, 738

Interstitial fluid: Fluid in the tissues that fills the spaces between cells, 60

Interventricular septum, 463, 464

Intervertebral articulations, 200–202

Intervertebral disc: Fibrocartilage pad between the bodies of successive vertebrae that acts as a shock absorber, 183, 200

Intestines, 412

Intracellular fluid (ICF), 717

Intracerebral hemorrhage (ICH), 331

Intramembranous ossification: The formation of bone within a connective tissue without the prior development of a cartilaginous model, 162

Intramuscular injections, 250

Intraosseous (IO) route of medication administration, 159

Intrauterine device (IUD), 764

Intrinsic pathway: A pathway of the clotting system within the bloodstream that begins with the activation of platelets and ends with the activation of Factor X, forming prothrombinase, 450

Invasion, 90

Inversion, 199

IO route of medication administration, 159

Iodine, 27

Ion pumps, 69

Ionic bond: Molecular bond created by the attraction between ions with opposite charges, 28–29

Ionization: Dissociation; the breakdown of a molecule in solution to form ions, 35

Iris: A contractile structure made up of smooth muscle that forms the colored portion of the eye, 357

Iron, 27, 681

Iron deficiency anemia, 438

Irregular bones, 158

IRV, 595

Ischemic strokes, 331

Ischiocavernosus, 248

Ischium, 190

Islets of Langerhans, 410

Isometric contraction: A muscular contraction characterized by rising tension production but no change in length, 228

INDEX

Isotonic contraction: A muscular contraction during which tension climbs and then remains stable as the muscle shortens, 228

Isotonic solutions, 68, 70

Isotopes: Forms of an element whose atoms contain the same number of protons but different numbers of neutrons (and thus differ in atomic weight), 27

IUD, 764

IV fluid therapy, 70–72

J

Jaundice, 135, 438

Jejunum: The middle portion of the small intestine, 631

Joint capsule: Dense collagen fiber sleeve that surrounds a joint and provides protection and stabilization; also called articular capsule, 196

Joint movements, 197–199

Jugular notch, 186

Juvenile-onset diabetes, 413

Juxtaglomerular apparatus: The macula densa and the juxtaglomerular cells; a complex responsible for the release of renin and erythropoietin, 701

Juxtamedullary nephrons, 697

K

Kappa receptors, 347

Karyotype, 798

kcal, 684

Keloid, 145, 149

Keratin: Tough, fibrous protein component of nails, hair, calluses, and the general integumentary surface, 133

Keratinized, 133

Keratinocytes, 130

Kernig's sign, 290

Ketoacidosis, 677

Ketone bodies: Organic acids produced during the catabolism of lipids and certain amino acids; acetone is one example, 674, 676

Ketosis, 677

Kidney: A component of the urinary system; an organ functioning in the regulation of plasma composition, including the excretion of wastes and the maintenance of normal fluid and electrolyte balance, 694–702

Kidney function, 707–712

Kidney lobe, 697

Kidney stones, 714–715

Kidney transplant, 712

Killer T cells, 553–554

Kilocalorie (kcal): The amount of heat required to raise the temperature of a kilogram of water 1°C, 684

Kinetic energy, 31

Klinefelter syndrome, 805

Knee jerk reflex, 315

Knee joint, 204–205

Korsakoff's syndrome, 683

Krebs cycle, 230, 688

Kupffer cells: Phagocytic cells of the liver sinusoids, 640

Kuru, 291

L

Labia: Lips; labia majora and minora are components of the female external genitalia, 620

Labia majora, 755

Labia minora, 755

Labor, 790–792

Labor contractions, 789

Laboratory values, 703

Laceration, 145

Lacrimal apparatus, 354

Lacrimal bones, 180

Lacrimal caruncle, 354

Lacrimal gland: Tear gland on the dorsolateral surface of the eye, 354

Lactated Ringer, 70

Lactation: The production of milk by the mammary glands, 755

Lacteal: A terminal lymphatic within an intestinal villus, 632

Lactic acid recycling, 231

Lactic dehydrogenase (LDH), 236

Lactiferous duct, 755

Lactiferous sinus: An expanded portion of a lactiferous duct adjacent to the nipple of a breast, 756

Lactose intolerance, 654

Lambdoid suture: Synarthrotic articulation between the parietal and occipital bones of the cranium, 177

Lamellated corpuscles, 348

Langer's lines, 131

Large intestine: The terminal portions of the intestinal tract, consisting of the colon, the rectum, and the anorectal canal, 617, 646–650

Large veins, 492

Laryngopharynx: Division of the pharynx inferior to the epiglottis and superior to the esophagus, 579

Larynx: A complex cartilaginous structure that surrounds and protects the glottis and vocal cords; the superior margin is bound to the hyoid bone, and the inferior margin is bound to the trachea, 580–581

Lateral, 18

Lateral canthus, 354

Lateral epicondyle, 189

Lateral malleolus, 193

Lateral sulcus, 300

Latissimus dorsi, 250

LCIS, 756

LDH, 236

LDLs, 675

LeFort I fracture, 171, 172

LeFort II fracture, 171, 172

Left common carotid artery, 513

Left lower quadrant (LLQ), 15

Left primary bronchus, 581

Left subclavian artery, 513

Left upper quadrant (LUQ), 15

Lens: The transparent body lying behind the iris and pupil and in front of the vitreous humor, 359–360

Lentiform nucleus, 305

Leptin, 418

Lesser omentum: A small pocket in the mesentery that connects the lesser curvature of the stomach to the liver, 625

Lesser trochanter, 192, 193

Lesser tubercle, 188

Leukemia: A malignant disease of the blood-forming tissues, 446

Leukocyte: A white blood cell, 433

Leukocytosis, 446

Leukopenia, 446

Levator ani, 248

Levator scapulae, 250

Levels of organization, 4–6

LH. *See* Luteinizing hormone (LH)

Lifting, 246

Ligament: Dense band of connective tissue fibers that attach one bone to another, 112, 196

Ligands, 73

Light micrograph (LM), 58

Light microscopy, 58

Light refraction, 361–362

Limb replantation, 146–147

Limbic system: Group of nuclei and centers in the cerebrum and diencephalon that are involved with emotional states, memories, and behavioral drives, 306

Linea aspera, 192

Lingual frenulum: An epithelial fold that attaches the inferior surface of the tongue to the floor of the mouth, 620

Lipid: An organic compound containing carbons, hydrogens, and oxygens in a ratio that does not approximate 1:2:1; includes fats, oils, and waxes, 41–43

Lipid catabolism, 673–674

Lipid digestion, 652

Lipid metabolism, 673–676

Lipid synthesis, 675

Lipogenesis, 675

Lipolysis: The catabolism of lipids as a source of energy, 673

Lipoprotein: A compound containing a relatively small lipid bound to a protein, 431, 675–676

Liver: An organ of the digestive system with varied and vital functions, including the production of plasma proteins, the excretion of bile, the storage of energy reserves, the detoxification of poisons, and the interconversion of nutrients, 617

Liver transplantation, 643

LLQ, 15

LM, 58

LMWHs, 452

Lobular carcinoma in situ (LCIS), 756

Lobule: The basic organizational unit of the liver at the histological level, 583

Lockjaw, 222

Logarithm, 39

Long bones, 158

Long-term memories, 305

Longissimus, 244

Longitudinal fissure, 300

Loop of Henle, 697, 701

Loose connective tissue: A loosely organized, easily distorted connective tissue containing several fiber types, a varied population of cells, and a viscous ground substance, 110–112

Low-density lipoproteins (LDLs), 675

Lower limb, 192–194

Low-molecular-weight heparins (LMWHs), 452

Lumbar arteries, 519

Lumbar plexus, 312, 313

Lumbar puncture, 290

Lumbar region, 182, 184

Lumbar vertebrae, 182, 184

Lung cancer, 609

Lung volumes/capacities, 593–595

Lunula, 143

LUQ, 15

Luteal phase, 750

Luteinizing hormone (LH): Anterior pituitary hormone that in females assists FSH in follicle stimulation, triggers ovulation, and promotes the maintenance and secretion of the endometrial glands; in males, stimulates spermatogenesis; formerly known as interstitial cell-stimulating hormone in males, 396, 400, 746, 757

Lymph nodes, 543

Lymphadenopathy, 544

Lymphatic capillaries, 539

Lymphatic ducts, 540

Lymphatic system, 8, 537

Lymphatic system and immunity, 536–572

  aging, 564–565

  allergies, 563–564, 567–568

  anatomical barriers, 537

  B cells, 541

  cell participation, 561

  complement system, 548

  components and functions of, 538–546

  fever, 549

  functions of lymphatic system, 539

  hormones, 561–562

  immune surveillance, 548

  immunity, 556

  immunization, 556

  inflammation, 548

  interferon, 548

  lymphatic vessels, 539–540

  lymphocytes, 540–541

  lymphoid nodules, 541

  lymphoid organs, 543–546

  NK cells, 541, 542, 561

  phagocytes, 546–548

  physical barriers, 546

  spleen, 544

  T cells, 540, 553–554

  thymus, 543–544

Lymphatic vessels, 538

Lymphedema, 540

Lymphocyte: A cell of the lymphatic system that participates in the immune response, 445, 537

Lymphoid nodules, 538, 541

Lymphoid organs, 538–541

Lymphoid tissues: loose connective tissues dominated by lymphocytes, 541

Lymphopoiesis: The production of lymphocytes, 447, 541

INDEX

INDEX

INDEX

INDEX

Illustration Credits

Chapter 1 **Chapter Opener** © Taxi/Getty Images **1-07** CMSP/Custom Medical Stock Photo **1-10** Edward Dickinson, MD **1-CN-01** Omikron/Science Source **01-CN-02** Biophoto Associates/Science Source **01-CN-03** CMSP/Custom Medical Stock Photo **01-CN-04** Dr. Kathleen Welch/Frederic Martini **01-CN-05** Dr. Kathleen Welch/Frederic Martini **01-CN-06** National Institute on Aging/NIH/Science Source **01-CN-07** Chad Ehlers/Alamy Stock Photo **01-CN-08** ICVI-CCN/Voisin/Science Source **01-CN-09** Alexander Tsiara/Science Source

Chapter 2 **Chapter Opener** © Taxi/Getty Images **2-04** GYSSELS/BSIP SA/Alamy Stock Photo **02-CN-01** Stockbyte/Getty Images **02-CN-02** Madlen/Shutterstock **2-24** Bryan Bledsoe

Chapter 3 **Chapter Opener** © Taxi/Getty Images **03-07a** Steve Gschmeissner/Science Source **03-07b** David M. Phillips/Science Source **03-07c** Steve Gschmeissner/Science Source **03-16** Transmission Electron Micrograph of Exocytosis, courtesy of Dr. Birgit H. Satir **03-17** Bill Longcore/Science Source **03-18** PhD Alvin Telser/Cultura Science/Getty Images

Chapter 4 **Chapter Opener** © Taxi/Getty Images **04-01-01** Frederic Martini **04-01-02** Biophoto Associates/Science Source **04-04-03** Frederic Martini **04-05-01** Frederic Martini **04-06** Image & © Dr. H. Jastrow from Dr. Jastrow's electron microscopic atlas http://www.drjastrow.de **04-CN-01** Davis, Joeff. Print. **04-09c** Micrograph source material provided by VWR-Ward's Science **04-10b** Frederic Martini **04-11b** Biophoto Associates/Science Source **04-16-01** Donald P Oehman/Shutterstock **04-16-02** Leah-Anne Thompson/Shutterstock

Chapter 5 **Chapter Opener** © Taxi/Getty Images **05-04-03** Cloud Hill Imaging **05-CN-01** Van D Bucher/Science Source/Getty Images **05-CN-02** Hriana/Shutterstock **05-06-01** Science Photo Library/Alamy Stock Photo **05-06-02** D. Kucharski K. Kucharska/Shutterstock **05-07-01** Beneda Miroslav/Shutterstock **05-07-02** bilanol/123RF **05-08** Michael Abbey/Science Source **05-CN-03** herkisi/E+/Getty Images **05-09** Frederic Martini **05-12** William C. Ober, M.D. **05-13** David Effron **05-14** David Effron **05-15a** Edward Dickinson, MD **05-15b** Edward Dickinson, MD **5-16** Edward Dickinson, MD **05-17** Edward Dickinson, MD **05-18** Edward Dickinson, MD **05-19a** Edward Dickinson, MD **05-19b** Edward Dickinson, MD **05-19c** Edward Dickinson, MD **05-21** Scott Camazine/Alamy Stock Photo **05-22** Edward Dickinson, MD **05-23** David Effron **05-25** Dr M.A. Ansary/Science Source

Chapter 6 **Chapter Opener** © Taxi/Getty Images **06-06** Pyng Medical Corp. **06-07** Sgt. Alex Manne/AB Forces News Collection/Alamy Stock Photo **06-CN-01** fotografixx/iStock/Getty Images **06-CN-02** Frederic Martini **06-CN-03** English/Custom Medical Stock Photo **06-CN-04** Zephyr/Science Source **06-CN-05** SIU Biomed Com/Custom Medical Stock Photo **06-CN-07** Image reprinted with permission from Charles T. Mehlman, DO, MPH, Cincinnati Children's Hospital Medical Center, published by Medscape Drugs & Diseases (http://emedicine.medscape.com/), 2015, available at: http://emedicine.medscape.com/article/1260663-overview. **06-CN-08** Frederic Martini **06-CN-09** Scott Camazine/Science Source **06-CN-10** Living Art Enterprises, LLC/Science Source **06-CN-11** kameel/123RF **06-13-01** Edward Dickinson, MD **06-13-02** Edward Dickinson, MD **06-28** William C. Ober, M.D. **06-CN-12** Antonia Reeve/Science Source **06-CN-13** StanRohrer/E+/Getty Images

Chapter 7 **Chapter Opener** © Taxi/Getty Images **07-CN-01** Thanasak Kusolvisitkul/123RF **07-CN-02** Peter Arnold, Inc./Alamy Stock Photo **07-05** pkline/E+/Getty Images **07-11b** Frederic Martini **07-14** William C. Ober, M.D. **07-CN-03** Levent Konuk/Shutterstock **07-24a** William C. Ober, M.D. **07-24b** William C. Ober, M.D.

Chapter 8 **Chapter Opener** © Taxi/Getty Images **08-05a** Biophoto Associates/Science Source **08-05b** Don W. Fawcett/Science Source **08-16** Biophoto Associates/Science Source **08-18b** Frederic Martini **08-19** VideoSurgery/Science Source **08-24** Images & Stories/Alamy Stock Photo **08-26** Science Photo Library/Getty Images **08-CN-01** Eleni Seitanidou/123RF **08-CN-02** Cecilia Magill/Science Source **08-CN-03** KirVKV/123RF **08-CN-04** mevans/E+/Getty Images

Chapter 9 **Chapter Opener** © Taxi/Getty Images **09-11-01** Ed Reschke/Photolibrary/Getty Images **09-11-02** Keith/Custom Medical Stock Publishers **09-14** BSIP SA/Alamy Stock Photo **09-CN-01** Clinical Photography, Central Manchester University Hospitals NHS Foundation Trust, UK/Science Source **09-17-01** Frederic Martini **09-17-02** Jose Oto/BSIP SA/Alamy Stock Photo **09-18** PRISMA ARCHIVO/Alamy Stock Photo **09-CN-02** Blend Boost/DreamPictures/Vstock/AGE Fotostock **09-CN-03** Csaba Deli/Shutterstock

09-23 David Effron **09-24** David Effron **09-25** David Effron **09-31** Biophoto Associates/Science Source **09-CN-04** New vave/Shutterstock

Chapter 10 **Chapter Opener** © Taxi/Getty Images **10-09-01** William C. Ober, M.D. **TBL10-02** "American Thyroid Association Guidelines for Detection of Thyroid Dysfunction." Archives of Internal Medicine 160 (2000): 1573–75. **10-16** Biophoto Associates/Science Source **10-15-02** Biophoto Associates/Science Source **10-19** David Effron **10-CN-01** Mikhail Kokhanchikov/iStock/Getty Images **10-20** ROBERTO SCHMIDT/AFP/Getty Images **10-CN-02** Mediscan/Alamy Stock Photo **10-CN-03** Camazine Scott/Science Source/Getty Images **10-CN-04** Incredible Features/Barcroft Media/Getty Images **10-CN-05** Custom Medical Stock Publishers **10-CN-06** Biophoto Associates/Science Source

Chapter 11 **Chapter Opener** © Taxi/Getty Images **11-01** Dizzy/iStock/Getty Images **11-02a** Frederic Martini **11-02b** Cheryl Power/Science Source **11-CN-01** Eye of Science/Science Source **11-07** Karen E. Petersen, Dept. of Biology, University of Washington **11-10** Mediscan/Alamy Stock Photo

Chapter 12 **Chapter Opener** © Taxi/Getty Images **12-06-01** Biophoto Associates/Science Source **12-06-02** SPL/Science Source **12-08** David Effron **12-10** Bryan Bledsoe **12-11** SPL/Science Source **12-17** Bryan Bledsoe **12-20a** Larry Mulvehill/Science Source **12-CN-01** Maria Dubova/123RF

Chapter 13 **Chapter Opener** © Taxi/Getty Images **13-01** Biophoto Associates/Science Source **13-CN-01** Martin M. Rotker/Science Source **13-CN-02** Ed Reschke/Photolibrary/Getty Images **13-CN-03** B&B photos/Custom Medical Stock Photo **13-03** Biophoto Associates/Science Source **13-07b** Rido/Shutterstock **13-CN-04** William C. Ober, M.D.

Chapter 14 **Chapter Opener** © Taxi/Getty Images **14-02** Frederic Martini **14-05** Biophoto Associates/Science Source **14-CN-01** Dr. P. Marazzi/Science Source **14-18a** Tim Mainiero/Shutterstock **14-18b** Organica/Alamy Stock Photo **14-18c** ShutterstockProfessional/Shutterstock **14-19a** Edward Dickinson, MD **14-19b** Edward Dickinson, MD **14-20** Charles Stewart, MD, FACEP, FAAEM

Chapter 15 **Chapter Opener** © Taxi/Getty Images **15-02b** Photo Insolite Realite/Science Source **15-03** William C. Ober, M.D. **15-04e** CNRI/Science Source **15-CN-01** Science Photo Library/Getty Images **15-11** Vortran Medical Technology **15-CN-02** Khoroshunova Olga/Shutterstock **15-CN-03** Arthur Glauberman/Science Source

Chapter 16 **Chapter Opener** © Taxi/Getty Images **16-12** M.I. Walker/Science Source **16-14c** Frederic Martini **16-25** iStock/Getty Images **16-CN-01** Will & Deni McIntyre/Science Source

Chapter 17 **Chapter Opener** © Taxi/Getty Images **17-CN-01** dehooks/iStock/Getty Images **17-11** U.S. DEPARTMENT OF AGRICULTURE **17-13** Andy Nowack/iStock/Getty Images **17-14** slobo/E+/Getty Images

Chapter 18 **Chapter Opener** © Taxi/Getty Images **18-06** Steve Gschmeissner/Science Source **18-12** Dr. E. Walker/Science Source **18-18** David Effron

Chapter 19 **Chapter Opener** © Taxi/Getty Images **19-10-01** Frederic Martini **19-10-02** Frederic Martini **19-10-03** Jacques Testart/ARFIV/Science Source **19-10-04** Frederic Martini **19-10-05** Claude Edelmann/Science Source **19-10-06** BSIP/AGE Fotostock **19-CN-01** Peter Ardito/Photolibrary/Getty Images

Chapter 20 **Chapter Opener** © Taxi/Getty Images **20-01** Francis Leroy/Custom Medical Stock Photo **20-05** Lennart Nilsson/Tidningarnas Telelgrambyra AB **20-07a** Lennart Nilsson/Tidningarnas Telelgrambyra AB **20-07b** Lennart Nilsson/Tidningarnas Telelgrambyra AB **20-07c** Lennart Nilsson/Tidningarnas Telelgrambyra AB **20-08a** Lennart Nilsson/Tidningarnas Telelgrambyra AB **20-08b** Molly Ward/Science Source **20-14-01** Victoria Penafiel/Moment/Getty Images **20-14-02** jaroo/iStock/Getty Images **20-14-03** jaroon/E+/Getty Images **20-14-04** jhorrocks/E+/Getty Images **20-14-05** Jacob Wackerhausen/iStock/Getty Images **20-15** Bryan Bledsoe **20-17** CNRI/Science Source **20-CN-01** CNRI/Science Source

Appendix 1 **A01-01** Michal Heron

Appendix 2 **A01-03** Michal Heron

All chapters ayzek/Shutterstock

FM **FM-01** Bryan Bledsoe **FM-02** Frederic Martini **FM-03** Edwin F. Bartholomew **FM-04** William C. Ober, M.D. **FM-05** Claire E. Ober **FM-06** Kathleen Welch **FM-07** Ralph T. Hutchings

CLINICAL NOTES IN ANATOMY & PHYSIOLOGY FOR EMERGENCY CARE
The following topics appear throughout the text as Clinical Notes

FOREIGN WORD ROOTS, PREFIXES, SUFFIXES, AND COMBINING FORMS

Each entry starts with the commonly encountered form or forms of the prefix, suffix, or combining form followed by the word root (shown in italics) with its English translation. One example is given to demonstrate the use of each entry.

a-, *a-,* without: avascular
ab-, *ab,* from: abduct
-ac, *-akos,* pertaining to: cardiac
acr-, *akron,* extremity: acromegaly
ad-, *ad,* to, toward: adduct
aden-, adeno-, *adenos,* gland: adenoid
adip-, *adipos,* fat: adipocytes
aer-, *aeros,* air: aerobic respiration
af-, *ad,* toward: afferent
-al, *-alis,* pertaining to: brachial
alb-, *albicans,* white: albino
-algia, *algos,* pain: neuralgia
allo-, *allos,* other: allograft
ana-, *ana,* up, back: anaphase
andro-, *andros,* male: androgen
angio-, *angeion,* vessel: angiogram
ante-, *ante,* before: antebrachial
anti-, ant-, *anti,* against: antibiotic
apo-, *apo,* from: apocrine
arachn-, *arachne,* spider: arachnoid
arter-, *arteria,* artery: arterial
arthro-, *arthros,* joint: arthroscopy
-asis, -asia, *asis,* state, condition: homeostasis
astro-, *aster,* star: astrocyte
atel-, *ateles,* imperfect: atelectasis
aur-, *auris,* ear: auricle
auto-, *auto,* self: autonomic
baro-, *baros,* pressure: baroreceptor
bi-, *bi-,* two: bifurcate
bili-, *bilis,* bile: bilirubin
bio-, *bios,* life: biology
blast-, -blast, *blastos,* precursor: blastocyst
brachi-, *brachium,* arm: brachiocephalic
brachy-, *brachys,* short: brachydactyly
brady-, *bradys,* slow: bradycardia
bronch-, *bronchus,* windpipe, airway: bronchial
carcin-, *karkinos,* cancer: carcinoma
cardi-, cardio-, -cardia, *kardia,* heart: cardiac
-cele, *kele,* tumor, hernia, or swelling: blastocoele
-centesis, *kentesis,* puncture: thoracocentesis
cephal-, *cephalos,* head: brachiocephalic
cerebr-, *cerebros,* brain: cerebral hemispheres
cerebro-, *cerebrum,* brain: cerebrospinal fluid
cervic-, *cervicis,* neck: cervical vertebrae
chole-, *chole,* bile: cholecystitis
chondro-, *chondros,* cartilage: chondrocyte
chrom-, chromo-, *chroma,* color: chromatin
circum-, *circum,* around: circumduction
-clast, *klastos,* broken: osteoclast
colo-, *kolon,* colon: colonoscopy
contra-, *contra,* against: contralateral
corp-, *corpus,* body: corpuscle
cortic-, *cortex,* rind or bark: corticospinal
cost-, *costa,* rib: costal
cranio-, *cranium,* skull: craniosacral
cribr-, *cribrum,* sieve: cribriform
-crine, *krinein,* to secrete: endocrine
cut-, *cutts,* skin: cutaneous
cyan-, *kyanos,* blue: cyanosis

cyst-, -cyst, *kystis,* sac: blastocyst
cyt-, cyto-, *kyton,* a hollow cell: cytology
de-, *de,* from, away: deactivation
dendr-, *dendron,* tree: dendrite
dent-, *dentes,* teeth: dentition
derm-, *derma,* skin: dermis
desmo-, *desmos,* band: desmosome
di-, *dis,* twice: disaccharide
dia-, *dia,* through: diameter
digit-, *digit,* a finger or toe: digital
dipl-, *diploos,* double: diploid
dis-, *des,* apart, away from: disability
diure-, *diourein,* to urinate: diuresis
dys-, *dys-,* painful: dysmenorrhea
-ectasis, *ektasis,* expansion: atelectasis
ecto-, *ektos,* outside: ectoderm
-ectomy, *ektome,* excision: appendectomy
ef-, *ex,* away from: efferent
emmetro-, *emmetros,* in proper measure: emmetropia
encephalo-, *enkephalos,* brain: encephalitis
end-, endo-, *endos,* inside: endometrium
entero-, *enteron,* intestine: enteric
epi-, *epi,* on: epimysium
erythema-, *erythema,* flushed (skin): erythematosis
erythro-, *erythros,* red: erythrocyte
ex-, *ex,* out, away from: exocytosis
extra-, outside, beyond, in addition: extracellular
ferr-, *ferrum,* iron: transferrin
fil-, *filum,* thread: filament
-form, *-formis,* shape: fusiform
gastr-, *gaster,* stomach: gastrointestinal
-gen, -genic, *gennan,* to produce: mutagen
genicula-, *geniculum,* kneelike structure: geniculate nuclei
gest-, *gesto,* to bear: gestation
glosso-, -glossus, *glossus,* tongue: hypoglossal
glyco-, *glykys,* sugar: glycogen
-gram, *gramma,* record: myogram
gran-, *granulum,* grain: granulocyte
-graph, -graphia, graphein, to write, record: electroencephalograph
gyne-, gyno-, *gynaikos,* woman: gynecologist
hem-, hemato-, *haima,* blood: hemopoiesis
hemi-, *hemi-,* half: hemisphere
hepato-, *hepaticus,* liver: hepatocyte
hetero-, *heteros,* other: heterozygous
histo-, *histos,* tissue: histology
holo-, *holos,* entire: holocrine
homeo-, homo-, *homos,* same: homeostasis
hyal-, hyalo-, *hyalos,* glass: hyaline
hydro-, *hydros,* water: hydrolysis
hyo-, *hyoeides,* U-shaped: hyoid
hyper-, *hyper,* above: hyperpolarization
hypo-, *hypo,* under: hypothyroid
hyster-, *hystera,* uterus: hysterectomy
-ia, state or condition: insomnia
idi-, *idios,* one's own: idiopathic
ile-, *ileum:* ileocecal valve
ili-, ilio-, *ilium,* flank, groin: iliac
in-, *in,* within, or denoting negative effect: inactivate